EMERGENCY MEDICINE
H A N D B O O K
Critical Concepts for Clinical Practice

Lynn P. Roppolo, MD
Assistant Professor
Assistant Residency Director
Division of Emergency Medicine
University of Texas Southwestern Medical Center
Parkland Health & Hospital System
Dallas, Texas

Daniel Davis, MD
Associate Professor
Department of Emergency Medicine
University of California San Diego Medical Center
San Diego, California

Sean P. Kelly, MD
Attending Physician
Department of Emergency Medicine
Beth Israel Deaconess Medical Center
Instructor
Harvard Medical School
Boston, Massachusetts

Peter Rosen, MD
Attending Physician
Department of Emergency Medicine
Beth Israel Deaconess Medical Center
Boston, Massachusetts

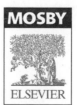

MOSBY

ELSEVIER

MOSBY
ELSEVIER

1600 John F. Kennedy Blvd.
Suite 1800
Philadelphia, PA 19103-2899

Notice

Knowledge and best practice in this field are constantly changing. As new
research and experience broaden our knowledge, changes in practice, treatment
and drug therapy may become necessary or appropriate. Readers are advised to
check the most current information provided (i) on procedures featured or (ii) by
the manufacturer of each product to be administered, to verify the recommended
dose or formula, the method and duration of administration, and contraindications.
It is the responsibility of the practitioner, relying on their own experience and
knowledge of the patient, to make diagnoses, to determine dosages and the best
treatment for each individual patient, and to take all appropriate safety
precautions. To the fullest extent of the law, neither the Publisher nor the Editors
assumes any liability for any injury and/or damage to persons or property arising
out or related to any use of the material contained in this book.

The Publisher

Library of Congress Cataloging-in-Publication Data

Emergency medicine handbook/Lynn Roppolo ... [et al.].
    p. cm.
  ISBN 0-323-03729-1
    1. Emergency medicine—Handbooks, manuals, etc. 2. Medical
emergencies—Handbooks, manuals, etc. I. Roppolo, Lynn.
  RC86.7.E573 2007
  616.02'5—dc22   2006048140

Acquisitions Editor: Todd Hummel
Developmental Editor: Jean Nevius
Editorial Assistant: Martha Limbach
Project Manager: David Saltzberg
Design Direction: Steve Stave

Printed in China

Last digit is the print number: 9 8 7 6 5 4 3 2 1

Working together to grow
libraries in developing countries
www.elsevier.com | www.bookaid.org | www.sabre.org

ELSEVIER   BOOK AID International   Sabre Foundation

Dedication

I would like to thank my husband, Mark, my children (JP and the triplets), and my parents who have helped me realize the true meaning of life. To my mentors, especially Peter Rosen, for their encouragement and support. To the residents and students in Emergency Medicine who continue to inspire me . . . they are our future. May this book help new learners achieve a baseline foundation of clinical competence to care for our unique population of patients.

Lynn P. Roppolo, MD

I dedicate this book to our mentors, who prepared a path so that we might succeed; our peers, who are challenged daily by the trickery of illness and injury; and our students, who will continue to navigate through the uncharted waters that lie ahead.

Daniel Davis, MD

I hope this book helps it's readers learn to trust in themselves and the science and art of practicing Emergency Medicine. I would like to thank my wife, Dara, for her support, infinite patience, and understanding, as well as my children, Jaida and Piper, for their inspiration and boundless energy.

Sean P. Kelly, MD

I dedicate this book to the students and residents who are attempting to become fluent in the language of Emergency Medicine. I hope this book helps in the journey to acquire self-confidence and competency.

Peter Rosen, MD

Preface

This book is meant for the newcomer to Emergency Medicine: the student who wishes an introduction to the field and an exposure to its responsibilities as well as the resident who has chosen the field for specialty training. It is also meant as an overview for those outside of the field who wish to know something about our discipline: how we practice, how we think, and what responsibilities are our concerns.

The act of introducing the specialty of Emergency Medicine to students and residents in training programs can serve to remind the more seasoned practitioners that we have great expectations, which may be impossible to realize without helping the students understand our approach to the patient, how we think in Emergency Medicine, and most importantly, what we expect the novices to know.

Of course, we immediately realize that it is the last category that is most unrealistic, based upon how much we forget about our own experiences as students, and how much our experiences in medical school, residency training, and postgraduate work have produced irreversible changes in us. It is exactly comparable to expecting someone to be fluent in a foreign language without special study, training, and experience. This book is our effort to introduce the student, emergency physician-in-training, and non-emergency physician to not only our language, but our logic, our style of clinical thinking, and our sense of the most important responsibilities.

There are many excellent textbooks of Emergency Medicine, but by the time of the editions that they now present, they are more like encyclopedias than places to begin the study of a new language. It is not only unrealistic to expect newcomers to have read the Rosen or Tintinalli text before they come on service in the Emergency Department (ED), but it is the wrong way to read these books. They should be used to read in depth about a given problem, to prepare a report or a lecture, or to find a reliable source of the evidence upon which these texts are based.

There are some other books that are much more condensed, such as the Five Minute Consultation in Emergency Medicine and the several reference pocket books that are currently available. They are terse, succinct, and well-focused. This is, in fact, the very problem they present for the student and new resident. One must already be fluent in the language of Emergency Medicine, and one must already know quite a bit about the subject to obtain the useful mnemonic advice that these texts provide.

Therefore we decided to collect what it is that we want our newcomers to begin with; an oversight into **how** we think, as well as **what** we think. We want to overcome the depressing sensation of being lost, when everyone else seems to have a role and knows what to do. We want to make our students and residents feel part of our operation, to behave and feel like colleagues, not outsiders, and to have a foundation of information and language upon which they can build their fluency and expertise in Emergency Medicine.

It is impossible to communicate all these attitudes and facts without ending up with a sizable book. Our goal is not to have something every student and resident will have read before starting on the rotation, but something they can repeatedly turn to throughout their rotations, and through the subsequent course of their education to become familiar with our language.

We have attempted to be directive. This is not the place to dissect controversy, nor is it the place for wavering over decisions. We want the student and resident to learn that decisions have to be made, actions taken, and treatments given in a real world time frame that often does not permit long reflection. This book therefore represents our best knowledge and the kinds of solutions that we have chosen to solve controversy. We have tried always to communicate these ideas in recognizable forms as opposed to falling back on legend and jargon. We have tried never to tell our learners to have that all-time obfuscating jargon: "a high index of suspicion," but rather what to look for, and what actions to take.

Diagnostic accuracy is always difficult, and the hardest part of our responsibility lies in knowing what to look for, what questions to pose, and **HOW TO START!**

It is certainly true that the methodology of medical decision-making in Emergency Medicine must be different from that existing in other specialties. The diagnosis is of secondary importance, and may never be revealed in the ED. We must deal with patients whose disease state resembles that of thousands of other problems, and learn how to think on dual levels of concern: first, is there a life threat, and how must one intervene to protect the patient; and second, what is probable, and how must it be managed? Every patient then becomes a calculus problem of two variables: the statistically probable and probably not serious problem, versus the statistically rare but very serious problem.

We are further constrained by the task of performing a logical improbability: you cannot prove a negative, but that is precisely what we must do. You cannot admit every patient, you cannot order every possible diagnostic test, every therapy has a cost as well as a benefit, and we often do not have time for the disease state to declare itself, and present the "classical" signs and symptoms. What then represents adequate negative evidence? How far must we pursue the statistically improbable? What does help us to distinguish between diseases in their earliest manifestations?

These are the questions that befuddle even the most experienced emergency physicians, and our goal in this text is to try to provide a road map to start with, and to provide definitive answers, and not to present all sides to every controversy.

There is, of course, repetition throughout the book, because the beginner is not going to be capable of recognizing the importance of single facts. The book, however, will present many important traps, pitfalls, and dangers that we must try to avoid, and our suggested road maps to escape them.

Finally, this book expresses our desire to reinforce the humanity, ideals, and desires for beneficence that we have always found in our students and residents. Over time, and with life's pressure, we often appear cynical and uncaring, and this is often mistakenly thought to represent sophistication and experience.

We wish to remind our newcomers, and ourselves as well, that Emergency Medicine is important; that we have millions of hurt, frightened, and unstable people for whom we are responsible. That what we do is important, and can make a difference. That all of what we do rests upon what Lewis Thomas (*The Youngest Science*, 1983) referred to as the "gift of affection" and our patients should feel that WE CARE!

Lynn P. Roppolo
Daniel Davis
Sean P. Kelly
Peter Rosen

Contributors

Christopher S. Amato, MD
Attending Physician
Department of Emergency Medicine
Morristown Memorial Hospital
Morristown, New Jersey

Leigh P. Anderson, MD
Resident Physician
Emergency Department
Maricopa Medical Center
Phoenix, Arizona

Philip D. Anderson, MD
Assistant Professor in Medicine
Harvard Medical School
Attending Physician
Department of Emergency Medicine
Beth Israel Deaconess Medical
  Center
Boston, Massachusetts

Christian Arbelaez, MD, MPH
Instructor of Medicine
Harvard Medical School
Attending Physician
Department of Emergency Medicine
Brigham and Women's Hospital
Boston, Massachusetts

Deepta S. Atre, MD
Resident Physician
Department of Emergency Medicine
Mayo Clinic
Rochester, Minnesota

Daniel L. Bamber
Medical Student
University of California San Diego
  School of Medicine
La Jolla, California

Michael Barr
Medical Student
University of California San Diego
  School of Medicine
La Jolla, California

Adam Z. Barkin, MD
Instructor
Department of Medicine
Harvard Medical School
Attending Physician
Department of Emergency Medicine
Beth Israel Deaconess Medical Center
Boston, Massachusetts

Rebeka Barth
Medical Student
University of California San Diego
  School of Medicine
La Jolla, California

Nelsson H. Becerra, MD
Resident Physician
Department of Emergency Medicine
Thomas Jefferson University Hospital
Philadelphia, Pennsylvania

Jeff Beeson, DO
Resident Physician
Division of Emergency Medicine
University of Texas Southwestern
  Medical Center
Parkland Health & Hospital System
Dallas, Texas

Diane M. Birnbaumer, MD
Professor of Clinical Medicine
Department of Medicine
David Geffen School of Medicine at
  UCLA

Los Angeles
Associate Residency Director
Department of Emergency Medicine
Harbor-UCLA Medical Center
Torrance, California

Andra L. Blomkalns, MD
Assistant Professor
Residency Program Director
Department of Emergency Medicine
University of Cincinnati Medical Center
Vice President of Education
Emergency Medicine Resident Program
Vanguard Medical
Cincinnati, Ohio

Eduardo Borquez
Medical Student
Harvard Medical School
Boston, Massachusetts

Craig Reece Brockman II, MD
Clinical Instructor
Division of Emergency Medicine
University of Texas Southwestern
  Medical Center
Parkland Health & Hospital System
Dallas, Texas

David P. Bryant, DO
Clinical Assistant Professor of Medicine
Department of Medicine
Section of Emergency Medicine
Louisiana State University Health
  Science Center in New Orleans
New Orleans

Jeremy J. Brywczynski, MD
Resident Physician
Department of Emergency Medicine
Vanderbilt University Medical Center
Nashville, Tennessee

Colleen Buono, MD
Emergency Medical Services and
  Disaster Fellow
Clinical Faculty
Department of Emergency Medicine
University of California, San Diego
San Diego, California

Colleen J. Campbell, MD
Associate Professor
Department of Emergency Medicine
University of California San Diego
San Diego, California

Andrew J. Capraro, MD
Instructor in Pediatrics
Department of Medicine
Harvard Medical School
Attending Physician
Division of Emergency Medicine
Department of Medicine
Children's Hospital of Boston
Boston, Massachusetts

Jennifer J. Casaletto, MD
Assistant Professor of Clinical
  Emergency Medicine
Department of Emergency Medicine
Maricopa Medical Center
Phoenix, Arizona

Tom Catron
Medical Student
University of California San Diego
  School of Medicine
La Jolla, California

Theodore C. Chan, MD
Professor of Clinical Medicine
Department of Emergency Medicine
University of California Medical Center
San Diego, California

Kerlen Chee, MD
Resident Physician
Department of Emergency Medicine
Brown Medical School
Providence, Rhode Island

Anna I. Cheh, MD
Resident Physician
Division of Emergency Medicine
Harvard Affiliated Emergency Medicine
  Residency
Beth Israel Deaconess Medical Center
Boston, Massachusetts

Emmie A. Chen, MD
Department of Emergency Medicine
J.H. Stroger Hospital of Cook County
Chicago, Illinois

Wenlan Cheng, MD
Division of Emergency Medicine
University of Texas Southwestern
    Medical Center
Parkland Health & Hospital System
Dallas, Texas

Stephen John Cico, MD
Assistant Professor
Department of Emergency Medicine,
    Internal Medicine & Pediatrics
Vanderbilt University
Attending Physician
Vanderbilt University Medical Center &
    Vanderbilt Children's Hospital
Nashville, Tennessee

Jason N. Collins, MD
Division of Emergency Medicine
University of Texas Southwestern
    Medical Center
Parkland Health & Hospital System
Dallas, Texas

Matthew Cook, MD
Toxicology Fellow
Department of Emergency Medicine
University of California San Diego
    Medical Center
San Diego, California

Theodore J. Corbin, MD
Instructor
Department of Emergency Medicine
Jefferson Medical College
Medical Director
Jefferson Community Violence
    Prevention
Department of Emergency Medicine
Thomas Jefferson University Hospital
Philadelphia, Pennsylvania

Chalene A. Corinaldi, MD
Director, Emergency Ultrasound
Department of Emergency Medicine
Good Shepherd Medical Center
Longview, Texas
Clinical Assistant Professor
Division of Emergency Medicine
University of Texas Southwestern
    Medical Center
Parkland Health & Hospital System
Dallas, Texas

Joshua M. Cott, MD
Resident Physician
Department of Emergency Medicine
Rhode Island Hospital
The Miriam Hospital
Providence, Rhode Island

Christopher S. Courtney, MD
Department of Emergency Medicine
Maricopa Medical Center
Phoenix, Arizona

Edward P. Curcio, III, MD
Instructor in Medicine
Division of Emergency Medicine
Harvard Medical School
Boston, Massachusetts
Attending
Department of Emergency Medicine
Mount Auburn Hospital
Cambridge, Massachusetts
Instructor
Department of Emergency Medicine
University of Massachusetts Medical
    School
Worcester, Massachusetts

Daniel Davis, MD
Associate Professor
Department of Emergency Medicine
University of California San Diego
    Medical Center
San Diego, California

David Davis, MD
Assistant Clinical Professor
Department of Emergency Medicine
Duke University Medical Center
Durham, North Carolina

Griffin L. Davis, MD, MPH
Assistant Professor
Department of Emergency Medicine
Georgetown University School of
  Medicine
Attending Physician
Department of Emergency Medicine
Washington Hospital Center
Georgetown University Hospital
Washington, District of Columbia

Martin de Kort, MD
Resident Physician
Department of Emergency Medicine
Maricopa Medical Center
Phoenix, Arizona

Jennifer E. Delapeña, MD
Resident Physician
Department of Emergency Medicine
Harvard Affiliated Emergency Medicine
  Residency
Beth Israel Deaconess Medical Center
Boston, Massachusetts

Jeffrey Druck, MD
Assistant Professor
Department of Surgery
Division of Emergency Medicine
University of Colorado
Emergency Department Physician
Department of Surgery
Division of Emergency Medicine
University of Colorado Hospital
Denver, Colorado

Christopher L. Dunnahoo, MD
Clinical Instructor
Department of Emergency Medicine
Vanderbilt University Medical Center
Nashville, Tennessee

Cristina Maria Estrada, MD
Fellow and Clinical Instructor, Pediatric
  Emergency Medicine
Department of Emergency Medicine
  and Pediatrics
Vanderbilt University Medical Center
Nashville, Tennessee

Jeffrey A. Evans, MD
Department of Medicine
Division of Emergency Medicine
Harvard Medical School
Boston
Attending Physician
Department of Emergency Medicine
Mount Auburn Hospital
Cambridge, Massachusetts

Brenna M. Farmer, MD
Resident Physician
Department of Emergency Medicine
Vanderbilt University School of
  Medicine
PGY2 Emergency Medicine Resident
Department of Emergency Medicine
Vanderbilt University Medical Center
Nashville, Tennessee

Christopher M. Fischer, MD
Chief Resident
Department of Emergency Medicine
Harvard Affiliated Emergency Medicine
  Residency
Beth Israel Deaconess Medical Center
Boston, Massachusetts

Garry F. Gagnon, MD
Resident Physician
Division of Emergency Medicine
University of Texas Southwestern
  Medical Center
Parkland Health & Hospital System
Dallas, Texas

Andrew Garff
Resident Physician
Department of Emergency Medicine
Maricopa Medical Center
Phoenix, Arizone

Kulleni Gebreyes, MD
Assistant Professor
Emergency Department
Georgetown University Hospital
Assistant Residency Director
Emergency Department
Washington Hospital Center
Washington, District of Columbia

Ali Ghobadi, MD
Resident Physician
Department of Emergency Medicine
University of California Irvine Medical
 Center
Orange, California

Eugene Gicheru, MD
Division of Emergency Medicine
University of Texas Southwestern
 Medical Center
Parkland Health & Hospital System
Dallas, Texas

Timothy G. Givens, MD
Associate Professor
Department of Emergency Medicine
 and Pediatrics
Vanderbilt University School of
 Medicine
Associate Medical Director
Emergency Department
Monroe Carell, Jr. Children's Hospital
 at Vanderbilt
Nashville, Tennessee

Autumn Graham, MD
Department of Emergency Medicine
University of Cincinnati
Cincinnati, Ohio

Eric A. Gross, MD
Assistant Professor of Clinical
 Emergency Medicine
Associate Residency Director
Department of Emergency Medicine
Maricopa Medical Center
Phoenix, Arizona

Shamai A. Grossman, MD, MS
Assistant Professor of Medicine
Harvard Medical School
Director of the Clinical Decision Unit
 and Cardiac Emergency Center
Department of Emergency Medicine
Beth Israel Deaconess Medical Center
Boston, Massachusetts

Ian R. Grover, MD
Assistant Clinical Professor of Medicine
Department of Emergency Medicine
University of California San Diego
 Medical Center
San Diego, California

Pilar Guerrero, MD
Assistant Professor of Emergency
 Medicine
John H. Stroger Jr. Cook County
 Hospital
Chicago, Illinois

Shireen Victoria Guide, MD
Resident Physician
Department of Dermatology
University of Texas Southwestern
 Medical Center
Parkland Health & Hospital System
Dallas, Texas

Kama Z. Guluma, MD
Assistant Professor
Department of Emergency Medicine
University of California San Diego
 Medical Center
San Diego, California

Deborah Gutman, MD, MPH
Clinical Assistant Professor
Assistant Residency Director
Department of Emergency Medicine
Brown University
Attending Physician
Department of Emergency Medicine
Rhode Island Hospital
Providence, Rhode Island

Tenagne Haile-Mariam, MD
Assistant Professor
Department of Emergency Medicine
The George Washington School of
  Medicine
Washington, District of Columbia

Heather S. Hammerstedt, MD
Resident Physician
Department of Emergency Medicine
Harvard Affiliated Emergency Medicine
  Residency
Beth Israel Deaconess Medical Center
Boston, Massachusetts

Khary Harmon, MD
Resident Physician
Department of Emergency Medicine
Vanderbilt University Medical Center
Nashville, Tennessee

Neil Harris, MD
Clinical Instructor
Department of Emergency Medicine
Vanderbilt University
Nashville, Tennessee
Staff Physician
Department of Emergency Medicine
Northwest Tucson Emergency
  Physicians
Northwest Medical Center
Tucson, Arizona

H. Gene Hern, Jr., MD, MS
Assistant Clinical Professor of Medicine
University of California San Francisco
Associate Residency Director
Deparment of Emergency Medicine
Alameda County Medical Center –
  Highland General Hospital
Oakland, California

Eugene W. Hu, MD
Resident Physician
Department of Emergency Medicine
Loma Linda University Medical Center
Loma Linda, California

Alec Tuan Huynh, MD
Resident Physician
Department of Emergency Medicine
University of California San Diego
  Medical Center
San Diego, California

James Hwang, MD
Resident Physician
Department of Emergency Medicine
University of California San Diego
  Medical Center
San Diego, California

Ahamed H. Idris, MD
Professor of Surgery and Medicine
Division of Emergency Medicine
Director and Principal Investigator
Dallas Center for Resuscitation Research
University of Texas Southwestern
  Medical Center
Parkland Health & Hospital System
Dallas, Texas

Jason Imperato, MD
Instructor of Emergency Medicine
Department of Emergency Medicine
Harvard Medical School
Boston, Massachusetts
Instructor of Emergency Medicine
Department of Emergency Medicine
Mount Auburn Hospital
Cambridge, Massachusetts

Paul Ishimine, MD
Assistant Professor
Department of Emergency Medicine
University of California San Diego
  Medical Center
San Diego, California

Richard B. Ismach, MD, MPH
Adjunct Assistant Professor
Attending Emergency Physician
Department of Emergency Medicine
Oregon Health and Science University
Staff Emergency Physician
Department of Emergency Medicine

Portland Veterans' Affairs Medical
  Center
Portland, Oregon

Colleen Johnson, MD
Clinical Instructor
Department of Medicine
Division of Emergency Medicine
University of California, San Francisco
San Francisco, California

Jennifer Serrano Johnson, MD
Resident Physician
Department of Emergency Medicine
University of California San Diego
  Medical Center
San Diego, California

Amy Kahn, MD
Chief Resident
Division of Emergency Medicine
University of Texas Southwestern
  Medical Center
Parkland Health & Hospital System
Dallas, Texas

Andy Kahn, MD
Education Chief Resident
Division of Emergency Medicine
University of Texas Southwestern
  Medical Center
Parkland Health & Hospital System
Dallas, Texas

Tarina Lee Kang, MD
Resident Physician
Department of Emergency Medicine
Harvard Affiliated Emergency Medicine
  Residency
Beth Israel Deaconess Medical Center
Boston, Massachusetts

Sean P. Kelly, MD
Instructor of Medicine
Department of Emergency Medicine
Harvard Medical School
Attending Physician and Associate
  Director of Graduate Medical
  Education

Department of Emergency Medicine
Beth Israel Deaconess Medical Center
Boston, Massachusetts

Mamata Kene, MD
Resident Physician
Department of Emergency Medicine
University of California San Diego
  Medical Center
San Diego, California

Angela J. Kennedy, DO
Resident Physician
Division of Emergency Medicine
University of Texas Southwestern
  Medical Center
Parkland Health & Hospital System
Dallas, Texas

Christine Keyes, MD
Resident Physician
Department of Emergency Medicine
Vanderbilt University Medical Center
Nashville, Tennessee

James Killeen, MD
Assistant Clinical Professor of Medicine
Department of Emergency Medicine
University of California San Diego
  Medical Center
San Diego, California

Kelly R. Klein, MD
Assistant Professor
Division of Emergency Medicine
University of Texas Southwestern
  Medical Center
Parkland Health & Hospital System
Dallas, Texas

Kurt C. Kleinschmidt, MD
Associate Professor
Associate Medical Director
Toxicology Fellowship Director
Division of Emergency Medicine
University of Texas Southwestern
  Medical Center
Parkland Health & Hospital System
Dallas, Texas

P.J. Konicki, DO
Director
Emergency Ultrasound Fellowship
Assistant Professor
Department of Emergency Medicine
Christ Medical Center
Oak Lawn, Illinois

Brian Alan Krakover, MD
Clinical Instructor
Government Emergency Medical
  Security Services Fellow
Division of Emergency Medicine
University of Texas Southwestern
  Medical Center
Parkland Health & Hospital System
Dallas, Texas

Lara K. Kulchycki, MD
Attending Phisician
Emergency Medicine
Beth Israel Deaconess Medical Center
Boston, Massachusetts

Gregory Kutsen, MD
Department of Surgery
University of Texas Southwestern
  Medical Center
Parkland Health & Hospital System
Dallas, Texas

Amanda S. Lake, MD
Resident Physician
Department of Emergency Medicine
Maricopa Medical Center
Phoenix, Arizona

Hollynn Larrabee, MD
Assistant Residency Director
Director of Resident EMS Education
Department of Emergency Medicine
University of Cincinnati Medical Center
Cincinnati, Ohio

Lois K. Lee, MD, MPH
Instructor of Pediatrics
Department of Pediatrics
Harvard Medical School
Staff Attending Physician

Department of Emergency Medicine
Children's Hospital Boston
Boston, Massachusetts

Saul D. Levine, MD
Resident Physician
Department of Emergency Medicine
University of California San Diego
  Medical Center
San Diego, California

Steve Lim, MD
Resident Physician
Department of Emergency Medicine
Louisiana State University – Charity
  Hospital
New Orleans, Louisiana

Lisa G. Lowe, MD
Resident Physician
Department of Emergency Medicine
University of California San Diego
  Medical Center
San Diego, California

Samuel D. Luber, MD, MPH
Assistant Professor
Assistant Residency Director
Division of Emergency Medicine
University of Texas Southwestern
  Medical Center
Parkland Health & Hospital System
Dallas, Texas

Binh T. Ly, MD
Associate Clinical Professor of
  Medicine
Assistant Residency Director
Department of Emergency Medicine
University of California San Diego
  Medical Center
San Diego, California

Laura Macnow, MD
Instructor
Department of Medicine
Harvard Medical School
Attending Physician
Department of Emergency Medicine

Beth Israel Deaconess Medical Center
Boston, Massachusetts

E. Gregory Marchand, MD
Assistant Professor of Clinical
  Emergency Medicine
Department of Emergency Medicine
Georgetown University
Associate Medical Director
MedSTAR Transport Services
Department of Emergency Medicine
Washington Hospital Center
Washington, District of Columbia

Joy Martin, MD
Assistant Clinical Professor
Department of Surgery
Division of Emergency Medicine
Duke University
Durham, North Carolina

Joseph N. Martinez, MD
Assistant Professor
Division of Emergency Medicine
University of Texas Southwestern
  Medical Center
Parkland Health & Hospital System
Dallas, Texas

Chilembwe Mason, MD
Chief Resident
Department of Emergency Medicine
St. Luke's – Roosevelt Hospital
Columbia College of Physicians and
  Surgeons
New York, New York

Barbara A. Masser, MD
Instructor in Medicine
Department of Emergency Medicine
Harvard Medical School
Attending Faculty
Department of Emergency Medicine
Beth Israel Deaconess Medical Center
Boston, Massachusetts

Larissa S. May
Chief Resident
Department of Emergency Medicine

The George Washington University
Washington, District of Columbia

Christopher M. McCarthy, MD
Resident Physician
Department of Emergency Medicine
Harvard Affiliated Emergency Medicine
  Residency
Beth Israel Deaconess Medical Center
Boston, Massachusetts

Nicole Streiff McCoin, MD
Chief Resident
Department of Emergency Medicine
Vanderbilt University Medical Center
Nashville, Tennessee

Daniel C. McGillicuddy, MD
Instructor of Medicine
Department of Medicine
Harvard Medical School
Attending Physician
Department of Emergency Medicine
Beth Israel Deaconess Medical Center
Boston, Massachusetts

Michelle McMahon-Downer,
MD
Resident Physician
Department of Emergency Medicine
Brown Medical School
Resident
Department of Emergency Medicine
Rhode Island Hospital
Providence, Rhode Island

Patrick Meehan, MD
Department of Emergency Medicine
INOVA Fair Oaks Hospital
Fairfax, Virginia

Nikolas Mendrygal, MD
Division of Emergency Medicine
University of Texas Southwestern
  Medical Center
Parkland Health & Hospital System
Dallas, Texas

Roland C. Merchant, MD, MPH

Assistant Physician
Department of Emergency Medicine
  and Community Health
Brown Medical School
Attending Physician
Department of Emergency Medicine
Rhode Island Hospital
Providence, Rhode Island

Adam H. Miller, MD, MSc

Assistant Professor
Division of Emergency Medicine
University of Texas Southwestern
  Medical Center
Parkland Health & Hospital System
Dallas, Texas

Greg Miller, MD

Department of Emergency Medicine
Harbor-UCLA Medical Center
Torrance, California

Lisa D. Mills, MD

Assistant Professor
Division of Emergency Medicine
  Ultrasound
Section of Emergency Medicine
Louisiana State University at New
  Orleans
Tulane University
New Orleans, Louisiana

Trevor J. Mills, MD, MPH

Associate Clinical Professor
Residency Program Director
Department of Emergency Medicine
  Residency
Louisiana State University Health
  Sciences Center
Charity Hospital
Section of Emergency Medicine
LSU School of Public Health
New Orleans, Louisiana

Daniel S. Moore, MD

Assistant Professor
Department of Radiology

Medical Director of Emergency
  Radiology
University of Texas Southwestern
  Medical Center
Parkland Health & Hospital System
Dallas, Texas

Granville A. Morse, III, MD

Resident Physician
Department of Emergency Medicine
Louisiana State University Health
  Sciences Center – New Orleans
New Orleans, Louisiana

Elysia Moschos, MD

Assistant Professor
Department of Obstetrics and
  Gynecology
University of Texas Southwestern
  Medical Center
Parkland Health & Hospital System
Dallas, Texas

Scott B. Murray, MD

Chief Resident
Department of Emergency Medicine
Harvard Affiliated Emergency Medicine
  Residency
Beth Israel Deaconess Medical Center
Boston, Massachusetts

James A. Nelson, MD

Resident Physician
Department of Emergency Medicine
University of California San Diego
  Medical Center
San Diego, California

Michael J. Nelson, MD

Clinical Instructor
Emergency Medicine
Harvard Medical School
Attending Physician
Department of Emergency Medicine
Mount Auburn Hospital
Cambridge, Massachusetts

Ellen J. O'Connell, MD
Assistant Professor
Fellow, Medical Toxicology
Division of Emergency Medicine
University of Texas Southwestern
   Medical Center
Parkland Health & Hospital System
Dallas, Texas

Oreoluwa T. Ogunji, MD
Resident Physician
Division of Emergency Medicine
University of Texas Southwestern
   Medical Center
Parkland Health & Hospital System
Dallas, Texas

Heather S. Owen, MD
Resident Physician
Division of Emergency Medicine
University of Texas Southwestern
   Medical Center
Parkland Health & Hospital System
Dallas, Texas

Peter D. Panagos, MD
Assistant Professor
Department of Emergency Medicine
Brown Medical School
Attending Physician
Department of Emergency Medicine
Rhode Island Hospital
The Miriam Hospital
Providence, Rhode Island

Raj J. Patel, MD
Resident Physician
Department of Emergency Medicine
University of California San Diego
   Medical Center
San Diego, California

Jeremy Peay, MD
Resident Physician
Department of Emergency Medicine
University of California San Diego
   Medical Center
San Diego, California

Jayson Pereira, MD
Chief Resident
Department of Emergency Medicine
Harvard Affiliated Emergency Medicine
   Residency
Beth Israel Deaconess Medical Center
Boston, Massachusetts

Dirk Alan Perritt, MD
Resident Physician
Division of Emergency Medicine
University of Texas Southwestern
   Medical Center
Parkland Health & Hospital System
Dallas, Texas

Aaron Pessl, MD
Resident Physician
Department of Emergency Medicine
University of California San Diego
   Medical Center
San Diego, California

Bruno Petinaux, MD
Assistant Professor
Department of Emergency Medicine
George Washington University
Washington, District of Columbia

John Pettini, MD
Division of Emergency Medicine
University of Texas Southwestern
   Medical Center
Parkland Health & Hospital System
Dallas, Texas

Kelly Pettit, MD
Resident Physician
Department of Emergency Medicine
University of California San Diego
   Medical Center
San Diego, California

Riva L. Rahl, MD
Division of Emergency Medicine
University of Texas Southwestern
   Medical Center
Staff Physician

Department of Internal Medicine/
  Preventive Medicine
Cooper Clinic
Dallas, Texas

Juan Reynoso
Medical Student
University of California San Diego
  School of Medicine
La Jolla, California

Stephanie Horn Richling, MD
Clinical Fellow
Department of Emergency Medicine/
  Pediatrics
Vanderbilt University Medical Center
Nashville, Tennessee

Steven Riley, MD
Assistant Professor of Emergency
  Medicine and Pediatrics
Department of Emergency Medicine
Vanderbilt University Medical Center
Nashville, Tennessee

Colleen N. Roche, MD
Assistant Professor
Associate Residency Director
Department of Emergency Medicine
The George Washington University
Washington, District of Columbia

Lynn P. Roppolo, MD
Assistant Professor
Assistant Residency Director
Division of Emergency Medicine
University of Texas Southwestern
  Medical Center
Parkland Health & Hospital System
Dallas, Texas

Carlo L. Rosen, MD
Assistant Professor
Department of Medicine
Harvard Medical School
Residency Program Director
Beth Israel Deaconess Medical Center
  Harvard Affiliated Emergency
  Medicine Residency

Beth Israel Deaconess Medical Center
Boston, Massachusetts

Peter Rosen, MD
Attending Physician
Department of Emergency Medicine
Beth Israel Deaconess Medical Center
Boston, Massachusetts

Stephan E. Russ, MD
Chief Resident
Department of Emergency Medicine
Vanderbilt University Medical Center
Nashville, Tennessee

Leon D. Sanchez, MD, MPH
Instructor in Medicine
Harvard Medical School
Attending
Department of Emergency Medicine
Beth Israel Deaconess Medical Center
Boston, Massachusetts

John Sarko, MD
Clinical Assistant Professor of
  Emergency Medicine
Department of Emergency Medicine
University of Arizona School of
  Medicine
Tucson
Clinical Attending Physician
Department of Emergency Medicine
Maricopa Medical Center
Phoenix, Arizona

Shari Schabowski, MD
Senior Faculty
Department of Emergency Medicine
JHS Cook County Hospital
Assistant Professor
Rush Medical College
Chicago, Illinois

Aaron Schneir, MD
Assistant Professor
Department of Emergency Medicine
University of California San Diego
  Medical Center
San Diego, California

Chuck Seamens, MD
Assistant Professor
Department of Emergency Medicine
Vanderbilt University Medical Center
Nashville, Tennessee

Kaushal H. Shah, MD
Director of Medical Student Education
Department of Emergency Medicine
St. Luke's – Roosevelt Hospital
Columbia College of Physicians and
    Surgeons
New York, New York

Purvi Shah, MD
Division of Emergency Medicine
University of Texas Southwestern
    Medical Center
Parkland Health & Hospital System
Dallas, Texas

Sam H. Shen, MD, MBA
Resident Physician
Department of Emergency Medicine
Harvard Affiliated Emergency Medicine
    Residency
Beth Israel Deaconess Medical Center
Boston, Massachusetts

Stephen V. Sherick
Medical Student
Department of Emergency Medicine
University of Colorado School of
    Medicine
Denver, Colorado

Suneet Singh, MD
Division of Emergency Medicine
University of Texas Southwestern
    Medical Center
Parkland Health & Hospital System
Dallas, Texas

Christian M. Sloane, MD
Assistant Clinical Professor
Department of Emergency Medicine
University of California San Diego
    Medical Center
San Diego, California

Corey M. Slovis, MD
Professor of Emergency Medicine and
    Medicine
Chairman, Department of Emergency
    Medicine
Vanderbilt University School of Medicine
Medical Director
Metro Nashville Fire Department
Nashville, Tennessee

Clay B. Smith, MD
Assistant Professor of Emergency
    Medicine, Internal Medicine, and
    Pediatrics
Department of Emergency Medicine
Vanderbilt University Medical Center
Nashville, Tennessee

Dionne Smith, MD
Division of Emergency Medicine
University of Texas Southwestern
    Medical Center
Parkland Health & Hospital System
Dallas, Texas

Dustin D. Smith, MD
Assistant Professor
Associate Residency Director
Department of Emergency Medicine
Loma Linda University Medical Center
Loma Linda, California

Jennifer C. Smith, MD
Department of Emergency Medicine
Loma Linda University Medical Center
Loma Linda, California

Jaime T. Snarski, MD
Resident Physician
Emergency Medicine Residency
Duke University Medical Center
Durham, North Carolina

Camie J. Sorensen, MD, MPH
Resident Physician
Department of Emergency Medicine
Harvard Affiliated Emergency Medicine
    Residency
Beth Israel Deaconess Medical Center
Boston, Massachusetts

Jeremy Spinks, MD
Resident Physician
Division of Emergency Medicine
University of Texas Southwestern
  Medical Center
Parkland Health & Hospital System
Dallas, Texas

Lawrence B. Stack, MD
Associate Professor
Emergency Medicine
Vanderbilt University Medical Center
Associate Professor
Emergency Medicine
Vanderbilt Hospital
Nashville, Tennessee

J. Scott Stephens, MD
Resident Physician
Department of Radiology
University of Texas Southwestern
  Medical Center
Parkland Health & Hospital System
Dallas, Texas

Andrew Sucov, MD
Assistant Professor
Department of Emergency Medicine
Brown Medical School
Medical Director
Department of Emergency Medicine
Department of Quality Management
Rhode Island Hospital
Providence, Rhode Island

Daniel E. Surdam, MD
Division of Emergency Medicine
University of Texas Southwestern
  Medical Center
Parkland Health & Hospital System
Dallas, Texas

Traci Thoureen, MD
Assistant Professor
Division of Emergency Medicine
University of Maryland
Baltimore, Maryland

M. Olivia Titus, MD
Assistant Professor
Department of Pediatrics and Pediatric
  Emergency Medicine
Division of Pediatric Emergency
  Medicine and Critical Care
Medical University of South Carolina
Charleston, South Carolina

Gerard M. Toso, MD
Resident Physician
Department of Emergency Medicine
Brown Medical School
Providence, Rhode Island

Edward Ullman, MD
Clinical Instructor
Department of Medicine
Harvard University
Attending Physician
Department of Emergency Medicine
Beth Israel Deaconess Medical Center
Boston, Massachusetts

Karen Van Hoesen, MD
Associate Professor
Department of Emergency Medicine
University of California San Diego
  Medical Center
San Diego, California

Larissa I. Velez, MD
Assistant Professor
Associate Residency Director
Division of Emergency Medicine
University of Texas Southwestern
  Medical Center
Parkland Health & Hospital System
Staff Toxicologist
North Texas Poison Center
Dallas, Texas

Gary M. Vilke, MD
Professor of Clinical Medicine
Director of Clinical Research
Department of Emergency Medicine
University of California San Diego
  Medical Center
San Diego, California

Rais Vohra, MD
Toxicology Fellow
Department of Emergency Medicine
University of California San Diego
  Medical Center
San Diego, California

Wame N. Waggenspack, Jr., MD
Division of Emergency Medicine
University of Texas Southwestern
  Medical Center
Parkland Health & Hospital System
Dallas, Texas

Benjamin K. Wakamatsu, MD
Resident Physician
Department of Emergency Medicine
Loma Linda University Medical Center
Loma Linda, California

Brian William Walsh, MD, MBA
Faculty
Department of Emergency Medicine
Morristown Memorial Hospital
Morristown, New Jersey

Alan Weir, MD
Resident Physician
Division of Emergency Medicine
University of Texas Southwestern
  Medical Center
Parkland Health & Hospital System
Dallas, Texas

William A. Wittlake, MD
Associate Professor and Chair
Department of Emergency Medicine
Loma Linda University
Chief of Service
Department of Emergency Medicine
Loma Linda University Medical Center
  and Children's Hospital
Loma Linda, California

Peter Witucki, MD
Assistant Clinical Professor of Medicine
Department of Emergency Medicine
University of California San Diego
  Medical Center
San Diego, California

Richard E. Wolfe, MD
Associate Professor of Medicine
Department of Medicine
Harvard Medical School
Chief of Emergency Medicine
Department of Emergency Medicine
Beth Israel Deaconess Medical Center
Boston, Massachusetts

Michael M. Woodruff, MD
Instructor in Medicine
Department of Medicine
Harvard Medical School
Attending Physician
Department of Emergency Medicine
Beth Israel Deaconess Medical Center
Boston, Massachusetts

Adam Wos, MD
Resident Physician
Department of Emergency Medicine
University of California San Diego
  Medical Center
San Diego, California

Sandra S. Yoon, MD
Resident Physician
Department of Emergency Medicine
Harvard Affiliated Emergency Medicine
  Residency
Beth Israel Deaconess Medical Center
Boston, Massachusetts

Julie A. Zeller, MD
Resident Physician
Department of Emergency Medicine
Harvard Affiliated Emergency Medicine
  Residency
Beth Israel Deaconess Medical Center
Boston, Massachusetts

Contents

EMERGENCY DEPARTMENT ORIENTATION (FOR STUDENTS, INTERNS, AND ROTATING RESIDENTS)

CHAPTER 1

Overview of the Emergency Department

Scott B. Murray ■ Heather S. Hammerstedt ■ Sean P. Kelly

Welcome to the emergency department (ED)! It may seem chaotic, but everything serves a purpose, and everyone has a role to play in order to function as a team. Understanding the basic setup and personnel staffing will enhance your ability to provide good patient care and help you have a worthwhile and educational experience.

Departmental Organization

Many departments will have subsections divided by function or acuity.

Prehospital personnel. For many patients, care starts before arriving at the ED. Refer to Chapter 89 for a detailed description of prehospital services. The best practice is to speak with the prehospital personnel whenever possible, because limited information may be available from the patient.

Triage. A rapid history and physical examination with vital signs is used to prioritize patient evaluation by acuity and availability of resources in the ED. Most ED triage systems try to prioritize acute problems over minor ones, and incorporate such factors as room availability, level of care needed, and staffing.

Waiting room. The wait is uncomfortable, boring, and frustrating—be conscious of this, apologize for the wait, and kindly explain any delays. Also, remember that patients may be sicker than they initially appeared at triage, or than they think they are, or their health may have worsened while waiting to be seen.

Resuscitation room. This area is reserved for critically ill medical and trauma patients. Often this is where resuscitation equipment is stored (i.e., airway equipment, defibrillator, code drugs, etc.).

Acute area. For emergent but relatively stable patients.

Express/fast-track. For relatively simple and straightforward cases in which patients are likely to be discharged. While working here, remain vigilant for sick patients who have been incorrectly designated as fast-track patients; triage is not a perfect science.

Pediatrics or psychiatry. Some departments have separate areas for these populations.

Observation units. Patients requiring more than several hours of diagnostics or therapy can be placed in an observation or "clinical decision-making" unit located within the ED, rather than being admitted to the hospital. Policies vary according to institution, but generally this unit is considered appropriate for straightforward patients requiring less than 24 hours of care who can be safely discharged home afterwards. Typical patients are those with low-risk chest pain or cellulitis requiring a few doses of antibiotics.

Ancillary services/radiology. Each hospital will have its own organization for emergency ("stat") laboratory studies and radiology services. Find out promptly where everything is located, how to obtain laboratory and radiologic studies, and how to get results. Know what you are looking for when you order a test. Do not order a test if it will not alter your management or disposition. Remember the golden rule of NEVER SENDING AN UNSTABLE PATIENT TO RADIOLOGY. Request portable radiologic studies, bedside ultrasound examinations or other tests if possible, and control the airway and adequately resuscitate the patient before sending the patient to the radiology department. If you do decide to send a sick patient to radiology, ensure that the patient is adequately monitored and transported to radiology with the necessary emergency equipment.

Personnel

Registered Nurse and Licensed Practical/Vocational Nurse. Nurses can be a valuable resource for patient care. Many of them have a wealth of knowledge and experience. Always talk with nurses about the patients they are caring for and review their nursing documentation. LISTEN TO THE NURSES. They often have insights a physician might miss. Many departments have protocols allowing nurses to draw blood; order radiologic studies; and obtain urine specimens, IV access, or electrocardiograms (EKGs) before the physician's evaluation. Nurses may be caring for multiple patients. Notify nurses when you order an intervention that is time critical. Be a team player and help out the nurses when it is feasible to do so.

Nursing assistants and ED technicians. These are medically trained personnel without formal nursing training. Their scope of practice varies between institutions, but can include obtaining supplies, drawing blood, splinting, assisting with procedures, and fitting crutches. These individuals are NOT licensed to give medications or start IV lines.

Unit coordinators/clerks/secretaries. These are the personnel responsible for communications flow (pages, faxes, telephone calls), charts, and other paperwork.

Physician assistants and nurse practitioners. These are mid-level providers or physician "extenders" who are able to examine patients and prescribe medications under a supervising physician's license. These professionals may be a valuable resource in some institutions. Physician assistants have 2 years of academic and clinical training after undergraduate training. Nurse practitioners are registered nurses with a master's degree in nursing.

Security. These are the personnel selected to protect the staff and patients, as well as maintain safety and security in the ED.

Psychiatry. Most institutions have a system in which there is a social worker, case manager, or psychiatry resident in the ED or on call to evaluate psychiatric patients. Some hospitals may have a separate psychiatric ED; however, patients often require medical clearance in the main ED.

Social workers and case managers. These are personnel trained to assist patients and caregivers with social or financial concerns such as the proper level of care needed for the patient to perform activities of daily living or placement in rehabilitation centers or nursing homes.

What to do/ find out on your first day in the Emergency Department

First, introduce yourself to the attending physician and senior resident and let them know who you are and what level of training you represent. See Box 1–1 for a quick list of the most important questions to ask.

BOX 1–1   Things to Know on the First Day in the Emergency Department

Which patients are you allowed to see, and how can you sign up for them?

To whom do you present?

How can you contact the attending emergency physician if a patient is really sick?

Who do you go to if you need help?

How can you find out which nurse is taking care of a patient?

How do you document appropriately on the emergency department chart?

Where are the nurse's notes located?

How do you order diagnostic tests (blood work, urine tests, radiologic studies) and obtain results of tests?

How can you view radiologic studies, and is there a radiologist available to help interpret results?

How do you obtain medical records?

How do you order medications?

How do you discharge and admit patients?

What is the appropriate dress for the department (scrubs, shirt and tie, etc)?

Where do you find the code cart, sutures, splint materials, intravenous line supplies, and blood tubes?

What learning resources are immediately available in the emergency department (i.e., internet access, reference books)?

Where is a safe and secure place to put your personal belongings?

CHAPTER 2

General Approach to the Emergency Department Patient

HEATHER S. HAMMERSTEDT ■ SCOTT B. MURRAY ■ SEAN P. KELLY

The Chart

Look quickly for the following things that will help you frame your thoughts and questions before you have even seen the patient: age, sex, chief complaint, vital signs, triage history, and diagnostics obtained or treatment given before your evaluation. Identify any *red flags* (e.g., low oxygen saturation, abnormal vital signs, fever, elderly, concerning chief complaint, etc.) that may make you more concerned for serious pathology. Your questions and physical examination should be directed at potentially life-threatening problems first. Any patient who is hemodynamically unstable or has significant respiratory compromise should be in a resuscitation area. The ED attending or senior EM resident should be called immediately to the bedside if not already present.

Vital Signs

Temperature, heart rate, blood pressure, respiratory rate, and oxygen saturation.
■ Make sure that all five vital signs are available. If not, measure them yourself.
■ Vital signs are truly VITAL. Often when there is no available history, they will be enough for you to treat and resuscitate an acutely distressed patient.
■ Decode the vital signs! Think of it like a puzzle. A sinus tachycardia, for example, must be explained and treated BEFORE a patient is discharged from the ED. It may be the result of pain, anxiety, or hypovolemia that can be easily resolved in the ED with intravenous (IV) fluids and analgesia. However, an unresolved and unexplained tachycardia should not be ignored and warrants further investigation. For example, the tachycardia could be secondary to something more concerning such as a pulmonary embolism, myocarditis, or endocarditis.
■ Vital sign pearls and pitfalls: An oral temperature in a patient with tachypnea may be falsely low; obtain rectal temperatures in these patients. A low normal blood pressure (i.e., systolic blood pressure of 90-100 mm Hg) in a patient who is at baseline hypertensive is NOT a normal vital sign. A normal heart rate in a patient on a beta-blocker should NOT be reassuring; they may not develop a reflex tachycardia in response to hypotension or infection.

Table 2-1   Orthostatic Vital Signs

	How to Measure	Orthostatic Positive
(O+ lying down)	Patient supine for 2 full minutes	This represents the control HR, BP
(♀ standing)	Patient standing for 2 full minutes	⇑ HR >20 ⇓ SBP >20 mmHg ⇓ DBP >10–20 mmHg Near syncope

BP, blood pressure; bpm, beats per minute; HR, heart rate.

■ Orthostatic vital signs: The accuracy of these measurements is low, and they should not be obtained in any patient who is already hypotensive or having a tachycardia. They are often still used to detect hypovolemia since young, healthy patients with positive orthostatics are usually truly hypovolemic. Note that patients who are not orthostatic by vital signs may still be hypovolemic. The elderly patient may be orthostatic, even if not hypovolemic due to autonomic insufficiency or medications. Table 2–1 demonstrates how to measure and interpret these results.

Approach to the Patient Encounter
General

■ If a patient appears sick, get appropriate help and proceed directly to the assessment and management of the ABCs (*a*irway, *b*reathing, *c*irculation). Each and every time you approach any patient, the ABCs are the first assessment you make—sometimes even from across the room. Refer to Section 2 for "Life Threatening Emergencies."
■ Remember that your patient is not just ill, but may be nervous and uncomfortable in a new environment that is often intimidating and chaotic to most laypersons.
■ *Physical contact*, whether it is by shaking hands or touching someone's shoulder, may speed up the patient–provider relationship and allow the patient to relax. Be conscious of cultural differences when making contact.
■ *Sitting down* for the patient interview makes it seem like you are there longer than you really are.
■ *Apologize* for the patient's wait, even if you do not know how long they waited.
■ *Avoid jargon*. Explain basic pathophysiology. You are a teacher as well as a physician. Use drawings and layman's terms, but do not be condescending.
■ *Respect the patient's right to privacy:* Do not discuss the patient's medical information in front of other patients. This is especially true for HIV status, sexual history, recreational drug use, bowel and bladder function, breast masses, and genital problems. Do not physically expose the patients. Keep the patient covered as much as possible and perform physical examinations of private areas (i.e., genitals, breasts, buttocks,

extensive wounds) in an enclosed room and with an appropriate chaperone.

Talking to the Patient

■ KNOCK first before entering the room!! Smile, introduce yourself, and shake hands with your patient. Verify the patient's identity by asking the patient to say his or her name *and check the patient's identification (ID) band*.
■ For the first minute of the patient encounter, let the patient talk *without interruption*; it will allow the patient to get his or her most important concerns out in a manner that makes sense to the patient, and feel like his or her concerns are validated. Interrupting the patient early in the encounter will be perceived as impolite, and is actually unlikely to speed up your encounter much at all. Use this opportunity to observe the patient, and to make a few important emergency medicine distinctions such as the following:
   ■ *Sick or not sick?* This distinction is sometimes obvious, but it may take experience to spot subtle illness in other situations. Look for red flags such as the general appearance of the patient, abnormalities in vital signs, respiratory distress, alteration in mental status, or concerning complaints (e.g., chest pain, hematemesis, and syncope). In "sick" patients, the history and physical examination should be done simultaneously with emergent studies or interventions (e.g., EKG, IV access).
   ■ *Is there anything I need to do right NOW?* Emergency medicine is different from other specialties in that sometimes, such as with a sick patient, it is necessary to ACT before collecting more information. Examples include starting high-flow oxygen, placing the patient on a monitor, obtaining IV access, performing an EKG, or administering medications for vital sign abnormalities or altered mental status.

History and Physical Examination

Unlike other specialties, the emergency medicine history and physical examination are focused events and the differential diagnosis rapidly evolves as information is obtained.

■ Ask questions pertaining to the patient's chief complaint.
■ Be flexible and prepared to adjust your differential diagnosis, line of questioning, and physical examination as the patient encounter progresses.
■ Allow your questions to help you form a differential diagnosis while you are still in the room.
■ Remember that the history can be taken simultaneously with your physical examination if necessary, especially for your review of systems.
■ Be resourceful in obtaining a history. Prehospital personnel, family, nursing home staff, and old hospital records can be excellent sources of information.
■ Obtain the eight characteristics of a chief complaint and essential information found in the acronym "OLD CARRTS" (Table 2–2).

Table 2–2 Essential Characteristics of Chief Complaint (OLD CARRTS)

Onset: Did symptoms develop suddenly or gradually (years/days/hours)? What was the patient doing when the symptom started?
Location: What is affected? Where does it hurt?
Duration: Constant, intermittent, waxing/waning, crescendo/decrescendo.
Character: Pain → sharp, pressure, dull, achy, burning, crampy, heavy, similarity to previous episodes. Cough: dry, staccato, hacking, productive. Describe appearance of stool or emesis.
Associated symptoms: What other factors occur in same time period?
Radiation: Is there referred pain? Does the pain radiate anywhere? Is there pain anywhere else?
Relieving/exacerbating factors: What makes it better or worse (e.g., food, breathing, body position)?
Treatment: Treatment taken or given for the presenting condition.
Severity: Scale of 1 to 10 for pain. Frequency of stool, emesis, cough, fever.

Table 2–3 "AMPLE History"

Allergies: Drug allergies or reactions to contrast dye.
Medications: Medications, including prescription and over-the-counter.
Past medical history: Be complete but focus on previous medical problems that are relevant to the chief complaint, such as cardiac risk factors for patients with chest pain or previous ankle injury in someone with new ankle pain.
Last: Last meal, tetanus immunization, bowel movement, menstrual period, or whatever is appropriate for that case.
Events: Events leading up to presentation. History of present illness.

■ Also be aware of the AMPLE mnemonic that many prehospital personnel and emergency physicians use to obtain a rapid and focused history, which is particularly useful in potentially critical situations. (Table 2–3).
■ A more focused physical examination can be done on patients with benign and focal problems such as a simple laceration or ankle sprain.
■ A more complete physical examination is indicated in most other patients, especially if they are very young or old, are ill-appearing, are inaccurate historians, have an altered mental status, have significant co-morbid medical conditions, or have concerning complaints. The ABCs should always be assessed first, followed by a more detailed examination progressing in a *head-to-toe* fashion. Females with lower abdominal pain require a pelvic examination with a chaperone present. Most patients presenting with abdominal pain should have a rectal examination. Any information of a confidential nature or anything that physically exposes the patient should be done in an enclosed room.

Differential Diagnosis

Formulating a differential diagnosis in emergency medicine is a somewhat different process than that which occurs in other specialties. Due to high levels of acuity and the necessity to diagnose and treat early in the patient course, the clinician should begin formulating the differential diagnosis DURING the initial assessment of the patient. This will also help focus the history and physical examination on areas that require the most attention. The differential diagnosis should have the following characteristics:

■ Dynamic: broadens and narrows with each new clue the patient gives you and directs you to your next question.
■ Each differential diagnosis list should include the following components:
  ■ Critical or life-threatening: What is the worst-case scenario? What disease can you not afford to miss in this patient?
  ■ Emergent: not immediately life-threatening, but requires prompt attention.
  ■ Non-emergent: not a true emergency and treatment may be delayed; however, problems such as these commonly present to the ED and should be treated appropriately.
■ Many times, a definitive diagnosis is not made in the ED, but life threats are ruled out. Ruling out life threats can occur by simple history-taking and physical examination or by laboratory or radiologic tests.
■ When you walk out of a patient's room, have a good idea of what the problem is and a short list of life-threatening conditions that you have already ruled out clinically or that you will rule out with ancillary testing.

Initial Management of the Patient

Concurrently with the history and physical examination, begin to order the essential tests and therapeutic interventions to diagnose and treat the patient.

■ Laboratory tests, radiologic studies, IV fluids, medications, consultations, procedures, initial stabilization, and treatments.
■ Plan ahead: If test "A" is positive, the patient will be admitted. If it is negative, the patient will be discharged. If indeterminate, order test "B" and obtain a consult.

Always remember the *ten commandments* of emergency medicine management (Box 2-1).

Follow-up and Keeping the Patient Satisfied

As previously mentioned, the ED is a difficult place to be a patient. There are long waits both before and after seeing a physician. Often during these times, patients have no idea what is happening around them. A few pointers:

■ *Ask if there are questions,* and tell the patient that he or she should let you know if any come up.
■ *Provide reassurance* when you can, but do not commit to certainty of a diagnosis/disposition before talking to the attending physician.
■ *Explain* to the patient what will be happening while they are waiting (laboratory or radiologic studies, consults, medications), the role of the other doctors coming into their room (senior resident, attending

---

BOX 2–1   Ten Commandments of Emergency Medicine

- Secure the ABCs
- Do the DON'T (*D*extrose, *O*xygen, *N*aloxone, *T*hiamine) for patients with altered mental status.
- Get a pregnancy test in all women of child-bearing age.
- Assume the worst-case scenario when considering patient diagnosis.
- Do not send unstable patients to radiology.
- Look for common red flags that should raise awareness for the presence of serious pathology. Examples include multiple ED visits, abnormal vital signs, extremes of age, and immunocompromise.
- Trust no one, believe nothing (not even yourself), avoid premature closure.
- Learn from your mistakes.
- Do unto others as you would your family.
- Always err on the side of the patient.

Adapted from: Wrenn K, Slovis CM. The ten commandments of emergency medicine. Ann Emerg Med 1991; 20(10): 1146–7.

physicians, consultants), and reassure them that while you are not in the room it does not mean that they are being neglected, but that tests are being performed and evaluated and treatments being undertaken. Give patients realistic time expectations.

- *Advise* the patient and family to let the nurse or the physician know if they need anything or *if their current situation changes* (new symptoms, resolution, etc.).
- *Follow-up on any patient interventions.* Critically ill patients will need very frequent reassessments. Stable patients who receive a pain medication for pain relief should be reassessed 30 to 60 minutes after the pain medication is given.
- *Follow-up closely on all diagnostic tests* to ensure they were performed and that the results are received in a timely fashion. Inquire about how long it usually takes to receive results. Any significant delay in receiving the result of a particular study should be investigated. The results of all studies do not need to be back before a decision on the disposition of a patient is made, especially if the patient needs to be admitted. The admitting physician can follow-up on the remaining studies, or the patient's primary care physician can follow-up on laboratory studies that may not be available in a timely fashion (i.e., send-out laboratory studies), should the patient be discharged home.
- *Inform* the patient or family of any updates or changes in status (results, new tests, new consults, admission, and discharge).

CHAPTER 3

Communicating Information

SCOTT B. MURRAY ■ HEATHER S. HAMMERSTEDT ■ SEAN P. KELLY

Clear and succinct communication is essential in emergency medicine. Speaking with primary care physicians (PCPs), patients, emergency department (ED) attending physicians, and consultants requires communicating the same information in different ways.

Communicating with Emergency Department Attending Physicians

- Summarize.
- Be concise and definite.
- Prioritize, and stay focused on pertinent positives and negatives.
- Attempt to be binary (yes or no) regarding the presence of symptoms and signs.
- Paint a picture of what you think is going on and what you are trying to convey.
- Remember that it is more important in emergency medicine to rule out life-threatening diagnoses, rather than to rule in less urgent diagnoses.
- Actively seek feedback regarding your presentation technique (from senior emergency medicine residents and attending physicians) and modify your approach as needed.

Initial Patient Presentation

This is more focused and directed than in other environments. It is okay to include vital information wherever it most logically fits in the presentation. You should be able to not only *tell* a story in a manner that makes sense to the listener, but *sell* the story so you are convincing.

- *Age, gender, and chief complaint.* This should be at the beginning of every presentation.
- *Critical medical history.* Present key pieces of information that will radically alter management. For example, provide cardiac risk factors in a patient complaining of chest pain.
- *History of present illness (HPI).* This should contain the eight features of any chief complaint (see Table 2–2). Only list relevant information, including pertinent positives and negatives. This is not the time to prove your thoroughness at the HPI. Questions can be asked of you at the end of the presentation. If patients present with two separate processes, present each chief complaint and HPI separately. Always include data that make life-threatening diseases more or less likely.

- **Medical history, review of systems, family history and social history.** Chronic disease processes or systemic complaints are relevant only if they alter the differential diagnosis or management. Any relevant family history or social history should also be mentioned.
- **Medications.** These are generally not important to present unless they change management, but they should be completely documented on the chart. For example, warfarin in a patient who fell, or who has bleeding.
- **Allergies.** Mention only if you think the patient needs a specific medication or potential contrast allergy for a contrast-enhanced CT study. For example, a patient with an infection who has an antibiotic allergy.
- **Pertinent physical examination.** Report all vital signs, and whether the patient is ill-appearing, in distress or looks well and comfortable. Report all abnormal findings, even if they seem unrelated. They may be relevant to the attending. Report pertinent negative findings if they help rule out items on the differential diagnoses. For example, no photophobia or meningismus in a patient with headache, or no costovertebral angle tenderness in a patient with dysuria.
- **Tests.** Include any laboratory studies, imaging, electrocardiogram (EKG), or other test already performed. Have baseline comparison values ready for any abnormal study result (e.g., old EKG, prior creatinine level). If a testing result is normal, it is permitted to simply state "normal." There is no need to list all individual results unless specifically asked.
- **Differential diagnosis.** List the most life-threatening (or critical) and the most likely (common) diagnoses. State clearly how you plan to exclude life threats on your differential with history and physical examination data or ancillary tests.
- **Treatment.** This may begin before the final diagnosis is made as the consequences of starting treatment too late can be fatal. For example, a hypotensive, febrile patient with respiratory complaints should receive IV fluids and empiric antibiotics before a chest X-ray confirms the diagnosis of pneumonia.

Sign-Out

- This is the communication between physicians working in the emergency department at shift change. It should convey how you would want your patients to be treated in your absence. Sign-out should include the following: the diagnosis or clinical impression in three sentences or less; tests that are pending; and plan of action when they return. For example, "If the abdominal CT scan has normal findings, then discharge. If positive, then consult surgery." It should also include the patient's response to treatment requiring follow-up. For example, "If patient tolerates oral fluids after antiemetics, then discharge." It is bad etiquette to sign-out procedures, rectal and pelvic examinations, calling consultants and PCPs, or discharge paperwork in a patient who will be leaving soon. However, a procedure may be signed out if it is impossible to perform the procedure due to circumstances beyond your control. For example, a patient with AIDS and a headache who needs a lumbar puncture but the head CT (to rule out a mass lesion) has not been done yet.

Communicating with Consultants

- Consultants are busy. Be brief and unambiguous about what you need them to do. Remember, you should be able to not only *tell* a story in a manner that makes sense to the listener, but *sell* the story so that you are convincing. Consider in advance your response to any possible concerns a consultant may have to convince him or her to do what you are asking them to do.
- Establish good rapport early and make the consultant feel welcome in the ED. Offer any further assistance as needed.
- Consultants offer valuable advice, but ultimately, the emergency physician is the doctor responsible for the patient's well-being and ultimate disposition. The emergency physician is not required to follow the consultant's advice, especially if he or she believes a consultant's recommendation is not safe or necessary.
- The most common challenge is the refusal of a consultant to see a patient in a timely manner. Acknowledge how busy they are, that they are the expert in this particular field, the problem is beyond your scope of practice, or only they are able to provide a needed intervention (e.g., endoscopy, catheterization, and so forth).
- Box 3–1 summarizes "how to call a consult" from the ED.

Communicating with the Primary Care Physician

Primary care physicians (PCPs) are great resources of information about their patients and are very important in arranging follow-up for patients you discharge.

- ***Calling PCPs.*** A PCP should be called when you need more patient information (old EKG or test results), when the patient will be admitted,

---

BOX 3–1 How to Call a Consult

- Before calling, determine with ED attending: correct person to call, clinical question or procedure being requested, and time period for evaluation.
- Have the patient's chart and any other relevant information readily available
- Introduce yourself and position (student, resident, etc.)
- Thank consultant for calling back in timely fashion
- Be very clear what you need the consultant to do: to come emergently to the ED, arrange outpatient follow-up, or advise over the phone regarding management.
- Give patient's name, medical record number, room number
- Give the brief HPI: one or two sentences to summarize patient's case
- Thank consultant again and verify the advice, and time he or she will see patient or come to the ED

or when the patient will be discharged and specific new treatment is initiated or close follow-up of the patient or pending tests is needed.

- *Admitting a patient.* Generally PCPs want to know more details over the phone than consultants. Follow the same general format as when speaking with consultants (Box 3–1). End the conversation by agreeing upon the following: floor or service the patient will be admitted to, under whose name (admit to the PCP, on-call physician, or hospitalist service), any consults the PCP wishes you to call emergently, and any further workup or treatment the PCP recommends. If the PCP disagrees with the planned patient disposition, have the attending emergency physician speak with him or her.

Communicating with Patients and Family

Refer to Chapter 2 for the general approach to emergency patient. This section will cover some common and potentially difficult interactions for the care provider.

Delivering Bad News

- There is a significant chance that a patient's course will result in serious diagnosis, complication, or death.
- It is the responsibility of the physician primarily taking care of the patient to discuss these findings with the patient or family. Do not wait for someone else to do this, and do not be paternalistic and assume that it is better for the patient not to know.
- Make eye contact. It is okay to touch the patient's arm or shoulder if it seems appropriate.
- State clearly and simply, without jargon, what the problem is in a delicate and sensitive manner. Do not give a definitive diagnosis if the diagnosis is not certain or additional tests will need to be performed to confirm the diagnosis. For example, if a pancreatic mass found on CT scan is concerning for cancer, do not abruptly tell the patient that you have found a pancreatic cancer. A better approach would be to tell the patient that a pancreatic mass was found on CT scan, and additional studies will need to be performed to determine what it is.
- Many people stop listening as soon as they hear bad news. It may be helpful to do the following: Try to educate the patient/family on medical terms, describe the next steps in care, describe any consultants that may be involved in the case, attempt to answer all questions, and offer hope if it exists, but be realistic.
- It may be appropriate to give the patient and family time alone, but offer to return shortly. Remember to return! You may have to repeat much of the information again.

Notifying Families of Death

- It is the responsibility of the physician primarily taking care of the patient to discuss this with the family. The physician should not go alone but instead should be accompanied by either a nurse, social worker, chaplain, or other support staff to aid the family.

- Follow the same suggestions as in the prior section.
- Avoid euphemisms such as *passed away*, *moved on*, and *no longer with us*. Use concrete terms such as *dead* or *died*.
- Do not take blame nor blame the death on anyone.
- Bring the family to a quiet, private area where they can sit and be alone. Introduce yourself to all involved. Begin with what precipitated the visit (e.g., automobile collision, heart attack) and what happened as a result (e.g., too much blood was lost, the heart could not pump anymore). Explain that despite all your efforts, the patient died. For example, "We tried to breathe for her, gave medications and blood, shocked the heart." Use the patient's name. Families may ask for specifics; knowing what you did to try to save the patient is comforting to some.

Hostile or Confrontational Patients or Family

Some patients or families may be upset with you before you have even met them. Long waiting times, prior health care experiences, family issues, or personality conflicts may cause problems on this current visit.

- Apologize for any delay, noting how busy it has been.
- Avoid arguing.
- Address the conflict head on, or it will obstruct the remainder of your time with the patient.
- Use neutral, nonaccusatory language.
- Allow patients and family members to vent pent-up frustrations.
- Verbally praise patients and family members for something they have done to offer support.
- Validate their willingness to wait for care or support their family member despite the difficulties they are facing.

Multiple Unrelated Problems, Chronic Problems, and Nonemergent Problems

- *Nonemergent and chronic problems.* The ED is the safety net for those not properly cared for in the medical system; advocate for those who have no one who will care for them. Either care for the problem, or arrange for someone else to do it.
- *Multiple problems (the "hidden" agenda).* Search for an underlying problem being masqueraded as multiple complaints such as a history of abuse or psychiatric disorder. Ask the patient if he or she feels safe at home. Inquire about symptoms of depression and any threat to self or others.

Intoxicated or Psychiatrically Altered Patient

- Patients who are not capable of making safe decisions cannot leave on their own as they are at risk to self or others.
- Remember your safety: Keep yourself positioned between the door and the patient, to exit quickly. Avoid fast, threatening arm motions or crossing your arms. Keep your hands by your sides, palms toward the patient. Do not touch the patient.
- Gain trust by explaining what will happen step by step during the ED visit.

- Be polite, friendly, caring, calm, reassuring, and professional.
- Do not argue with the patient or escalate the situation.
- Set firm limits and do not waiver on rules.
- Safety first. Get help if the situation worsens or seems to be escalating. In many cases, physical or chemical restraints may be necessary. Follow the necessary policies and procedures at your institution for using these techniques.
- Refer to Chapter 70 (Psychiatric Emergencies) for a more detailed discussion.

Documentation

- The ED chart is a durable form of communication that conveys the thoughts and clinical findings of those caring for the patient. The chart is also a medical-legal document and billing record.
- Refer to Appendix 3 for ED documentations procedures.

How to Admit or Discharge a Patient

As soon as disposition becomes clear, make sure you let the patient and family know the plan. The patient has had a long anxious wait, and can be understandably upset when he or she learns from someone other than you about the decision for admission or discharge.

Admission

Notification of admission:
- Notify the nurse, who will usually call report to the nurses on the floor.
- Notify the person responsible for assigning the patient a bed. Communicate what type of bed or floor the patient requires. Find out if any admission paperwork needs to be filled out.
- Notify the admitting resident (if applicable), PCP, or the physician who will assume care of the patient.

Holding orders. These are temporary orders for stable admitted patients who have a floor bed, but have not been seen by the admitting physician or team. This allows an ED bed to become available more quickly for evaluation of a new patient. These orders should be limited to only necessary treatment and include the following: admitting diagnosis, vital sign frequency, essential medications, intravenous access, oral intake status, code status, allergies, and physician to call and pager number upon patient arrival to floor.

Discharging a Patient

Patients may erroneously interpret being discharged as meaning that they are not ill, and may not pay attention to further disease progression. Patients may not recall details of verbal discharge instructions. Thus, it is important to detail in writing the discharge plan in layman's terms.
- ***Brief summary of ED visit.*** Results of tests.

- *Diagnosis if known or impression.* This should be written so the patient understands the meaning. For example, "broken elbow," not "supracondylar fracture," although medical terms may be written in addition to laymen's terms.
- *Treatment and instructions.* Briefly mention any therapy provided in the ED. Give a detailed description of therapy required upon ED discharge in terms that are easily understandable to the patient. For orthopedic injuries or wound care, include weight-bearing status, splint or wound care, and number of sutures placed and timeline for removal. Include medications to be taken. Remember to remind patients who are taking narcotics and benzodiazepines not to drink alcohol or drive. Patients on narcotic/acetaminophen combinations should be warned not to take extra acetaminophen.
- *Warning signs.* Describe the symptoms and signs for which the patient should return to the ED. They should be inclusive but pertinent, such as a list of life threats or worsening disease state related to the patient diagnosis. Because not all complications can be anticipated, it is good practice to advise patients to call their physician or return to the ED for "any new or worrisome symptoms." Many EDs have prefabricated instruction sheets for specific diagnoses in multiple languages.
- *Follow-up plan.* If safe patient care mandates a short timeframe for follow-up, schedule the appointment yourself or call the PCP to follow-up. The following should be documented on patient discharge instruction from the ED: who (PCP or specialist), when (within what time period), where, and how (contact phone number).

LIFE-THREATENING EMERGENCIES

CHAPTER 4

General Approach to Life-Threatening Emergencies

COLLEEN BUONO ■ DANIEL DAVIS ■ REBEKA BARTH

Overview

Any patient presenting to the emergency department (ED) who appears ill, is in respiratory distress, is hypoxic, has significantly decreased mental status, or is hemodynamically unstable should alert the physician to a potentially life-threatening problem requiring immediate attention.

Evaluation of vital signs, historical data, and physical examination findings should occur simultaneously while initial stabilizing interventions are being performed.

The initial assessment should begin immediately upon arrival with a primary survey using the ABCDE approach: *a*irway, *b*reathing, *c*irculation, *d*isability (discussed below), and *e*xposure. Issues with regard to airway, breathing, and circulation should be addressed immediately with therapeutic interventions. As the patient becomes stabilized or as time permits, the secondary survey should begin. This includes a detailed history and physical examination, ancillary studies, and additional interventions. Reassessment of airway, breathing, and circulation should be performed over the duration of the ED stay, after each intervention, and with any change in status.

An electrocardiogram (EKG) and portable chest radiograph should be ordered, especially for patients with chest pain or shortness of breath. An EKG is not only helpful in the detection of cardiac ischemia or dysrhythmias, but may provide a clinical clue for other pathology such as electrolyte abnormalities or a toxicologic ingestion. Blood should be obtained for laboratory studies and a finger-stick glucose level should be determined quickly especially in a patient with an altered mental status. If available, a bedside hemoglobin level should be obtained. A pregnancy test should be performed on all females of reproductive age. A more liberal use of diagnostic studies are often required in these patients.

The differential diagnosis should be narrowed quickly to identify potentially life-threatening causes and correctable pathology.

Take note of underlying medical conditions, using the medication list, old medical records, information from prehospital providers, family, and friends, and any physical examination findings as clues to the diagnosis. Do not forget to ask about code status especially if the need for aggressive resuscitation measures are immediately imminent. Pediatric resuscitation is discussed in Chapter 74.

Airway

- *General.* The airway should be evaluated for patency and the ability of the patient to protect his or her airway.
- *Historical clues.* Ask about choking prior to unconsciousness, trauma, recent illness, infection, fever, or immunocompromised status. Inquire about oropharyngeal masses, weakness, or swallowing problems. Consider the presence of recreational drugs, exposures, or medications that depress mental status.
- *Assessment.* An alert, talking patient, with no facial swelling or deformity, no excessive secretions, and no stridor, drooling, or choking, most likely has an intact airway. There is no reliable measure of the ability to protect the airway. Indirect measures of level of consciousness, such as Glasgow Coma Scale score (Appendix 2) and bispectral electroencephalogram, are used as surrogates. The absence of a gag or cough reflex and difficulty with secretions are concerning for an unprotected airway. A gradual rise in end-tidal carbon dioxide level may indicate worsening mental status and the inability to protect the airway. Refer to Chapter 5 for a more detailed discussion of airway assessment.
- *Intervention.* Endotracheal intubation is the standard of care for airway protection. Any suspicion for foreign body obstruction requires immediate attention for confirmation and possible emergent removal (see Chapter 5).

Breathing

- *General.* Adequate oxygenation indicates appropriate tissue delivery of oxygen to meet the metabolic needs. The effectiveness of ventilation can be assessed clinically and with carbon dioxide measurements.
- *Historical clues.* Inquire about the presence of underlying cardio-pulmonary disease. The routine use of inhalers or supplemental oxygen is an important clue. Assess for a history of trauma, recent illness, infection, fever, immunocompromised status, missed medications, or dietary indiscretions. Inquire about the presence of underlying neuromuscular or pulmonary disease. Consider the presence of recreational drugs or medications that suppress respiratory drive.
- *Assessment.* Central cyanosis, such as with the lips or tongue, suggests inadequate oxygenation, and is more reliable than peripheral cyanosis, which may be present in low-flow states or with hypothermia. The presence of rales or rhonchi on auscultation may help localize the cause of hypoxia (e.g., pulmonary edema, pneumonia). Dullness to percussion indicates a pleural effusion or hemothorax. Tracheal deviation (e.g., tension pneumothorax) or jugular venous distention (e.g., pneumothorax,

cardiac tamponade, congestive heart failure) may also suggest specific diagnoses that produce hypoxia. Pulse oximetry is the most reliable continuous measure of oxygenation, with a low oxygen saturation (<95%) value indicating a problem with delivery of oxygen to the blood stream. Potential causes include pneumonia, pulmonary edema, pulmonary embolism, severe bronchospasm, and pneumothorax. Pulse oximetry is often unreliable in the presence of profound hypotension. An arterial blood gas analysis will give the most accurate measure of circulatory oxygenation status. Other laboratory tests, such as base deficit, serum lactate level, and the arterial–venous oxygenation difference, suggest tissue oxygen delivery. Chest radiography is useful in differentiating various causes of hypoxemia. The physical examination should assess for ventilation rate and tidal volume as well as air movement. The use of accessory muscles for breathing suggests respiratory failure. Serum carbon dioxide can be measured directly (arterial blood gas PCO_2) or indirectly (end-tidal CO_2). Obtundation may be a sign of hypercapnia due to respiratory failure.

- ■ *Intervention.* With documented or suspected hypoxemia, supplemental oxygen should be delivered via nasal cannula or face mask. Caution should be taken in patients who are dependent on hypoxic respiratory drive for ventilation, such as those with profound chronic obstructive pulmonary disease but high-flow oxygen should not be withheld in the setting of severe hypoxia (SaO_2 <90%) and respiratory distress. Address reversible causes of ventilatory compromise. Ventilatory support with continuous positive airway pressure (CPAP) or biphasic positive airway pressure (BiPAP) may be initiated in the ED in alert, cooperative patients who can handle their own secretions. Endotracheal intubation and mechanical ventilation represent definitive management of profound or resistant hypoxemia (see Chapter 5). Emergent needle decompression followed by tube thoracostomy are indicated for suspected or documented tension pneumothorax (hypotension, unilateral decreased breath sounds, tracheal deviation). This is a clinical diagnosis.

Circulation

- ■ *General.* Hypotension is most commonly seen in the setting of sepsis, decreased circulating blood volume, or pump failure. Less common causes include anaphylaxis and neurogenic shock (see Chapter 7).
- ■ *Historical clues.* Altered mental status, dizziness, and confusion are all symptoms of hypoperfusion. Assess for complaints of chest pain or shortness of breath (congestive heart failure or acute myocardial infarction with cardiogenic shock, aortic dissection, pulmonary embolism, tension pneumothorax), abdominal pain (ruptured abdominal aortic aneurysm, ectopic pregnancy, perforated viscous), or bleeding (gastrointestinal bleeding, menorrhagia, ectopic pregnancy). Assess for a history of trauma to the chest, autoimmune or renal disease to suggest pericardial effusion, coronary artery disease, or previous valvulopathy. Obtain a medication history to determine potential toxicities. Ascertain a history of underlying medical disease or social habits that may increase risk for sepsis or hemorrhage, including bleeding disorders, immunocompromised status,

renal disease, liver disease, diabetes, or intravenous drug use. Identify risk factors for pulmonary embolus (personal or family history of clotting disorders, malignancy, immobilization, recent trauma or myocardial infarction, certain medications).

■ *Assessment.* Vital signs (blood pressure and heart rate) are the most reliable, rapid assessment of perfusion. In addition, the presence of peripheral pulses and pulse quality can give a rough estimate of systolic blood pressure. The radial pulse may not be palpable if the systolic blood pressure is less than 80 mm Hg. The carotid pulse may not be palpable if the systolic blood pressure is less than 60 mm Hg. Examine the lungs (rales in congestive heart failure), heart (gallop in congestive heart failure; muffled in pericardial effusion), and jugular venous pressure (elevated in pericardial tamponade or congestive heart failure; decreased in hypovolemia). Skin findings, such as delayed capillary refill or cyanosis, are important indicators of hypoperfusion. Also examine the skin and mucous membrane for pallor (anemia) and moisture (volume status). Assessment of mental status can indicate adequacy of cerebral perfusion as well as the need for active airway intervention. The three-lead EKG is critical in demonstrating underlying rhythm and monitoring rate. A 12-lead EKG can give additional information about myocardial ischemia or other cardiopulmonary pathology. Serum markers may indicate focal (creatine kinase-MB, troponin for cardiac ischemia) or global ischemia (base deficit, lactate).

■ *Intervention.* Any patient with hypoperfusion should have two large-bore IVs (16–18 gauge). If peripheral venous access is impossible, central venous access (femoral, internal jugular, or subclavian vein) should be obtained. A cordis or introducer catheter is preferred for large-volume infusion as the triple-lumen catheters are too small to permit rapid high-volume infusion. Other alternatives include an interosseous catheter (anterior tibia) or venous cutdown using the saphenous vein. Isotonic (Lactated Ringers solution or normal saline) IV fluids should be considered the mainstay of treatment for hypoperfusion. Pressor therapy should be secondary, and should be given after 2 L of isotonic fluids are given in the presence of hypotension unless the patient is in cardiogenic shock. Specific therapy depends on the diagnosis that is strongly suspected. This includes inotropes for cardiogenic shock, thrombolytics for massive pulmonary embolus, needle decompression and tube thoracostomy for tension pneumothorax, blood transfusion for hemorrhagic shock, or surgery (ruptured ectopic, perforated viscous). Invasive monitoring, either measuring central venous pressure or using Swan-Ganz catheterization, should be used to guide therapy, but is not typically performed in the ED. Balloon-pump insertion should be performed as a temporizing measure with cardiac pump failure. Advanced cardiac life support should be used to guide therapy for specific dysrhythmias (see Chapter 6).

Disability

■ *General.* A rapid neurologic examination is necessary in critical patients for documentation and identification of a potential etiology. Focal neurologic deficits suggest intracranial or spinal cord pathology. A global assessment of consciousness should be performed immediately and repeated frequently on critically ill patients.

■ *Historical clues.* Ascertain a medical history of hypertension, stroke, or cardiovascular disease. Determine whether antecedent symptoms, such as headache, focal weakness, seizures, fevers, or trauma, were present. Also determine the progression of symptoms. The history is critical in determining a potential etiology for altered mental status. This includes a medical history, such as hypertension, stroke, seizures, liver disease, or diabetes. Medications and drug use are often the cause of altered mental status. These include substances that alter level of consciousness directly (opioids or benzodiazepines) or indirectly (oral diabetes agents).

■ *Assessment.* A core temperature should be noted to identify hyper- or hypothermia. Fingerstick glucose level should be determined on all patients with altered mental status or neurologic deficit. The *universal antidotes*, also know as a "coma cocktail" (DON'T: dextrose, oxygen, naloxone, thiamine) should be used for diagnosis and treatment in patients with altered mental status. A rapid neurologic assessment should be performed using the AVPU method or Glasgow Coma Scale or GCS score. The GCS score is described in Appendix 2. AVPU stands for the following: **A**wake, responds to **V**erbal stimuli, responds to **P**ain, or is **U**nresponsive. Asymmetry is concerning for intracranial pathology. Pinpoint pupils are classically seen with opioid overdose. The neurologic assessment should be repeated frequently. Imaging with a non-contrast head CT scan should be performed to rapidly identify causes for altered mental status that require immediate neurosurgical intervention. Patients who are hemodynamically unstable or have an unprotected airway should not leave the ED until stabilized. Initial diagnostic studies for patients with an altered mental status include a urine toxicology screen, routine chemistries, ammonia, and an EKG. An arterial blood gas level may be needed to determine acid-base status or if concerned for CO_2 retention or hypoxia. A lumbar puncture should be performed with altered mental status of possible infectious etiology, concern for subarachnoid hemorrhage, or if no specific diagnosis is reached and the patient continues to have an altered mental status.

■ *Intervention.* Addressing airway, breathing, and circulation should be the first priority. Rapid diagnosis is critical to determining whether there is an indication for thrombolytic therapy, or the need for hemorrhage control in patients with an intracranial bleed (to include reversal of anticoagulants, activated factor VIIa, or prothrombin complex concentrate). Early neurology consultation should be done for acute stroke. Evidence of increased intracranial pressure, including altered mental status with a unilateral fixed and dilated pupil, is an indication for the initiation of intracranial pressure therapy. This includes gentle hyperventilation (CO_2 of 30–35 mm Hg), mannitol or hypertonic saline, and head elevation. Early neurosurgical consultation should be initiated. Early antibiotic therapy should be administered if meningitis is suspected, even before laboratory testing is complete or lumbar puncture is performed.

Teaching Points

All critically ill patients need immediate evaluation and frequent re-evaluation as to their clinical status. If there is any possibility of a critical disease being present, an immediate determination of the ABCs is appropriate.

Any patient who has altered vital signs or an altered mental status should have a fingerstick glucose level determined or be empirically given the universal antidotes (DON'T: dextrose, oxygen, naloxone, thiamine). Such patients should be evaluated for active airway management.

Be alert to time-constrained diseases such as tension pneumothorax, pericardial tamponade, cerebral herniation syndromes, and inadequate tissue and organ perfusion.

CHAPTER   **5**

Airway Management

MAMATA KENE ■ DANIEL DAVIS

Overview

A managed airway is one that allows successful ventilation and oxygenation as well as one that protects the respiratory tree from compromise by foreign body or aspiration. Assessment and management of the airway and ventilation, both in resuscitation and the acute management of medical patients, are critical issues in emergency medicine.

Initial Approach to the Patient
General

■ Continuous pulse oximetry and cardiac monitoring should be performed on any patient with possible airway or respiratory compromise. A good wave form suggests the reading is accurate. In situations where poor peripheral perfusion exists (i.e., shock), the reading is often not reliable and an arterial blood gas may be more helpful. Central placement of the pulse oximetry probe (e.g., ear, nose, or forehead) may improve accuracy in low perfusion states. Intravenous (IV) access should be immediately obtained for the administration of medications.

Patient Assessment

- *Airway.* The first assessment when patients present to the emergency department (ED) should be their ability to maintain a patent airway. Most often, this can be confirmed by having the patient speak. Simple questioning such as asking the name, location, and date should suffice for this initial assessment. This will also allow assessment of the patient's level of alertness, ability to phonate, and handle oral secretions. A detailed examination of the external face, oral cavity, neck, and mouth should follow, looking for any abnormality that may interfere with the passage of air or direct laryngoscopy. Several assessments have been described that may help to predict the presence of a difficult airway and are listed in Table 5–1. Also assess the patency of the nares. The presence of subcutaneous emphysema (a crackling sensation upon palpation of the soft tissues) is concerning for disruption of an air-filled passage such as from trauma to the airway, pneumothorax, or esophageal rupture. In the comatose patient, a gag reflex and the ability of a patient to handle oral secretions are used in evaluating protective reflexes.

- *Respiratory pattern.* Stridor is often audible without a stethoscope and is concerning for upper airway obstruction. Assess chest movement for symmetry. Paradoxical movement may be seen in a flail chest in which the flail segment expands during exhalation and is depressed during inhalation with respect to the unaffected parts of the chest cavity. Asymmetric movement of the chest may be seen in patients with a pneumothorax. Diaphragmatic breathing may be noted in patients with a spinal cord injury. During inspiration, there is little movement of the chest, but expansion of the abdominal cavity is occurring due to the descent of the diaphragm.

- *Breath sounds.* Auscultation of the chest will assist in determining the adequacy of air exchange in the lungs. Breath sounds that are decreased on one side suggest a hemothorax, pneumothorax, pleural effusion, or other pulmonary process. Assess for adventitious sounds such as wheezing (e.g., asthma or chronic obstructive pulmonary disease [COPD]), rales (e.g., pulmonary edema), or gurgling (e.g., aspiration). Diminished breath sounds are more concerning in the asthmatic patient in respiratory distress than diffuse wheezes readily heard throughout the lung fields as this is more indicative of poor gas exchange and a tiring patient who needs more aggressive therapy.

- *Other.* The clinical assessment should include the patient's level of consciousness and degree of fatigue secondary to laborious breathing. The severity of coexisting conditions or injuries should also be assessed.

Who Needs Active Airway Management?

The indications fall into three general categories:

- Failure of airway maintenance: obstruction or inability to protect airway (e.g., loss of airway reflexes).
- Failure of oxygenation (evidence of tissue hypoxemia/impaired oxygen delivery) or ventilation (hypercarbia).

Table 5–1 Assessments for Predicting the Difficult Airway

	Assessment	Concern
External face	Facial hair	May prevent adequate seal of face mask.
	Face shape	Abnormal face shape or trauma may prevent adequate seal of face mask and may make intubation difficult.
Oral cavity	Oral pharynx	Oral intubation will be difficult if unable to fit at least three of the patient's fingers between the upper and lower teeth. Any swelling, mass lesions, secretions, and bleeding may also make intubation difficult.
	Teeth	Edentulous people are easier to intubate but may have a poor seal with the bag-valve-mask. Buck teeth or prominent central incisors may make intubation difficult. Take caution with broken or fragile teeth that may break off during laryngoscopy and lodge in the airway.
Neck	Short bull neck	May make visualization of the glottic opening very difficult.
	Immobility	Unable to optimally align the oral, pharyngeal, and laryngeal axis. Visualization of the glottic opening is more difficult.
	Mass	May cause an obstructing lesion or distort anatomic landmarks for intubation.
Measurements	Thyroid notch to mentum	If less than two fingers fit in this space, larynx may not be low enough to permit visualization by oral route.
	Mentum to hyoid	Measurement of the mandibular space for access to the airway. If less than three fingers fit into this space, the tongue may get in the way.
	Mallampati score*	The patient should open the mouth as wide as possible and stick out the tongue. There may be moderate (class III) to severe difficulty (class IV) in visualizing the glottic opening if most of the uvula is not visualized.

*A class I Mallampati score indicates complete visualization of the oropharynx, including the tonsillar pillars which are not visualized in a class II. The soft palate and base of the uvula are visualized in a class III. Only the hard palate is seen in a class IV. Most individuals are class I and class II. There is usually no difficulty with visualizing the glottic opening in these patients.

■ Anticipated clinical course: a patient may require immediate intubation because the disease state can be predicted to produce obstruction or ventilatory failure (e.g., third degree burns or Ludwig's angina).

Within these categories are patients who need a definitive, immediate, life-saving intervention and patients who may benefit from basic noninvasive adjunctive measures to maintain adequate oxygenation and ventilation.

Clinical Decision Making

- The decision to intubate emergently is a clinical one, and should not be delayed pending diagnostic studies such as a chest radiograph or arterial blood gas. Immediate intubation is indicated for patients who are unable to protect the airway. The exception is those patients with an immediately reversible condition, such as opioid overdose or reversible cardiac dysrhythmia. Intubation may be avoided in some patients who initially present with respiratory distress and hypoxia if they respond to aggressive therapy with noninvasive ventilation or pharmacotherapy (e.g., asthma, pulmonary edema).
- For patients who do not require immediate intubation, time may allow for initial diagnostic studies while waiting for pharmacotherapy and basic noninvasive measures to take effect. These studies include arterial blood gas, chest radiographs, and soft-tissue lateral radiograph of the neck (e.g., epiglottitis).

Basic Noninvasive Measures
Supplemental Oxygen

- *Indications.* Oxygen should be administered to any patient with respiratory distress, hypoxia, or potential airway or respiratory compromise.
- *Technique.* A nonrebreather (NRB) mask or nasal cannula is placed over the face or nares. Any patient requiring intubation should be placed on a NRB immediately to provide an adequate oxygen reservoir during the intubation procedure.
- *Advantages.* The NRB with reservoir allows theoretical delivery of 100% oxygen; in practice this figure is closer to 75%. A nasal cannula or simple face mask delivers about 26% oxygen flow.
- *Disadvantages.* This strategy does not provide airway protection. Patients who are dependent on hypoxic respiratory drive (e.g., COPD) may develop respiratory arrest if given high flow oxygen therapy.

Nasopharyngeal Airway

- *Indications.* The nasopharyngeal airway (NPA) is a method to open the airway in a patient who requires bag-valve-mask (BVM) ventilation. To maximize BVM, one NPA can be placed in each naris in addition to an oral pharyngeal airway (OPA). It is also useful for the patient with active gag reflexes who is somnolent but still spontaneously breathing effectively (e.g., overdose patient) and to facilitate nasotracheal suctioning in a patient with copious secretions.
- *Technique.* Apply lidocaine gel or sterile lubricant to the airway tip, then direct the airway posteriorly avoiding trauma to the nasal septum. The ideal length is measured from the nares to tragus of the ear.
- *Advantages.* The NPA opens the upper airway for spontaneous or BVM ventilation and can be used in patients with an intact gag reflex.
- *Disadvantages.* The NPA does not protect against aspiration and is only an adjunct.

Oropharyngeal Airway (OPA)

- **Indications.** The OPA is another means to open the airway in a patient with *absent* upper airway reflexes to facilitate BVM ventilation. Patients who are able to tolerate an OPA require endotracheal intubation for airway protection.
- **Technique.** Direct the concave portion cephalad over the tongue and rotate 180 degrees, or insert with the concave portion caudad over the tongue while depressing the tongue with a tongue blade. Alternatively, the OPA can be placed directly with the concave portion over the tongue while the tongue is depressed with a tongue blade. The ideal length is measured from the patient's lips to the tragus of the ear.
- **Advantages.** The OPA opens the upper airway for effective BVM ventilation.
- **Disadvantages.** The OPA does not protect against aspiration, and is only an adjunct until endotracheal intubation can be instituted. Its use may be precluded by an active gag reflex.

Bag-Valve-Mask (BVM)

- **Indications.** In the spontaneously breathing patient, BVM ventilation is used to augment the patient's breathing. In the apneic patient, this is used as a temporizing measure while preparations for intubation are made. This is the first rescue device for a failed intubation.
- **Technique.** The patient should be placed in the sniffing position with slight flexion of the neck, with the head extended on the neck in order to optimize the alignment of the oral, pharyngeal, and laryngeal axes (Figure 5–1). In patients with suspected cervical spine injury, the c-spine should be placed in neutral position. The operator must establish an effective seal, compress the bag, and allow for adequate inspiration and expiration. A two-person approach is more successful due to the difficulty in maintaining a proper seal. Place the mask initially on the nasal bridge, then lower it down onto the malar eminences and lower alveolar ridge to completely cover the nose and mouth. The thumb and index finger of one hand are used to apply pressure to the mask, and to obtain a seal on the face. The long, ring, and little fingers of this same hand should be used to maximally elevate the mandible (i.e., jaw thrust) to help keep the airway open. Insertion of an OPA or NPA may help with upper airway obstruction during BVM ventilation. A jaw thrust may also facilitate opening of the airway. Ideal rate and tidal volume are 8-12 breaths per minute and 500 to 700 ml per breath, being careful not to overventilate the patient. Effective BVM ventilation is noted by feeling resistance in the bag, low resistance to ventilation of the patient, the rise and fall of the chest, no gastric distention, and improvement in oxygen saturation.
- **Advantages.** The BVM can provide adequate ventilation without requiring active airway management.
- **Disadvantages.** A BVM is not a controlled airway, and may lead to gastric insufflation and regurgitation. Cricoid pressure (i.e., Sellick maneuver) can be used to prevent gastric insufflation and divert air into

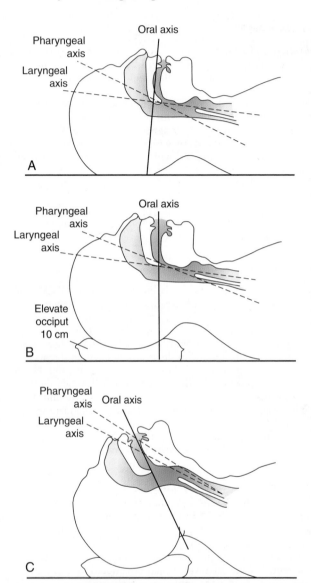

Figure 5–1. Head positioning for endotracheal intubation. **A,** Neutral position. **B,** Head elevated. **C,** "Sniffing" position, with flexed neck and extended head. Note how flexing the neck and extending the head to line up the various axes allows for intubation. This position creates the shortest distance and straightest line between the teeth and vocal cords. *(From Clinical Procedures in Emergency Medicine, Philadelphia: WB Saunders, 2004, p. 73.)*

the lungs. If the patient is actively vomiting, release cricoid pressure, turn the patient to the side (log roll if there is concern for spinal injury), and suction the oral cavity. These patients may need intubation using RSI (see below) for airway protection. Patient anxiety or discomfort limits its use if the patient is awake.

Noninvasive Positive-Pressure Ventilation Via Continuous Positive Airway Pressure or Biphasic Positive Airway Pressure

- ■ *Indications.* Noninvasive positive-pressure ventilation (NIPPV) via continuous positive airway pressure (CPAP) or biphasic positive airway pressure (BiPAP) is a technique in which patients must have a patent airway, spontaneous respirations, and be conscious and cooperative. Typical ED patients who are eligible for NIPPV include those with status asthmaticus, congestive heart failure (CHF), COPD exacerbation, pneumonia, or mild postextubation stridor.
- ■ *Technique.* CPAP requires a mask over the nose and mouth, and delivers a constant low level of positive airway pressure (usually 10 cm H_2O) during inspiratory and expiratory phases. BiPAP can be delivered through a mask covering the nose, and alternates between a higher inspiratory pressure (10-12 cm H_2O) and lower expiratory positive pressure (5 cm H_2O).
- ■ *Advantages.* BiPAP or CPAP facilitate airway opening, including the alveoli, support respiration to prevent fatigue, and improve gas exchange.
- ■ *Disadvantages.* This does not provide airway protection. Patient anxiety or discomfort may limit successful use.

Endotracheal Intubation and Rapid-Sequence Induction (RSI)
General

- ■ A *definitive airway* is defined as the placement of a cuffed endotracheal tube (ETT) within the trachea to maximize oxygenation and ventilation and minimize the potential for aspiration.
- ■ Once the decision to intubate is made, several approaches are available. An "awake" oral intubation can be performed on the spontaneously breathing, conscious, or semiconscious patient, and is most commonly used today when paralytic agents are contraindicated. Blind nasotracheal intubation is another method of intubation used in the ED. The procedure requires a spontaneously breathing patient, but is now used infrequently in most EDs since the advent of rapid-sequence intubation (RSI). Various sedative and topical agents are used to facilitate both of these methods of intubation.
- ■ RSI establishes an active controlled airway using pharmacologic adjuncts that induce unconsciousness and paralysis in order to facilitate laryngoscopy and intubation as well as minimize adverse consequences associated with the procedure.
- ■ Acute complications of endotracheal intubation include tube misplacement, desaturation, bradycardia, and injury to the soft tissues of the hypopharynx and larynx. Prolonged high-pressure ventilation can result in barotrauma (pneumothorax, pneumomediastinum, and subcutaneous emphysema.) This is especially important to prevent in the child.

Rapid-Sequence Intubation Technique (7 P's)

■ **Preparation.** Assess the patient for a difficult airway and likelihood of successful BVM ventilation (first rescue device in a failed intubation). The patient should be placed in a resuscitation room with continuous pulse oximetry and cardiac monitoring should be in place. The patient should have at least one well-functioning IV line. Test all airway equipment to be used for intubation (i.e., ETT cuff and laryngoscope). At least two blades and two ETTs (include one size smaller than the one to be used) should be readily available. In general, an 8.0- to 8.5-French tube should be used on adult men, and a 7.5- to 8.0-French tube should be used on adult women. If a difficult intubation is anticipated, smaller tubes and rescue airway devices should be available as well. A stylet should be used for all adult intubations to facilitate passage of the ETT. With the stylet in place, the ETT should be bent and formed into the shape of a "hockey" stick such that the tip of the ETT is facing upward to facilitate entry into the anterior placed glottic opening. Ensure that the stylet does not protrude through the distal end of the ETT or the small side port. The proximal end of the ETT should be bent over proximal to the ETT adapter. Ensure that the stylet can be easily removed from the ETT.

■ **Preoxygenation.** This is achieved with NRB or BVM and 100% oxygen for at least 5 minutes to create an oxygen reservoir so that the patient can tolerate the several minutes of apnea during the intubation procedure itself. Children, obese individuals, and critically ill patients have less reserve and desaturate more rapidly than other patients.

■ **Pretreatment.** Pretreatment agents are often included in the RSI protocol to reduce the adverse physiologic consequences of laryngoscopy. The mnemonic for the agents typically used is LOAD: *l*idocaine, *o*pioids, *a*tropine, and a *d*efasiculating dose of a paralytic agent. The administration of 1.5 mg/kg of lidocaine helps to attenuate the cardiovascular response to intubation, suppress the cough reflex, and mitigate the increase in intracranial pressure (ICP) response to intubation. Opioids, specifically fentanyl, may significantly attenuate the sympathetic response to intubation. Fentanyl has the greatest utility in patients with conditions at risk of worsening from increasing blood pressure or vascular shear forces (e.g., aneurysm or penetrating vascular trauma patient) associated with laryngoscopy. Fentanyl also has the added benefit of sedation and analgesia; however, caution must be used in blunting the sympathetic response in a patient in shock who is dependent on a sympathetic drive for cardiovascular stability. Atropine is recommended in children younger than 5 to 10 years to blunt the potential vagal response of bradycardia resulting from laryngoscopy and the use of succinylcholine. Because repeated doses of succinylcholine may lead to asystole in adults, atropine should be considered in this patient population as well. A defasiculating dose of a nondepolarizing paralytic agent (e.g., vecuronium) may be given before succinylcholine to reduce the fasciculations associated with its administration and the associated increase in ICP. Beta-blockers, particularly esmolol, may also reduce the incidence and severity of the hypertensive and tachycardic responses

Table 5–2 Summary of Rapid-Sequence Intubation Agents

Pretreatment Agents	Dose	Comment
Lidocaine	1.5 mg/kg	Increased ICP
Opioid (fentanyl)	3 µg/kg	Sympathetic stimulation of laryngoscopy; increased ICP
Atropine	0.02 mg/kg	Pediatric patients or repeated doses of succinylcholine in adults. Minimum dose is 0.5 mg IV.
Defasiculating agents (vecuronium)	0.01 mg/kg	Increased ICP
Beta-blocker (esmolol)	2 mg/kg	Sympathetic stimulation of laryngoscopy

Induction Agents	Dose	Comment
Etomidate	0.3 mg/kg	Advantage: Rapid onset, short duration, protection from myocardial and cerebral ischemia, minimal histamine release, and stable hemodynamic profile Disadvantage: Lack of blunting of the sympathetic response to intubation, high incidence of myoclonus, nausea and vomiting, potential activation of seizures in patients with epileptogenic foci, and impaired glucocorticoid response to stress
Ketamine	1–2 mg/kg	Advantage: Bronchodilator effect for severe asthmatics; may use for hemodynamically unstable if no concern for increased ICP Disadvantage: Cardiovascular stimulation, bronchodilation, and increases ICP
Propofol	2.5 mg/kg	Advantage: Profound amnesic properties and reliable prompt awakening; ideal agent in which frequent neurologic assessments are warranted; attenuates potential rises in ICP; may depress pharyngeal and laryngeal muscle tone and reflexes Disadvantage: May decrease cerebral perfusion pressure; may cause myocardial depression
Thiopental	3–5 mg/kg	Advantage: Cerebroprotective; favorable induction agent for patients with status epilepticus or increased ICP; causes cerebral vasoconstriction, reduces cerebral blood volume. Disadvantage: Hypotension.

Continued

Table 5–2 Summary of Rapid-Sequence Intubation Agents—*cont'd*

Paralytic Agents	Dose	Comment
Midazolam	0.2–0.3 mg/kg	Advantage: Anticonvulsant activity Disadvantage: May cause hypotension at high doses
Succinylcholine (Sch)	1.5 mg/kg	It actually acts as an agonist at the acetylcholine receptor, and causes prolonged depolarization resulting in muscle relaxation after a brief period of fasciculation. Advantage: Very rapid onset of action and short duration Disadvantage: Hyperkalemia, increased ICP, malignant hyperthermia. Certain disease states cause an exaggerated release of potassium in response to succinylcholine that is due to an up-regulation of acetylcholine receptors: spinal cord injury, stroke, muscular dystrophy, multiple sclerosis, Guillain-Barré syndrome, and other conditions that cause prolonged immobility.
Rocuronium	1 mg/kg	Nondepolarizing agent that blocks the acetylcholine receptor at the neuromuscular junction. Advantage: Nondepolarizing agent; does not increase potassium or cause increased ICP Disadvantage: Long onset and offset
Vecuronium	0.1 mg/kg	Same as rocuronium but longer onset time and duration.

ICP, intracranial pressure.

to tracheal manipulation. The pretreatment agents should be given approximately 3 minutes prior to laryngoscopy. The most common agents are listed in Table 5–2.

- *Paralysis with induction.* Induction agents are usually given just before the paralytic agent to *induce* unconsciousness. The most useful induction and paralytic agents have a quick onset and rapid offset. The most commonly used agents are listed in Table 5–2.
- *Protection and positioning.* The Sellick maneuver (cricoid cartilage pressure) may be applied with the administration of the induction agent to prevent passive regurgitation. This should be released if the patient starts to vomit (if actively vomiting, the patient is not adequately paralyzed), or if it obscures the airway anatomy. Patient positioning is the same as that described under BVM technique (Figure 5–1).
- *Placement with proof.* The procedure for direct laryngoscopy is described in Figure 5–2. Direct laryngoscopy should include external laryngeal manipulation to optimize visualization of the glottis. The BURP

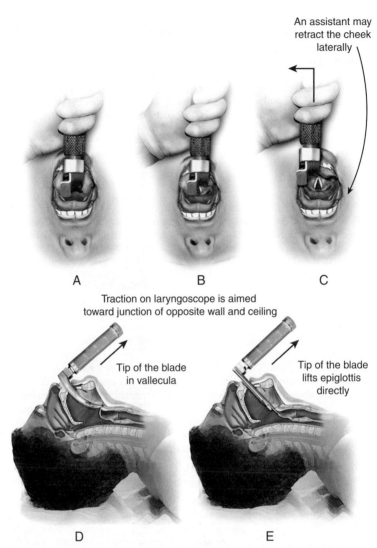

An assistant may retract the cheek laterally

A B C

Traction on laryngoscope is aimed toward junction of opposite wall and ceiling

Tip of the blade in vallecula

Tip of the blade lifts epiglottis directly

D E

Figure 5-2. Direct laryngoscopy technique. **A,** Incorrect technique: laryngoscope blade under the middle of the tongue, with the sides of the tongue hanging down and obscurring the glottis. **B,** Incorrect technique: Tongue not pushed far enough to the left, obscuring the glottis. **C,** Correct blade position with tongue elevated and to the left. **D,** Use of the curved (MacIntosh) laryngoscope blade with the tip in the vallecula with secondary elevation of the epiglottis. **E,** Use of the straight (Miller) blade with tip directly elevating the epiglottis. *(From Clinical Procedures in Emergency Medicine, Philadelphia: WB Saunders, 2004, p. 76.)*

(*b*ackward, *u*pward, and *r*ightward *p*ressure of the larynx) maneuver may improve the laryngoscopic view. The BURP maneuver can be initially performed by the intubator and maintained by the individual holding cricoid pressure. Endotracheal tube placement is confirmed by direct visualization of the ETT passing through the cords, bilateral breath sounds with absence of gurgling over the epigastrium, condensation within the ETT corresponding with exhalation, rise and fall of the chest with bagging, improvement in pulse oximetry, CO_2 detection (Yes for "yellow" if in the trachea, or will remain purple if in the esophagus when using qualitative or colorimetric detectors; quantitative measurement of CO_2 are also available), or an aspiration device (easy aspiration or re-expansion occurs if the ETT is in the trachea). A chest radiograph should be obtained to assess pulmonary status and confirm that the ETT is midline and located 2 cm above the carina. It cannot confirm that the ETT is within the trachea.

■ *Postintubation management.* The patient requires continued sedation and monitoring of ventilation, oxygenation, and hemodynamic stability. Initial ventilator settings are listed in Table 5–3. Bradycardia with hypoxia should be assumed to be due to an esophageal intubation until proven otherwise (by direct visualization of the endotracheal tube within the glottic opening). Hypertension is usually due to inadequate sedation or pain management. Long acting sedation should be administered with a benzodiazepine and a competitive neuromuscular blocking agent or propofol (if the patient is not hypotensive). An opioid analgesic may be added for patient comfort. Hypotension following intubation may be due to induction agents, hypovolemia, or may be cardiogenic, and should be treated with fluid boluses. Hypotension in the setting of high peak inspiratory pressures (PIPS) may be due to decreased venous return or the more concerning tension pneumothorax. A tension pneumothorax is manifested by increased resistance to BVM, unilateral decreased breath sounds, and hypoxia. Decreased venous return is seen in patients with high intrathoracic pressures, and is treated with fluid boluses, bronchodilators, increasing expiratory time, decreased tidal volumes.

Rescue Airway Techniques

Basic principle. Failure of endotracheal intubation is defined as three un-successful attempts by the most skilled operator present. The first rescue technique for a failed intubation is BVM. If the patient is able to be oxygenated with BVM, there are several rescue airway techniques available, a few of which are described below. If the patient cannot be intubated or may be oxygenated using BVM, a Combitube or laryngeal mask airway should be attempted to maintain oxygenation if no obstruction exists. If this is not successful, a surgical airway is required. A cricothyrotomy is the surgical airway of choice used by emergency physicians. The choice of a rescue strategy should be guided by ability to maintain oxygenation and operator comfort with various techniques.

Combitube

■ *Insertion.* The device can be inserted in any position. After lifting the jaw and tongue upward with the nondominant hand, the Combitube is

Table 5–3 Initial Ventilator Settings (General)

Parameter	Setting	Comment
Tidal volume (V_T) Respiratory rate (RR) or frequency (f)	8-10 ml/kg	The volume in single breath. Lower tidal volumes used in ARDS (adult respiratory distress syndrome) and obstructive pulmonary diseases.
	8–12 breaths/ minute	This should be higher in children children and situations in which CO_2 production is increased (i.e., acidosis)
Fractional concentration of inspired oxygen (F_iO_2)	100% or 1.0 v	This should be weaned as soon as possible to the lowest amount of oxygen required to maintain an oxygen saturation of at least 95%.
Positive end-expiratory pressure (PEEP);	0-5 cm H_2O (5 cm H_2O is physiologic)	May be added to maintain pressure in alveoli to prevent collapse of the small airways. May be useful in hypoxemia and enable decreased oxygen requirements but may cause a decreased venous return and cardiac output. May also worsen barotrauma or further increase ICP (intracranial pressure).
Ventilation mode	Continuous mechanical ventilation	Also called assist control mode. Usually for patients who have no spontaneous respiratory activity of their own or are barely breathing. The patient receives a minimum number of breaths each minute at a preset tidal volume. If the patient takes a spontaneous breath, it will trigger the ventilator to give an assisted breath at the preset tidal volume.
	Synchronized intermittent mechanical ventilation	This is for patients who are able to breath on their own but require some assistance. Patients receive a minimum number of breaths at a preset tidal volume but are also able to breath on their own between these breaths without ventilator assistance.
	Continuous positive airway pressure	For patients who are breathing spontaneously on their own. Various forms of pressure support may be added to decrease the work of breathing.

inserted in the midline, allowing the curve of the device to follow the curved path of the airway until the alveolar ridge is opposite the imprinted bands on the device. Inflate the proximal, large cuff (blue) then the distal smaller cuff (white) with the indicated amount of air (usually 100 ml for the large cuff and 5 to 10 ml for the small cuff). Ventilation to either the proximal port (if esophageally inserted, which is most common) or distal port (if endotracheally inserted, rare) allows oxygen delivery to the respiratory tree. When suctioning the patient through the Combitube, always introduce the suction catheter through the white tube. Because the Combitube will usually be in the esophagus, most of the suctioning through the tube will be from the stomach, and will result in decreased gastric distension. In the event that the Combitube is in the trachea, suctioning of the patient's airway will result. For removal, completely deflate the blue balloon then the white balloon. Have suction readily available.

- **Advantages.** The Combitube is successful as a temporizing measure when endotracheal intubation attempts are unsuccessful. It is a blind technique although a laryngoscope may be used to facilitate insertion.
- **Disadvantages.** The Combitube does not protect against aspiration nor does it allow high-pressure ventilation as may be necessary with severe reactive airways disease or ARDS.
- **Complications.** Excessive force with insertion can cause trauma to the airway or esophagus. Aspiration is always a concern.

Laryngeal Mask Airway
- **Insertion.** The laryngeal mask airway (LMA) is placed blindly by directing the mask portion posteriorly with a 180-degree rotation; upon insertion into the posterior pharynx, the tube is rotated and the laryngeal mask inflated.
- **Advantages.** The LMA is successful as a temporizing measure when endotracheal intubation attempts are unsuccessful. Intubating LMAs allows for placement of an ETT.
- **Disadvantages.** The LMA does not protect against aspiration nor does it allow high-pressure ventilation as may be necessary with severe reactive airways disease or respiratory insufficiency (adult respiratory distress syndrome [ARDS]).
- **Complications.** Complete airway obstruction and aspiration.

Nasotracheal Intubation (NTI)
- **Insertion.** The patient is placed semi-upright with the neck slightly extended and the nares are sprayed with a topical vasoconstrictor to minimize epistaxis. The ETT should be 0.5 to 1 mm smaller than for orotracheal intubation. The nasotracheal tube is advanced posteriorly toward the occiput, with gentle rotation to bypass any obstructions encountered; insertion should be coordinated with inspiration. Placement of a nasal trumpet prior to NTI may help prime the nares.
- **Advantages.** Nasotracheal intubation may be used in patients who cannot tolerate the positioning or paralysis necessary for RSI.
- **Disadvantages.** This technique is often unsuccessful in an apneic patient. It has a lower success rate than oral intubation. It should not be used in

patients with complex or extensive nasal or mid-facial fractures, or severe cervical arthritis.

- ■ ***Complications.*** Nasal trauma, epistaxis, nasopharyngeal perforation; cribriform plate penetration, and esophageal intubation.

Fiberoptic Intubation

- ■ ***Insertion.*** The fiberoptic scope is lubricated (to facilitate easy removal through the ETT) and placed through the ETT lumen. The traditional fiberoptic scope has a control lever to manipulate the distal tip: forward and backward movement is achieved; rotational movement is done by rotating the wrist. Rotate both the ETT and the scope as one unit. The intubator should stand at the head of the bed. The scope is advanced through the cords during inspiration and into the trachea but avoiding the carina (stimulates coughing). The ETT is passed over the scope and into the trachea; the fiberoptic scope is then removed.
- ■ ***Advantages.*** This is a very helpful technique for a predicted difficult airway in which direct visualization of the glottic opening is limited or impossible.
- ■ ***Disadvantages.*** Excessive blood and secretions in the airway may obstruct the view. The procedure may take more time especially in inexperienced hands, and patients are not able to be oxygenated or ventilated during this time.

Gum-Elastic Bougie

- ■ ***Insertion.*** This is a semirigid stylet that can be shaped and anteriorly directed for localization of the trachea. An endotracheal tube is then advanced over the gum elastic bougie to achieve intubation.
- ■ ***Advantages.*** This technique may be helpful in patients with anterior laryngeal anatomy in which direct visualization of the glottic opening is limited.
- ■ ***Disadvantages.*** Without direct visualization, esophageal intubation remains possible, and the stylet may cause soft tissue trauma.

Retrograde Tracheal Intubation

- ■ ***Technique.*** A needle is inserted into the cricothyroid membrane and directed cephalad 30 to 45 degrees from horizontal; a guide wire is passed cephalad through the needle to the oropharynx, and the ETT advanced over the guide wire.
- ■ ***Advantages.*** Using a guide wire ensures accurate placement of the ETT.
- ■ ***Disadvantages.*** Requires more time to perform than cricothyrotomy.
- ■ ***Complications.*** Laceration to the oropharyngeal structures by the guide wire and failure to place the ETT, as well as difficulties in finding the guide wire in the face of secretions or oral bleeding.

Surgical Airways

Basic principle. Surgical airways are indicated as a rescue technique (especially in the patient who is unable to be intubated or ventilated by BVM). For patients who have distorted airway anatomy or injuries, the most likely scenarios include facial trauma or upper airway obstruction that make surgical airway the preferred approach.

Cricothyrotomy

■ *Technique.* A vertical scalpel incision is made from the level of the thyroid cartilage to about 1 cm above the sternal notch. The cricothyroid membrane is visualized (or palpated if bleeding obsures visualization) following blunt dissection with curved hemostats and incised horizontally with a #11 scalpel blade. The laryngeal structures are stabilized with a tracheal hook, and the membrane incision is dilated with a Trousseau dilator. The Shiley #4 (cuffed tube) or a cut down ETT is then advanced and directed inferiorly (Figure 5–3). There are several percutaneous cricothyrotomy kits now available using a method similar to the Seldinger technique for vascular catheter placement.

■ *Advantages.* The open technique allows airway access when the trachea cannot be intubated.

■ *Disadvantages.* This operation cannot be performed on children who are under age 8, or older children who are very small.

■ *Complications.* Complications include bleeding, soft tissue damage, subcutaneous or supraglottic tube placement, scarring, superior laryngeal nerve damage, or pneumothorax.

Tracheostomy

■ *Technique.* This technique is indicated in children too small for safe cricothyrotomy, for any diseases that destroy the upper airway anatomy, and for penetrating injuries of the upper Zone 2 neck that produce too much hemorrhage to safely perform cricothyrotomy. The technique is similar to cricothyrotomy, except that the trachea is exposed at the level of the second tracheal ring. The thyroid isthmus may interfere with performance, and require division between clamps.

■ *Advantages.* A larger Shiley tube can be used, and the technique is applicable to very small tracheas.

■ *Disadvantages.* This is technically much harder to perform than cricothyrotomy, and has more serious potential complications. It is typically beyond the scope of emergency medicine practice.

■ *Complications.* The risk of damage to parathyroid glands, recurrent laryngeal nerve, jugular vein, and carotid artery is greater than with cricothyrotomy.

Needle Cricothyrotomy or Jet Insufflation

■ *Technique.* A 12- or 14-gauge angiocatheter is advanced over a needle into the cricothyroid membrane, and then jet insufflation is used to ventilate (high pressure air flow, 1:10 to 1:15 inspiratory to expiratory ratio). There is a variation of this technique using a Cook Catheter kit that allows insertion of a larger tube. This tube is not cuffed, and insertion is difficult if there is any airway anatomic distortion.

■ *Advantages.* This method can be used in children, in whom the larynx is more susceptible to damage from surgical cricothyrotomy.

■ *Disadvantages.* This technique is inadequate for prolonged ventilation, especially in adults. The equipment is difficult to set up, especially when used infrequently.

■ *Complications.* Damage to soft tissue structures and failure to adequately ventilate; in the presence of upper airway obstruction, this can lead to tension pneumomediastinum or tension pneumothorax.

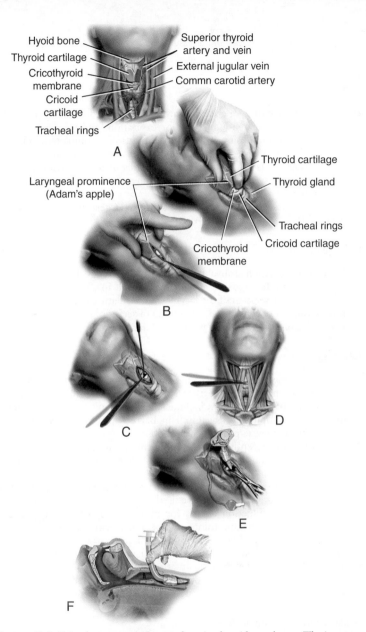

Figure 5–3. Cricothyrotomy. **A,** Locate the cricothyroid membrane. The insert shows further anatomic details of the region. **B,** A longitudinal skin incision is made over the cricothyroid membrane. **C,** The larynx is stabilized with the thumb and middle finger or a tracheal hook (held in the nondominant hand) while an incision is made in the cricothyroid membrane. **D,** The surrounding anatomy of the neck is shown, with the incision being made in the cricothyroid membrane. **E,** After the incision in the cricothyroid membrane is widened using hemostats, curved Mayo scissors, or the blunt end of the scalpel, the tracheostomy tube is inserted between the curved hemostats or tracheal dilator. **F,** Lateral view, showing insertion of the tracheostomy tube. *(From Clinical Procedures in Emergency Medicine, Philadelphia: WB Saunders, 2004, p. 120.)*

Labels in figure:

- Hyoid bone
- Thyroid cartilage
- Cricothyroid membrane
- Cricoid cartilage
- Tracheal rings
- Superior thyroid artery and vein
- External jugular vein
- Commn carotid artery
- A
- Laryngeal prominence (Adam's apple)
- Thyroid cartilage
- Thyroid gland
- Tracheal rings
- Cricoid cartilage
- Cricothyroid membrane
- B
- C
- D
- E
- F

Special Situations
Asthma

- The inspiratory time of the respiratory cycle should be short (i.e., rapid peak flow) to allow enough time for expiration, and to avoid stacking breaths (i.e., inspiration begins before expiration is completed). The rate should also be slow enough to allow time for expiration. Permissive hypercapnea is used in intubated asthmatics to avoid having too high a level of airway pressures and subsequent barotrauma or decreased cardiac output.
- These patients should be intubated with the largest diameter ETT that is possible.

Laryngospasm

- Inadequate sedation, saliva levels, and oropharyngeal instrumentation can precipitate laryngospasm, which can result in an obstructed airway. This involuntary spasm of the laryngeal musculature may be ablated with positive-pressure ventilation, suctioning of secretions, cessation of airway manipulation, jaw thrust, or neuromuscular blockade.

Neurologic

- Certain disease states cause an exaggerated release of potassium in response to succinylcholine that is due to an up-regulation of acetylcholine receptors. Examples include spinal cord injury, stroke, muscular dystrophy, multiple sclerosis, Guillain-Barré syndrome (GBS), and other conditions that cause prolonged immobility.
- The period of susceptibility to succinylcholine-induced hyperkalemia is not well defined but its use appears to be safe within the first 24 hours of an acute insult.
- In patients with GBS or myasthenia gravis, lower doses of short-acting nondepolarizing agents should be used.
- The preferred induction agents for intubating a patient experiencing seizures include sodium thiopental or midazolam due to their anticonvulsant activity. The effect of etomidate on the seizing patient is unclear. It also causes myoclonus, which may be mistaken for seizure activity. It may still be given in situations in which the presence of hypotension precludes the use of other agents. Pretreatment with lidocaine should be used if increased intracranial pressure is suspected.

Sepsis or Hypermetabolic State

- In states of increased physiologic oxygen consumption such as sepsis or diabetic ketoacidosis, there may be no impediment to oxygenation or ventilation, but fatigue may occur and ultimately necessitate airway management.
- With profound acidosis, ventilation must be increased to prevent worsening acidosis, and since the patient cannot sustain the work of respiration, ventilation will fail. These patients are also prone to develop ARDS; early intubation is prudent.

Trauma

- One indication for active airway management in the trauma patient is an injury that has the potential for altering the normal airway anatomy either from traumatic distortion, direct airway injury (subcutaneous air) or vascular injury (bleeding or expanding neck hematoma). Intubation should ideally be carried out before significant distortion occurs which would make intubation much more difficult.
- Any patient who has altered mental status, Glasgow Coma Score 8 or less should have active airway management.
- Any patient with shock from traumatic injuries should have active airway management.
- Any patient whose ventilatory status is failing (e.g., patients who cannot tolerate the work of breathing) or patients who do not respond to correction of intrathoracic pressures or chest wall stabilization should have active airway management.
- In the event of tracheal separation, an airway can be obtained by grasping the distal stump before opening the pretracheal fascia.

Burns

- Inhalational injuries in burn patients may cause impending airway edema, so early intubation for expectant management may be appropriate. Clues to the need for active airway management are severe facial and neck burns, especially a circumferential neck burn; being burned inside a closed area; nasal or oral soot or burns in the pharynx; chemical burns of the nose or mouth. When possible, early bronchoscopy may reveal an absence of tracheal burns and therefore obviate the need for intubation. If not possible, it is prudent to proceed with an RSI endotracheal intubation. With massive facial swelling and interference with respiration, it may be necessary to perform a cricothyrotomy to achieve active airway control even if the operation has to be performed through burned tissue.
- Severely burned patients will have elevated potassium levels, but only after 24 to 48 hours; therefore succinylcholine should be used with caution as a paralyzing agent after this period of time has elapsed.

Foreign Body Aspiration

- *Partial obstruction.* If the patient is breathing spontaneously with good oxygenation, preparations should be made to have the foreign body removed in the operating room. If this is not possible, a very careful attempt to remove the foreign body in the ED may be performed under sedation using topical anesthesia to facilitate direct laryngoscopy. Magill forceps are used to retrieve the foreign body. A gynecologic tenaculum or towel clip may be required to remove some foreign bodies (e.g., balls). Another possibility is to pass a Foley catheter with a 30-ml balloon distal to the foreign body, inflate the balloon, and use it to pull the foreign body upward for retrieval.
- *Complete obstruction in a conscious patient.* In patients older than 1 year, the Heimlich maneuver or subdiaphragmatic thrusts are used. Chest thrusts are recommended only in adults who are markedly obese or

in late pregnancy. Infants younger than 1 year should receive a series of four back blows delivered between the shoulder blades, followed by four chest thrusts. Abdominal thrusts should not be administered because of concern of injury to abdominal organs. Blind finger sweeps are not performed in infants or children, as this may jam the object further into the airway. The Heimlich maneuver should be repeated until the foreign body is expelled or the patient loses consciousness.

■ ***Complete obstruction in an unconscious patient.*** If the patient is unconscious, immediate removal of the foreign body should be performed under direct laryngoscopy in the ED as mentioned above. A single dose of succinylcholine may be used to facilitate removal. Any foreign body above the glottis should be easily visualized for removal. If the foreign body cannot be removed, immediate cricothyrotomy is indicated. If the foreign body appears to be within the subglottic space or trachea and cannot be removed, an attempt to dislodge it with an endotracheal tube into a main stem bronchus may allow ventilation of the other lung. If an obstructing foreign body is distal to the vocal cords and cannot be visualized by direct laryngoscopy, cricothyrotomy is of no benefit and should not be performed.

Pediatric Airway Management

■ Cardiopulmonary failure in children is most often secondary to respiratory compromise, thus actively managing the pediatric airway will be helpful to achieve successful resuscitation.

■ See Chapter 74, "Pediatric Resuscitation" for a more detailed discuss on pediatric airway and ventilation management.

Teaching Points

Active airway management is the key responsibility in the management of critical patients. It is useful to think through the indications for mandatory intubation, learn how to recognize them clinically, and practice the technical skills necessary to accomplish this important task.

Any condition that alters the patient's ability to protect the airway, such as a head injury (GCS Score of 8 or less), should have active airway management.

Do not rely on levels of P_{O_2} or P_{CO_2} because it may be appropriate to intubate the patient before these levels are abnormal, and abnormal levels may be correctable easily without intubation.

Suggested Readings

Butler KH, Clyne B. Management of the difficult airway: alternative airway techniques and adjuncts. Emerg Med Clin North Am 2003;21:259–289.

Walls RM, Luten RC, Murphy MF, Schneider RE. Manual of Emergency Airway Management (2nd edition). Philadelphia: Lippincott, Williams & Wilkins, 2004.

Walls RM. Airway. In: Marx JA, Hockberger R, Walls RM, et al. Rosen's Emergency Medicine: Concepts and Clinical Practice (6th edition). Philadelphia: Mosby, 2006, pp 2–26.

Orebaugh SL. Initiation of mechanical ventilation in the emergency department. Am J Emerg Med 1996;14:59–69.

CHAPTER 6

Advanced Cardiac Life Support

Eugene Gicheru ■ Ahamed H. Idris

Overview

- For 75% of patients with sudden unexpected nontraumatic death, the cause of death is attributed to cardiovascular disease, with the remaining 25% caused by noncardiac causes. Most cardiac arrests occur in the out-of-hospital setting, and are due to a ventricular tachydysrhythmia, either pulseless ventricular tachycardia (VT) or primary ventricular fibrillation (VF). Coronary artery disease is usually the underlying cause of death for patients who die suddenly from VF.
- Cardiac output generated by standard chest compressions is at best less than 30% of baseline, and decreases precipitously with both time to initiation and duration of chest compressions. Immediate resuscitative efforts are necessary to preserve perfusion to vital organs. Brain death occurs after 5 to 10 minutes of anoxia. The heart is the second most susceptible organ to ischemic injury. In the clinical setting, survival of neurologically intact individuals rarely occurs after durations of untreated cardiac arrest longer than 10 minutes.
- The American Heart Association has developed Advanced Cardiac Life Support (ACLS) guidelines. These guidelines provide evidence-based protocols for the initial management of patients presenting with a variety of dysrhythmias including those causing sudden cardiac death. The ACLS protocols are updated every 4 years and are used throughout most of this chapter.
- The team leader of any resuscitative effort is primarily responsible for ensuring the following: patient priorities are addressed immediately (i.e., ABCs), ACLS protocols are being followed (correct drug, indication, and timing), and cerebral perfusion is optimized (correct and timely use of pacemaker and defibrillator with minimal interruption in chest compressions). The team leader should be able to direct others during a resuscitation attempt.

Initial Diagnostic Approach
General

Initial diagnostic efforts are clinical and include immediate attention to the ABCs as discussed in Chapter 4, "General Approach to Life-Threatening Emergencies," and Chapter 5, "Airway Management."

- The patient should be on placed in a resuscitation room fully stocked with airway equipment, ACLS medications, and a defibrillator. The focus of the primary survey includes an initial assessment of the ABCs and the need for immediate defibrillation. The patient should be completely disrobed, large-bore intravenous (IV) access should be obtained, and continuous cardiac monitoring and pulse oximetry should be performed. Oxygen saturation by pulse oximeter may not register in the underperfused patient.
- The secondary survey includes a search for any reversible causes that can be treated. A more detailed physical examination and diagnostic studies are performed as the situation permits.

EKG

- An electrocardiogram (EKG) should be obtained on all patients except those without a pulse for whom resuscitative efforts are the priority.
- A rhythm strip should be printed for every rhythm change noted, including asystole (after the rhythm is noted in two different leads).

Refer to Chapter 87, "EKG Interpretation."

Laboratory

- Studies are of limited use if the patient is in cardiac arrest, however, bedside blood glucose, hemoglobin, and arterial blood gas levels with an emergent (stat) potassium level can be quickly checked.
- The following laboratory studies should be performed only after the patient has been successfully resuscitated: complete blood count (CBC); electrolytes including calcium, magnesium, and phosphorus; renal function studies (blood urea nitrogen [BUN] and creatinine levels), coagulation panel, cardiac enzymes, liver function tests, and urinalysis. Other tests include therapeutic drug levels (i.e., digoxin) and toxicology screen as indicated.
- A sample for type and cross match should be sent if hemorrhage is suspected.

Radiography

- Radiographic studies are contraindicated in the pulseless patient to avoid any delays or interruptions in chest compressions.

- A bedside Doppler or ultrasound study can help determine the presence of a pulse or cardiac activity, respectively, in the patient with pulseless electrical activity (PEA). A bedside ultrasound may also detect pericardial tamponade.
- If resuscitation is successful, obtain a portable chest radiograph to evaluate for cardiac or pulmonary pathology, line placement, and endotracheal tube position.

Emergency Department Management Overview
General

- In any patient, the first priority in management is for the ABCs. A bag-valve mask should be used to provide 100% oxygen in the pulseless or minimally breathing patient as soon as possible, and intubation carried out quickly.
- Any patient without a pulse will have one of the following underlying rhythms: VF, VT, asystole, PEA.
- During the primary survey, any patient without a pulse (regardless of the underlying rhythm) should receive immediate cardiopulmonary resuscitation (open the airway, provide positive-pressure ventilation, and chest compressions) while preparations are made to intubate, defibrillate, pace, or administer appropriate medications. The person performing chest compressions should push hard and fast, allowing the chest to completely return to the normal position after each compression in order to allow better cardiac filling. In the adult patient, the rate should be at least 100 compressions per minute and the depth should be at least $1^{1}/_{2}$ to 2 inches. Interruptions in chest compressions should be kept to a minimum. The rhythm should be identified on the bedside cardiac monitor. Instead of checking the rhythm or pulse immediately after shock delivery, rescuers should immediately resume CPR, beginning with chest compressions, and should check the rhythm after 5 cycles (or about 2 minutes) of CPR.
- Immediate defibrillation should be performed for pulseless patients with VF or VT on the monitor. Asystole should always be checked in two leads. Causes of PEA should be sought and interventions should be made (Table 6–1).
- For any patient with a pulse, evaluate for signs or symptoms of cardiac hypoperfusion (hemodynamic instability, ischemic chest pain, lightheadedness), and obtain a 12-lead EKG (see Chapter 87). Hemodynamically unstable patients require immediate intervention (i.e., cardioversion for a tachydysrhythmia).

Medications

- A list of medications commonly used in ACLS is provided in Table 6–2.
- Alert patients requiring transthoracic pacing or cardioversion should be sedated with IV medications. Midazolam (0.05-0.1 mg/kg) in combination with fentanyl (1-2 μg/kg), are commonly used. Other agents include etomidate (0.15 mg/kg), methohexital (1 mg/kg), propofol (0.5-0.8 mg/kg over 3-5 minutes), and thiopental (3 mg/kg). All the drugs except etomidate cause a small drop in blood pressure.

Table 6–1   Differential Diagnosis for Pulseless Electrical Activity (5 H's, 5 T's)

Diagnosis	Physical Finding	Treatment
Hypothermia	Core temperature	Hypothermia algorithm
H⁺ (acidosis)	Diabetic/renal patient, ABG	Sodium bicarbonate, hyperventilation
Hypoxia	Airway, cyanosis, ABG	Oxygen, ventilation
Hypovolemia	Collapsed vasculature, signs of hemorrhage	Fluids, blood products
Hyperkalemia	Renal patient, EKG, serum K level	Sodium bicarbonate, calcium chloride, nebulized albuterol albuterol nebulizer, insulin/glucose, diuresis, kayexalate, dialysis
Thrombosis (pulmonary embolism)	No pulse w/CPR, JVD	Thrombolytics, thoracotomy
Tension pneumothorax	No pulse w/CPR, JVD, tracheal deviation	Thoracostomy
Tamponade (cardiac)	No pulse w/CPR, JVD, narrow pulse pressure prior to arrest	Pericardiocentesis
Thrombosis (massive MI)	History, EKG	Acute coronary syndrome algorithm
Tablets (drug overdose)	Medications, illicit drug use	Identify and treat accordingly. Some drugs may require alkalinization (i.e., phenobarbital, aspirin, tricyclics and class 1 antidysrhythmics).

ABG, arterial blood gas; CPR, cardiopulmonary resuscitation; EKG, electrocardiogram; JVD, jugular venous distention; K, potassium; MI, myocardial infarction.

Emergency Department Interventions

- Airway management is discussed in Chapter 5.
- ***Mechanical ventilation.*** In the pulseless patient, overventilation should be avoided. Due to the significantly reduced cardiac output, blood flow returning to the heart is severely diminished resulting in less carbon dioxide being delivered to the lungs and thus, less carbon dioxide needing to be exhaled. Furthermore, overventilation can reduce cardiac output even more by increasing intrathoracic pressures. It may also inadvertently cause a respiratory alkalosis that can decrease oxygen delivery to the tissues even further. Healthcare providers performing single- or 2-rescuer in adults or single rescuer CPR in children should use a 30:2 compression-ventilation ratio (30 compressions and 2 breaths) and those

Table 6–2   Selected ACLS Medications

Medication	Mechanism of Action	IV Dose	Indication	Comment
Adenosine	Blocks AV node conduction	6 mg rapid IVP over 1–3 s Repeat 12 mg rapid IVP twice Allow 1–2 min between doses	Narrow-complex tachycardias or SVT with aberrancy	Follow with normal saline bolus of 20 ml May precipitate faster rate in WPW
Amiodarone	Class III antidysrhythmic	VF/pulseless VT: 300 mg IVP, Repeat 150 mg IVP in 3–5 min. Unstable tachycardias: Load: 150 mg IVP then 1 mg/min for 6 h followed by 0.5 mg/min for 18 h	Refractory VF/ pulseless VT, wide-complex, preexcitation (e.g., WPW), reentry (e.g., SVT) tachycardias	Maximum dose 2.2 g over 24 h; may cause pneumonitis. Major side effects include hypotension and bradycardia.
Atropine	Antimuscarinic	0.5–1 mg IV every 3–5 min	Asystole, bradycardias	Maximum dose 0.04 mg/kg. Ineffective in the denervated heart (i.e., heart transplant).
Calcium	Positive inotrope	Calcium chloride 10% solution, 5 to 10 mL IV preferably in a central vein. For peripheral venous access, use calcium gluconate: 1 gram in 50 mL of D_5W	No indication in cardiac arrest. Indicated for hyperkalemia, calcium channel blocker toxicity, or ionized hypocalcemia (e.g., after blood transfusion)	

Continued

Table 6–2 Selected ACLS Medications—*cont'd*

Medication	Mechanism of Action	IV Dose	Indication	Comment
Diltiazem	Calcium channel blocker	15–20 mg (0.25 mg/kg) IV over 2 min; repeat 20–25 mg (0.35 mg/kg) IV after 10 min Maintenance infusion: 5–15 mg/h, titrated to HR.	Atrial fibrillation, atrial flutter	Monitor for hypotension. Use with caution with concurrent use of other nodal blocking agents (i.e., β blockers) and digoxin.
Epinephrine	Potent non-selective α_1 and β_2 agonist	1 mg IV every 3–5 minutes	VF/pulseless VT, PEA, asystole	
Isoproterenol	Synthetic $\beta_1\beta_2$ agonist	Infusion: 2–10 µg/min	Refractory bradydysrhythmias	Can precipitate myocardial ischemia due to increased O_2 demand
Lidocaine	Class Ib antidysrhythmic	1–1.5 mg/kg IVP Repeat 0.5–0.75 mg/kg IVP in 5–10 min. Infusion of 1 to 4 mg/min. Maintenance: 1–4 mg/min	Refractory VF and VT if ventricular function preserved.	Maximum dose 3 mg/kg. Give slowly if patient is awake. Toxicity and side effects: slurred speech, altered consciousness, muscle twitching, seizures, and bradycardia.
Magnesium Sulfate	Natural calcium channel blocker, maintains intracellular potassium, and magnesium repletion.	1–2 g diluted in D_5W IVP over 5 to 60 min.	Polymorphic VT, torsades de pointes	If torsades without cardiac arrest may follow with 0.5–1 g/h IV Monitor for hypotension and hypermagnesemia

Table 6–2 Selected ACLS Medications—*cont'd*

Medication	Mechanism of Action	IV Dose	Indication	Comment
Metoprolol	β₁ selective beta-blocker	5 mg IV every 5 min for three doses	Atrial fibrillation, Atrial flutter	Contraindicated if ↓BP, ↓HR or WPW
Procainamide	Class Ia anti-dysrhythmic	Infusion: 20 mg/min IV	VT, atrial fibrillation, atrial flutter, pre-excitation (e.g., WPW), and AV reentrant narrow-complex tachycardias (i.e., SVT) with preserved ventricular function	Maximum dose 17 mg/kg. Discontinue if the QRS is prolonged >50%, hypotension ensues, or dysrhythmia suppressed.
Sodium bicarbonate	Buffering agent	1 mEq/kg IV	Pre-existing metabolic acidosis, tricyclic antidepressant overdose, and hyperkalemia	
Vasopressin	Nonadrenergic peripheral vasoconstrictor	40 U, IV or IO in cardiac arrest	May replace either the first or second dose of epinephrine in pulseless arrest. Also used for vasodilatory shock (i.e., sepsis) when conventional vasopressor drugs are ineffective.	

Drug that can be placed in the ETT in the event that there is no IV access include narcan, atropine, valium, epinephrine, and lidocaine (NAVEL). The dose is typically twice the IV dose and should be administered with 10 mL of normal saline.

AV, atrioventricular; BP, blood pressure; HR, heart rate; K, potassium; Na, sodium; NS, normal saline; IVP, intravenous push; IV, intravenous; S-A, sinoatrial; VF, ventricular fibrillation; VT, ventricular tachycardia; WPW, Wolf Parkinson White. See Chapter 90.3 for a more detailed listing of cardiovascular medications.

performing 2-rescuer CPR in children should use a 15:2 compression-ventilation ratio until an advanced airway is in place. In a pulseless patient in the hospital setting, assisted ventilation should be given manually with the aid of BVM at a rate of 8 to 10 breaths per minute or one breath every 6 to 8 seconds in the adult patient. If there is return of spontaneous circulation, the endotracheal tube should be connected to a mechanical ventilator. Ventilatory settings can then be adjusted based on results of arterial blood gas analysis.

- **Defibrillation versus cardioversion.** If the patient is in VF or pulseless VT, attach the defibrillator and shock. There should be only 1 shock, instead of 3 stacked shocks, and the shock should be given within 10 seconds of the last chest compression. Begin with 120 to 200 J for manual biphasic defibrilators and 360 J for monophasic defibrillators. Immediately after shock delivery, resume CPR beginning with chest compressions and continue for 5 cycles (about 2 minutes if an advanced airway is in place), then check the rhythm. Patients who have been in VF for more than several minutes will benefit from measures to improve cardiac perfusion (chest compressions and IV epinephrine) before the initial shock is delivered. Cardioversion is performed in the patient who has a pulse but is either hemodynamically unstable or is refractory to pharmacologic therapy. To perform cardioversion, place in synchronized mode before delivering the shock due to the risk of inducing VF when the shock is delivered on a T wave. For patients with monomorphic VT (regular form and rate) and a pulse, the initial shock is 100 J and is increased in a stepwise fashion (up to 360 J) if there is no response. For polymorphic VT and a pulse, treat as VF with unsynchronized shocks if the patient is unstable. The initial recommended dose for cardioversion of atrial fibrillation is 100 J to 200 J with a monophasic waveform and 100 J to 120 J with a biphasic waveform. Initial energy for cardioversion of atrial flutter and other supraventricular tachycardias (SVTs) is 50 J to 100 J.

- **Chest compressions.** Effective chest compressions (i.e., push hard and fast) are critical to providing blood flow during CPR. Interruptions in chest compressions should be avoided as much as possible. The team leader must ensure that adequate delivery of chest compressions noted by proper hand placement in the middle of the sternum just above the xyphoid process, a depth of 1.5 to 2 inches, a rate of 100 chest compressions per minute, a palpable femoral or carotid pulse (or by Doppler), and a good wave form on the cardiac monitor. The chest should be allowed to recoil completely after each compression, and allow equal compression and relaxation times.

- **Pacing.** If the patient is recently converted to asystole from a perfusing rhythm or is hypotensive secondary to bradycardia or other form of heart block, attach the transthoracic pacemaker and attempt external pacing.

●●● Refer to Chapter 91,"Procedures," for transthoracic and transvenous
●●● pacing procedures.
●●●

- **IV access.** Central venous IV access is ideal in patients requiring CPR primarily because of quicker access to the central circulation and less venous irritation by vasoactive drugs. If the patient will require large volume fluid resuscitation, a Cordis (also known as an introducer) should be placed. A triple-lumen catheter has a lumen that is too narrow for large volume infusion and should not be used in these situations. However, if the patient will primarily require vasopressors and not large volume IV fluid administration, central venous IV access with a triple-lumen catheter should be adequate. Two large-bore IVs placed in the antecubital fossa or external jugular vein are appropriate in the immediate resuscitative period. A saphenous venous cutdown should be performed if peripheral or central IV access is not possible. The intraosseous route can be utilized in adults as well as children.

■ *IV fluid administration.* Normal saline or lactated ringer's should be infused with the IV tubing wide open if the patient is hypovolemic or hypotensive. Give O-negative blood to the patient who has suffered cardiac arrest due to hemorrhage. A rapid infuser and warmer should be used for resuscitations requiring large volumes of fluid.

■ *Foley catheter.* This should be placed once spontaneous return of circulation is achieved to adequately monitor urine output.

■ *Nasogastric tube.* This should be placed on all patients requiring intubation.

Disposition

■ *Terminating a code.* Determine if the patient has a *do not resuscitate* (DNR) order, living will, or durable power of attorney. Assess the quality of resuscitation, underlying circumstances, and what was the presenting rhythm (asystole has a worse prognosis than PEA). If resuscitation is still unsuccessful and any additional resuscitative efforts seem futile, terminate the resuscitation. When the physician has decided to terminate resuscitation, the family should be asked to meet in a private family room. The chaplain and preferably the nurse assigned to the patient should accompany the physician to meet with the family. See Chapter 3, "Communiucating Information".

■ *Disposition of a deceased patient in the ED.* The medical examiner should be contacted regarding all deaths that occur in the ED. The medical examiner's office determines if an autopsy is mandatory and when to release the body to an undertaker.

■ *Admission.* Most patients requiring ACLS interventions require admission to an intensive care setting. Stable patients may be admitted to a monitored setting with a lower level of care (e.g., new-onset, rate-controlled AF).

■ *Discharge.* Otherwise healthy patients with a benign dysrhythmia that is easily resolved in the ED may be discharged with close follow-up after a brief period of observation in the ED if they remain stable and are asymptomatic (e.g., SVT).

Specific Problems

Figure 6–1: Algorithm 1, ACLS pulseless arrest.
Figure 6–2: Algorithm 2, ACLS tachycardia.
Figure 6–3: Algorithm 3, ACLS bradycardia.

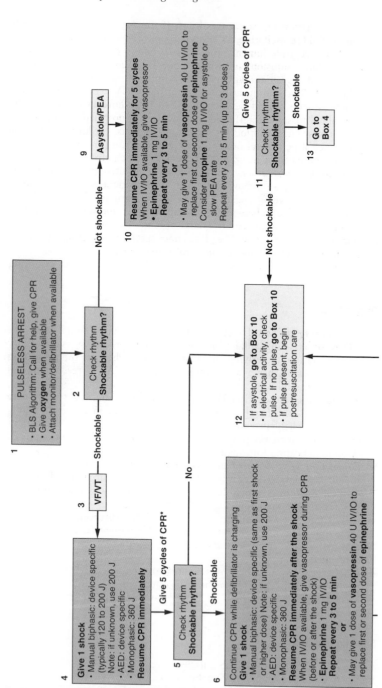

1

PULSELESS ARREST
· BLS Algorithm: Call for help, give CPR
· Give **oxygen** when available
· Attach monitor/defibrillator when available

2

Check rhythm
Shockable rhythm?

3   VF/VT — Shockable

9   Asystole/PEA — Not shockable

4

Give 1 shock
· Manual biphasic: device specific
  (typically 120 to 200 J)
  Note: if unknown, use 200 J
· AED: device specific
· Monophasic: 360 J
Resume CPR immediately

Give 5 cycles of CPR*

5

Check rhythm
Shockable rhythm?

Shockable

No

6

Continue CPR while defibrillator is charging
Give 1 shock
· Manual biphasic: device specific (same as first shock
  or higher dose) Note: if unknown, use 200 J
· AED: device specific
· Monophasic: 360 J
Resume CPR immediately after the shock
When IV/IO available, give vasopressor during CPR
  (before or after the shock)
· **Epinephrine** 1 mg IV/IO
  Repeat every 3 to 5 min
  or
· May give 1 dose of **vasopressin** 40 U IV/IO to
  replace first or second dose of **epinephrine**

10

Resume CPR immediately for 5 cycles
When IV/IO available, give vasopressor
· **Epinephrine** 1 mg IV/IO
  Repeat every 3 to 5 min
  or
· May give 1 dose of **vasopressin** 40 U IV/IO to
  replace first or second dose of **epinephrine**
Consider **atropine** 1 mg IV/IO for asystole or
  slow PEA rate
Repeat every 3 to 5 min (up to 3 doses)

Give 5 cycles of CPR*

11

Check rhythm
Shockable rhythm? — Shockable

Not shockable

13   Go to Box 4

12

· If asystole, **go to Box 10**
· If electrical activity, check
  pulse, **go to Box 10**
· If pulse present, begin
  postresuscitation care

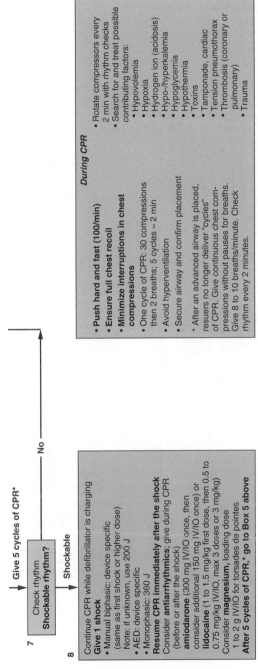

During CPR

- **Push hard and fast (100/min)**
- **Ensure full chest recoil**
- **Minimize interruptions in chest compressions**
  - One cycle of CPR: 30 compressions then 2 breaths; 5 cycles = 2 min
  - Avoid hyperventilation
  - Secure airway and confirm placement
  - * After an advanced airway is placed, resuers no longer deliver "cycles" of CPR. Give continuous chest compressions without pauses for breaths. Give 8 to 10 breaths/minute. Check rhythm every 2 minutes.
- Rotate compressors every 2 min with rhythm checks
- Search for and treat possible contributing factors:
  - Hypovolemia
  - Hypoxia
  - Hydrogen ion (acidosis)
  - Hypo-/hyperkalemia
  - Hypoglycemia
  - Hypothermia
  - Toxins
  - Tamponade, cardiac
  - Tension pneumothorax
  - Thrombosis (coronary or pulmonary)
  - Trauma

7 Check rhythm
Shockable rhythm?

Give 5 cycles of CPR*

— No —

Shockable

8 Continue CPR while defibrillator is charging
Give 1 shock
- Manual biphasic: device specific (same as first shock or higher dose)
Note: if unknown, use 200 J
- AED: device specific
- Monophasic: 360 J
Resume CPR immediately after the shock
Consider **antiarrhythmics**; give during CPR (before or after the shock)
amiodarone (300 mg IV/IO once, then consider additional 150 mg IV/IO once) or **lidocaine** (1 to 1.5 mg/kg first dose, then 0.5 to 0.75 mg/kg IV/IO, max 3 doses or 3 mg/kg)
Consider **magnesium**, loading dose 1 to 2 g IV/IO for torsades de pointes
After 5 cycles of CPR,* go to Box 5 above

Figure 6–1. Algorithm 1, ACLS pulseless arrest. *Used with permission: 2005 American Heart Association Guidelines for Cardiopulmonary Resuscitation and Emergency Cardiovascular Care, Part 4: Adult Basic Life Support. Circulation. 2005;112(suppl. IV):IV 59–189 © 2005, American Heart Association.*

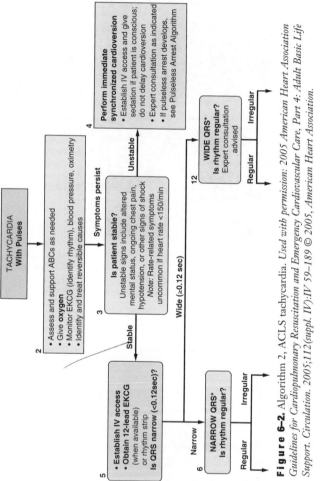

Figure 6-2. Algorithm 2, ACLS tachycardia. *Used with permission: 2005 American Heart Association Guidelines for Cardiopulmonary Resuscitation and Emergency Cardiovascular Care, Part 4: Adult Basic Life Support. Circulation. 2005;112(suppl. IV):IV 59–189 © 2005, American Heart Association.*

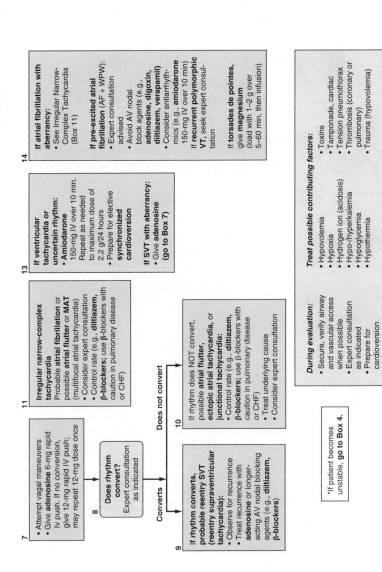

Figure 6-2. *continued.*

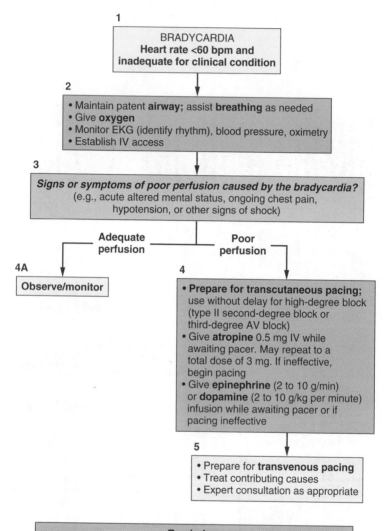

1

BRADYCARDIA
**Heart rate <60 bpm and
inadequate for clinical condition**

2

- Maintain patent **airway**; assist **breathing** as needed
- Give **oxygen**
- Monitor EKG (identify rhythm), blood pressure, oximetry
- Establish IV access

3

Signs or symptoms of poor perfusion caused by the bradycardia?
(e.g., acute altered mental status, ongoing chest pain,
hypotension, or other signs of shock)

**Adequate
perfusion**

**Poor
perfusion**

4A

Observe/monitor

4

- **Prepare for transcutaneous pacing;**
  use without delay for high-degree block
  (type II second-degree block or
  third-degree AV block)
- Give **atropine** 0.5 mg IV while
  awaiting pacer. May repeat to a
  total dose of 3 mg. If ineffective,
  begin pacing
- Give **epinephrine** (2 to 10 g/min)
  or **dopamine** (2 to 10 g/kg per minute)
  infusion while awaiting pacer or if
  pacing ineffective

5

- Prepare for **transvenous pacing**
- Treat contributing causes
- Expert consultation as appropriate

Reminders

- If pulseless arrest develops, go to Pulseless Arrest Algorithm
- Search for and treat possible contributing factors:

  - Hypovolemia
  - Hypoxia
  - Hydrogen ion (acidosis)
  - Hypo-/hyperkalemia
  - Hypoglycemia
  - Hypothermia

  - Toxins
  - Tamponade, cardiac
  - Tension pneumothorax
  - Thrombosis (coronary or pulmonary)
  - Trauma (hypovolemia, increased ICP)

Figure 6–3. Algorithm 3, ACLS bradycardia. *Used with permission: 2005 American
Heart Association Guidelines for Cardiopulmonary Resuscitation and
Emergency Cardiovascular Care, Part 4: Adult Basic Life Support. Circulation.
2005;112(suppl. IV):IV 59–189 © 2005, American Heart Association.*

Special Considerations
Hypothermia

- Hypothermia is defined as a core temperature of less than 35° C (95° F)
- Rewarming techniques should be initiated (passive, active external, active core).
- Ventilate with warm, humidified oxygen. Limit shocks for VF/pulseless VT to three maximum or a single maximum shock with the new waveform defibrillators. Limit movement of patient.
- Follow rhythm appropriate algorithm as detailed in this chapter.

Refer to Chapter 65, "Environmental Emergencies."

Pediatric

- The vast majority of cardiopulmonary arrests in the pediatric patient are due to respiratory arrest or hypoxia from shock.
- Rhythm disturbances are usually secondary to hypoxia rather than a primary cardiac cause.

Refer to Chapter 74, "Pediatric Advanced Cardiac Life Support."

Trauma

- Resuscitation is futile in patients arriving in the ED in arrest after blunt trauma.
- ED thoracotomy is indicated for penetrating chest trauma in arrested patients. It is not useful for penetrating wounds to the abdomen, head, or extremities.
- The focus should be on resuscitation (i.e., airway management, IV fluids, blood products) and control of hemorrhage.
- Follow the rhythm appropriate algorithm as detailed in this chapter.

Refer to Chapter 8, "General Approach to Trauma."

Pregnancy

- The leading causes of maternal death are pulmonary embolism, hemorrhage, pregnancy induced hypertension, and infection.
- Before 24 weeks of gestation, resuscitative efforts should focus on the mother and standard ACLS protocol should be followed.
- After 24 weeks of gestation (the uterine fundus is palpable at the umbilicus at 20 weeks), perform a perimortem cesarean delivery if no perfusing rhythm is obtained within 2 to 3 minutes.
- Maternal CPR should be continued throughout resuscitation and delivery.

Automated Implantable Cardioverter-Defibrillator

- If defibrillation is necessary, do not place the paddles over the automated implantable cardioverter-defibrillator (AICD).
- Deactivate the AICD by placing a donut-shaped magnet over the right upper quadrant or left lower quadrant (depending on pacemaker) of the AICD for 30 seconds. Some pacemakers require the magnet be taped to it for deactivation.
- Follow standard ACLS protocol as outlined in this chapter.

Teaching Points

Cardiac arrest is common, and when witnessed, has a better prognosis if the initiating rhythm is ventricular tachycardia or ventricular fibrillation. Immediate ACLS is useful, and it is helpful to know the algorithms for efficient response.

For tachycardia, unless it is a sinus tachycardia, such as from hemorrhage, if the patient is unstable, immediate cardioversion is the optimal approach.

For bradycardia, if the patient does not immediately respond to oxygen, try atropine, and if no response, use an external pacer.

Children rarely arrest from cardiac causes. They primarily experience cardiac arrest as a result of hypoxia from shock or pulmonary failure. Children often become bradycardic immediately before cardiac arrest, and they need oxygen, not atropine or pacing.

Traumatic cardiac arrest from blunt trauma is almost always fatal, and if the patient arrives in the ED in arrest, will not respond to thoracotomy. If there is penetrating chest trauma, thoracotomy has a reasonable chance for success depending on the extent of the penetrating trauma pathology.

Suggested Readings

2005 American Heart Association Guidelines for Cardiopulmonary Resuscitation and Emergency Cardiovascular Care. In Circulation: Volume 112, Issue 24 Supplement; December 13, 2005.

CHAPTER 7

Shock

RICHARD E. WOLFE ■ CHRISTOPHER M. FISCHER

Overview

- Shock is a state of organ hypoperfusion caused by a variety of failures of the body's normal homeostatic mechanisms.
- Untreated shock usually progresses from inadequate perfusion to systemic inflammation, permanent organ dysfunction, and death.
- The organs most susceptible to hypoperfusion and resulting dysfunction include the brain, kidneys, gastrointestinal (GI) tract, and immune system.
- Early recognition of inadequate organ perfusion and the inciting causes is critical to arresting the inevitable downward progression and resulting death. Patient anxiety, tachycardia, tachypnea, fevers, poor capillary refill, skin pallor, and fatigue may all be signs or symptoms of impending shock. Late findings in shock are hypotension, oliguria, and altered mental status.
- Table 7–1 summarizes the different types of shock.
- The role of the emergency physician is early recognition, initiation of stabilization interventions, and early consultation for definitive care.

Initial Approach

- Recognition of the early clinical presentation of shock is the first and most important step. Aggressive management directed toward maintaining perfusion should precede specific identification of the cause. Once the cause is identified, specific therapies addressing it should be added, and the general approach should be appropriately tailored.
- Patients in shock are critically ill, and should be placed in a resuscitation area. While the physician is assessing the patient, two large-bore intravenous (IV) lines (at least 16-guage) should be placed, continuous pulse oximetry and cardiac monitoring should be applied, and supplemental oxygen should be given. Oxygen helps augment end-organ perfusion. Pulse oximetry is often inaccurate or unobtainable in low-flow states. Early measures should be undertaken to ensure adequate oxygenation and ventilation. Endotracheal intubation and mechanical ventilation should be performed early in these patients to reduce the metabolic demands of the work of respiration.

Table 7–1 Types of Shock

Type of Shock	Risk Factors	Clinical Presentation	Management
Hypovolemic: traumatic	Trauma	Anxiety, poor peripheral perfusion, hypotension, tachycardia (despite crystalloids), may have positive FAST, chest radiograph, or other obvious injuries	Crystalloids, PRBCs, oxygenation, identify source of bleeding, operative repair
Hypovolemic: nontraumatic	Dehydration, GI bleed	Anxiety, poor peripheral perfusion, hypotension, tachycardia	Crystalloids, PRBCs, oxygen, decrease fluid losses, identify source of GI bleeding
Cardiogenic	MI, valvular dysfunction, PE	Chest pain, dyspnea, JVD, pulmonary edema, abnormal heart sounds & murmurs, peripheral edema, EKG abnormalities	Intubation, oxygenation, vasopressors, emergent revascularization
Vasogenic: septic	Infection	Fever or hypothermia, peripheral vasoconstriction, altered mental status, tachycardia, tachypnea, localizing signs or symptoms of infection	Early goal-directed therapy and broad-spectrum empiric IV antibiotics
Vasogenic: anaphylactic	Exposure to allergen	Urticaria, angioedema, diffuse erythema, bronchospasm, laryngeal edema, hyperperistalsis, and hypotension	Airway management, epinephrine, H_1 and H_2 blockers, steroids, beta-agonists
Vasogenic: neurogenic	Spinal cord trauma	Hypotension, lack of reflex tachycardia, poor response to crystalloids, spinal cord trauma, paralysis, paresthesias	Crystalloids, vasopressors if needed, and other causes of shock excluded

GI, gastrointestinal; FAST, focused assessment for sonography in trauma; H, histamine; JVD, jugular venous distention; MI, myocardial infarction; PE, pulmonary embolism; PRBCs, packed red blood cells.

- A urinary catheter should be placed to monitor urinary output, which is a sign of adequate kidney (end-organ) perfusion.
- If peripheral venous access is impossible, central venous access (femoral vein, internal jugular, or subclavian) should be obtained. A cordis or introducer catheter is preferred for large-volume infusion as the triple-

lumen catheters are too small. Other alternatives include an interosseous catheter (anterior tibia) or venous cutdown (saphenous vein). A central venous line to monitor central venous pressures (CVP) can also help guide resuscitation efforts, but this capability may not be available in some EDs. A complete blood count (CBC), and a blood type and cross-match should be sent. Blood cultures should be obtained when sepsis is the source of shock. Serum lactic acid levels should be obtained. Lactate is a by-product of anaerobic metabolism. Lactate is often considered a measure of tissue hypoxia. Electrolyte levels, a blood glucose level, renal function tests, liver function tests, a urinalysis, a urinary culture, and coagulation studies are all indicated in cases of undifferentiated shock. A urine pregnancy test should be ordered on all women of reproductive age.

- An EKG is important in excluding myocardial dysfunction as a cause or complication of inadequate perfusion.
- All patients in shock should be admitted to a critical care setting.

Specific Problems
Cardiogenic Shock

- *Epidemiology and risk factors.* Cardiogenic shock occurs when there is evidence of organ hypoperfusion due to decreased cardiac output and myocardial dysfunction despite adequate intravascular volume. The leading cause of nontraumatic cardiogenic shock is acute myocardial infarction (AMI). Other causes include small infarctions in patients with compromised baseline function, acute mitral regurgitation, ventricular wall or septal rupture, myocarditis, end-stage cardiomyopathy, valvular heart disease, and hypertrophic obstructive cardiomyopathy. Indirect causes are from pulmonary embolism (PE), aortic dissection, pericardial tamponade, or vascular disease. The mortality is very high (50%-80%).
- *Pathophysiology.* Myocardial ischemia causes pump dysfunction, which progresses to pump failure, followed by compensatory sympathetic activation, which can increase myocardial demand and worsen ongoing ischemia.
- *Clinical presentation.* Jugular venous distention (JVD) is common. The absence of JVD should lead to an investigation of the patient's volume status. Abnormal heart sounds (murmurs, S_3, S_4) may be present and represent cardiac dysfunction. Careful auscultation of the lungs is necessary—pulmonary edema in the setting of hypotension is highly suggestive of cardiogenic shock. Peripheral edema may suggest right-sided heart failure.
- *Diagnostic testing.* An EKG is obtained to look for the changes of an ST elevation myocardial infarction. Cardiac enzymes can help establish the diagnosis of AMI (see Chapter 22). A chest radiograph should be obtained early in the clinical course to assess for pulmonary edema or tension pneumothorax. A bedside ultrasound can be used to assess for pericardial fluid and tamponade.
- *ED management.* Endotracheal intubation and mechanical ventilation should be performed as soon as pump failure is recognized and the patient is in respiratory distress. Optimizing myocardial contractility and

pump function is also important. Aortic balloon pump assistance may be utilized, as well as emergency coronary artery bypass surgery. Vasopressors such as dopamine or dobutamine are helpful in providing inotropic support until revascularization is available. Dobutamine is an almost pure inotropic agent, with primarily β_1-agonist effects, that increases cardiac contractility. It also provides some relatively weak β_2-mediated peripheral vasodilation that might reduce systemic vascular resistance and afterload and improve tissue perfusion; however, dobutamine may cause hypotension, and thus is often combined with dopamine. At intermediate doses (i.e., 5-10 μg/kg/ min IV), the β_1-agonist effect of dopamine assists by improving myocardial contractility, cardiac output, and enhancing conduction in the heart. At higher doses (i.e., 10-20 μg/kg/min IV or more), the α-agonist effect increases peripheral vasoconstriction and central blood pressure (BP). Cardiac dysrhythmias should be treated as indicated (see Chapter 6). Tension pneumothorax, a clinical diagnosis, should be treated with needle decompression followed by tube thoracostomy (see Chapter 91).

Hypovolemic Shock: Nontraumatic

- **Epidemiology and risk factors.** The major causes of nontraumatic hypovolemic shock are vomiting, diarrhea, dehydration, or hemorrhage from a GI tract bleed, a ruptured abdominal aortic aneurysm (AAA) or other vascular sources of hemorrhage.
- **Pathophysiology.** Decreased blood volume causes underperfusion of end organs. Eventually, with falling blood volumes, oxygen-carrying capacity is reduced to levels inadequate to meet the metabolic demands of organs. In addition, a systemic inflammatory response occurs. The body tries to compensate for these insults by sympathetic activation, resulting in increased heart rate, peripheral vasoconstriction, and an increased force of cardiac contraction. These changes are variable from person to person and dependent on many factors (i.e., co-morbidities, medications, rate of blood loss).
- **Clinical presentation.** Important historical clues that may help direct management include duration and frequency of vomiting or diarrhea, preceding illnesses, presence of bloody or dark stools, use of nonsteroidal anti-inflammatory medications (that predispose to GI hemorrhage), and presence of chest or back pain (that suggest an aortic dissection or aneurysm). The peripheral skin may become pale, cool, diaphoretic, or mottled, with sluggish capillary refill. Vital signs may be normal in early hypovolemic shock. Tachycardia may be present initially, followed by a slight increase in the diastolic BP, causing the pulse pressure (difference between systolic and diastolic BP) to narrow. After approximately one third of the total blood volume is acutely lost, ventricular filling is compromised and cardiac output drops, followed by a reduction in systolic BP.
- **Diagnostic testing.** Elevated hemoglobin and hematocrit levels can indicate hemoconcentration from hypovolemia, as can an elevated blood urea nitrogen (BUN)–to-creatinine ratio. Note that the hemoglobin or hematocrit level may not reflect acute blood loss. Obtain blood immediately for type and cross-match. The lactate level is generally

greater than 4.0 mmol/L (due to hypoperfusion), and the $PaCO_2$ is less than 35 mm Hg (increased minute ventilation to normalize the pH). Bedside ultrasound can be used to assess the abdominal aorta, and should be part of the diagnostic algorithm in any patient with undifferentiated shock. An enlarged abdominal aorta (>3 cm) with or without free fluid on ultrasound in the setting of hypotension is concerning for a ruptured AAA. These patients require emergent vascular surgery consultation for surgical management.

■ ***ED management.*** If vital signs remain abnormal after 2 L of crystalloid, transfusion of packed red blood cells (PRBCs) should be started. If GI bleeding is suspected, a rectal examination should be performed to determine the presence of gross or occult blood. Nasogastric (NG) lavage should be performed early in the patient's course to determine if there is an active upper GI source of the bleeding. Gastroenterology should be involved for a more invasive investigation of the source of GI bleeding (esophagogastroduodenoscopy [EGD], colonoscopy, tagged RBC scan, as available) (see Chapter 34). If a ruptured AAA is suspected, as long as the patient is conscious and has adequate peripheral perfusion, euvolemic resuscitation should be deferred until the patient has been transported to the operating room. Increasing blood pressure without control of the aneurysm may lead to loss of retroperitoneal tamponade with further bleeding, profound hypotension, and death.

■ ***Helpful hints and pitfalls.*** The heart rate and blood pressure responses to hemorrhage are variable, so no firm conclusion can be made at the bedside about the presence or absence of hemorrhagic shock simply by evaluating the heart rate and BP.

Hypovolemic Shock: Traumatic

■ ***Epidemiology and risk factors.*** Hypovolemic shock is the leading cause of death in trauma patients. Ongoing blood loss resulting in hypovolemic shock is usually located in one of three body cavities: the chest, the abdomen, or the retroperitoneum. Although significant hemorrhage can occur with long bone fractures, this bleeding is usually more limited. In the infant, intracranial bleeding can also produce shock. Severe burn injury can cause an increase in capillary permeability resulting in an egress of fluid from the intravascular space to adjacent tissues. In addition, inordinate amounts of fluid are lost by evaporation from the damaged surface that is no longer able to retain water. This increase in capillary permeability, coupled with evaporative water loss, causes hypovolemic shock.

■ ***Pathophysiology.*** See "Hypovolemic Shock: Nontraumatic."

■ ***Clinical presentation.*** The patient may initially present with tachycardia and tachypnea (early signs of shock); however, other causes include pain, anxiety, acidosis, or primary cardiac or pulmonary injuries. The absence of tachycardia does not rule out significant blood loss after trauma. Refer to Section III for specific traumatic injuries.

■ ***Diagnostic testing.*** Hypotension in a trauma patient warrants an investigation of the most concerning and likely sources of bleeding: the chest, the abdomen, and the retroperitoneum. The investigation should include a focused assessment for sonography in trauma (FAST) for hemoperitoneum and pericardial effusion. When hypotension accompanies significant blunt trauma and is unexplained, intraperitoneal hemorrhage should be assumed until it is excluded. A known extra-abdominal source of hemorrhage (e.g., chest) does not mitigate the need to evaluate the peritoneal cavity. A head injury alone usually does not explain shock except in the very small infant for whom traumatic intracranial or extracranial (e.g., cephalohematoma) blood may be proportionally substantial. The initial hemoglobin and hematocrit levels may be normal in hemorrhagic shock because whole blood is lost. Blood type and cross-match is still needed. An EKG need not be routinely obtained in all trauma patients unless chest trauma, cardiac injury, a precipitating cardiac event or dysrhythmia is present, or the patient is elderly with the potential to develop a cardiac ischemic just from the fall in blood pressure.

■ *ED management.* Advanced trauma life support (ATLS) guidelines should be followed (see Section III). Aggressive IV fluid resuscitation with crystalloid solutions (normal saline or lactated ringer's solution) and blood, along with rapid identification and control of hemorrhage are the mainstays to trauma care. Two liters of crystalloid (or boluses of 20 ml/kg in children; up to 50 ml/kg) should be rapidly infused in any hemodynamically unstable trauma patient, followed by the rapid infusion of PRBCs. Although cross-matched blood is preferred, O-negative or type-specific blood may be necessary, depending on the clinical situation. Direct pressure should be applied to any external bleeding.

■ *Helpful hints and pitfalls.* Other causes for hypotension in the trauma patient such as pericardial tamponade or tension pneumothorax require immediate attention. Young patients often maintain normal vital signs even with significant injury. Pulse is the most important early indicator of hypovolemic shock in pediatric trauma patients.

Vasogenic: Anaphylactic Shock

■ *Epidemiology and risk factors.* Anaphylactic shock is caused most commonly by food allergies. Peanuts, tree nuts, shellfish, fish, milk, eggs, soy, and wheat account for 90% of food anaphylaxis; medications (most commonly aspirin and beta-lactam antibiotics), latex, contrast media, insect stings, or exercise may also lead to anaphylaxis. Idiopathic anaphylaxis is an increasingly encountered entity.

■ *Pathophysiology.* Anaphylaxis results from the sudden degranulation of mast cells and basophils. Although the precise mechanisms can be mediated by immunologic mechanisms or may be independent of the immune system (anaphylactoid reactions), the clinical symptoms are identical. Mast cell and basophil degranulation results in the release of preformed vasoactive substances including histamine, along with a host of cytokines. The most important clinical manifestations are caused by the activation of histamine receptors (H_1 and H_2). The organ systems most directly affected are the heart, lungs, and circulatory system. As a result of the effects on vascular permeability, there can be a transfer of 50% of the intravascular fluid into the extravascular space within 10 minutes.

- *Clinical presentation.* Most patients present with a known exposure, although a known history of sensitization may be lacking. Most develop symptoms within 5 to 30 minutes of exposure, although delays in presentation of several hours have been rarely reported. The most commonly encountered findings are urticaria, angioedema, diffuse erythema, bronchospasm, laryngeal edema, hyperperistalsis, and hypotension. In the case of β-adrenergic blockade, those taking beta blockers may be more likely to experience severe symptoms of anaphylaxis that may manifest as paradoxical bradycardia, profound hypotension, and severe bronchospasm.

- *Diagnostic testing.* Laboratory testing has no role in establishing the diagnosis. An EKG should be obtained during treatment. Myocardial ischemia, conduction abnormalities, and atrial and ventricular dysrhythmias have all been reported in cases of severe anaphylaxis.

- *ED management.* Epinephrine is the cornerstone of treatment. Histamine receptor antagonists and corticosteroids should also be given. Refer to Chapter 19 (Allergic Reactions under "Emergency Management Overview") for a more detailed discussion of therapy. Inhaled beta-agonists (e.g., albuterol) may help with respiratory compromise. Patients with severe bronchospasm, obvious respiratory distress, and hypotension, may require mechanical ventilation. Ketamine is a good induction agent during intubation due to its bronchodilatory effect. Isopropteronol may be used in treatment of patients on beta blockers.

- *Helpful hints and pitfalls.* Epinephrine should be given if the patient has any evidence of airway compromise, respiratory distress or anaphylaxis.

Vasogenic: Neurogenic Shock

- *Epidemiology and risk factors.* This is a rare form of shock. Neurogenic shock usually results from a spinal cord injury above the level of T6. In the appropriate clinical setting, trauma patients should be evaluated for neurogenic shock after other causes of shock have been eliminated.

- *Pathophysiology.* Neurogenic shock refers to the loss of neurologic function and autonomic tone below the level of a spinal cord injury. Shock is secondary to the disruption of sympathetic outflow from T1-L2 and to unopposed vagal tone, leading to a decrease in vascular resistance with associated vascular dilatation, and a relative hypovolemia despite preserved blood volume. Spinal shock is a state of transient physiologic (rather than anatomic) reflex depression of cord function below the level of injury with associated loss of all sensorimotor functions. Spinal shock often coincides with neurogenic shock, which is evidenced by loss of autonomic control (bradycardia, vasodilation, and hypotension).

- *Clinical presentation.* The usual signs are a slow pulse and warm, dry skin. Patients with neurogenic shock have significant neurologic dysfunction, and should be examined for manifestations of this. Specifically, deep tendon reflexes, peripheral sensation, rectal tone, and the bulbocavernosus reflex should be evaluated. The examiner should perform a rectal examination, and at the same time, pull on the Foley catheter or squeeze the patient's penis. If the examiner feels tightening of the anal sphincter, the bulbocavernosus reflex is positive, indicating an intact spinal reflex circuit at the level of S3-S4. The bulbocavernosus reflex is often present in patients with neurogenic shock. It is usually absent in patients with *spinal shock* where the spinal cord is contused. Patients with spinal shock have a better prognosis than those with neurogenic shock. They sometimes have a spinal cord injury that is not permanent, and may regain some or all function within 48 to 72 hours. Patients with neurogenic shock almost always have significant, permanent spinal cord injury. They are also hypotensive and areflexic.

- **Diagnostic testing.** Appropriate imaging of the brain, spine, and spinal cord (including radiographs of the cervical, thoracic and lumbar spine, computed tomography (CT scan) of the head and cervical spine, and magnetic resonance imaging (MRI) of the brain, thoracic, lumbar, or sacral spine) should be obtained once the patient is hemodynamically stable.

- **ED management.** The hypotension accompanying neurogenic shock usually responds to crytalloids and placing the patient in trendelenburg position. Bradycardia secondary to increased vagal tone should be treated with atropine to increase heart rate and prevent sudden death. Pharmacologic vasoconstriction should be instituted promptly to increase spinal cord perfusion. The agents of choice are α_1-adrenergic specific, including phenylephrine and ephedrine. In the setting of trauma resuscitation, ephedrine is especially useful; one 10-mg bolus will increase vascular resistance for 3 to 4 hours. Persistent and severe hypotension should prompt immediate investigation into other possible causes of shock. Patients should be immobilized in a cervical collar and spinal precautions should be maintained at all times, especially during transfers and procedures. Spinal trauma is discussed more in Chapter 12.

- **Helpful hints and pitfalls.** Neurogenic shock can be differentiated from hypovolemic shock on the basis of the presence of relative bradycardia in neurogenic shock, as opposed to tachycardia and hypotension with hypovolemic shock.

Vasogenic: Septic Shock

- **Epidemiology and risk factors.** Sepsis is secondary to the presence of infection from a virus, bacteria, or fungus. The infection may result in a systemic inflammatory response, which can progress to septic shock if untreated (Table 7–2). Sepsis is the tenth most common cause of death in the United States and one of the most common causes of death in the intensive care unit. Patients at the extremes of age, with underlying chronic disease, or with immune deficiencies are at the highest risk of developing sepsis, although patients at all ages are susceptible.

- **Pathophysiology.** The vasogenic nature of septic shock results from the body's response to the systemic inflammatory response, which causes increased venous capacitance, causing a relative hypovolemia. In addition, capillary leak caused by vasoactive mediators worsens the hypovolemia. The same substances often cause myocardial depression, which worsens the resulting hypoperfusion.

- **Clinical presentation.** Patients or caregivers may relate a history of worsening systemic illness, fever, chills, fatigue, malaise, myalgias, or focal infectious symptoms such as cough, dysuria, nausea, vomiting, headache,

Table 7–2   Systemic Inflammatory Response Syndrome and Sepsis

Systemic inflammatory response syndrome (SIRS)

These guidelines must be evaluated in line with normal vital signs per age of the patient.

Two or more of the following:

Temperature >38° C or <36° C

Heart rate >90 beats per minute

Respiratory rate >20 breaths per minute or $PaCO_2$ <32 mm Hg

White blood cell count >12,000/mm³, <4000/mm³, or >10% band neutrophilia

Sepsis syndrome

SIRS associated with organ dysfunction or hypotension; organ dysfunction may include presence of lactic acidosis, oliguria, or altered mental status.

Septic shock

SIRS with hypotension despite adequate fluid resuscitation

or stiff neck. Patients may show evidence of systemic hypoperfusion, including peripheral vasoconstriction; cool, pale, or mottled skin; altered mental status; tachycardia, tachypnea; and oliguria. Either fever, sometimes higher than 104° F, or hypothermia may be present.

■ *Diagnostic testing.* Blood cultures should be obtained, preferably before antibiotic administration. A CBC, chemistry panel, and serum lactate level should be obtained. Urinalysis and culture should be sent to assess for urinary tract infection and urosepsis. A chest radiograph should be obtained to assess for pneumonia or adult respiratory distress syndrome (ARDS).

■ *ED management.* Initial resuscitative measures should target a central venous pressure of 8 to 12 mm Hg, a mean arterial pressure of 65 mm Hg, and a urine output of 0.5 ml/kg per hour. Broad-spectrum antibiotics should be initiated (preferably after cultures are obtained) early in the clinical course and should be directed at the most likely cause for sepsis (Table 7–3). Aggressive hemodynamic support should begin with crystalloids such as normal saline. Dobutamine may be used to increase cardiac output. If used in the presence of low blood pressure, it should be combined with vasopressor therapy (e.g., norepinephrine). IV corticosteroids (hydrocortisone 200 to 300 mg/d) are recommended in patients with septic shock who, despite adequate fluid replacement, require vasopressor therapy to maintain adequate blood pressure. Steroids should be continued if the random cortisol concentration obtained during the period of shock is less than 25 µg/dl. Once tissue hypoperfusion has resolved and in the absence of extenuating circumstances, such as significant coronary artery disease, acute hemorrhage, or lactic acidosis, red blood cell transfusion should occur only when hemoglobin decreases to below 7.0 g/dl (<70 g/L) to target a hemoglobin of 7.0 to 9.0 g/dl. Recombinant human-activated protein C (rhAPC) is recommended in patients at high risk of death (sepsis-induced multiple organ failure, septic shock, or sepsis-induced ARDS) and with no absolute contraindication

Table 7-3   Guidelines for Empiric Antibiotic Selection in Severe Sepsis and Septic Shock

	Suspected Source of Sepsis				
	Lung	Abdomen	Skin/Soft Tissue	Urinary Tract	Central Nervous System
Major community-acquired pathogens	*Streptococcus pneumoniae,* *Haemophilus influenzae, Legionella species, Chlamydia pneumoniae, Pneumocystis carinii*	*Escherichia coli, Bacteroides fragilis*	*Group A streptococcus, Staphylococcus aureus, Clostridium species,* Polymicrobial: enteric gram-negative rods, *Pseudomonas aeruginosa,* anaerobes, *staphylococci*	*E. coli, Klebsiella species, Enterobacter species, Proteus species*	*S. pneumoniae,* *Neisseria meningitidis, Listeria monocytogenes, E. coli, H. influenzae*
Empiric antibiotic therapy	Macrolide and third-generation cephalosporin or levofloxacin	Imipenem-cilastatin or piperacillin-tazobactam with or without aminoglycoside	Vancomycin with or without imipenem-cilastatin or piperacillin-tazobactam	Ciprofloxacin with or without aminoglycoside	Vancomycin and third-generation cephalosporin or meropenem
Major nosocomial pathogens[†]	Aerobic gram-negative bacilli	Aerobic gram-negative rods, anaerobes, *Candida species*	*S. aureus,* aerobic gram-negative rods	Aerobic gram-negative rods, enterococci	*P. aeruginosa, E. coli, Klebsiella species, Staphylococcus species*
Empiric antibiotic therapy	Cefipime or imipenem-cilastatin with aminoglycoside	Imipenem-cilastatin with or without aminoglycoside, or piperacillin-tazobactam with or without amphotericin B	Vancomycin plus cefipime	Vancomycin plus cefipime	Cefipime or meropenem plus vancomycin

*Empiric antibiotic selection for invasive pneumococcal disease should be based on known antibiotic susceptibility patterns in the community. High-level penicillin resistance among pneumococcal isolates is increasing. Resistance to third-generation cephalosporins and quinolones has been reported.

[†]Empiric antibiotic selection for hospital-acquired sepsis should be based on antibiotic resistance patterns for bacteria from each specific institution or intensive care unit. Antibiotic regimen can be modified after 48 to 72 hours, based on culture and antibiotic susceptibility results.

From Gando S, Nanzaki S, Sasaki S, et al. *Crit Care Med* 1998;26:2005–2009.

related to bleeding risk. Activated protein C has antithrombotic, anti-inflammatory, and profibrinolytic properties and has been found to reduce mortality in patients with severe sepsis. Surgery should be promptly consulted for surgical disease. Early goal-directed therapy is a new innovative protocol for the initial management of sepsis that has been found to significantly improve mortality. Patients require the insertion of a special central venous catheter capable of measuring central venous oxygen saturation. Central venous pressure, mean arterial pressure, the hematocrit level, and central venous oxygen saturation are optimized using crystalloids, vasopressors, PRBCs, and vasoactive agents according to a specific set of parameters.

■ *Helpful hints and pitfalls.* Early goal-directed therapy is resource intensive, and activated protein C is expensive. If available, these resources should be used on selected patients who may benefit the most from these therapies.

Teaching Points

Shock has a variety of causes, but the end result is a failure of tissue perfusion. This results in tissue hypoxia and an accumulation of metabolic waste products. This in turn produces a cascade of cellular function failures that ultimately lead to apoptosis, organ failure, and organism death. Aggressive management and reversal of these cellular failures is the key to lowering morbidity and mortality.

Suggested Readings

Balk RA. Optimum treatment of severe sepsis and septic shock: evidence in support of the recommendations. Dis Mon 2004;50:168–213.

Richards CF, Mayberry JC. Initial management of the trauma patient. Crit Care Clin 2004;20:1–11.

Rivers E, Nguyen B, Havstad S, et al. Early goal-directed therapy in the treatment of severe sepsis and septic shock. N Eng J Med 2001;345:1368–1377.

Schwarz A. Shock. EMedicine. Last updated October 19, 2004. Accessed September 23, 2005. *http://www.emedicine.com/ped/topic3047.htm*

TRAUMA

CHAPTER 8

General Approach to Trauma

CHRISTIAN M. SLOANE ■ AARON PESSL

Overview

- Trauma is the leading cause of death in patients younger than 45 years, and is the fourth leading cause of death in adults over all. Traumatic injury causes more deaths in children and adolescents, aged 1 to 19, than all other diseases combined. The leading cause of injury in the United States is the motor vehicle collision (MVC). The "golden hours" after significant traumatic injuries is the period of time where rapid assessment and resuscitation can make a significant difference in morbidity and mortality.

- All trauma patients must be *systematically and thoroughly* assessed with a diligent search for underlying injuries. Young, previously healthy patients may mask the seriousness of their traumatic injuries until just before they arrest.

- Advanced trauma life support (ATLS) is a standardized protocol for evaluation of the trauma patient. The most immediate life-threatening conditions are aggressively identified and addressed in the order of their risk potential. The objectives of the initial evaluation of the trauma patient are (a) to stabilize the trauma patient, (b) to identify life-threatening injuries and to initiate adequate supportive therapy, and (c) to efficiently and rapidly organize either definitive therapy or transfer to a facility that provides definitive therapy.

- The scope of prehospital care of the trauma patient includes airway management, control of external bleeding, immobilization of the spine, needle decompression of suspected tension pneumothorax, and splinting of major extremity fractures. Any delays in transport to a hospital are to be avoided. Prehospital personnel use well-defined mechanistic, anatomic, and physiologic criteria to determine if transport to a designated trauma center is needed. The type of trauma activation depends on the mechanism of injury and patient presentation. One example is located in Table 8–1.

- Trauma centers typically have predetermined response teams with defined roles so that multiple therapeutic and diagnostic procedures can be performed simultaneously. One physician is the designated team leader who does the assessment of the patient, orders and interprets diagnostic studies, and prioritizes therapeutic concerns. The team leader ensures that life-threatening problems are addressed immediately.

Table 8–1   Trauma Activation

Full response	Systolic BP <90 mm Hg
	Decreased LOC (GCS <10)
	Penetrating injuries to torso
	Penetrating injuries to head and neck
	RTS <11
	Actual or potential airway compromise
	Amputation proximal to wrist or ankle
	Traumatic cardiac arrests
Modified response	High-energy mechanism including but not limited to:
	• MVC at highway speed
	• MVC with ejection from vehicle
	• MVC with rollover crash
	• Pedestrian hit by vehicle
	• Motorcycle crash
	• Falls > 20 feet (2 stories or greater)
	Nonsuperficial penetrating injury proximal to knee or elbow.
	Patients older than 70 years with the following:
	• Any MVC mechanism
	• Any fall, except from standing
	Presence of, or suspected, compartment syndrome
	Two or more long-bone fractures
	Active hemorrhage from any wound with orthostatic hypotension
	Suspected spine fractures:
	• Motor or sensory loss associated with a traumatic event
	• Bone deformity of axial spine
	Patients with traumatic brain injury and:
	• GCS between 11 and 13
	• GCS > 14 and > 2 organ system injuries

BP, blood pressure; GCS, Glasgow Coma Scale; LOC, loss of consciousness; MVC, motor vehicle crash; RTS, Revised Trauma Score (calculation based on respiratory rate, systolic BP, and GCS).

■ The following discussion addresses the approach to trauma patients who have a significant mechanism of injury or concerning presentation in which the potential for multiple traumatic injuries is high.

Initial Diagnostic Approach
General

■ While the team leader (a physician) is conducting the primary survey, other team members should obtain intravenous (IV) access (two large-bore 16 gauge), place the patient on a continuous cardiac and pulse oximetry monitoring, and provide supplemental oxygen.

■ *Primary survey.* The initial, rapid evaluation of the trauma patient is called the primary survey. This includes a complete assessment of vital signs, the ABCDEs (*A*irway, *B*reathing, *C*irculation, *D*isability and

*E*xposure/*E*nvironment) of trauma care, and the orderly identification and concomitant treatment of life-threatening conditions. Although components of the primary survey are described sequentially, some components may be performed simultaneously. Adjuncts to the primary survey include monitoring devices (cardiac, pulse oximetry), insertion of urinary and gastric catheters, and critical diagnostic studies.

■ *Secondary survey.* A detailed history is now obtained. A useful mnemonic is the AMPLE history: **A**llergies, **M**edications, **P**ast illnesses/**P**regnancy, **L**ast meal, **E**vents/**E**nvironment related to the injury (AMPLE). A head-to-toe examination of the patient that begins after the primary survey has been completed, with resuscitative efforts underway and when the patient is beginning to show normalization of vital signs. The secondary survey also includes a reassessment of all vital signs. Adjuncts to the secondary survey include specialized diagnostic studies such as additional x-rays of the spine and CT scans.

■ *Trauma history.* During the secondary survey a detailed history should be obtained from the patient, witnesses, and paramedics. It should include the mechanism and sites of apparent injury, damage to vehicles involved including windshield starring, injuries to other people involved in the trauma (e.g., death of another crash victim strongly correlates with serious injuries in the other people involved), passenger compartment intrusion, seat belt use, and airbag deployment. Additionally, any blood loss on scene, descriptions of weapons used, and vital signs recorded at the scene should be included in the trauma history. Medical history, medications, allergies, and the use of alcohol or illicit drugs are also very useful to obtain as they may not be available should the patient experience deterioration.

■ If at any time during the secondary survey the patient's clinical status deteriorates, the examiner should return to the elements of the primary survey.

Laboratory

■ A baseline hemoglobin or hematocrit level is useful on arrival. However, in acute hemorrhage, the hematocrit may be normal initially until volume losses have been replaced with saline or the patient has had time to reconstitute plasma volume. A urinalysis is useful to exclude occult hematuria. Depending on the severity of the injury, other studies may include arterial blood gas levels, complete blood count, electrolytes with blood urea nitrogen and creatinine, lipase, coagulation studies, type and screen or type and cross for blood products, cardiac markers, and a lactate level. Parameters such as blood lactate levels and base deficit on an arterial blood gas may help identify patients who are severely injured. Blood lactate appears to be a good marker not only for severity of the shock insult, but also for survival. Patients with altered levels of consciousness may require a urine toxicology screen and serum ethanol level. A bedside glucose level should be checked on all patients with alterations in consciousness. A urine pregnancy test should be ordered on all women of reproductive age.

Radiography

- If possible, imaging should occur during resuscitation, and should be performed in the resuscitation area simultaneously with assessment and subsequent treatment. However, the ABCs should be addressed prior to any imaging studies (i.e., secure the airway, decompress a tension pneumothorax, and initiate fluid resuscitation).
- A portable chest film is usually the only radiograph necessary in cases of penetrating torso trauma. A chest tube should be placed prior to obtaining chest films if there is concern for a tension pneumothorax. Routine emergent radiographs in patients with blunt injury include portable radiographs of the anteroposterior chest, anteroposterior pelvis, and lateral cervical spine film.
- Focused assessment with sonography for trauma (FAST) is commonly performed on all patients with major trauma to look for free fluid in the abdomen (see Chapter 93). Other studies in the initial trauma evaluation include computed tomography (CT scan), diagnostic peritoneal lavage, contrast urography, and angiography.
- Patients with an unprotected airway or hypotension should not be sent to the CT scanner. Unstable patients may require operative intervention with less precise imaging modalities, such as FAST examination or diagnostic peritoneal lavage (DPL) rather than CT scan or angiography.

EKG

- *Electrocardiogram (EKG) monitoring.* Monitor for dysrhythmias that may indicate blunt cardiac injury, a tachycardia that may represent ongoing hemorrhage, or other EKG changes that may be a manifestation of underlying medical pathology.

Emergency Department Management Overview
General

- Problems identified during the primary survey of the evaluation are managed immediately and will be briefly discussed here.
- A detailed discussion of specific injuries are discussed in the remaining chapters in this section.

Primary Survey: A-B-C-D-E

Airway
- *General.* The initial approach to airway management is simultaneous assessment and management of the adequacy of airway patency, oxygenation, and ventilation. Protection of the spine and the spinal cord must be maintained; cervical spine injury should be assumed in any patient with multisystem trauma, altered level of consciousness, or a blunt injury above the clavicle. Evaluate for airway foreign body or obstruction, gag reflex, obvious head and neck trauma, pooling of secretions, tracheal deviation, and the presence and quality of breath

sounds are immediately assessed on physical examination. Patients with a severe head injury and a Glasgow Coma Scale (GCS) of 8 or less require the placement of a definitive airway.

- **Interventions.** Airway management techniques and rapid sequence intubation are covered in detail in Chapter 5.
- **Pearls.** In patients with facial or neck trauma, it is far better to intubate early before signs of respiratory distress while there is relatively normal anatomy, than to wait and subsequently find the airway so distorted that active management becomes difficult or impossible.

Breathing

- **General.** Airway patency alone does not ensure adequate ventilation. Ventilation requires adequate function of the lungs, chest wall, and diaphragm; adequate gas exchange in the lungs is necessary to maximize oxygenation and carbon dioxide elimination.
- **Interventions.** One hundred percent oxygen is administered via face mask or with a bag-valve-mask with attached oxygen reservoir. Needle decompression followed by tube thoracostomy is indicated for tension pneumothorax. Open pneumothorax is treated with prompt closure of the chest wall defect with a sterile occlusive dressing taped on three sides to allow air to escape, with tube thoracostomy remote from the defect. Flail chest is treated with re-expansion of the lung along with tracheal intubation and ventilation if necessary, and always with appropriate analgesia.
- **Pearls.** Worsening of the patient's ventilation status with intubation and bag-valve ventilation may indicate that a pneumothorax or tension pneumothorax is the underlying problem. Increasing respiratory rate and progressively shallow respirations are subtle signs of chest injury or hypoxia. Children often become bradypneic before respiratory arrest, and a slowing respiratory rate in an adult may indicate the onset of a cerebral herniation syndrome.

Circulation

- **General.** Hypotension after traumatic injury must be considered to be hypovolemic in origin until proven otherwise. Vital signs and cardiac monitoring are helpful only if they are done repeatedly. For patients presenting in shock, a thorough search for a source of bleeding must be conducted. Significant blood loss is usually located in one of the following body cavities or spaces: chest, abdomen, pelvis, retroperitoneum, thigh, or street.
- **Interventions.** Two large-bore peripheral IV catheters (16 gauge preferred in adults) are usually sufficient. Place a central line (cordis or introducer catheter and NOT a triple lumen) if unable to obtain peripheral access. Patients in profound shock often require venous cutdowns. Start resuscitation with 2 L of warmed crystalloid fluids, and repeat the infusion with up to 50 ml/kg of fluid. If there is no response, or signs of ongoing hemorrhage, commence transfusion with O-negative or type-specific blood. Control external hemorrhage with direct pressure and pneumatic splinting as necessary. Scalp hemorrhage can be controlled with a figure-8 or running 3-0 Ethilon suture or Raney clips. Hemorrhage from an extremity wound can often be controlled with direct pressure, plus elevation of the extremity. Avoid blind clamping of

bleeding vessels. Lower extremity tourniquets often are a source of increased hemorrhage because they are often inflated above venous but below arterial pressure. Massive hemothorax with chest tube output of greater than 1500 mL of blood on initial placement, or ongoing bleeding greater than 200 mL per hour for 2 to 4 hours is an indication for operative exploration thoracotomy. Pericardiocentesis is performed for cases of cardiac tamponade. Removal of as little as 15 mL to 20 mL of fluid by pericardiocentesis may result in immediate hemodynamic improvement until the patient can be transported to the operating room for thoracotomy, pericardiotomy, and repair of the injured heart.

- *Pearls.* Not all patients have a *normal* response to volume loss. Absence of tachycardia should not reassure the clinician about the absence of significant blood loss after trauma. Medications, i.e., beta-blockers, may blunt the normal tachycardic response. The young or well-trained athletes with baseline bradycardia may initially have a heart rate within normal limits in the face of hypovolemia. The pregnant woman has an expanded blood volume, and may not develop tachycardia before a large volume depletion. Pediatric patients have a large physiologic reserve, and therefore show few early signs of volume depletion. Elderly patients have a decreased ability to mount a heart rate response to volume loss, and may not initially exhibit tachycardia especially if they are taking beta blocking medication. See Special Considerations.

Disability

- *General.* Perform a rapid focused neurologic examination at the end of the primary survey, assessing level of consciousness, pupil size and reactivity, reflexes, and gross motor and sensory examinations. A rectal examination will provide evidence of anal sphincter tone and sensation, and will provide an early clue to the integrity of spinal cord function. Assess the level of consciousness using the Glasgow Coma Scale (Appendix 2) or the AVPU mnemonic (Alert, responds to Verbal, responds to Pain, Unresponsive). Determine the pupil sizes and reactivity. Assess motor strength in all extremities. Test pain sensation on the trunk and extremities, and if absent, determine the level of loss. Imaging studies are directed toward evaluting causes for altered mental status or neurologic deficit. A bedside glucose should be rapidly checked on all altered patients.
- *Interventions.* Undertake active airway management for patients with head injury: e.g., a GCS of 8 or less, and for any patient whose airway may become distorted by the trauma. Intubate any patient in shock, as well as any patient with deterioration of ventilation.
- *Pearls.* Patients with closed head injury can deteriorate rapidly. Any decrease in level of consciousness may indicate decreased cerebral oxygenation or traumatic central nervous system injury. A short lucid period may follow head injury with epidural hematoma before rapid deterioration. Hypotension with a normal or slow heart rate may be present with an acute spinal cord injury.

Exposure

- *General.* Completely undress the trauma patient in a warm resuscitation area to evaluate for other injuries, while maintaining patient body temperature. If the patient has been injured in low- or high-temperature environments, core temperature assessment with rectal temperature should be done.

■ ***Interventions.*** Treatment for hypo- or hyperthermia is discussed in Chapter 65. Interventions for extremity injuries are discussed in Chapter 17. Wound care is discussed in Chapter 94.

■ ***Pearls.*** Hypothermia may be present when the patient arrives, may develop rapidly while the patient is uncovered and examined, or may develop with the administration of room-temperature IV fluids or refrigerated blood products.

ED interventions

■ Airway management: See Chapter 5.
■ Fractures reduction and splinting: See Chapter 17.
■ Procedures: thoracotomy, thoracentesis, diagnostic peritoneal lavage, central venous access, venous cutdown. See Chapter 91.
■ Wound care: See Chapter 94.

Disposition

■ ***Consultation.*** Early consultation with specialists is important to address acute life threats. Consultation with trauma surgeons is automatic in many institutions when certain threshold criteria are met. Neurosurgery needs to be involved early for head injury requiring possible surgical intervention or intracranial pressure monitoring. Orthopedic consultation is required for fractures and major musculoskeletal injuries. Other consultants are required, as needed depending on the organ system or region of the body involved.

■ ***Admission.*** Unstable vital signs, multisystem trauma, and significant injury are generally agreed upon admission criteria. Trauma patients are best admitted to a trauma service with appropriate consultation.

■ ***Discharge.*** Stable vitals after observation, minor injuries only, isolated system trauma, minor mechanisms with negative workups and good sociologic follow-up capability are all necessary to enable a safe discharge.

Special Considerations
Pediatrics

■ Although the differences in anatomy, physiology, and psychology of the pediatric trauma patient call for some modification of the evaluation and treatment, the overall priorities of care and management are the same as for adults. Quantities of blood, fluids, medications, injury patterns, and the degree and rapidity of heat loss all differ in the pediatric patient, but the general approach to the trauma patient remains the same. The Broselow tape contains a quick reference to doses of medications and sizes of resuscitation equipment based on the child's length. It should be readily available for any pediatric resuscitation. Another important consideration in the pediatric trauma patient is the possibility of nonaccidental trauma, or child abuse (see Chapter 82).

- Children younger than 6 months are obligate nose breathers; therefore any facial trauma or blood in the nasopharynx can cause significant respiratory distress. Nasal flaring, grunting, retractions, tachypnea, and accessory muscle use must be recognized in the dyspneic pediatric patient. Airway management can be difficult secondary to a relatively larger tongue and a more cephalad location of the larynx. The indications for endotracheal intubation remain the same for pediatric and adult trauma patients (see Chapter 5). Pediatric resuscitation is discussed in more detail in Chapter 74.
- Tachycardia is the most sensitive sign of volume loss, with hypotension being a late sign of shock and thus ominous when observed. Vascular access can be challenging and the early placement of interosseous cannulation should be utilized rather than spending long times trying to establish a peripheral access. IV fluid resuscitation should be administered with two 20-ml/kg boluses of crystalloid, followed by a 10-ml/kg bolus, and then administration of packed red blood cells at 10 ml/kg if there is no improvement or a worsening after an initial response to crystalloid.
- The ratio of surface area to mass in the pediatric patient is greater than that in adults, putting the pediatric patient at greater risk of hypothermia.
- The pediatric patient has a more compliant chest wall, and therefore may have serious underlying thoracic injury without external evidence of trauma. Similarly, the existence of external trauma to the chest, such as a fractured rib, is a very sensitive indicator of intrathoracic trauma. In the infant, intracranial bleeding can also produce shock.
- Disposition of the pediatric trauma patient is difficult, and the emergency physician should never be reluctant to admit to the hospital or transfer to a pediatric trauma center. Social services should be contacted and reporting to child protective services is mandatory for any suspicion of nonaccidental trauma.

Elderly

- Falls are the most common accidental injury in the over-75 age group and the second most common injury in the 65- to 75-year-old group. Motor vehicle crashes and being struck by automobiles account for most elderly patient presentations to trauma centers in the United States. The geriatric trauma patient often has a significant past medical history that must be taken into account during the assessment and treatment. Falls are often the result of syncope from a variety of cardiac and metabolic causes, and early cardiac monitoring is essential. A normal heart rate may be deceiving in the geriatric patient, as the normal tachycardic response to hypovolemia, pain, and anxiety may be blunted by medications such at beta-blockers.
- Airway management may be difficult secondary to anatomic variations and cervical spine arthritis. Subdural hemorrhages occur more frequently in elderly patients, and a more liberal use of CT scanning is therefore justified. Do not assume that alterations in mental status are due to senility and represent the patient's level of function before the trauma. Thoracic injury, including rib fractures, can lead to significant respiratory

decompensation in patients with limited O_2 reserves, and early ABG analysis is warranted. Orthopedic injuries such as hip, pelvic, and long bone fractures can be the sole etiology for hypovolemia in the elderly patient.

- The elderly require early and liberal use of packed red blood cells; however, precautions should be taken to avoid fluid overload. Early invasive monitoring is also useful, as with children. It is prudent to admit the elderly patient to a monitored care unit because so many will deteriorate from what appear to be minor injuries.

Women and Pregnancy

- A pregnant trauma patient represents two patients requiring rapid evaluation and treatment. Trauma is the leading cause of nonobstetrical mortality in pregnant women, and has a high incidence of associated placental abruption, preterm labor, fetal–maternal hemorrhage, and miscarriage.
- The physiologic changes of pregnancy make it difficult to determine if tachycardia and hypotension represent ongoing blood loss or normal vital signs of pregnancy. Typically, heart rate increases ten to twenty beats per minute, blood pressure drops 10 to 15 mm Hg, and blood volume increases by up to 50%. Patients can lose 30% to 35% of circulating blood volume before manifesting any clinical evidence of shock, and at this point, blood flow to the placenta may already be compromised.

Teaching Points

Caring for the multiple trauma patient is a unique responsibility and challenge. It requires an organized methodical approach to assessment, stabilization, diagnosis, and management. Common errors are made in the underassessment of the individual patient because prior to trauma the patient is young and healthy, and does not show signs and symptoms of internal injuries until late in the course. It is not possible to recognize many internal injuries early after trauma, and it is necessary to pay close attention to the mechanism of injury and other signs that correlate with serious injuries that can be found in the field (e.g., the death of someone at the scene from a motor vehicle crash).

Trauma is best managed by a team approach that is efficient, compulsive, and thorough. It requires frequent reassessment of the patient, and observation over time, but also objective evaluations of the hidden cavities for hemorrhage whenever there is a significant mechanism.

Suggested Readings

ATLS, Advanced Trauma Life Support Program for Doctors, (ATLS) (7th edition). The Chicago: American College of Surgeons: Chicago, 2004.

Dries DJ, Hays W. Initial evaluation of the trauma patient. eMedicine. Last update July 28, 2005, accessed September 25, 2005. Available at *http://www.emedicine.com/med/topic3221.htm*

Richards CF, Mayberry JC. Initial management of the trauma patient. Crit Care Clin 2004;20:1–11.

Shah AJ, Kilcline BA. Trauma in pregnancy. Emerg Med Clin N Am 2003;21:615–629.

Stafford PW, Blinman TA, Nance ML. Practical points in evaluation and resuscitation of the injured child. Surg Clin N Am 2002;82:273–301.

Shoenberger JM, Houpt JC, Swadron SP. Occult trauma in high-risk populations. Emerg Med Clin North Am 2003;21:1145–1163.

CHAPTER   **9**

Head Injury

MARTIN DE KORT ■ **ANDREW GARFF** ■ **JENNIFER J. CASALETTO**

 Red Flags

Age < 2 or > 60 y ● Acute intoxication ● Physiologic or pharmacologic anticoagulation ● Post-traumatic seizure ● Severe headache ● Recurrent vomiting ● Loss of consciousness ● Glasgow Coma Scale < 13 ● Vital sign abnormalities especially elevated blood pressure and bradycardia, and decreased respiratory effort (Cushing reflex*) ● Anisocoria or ipsilateral unreactive pupil ● Focal neurologic deficit

A specific response to acute, potentially lethal rises in intracranial pressure.

Overview

■ The incidence of traumatic brain injury (TBI) is unknown; however, it is responsible for 40% of trauma-related deaths. TBI is the leading cause of death in patients younger than 25 years. Beware of historical and physical examination "Red Flags" indicating the potential for severe head injury (see Box).

■ Motor vehicle crashes (MVCs) are the leading cause of TBI in the United States, followed by falls and firearms. Alcohol is often associated with each of the leading causes of TBI.

■ The Glasgow Coma Scale (GCS) is a standard scoring system that is used to define altered mentation in head trauma patients (see Appendix 2). Eighty percent of TBI is mild (GCS 13-15), 10% moderate (GCS 9-12), and 10% severe (GCS 3-8). Patients should be hemodynamically stable and fully resuscitated, with evacuation of all surgical lesions, and not intoxicated for the GCS to be used to predict mortality.

■ The traumatized brain is vulnerable to secondary insult from hypotension, hypoxia, or hypocapnia due to overaggressive hyperventilation. Every effort should be made to prevent further injury by reducing elevated intracranial pressure (ICP), maintaining normal intravascular volume, maintaining normal mean arterial blood pressure (MAP), and restoring normal oxygenation and normocapnia.

Initial Diagnostic Approach
General

■ Evaluate the ABCs (*a*irway, *b*reathing, and *c*irculation), and test for major neurologic disability (pupil reactivity, ability to move extremities). Briefly determine the patient's GCS on arrival in the ED. Although an initial GCS is not predictive of prognosis until all alcohol or other drugs have been metabolized, it is a useful baseline to which future determinations can be compared.

■ Begin cardiovascular monitoring and resuscitation, including supplemental oxygen and intravenous (IV) access, as 60% of severely head injured patients sustain multisystem trauma. Although hemorrhagic shock may result from head injury in young children, an alternate cause needs to be sought and treated in most adults.

■ The history should include the time of event, mechanism, alcohol or drug use, the patient's condition before the injury, duration of loss of consciousness, co-morbidities, and the use of anticoagulant medications.

■ The secondary survey should include a neurologic examination. A directed examination should identify life-threatening injuries and establish a baseline. A large fixed pupil suggests a herniation syndrome and is usually on the side of the expanding lesion. Traumatic mydriasis also presents with a fixed dilated pupil. Fixed, dilated pupils signify severe global brain injury. Check for rhythmic eye movements, indicating seizure activity, or gaze preference toward a mass lesion. The evaluation should also include examination of the other cranial nerves, motor strength and gross sensory assessments, and testing for deep tendon and pathologic reflexes (e.g., Babinski, rectal tone).

■ Decorticate posturing (flexion of upper extremities, extension of lower extremities) indicates injury above the midbrain. Decerebrate posturing (arms extended and adducted; legs extended and internally rotated) in response to noxious stimuli indicates a brainstem lesion and has a worse prognosis.

■ Specific maneuvers further characterize severe brain injury. Stimulation of the cornea is performed with a cotton wisp or applicator. Any observed eye closure in response to corneal stimulation indicates that the cranial nerve V-VII reflex arc remains intact and excludes the diagnosis of brain death. Testing of the oculocephalic reflex (doll's eyes) is contraindicated due to cervical spine precautions. An intact oculocephalic reflex (eye movements are in a direction opposite to head turning) demonstrates the functional integrity of a large portion of the brainstem. The oculo-vestibular reflex (caloric stimulation) is a stronger stimulation to the brainstem. The normal response is a transient slow deviation of gaze toward the side of the stimulus (brainstem mediated; eyes toward the "ice") followed by a quick saccadic correction back to the midline (cortical mediated)

- The head and neck should be carefully examined for any evidence of trauma. Basilar skull fractures are often diagnosed by clinical evaluation for the presence of blood in the ear canal, hemotympanum, rhinorrhea, otorrhea, Battle's sign (retroauricular hematoma), Raccoon's sign (periorbital ecchymosis), or cranial nerve deficits.

Laboratory

- Immediately perform rapid glucose testing to rule out a confounding etiology. Alcohol and drug screening may also reveal confounders.
- Platelet levels and coagulation profiles are necessary in patients with a GCS less than 8, due to high risk of DIC, to identify the presence of a coagulopathy, and in patients likely to require intracranial procedures.

Radiography

- *Plain films.* Plain films are helpful in patients with penetrating head injuries from impalement or a penetrating object. A skull radiograph will show the size of the object, the angle of impalement, and the depth of penetration.
- *Computed tomography.* A non–contrast-enhanced computed tomography (CT scan) is indicated for patients with a GCS less than 15 as well as those with a GCS of 15 and loss of consciousness for more than 5 minutes, severe headache, recurrent vomiting, or clinical intoxication with physical evidence of head injury, a wound that might suggest a depressed skull fracture, any patient who is hemophiliac or who is on anticoagulant medications, or any patient with no witnessed loss of consciousness or diminished neurologic function whose neurologic function is becoming abnormal. A CT scan can be performed quickly with continued patient monitoring. It identifies bony injury, intracranial hemorrhage, cerebral edema, hydrocephalus, and mass effect. Patient movement and foreign bodies degrade images.
- *Magnetic resonance imaging.* Magnetic resonance imaging (MRI) has no role in the diagnosis of acute TBI because it is time-consuming, does not allow adequate patient monitoring, and is less accurate than a CT scan for intracranial hemorrhage. It may be used later in a patient's care to identify diffuse axonal injury, gray matter injury, or brainstem lesions.

Emergency Department Management Overview
General

- The ABCs should be addressed. Establish two IV lines, place the patient on a monitor, and give supplementary oxygen to any patient who is being evaluated after major trauma.

- *Airway management.* Patients with an initial GCS of 8 or less or a decreasing level of consciousness should undergo intubation to protect the airway. If possible, conduct a directed neurologic examination before intubation. Rapid-sequence intubation (RSI) with cervical spine precautions is the preferred method of airway control. To minimize any ICP increase associated with laryngeal stimulation, premedicate with lidocaine and fentanyl. Etomidate and succinylcholine are most commonly used for induction and paralysis, respectively. A defasiculating dose of a nondepolarizing paralytic agent (e.g., vecuronium 0.1 mg/kg lV) may be given before succinylcholine to reduce the fasciculations associated with its administration and the associated increase in ICP.
- *Cardiovascular resuscitation.* Hypotension decreases cerebral perfusion, doubling morbidity and mortality in head-injured patients. Use nonglucose-containing, isotonic fluid to resuscitate hypotensive patients regardless of ICP. Anemia decreases oxygen-carrying capacity and increases mortality; transfuse if the hemoglobin drops below 8 g/dl in the young healthy adult or 10 g/dl in the elderly or individuals with underlying cardiac disease.
- *Cerebral resuscitation.* Hypoxia (PaO_2 <60) doubles morbidity and mortality in severe TBI; therefore, initiate supplemental oxygen upon arrival. Compensatory mechanisms allow 50 to 100 ml of additional intracranial volume, after which ICP rises. Increased ICP compromises cerebral perfusion pressure (CPP = MAP – ICP [cerebral perfusion pressure = mean arterial pressure – intracranial pressure]) leading to loss of autoregulation, further ICP increase, and impending cerebral herniation. Hyperventilation to an end-tidal CO_2 of 30 to 35 mm Hg induces cerebral vasoconstriction within seconds, lowering ICP by as much as 25%; however, this is only a temporizing measure. Levels below 30 mm Hg cause cerebral vasoconstriction and ischemia.
- *Monitoring.* Vital sign, pulse oximetry, end-tidal CO_2, cardiac output, urine output, and GCS monitoring are required to evaluate patients with TBI and to prevent secondary brain injury. Continuous mixed venous oxygen saturation (SvO_2) has recently been added to monitoring of patients with brain injury because an SvO_2 of less than 50% indicates ongoing cerebral ischemia; however, this is not routinely performed in the ED setting. In severe TBI, continuous ICP monitoring is essential, as effective management of ICP decreases morbidity and mortality.

Medications

- *Osmotic agents and diuretics.* Use mannitol (0.25 to 1 g/kg) to reduce cerebral edema and ICP in patients with increased ICP or signs of herniation. Mannitol acts within 60 minutes and lasts 6 hours. Furosemide may also be used, but repeated use risks dehydration and hypokalemia. Hypertonic saline has been found to decrease ICP without adversely affecting hemodynamic status.
- *Steroids.* These are not helpful in TBI.
- *Sedatives.* Sedating patients decreases ICP via reduced metabolic demand, ventilator asynchrony, and sympathetic response. Propofol is ideal in the normotensive patient due to its ease of titration and short half-life, which allows for neurologic reassessment.

- *Paralytics.* Paralytics may be required when hypotension does not allow for adequate sedation to prevent ventilator asynchrony and movements resulting in increased ICP.
- *Anticonvulsants.* Treat actively seizing patients with benzodiazepines. Phenytoin prophylaxis is indicated in patients with depressed skull fracture, intracranial hemorrhage, posttraumatic seizure, or penetrating injury. The presence of seizures has no prognostic value. Long-term prophylactic anticonvulsant use does not change the incidence of post-traumatic epilepsy.

Emergency Department Interventions
Surgical

- Emergent craniotomy indications include an expanding mass lesion, penetrating skull injury, depressed skull fracture, and clinical deterioration in a patient with a mass lesion. Rarely, an emergency burr hole in the temporal bone is made in cases of active herniation or expanding mass lesion that has been produced by an epidural hematoma.

Consultation

- Know institution specific capabilities for neurosurgical consultation.
- Neurosurgery consultation is prudent for all patients with intracranial pathology that may require emergent surgical intervention or ICP monitoring.

Disposition

- Stabilize and transfer patients requiring neurosurgical care if none is locally available.
- Admit patients with a GCS below 15, an abnormal neurologic evaluation, or an abnormal CT scan for serial neurologic examinations.
- Patients with a mild TBI, GCS 15, normal findings on head CT scan, and a normal neurologic examination may be discharged to the care of a responsible observer.

Specific Problems
Intracranial Hemorrhage
Epidural Hematoma

- *Background.* An epidural hematoma (EDH) occurs in people who have sustained blunt trauma to the head. Skull fracture overlying the middle meningeal artery is associated with 80% of EDHs; 40% of patients have multiple intracranial lesions.
- *Clinical presentation.* Symptoms develop within hours and often result in rapid deterioration. A patient may have a classic presentation that includes a brief loss of consciousness (LOC) followed by a lucid interval and return of altered level of consciousness; however, most patients present with decreased alertness, severe headache, dizziness, and nausea or vomiting. Rapid expansion may lead to herniation and resultant cardiac arrest.

- **Diagnostic testing.** The CT scan shows a biconvex, lenticular, hyperdense lesion with sharp margins on the surface of the brain that does not cross suture lines (Figure 9–1).
- **ED management.** Neurosurgery should be consulted for rapid evacuation of the EDH.
- **Helpful hints and pitfalls.** Only 30% of EDHs present classically; failure to recognize and treat promptly may prevent successful surgical intervention.

Intracerebral Hemorrhage

- **Background.** Intracerebral hemorrhage (ICH) occurs within the parenchyma via blunt or penetrating injury. Multiple ICHs are often encountered; 85% occur in the frontal and temporal lobes. ICH results from injury to arterioles caused by shearing and tensile forces as the brain moves along irregular skull surfaces.

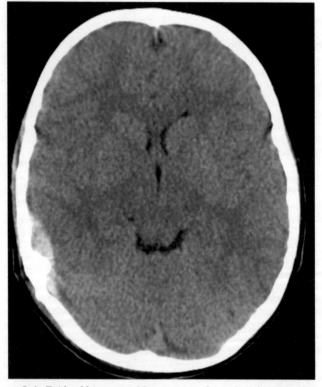

Figure 9–1. Epidural hematoma. Noncontrast-enhanced axial computed tomography image. *(Courtesy Jason Scott Stephens, M.D., The University of Texas Southwestern, Department of Radiology.)*

- *Clinical presentation.* Presentation ranges from asymptomatic to cerebral herniation and is determined by size, location, and rate of bleeding. Seizures can complicate the course.
- *Diagnostic testing.* Hours to days after injury, the CT scan shows a well-defined hyperdense, homogenous lesion deep within the brain parenchyma.
- *ED management.* Neurosurgery should be consulted for possible ICP monitoring or operative intervention.
- *Helpful hints and pitfalls.* Failure to control hypertension may result in increased bleeding. Bleeding into the ventricles or in the cerebellum increases mortality.

Subarachnoid Hemorrhage

- *Background.* Subarachnoid hemorrhage (SAH) occurs in blunt or penetrating head injury and is the most common CT scan abnormality in TBI. Half of these patients have associated intracranial hemorrhages. SAH occurs when blood vessels within the subarachnoid space are lacerated leading to the accumulation of blood within the cerebrospinal fluid (CSF) and meningeal intima.
- *Clinical presentation.* This depends on the size of the hemorrhage; however, headache, photophobia, and decreased consciousness are common findings. Patients with SAH are more likely to be hypotensive, hypoxic and have higher ICP.
- *Diagnostic testing.* CT scan reveals hyperdensity in the basal cisterns and sulci (see Chapter 35).
- *ED management.* Nimodipine may be used to reduce or prevent vasospasm if blood pressure and other injuries allow.
- *Helpful hints and pitfalls.* Complications of SAH include rebleeding, hydrocephalus, delayed cerebral ischemia associated with cerebral vasospasm, and seizures.

Subdural Hematoma

- *Background.* Subdural hematoma (SDH) is more common than EDH and has a higher mortality. SDH occurs via an acceleration–deceleration mechanism, leaving elderly and alcoholic patients at greatest risk due to brain atrophy. SDH in children is caused by child abuse until proven otherwise. SDH results from rupture of superficial bridging veins as the brain moves relative to the skull, leading to bleeding between the dura and arachnoid.
- *Clinical presentation.* SDH is classified on the basis of the time elapsed between injury and symptoms. Acute SDH is symptomatic within 24 hours, most often with decreased consciousness. At least half of these patients have a lucid interval after injury, followed by declining mental status. Subacute SDH presents with headache, weakness, or altered consciousness 24 hours to 2 weeks after injury. Chronic SDH presents more than 2 weeks from injury; 50% of patients have unilateral weakness or altered consciousness.
- *Diagnostic testing.* Noncontrast CT scan is the study of choice, but findings vary. Acute SDH usually appears as a hyperdense, crescent-shaped

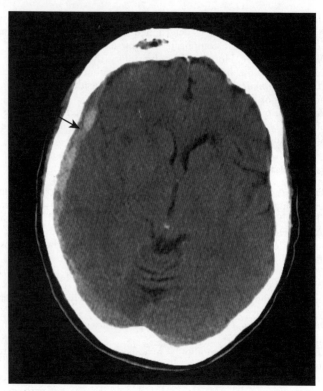

Figure 9–2. Subdural hematoma. Noncontrast-enhanced axial computed tomography image. Hyperdense crescent-shaped SDH that extends beyond suture lines unlike an EDH.

lesion on the surface of the brain extending across suture lines (Figure 9–2), but may be found along the tentorium. Subacute and chronic SDHs appear as hypodense, isodense, or mixed-density lesions.

- *ED management.* Acute and subacute SDHs are managed surgically depending on size and the patient's signs and symptoms.
- *Helpful hints and pitfalls.* Isodense lesions are easily missed on a CT scan and may require addition of IV contrast as well as careful examination for subtle effacement of the sulci and ventricular compression. Spontaneous rebleeding and seizures are common complications.

Other Intracranial Injuries
Cerebral Contusion

- *Background.* Cerebral contusions are the most common CT abnormality in mild head trauma, usually occurring with rapid-deceleration injuries or direct blows. Contusions are the result of parenchymal vessel injury, most often in the frontal and temporal lobes, which strike bony irregularities along the skull base.

- *Clinical presentation.* Contusions may present as brief LOC or a subtle decrease in alertness. Coma is rare. Declining consciousness may occur as edema increases in the hours after injury.
- *Diagnostic testing.* A CT scan may reveal areas of punctate hemorrhage or edema in the acute setting. MRI is more sensitive and accurate than a CT scan for detecting contusions. MRI findings typically demonstrate the lesions from the onset of injury, but many facilities cannot perform MRI on an emergent basis.
- *ED management.* Neurosurgery should be consulted and the patient should be admitted for observation and serial neurologic examinations.
- *Helpful hints and pitfalls.* Many patients do well and have an uneventful recovery. However, others may have significant neurologic problems such as increased ICP, posttraumatic seizures, and focal deficits. Look for contracoup injury on the opposite side of impact.

Concussion

- *Background.* Concussion is a traumatically induced brief disruption of neurologic function. This accompanies 75% of TBI and is most commonly sustained during contact sports. The mechanism of injury is not well understood, but may be due to axonal stretching and neurotransmitter alterations.
- *Clinical presentation.* A concussion presents with altered alertness (GCS 13-15) and amnesia to events surrounding the traumatic episode or transient loss of other neurologic functions. Postconcussive syndrome affects 25% of patients, may follow a concussion or other types of head injuries, and may last up to 6 months. It may include headache (particularly with exertion), dizziness, fatigue, irritability, ataxia, and impaired memory and concentration.
- *Diagnostic testing.* There are no consistent CT scan findings for a concussion.
- *ED management.* Discharge to a responsible observer and give head injury precautions and instructions to avoid contact sports until follow-up and clearance by a physician.
- *Helpful hints and pitfalls.* Second-impact syndrome is defined as a fatal, uncontrollable increase in ICP secondary to diffuse brain swelling. The swelling occurs after a blow to the head that is sustained before full recovery from a previous injury to the head.

Diffuse Axonal Injury

- *Background.* Diffuse axonal injury (DAI) follows rapid acceleration-deceleration injuries. DAI is classified by coma length: mild (6-24 hours), moderate (>24 hours), and severe (prolonged). It results from shearing forces that disrupt axonal fibers throughout the brain.
- *Clinical presentation.* The patient is comatose with a nonfocal neurologic examination. Seizures and prolonged or permanent coma may result.

- *Diagnostic testing.* The CT scan findings are nonspecific, but may include loss of gray–white interface, edema, or sulcal effacement. An MRI is more sensitive after the acute phase.
- *ED management.* Admit for serial observation and possible ICP monitoring.
- *Helpful hints and pitfalls.* Increasing coma length predicts increased morbidity and mortality.

Penetrating Injuries

- *Background.* Penetrating injury, specifically firearms, account for most deaths due to TBI in the United States; 76% of affected patients are pronounced dead at the scene. Tangential wounds often do not penetrate the skull, but result in cerebral contusions at the initial site of impact. Penetration of the cranial vault can cause massive intracranial damage due to direct injury, cavitation injury, and depressed skull fragments.
- *Clinical presentation.* Presentation depends on the mechanism and location of the injury. Signs of self-inflicted gunshot wounds include a large, stellate entry wound with powder burns most often seen on the side of the dominant hand of the patient. Infectious complications such as meningitis, abscess or empyema, and osteomyelitis complicate penetrating injury.
- *Diagnostic testing.* CT scan can provide data on cranial vault penetration, skull fracture, contusion, pneumocephaly, and missile tract. Plain radiographs can be useful in impalement injury to show the size, angle, and depth of penetration. Angiography may be appropriate to aid in determining the involvement of vascular structures.
- *ED management.* Impaled objects should be removed intraoperatively, not in the ED. Use prophylactic antibiotics and antiepileptics with intracranial penetration injury.
- *Helpful hints and pitfalls.* Small penetrating injuries such as low caliber gunshots can be easily missed when covered by hair.

Extracranial Injury
Scalp Laceration

- *Background.* Scalp lacerations and hematomas account for 85% of ED visits for head trauma. The scalp is vascular and lacerations may lead to significant hemorrhage.
- *Clinical presentation.* Presentation depends upon the presence of underlying injury, the mechanism of injury, and the extent of laceration.
- *Diagnostic testing.* Plain films can aid in identifying the presence of foreign bodies or cranial vault penetration. They need not be obtained if there are already indications for a CT scan.
- *ED management.* Obtain hemostasis with direct pressure or the use of Raney clips to compress the edges of the scalp laceration, lidocaine with epinephrine, or ligation of vessels. Sterilely irrigate and explore for foreign bodies, galea injury, or skull involvement. When possible, repair the galea with 3-0 nylon; staple or suture the remaining laceration. A

continuous or running suture (or figure-of-8 suture; see Chapter 94) of the scalp laceration can also be used to control the hemorrhage while the patient is still being evaluated.

■ *Helpful hints and pitfalls.* It may be necessary to clip or shave the hair to find the source and site of the scalp laceration. The capability of large hemorrhage is often underestimated with a scalp laceration, which can lead to hypotension even in an adult. This is particularly likely with the alcoholic patient who may have been unconscious for some time before being discovered and who may not be actively bleeding when finally found. Infections are uncommon unless there is gross contamination.

Skull Fracture

■ *Background.* Skull fractures result from direct blows; they are found in 60% of moderate and severe TBI. Fractures are classified as linear, depressed, basilar, and open. A fracture can lead to local cerebral contusion or hemorrhage.

■ *Clinical presentation.* The clinical presentation varies depending on underlying TBI. Basilar skull fractures may present with loss of ipsilateral vestibulocochlear or facial nerve function, CSF leakage, hemotympanum, Battle's sign, or Raccoon's eyes.

■ *Diagnostic testing.* A CT scan may reveal the fracture, pneumocephaly, and underlying brain injury. A basilar fracture may be revealed by an air fluid level in the sphenoid sinus in the lateral cervical spine film.

■ *ED management.* Most fractures will require that the patient be admitted to the hospital, with the exception of linear fractures in an asymptomatic adult. Isolated, closed-linear fractures require no specific intervention. Depressed fractures larger than 5 mm require elevation, anticonvulsants, and administration of antibiotics if they are open. Open fractures require irrigation, debridement, and antibiotics.

■ *Helpful hints and pitfalls.* The risk of cervical spine injury in patients with TBI doubles in the presence of a skull fracture. Meningitis can develop after otorrhea or rhinorrhea, but cannot be prevented by antibiotic prophylaxis. Basilar fracture can result in a delayed-onset neuropraxia of cranial nerves VII and VIII that may benefit from steroid administration. Associated internal carotid injury can result in arterial dissection of carotid or vertebral arteries.

Special Considerations
Pediatrics

■ Children sustain fewer ICHs, but more cerebral edema and DAI.
■ Mental status changes are difficult to detect; beware of irritability.
■ The incidence of posttraumatic seizures after TBI is higher in children than adults.
■ Search for child abuse; up to 66% of head injuries in children are intentional. Skull fractures in children should trigger a search for nonaccidental trauma.
■ Intracranial pathology is more likely to be found in children in the presence of skull fracture.

- Shaken-baby syndrome often does not present with external signs of trauma. Note irritability and vomiting. Look for rib fractures, SDHs, and retinal hemorrhages.
- Hypovolemic hypotension secondary to intracranial bleeding can occur in children.

Elderly

- Head injury is the most common cause of mortality in elderly (those older than 60) trauma victims.
- The elderly have an increased risk of SDH and ensuing mortality due to brain atrophy.
- EDHs are less common as the dura adheres to the skull.

Woman and Pregnancy

- Consider domestic violence; 10% to 20% of women are abused during pregnancy.
- Shield abdomen when possible for imaging studies of the head.

Teaching Points

All patients with head injury require serial neurologic examinations especially in patients with moderate to severe injury. Any neurologic deterioration requires reassessment of the ABCs, early intubation, and repeat imaging. Any concern for herniation requires securing the airway, hyperventilation as a temporizing measure, administration of mannitol, and emergent neurosurgical interventions.

Measures should be taken in the prehospital care environment and the ED setting to prevent secondary insult to the brain in patients with moderate to severe brain injury.

Suggested Readings

Chesnut RM. The management of severe traumatic brain injury. Emerg Med Clin North Am 1997;15:581–604.

Dawodu ST. Traumatic brain injury: definition, epidemiology, pathophysiology. eMedicine 2004 Jul. Retrieved January 20, 2005 from *http://www.emedicine.com/ pmr/topic212.htm*.

Heegaard WS. Biros MH. Head. In: Marx JA (editor). Rosen's Emergency Medicine: Concepts and Clinical Practice (6th edition). Philadelphia: Mosby, 2006, pp. 349–382.

Zink BJ, Lanter PL. Traumatic brain injury. In: Ferrera PC, Colucciello SA, Marx JA, Verdile VP, Gibbs MA (editors). Trauma Management: An Emergency Medicine Approach. St Louis: Mosby, 2001, pp. 127–150.

Zink BJ. Traumatic brain injury. Emerg Med Clin North Am 1996;14:115–150.

Jagoda AS, Cantrill SV, Wears RL, et al. Clinical policy: neuroimaging and decisionmaking in adult mild traumatic brain injury in the acute setting. Ann Emerg Med 2002;40:231–249.

CHAPTER 10

Maxillofacial Injury

AMANDA S. LAKE ■ JENNIFER J. CASALETTO

Red Flags

Airway compromise • Nasal or pharyngeal hemorrhage • Blindness, afferent pupillary defect, or diplopia • Cerebrospinal fluid rhinorrhea or otorrhea • Pediatric or elder abuse and domestic violence

Overview

■ Maxillofacial injury can be dramatic, but should not distract from significant injuries to other organ systems.

■ Seventy percent of maxillofacial fractures result from assaults, with the remainder due to falls, motor vehicle collisions, and sports injuries.

■ The primary concern with facial injury is the status of the airway. The history and physical examination may reveal some clues and red flags for concerning injuries (see Box).

■ The facial skeleton (Figure 10–1) is divided into three geographic regions. The upper third spans the area above the superior orbital rim. The middle third extends from the superior orbital rim to the maxillary teeth. The lower third consists of the mandibular region.

■ The ophthalmic, maxillary, and mandibular divisions of the trigeminal nerve provide sensation to the face from the superior to inferior aspect, respectively. Supraorbital (frontal), infraorbital (cheek), superior and inferior alveolar (gingiva and teeth), and mental (chin) nerve branches are most often injured.

Initial Diagnostic Approach
General

■ Always begin by assessing the ABCs (*a*irway, *b*reathing, *c*irculation) as discussed in Chapter 8. Ensure the airway is patent by having the patient speak. Assess the airway for the presence of blood, foreign body (broken teeth), swelling, or traumatic disfigurement that may occlude the airway or impede visualization of the glottic opening should the patient require intubation.

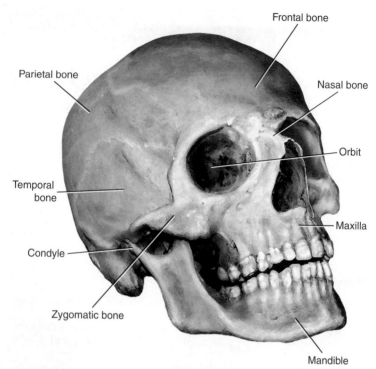

Figure 10–1. Facial skeleton. *(From Rosen's Emergency Medicine: Concepts and Clinical Practice (5th edition). St. Louis, MO: Mosby, 2002, p. 323.)*

- Approximately 40% of patients suffering facial fractures have concomitant closed head injury.
- Useful historical details are the location of facial pain, visual changes, facial numbness, painful mandibular movement, and presence of malocclusion.
- The physical examination can help to identify 90% of clinically significant fractures in patients who can cooperate and who are not impaired by drug, alcohol, or competing injuries. Inspect for facial swelling. Recognize facial asymmetry, which may be enhanced by facial expressions. Palpate facial structures, evaluating for tenderness, anesthesia, bony defects, crepitus, and false motion.
  - *Cranial nerves.* See Appendix 2.
  - *Eyes and orbits.* Evaluate the cornea, conjunctivae, eyelids, visual acuity, visual fields, extraocular movements, and papillary response. Note the presence of hypertelorism (wide separation of the eyes or an increased interorbital distance) and periorbital ecchymosis. A slit lamp examination is required to evaluate for lens dislocation and anterior chamber pathology. Facial injury may be associated with retinal detachment and ruptured globe (see Chapter 69).

- *Nose.* Check for position and integrity of the nasal septum, septal hematoma, and cerebrospinal fluid (CSF) rhinorrhea. CSF rhinorrhea is suspected when bloody but semiserous nasal discharge persists after the original trauma. It may have been triggered by coughing, sneezing, or the patient sitting up. The liquid forms a double-ring sign (or halo sign) on filter paper or a dressing. The presence of CSF is indicative of cribriform plate disruption and defines the presence of a basilar skull fracture. Palpate for deformity, step-offs, or crepitus.
- *Ears.* Examine for soft-tissue injury including a perichondral hematoma. Remember to look behind the ear to avoid missing a laceration. Inspect the inside of the ear for hemotypanum, otorrhea, or tympanic membrane rupture. Persistent oozing from the ear canal should suggest otorrhea and a basilar skull fracture. A common error is to think this secretion has been caused by an external laceration that has run into the ear canal.
- *Mouth and jaw.* Observe for jaw deviation. Test for malocclusion by having the patient open and close the mouth, by biting down, and eliciting whether the motion and the bite feel normal. Perform an intraoral examination, noting hematomas, lacerations, or dental injuries. Evaluate maxillary and mandibular stability by grasping each alveolar ridge and assessing motion.

Radiography

- *Plain films.* A facial series consists of the Waters (occipitomental), Caldwell (occipitofrontal), and lateral projections. The Waters view is best for the evaluation of the maxilla, maxillary sinuses, orbital floors and inferior rims, and zygomatic bones. Zygomatic arches are best evaluated on the submentovertex (jug-handle) view. Mandibular fractures are best evaluated via panoramic radiographs. If panorex views are not available, a mandible series can be ordered.
- *Computed tomography.* The CT scan is useful in the definition of the true extent of bony injuries and to evaluate for concomitant intracranial injuries. In many institutions, CT scans have replaced plain films in the evaluation of maxillofacial trauma. It is also useful for the evaluation of the temporomandibular joint (TMJ) or mandibular condyle if a panorex is not available. To fully evaluate the horizontal facial structures (e.g., orbital floor), a CT scan is performed in a coronal plane (in addition to axial images), using 1-mm cuts. This requires that the patient be able to flex and extend the cervical spine, and also requires a relatively long scanning time. Because this is often not possible in the initial evaluation of the trauma patient, a full delineation of any maxillofacial fracture often must be deferred. Three-dimensional CT scan reconstruction may also be available at some centers.
- Take note of the "three S's," which indicate fracture: sinuses (fluid filled, herniated orbital contents), symmetry, and subcutaneous air.

● ● ● See Chapter 92, "Radiology," for normal axial and coronal images of the
● ● ● face.

Emergency Department Management Overview
General

- *Airway and breathing.* Patients with facial injury may be unable to maintain a patent airway as a direct result of injury or secondary to blood, soft tissue swelling, or vomitus. Initial management includes removal of loose material in the oropharynx manually and via suction. If there are no other injuries that would mandate a supine position, the airway can often be cleared by allowing the patient to sit up and lean forward, and at times, self-administer an oral suction unit. If the airway must be controlled, orotracheal intubation is preferred. Nasotracheal intubation is contraindicated with mid-face injury due to concern for cribriform plate disruption. If the hemorrhage or anatomic distortion interferes with adequate visualization of the mouth and larynx, a surgical airway (e.g., cricothyrotomy) may be necessary.
- *Circulation.* Hemorrhage resulting from facial trauma is initially managed with direct pressure. Hemorrhagic shock resulting from facial injury is extremely rare. Seek and treat alternative etiologies of shock prior to continuing management.
- *Other.* Consider coexisting head, cervical spine, or torso injuries. Stabilize all life-threatening injuries before continuing with facial fracture management.

Medications

- *Antibiotics.* In the past, antibiotics were administered for a possible open skull fracture (CSF leak or intracranial air). Prophylactic antibiotics such as ceftriaxone or a penicillinase-resistant penicillin were often given. However, this practice has not been found to reduce the incidence of meningitis or brain abscess. Any contaminated wound (human or animal bite) should receive antibiotics (see Chapter 90.2).
- *Tetanus.* Update appropriately for patients with open wounds.
- *Analgesia.* Administer as needed with special caution to avoid oversedating the patient who may have an associated head injury (see Chapter 90).

Emergency Department Interventions

- *Difficult intubation.* If the tongue obstructs airway access, grasp the distal tongue with a towel clip or place a suture through it and lift it from the hypopharynx. If severe injury makes the hypopharynx difficult to locate, secure the airway using available rescue devices as time and resources allow (e.g., Bullard laryngoscope, bougie). Otherwise, the patient will require an emergency cricothyrotomy (See Chapter 6).
- *Uncontrolled hemorrhage.* Due to the vascular nature of the face, direct pressure may not succeed in controlling hemorrhage. Do not blindly clamp, because vital structures such as the facial nerve and salivary ducts run in close proximity to facial vessels. Tamponade uncontrolled nasal bleeding via inflation of a Foley balloon (or other commercial device) in the posterior nasal region. Bleeding associated with Le Fort fractures may require posterior pharynx packing after the airway has been secured.

In rare cases, manual reduction of mid-face fractures performed by grasping and aligning the hard palate may be helpful in slowing the hemorrhage.

■ *Wound care.* Closure of most relatively clean facial lacerations may be delayed up to 24 hours. Hemostasis should be controlled immediately with irrigation and temporary approximation. Consultation with a specialist should be made for wounds in which adequate anesthesia in the ED is unable to be achieved, wounds involving underlying structures (nerves), wounds that may require delayed primary closure (open for more than 24 hours, gross contamination more than 6 hours old, foreign body that cannot be removed), and other complicated lacerations that the ED physician is unable to repair.

> Refer to Chapter 94, "Wound Care."

Disposition

■ *Consultation.* Arrange urgent consultation versus outpatient follow-up based on the injury. Multiple subspecialties care for facial injuries including neurosurgery, plastic/maxillofacial surgery, otolaryngology, oral surgery, and ophthalmology. Their availability will vary according to individual institutional staffing patterns.

■ *Admission.* Patients requiring emergent surgery, have complicating injuries, or are unable to tolerate oral fluids should be admitted.

■ *Discharge.* The majority of patients with isolated and uncomplicated maxillofacial trauma do not require admission, but require close outpatient follow-up, analgesia, and antibiotics as indicated.

Specific Problems
Mandibular Fractures

■ *Background.* Mandibular fractures are the second most common facial fracture. Because the mandible is a hemi-ring bone, it rarely breaks in a single place, although the position of a second fracture can be clinically subtle. The body, angle, and condyle are the most commonly involved segments (Figure 10–2). Mandibular body and angle fractures result from side impact forces most often sustained during an altercation. Condyle and symphysis fractures result from head-on forces, such as during a motor vehicle collision (MVC).

■ *Clinical presentation.* There may be jaw deviation or asymmetry; the chin deviates toward a fracture. When the patient opens and closes the jaw, pain, trismus, malocclusion, or crepitus along the mandible or against the posterior aspect of the tragus may be elicited. There may be associated lacerations, a step-off in dentition, or sublingual ecchymosis. Sensory deficits in the inferior alveolar and mental nerve distributions may be present. Finally, when the patient bites down on a tongue blade placed between the upper and lower incisors and the blade is twisted, the patient typically cannot bite hard enough to allow the examiner to break the tongue blade if a mandibular fracture is present.

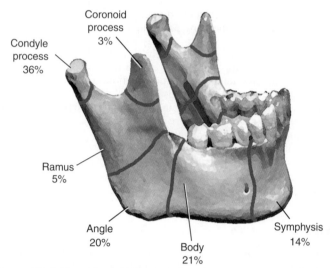

Figure 10–2. Types of mandibular fracture and frequency of fracture sites. *(From Rosen's Emergency Medicine: Concepts and Clinical Practice (5th edition). St. Louis, MO: Mosby, 2002, p. 326.)*

- *Diagnostic testing.* A panorex view is the best imaging study with which to demonstrate a mandibular fracture if the condyles are included. If panorex views are not available, anteroposterior and lateral views of the mandible can exclude fractures outside the condyles. A Townes view allows evaluation of the condyles. A CT scan can be used if the plain films are not diagnostic.
- *ED management.* Hospital admission is required for patients with open mandibular fractures for intravenous (IV) antibiotics and operative fixation. Penicillin remains the antibiotic of choice. Clindamycin can be used for patients allergic to penicillin. Closed-fracture management includes analgesics, liquid or blended diet, and consultation with a facial surgeon.
- *Helpful hints and pitfalls.* Airway management is crucial, as the tongue may occlude the pharynx. Significant hemorrhage may occur in open fractures.

Mandibular or Temporomandibular Joint Dislocations

- *Background.* Mandibular dislocations can be unilateral or bilateral. Dislocations are unlikely to be associated with mandibular fractures in adults, but are rarely seen without fracture in children. Mandibular dislocation may result from trauma, seizure activity, or extreme jaw opening. The condyle lies anterior to the glenoid fossa and is prevented from relocating by masseter spasm.
- *Clinical presentation.* There may be chin deviation away from a unilateral dislocation or forward placement of the mandible in a bilateral

dislocation. The patient will be unable to close the mouth. Palpate for a depression in the preauricular region.

- **Diagnostic testing.** Obtain panorex and Townes views to evaluate for fracture.
- **ED management.** Temporomandibular (TMJ) dislocations can be reduced following benzodiazepine administration to lessen muscular spasm. With the patient in a sitting position, reduce the dislocation by placing each thumb on the corresponding inferior third molar with fingers curled under the mandible. Apply downward pressure on the molars with concomitant upward pressure on the symphysis, followed by minimal posterior pressure. The mandible often reduces with a forceful snap; therefore it is prudent to have a bite block in place so the reducing fingers will not be bitten. Isolated TMJ dislocations that are reduced successfully can be discharged with analgesics, liquid or blended diet, avoidance of extreme jaw opening, and follow-up.
- **Helpful hints and pitfalls.** Repeated dislocations are frequent within several days in cases of overuse. Buccolingual phenothiazine reactions can masquerade as TMJ dislocations.

Maxillary (Le Fort) Fractures

- **Background.** Because it requires significant force to produce a maxillary fracture, they are almost always associated with multisystem trauma. Fractures of the maxilla are described using the Le Fort classification (Table 10–1 and Figure 10–3). Maxillary fractures usually result from high-speed MVCs.

Table 10–1 Types of Le Fort Fracture

Le Fort Classification	Physical Examination Findings	Structures Involved
Type I Palatofacial disjunction	Abnormal motion of the alveolar ridge and hard palate	Horizontal fracture through the maxilla at the level of the nasal fossa
Type II Pyramidal disjunction	Abnormal motion of the mid-face, nasal, and alveolar structures	Pyramidal fracture separating the maxilla, nasal bones, and infraorbital rim from the orbital and zygomatic complex
Type III Craniofacial disjunction	All facial structures mobile from the base of the skull	Fracture separates the maxilla, naso-ethmoid-orbital complex, and zygoma from the cranium

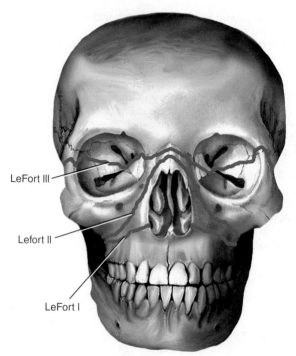

LeFort III

Lefort II

LeFort I

Figure 10–3. Le Fort classification of facial fractures. *(From Rosen's Emergency Medicine: Concepts and Clinical Practice (5th edition). St. Louis, MO: Mosby, 2002, p. 325.)*

- **Clinical presentation.** There may be significant soft-tissue injury, swelling, and mid-face mobility. Facial lengthening or asymmetry may be present. Mid-face mobility can be tested by grasping the hard palate; impacted and greenstick fractures may not be mobile. Malocclusion and CSF rhinorrhea may be present. Sensation in the distribution of the infraorbital and superior alveolar nerve may be compromised. Visual acuity and extraocular motions may be affected.
- **Diagnostic testing.** A facial CT scan is the best imaging study.
- **ED management.** Ensure that the airway and hemorrhage are controlled. Evaluate for concomitant life-threatening injuries. Admit under the care of a facial surgeon for operative repair.
- **Helpful hints and pitfalls.** Airway compromise is common. Nasal intubation is contraindicated. Rapid sequence intubation may be difficult due to hemorrhage or anatomic deformity, and cricothyrotomy may be necessary if the patient cannot sit up and lean forward. Hemorrhage is common. Use manual closed reduction of the fracture and bilateral anterior and posterior nasal packing to attempt control; angiographic embolization may be needed in rare cases. Nearly all patients have associated severe injuries. There is a high incidence of blindness with Le

Fort III fractures. Le Fort fractures are not usually seen in pure forms, but in combinations.

Nasal Injuries

- *Background.* Nasal fractures are the most common facial fracture due to the position of the nose as well as the smaller amount of force required to cause a fracture. Nasal fractures are most often the result of a direct or lateral blow.
- *Clinical presentation.* Epistaxis, nasal deformity, edema, hypermotility, septal deviation, step-offs, and crepitus may be present. All patients should be evaluated for the presence of a septal hematoma.
- *Diagnostic testing.* This is a clinical diagnosis. Plain films are unnecessary. In cases involving more severe trauma and in which there is physical evidence of other facial fractures, computed tomography should be employed to assess the extent of bony injury.
- *ED management.* Patients with significant deformity and minimal swelling may undergo reduction acutely if there are no other more serious injuries. Those with significant swelling, cosmesis issues, or septal deviation–induced obstruction may need acute consultation, but the facial consultant will decide whether to repair acutely or after follow-up. Significant epistaxis can be managed with direct pressure, topical vasoconstrictors, packing, and reduction of the fracture. Most nasal hemorrhage will not be persistent, if oozing of a bloody fluid persists, look for a cerebrospinal fluid leak. Septal hematomas must be incised and drained to prevent infection and septal necrosis. Pack the nares after drainage to prevent reaccumulation. For those patients who will be discharged to home, instruct the patient to elevate the head of the bed, use topical nasal decongestants for 3 days after the injury, apply ice, take analgesics for pain, and avoid blowing the nose. A follow-up appointment should be arranged with a consultant (otolaryngologist or plastic surgeon) in 5 to 7 days and earlier in children (4 days).
- *Helpful hints and pitfalls.* Anosmia or CSF rhinorrhea indicates cribriform plate disruption. This represents basilar skull fracture. The patient should have a CT scan and will often require admission to the hospital and observation for the development of complications such as meningitis. Prophylactic antibiotics do not lower the incidence of this complication.

Naso-Ethmoid-Orbital Injuries

- *Background.* Naso-ethmoid-orbital (NEO) injuries are high-energy injuries that are often associated with multisystem trauma. NEO injury results from a direct blow to the bridge of the nose.
- *Clinical presentation.* Hypertelorism (i.e., increased distance between the orbits) may be present; normal intercanthal distance is 30 to 34 mm, or approximately the width of one orbit. There may be painful extraocular movement and medial canthal tenderness or crepitus. Check for CSF rhinorrhea.
- *Diagnostic testing.* CT scan is necessary; plain films will not reveal the fractures.

- ***ED management.*** These patients require hospital admission, neuro-surgical consultation, and most likely surgical repair.
- ***Helpful hints and pitfalls.*** Nasolacrimal duct injury is common and may be evidenced by epiphora (decreased tear elimination). Dural tears may be present. Medial canthal ligament rupture and medial rectus entrapment are complications seen with this injury.

Orbital Fractures

- ***Background.*** Orbital fractures are one of the most common types of facial fractures in patients with facial trauma. Orbital floor fractures are the most common type, as the orbital floor and medial orbital wall are the weakest portions of the orbit. A blowout fracture occurs when the orbital floor gives way, with possible herniation of orbital contents into the maxillary sinus. Fractures of the medial wall and orbital roof can also occur. Blowout fractures can only occur by objects with a radius of curvature of 5 cm or less due to the architecture of the orbital rim. Orbital fractures more commonly result more from blunt force transmitted from the globe to the orbit than from a direct blow to the orbital rim itself.
- ***Clinical presentation.*** These patients may have enophthalmos, impaired ocular movements, or diplopia from entrapment of the inferior rectus muscle. Diplopia is more commonly due to extraocular muscle injury than entrapment; however, entrapment must be ruled out. The presence of periorbital emphysema indicates communication of the orbit with a sinus. Infraorbital nerve anesthesia may be present. An orbital fracture is present if air fills the orbit when the patient blows the nose or sneezes. These patients require an ocular examination including a fundoscopic evaluation.
- ***Diagnostic testing.*** Diagnosis is made via a modified Waters view based on findings such as the hanging teardrop sign, which results from orbital contents herniation into the maxillary sinus (Figure 10–4). Depression of bony fragments into the maxillary sinus or orbital emphysema can also be used to diagnose orbital fracture via radiographs. Clouding or an air–fluid level in the maxillary sinus indicates orbital fracture. Obtain a CT scan in patients with diplopia, decreased extraocular motion, or enophthalmos.
- ***ED management.*** Emergent ophthalmology consultation is prudent in those patients with decreased vision or abnormalities on ocular examination. Increasing periorbital emphysema or retrobulbar hematoma resulting in increasing intraocular pressure and decreasing vision requires an emergent lateral canthotomy to preserve optic nerve function (see Chapter 69, under treatment for retrobulbar hemorrhage). Consultation with facial surgeons is most often nonurgent. Surgical repair of blowout fractures may be required for persistent diplopia or enophthalmos. Pain medication and decongestants should be prescribed. Patients should not blow the nose nor sneeze forcibly.
- ***Helpful hints and pitfalls.*** Associated ocular injury occurs in up to 30% of periorbital fractures, with associated globe rupture in 5% to 10% of orbital blowout fractures. Binocular diplopia spontaneously resolves in up to 80% of fractures, but inferior rectus entrapment often requires surgical repair.

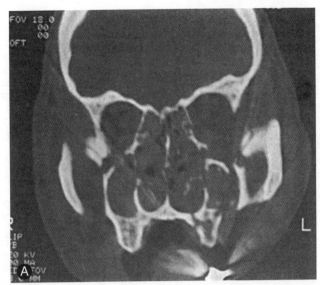

Figure 10–4. Waters view of facial bones: orbital blowout fracture. A fracture is noted through the inferior orbital rim (*arrow*). A convex mass is seen projecting through the roof of the maxillary sinus representing displaced periorbital tissues (*arrowheads*). An air–fluid level is present in the maxillary sinus (*curved arrow*) representing blood. (*From Structural Injuries of the Orbit. In: Albert D, Jakobiec F, et al. (eds): Principles and Practice of Ophthalmology, Saunders, 2000, figure 380-35.*

Tripod Fractures

- *Background.* The tripod fracture includes extension into the infraorbital rim and disruption of the zygomatic-frontal and zygomatic-temporal sutures. Tripod fractures are typically due to a direct blow to the temporal region with force transmitted medially and posteriorly.
- *Clinical presentation.* There may be malar (cheek) tenderness or flatness, periorbital edema, ecchymosis, diplopia, trismus, lateral subconjunctival hemorrhage, and decreased sensation in the distribution of the inferior orbital nerve. The patient should have visual acuity checked and be evaluated for integrity of extra-ocular movements.
- *Diagnostic testing.* Although fracture lines associated with tripod fractures are readily apparent on Waters view accompanied by depression

of the malar eminence and maxillary sinus opacification, a CT scan is required for complete evaluation of fracture extension, especially in regard to the orbital floor component.

- *ED management.* Tripod fractures require consultation with a facial surgeon for possible surgical correction. They do not necessarily require admission, but prompt follow-up with adequate analgesia provided.
- *Helpful hints and pitfalls.* Trismus may result from trapping of the masseter muscle beneath the fracture site. Malocclusion is due to fracture fragment impingement on the coranoid process. Diplopia occurs in 30% due to entrapment or direct muscular injury. Concomitant globe injury takes place in 5%.

Zygomatic Arch Fractures

- *Background.* Zygomatic arch fracture is the third most common facial fracture following nasal and mandibular fractures. These occur most often in young men as a result of assault, MVC, or sports injuries. Zygomatic arch fracture results from a direct blow to the lateral face.
- *Clinical presentation.* Malar flattening, deformity, tenderness, crepitus, and limited mandibular motion may be present. Depression of a zygomatic arch fracture may lead to trismus. Look for an accompanying laceration that mandates treatment as an open fracture.
- *Diagnostic testing.* Isolated arch fractures are diagnosed via the submentovertex view.
- *ED management.* Patients with depressed arch fractures and trismus should have urgent facial surgical consultation, and may be admitted for elevation of the fracture. Those without limitation of their range of motion can usually be followed as outpatients.
- *Helpful hints and pitfalls.* Extensive edema may obscure malar flattening. As in tripod fractures, trismus and malocclusion may occur.

Special Considerations
Pediatrics

- Fewer than 10% of all facial trauma injuries are seen in children.
- Falls are the most common etiology. Young children more commonly injure the upper face, whereas older children injure the lower face.
- Nonaccidental trauma must be considered in all children with facial trauma, especially those with skull fractures or frenulum injury.
- Cricothyrotomy is contraindicated in children younger than 8 years or in any child whose cricothyroid space looks too small to accept a cuffed Shiley tube (size ranges from 3 to an adult size 7 mm, but most institutions will not have them readily available if they do not routinely care for small children). Transtracheal jet ventilation via needle cricothyrostomy may allow for temporary airway control until formal tracheotomy can be performed.
- There is increased association with intracranial injury in children.

Woman and Pregnancy

■ Consider domestic violence; 10% to 20% of women are abused during pregnancy. More than 25% of facial trauma in women is the result of domestic violence.

Teaching Points

Patients with significant facial trauma require immediate attention to the airway because it may be compromised from bleeding, traumatic disfigurement, foreign body, or other causes of obstruction such as the tongue.

Very seldom does facial trauma cause shock. An aggressive search for other causes of shock must be identified.

Definitive management for patients with major facial trauma can be delayed for at least 24 hours while the patient is being stabilized for more concerning traumatic injuries.

Suggested Readings

Alonso LA, Purcell TB. Accuracy of the tongue blade test in patients with suspected mandibular fracture. J Emerg Med 1995;13:297–304.

Brady SM, McMann MA, Mazzoli RA, Bushley DM, Ainbinder DJ, Carroll RB. The diagnosis and management of orbital blowout fractures. Am J Emerg Med 2001;19:147–154.

Ellis E, Scott K. Assessment of patients with facial fractures. Emerg Med Clin North Amer 2000;18:411–47.

Ferrera PC, Colucciello SA, Marx JA, et al. Trauma management: an emergency medicine approach. St Louis: Mosby, 2001: pp 180–96.

Kucik CJ, Clenney T, Phelan J. Management of acute nasal fractures. Am Fam Physician 2004;70(7):1315–20.

Leipziger LS, Manson PN. Nasoethmoid orbital fractures. Clin Plast Surg 1992:19:167–93.

Lynham AJ, Hirst JP, Cosson JA, Chapman PJ, McEniery P. Emergency department management of maxillofacial trauma. Emerg Med Australasia 2004;16:7–12.

Mckay MP. Facial trauma. In: Marx JA, Hockberger RS, Walls RM, eds. Rosen's Emergency Medicine: Concepts and Clinical Practice. 6th ed. Philadelphia: Mosby, 2006:382–396.

CHAPTER 11

Neck Trauma

KAUSHAL H. SHAH ■ CHILEMBWE MASON

 Red Flags

Vascular	Expanding or pulsatile hematomas
	Uncontrolled, continued bleeding
	Arterial bruit
	Diminished carotid pulse
	Unstable vital signs
Airway	Difficulty breathing, respiratory distress
	Stridor
	Voice change (hoarseness, dysphonia)
	Hemoptysis
	Subcutaneous emphysema
Digestive tract	Drooling, dysphagia, odynophagia
	Subcutaneous emphysema
	Blood in oropharynx, hematemesis
Neurologic	Altered level of consciousness not due to head injury
	Horner's syndrome
	Cranial nerve deficits
	Lateralized neurologic deficit consistent with injury

Overview

Neck trauma is caused by three major mechanisms: blunt, penetrating, and strangulation or near-hanging.

Neck injuries are often categorized into injuries of the airway (laryngotracheal), digestive track (pharyngoesophageal), vascular system, and neurologic system. Look for "red flags" that require emergent attention (see Box). Patients with any "red flags" often require surgical exploration. Be prepared for a difficult airway in the setting of neck injuries. Serious, possibly life-threatening, injuries may have innocuous appearing wounds in the neck.

Anatomically, the neck is divided into *zones*, which has critical implications for management of penetrating neck trauma (Figure 11–1). Zone I extends superiorly from the sternal notch to the cricoid cartilage. Injury to this region has the highest mortality due to the presence of the great vessels and the difficult surgical approach. Zone

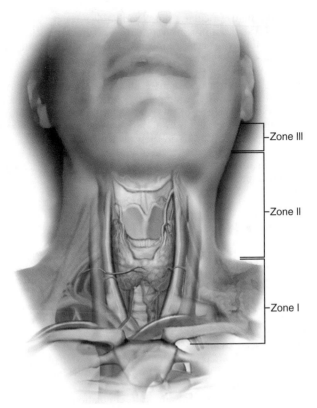

Figure 11–1. Zones of the neck.

II lies between the cricoid cartilage and the angle of the mandible. This is the most exposed region of the neck and allows for direct visualization to evaluate for underlying injury and control of bleeding. Zone III extends from the angle of the mandible to the base of the skull. In this region, it is difficult to achieve vascular control, and direct surgical exploration is often impossible. This is the region of the neck most likely to be associated with carotid dissection from even minor trauma.

Patients with penetrating zone II injuries require neck exploration often with surgical intervention if the platysma is violated. Patients with zone I and III injuries, and patients who are thought to be at low risk for significant injury undergo further diagnostic testing and are observed if the studies are negative.

The neck is also divided anatomically into two triangles. The anterior triangle is bordered anteriorly by the midline, posteriorly by the lateral border of the sternocleidomastoid muscle, and superiorly by the lower edge of the mandible. This triangle is packed with vital structures such as the neurovascular and aerodigestive tracts. The posterior triangle is located within the boundaries of the sternocleidomastoid muscle anteriorly, the clavicle inferiorly and the anterior border of the trapezius muscle posteriorly. Injury to this region is less likely to involve major vital structures.

The platysma muscle is superficially located over the anterolateral neck. Major vascular and aerodigestive structures in the neck are deep to the platysma. Violation of the platysma muscle in penetrating neck trauma requires surgical exploration because it is associated with an increased incidence of injury to these structures.

The pretracheal fascia travels behind the sternum and inserts on the anterior pericardium. This anatomic relationship connects the neck to the mediastinum. Mediastinitis may result from a missed aerodigestive injury.

Initial Diagnostic Approach
General

- The general approach to a patient with neck trauma begins with the primary survey and the ABCs (*a*irway, *b*reathing, and *c*irculation) as discussed in Chapter 8. The immediate assessment should identify any airway compromise, hypotension, or active bleeding. Airway compromise may be due to direct injury to the larynx or trachea, expanding neck hematoma, bleeding into the airway, or traumatic disfigurement from associated facial trauma. Penetrating zone II injuries require surgical exploration (without probing) to determine if the platysma has been violated. Angiography is required for zone I and III injuries in all but the most unstable patients.
- A more detailed history and physical examination should be performed during the secondary survey. Stable patients should be assessed for any aerodigestive or neurovascular compromise. The patient must be reassessed frequently for potential airway compromise or developing neurologic deficit.

Laboratory

- Order standard trauma blood studies including blood type and cross-matching.

Radiography

- See discussion under each specific problem for recommended diagnostic testing.

Emergency Department Management Overview
General

- The ABCs should be addressed. Airway management is the highest priority, along with cervical spine immobilization.

- Any evidence of bleeding must be controlled initially with direct pressure. Blind clamping should not be performed to avoid iatrogenic injury to neurovascular structures in the neck.
- IV access should preferably be placed on the noninjured side until vascular injury can be excluded.

Medications

- Prophylactic antibiotics are given in patients thought to be at risk for contamination of soft tissues with aerodigestive perforation. Mixed aerobic and anaerobic coverage is needed (e.g., clindamycin 600 mg IV every six hours).
- Tetanus prophylaxis should be given as indicated.

Emergency Department Interventions

- Early control of the airway prior to anatomic distortion or airway distress is the highest priority. It is more prudent to intubate before there are signs of airway compromise, because there will be less anatomic distortion. Oral intubation with rapid sequence intubation is safe for most patients; however, caution should be taken in the use of paralytics as these patients may be difficult to intubate.
- Nasogastric tubes should be inserted only if absolutely necessary, as the retching associated with the procedure may dislodge a clot and cause massive bleeding.

Disposition

- *Consultation.* A surgeon should be consulted for penetrating neck injury, suspected aerodigestive injury or neurovascular injury.
- *Admission.* Admission is prudent for all patients with platysma violation, potential for airway compromise, presence of a hematoma (whether or not it is expanding), voice changes, aerodigestive injury, neurologic deficits, suspected carotid or vertebral dissection, and for psychosocial considerations (e.g., near hanging). Patients with alcohol or substance abuse need to be observed until they can metabolize the ingested substance since it will interfere with accurate assessment of stability.
- *Discharge.* Stable asymptomatic patients with no other significant injuries and no significant mechanism concerning for injury can be discharged home.

Specific Problems by Mechanism
Blunt

- *Background.* Blunt neck trauma can produce a direct blow to the airway, hyperextension of the neck, or increased intraluminal pressure injuries. Most injuries result from motor vehicle crashes, violent attacks, or sports-related injuries. Aerodigestive injuries are less common with blunt trauma than with penetrating trauma. Blunt injury to the larynx, trachea, or carotid arteries often has a subtle presentation.

- *Clinical presentation.* Dysphonia, dyspnea, stridor, hemoptysis, subcutaneous emphysema, bony crepitus, neck tenderness or pain over the larynx should prompt further testing. Carotid pulses and the presence of bruits should be assessed, as well as neurologic signs or symptoms that may suggest dissection. Unfortunately, these may be delayed for many hours, and dissection can follow very trivial trauma.

- *Diagnostic testing.* A chest radiograph and cervical films (anteroposterior and lateral) will allow diagnosis of cervical injury and evaluation for extraluminal air or edema. A computed tomography (CT scan) is a useful study because it is quick, readily obtainable, and provides detailed information about laryngeal integrity and the surrounding region. Direct laryngoscopy or flexible nasopharyngoscopy can show hypopharyngeal tears, but are not useful for seeing more distal injuries. Duplex ultrasonography is useful for evaluating cervical vascular injury, but often cannot identify zone I and III injuries. Arteriography is the best imaging study for finding vascular injuries such as dissection in the carotid or vertebral arteries.

- *ED management.* With strong blows to the neck (such as running into a chain while riding a motorcycle), there is a possibility for laryngotracheal disruption. These patients are often impossible to intubate orally, and cricothyrotomy is ineffective because the disruption is often below the level of the cricoid cartilage; thus tracheostomy will be necessary. If a surgical airway is attempted, it is prudent to stabilize the distal tracheal segment with a towel clip before opening the anterior cervical fascia to prevent the distal trachea from falling into the mediastinum where it cannot be accessed for intubation. Most patients with blunt neck trauma will require admission to the hospital for observation unless the mechanism was trivial and there are no symptoms of voice change, hematoma, cervical spine injuries, and concomitant injuries.

- *Helpful hints and pitfalls.* Associated cervical spine injuries should always be considered with blunt neck trauma. Vascular injuries resulting from blunt trauma are often missed because their signs and symptoms often present in a delayed fashion and prevent detection at a time that treatment is possible. Cervical collars can obscure impending airway compromise (hematomas) and other signs of injury if not removed periodically to allow for serial examinations.

Penetrating

- *Background.* Penetrating neck trauma results from gunshot wounds, stabbings or other impalements (glass, shrapnel, dog bites). Zone I and III injuries are more difficult to manage and often require diagnostic testing to determine the best surgical approach.

- *Clinical presentation.* Any violation of the platysma muscle may be associated with injury to significant underlying structures. Dysphonia and dyspnea are indicators of potentially serious laryngeal injury and require further diagnostic testing and urgent airway evaluation. Absence of the carotid pulse, presence of a bruit, or hematoma formation are all concerning for vascular injury.

- *Diagnostic testing.* Platysmal penetration must be established visually; a cotton tip applicator or hemostat cannot reveal the depth of a penetration. A violation of the platysma mandates a surgical consultation with further diagnostic studies or surgical exploration. Obtain a chest radiograph and neck films (anteroposterior and lateral) to evaluate for associated injury. A CT scan can assess vital structures such as the vascular system (although it may miss lethal lesions such as pseudo-aneurysms). Duplex ultrasonography has the ability to exclude cervical vascular injury but is not as accurate in the assessment of zone I and III injuries when compared to arteriography. Arteriography is the most accurate imaging study to demonstrate vascular injuries to the carotid, vertebral, and basilar arteries. It is less accurate for venous injuries. Patients not requiring operative exploration may need to have the aerodigestive track evaluated with bronchoscopy, upper endoscopy, or esophagography to exclude injury.

- *EM management.* Airway management is the highest priority, along with cervical spine immobilization. It is more prudent to intubate before there are signs of airway compromise, because there will be less anatomic distortion. This is especially true for gunshot wounds. Surgical airways are best avoided when the penetrating injury is in zone II, making it even more imperative to obtain airway control before anatomic distortion and signs and symptoms of airway compromise. Intravenous access is best placed on the noninjured side, avoiding the ipsilateral neck or upper extremity until a vascular injury has been excluded. Evidence of cerebral ischemia as manifested by profound alteration in consciousness or stroke-like symptoms should suggest injury to the cervical vessels. Dissection can occur in the vertebral or carotid arteries, even in children and healthy young adults. Avoid maneuvers that stimulate retching or gagging and any direct probing of injuries to avoid dislodging a hematoma. Stable patients with penetrating wounds can be managed with selective surgical exploration. Do not extract impaled objects; this should be done in the operating room.

- *Helpful hints and pitfalls.* Examination of all penetrating neck wounds should document the zone (s) of injury and the presence of platysma muscle violation (without probing), when this can be determined visually. The leading cause of immediate death from neck trauma is exsanguination secondary to vascular injury. The leading cause of delayed death from neck trauma is esophageal injury. These are rare and insidious injuries but associated with high mortality rates if missed.

Strangulation and Near-Hanging

- *Background.* A strangulation attempt is often an injury of domestic violence, and is extremely serious because there is a high subsequent mortality in the victims. Hanging is categorized as complete or incomplete. Complete hanging refers to the presence of a ligature around the victim's neck and a subsequent drop, resulting in the victim being freely suspended. Incomplete hanging refers to the partial suspension of the victim's body with some part still in contact with the ground. Hangings with adequate fall distance (this must be at least the length of the patient's body,) result in forceful distraction of the head from the neck and body. This leads to high cervical fractures, complete cord transection, and death. If there is an inadequate fall distance, the ligature or external force initially applied causes venous congestion with stasis of cerebral blood flow leading to unconsciousness, causing the victim to become limp, which allows for complete arterial occlusion and brain injury or death.

- *Clinical presentation.* There may be airway edema, bronchopneumonia and adult respiratory distress syndrome (ARDS). These complications are responsible for most in-hospital deaths after incomplete hangings. Petechial hemorrhages are often found in the conjunctiva, mucous membranes and the skin cephalad to the ligature marks. They are often found in asphyxial deaths. Laryngeal, thyroid and hyoid bone fractures are found most commonly in cases of manual strangulation. Vascular injury leading to delayed neurologic sequelae after near-hanging is less common.
- *Diagnostic testing.* Cervical spine radiographs are indicated to rule out fracture, but are not necessary if there has been no drop. A chest radiograph is indicated to rule out a pneumothorax and other lung pathology, including ARDS, pulmonary edema, and aspiration pneumonitis. Carotid vascular studies should be considered in patients with unexplained focal or global neurologic deficits.
- *EM management.* The airway should be aggressively managed as has already been described. Positive end-expiratory pressure (PEEP) is often necessary when pulmonary edema or ARDS develops. The altered or comatose patient may have cerebral edema with elevated intracranial pressure requiring treatment (see Chapter 9). Phenytoin has a cerebroprotective effect, and may help decrease the development of centroneurogenic ARDS.
- *Helpful hints and pitfalls.* Near-hanging/strangulation patients who are comatose may have elevated intracranial pressure. Pulmonary complications are the leading cause of in-hospital death. The victim of domestic violence who has survived strangulation is at great risk for further violence.

Specific Problems by Type of injury
Esophageal Perforation

- *Background.* Esophageal injury is rare, and occurs more often in patients with penetrating trauma. It is the most frequently missed injury of the neck.
- *Clinical presentation.* Patients may present with shortness of breath, stridor, cough, neck pain (including pain with passive neck movement), hematemesis, odynophagia, or subcutaneous emphysema.
- *Diagnostic testing.* The combination of contrast swallow and endoscopy are often required to diagnose this injury. Plain films may reveal esophageal perforation if pneumomediastinum or retropharyngeal air is present.
- *EM management.* Broad-spectrum antibiotics should be administered, the patient should be kept NPO, and surgery should be consulted for exploration.
- *Helpful hints and pitfalls.* Any delay in diagnosis and management should be avoided due to the serious consequence from a delayed presentation.

Laryngotracheal Injury

- *Background.* Most of these injuries are due to blunt trauma. Associated cervical spine injuries may occur.
- *Clinical presentation.* Bubbling from the wound may be present. The patient may complain of dysphonia, stridor, hemoptysis, dyspnea, hemoptysis, subcutaneous emphysema, bone crepitus, and neck tenderness over the larynx.
- *Diagnostic testing.* Plain films may reveal extraluminal air, swelling, or a fracture of the laryngeal structures. Direct laryngoscopy or flexible nasopharyngoscopy is required to evaluate the larynx. A CT scan can be helpful to identify fractures or a surrounding hematoma but is not routinely used for penetrating trauma. A surgeon should be consulted for possible exploration.
- *EM management.* The airway should be managed as discussed under "Blunt" neck trauma. However, orotracheal intubation may complete a partial tear or create a false passage. Tracheostomy should be performed on patients with complete tears.
- *Helpful hints and pitfalls.* Blunt injuries can be easily overlooked, especially in the presence of multisystem trauma.

Vascular Injury

- *Background.* Extravasation from vascular injury is the most common cause of death after penetrating trauma. Vascular injury from blunt trauma is rare. The jugular vein is the most commonly injured vessel while the common carotid artery is the most commonly injured artery. Blunt trauma to the cervical vessels can cause intimal tears, thrombosis (with possible embolization), dissection, and pseudoaneurysm. The most common mechanism for blunt internal carotid artery injury is sudden, forceful hyperextension with lateral rotation of the neck. In penetrating trauma, vascular injury is due to direct penetration.
- *Clinical presentation.* Findings include a pulsatile or expanding hematoma, bruits, pulse deficit, hemothorax, and neurologic deficits. Neurologic deficits are found in patients with a delayed presentation of a vascular injury and include Horner's syndrome, and a focal or global neurological deficit. A transient ischemic attack (TIA) may result from the release of small emboli from the injured vessel. Serial examinations should evaluate for any airway, vascular compromise and neurologic deficits. Shock may be present from massive blood loss or an air embolism.
- *Diagnostic testing.* Arteriography remains the gold standard for detecting these injuries. Duplex ultrasonography can be used to evaluate for cervical vascular injury but is limited in detecting zone I and III injuries. A chest radiograph should be ordered to evaluate the mediastinum and the lungs (e.g., hemothorax or pneumothorax). Plain films of the neck are useful to determine the bullet trajectory or to evaluate for other foreign body. A CT scan and magnetic resonance angiography have also been used but are not as reliable as arteriography.
- *EM management.* A surgeon should be consulted for possible vascular repair. Anticoagulation is occasionally used. Patients with vascular

injuries should be admitted to the hospital. Stable patients who do not require an emergent operative intervention should be admitted for observation.

- *Helpful hints and pitfalls.* The diagnosis of vascular injury from blunt trauma is often delayed due to the late presentation of neurologic findings and the rare incidence of their occurrence. Venous air embolism occurs when air enters the injured vessel and is life-threatening if undetected. If suspected the patient should be in Trendelenberg position. If in cardiac arrest, an emergency thoracotomy should be performed with cross-clamping of the aorta and the right ventricle should be aspirated for air.

Teaching Points

Neck trauma is a source of potential major life-threatening injury because of the density of critical anatomy. Unfortunately, early symptoms and signs may not reflect the seriousness of the trauma, and the delay in onset of symptoms makes it difficult or impossible to predict who will have the most serious consequences. The zones of the neck are useful in predicting some of the injuries, but do not always reveal injuries that cross more than one zone. Penetrating injuries can appear deceptively mild, but if the platysma is penetrated (this should be determined by visual observation), the patient requires a more extensive workup, and possible surgical exploration. Alterations of voice, the presence of hematoma, and the mechanism of injury (e.g., gunshot wound) all mandate aggressive workup and management.

The airway is at special risk with cervical injury, and active management must be aggressive and timely. It is preferable to actively manage the airway before the patient has developed anatomic distortion or signs and symptoms of respiratory distress.

Both blunt and penetrating traumas place the carotid and vertebral arteries at risk, even with surprisingly mild mechanisms of injury. There may be a long delay before the onset of symptoms. Close observation of these patients, and sometimes early angiography may be the only way to find a dissection at a time when it is still treatable.

Suggested Readings

Carducci B, Lowe RA, Dalsey W. Penetrating neck trauma: consensus and controversies. Ann Emerg Med 1986;15(2):208–215.

Hoyt DB, Coimbra R, Potenza B. Management of acute trauma. In: Townsend CM, Beauchamp RD, Evers BM, Mattox KL. Sabiston Textbook of Surgery (17th ed). Philadelphia: Elsevier, pp 483–531.

Kendall JL, Anglin D, Demetriades D. Penetrating neck trauma. Emerg Med Clin North Am 1998;16:85–105.

Mandavia DP, Qualls S, Rokos I. Emergency airway management in penetrating neck injury. Ann Emerg Med 2000;35:221–225.

Newton K. Neck. In: Marx JA, Hockberger RS, Walls RM (editors). Rosen's Emergency Medicine: Concepts and Clinical Practice (6th ed). Philadelphia: Mosby, 2006: 441–453.

CHAPTER 12

Spine Trauma

JENNIFER SERRANO JOHNSON ■ COLLEEN J. CAMPBELL

 Red Flags

Inability to evaluate a trauma patient due to altered mental status, intoxication, or competing pain ● Midline neck pain ● Neurologic deficit

Overview

Aggressively search for spinal injury. Look for "red flags" (see Box) when evaluating any trauma patient.

The spine consists of 26 bony vertebrae: 7 cervical, 12 thoracic, 5 lumbar, the sacrum (5 bones fused into one), and the coccyx (3 to 5 fused bones) (Figure 12–1). The spinal cord extends from the mid brain at the base of the skull to the second lumbar vertebrae. Each vertebral body (the largest part of the vertebra) is separated by an intervertebral disc. Each intervertebral disc is made up of two parts: the annulus fibrosis (outer portion) and the nucleus pulposus (inner portion).

To assist in classification of injury stability, the spine is often divided into three anatomic columns: anterior, middle, and posterior. See Figure 12–2. The *anterior column* is composed of the anterior half of the vertebral bodies, the anterior portion of the annulus fibrosus, and anterior longitudinal ligament. The *middle column* is composed of the posterior half of the vertebral body, posterior half of the annulus, and the posterior longitudinal ligament. The *posterior column* is the bony arch formed by the pedicles, transverse processes, articulating facets, laminae, and spinous processes and is held in place by the posterior ligamentous complex (supraspinous ligament, interspinous ligament, infraspinous ligament, ligamentum flavum, and facet joint capsules). When there is disruption of at least two columns, the injury is *unstable*.

A *complete* neurologic lesion is defined by the absence of sensory and motor function below the level of injury and including the lowest sacral segment. If any sensory or motor function is present below the level of injury, the lesion is labeled as *incomplete*.

Spinal shock results from concussive injury to the spinal cord that causes total neurologic dysfunction distal to the site of injury. This

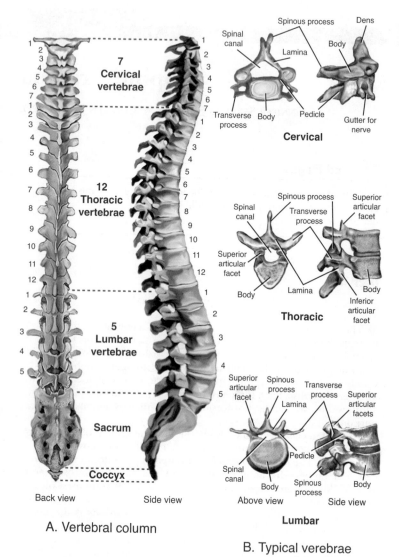

Figure 12–1. Anatomy of the spine: vertebral column and typical vertebrae. (*From Hockberger RS, Kaji AH, Newton EJ. Spine. In: Marx JA, Hockberger RS, Walls RM (editors). Rosen's Emergency Medicine: Concepts and Clinical Practice (6th ed). Philadelphia: Mosby, 2006, p. 400.*)

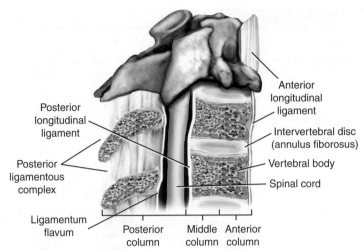

Figure 12–2. Structures composing the anterior, middle, and posterior columns of the spine.

clinical syndrome is associated with flaccid paralysis, loss of all sensory input, loss of deep tendon reflexes, and loss of bladder and rectal tone. It usually lasts less than 24 hours, but occasionally lasts several days. Spinal shock may be accompanied by a disruption in sympathetic outflow to the peripheral vasculature resulting in unopposed vagal tone in the heart and blood vessels. This phenomenon, known as *neurogenic shock*, is characterized by hypotension, bradycardia, warm extremities, and normal urine output. The bulbocavernosus reflex may be lost in spinal shock, but returns following the spinal shock, phase of injury. Increased muscle tone and hyperreflexia follow later.

Minor injuries are those that are localized to a distinct part of the spinal column, and do not cause instability. Major injuries can be classified into four distinct categories: (a) compression (wedge) fractures, (b) burst fractures, (c) flexion–distraction (seatbelt-type) fractures, and (d) fracture–dislocations. Table 12–1 summarizes unstable and stable spinal injuries. A more detailed discussion is provided below.

Initial Diagnostic Approach
General

- All trauma patients must initially be assessed using the basic ABC (*a*irway, *b*reathing, and *c*irculation) approach as discussed in Chapter 8.
- Any multiple trauma patient should be searched for spinal injury, and should have spinal cord immobilization with a hard cervical collar and long spine board until stability of the entire spine has been confirmed.

Table 12–1   Unstable and Stable Spinal Injuries

Injury Type	Unstable	Stable
Malalignment injuries	Bilateral facet dislocation Transverse ligament disruption Atlantoaxial dislocation Occipitoatlantal dissociation Hyperextension dislocation Anterior subluxation	Unilateral facet dislocation

Fractures	*Cervical spine*
	Jefferson fracture
	Burst fracture
	C1 posterior neural arch
	C1 anterior arch fracture
	Odontoid fracture
	Hangman fracture
	Flexion teardrop fracture
	Extension teardrop fracture
	Hyperextension fracture/
	  dislocation
	Wedge fracture with posterior
	  ligament disruption
	Thoracolumbar spine
	Burst fracture
	Compression fracture with
	  >50% loss of vertebral
	body height
	Flexion distraction injuries
	Flexion dislocation injuries
		Cervical spine
		Simple wedge fracture
		Clay-shoveler fracture
		Pillar fracture
		Transverse process
		Laminar fracture
		Uncinate process fracture
		Thoracolumbar spine
		Tranverse process fracture
		Spinous process fracture
		Pars interarticularis fracture
		Compression fracture with
		  <50% loss of vertebral
		  body height

Spinal immobilization should take place concurrent with other emergent interventions. During the primary and secondary surveys, care should be taken to ensure that the cervical spine remains in a neutral flexion–extension position, and that the head and neck move in unison with the trunk, especially during rolling the patient to examine the back.

- **History.** Assess the patient's baseline level of functioning and any gross neurologic dysfunction at the time of the accident from the patient or by report from field personnel, as well as the mechanism of injury.
- **Physical examination.** Findings that suggest spinal cord injury include abdominal breathing, Horner's syndrome, asymmetric extremity movement, or priapism. The diaphragm is innervated by the phrenic nerve (C3-C5), whereas the intercostal muscles of the rib cage are supplied by nerves that originate in the thoracic spine. Therefore abdominal breathing in the absence of thoracic breathing indicates an injury below the C5 level. Horner's syndrome results from damage to the cervical sympathetic chain, and is manifested by ipsilateral ptosis, miosis, and anhydrosis. Conduct a thorough motor and sensory examination to evaluate for disability or focal neurologic deficits Tables 12–2, 12–3, 12–4 and Figure 12–3). The final essential components of a complete

Table 12–2	Motor Grades
Score	Description
0	No visible or palpable contraction
1	Any visible or palpable contraction
2	Movement with gravity eliminated
3	Movement against gravity
4	Movement against gravity plus resistance
5	Normal power
NT	Not testable

Table 12–3	Sensory Grades
Score	Description
0	Absent, unable to distinguish sharp from dull
1	Impaired, able to distinguish but intensity is abnormal
2	Normal
NT	Not testable

Table 12–4	Sensory and Motor Examination: Lesion Localization	
Level of Lesion	Level of Loss of Sensation	Resulting Loss of Function
C2	Occiput	—
C3	Thyroid cartilage	—
C4	Suprasternal notch	Spontaneous breathing
C5	Below clavicle	Shrugging of shoulders
C6	Thumb	Flexion at elbow
C7	Index finger	Extension at elbow
C8	Small finger	Flexion of fingers (C8-T1)
T4	Nipple line	*
T10	Umbilicus	*
L1	Femoral pulse	Flexion at hip
L2	Medial thigh	Flexion at hip
L3	Medial thigh	Adduction at hip, knee flexion
L4	Knee	Abduction at hip
L5	Lateral calf	Dorsiflexion of foot
S1-S2	Lateral foot	Plantar flexion of foot
S2-S4	Perianal region±	Rectal sphincter tone

Localization of lesions in this area is best accomplished with the sensory examination

±*Sacral sparing, or preservation of sensation at the sacrum, in a patient with a spinal cord injury is a very good prognostic sign and should be carefully documented.*

neurologic examination include deep tendon and perineal reflex assessment. Perineal reflexes, including the cremasteric, anal wink, and bulbocavernosus, are essential components (Table 12–5). Priapism may occur transiently in males with complete spinal cord transection. When possible the neurologic examination should be completed before

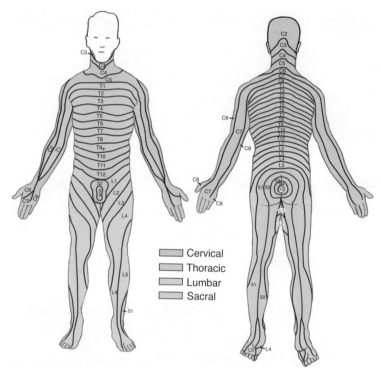

Figure 12–3. Sensory dermatomes. *(From Hockberger RS, Kirshenbaum KJ. Spine. In: Marx JA, Hockberger RS, Walls RM (editors). Rosen's Emergency Medicine: Concepts and Clinical Practice (6th ed). Philadelphia: Mosby, 2006, p. 400.)*

pharmacologic paralysis. The patient should be log-rolled and the entire spine should be examined. Note any areas of ecchymosis, hemorrhage, lacerations, abrasions, malalignment, point tenderness, or palpable gaps in the spinous processes.

■ Serial neurologic examinations are necessary to spot deteriorations.

Radiography

■ Any person who cannot be clinically cleared should undergo imaging of the cervical spine. Criteria for clinical clearance are listed in Box 12–1.
■ The imaging technique of choice will depend on the clinical circumstances, but the assessment of spinal injury typically begins with plain films.
■ *Plain films*:
  ■ *Cervical spine.* Classical radiologic clearance of the cervical spine begins with a lateral view. A cross-table lateral view can detect 70% to 80% of all traumatic cervical spine injuries. Be methodical and

Table 12–5 Perineal Reflex Assessment

Reflex	Location of Lesion	Stimulus	Normal Response	Abnormal Response
Cremasteric	T12–L1	Stroking the medial thigh proximal to distal	Upward motion of the scrotum	No motion of the scrotum
Anal wink	S2–S4	Stroking skin around anus	Anal sphincter contracts	No anal sphincter contraction
Bulbocavernosus*	S3–S4	Squeezing the penis in males, applying pressure to clitoris in females, or tugging the bladder catheter in either	Anal sphincter contracts	No anal sphincter contraction

The bulbocavernosus reflex is the last reflex to disappear in patients with spinal shock and the first to return with improvement.

BOX 12–1 Criteria for Clinical Clearance for Cervical Spine Injuries

Alert patient who has never lost consciousness
Not under the influence of drugs or alcohol
No cervical tenderness
No distracting injury
No neurologic deficit

---

complete when evaluating this image (Table 12–6, Figure 12–4). Today, many trauma centers are delaying obtaining plain films of the cervical spine and leaving the patient in a collar until a computed tomography (CT scan) is ordered or other more critical injuries have been stabilized. The full series consists of anteroposterior, lateral, and open mouth views. Some institutions also routinely obtain oblique views. If initial cervical spine plain film views are unsatisfactory in demonstrating the superior aspect of T1, special techniques such as traction on the arms to lower the shoulders or a swimmer's view (one arm raised next to the head, and the other is placed down alongside the waist) may be necessary. If there is concern for spinal injury (i.e., focal spinal tenderness) in the presence of normal plain films, a CT scan should be obtained.

Table 12–6 Tips for Interpreting Cervical Spine Films

Cross-table lateral view	"**ABCs**" of the lateral film: *a*lignment, *b*ony abnormalities, *c*artilage space assessment, and *s*oft tissues.
	• **Alignment** of vertebrae is assessed by examining the contour of three imaginary anatomic lines: anterior spinal line, posterior spinal line, and spinolaminal line. Any stepoffs or breaks in the contour of these lines suggests bony or ligamentous injury.
	• **Bony abnormalities** assessment includes not only looking for obvious fractures, but also looking for increased or decreased bone density. Increased density suggests a compression fracture or an osteoblastic metastatic lesion. Decreased density suggests diseased bone seen with osteoporosis, osteomalacia, or osteolytic metastatic lesions. These weak points are at increased risk for fractures.
	• **Cartilage space assessment** involves examination of regions of spine where critical supportive ligaments are found. Increases in these spaces may be the only clues to unstable dislocations. The three regions of most interest are the predental, intervertebral, and interspinous spaces. The **predental** space is located between the posterior aspect of the anterior arch of C1 and the anterior border of the odontoid. In adults it should measure <3 mm and in children <4 to 5 mm. The intervertebral and interspinous spaces should be equal anteriorly and posteriorly.
	• **Soft tissue (prevertebral)** space is examined for increased thickness or altered contour. Such soft-tissue changes are often related to acute hemorrhage, and are suggestive of acute cervical spine injury. The **retropharyngeal space**, located just anterior to the bodies of the cervical vertebrae and extending anteriorly to the posterior wall of the pharynx, should measure less than 7 mm at the level of C2, and less than 5 mm at the level of C3-C4. The **retrotracheal** space, located just anterior to the body of C6 and extending to the posterior wall of the trachea, should not exceed 22 mm in adults or 14 mm in children younger than 15 years.
Open mouth odontoid	Shows the odontoid and its relation to the lateral masses of C1. The dens should be centered between the C1 lateral masses, and the lateral masses of C1 should be directly over the lateral portions of C2. The normal lateral atlas-dens interval (LADI) should not exceed 2 mm on either side of the odontoid, and neither side should deviate more than 1 mm from the other. Rotation of the head may cause some displacement of the lateral masses and asymmetry of the LADI.
Anteroposterior view	Only effective in evaluating the lower cervical spine (C4 and below) because the structure of the face and mandible obscure the bony anatomy of C1-3. At all levels, alignment of the tips of the spinous processes should be checked as well as confirmation of midline tracheal and laryngeal air shadows. A line tracing the edges of the lateral masses should reveal a regular, undulating pattern. Angulation of the lateral cortex of the articular masses relative to the adjacent superior or inferior vertebrae is suggestive of fracture or dislocation.

Table 12–6	**Tips for Interpreting Cervical Spine Films—*cont'd***
Oblique view	Helpful for identifying fractures and dislocations of the facet joints, pedicles, and lateral masses. In a normal film, the overlapping elliptical-shaped laminae appear as "shingles on a roof" and the interlaminar spaces are equal. Disruptions of this orientation are helpful in confirming suspected posterior laminar fractures, unilateral facet dislocations, or real subluxation.
Flexion/extension view	Used to investigate for ligamentous injury. They should be obtained in (a) patients with normal mental status and normal neurologic examination who have a minor malalignment of their cervical spine on routine films or (b) patients with normal x-ray findings who complain of severe, persistent neck pain or spinal tenderness. In the acute setting, pain and spasm often cause flexion/extension views to be non-diagnostic because of limited mobility. Delayed views, after immobilization with a hard collar for 7-10 days, allow for muscle spasm to subside and often yield better results.

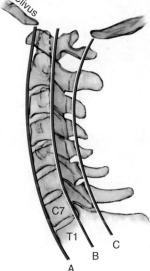

Figure 12–4. Spinal lines of cervical spine. **A,** Anterior spinal line. **B,** Posterior spinal line. **C,** Spinolaminal line. (*From Wiest P, Roth P. Fundamentals of Emergency Radiology. Philadelphia: WB Saunders, 1996, p. 23.*)

- *Thoracolumbar (T/L) spine.* Anteroposterior and lateral views should be obtained if there is midline tenderness to palpation, identified cervical spine injury, or focal neurologic signs or symptoms. Oblique views of the posterior lumbar elements in a normal patient form the figure of a Scotty dog (Figure 12–5). Spondylolysis is a defect in the pars articularis. Spondylolisthesis is the displacement of one vertebral body relative to the alignment of the normal vertebrae.
- *CT scan.* A CT scan is the diagnostic modality of choice for acute cervical injury. A CT scan is indicated for (a) all patients with suspected spinal fractures or dislocation identified on plain radiographs, (b) patients with incomplete visualization of the spinal column on conventional radiographs and, (c) high clinical probability of injury, despite a normal plain film survey. A CT scan does not demonstrate spinal cord or ligamentous injuries. These are seen better on magnetic resonance imaging (MRI). These injuries can be present without spinal column injury.
- *MRI/magnetic resonance angiography (MRA).* An MRI is the best modality for detecting ligamentous or disc injury. Ligamentous injury can be present without boney injury. An MRI can show acute cord hemorrhage, cord edema or contusion, and mixed cord injury. It should

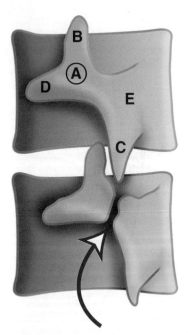

Figure 12–5. Posterior lumbar elements showing normal anatomy and spondylolyis. **A,** Pedicle. **B,** Superior facet. **C,** Inferior facet, **D,** Transverse process. **E,** Pars interarticularis. *(From Wiest P, Roth P. Fundamentals of Emergency Radiology. Philadelphia: WB Saunders, 1996, p. 37.)*

be performed urgently in any patient with an increasing neurologic deficit. An MRA can show injuries to the spinal artery such as arterial lacerations or delayed thrombosis.

Emergency Department Management Overview
General

- The ABCs should be addressed and spinal immobilization should be maintained until injury has been ruled out.
- *Prehospital care.* All major trauma patients are at risk for spinal injury. Protection and immobilization of the spine should be initiated at the site of injury and maintained until a spinal injury is ruled out or treated. Maintaining a neutral flexion–extension head position and neck alignment in pediatric patients requires making adjustments for their relatively larger heads. Children younger than 8 years should be accommodated by elevating the trunk and shoulders with padding or using a special pediatric spine board containing a cutout for the occiput.
- *Emergency department (ED) care.* If there are aspects of the history or physical examination that suggest a moderate to high risk of spine trauma, the immobilization apparatus should be left in place while the patients clothes are removed, associated injuries evaluated, and resuscitative measures performed. In alert patients who are not intoxicated and have no major distracting injuries, neck tenderness (initially by palpation in the midline followed by active range of motion of the neck), or neurologic deficits, the risk for spine fracture is so low that the patient can be removed from immobilization without further radiographic testing of the spine. The patient should be removed from the board as soon as practical. Skin breakdown and decubitus ulcers can begin within 1 hour of use. Transfer of the patient off the board should be performed using a sliding board or scoop system and a three-person logroll technique to prevent further injury.
- *Airway/breathing.* The best method of airway management for all trauma patients is orotracheal intubation with in-line stabilization (without distraction force) and cricoid pressure. When performed correctly, manual in-line stabilization is more effective for immobilization than leaving a cervical collar in place. Moreover, unless the collar is loosened or opened, it will interfere with the visualization of the glottis making intubation difficult or impossible.
- *Circulation.* The first-line treatment for hypotension in all trauma patients is rapid infusion of crystalloid fluid. This is also usually effective in treating mild isolated neurogenic shock. If the patient is unresponsive to initial fluid resuscitation, other more common causes of trauma-related hypotension (such as hemorrhagic shock, tension pneumothorax, and cardiac tamponade) should be searched for and treated. The diagnosis of neurogenic shock as the sole cause of hypotension is a diagnosis of exclusion. In severe cases of neurogenic shock, there is a danger of excessive fluid replacement, which can lead to heart failure and pulmonary edema. In these cases, placement of a pulmonary artery catheter to guide fluid administration can be very helpful but is not practical in the ED setting. Other options for hemodynamic support in these patients

include atropine due to increased vagal tone in neurogenic shock and pressor medications such as phenylephrine (alpha 1-agonist).

Medications

- ■ *Steroids.* High-dose methylprednisolone may be administered in patients with evidence of blunt spinal cord injury who present within 8 hours of injury; however, this treatment is controversial. An initial loading dose of 30 mg/kg IV is followed by a maintenance infusion of 5.4 mg/kg/h. This maintenance infusion is continued for 24 hours in patients being treated within 3 hours of injury and for 48 hours for those patients presenting within 3 to 8 hours of injury. High-dose corticosteroids have not been proven to be of benefit in penetrating spinal cord trauma, but is still recommended by some neurosurgeons.
- ■ *Atropine.* A dose of 0.5 to 1 mg IV should be given for bradycardia associated with spinal shock.
- ■ *Vasopressors.* Alpha-1 agonist adrenergic–specific agents such as phenylephrine (50 µg IV bolus then 100 µg/min IV) or ephedrine (10 mg IV) should be used in the presence of spinal shock.

Emergency Department Interventions

- ■ *Foley catheter.* A Foley catheter should be placed to help monitor fluid status and relieve bladder distention from urinary retention secondary to cord injury.
- ■ *Nasogastric tube.* A nasogastric tube should be placed to manage adynamic ileus (a common complication of spinal cord injury). A tube should be placed in unconscious or intoxicated patients unless there are facial injuries that would make placement unsafe.
- ■ *Spinal precautions.* These should be maintained in all patients with altered mentation until the presence of a spinal injury can be excluded clinically or radiographically. In combative patients this may require sedation or intubation and chemical paralysis.

Disposition

- ■ *Consultation.* Spine consultation, from an orthopedic surgeon or neurosurgeon, should occur emergently for any patient with an abnormal neurologic examination or with evidence of fracture or malalignment on imaging studies.
- ■ *Transfer.* In rural hospitals that transfer severe trauma patients, the primary and secondary survey should be completed, a nasogastric tube and Foley catheter should be inserted, the resuscitating physician should give report directly to the receiving physician, and copies of all diagnostic studies and imaging should accompany the patient.
- ■ *Admission.* Almost all patients with spinal fractures, whether unstable or stable, require hospitalization. Exceptions to this rule are isolated lumbar compression fractures less than 25% or spinous process fractures with no associated ligamentous instability or neurologic impairment.
- ■ *Discharge.* Patients with isolated musculoskeletal injuries of the spine with no associated neurologic deficits or radiographic abnormalities can

be discharged from the ED with pain medication and referral for follow-up evaluation.

Specific Problems: Cord Syndromes

- Injuries to the spinal cord can be described on the basis of the anatomic organization of the spinal cord (Figure 12–6).
- A complete spinal cord lesion results in total loss of sensory, autonomic (spinal shock or priapism), and motor innervation distal to the level of the injury. Reflexes may persist but may also be absent or abnormal.
- Incomplete cord syndromes are summarized in Table 12–7.

Specific Problems: Unstable Injuries in Cervical Spine
Atlantooccipital Dislocation

- ***Mechanism.*** This is a hyperextension and distraction mechanism such as that frequently seen in motor vehicle accidents.
- ***Description.*** Dislocation of the skull from the cervical spine is rare due to the strength of the supporting ligaments. These injuries are usually fatal, and are more common in children. The majority are anterior dislocations.
- ***Radiographic signs.*** The diagnosis is often subtle, and may be easily overlooked on routine radiographs. In a normal cervical spine with the head in neutral, the tip of the odontoid is in vertical alignment with the clivus (Figure 12–4). The normal distance between these two points in adult is 4 to 5 mm, and any increase in this distance is considered significant. In children, however, this distance may approach 10 mm.

Bilateral Facet Dislocation

- ***Mechanism.*** This is a hyperflexion injury.
- ***Description.*** This is a very unstable injury that results from complete disruption of all ligamentous structures of the spinal column. The result is anterior displacement of the entire spine segment above the level of injury.

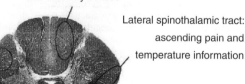

Figure 12–6. Spinal cord anatomy. (*From Perron AD, Huff JS. Spinal cord disorders. In: Marx JA, Hockberger RS, Walls RM (editors). Rosen's Emergency Medicine: Concepts and Clinical Practice (5th ed). St. Louis, MO: Mosby, 2002, p. 1497; Photomicrograph courtesy John Sundsten, Digital Anatomist Project, University of Washington.*)

Table 12–7 Cord Syndromes

Syndrome	Mechanism	Clinical Findings
Anterior cord	Hyperflexion injury	This injury causes damage to the corticospinal and spinothalamic pathways of the spinal column. • Incomplete motor paralysis • Loss of pain and temperature sensation distal to the level of injury • Preservation of vibration, light touch and position sense • Variable loss of sphincter tone
Brown-Sequard	Penetrating injury or lateral cord compression secondary to intervertebral disk protrusion, hematomas, or lateral mass fractures of the cervical spine	• Ipsilateral motor paralysis • Loss of proprioception and vibratory sense • Contralateral loss of pain and temperature sensation
Central cord	Hyperextension injury Often seen in elderly patients with preexisting spondylosis or degenerative arthritis.	This injury produces a contusion of the central portion of the spinal cord that results in an injury to the central gray matter and the most central portions of the corticospinal and spinothalamic tracts. • Weakness greater in the arms than the legs • Some loss of pain and temperature sensation (also greater in the upper extremities) • Bladder control is lost in more severe cases
Cauda equina	Most often secondary to midline lumbar disc herniation. Can also occur with traumatic fractures, spinal stenosis, tumors, or other compressive masses.	This syndrome results from compression of the lumbosacral peripheral nerve roots within the spinal canal. Symptoms are more often unilateral • Lower leg and back pain, bowel and bladder retention or incontinence • Weakness (may be of lower motor neuron type: decreased reflexes) • Incontinence, and numbness in the lower extremities • Saddle (perineal) anesthesia and a diminished rectal tone.

Table 12–7   Cord Syndromes—*cont'd*

Syndrome	Mechanism	Clinical Findings
Conus medullaris	Central disk herniation, neoplasm, trauma, or vascular insufficiency.	This is the terminal end of the spinal cord located at L1 in most adults. The clinical features often overlap with cauda equina syndrome but are more often bilateral. • Bladder or bowel incontinence • Weakness (may be of upper motor neuron type — increased tone and reflexes) • Saddle anesthesia

■ *Radiographic signs.* The lateral view reveals anterior displacement of the upper vertebrae greater than 50% of the width of the lower vertebral body.

Burst Fracture of the Cervical Spine

■ *Mechanism.* This injury results from vertical compression such as that created by a fall or hyperflexion.
■ *Description.* This injury is a shatter fracture of one or both of the vertebral body endplates that forces the nucleus pulposus of the intervertebral disk into the vertebral body. This type of fracture is often associated with retropulsion of bone and disk fragments into the spinal canal. If any fracture elements impinge on or penetrate the ventral surface of the spinal cord, anterior cord syndrome may result.
■ *Radiographic signs.* The lateral view shows a comminuted fracture of the vertebral body. The anteroposterior view reveals a vertical fracture and widening of the interpeduncular distance.

C1 Anterior Arch Fracture

■ *Mechanism.* This is a hyperextension injury.
■ *Description.* These are isolated fractures of the anterior arch of the atlas in which the odontoid is thrust against the anterior arch.
■ *Radiographic signs.* The lateral view reveals the fracture line as well as prevertebral soft-tissue swelling.

C1 Posterior Neural Arch Fracture

■ *Mechanism.* This is an extension injury.
■ *Description.* This mechanically stable fracture occurs when the posterior elements of C1 are compressed between the occiput and spinous process of C2 during forced hyperextension of the neck.
■ *Radiographic signs.* On lateral view this injury has much less associated prevertebral soft-tissue swelling than a Jefferson fracture.

Extension Teardrop Fracture

- *Mechanism.* This is a hyperextension injury.
- *Description.* This injury is an avulsion fracture of the anteroinferior portion of a vertebral body. The teardrop fragment is avulsed from the portion of the vertebral body where the anterior longitudinal ligament inserts. In younger adults, this injury tends to occur lower in the cervical spine. In this location massive prevertebral soft-tissue swelling or buckling of the ligamentum flavum into the spinal cord can lead to acute *central cord syndrome.*
- *Radiographic signs.* Lateral plain films reveal the characteristic *teardrop* fragment displaced anteriorly and inferiorly from its original anatomic position.

Flexion Teardrop Fracture

- *Mechanism.* This is a hyperflexion injury.
- *Description.* This highly unstable, hyperflexion injury is the most severe and devastating fracture of the cervical spine. Fracture of the antero-inferior corner of the involved vertebral body and subluxation or dislocation of the interfacetal joints characterizes the injury. Complete ligamentous and bony disruption occur at the level of injury. Severe neurologic compromise is very common. This fracture has a very high association with *anterior cord syndrome.*
- *Radiographic signs.* Lateral plain films reveal kyphosis with widening or fanning of posterior ligamentous structures as well as a large, commonly comminuted, anteriorly displaced wedge–shaped fracture fragment (teardrop) of the anterior aspect of the vertebral body.

Hangman's Fracture

- *Mechanism.* This is an extension injury.
- *Description.* Also known as *traumatic spondylolysis of C2*, this fracture of the pedicles of the axis is the result of extreme hyperextension that occurs with rapid deceleration. This unstable fracture may or may not be associated with anterior displacement of C2 on C3. Fortunately, because the diameter of the spinal canal is largest at the C2 level and the bilateral pedicle fractures allow the spine to decompress spontaneously, spinal cord damage with this injury either does not occur or is minimal.
- *Radiographic signs.* In the cross-table lateral view, the spinolaminal line connecting C1 with C3 should pass within 1 mm of the spinolaminal junction of C2. Displacement of more than 1 mm suggests anterior or posterior displacement of the odontoid or a hangman's fracture.

Jefferson Fracture

- *Mechanism.* This is a vertical compression injury.
- *Description.* This burst fracture of C1 is the result of an axial load transmitted from a direct blow to the top of the head. The downward force of the occipital condyles onto the lateral masses of the atlas drives the lateral masses outward, resulting in fractures of the anterior and posterior arches

of C1. In severe cases, this injury is often associated with rupture of the transverse ligament. Despite extreme mechanical instability, due to the large amount of central canal space in this region of the spine, patients with Jefferson fractures may still be neurologically intact.

■ *Radiographic signs.* On the cross-table lateral view, a widening of the predental space (>3 mm in adults or >5 mm in children) suggests a Jefferson fracture of C1. In the AP view, the lateral margins of C1 lie lateral to the margins of the articular pillars of C2.

Odontoid Fracture

■ *Mechanism.* The mechanism varies.
■ *Description.* Odontoid fractures occur in combination with one third of all fractures of the ring of C1, and are the most common subtype of C2 fractures. Classification of this injury is based on location of the fracture line (see below). Although type I odontoid fractures are considered mechanically stable, they have a high association with C1 to C2 ligamentous injury and resultant atlantoaxial dislocation. They should be treated as potentially unstable injuries.
■ *Radiographic signs.* Type I injuries are avulsion fractures of the lateral tip by the alar ligament. Type II injuries, which are the most common, are located at the waist of the odontoid in an area covered by the transverse ligament. Type III injuries extend caudally into the cancellous bone of the axis.

Specific Problems: Unstable Injuries in Thoracolumbar Spine
Burst Fracture of the Thoracolumbar Spine

■ *Mechanism.* This is due to axial loading such as that created by a fall landing on one's feet.
■ *Description.* This vertical compression fracture of the vertebral body. The mechanical stability of this fracture is markedly decreased when there is associated posterior column disruption.
■ *Radiographic signs.* The lateral view demonstrates decreased vertebral body height both anteriorly and posteriorly. The anteroposterior view demonstrates increased interpediculate distance.

Flexion–Distraction Injuries (Thoracolumbar Spine)

■ *Mechanism.* This is typically due to a head-on motor crash wearing a lap seatbelt only.
■ *Description.* If the axis of flexion lies anterior to the anterior longitudinal ligament, the result is a classic *Chance fracture*, producing horizontal fractures through the posterior and middle column bony elements along with disruption of the supraspinous ligament. When the axis of flexion occurs posterior to the anterior longitudinal ligament, an associated wedge compression fracture may occur, producing a more unstable injury. The incidence of severe, life-threatening intra-abdominal damage occurring with this type of spine injury is very high (50%-67%), and such injuries should be sought.

- *Radiographic signs.* The AP view shows an increase in the interspinous distance and possible horizontal fracture lines through the pedicles, transverse processes, and pars interarticularis

Wedge Fracture (Cervical Spine)

- *Mechanism.* This is a hyperflexion injury.
- *Description.* A fracture of the superior endplate of a vertebral body resulting from compression between two other vertebrae. The inferior endplate of the vertebral body remains intact. An isolated simple wedge fracture with less than 50% loss of the vertebral body height is considered a stable fracture. Severe wedge fractures (>50% loss of vertebral body height) and multiple adjacent wedge fractures have an increased risk of posterior element disruption, and are unstable injuries. Plain films often underestimate the extent of the injury, and often when the patient has significant pain, or is elderly, it is prudent to obtain a CT scan to see the true extent of the injury.
- *Radiographic signs.* Anteroposterior and lateral plain films may reveal a decreased vertebral body height along the anterior border. The bony impaction that occurs from a fracture of the superior endplate leads to an increased density of the vertebral body and prevertebral soft-tissue swelling. If associated with a posterior element disruption, an increased interspinous distance may be seen.

Wedge Compression Fracture (Thoracolumbar Spine)

- *Mechanism.* Anterior or lateral flexion causes this injury.
- *Description.* This flexion compression fracture of the vertebral body results in anterior column disruption with varying degrees of middle and posterior column disruption. Approximately 10% to 15% of patients presenting with calcaneal fractures after a fall have associated compression fractures of the thoracolumbar spine. Unstable fractures include a loss of vertebral height of greater than 50% or angulation of the thoracolumbar junction of greater than 20 degrees.
- *Radiographic signs.* The lateral view demonstrates diminished anterior height of the vertebral body, with a normal posterior height.

Specific Problems: Stable Injuries in Spinal Trauma
Clay-Shoveler's Fracture

- *Mechanism.* Extreme forced hyperflexion causes this injury.
- *Description.* This injury is an oblique avulsion fracture of the base of the spinous process of one of the lower cervical vertebrae. This injury may be the result of a direct blow to the spinous process, or from a sudden deceleration motor crash or direct occipital trauma leading to forced flexion. This is an extremely stable fracture with no associated neurologic involvement and can be treated conservatively with rest, ice, analgesia, and early referral for outpatient follow-up.
- *Radiographic signs.* Lateral cervical spine views reveal the isolated avulsed bony fragment.

Tranverse Process Fracture

- *Mechanism.* This is a hyperflexion injury.
- *Description.* This is a stable fracture, which can occur secondary to lateral flexion stress. It may occur in association with severe injury anywhere in the spine, but in the lumbar area, there may be an isolated injury due to local trauma. This is the most common isolated fracture to the posterior elements.
- *Radiographic signs.* Displacement of the transverse process can be easily visualized on an anteroposterior plain film.

Unilateral Facet Dislocation

- *Mechanism.* Flexion and rotation produce this dislocation.
- *Description.* This injury occurs when a flexion and rotation force applied to the spinal column gets localized to a single facet joint. This facet joint then acts like a fulcrum about which the superior and inferior segments of the spinal column simultaneously bend and twist. The end result is a dislocation of a single facet joint. In the cervical region this type of injury is often not associated with fractures of the articular processes and is considered mechanically stable. In contrast, within the thoracolumbar region, this type of injury is often associated with fractures at the base of the inferior articular mass of the dislocated vertebrae or the superior articular mass of the inferior vertebra. A fracture–dislocation such as this allows the upper vertebrae to swing anteriorly on the lower and is unstable.
- *Radiographic signs.* The anteroposterior view will reveal displacement of the tips of the spinous processes away from midline pointing towards the direction of rotation. On the lateral view, at the level of injury, there is posterior displacement of the vertebra below (less than 50% the width of a vertebral body) relative to the vertebra above.

Special Considerations
Pediatrics

- *Anatomic differences.* The spinal cord moves up relative to the spine from birth at L3-L4 level to approximately 3 months of age, when it comes to rest at the adult level of L1-L2. Ossification begins at about 7 years, and this process is complete by age 21 to 25 years. The growth plate, or epiphysis, is almost always involved in fractures crossing the vertebral discs. These are similar to Salter I type fractures, and are seen through the vertebral endplates or synchondroses. The fracture pattern in children older than 11 years usually mirrors adult patterns more closely. Anatomic differences in the pediatric cervical spine alter the injury patterns seen following cervical spine trauma. The more elastic ligaments and horizontally oriented facet joints predispose children to subluxation without bony injury. Furthermore, proportionately larger heads combined with weak structural support from immature neck muscles and more elastic ligaments place children younger than 8 years at increased risk for upper cervical spine fractures. The large head acts as a fulcrum. This fulcrum starts in the upper cervical levels and changes progressively to lower levels as the pediatric cervical spine matures, until it reaches adult levels at C5 and C6. The result is that most injuries occur at the C1 to C3 levels in children younger than 8 years.

■ *Spinal cord injury without radiographic abnormality (SCIWORA).* Children's spines are more elastic than adults, and can be stretched in neonates 5 cm without rupture. The cord remains unelastic and can only be stretched 0.5 cm without damage. It is elongated in flexion and shortened in extension. SCIORWA is thought to occur in children much more commonly than adults because of the elastic character of the pediatric spine. SCIWORA may present with delayed neurologic deficits. Injuries to the cartilage endplates cannot be diagnosed by radiography, and may be seen in this group. Diagnosis is by an MRI, and treatment is usually immobilization alone. Only in the case of a progressive deficit requiring decompression would operative management be considered.

■ *Normal variants mimicking disease*
  ■ *Absent cervical lordosis.* A hard cervical collar often causes a benign loss of lordosis of the cervical spine in children. This change in normal contour is due to weak musculature and highly elastic ligaments, and is not necessarily indicative of bony or ligamentous injury as it is in adults.
  ■ *Increased predental soft tissue.* Children younger than 24 months may exhibit a physiologic widening of the prevertebral space during expiration. For this reason the upper limit of normal for the predental space in children is 5 mm, rather than 3 mm as in adults.
  ■ *Pseudosubluxation.* In infants and young children, immature muscular development results in a hypermobile spine, which often causes the appearance of subluxation of C2 on C3. This can be seen in 24% of children younger than 8 years at the C2 to C3 region. In flexion and extension, there is 50% more movement at C3 to C 4 in children younger than 8 years compared with adults. Pseudo-subluxation can be differentiated from a true dislocation by inspecting the relative position of the lamina of C2 on a lateral radiograph. Displacement of less than 5 mm posterior or anterior to a vertical line drawn between the posterior ring of C1 and the lamina of C3 is consistent with a pseudosubluxation. Displacements that are more than 5 mm are consistent with true subluxation. In the absence of a history of significant trauma, this injury is often caused by nonaccidental trauma (NAT).

Elderly

■ *Anatomic differences.* The degenerative changes that occur in the spine with age lead to an increased risk of fracture, and an increased risk of missed diagnosis. The increased stiffness of the lower cervical spine seen with degenerative changes allows for greater mobility in the upper cervical spine. Spinal cord injury consequently occurs twice as frequently in patients older than 65 years than those younger. The most common level of fracture of the cervical spine in the elderly is C2. This includes odontoid fractures.

■ Spine fractures are more difficult to identify in the setting of concomitant degenerative changes such as osteoporosis, spondylosis, and spondylolisthesis. This may explain why some studies have shown spine fractures to be missed much more commonly in the elderly. Any elderly patient requiring a head CT scan for blunt trauma, regardless of the head CT scan result, has a higher risk of cervical spine injury than in the nonhead-injured patient.

Preexisting Disease That Alters Spinal Anatomy

■ Minor trauma can lead to spinal cord injury in patients who have congenital or acquired stenosis of the spine or ligamentous instability. Rheumatoid arthritis, ankylosing spondylitis, and osteoarthritis can lead to ossification of the posterior longitudinal ligament and instability. Sudden forced extension of the cervical spine may cause spinal cord injury in patients with cervical osteoarthritis by causing the hypertrophied ligamentum flavum to buckle into the spinal cord. Achondroplasia is associated with congenital spinal stenosis, while spondylosis causes an acquired stenosis that predisposes to spinal cord injury.

Comatose Patients

■ In the comatose patient, the cervical spine cannot be cleared solely by use of plain radiographs. A CT scan using 2-mm cuts to C2 and at the C7 region can be completed at the same time the patient has a head CT scan. Although this will elucidate spinal fractures, it will not provide information regarding spinal stability. Although more expensive, MRI remains the safer and more sensitive test for spine trauma. This is especially true in the case of children, where SCIWORA remains a significant injury pattern. In the very young, in the very old, and in patients with significant preexisting disease of the spine, even minor trauma can produce injury. These patients require early and aggressive imaging studies with an MRI or CT scan to reveal the pathology. It is easy to forget about the spine in a child who needs comfort from other injuries, but they also are subject to thoracic and lumbar spinal injuries.

Teaching Points

Spinal column injury is one of the problems in emergency medicine for which the prognosis can be altered significantly by appropriate management. It is therefore important to physically manage the spine correctly in the field and in the ED.

The radiologic imaging clearances can await stabilization of more life-threatening injuries. Moreover, the thoracic and lumbar spine is readily imaged by CT scan of the chest and abdomen. The plain films are still useful once the patient has been stabilized.

Suggested Readings

Akbarnia BA. Pediatric spine fractures. Orthop Clin North Am 1999;30:521–536.

Bracken MB, Shepard MJ, Collins WF Jr, et al. Administration of methylprednisolone for 24 or 48 hours or tirilazad mesylate for 48 hours in the treatment of acute spinal cord injury. JAMA. 1997;277:1597–1604.

Brooks RA, Willett KM. Evaluation of the Oxford protocol for total spinal clearance in the unconscious trauma patient. J Trauma 2001;50:862–867.

Bub LD, Blacksmoker Cl, Mann FA, Lomoschitz FM. Cervical spine fractures in patients 65 years and older: A clinical prediction rule for blunt trauma. Radiology 2005;64:355–358.

Hoffman JR, Mower WR, Wolfson AB, Todd KH, Zucker MI. Validity of a set of clinical criteria to rule out injury to the cervical spine in patients with blunt trauma. National Emergency X-Radiography Utilization Study Group. N Engl J Med 2000;343:94–99.

Hockberger RS, Kaji AH, Newton EJ. Spine. In: Marx JA, Hockberger RS, Walls RM (editors). Rosen's Emergency Medicine: Concepts and Clinical Practice (6th ed). Philadelphia: Mosby, 2006, pp. 398–441.

Pollack CV, Hendey GW, Martin DR, et al. Use of flexion-extension radiographs of the cervical spine in blunt trauma. Ann Emerg Med 2001;38:8–11.

Stiell IG, Wells GA, Vandemheen KL, et al. The Canadian C-spine rule for radiography in alert and stable trauma patients. JAMA 2001;286:1841–1848.

Wagner R, Jagoda A. Spinal cord syndromes. Emerg Med Clin North Am 1997;15:699–711.

CHAPTER **13**

Chest Trauma

Saul D. Levine ■ Aaron Schneir ■ Ali Ghobadi

Red Flags

Chest pain • Respiratory distress • Hypoxia • Hypotension
• Obvious chest trauma, especially penetrating injury

Overview

Traumatic injuries to the chest are most commonly due to motor vehicle crashes, and account for up to 25% of deaths in the United States resulting from trauma. The immediate cause of death in these cases is mostly likely due to rupture of the myocardial wall or thoracic aorta. Early deaths (less than 2 hours after trauma) may be prevented by immediate life-saving interventions. The cause of such deaths includes tension pneumothorax, pericardial tamponade, airway obstruction, and hemorrhage.

Look for red flags (see Box) that require immediate attention. Anyone with chest trauma and hypotension should be immediately evaluated for tension pneumothorax, pericardial tamponade, or uncontrolled hemorrhage. These patients should have emergent interventions before radiographic studies are obtained. A tension pneumothorax is a clinical diagnosis. Bedside ultrasonography is now available to evaluate for pericardial tamponade.

Associated injuries are common, especially with blunt trauma. For example, fractures to the lower ribs should raise concern for associated intra-abdominal injuries. Fractures of the first three ribs may be associated with severe intrathoracic trauma.

Blunt and penetrating trauma to the chest generally have different injuries and approaches.

Initial Diagnostic Approach
General

- All trauma patients must initially be assessed using the basic ABC (*a*irway, *b*reathing, and *c*irculation) approach as discussed in Chapter 8.
- *History.* Inquire about the mechanism of injury, for example in a motor vehicle collision, the speed of both cars, extent of damage to the patient's car, (including steering wheel deformity), the use of seat belts, the deployment of airbags, and a report from emergency medical service (EMS) providers on scene.
- *Physical examination.* Assess the chest for injury with inspection, auscultation, palpitation, and percussion. Observe the respiratory rate, effort, and chest wall excursion. Changes in respiratory rate may be the first sign of impending ventilatory failure but are often missed because nobody has been counting respirations. Inspect the neck and abdomen for associated injury. The posterior thorax also must always be evaluated, but keep in mind spinal immobilization if indicated. Unlike penetrating abdominal wounds, penetrating chest wounds are generally not locally explored, nor should they ever be probed to avoid an exacerbation in bleeding or creation of a new pneumothorax. Flail segments (two or more ribs broken in two or more places) are difficult to see, especially when the segment is central, but are an important cause of ventilatory failure. Penetrating injuries may be hidden in the axilla, supraclavicular folds or beneath a pendulous breast. Palpate for tenderness, crepitance, or subcutaneous air.

Laboratory

- The most useful laboratory studies in a patient with significant chest trauma include arterial blood gas, hemoglobin, and type and screen for blood products.

EKG

■ An electrocardiogram (EKG) is useful to detect conduction disturbance, frequent ectopy, and ischemia, although abnormalities are more likely to represent concomitant disease than the result of the acute injury.

Radiography

■ *Plain films.* The chest radiograph is the mainstay of screening for chest trauma, but should be delayed in a patient with airway compromise or hemodynamic instability. DO NOT obtain a chest radiograph until the ABCs are secured. An upright chest radiograph is preferable but is often impossible to obtain safely early on in the evaluation.
■ *Ultrasound.* This is useful mainly in identifying pericardial fluid and massive hemothorax.
■ *Computed tomography (CT scan) of the chest.* This is the optimal imaging study in all stable patients with major chest trauma.
■ *Angiography.* This is rarely used but may be a useful adjunct for preoperative delineation of aortic injuries.

Emergency Department Management Overview
General

■ The ABCs should be addressed. Establish two large-bore intravenous (IV) lines, place the patient on a monitor, and give supplementary oxygen to any patient who is being evaluated after major trauma to maintain the oxygen saturation above 95%.

Medications

■ *Analgesia and sedation.* Do not delay early analgesia for patients. Give morphine 2 to 5 mg IV (or 0.1 mg/kg IV) every 5 to 10 minutes until the patient is comfortable. Fentanyl 50 to 100 mcg IV is an alternative agent. It has less histamine release than morphine and thus causes less hypotension. If the clinical situation permits, conscious sedation should be used for painful invasive procedures such as a tube thoracostomy. See Chapter 90.1.
■ *Antibiotics.* Antibiotics are not needed for thoracostomy or thoracotomy unless there has been penetrating injury of a contaminating nature.
■ *Tetanus prophylaxis.* Give tetanus toxoid and tetanus immune globin as indicated for open wounds.

Emergency Department Interventions

■ *Endotracheal intubation.* There are no absolute indications for intubation in chest trauma other than failure to respond to resuscitation, persistent shock, a rising respiratory rate along with a rising $P\text{CO}_2$, as well as for the management of injuries outside of the chest, especially head injury (Glasgow Coma Scale [GCS] below 8). Caution should be taken in patients who require both intubation and a thoracostomy for a pneumothorax, as the positive pressure ventilation that occurs after intubation may convert a simple pneumothorax into a tension pneumothorax. If the clinical situation permits, the thoracostomy should be performed first.

■ *Occlusion of open chest wound.* Conversion of an open to closed pneumothorax or control of a sucking chest wound is accomplished by placement of an occlusive dressing, such as petroleum gauze, over the wound. Sterile 4×4 gauze is applied over the occlusive dressing and secured on three sides. This should be followed by tube thoracostomy at a separate location as soon as circumstances permit.

■ *Needle thoracostomy.* Rapid insertion of 14- or 16-gauge IV catheter through the chest wall into the pleural space is done to convert a tension pneumothorax to an open pneumothorax. The optimal site is the fifth intercostal space (ICS) in the anterior axillary line. This avoids the large bulky mass of the pectoralis muscles. The second ICS, mid-axillary line, is also commonly used. Relief of a tension pneumothorax is appreciated by a release of air and clinical improvement in the oxygen saturation as well as cardiac output. This procedure must be followed by tube thoracostomy.

■ *Tube thoracostomy.* This procedure is described in Chapter 91. Use a 24- to 28-French chest tube for simple pneumothorax but a larger tube, 32 to 40 French (24-34 French in children), for a hemothorax. The distal end of the tube should be attached to a water-seal, fluid-collection suction device, and, if possible, to an autotransfusion device for a large hemothorax. Table 13–1 lists the indications for surgery based on findings of tube thoracostomy.

■ *Pericardiocentesis.* For suspected pericardial tamponade, see Chapter 91. An emergency thoracotomy or a pericardial window is preferred to pericardiocentesis if the patient is in cardiac arrest or is rapidly deteriorating. Although tachycardia is most commonly present with tamponade, sudden bradycardia may indicate impending arrest.

Table 13–1 Indications for Surgery After Tube Thoracostomy

Massive hemothorax, >1000-1500 ml initial drainage (or 20 cc/kg)
Continued bleeding
   >300-500 mL in first hour (or 7 cc/kg/hr)
   >200 mL/h for first 3 or more hours (or 4 cc/kg/hr)
Increasing size of hemothorax on chest film
Persistent hemothorax after two functioning tubes placed
Clotted hemothorax
Large air leak preventing effective ventilation
Persistent air leak after placement of second tube or inability to expand lung fully.
Resumption of shock after the patient has been successfully resuscitated.

From Kirsch TD, Mulligan JP. Tube thoracostomy. In: Roberts JR, Hedges JR (editors). Clinical Procedures in Emergency Medicine (4th ed). St. Louis, MO: WB Saunders, 2004, pp. 187–210.

- **Thoracotomy and internal open cardiac massage.** Thoracotomy is not useful for blunt traumatic arrest, nor is it useful if the patient did not have vital signs in the field. The procedure is warranted in penetrating trauma to the chest with acute loss of vital signs (see Chapter 91).
- **Nasogastric tube.** Gastric decompression is a useful adjunct after intubation to decrease risk of aspiration of gastric contents (see Chapter 91).

Disposition

- **Consultation.** Thoracic trauma is best approached in a systematic, multidisciplinary approach and, if at all possible, managed by a joint emergency medicine and trauma surgical team.
- **Operating room.** Hemodynamically unstable patients should go as soon as possible to the operating room for a thoracotomy or laparotomy. Surgical intervention for hemostasis is listed in Table 13–1.
- **Admission.** Most patients with blunt or penetrating thoracic trauma require admission for observation and treatment of associated injuries. Patients with rib fractures who cannot breathe deeply and cough well should be admitted. These patients may benefit from an epidural catheter for pain control and pulmonary toilet. Patients with EKG abnormalities (conduction disturbance, frequent ectopy, ischemia) or a persistent tachycardia should be admitted to a monitored setting. Any patient with a chest tube will require close observation and serial chest radiographs.
- **Discharge.** A patient with *blunt* or minor penetrating trauma may be considered for discharge if there is only an isolated injury, serious pathologic conditions have been excluded, and the patient is minimally symptomatic. If the clinically stable patient has rib fractures or *penetrating* injury, discharge may be considered if there have been two chest radiographs at least 6 hours apart demonstrating no pneumothorax, hemothorax, or pulmonary contusion. The patient must be able to breathe deeply and cough, have adequate pain control, and have an adequate social situation.

Specific Problems: Pneumothorax and Hemothorax
Massive Hemothorax

- **Background.** Massive hemothorax, defined as at least 1000 ml of blood in the pleural space, or either a 20 cc/kg hemothorax drained with the first thoracostomy, or a continued bleed of 7 cc/kg/hr in the first hour, can be caused by either blunt or penetrating trauma. Rib fractures and recent chest tube placement should alert the clinician to a possible bleeding intercostal artery. Rapid accumulation may occur since each hemithorax can accommodate 40% to 50% of the circulating blood volume.
- **Pathophysiology.** Hemodynamic and respiratory collapse is due to hypovolemia from bleeding, vena caval compression causing preload reduction, and hypoxia from lung collapse. Sources of bleeding include large thoracic vessels, lung parenchyma, and intercostal and internal mammary arteries, although intra-abdominal sources should also be ruled out.
- **History.** Patients usually present in extremis, although they may complain of dyspnea and chest pain.

■ *Physical examination.* This reveals shock, tachypnea, tachycardia, shallow breaths, and decreased breath sounds with dullness to percussion on the affected side.

■ *Diagnostic testing.* The only necessary test is a type and cross match for packed cells; all other blood parameters can be measured once the patient has begun to stabilize. DO NOT obtain a chest radiograph until ABCs are secured. Chest radiographs and ultrasound studies are useful to evaluate the size and presence of a hemothorax. An upright chest radiograph is preferred since supine films may miss up to 1 L of pleural fluid. A chest CT scan does have a role in evaluation of hemothorax, but a massive hemothorax should be treated with a tube thoracostomy and surgery in any hemodynamically unstable patient rather than placing an unstable patient in the CT scanner.

■ *ED management.* Immediate drainage with tube thoracostomy is indicated, and is often followed by surgical repair. Start immediate transfusion with O-negative blood (or type-specific if it can be obtained within 15 minutes) in the hemodynamically unstable patient. An autotransfusion device should be used in these patients.

■ *Helpful hints and pitfalls.* Intra-abdominal injury may be the bleeding source, especially if a diaphragmatic injury is suggested by the clinical presentation. Although only 5% of patients with hemothorax require operative repair, recognition of the ones who do require thoracotomy must be made early to have a successful outcome.

Open Pneumothorax

■ *Background.* Penetrating trauma or crush injury to the chest wall may result in this phenomenon, also known as *sucking chest wound.* The condition occurs when the pleural space directly communicates with the outer chest wall, and there is an opening large enough to enable bypass of the patient's upper airway. When the patient inspires, the negative intrathoracic pressure pulls air preferentially into the pleural space directly, rather than into the lungs through the trachea.

■ *History.* Patients usually present in extremis, although they may complain of dyspnea, chest pain, and a gurgling sensation in their chest wall.

■ *Physical examination.* Open chest wounds should not be explored locally.

■ *Diagnostic testing.* Do not obtain a chest radiograph until the ABCs are secured. The chest radiograph will probably show a pneumothorax after the lesion is occluded.

■ *ED management.* The patient's open wound should be occluded with an air-tight adherent dressing, such as petroleum gauze. The dressing should temporarily be affixed on three, not four, sides to permit expulsion of air and prevention of a tension pneumothorax. Place a thoracostomy tube as soon as possible.

■ *Helpful hints and pitfalls.* Probing an open chest wound reveals nothing useful, and may cause rapid bleeding. An open chest wound may still act as a one-way valve with subsequent tension pneumothorax. This and the preferential passage of air into the lower pressure pleural cavity without lung inflation are the reasons that open wounds need to be covered.

Simple Pneumothorax and Simple Hemothorax

- **Background.** Blunt or penetrating injury to the lung or chest wall may permit air (pneumothorax) or blood (hemothorax) to leak into the pleural space. The presence of air or blood in the pleural space reduces pulmonary function by increasing intrathoracic pressure and decreasing vital capacity. Decreased venous return may follow. A pneumothorax secondary to trauma is most commonly due to a rib fracture that lacerates the pleura. When no rib fracture is present, it may occur when the impact is delivered during full inspiration with a closed glottis such that intra-alveolar pressure is increased and causes alveoli rupture. A *simple* pneumothorax is present when there is no communication with the atmosphere or shift in the mediastinum or hypotension as direct result of the pneumothorax. A small pneumothorax occupies less than 15% of the hemithorax, and a large pneumothorax is greater than 60%. A small pneumothorax may also be defined as <3 cm distance from the apex-to-cupola, and a large pneumothorax is defined anything larger than 3 cm. A simple hemothorax is most commonly due to injured lung parenchyma. The most common vessels involved are the intercostals and internal mammary arteries.
- **History.** Patients will likely complain of pleuritic chest pain and dyspnea.
- **Physical examination.** This may demonstrate tachypnea, shallow breathing, respiratory distress or obvious deformity. Decreased breath sounds may be appreciated on auscultation.
- **Diagnostic testing.** Apical-lordotic films and exhalation films will increase the ability to show a small pneumothorax, but may hide much other pathology, so the initial chest radiograph for a trauma patient should be with good inhalation of all lung fields. Occult pneumothorax is a small pneumothorax identified on CT scan but not plain film. On chest x-ray, there is an absence of lung markings. There may be deviation of the trachea contralaterally. For hemothoraces, blunting of the costophrenic angle on an upright chest radiograph requires at least 200 to 300 ml of fluid. A supine film is less accurate. A CT scan or ultrasound study can aid in the diagnosis. Serial chest radiographs are performed to identify progression of size.
- **ED management.** A complete evaluation for associated injuries is mandatory. It is a critical and usually a clinical distinction between a simple hemo- or pneumothorax and the much more serious tension pneumothorax and massive hemothorax (see above). Chest tube placement is generally advised for traumatic hemo- and pneumothorax. Small pneumothoraces may be observed with serial imaging unless the patient cannot be closely observed or if the patient will be intubated and placed on mechanical ventilation.
- **Helpful hints and pitfalls.** A simple traumatic pneumothorax is at risk of converting to tension pneumothorax so close monitoring is essential.

Tension Pneumothorax

- **Background.** This entity can occur with blunt or penetrating chest trauma. Positive airway pressure may convert a simple pneumothorax to a tension pneumothorax.

- *Pathophysiology.* With a rupture in the visceral or parietal pleura, there will be an equalization of atmospheric and intrapleural pressure. A one-way valve of parietal or visceral pleura or the tracheobronchial tree permits inflow but not exhalation of air from the pleural cavity, and therefore the intrapleural pressure rises. The trapped air mechanically displaces structures to the unaffected side causing disruption of venous return to the heart and function of the contralateral lung. Hypoxia, decreased cardiac output, cardiovascular collapse, and cardiac arrest will follow if the tension pneumothorax is not quickly corrected.
- *History.* The diagnosis is made clinically. This patient is typically in severe distress from pain, has a thoracic injury, and often has dyspnea and air hunger.
- *Physical examination.* Tachypnea, tachycardia, diminished breath sounds, and hyperresonnance to percussion on the affected side are all early signs. Late signs include distention of neck veins, hypotension, hypoxia, and tracheal deviation to the contralateral side.
- *Diagnostic testing.* All imaging studies should be deferred until stabilization of the patient is achieved. DO NOT obtain a chest radiograph. If there is a clinical diagnosis of a tension pneumothorax, perform an immediate needle thoracostomy (decompression) followed by chest tube placement.
- *ED management.* Immediate needle thoracostomy (decompression) is warranted followed by tube thoracostomy. Bilateral needle thoracostomies should be performed if there is any doubt as to which hemithorax is involved.
- *Helpful hints and pitfalls.* The diagnosis of a tension pneumothorax is a clinical one. After bilateral needle thoracostomies in the chest trauma victim, persistence of hypoperfusion and distended neck veins should suggest cardiac tamponade. A patient with pulseless electrical activity (PEA) may have a tension pneumothorax.

Specific Problems: Other
Blunt Aortic and Great Vessel Injury

- *Background.* Rapid deceleration injuries such as a high-speed motor vehicle crash can lead to a tear or rupture of the great vessels of the chest. The aorta tends to tear at the isthmus between the left subclavian artery and the ligamentum arteriosum. Tears in the aorta start at the intima with subsequent progression outward, allowing blood to pass between layers creating a false lumen or pseudoaneurysm. The tear can also be full thickness but this usually leads to immediate death of the patient.
- *History.* Patients may have chest pain radiating to the back. There are patients who develop symptoms from mass effect of a pseudoaneurysm or hematoma including dyspnea, stridor or dysphagia, but this is usually seen in those who have delayed presentation.
- *Physical examination.* Patients may have no outward signs of chest trauma. Tachycardia, upper extremity hypertension, discrepancy in the pulses between the upper and lower extremities, and difference of systolic blood pressure (>20 mm Hg) between upper extremities may be present.

More rarely, a bruit may be heard across the precordium or there may be focal neurologic findings that suggest an aortic dissection.

■ *Diagnostic testing.* There may be ST and T wave changes if dissection involves the coronary arteries. Chest radiograph findings suggestive of aortic injury are listed in Table 13–2 and Figure 13–1. All of these are indirect evidence of a dissection, and the patient will require a CT scan angiogram or aortogram if stable enough. The chest radiograph may have normal findings in some cases, and further imaging studies are necessary in high risk patients (i.e., rapid deceleration injuries). Transesophageal ultrasound and magnetic resonance imaging (MRI) are capable of detecting vascular injury and aortic dissection, but neither are readily available, and MRI is not prudent in an unstable trauma patient.

■ *ED management.* Patients who are hemodynamically unstable require an immediate transfusion with O-negative blood, (or type-specific blood if available within 15 minutes). After identification of the vascular injury, keep systolic blood pressure under tight control (90-120 mm Hg). Avoid over-rescusitation. Operative repair is currently the common therapy, although endovascular stenting is an emerging management technique.

■ *Helpful hints and pitfalls.* There may be loss of spinal artery flow, and it is useful to document baseline neurologic function in the trauma room.

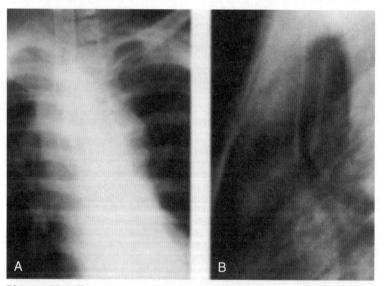

Figure 13–1. Traumatic aortic transection. **A,** Posteroanterior chest film showing widened upper mediastinum and displacement of the trachea (identified by endotracheal tube) to the right. **B,** The lateral film shows displacement and compression of the left main bronchus beyond the tip of the endotracheal tube. *(Courtesy D. J. Delany, MD.)*

Table 13–2 Chest Radiograph Findings Associated with Aortic Injury

Mediastinal width greater than 6 cm in the upright posteroanterior film, greater than 8 cm in the supine anteroposterior chest film, or greater than 7.5 cm at the aortic knob or a ratio of mediastinal width to chest width greater than 0.25 at the aortic knob

Opacification of the clear space between the aorta and pulmonary artery

Displaced nasogastric tube to the right

Widened paratracheal strip

Widened right paraspinal interface

Depression of left main stem bronchus below 40 degrees from the horizontal

Left hemothorax

Obliteration of the medial aspect of the left upper lobe apex (left apical pleural cap)

Deviation of the trachea to the right

Multiple rib fractures (fractures of the first and second ribs do not appear to be associated with increased risk compared with patients without these fractures)

Note: the chest radiograph findings may be entirely normal and further studies should be considered for patients at high risk (i.e., with a sudden deceleration mechanism of injury)

Blunt Myocardial Injury

- *Background.* This occurs with blunt trauma to the anterior chest, as in steering wheel injuries following motor vehicle crashes. It may also be seen after falls, auto–pedestrian injuries, and prolonged closed chest massage (cardiopulmonary resuscitation [CPR]). It is extremely rare for coronary artery occlusion to occur. Complications include dysrhythmia, cardiogenic shock, valve rupture, and tamponade from atrial tears.
- *History.* The mechanism of injury is helpful in suggesting this injury such as hitting the steering wheel, air bag deployment, and a lack of seat belt restraint. Patients may complain of chest pain or symptoms of shock or may be completely free of symptoms.
- *Physical examination.* One may encounter signs of chest trauma such as abrasions, contusions, flail segments or crepitance.
- *Diagnostic testing.* Serum cardiac markers may diagnose myocardial infarction but their use in diagnosing blunt cardiac injury is controversial as they offer no additional information beyond the EKG. An EKG is the best initial screening tool. A sinus tachycardia is the most common finding, but has many other etiologies. The patient may develop an acute dysrhythmia or conduction abnormalities that, in the proper clinical context, confirms the diagnosis. The only chest radiograph finding that suggests this injury is a sternal fracture, and this may only be visible on a lateral film. Echocardiography may reveal wall motion abnormalities, valve malfunction, and effusions.
- *ED management.* Associated injuries usually take precedence. Dysrhythmias are treated the same as in nontrauma patients. No prophylaxis for dysrhythmias is necessary. There is no consensus on which patients require hospital admission; therefore admission is usually based on the concomitant injuries. Even after a period of hospital observation, a small

number of patients develop late (5-7 days after trauma) deterioration and require admission to the hospital for cardiac monitoring, pain control, and hospital observation. Patients with an abnormal EKG or serum cardiac markers require admission to a monitored setting.

■ *Helpful hints and pitfalls.* Although the entity may be common, it is difficult to predict which patient will get into trouble. Most patients have a benign course. The best strategy is to concentrate on other important injuries, and monitor the patient for the appearance of dysrhythmias.

Diaphragmatic Injury

■ *Background.* Diaphragm tears can be caused by blunt or penetrating trauma although deceleration injury in a motor vehicle crash is the most common mechanism. Left-sided diaphragm injuries are more common, because the liver does exert some protection, but right-sided diaphragmatic injuries are also seen from high-speed auto crashes. Disruption of diaphragmatic integrity permits herniation of the abdominal contents into the chest because of the lower intrapleural pressure. Abdominal organs in the chest compromise breathing and circulation by encroaching on the lungs, airways, great vessels, and the heart and may interfere with the blood supply of the abdominal organ that herniates.

■ *History.* The patient may demonstrate significant respiratory distress, vomiting, or complain of chest or abdominal pain radiating to the shoulder.

■ *Physical examination.* The most helpful finding is auscultation of bowel sounds in the chest. One may also appreciate dullness to percussion of the thorax and decreased or absent breath sounds, simulating the appearance of a hemo- or pneumothorax. Either a scaphoid or distended abdomen may be observed. Patients may present in shock or sepsis, if visceral perforation has occurred.

■ *Diagnostic testing.* The EKG is not helpful but may reveal non-specific changes that can occur from a herniated organ pushing on the pericardial sac. The chest radiograph is a very useful imaging study, and may illustrate elevation of a hemidiaphragm or a bowel pattern in the chest. The findings on the plain film may be more revealing with a nasogastric tube in place (Figure 13–2). Gastrointestinal contrast studies are also very helpful, as are ultrasound, CT scan, and MRI. With right-sided tears, there may be a box-shaped mass in the right lower lobe that represents liver herniated into the chest. Thoracoscopy has been used to better visualize the diaphragm when the diagnosis is unconfirmed and laparotomy is not required.

■ *ED management.* Maintaining ventilation and oxygenation is critical because the patient may have significantly compromised ventilatory function. Nasogastric tube placement will help decompress herniating bowel and assist with the diagnosis (see above). Surgical consultation is necessary as definitive therapy requires a laparotomy.

■ *Helpful hints and pitfalls.* Because this entity may completely mimic a pneumothorax, it is prudent to sweep the pleural space with a finger before insertion of a thoracostomy tube. An intra-abdominal organ may take years to herniate; thus the patient may have mild and undiagnosed symptoms for long time before recognition.

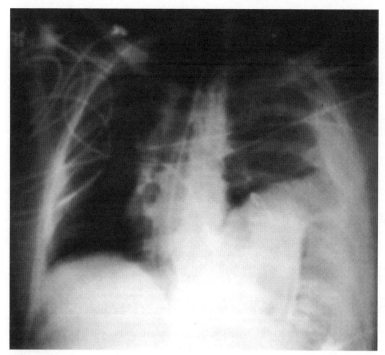

Figure 13–2. Traumatic diaphragmatic rupture. Chest radiograph in rupture of the left hemidiaphragm with apparent elevation of the hemidiaphragm, bowel herniating into the thorax, and a nasogastric tube coiled in the intrathoracic stomach. A left hemothorax is also present. *(Courtesy L. C. Morus, MD.)*

Esophageal Injury

- *Background.* This injury is only rarely seen in trauma patients due to the presence of severe concomitant injuries. This condition may also be seen in patients after foreign body ingestion, those who have esophageal stricture from any cause, and after iatrogenic injuries such as during insertion of esophageal obturator airways, Heimlich maneuvers, or esophageal stricture dilatation. Partial- or full-thickness injuries to the esophagus permit bacterial invasion and proliferation, causing mediastinitis and pneumomediastinum.
- *History.* Patients are likely to complain of chest pain, odynophagia, and dysphagia.
- *Physical examination.* The only physical finding that suggests this diagnosis is a Hamman's crunch sign, which is a crunching sound heard synchronously with the heart beat, as the heart beats against air-filled tissues.

- *Diagnostic testing.* There are no tests that reliably identify the injury. A plain chest radiograph may demonstrate mediastinal air or a pneumopericardium. A CT scan may also have normal findings and fail to demonstrate the injury unless it is a contrast scan and shows dye leakage. An esophagogram is a useful imaging study, and is usually initially performed with gastrograffin or other soluble contrast agents to avoid barium mediastinitis. Unfortunately, these agents are not as accurate as barium; therefore a barium study must often be performed to ensure the entity does not exist if the perforation has not been found with the soluble contrast agent. Esophagoscopy may be helpful but can also miss small tears in the esophagus.

- *ED management.* An effort should be made to insert a nasogastric tube, but do not persist if it will not pass. Administer broad-spectrum IV antibiotics therapy, give adequate pain control, and obtain early surgical consultation to arrange for a therapeutic thoracotomy. The earlier the mediastinitis is treated and the injury repaired, the lower the morbidity and mortality, but this is a very serious injury and often fatal even with optimal care.

- *Helpful hints and pitfalls.* Esophagoscopy and bronchoscopy may be done in concert because esophageal and tracheobronchial injuries tend to occur simultaneously.

Penetrating Injury to the Heart and Great Vessels of the Chest

- *Background.* Survival rates for this entity are actually higher than many other forms of severe chest trauma, but depend on size and location of injury, presence of tamponade, and prehospital time. Survival with meaningful neurologic recovery is rare unless the patient has vital signs in transport and on arrival to the ED.

- *History.* Information about the type and trajectory of the weapon used should be sought.

- *Physical examination.* Patients may present in respiratory distress or present with shock from hypovolemia or cardiac tamponade. Impaled objects should be removed in the operative room only. Do not probe any wounds. Signs of superior vena cava syndrome including facial edema or vascular engorgement are highly suggestive of a mediastinal hematoma. Auscultate the chest for the presence of a bruit that suggests a false aneurysm or fistula.

- *Diagnostic testing.* Obtain an ABG, hemoglobin, and type and screen. Commence immediate transfusion with O-negative blood (or type-specific blood if available within 15 minutes). The pericardium is not distensible with an acute effusion so the cardiac silhouette on chest radiograph may appear normal in acute cardiac tamponade. A large hemothorax or a central wound may indicate large vessel injury. Ultrasound may be useful to identify pericardial fluid and tamponade physiology.

- *ED management.* Firm, direct pressure on arterial bleeding is necessary. Reversal of hypotension with fluid resuscitation may be lifesaving, but definitive care is operative hemostasis.

- *Helpful hints and pitfalls.* The chest tube output may indicate injury that requires operative identification and repair. See Table 13–1.

Pulmonary Contusion

- *Background.* Although usually seen with blunt thoracic trauma, pulmonary contusion can occur around the path of a high-velocity missile. A pulmonary contusion is blunt damage to lung parenchyma without laceration, usually caused by a compression-decompression–type insult. Subsequently associated edema, inflammation, and hemorrhage cause a drop in pulmonary compliance. This may make the lung more likely to retain resuscitation fluids and develop a form of noncardiogenic pulmonary edema called *shock lung* or *congestive atelectasis.*
- *History.* The lung damage follows a history of blunt trauma, most commonly a motor vehicle collision or fall. Patients may complain of chest pain, dyspnea, or hemoptysis.
- *Physical examination.* This can be entirely normal, but also may reveal tachypnea, crackles, rhonchi, wheezes, or signs of respiratory distress.
- *Diagnostic testing.* The main utility of the laboratory is to follow the PCO_2; as this rises, it may indicate a failing ventilatory capacity that requires intubation, ventilation, and positive end-expiratory pressure (PEEP) support. A chest radiograph may reveal an area of opacification in various segments of the lung. Contusion occurs immediately but appreciation on plain film may be delayed by as much as 6 hours from the trauma. Moreover, there is no correlation between pulmonary dysfunction and the appearance of the chest radiograph. A chest CT scan can reveal changes much earlier than plain films, but also does not indicate pulmonary function.
- *ED management.* Treatment goals are maintenance of oxygenation and ventilation, and intervention with intubation, ventilation, and PEEP support if the patient shows a rising respiratory rate or PCO_2. These patients often have other critical injuries that must be aggressively identified and managed.
- *Helpful hints and pitfalls.* Aggressive hemodynamic monitoring is required in patients with any significant pulmonary contusion. Ventilatory support is improved by using high-frequency oscillation if available.

Rib Fractures and Flail Chest

- *Background.* Rib fractures occur commonly in patients with a moderate to severe mechanism of blunt trauma. Advanced age and osteoporosis increase the risk of fracture. Pain from rib fractures causes splinting and shallow breathing, which may lead to the development of atelectasis and subsequent pneumonia. A fractured rib can penetrate the lung or lacerate an intercostal artery causing a hemothorax or pneumothorax. Other significant complications include tension pneumothorax, massive hemothorax, pulmonary contusion, and major vascular injury. A segment of unstable chest wall may develop due to a double fracture (anterior and posterior) of two or more contiguous ribs. This results in paradoxical motion of the segment during respiration, called a *flail chest.*
- *History.* Usually a history of blunt thoracic trauma is provided but abdominal complaints are possible as well. Dyspnea and pleuritic chest pain are expected.

- **Physical examination.** This may reveal tachypnea, shallow breathing, respiratory distress, or obvious deformity. Rib fractures should be suspected with any focal tenderness of the chest wall.
- **Diagnostic testing.** An ABG may be necessary in some patients to determine if ventilation is adequate. The chest radiograph is the most common imaging study used to identify rib fractures, but is not always accurate. More fractures and associated complications can be seen on CT scan, but this is rarely needed to treat the patient with one or two fractured ribs. Dedicated rib radiograph series including oblique views may reveal additional fractures but usually do not change management and are rarely necessary.
- **ED management.** Pain control is the mainstay of treatment for rib fractures and flail chest. The goal of analgesia is to permit deep breathing and coughing. In some circumstances patient-controlled analgesia (PCA) or epidural analgesia may be required. Patients with co-morbid pulmonary disease may require more aggressive care, including ventilatory support. Identification of associated injuries is imperative, and subsequent imaging with CT scan of the chest is common. The patient with one or two rib fractures can be well managed with posterior intercostal blockade. If the patient is elderly, has co-morbid lung disease, has three or more fractures, or poor social circumstances, admission to the hospital will be necessary. Many patients with flail chest require no more than pain control, and their management is more dependent upon the ventilatory impact of the underlying pulmonary contusion, than with injury to the chest wall. It is useful to monitor respiratory rate and Pco_2. If these begin to rise, the patient will need active airway management and ventilatory support.
- **Helpful hints and pitfalls.** If there is clinical probability of a rib fracture, the diagnosis should be assumed and treated as such even if not seen on chest radiograph. Patients with first and second rib fractures frequently have poor outcomes from associated cardiovascular injury and bronchial tears. It requires a large amount of energy to fracture these protected ribs. Sternal fracture is also a marker of serious and life-threatening injury. The sternal fracture itself usually only requires analgesia, but the underlying myocardial contusion may produce clinical problems.

Tracheobronchial Injury

- **Background.** Blunt trauma with a rapid deceleration causes most of these injuries. The trauma produces partial or complete laceration of the intrathoracic or cervical trachea or the bronchial wall. This allows an abnormal communication between the airway and the mediastinum, soft tissue, and lung. Complications include chronic bronchopleural fistula, atelectasis, pneumothorax, and infection, including mediastinitis.
- **History.** Patients generally present with dyspnea, cough, and hemoptysis although the patient may be asymptomatic.
- **Physical examination.** Respiratory distress, tachypnea and subcutaneous emphysema are expected, and depending on the level of tracheal injury, may produce intermittent swelling of the neck with respiration. The

patient may display Hamman's sign, which is a crunching sound heard over the heart suggesting mediastinal air.

■ *Diagnostic testing.* Serial ABGs may give an early clue to diagnosis by identifying ventilatory failure. Persistent or large air leaks in a chest tube suggest tracheobronchial injury. The initial imaging study is usually a plain chest radiograph, which often shows a pneumothorax or pneumo-mediastinum, gas in soft tissue, or hyoid bone elevation (indicating tracheal transection.) A CT scan provides much more detail but may still miss small tears. In many patients, the injury becomes apparent only after tube thoracostomy fails to treat the pneumothorax, and the lung stays collapsed. The injury may be visualized by rigid or fiber optic bronchoscopy or seen on the CT scan. It cannot be directly visualized with a plain chest radiograph.

■ *ED management.* Aggressive airway management and ensuring adequate ventilation are necessary because the cause of death from this lesion is often airway obstruction with respiratory failure. High-frequency oscillatory ventilation may be helpful, especially if the site of the tear can be bypassed with an endotracheal tube, but many tears (over one third of the circumference) will require surgical repair.

■ *Helpful hints and pitfalls.* Look for this injury when the lung does not reexpand even with suction to the thoracostomy tube.

Traumatic Cardiac Tamponade

■ *Background.* Although much more common with penetrating injuries, tamponade can be seen after blunt injury as well. Blood accumulates in the pericardial sac and causes diminished venous return to the heart and poor cardiac output. Because traumatic tamponade, as opposed to uremic or viral pericarditic tamponade, is acute, the pericardium cannot hold as much volume before the patient gets into trouble.

■ *History.* Patients with acute cardiac tamponade are usually in extremis. They may complain of dyspnea, dizziness, chest pain, confusion, and a sense of impending doom.

■ *Physical examination.* Classically these patients present with Beck's triad of distended neck veins, hypotension, and muffled heart tones; however, the hypovolemia often seen in patients with penetrating chest trauma will obscure the jugular venous distention. Pulsus paradoxus (a drop of systolic blood pressure by more than 10-15 mm Hg with inspiration) or a Kussmaul sign (increased jugular venous distention with inspiration) may or may not be present.

■ *Diagnostic testing.* All such testing should be deferred until stabilization of the patient is ensured. An EKG may show tachycardia and electrical alternans, a phenomenon with alternating QRS voltage size from the heart moving in pericardial fluid; however, if tamponade is suspected, time to obtain an EKG should not be taken. A bedside ultrasound study will show pericardial fluid and collapsing atria and ventricles (see Chapter 93). Chest radiograph findings are likely to be normal and merely waste time because the pericardium is poorly compliant with an acute effusion.

- **ED management.** A pericardiocentesis or pericardial window can be lifesaving. An ED thoracotomy is indicated for patients with tamponade who are on the verge of cardiac arrest.
- **Helpful hints and pitfalls.** A positive response to pericardiocentesis is usually accompanied by return of about 10 to 20 ml of blood, but may be lifesaving after only 1or 2 ml. If larger quantities of blood are easily withdrawn it usually indicates aspiration from a ventricle.

Teaching Points

Thoracic trauma is common and often serious. In a stable patient, a chest radiograph may be the most helpful imaging study to establish the degree of injury and need for a procedure; however, in patients who are on the verge of cardiac arrest, specifically the patient with cardiac tamponade or tension pneumothorax, an aggressive effort to diminish the abnormal pleural or pericardial pressures must be made before confirmation with a radiologic study.

Whatever the pathology, the patient needs to be watched carefully for a rising respiratory rate, which is often a signal that there is a rising P_{CO_2} and a falling O_2 saturation. These patients need emergency active airway management.

In the presence of a pneumothorax, a tube thoracostomy should be placed simultaneously with or before intubation to prevent the development of a tension pneumothorax.

Suggested Readings

Branney SW, Moore EE, Feldhaus KM, Wolfe RE. Critical analysis of two decades of experience with postinjury emergency department thoracotomy in a regional trauma center. J Trauma 1998;45:87–94.

Calhoon JH, Grover FL, Trinkle JK. Chest trauma: approach and management. Clin Chest Med 1992;13:55–67.

Eckstein M, Henderson S. Thoracic trauma. In: Marx JA, Hockberger RS, Walls RM (editors). Rosen's Emergency Medicine: Concepts and Clinical Practice (6th ed). Philadelphia: Mosby, 2006, pp 453–488.

Holmes JF, Sokolove PE, Brant WE, Kuppermann N. A clinical decision rule for identifying children with thoracic injuries after blunt torso trauma. Ann Emerg Med 2002;39:492–499

Kirsch TD, Mulligan JP. Tube thoracostomy. In: Roberts JR, Hedges JR (editors). Clinical Procedures in Emergency Medicine (4th ed). St Louis, MO: WB Saunders, 2004,187–210.

Mansour KA (editor). Trauma to the diaphragm. Chest Surg Clin N Am 1997;7:373–383.

Sybrandy KC, Cramer MJ, Burgersdijk C. Diagnosing cardiac contusion: old wisdom and new insights. Heart 2003;89:485–489.

CHAPTER 14

Abdominal Trauma

JAMES A. NELSON ■ MICHAEL BARR ■ PETER WITUCKI

Red Flags

Hemodynamic instability ● Seat belt sign ● Shoulder pain ● Abdominal pain ● Pregnancy

Overview

Abdominal trauma includes multiple potential injuries with a variety of presentations. Look for "red flags" (see Box). Serious organ injury can present with minimal findings on physical examination. The diagnosis rests heavily on the astute clinician's ability to anticipate risk based on mechanism, as well as the appropriate use of advanced imaging studies. This is especially important in the patient with an altered level of consciousness or competing pain from another injury.

Injury to intra-abdominal structures can very quickly become life-threatening. The prompt diagnosis and management of these injuries must often take priority over traumatic injuries to other parts of the body.

Initial Diagnostic Approach
General

- All trauma patients must initially be assessed using the basic ABC (*a*irway, *b*reathing, and *c*irculation) approach as discussed in Chapter 8.
- Inquire about the mechanism of injury. For penetrating injuries, ask about the type of instrument, distance of the victim from the instrument, time of injury, number of shots or stab wounds, and blood loss at the scene. The prehospital course should also be obtained (vital signs and resuscitative measures).

Laboratory

- Studies may include a complete blood count (CBC), chemistry panel, coagulation panel, lipase, liver function tests (LFTs) and urinalysis. A urine pregnancy test should be performed on all females of reproductive age. Type and screen stable patients. Type and cross match unstable or potentially unstable patients. An alcohol and drug screen can be sent for patients who are altered.

■ Laboratory studies may be helpful but are not substitutes for good clinical assessments. For example, a hematocrit on these patients can provide a baseline value but may not be reflective of the degree of acute hemorrhage. Patients with pancreatic injury may have a normal lipase level. Likewise, an elevation of lipase in a patient with an abdominal injury may be due to other causes. Liver enzymes may be elevated from hepatic trauma but may be reflective of underlying liver disease. A metabolic acidosis in the setting of trauma is concerning for hemorrhagic shock, although normal values do not exclude abdominal injury.

Radiography

■ Hemodynamic stabilization takes precedence over any imaging studies.

■ *Plain films.* These may reveal free intraperitoneal air, which is indicative of hollow-organ injury (i.e., bowel perforation); however, free air is more readily seen on CT than plain films. Foreign bodies and missiles can also be identified. All entrance and exit wounds should be marked.

■ *Computed tomography (CT scan) of the abdomen and pelvis.* A CT scan is noninvasive but requires a hemodynamically stable patient. It can reveal intraperitoneal pathology, retroperitoneal injury, the source of intra-abdominal hemorrhage, and, occasionally, active bleeding. A CT scan can aid in evaluating the vertebral column and can be extended to visualize the thorax and pelvis. One advantage of the CT scan is the reduction of nontherapeutic laparotomies for self-limited injuries to the liver and spleen. Unfortunately, the CT scan is not accurate enough to detect injury to the pancreas, diaphragm, small bowel, and mesentery. Oral contrast is not used because the delay is potentially harmful, but IV contrast is essential to increase the ability of CT scans to identify hemorrhage.

■ *Ultrasound (US).* Ultrasonography has a primary role of detecting free intra-abdominal fluid and pericardial tamponade (see Chapter 93). It can show as little as 100 ml of intraperitoneal fluid. It can be rapidly performed at the bedside. However, it is not considered adequate to rule out solid-organ damage or injury to the retroperitoneum, bowel, or diaphragm. It is operator-dependent, and is not accurate in distinguishing blood from other intraperitoneal fluids such as ascites.

■ *Magnetic resonance imaging (MRI).* There is no role for MRI in the diagnosis of abdominal trauma, and its use is typically reserved for spinal injuries as well as difficult to diagnose diaphragmatic injuries (not acutely).

■ *Angiography.* This is typically reserved for the unstable patient with a pelvic fracture or splenic injury. It may also be used to further evaluate a patient in the setting of renal trauma when a vascular pedicle injury is suspected.

Diagnostic Peritoneal Lavage

■ In blunt trauma, diagnostic peritoneal lavage (DPL) is primarily indicated in the hemodynamically unstable patient who has multiple injuries.

A DPL can also better discern solid and hollow visceral injury better than US. A DPL can also be used in the diagnostic workup of a stab wound to the abdomen, lower chest, flank, or back to reveal intraperitoneal organ injury or an isolated diaphragmatic rupture. The procedure is described in Chapter 91.

- In blunt trauma and stab wounds to the anterior abdomen, flank, and back, a positive result consists of the following: aspiration of 10 ml or more of gross blood, >100,000 red blood cells (RBCs)/mm^3.
- For lower chest stab wound and gunshot wounds, the cutoff is 5,000 RBC/mm^3.
- Patients with equivocal findings should be observed for at least 24 hours. Many injuries will be from hollow viscera, and clinical manifestations should develop within that period.
- Elevated levels of peritoneal amylase may be indicative of small bowel or pancreatic injury. Other positive but less commonly documented DPL results include a positive Gram stain for food fibers or bacteria as well as the presence of fecal matter.

Emergency Department Management Overview
General

- The ABCs should be addressed. Establish two large-bore IV lines, place the patient on a monitor, and give supplementary oxygen to any patient who is being evaluated after major trauma to maintain the oxygen saturation >95%.

Medications

- *Analgesia.* Pain relief is appropriate for most injuries. Morphine sulfate 2 to 5 mg or 0.1 mg/kg IV is commonly used. Fentanyl 50 to 100 mcg IV is an alternative agent. It has less histamine release than morphine and thus causes less hypotension. Avoid medications with antiplatelet activity potential such as nonsteroidal anti-inflammatory drugs (NSAIDs).
- *Antibiotics.* Anaerobes and coliforms are the predominant organisms found in cases of intestinal perforation, and antibiotics active against these organisms should be given to decrease the incidence of intra-abdominal sepsis.

Emergency Department Interventions

- *Urinary catheter.* A Foley catheter should be inserted to monitor urine output in all patients with major trauma.
- *Wound care.* Cover any penetrating wound or eviscerations with a sterile dressing moistened with normal saline.

Disposition

- *Consultation.* A trauma surgeon should be consulted for any patient suspected of having a traumatic abdominal injury. The patient should be transferred to another facility if a trauma surgeon is unavailable.

- **Admission.** All patients with intra-abdominal injuries require admission for an emergent surgery or for observation. Patients with stab wounds that are found to be superficial to the abdominal cavity after wound exploration may be discharged to home.
- **Discharge.** Stable and reliable patients with no identifiable injury can be discharged to home.

Specific Problems: Blunt Abdominal Trauma

- **Background.** Blunt abdominal trauma carries greater morbidity and mortality than penetrating trauma because the injuries are often occult and more difficult to diagnose, and these injuries are often associated with significant trauma to other organ systems (i.e., head injuries). Motor vehicle crashes and auto–pedestrian collisions are the most common causes of blunt abdominal trauma accounting for approximately 50% to 75% of cases. The spleen is the most commonly damaged solid organ, followed by the liver and then the intestines. Splenic injury should be considered even with relatively minor trauma to the left upper quadrant or left costal margin, especially if the patient has a history of splenomegaly due to underlying disease. Traumatic pancreatic injuries often occur with duodenal injuries. The mechanism usually involves compression of this organ against the vertebral column.
- **Clinical presentation.** The seatbelt sign (contusion or abrasion across the lower abdomen) is found in fewer than one third of patients with abdominal injuries caused by solitary lap belts, but its presence is highly correlated with intraperitoneal pathology. Patients with splenic injuries often have left upper quadrant pain and occasionally pain in the left shoulder (Kehr's sign). Patients with hepatic injuries can have signs and symptoms ranging from hypotension to pain in the right upper quadrant to complete absence of symptoms at the time of presentation. Patients with hollow organ injuries often have nonspecific abdominal pain, and may have a blunt trauma mechanism that raises the possibility (e.g., a handlebar impalement or trauma from a seat belt).
- **Diagnostic testing.** For hepatic and splenic trauma, a CT scan with IV contrast is the best imaging modality for the identification of most injuries (Figures 14–1 and 14–2). Bedside ultrasound is useful in finding nonspecific free fluid in the abdomen in patients too unstable to travel to the CT scanner. Injuries to the bowel can sometimes be difficult to diagnose. A CT scan with IV contrast is the imaging modality of choice, but often has normal findings initially. The CT scan findings indicative of bowel injury include bowel edema, intraperitoneal free air gas, and abdominal free fluid in the absence of any solid organ injury. These findings often appear on repeated imaging in 12-24 hours. A US is usually not helpful, but may show nonspecific free fluid. An upright chest radiograph rarely shows free air under the diaphragm, and abdominal plain radiographs may show retroperitoneal air. A DPL may aid in the diagnosis. Pancreatic injuries are difficult to diagnose. Serum amylase levels may be elevated suggesting pancreatic injury, but this test is neither sensitive nor specific. A normal value does not rule out injury, as the

Free perihepatic fluid. Note how the fluid wraps
around the liver with a concave configuration.

Jagged low density
areas represent
lacerations of the
hepatic parenchyma

Free intraperitoneal
fluid collecting in
the hepatorenal
recess

Subcapsular hematoma
from recent blunt trauma.
Note how this fluid
collection has a convex
margin with the liver as
if it were pushing into
the liver parenchyma.

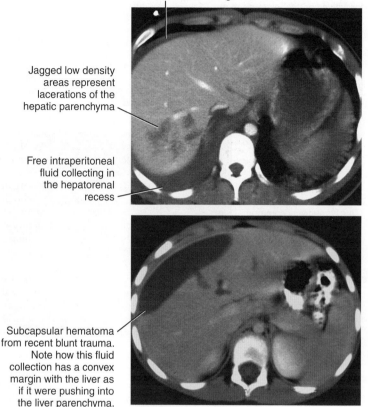

Figure 14–1. **A,** Liver laceration. **B,** Subcapsular hematoma. *(Courtesy Jason Scott Stephens, MD, The University of Texas Southwestern, Department of Radiology.)*

amylase level is only elevated 70% of the time in pancreatic injuries. A normal serum lipase does not rule out pancreatic injury. A CT scan with IV contrast is the imaging study of choice, but may be normal initially.

■ *ED management.* Some liver injuries can be managed nonoperatively; however hemodynamic instability mandates laparotomy. Management of these injuries in the ED involves hemodynamic support, surgical consultation, and admission to the hospital. Patients who are hemodynamically unstable, show a persistent drop in serial hematocrit despite transfusion, have progression of pain, or CT scan evidence of persistent bleeding require laparotomy. Persistent bleeding in a patient with a splenic injury may suggest that the patient is a candidate for angiography.

Contrast within the splenic artery. It is important to search for active contrast extravasation which indicates active bleeding during the time of scanning. Extravasation will typically appear as an irregular shaped area of high density (equal to the density of the aorta) within the perisplenic hematoma. This generally requires immediate embolization or surgery.

Splenic laceration appears as a jagged low density area within the spleen. The term splenic fracture is reserved for when a deep laceration extends from the splenic hilum to the outer capsule. Subcapsular hematomas can also occur and will appear as a fluid collection adjacent to the spleen and causing compression and flattening of the spleen. Also note delayed hemorrhage is not uncommon.

Contrast collecting within the gallbladder. This is relatively common and is a normal finding.

Perihepatic free fluid (hematoma). This patient also had a liver laceration which is not shown.

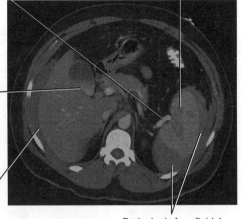

Perisplenic free fluid. In this case it represents, hematoma which will generally have a density measurement greater than 30 HU.

Figure 14–2. Splenic laceration with hemoperitoneum. *(Courtesy Jason Scott Stephens, MD, The University of Texas Southwestern, Department of Radiology.)*

Prophylactic antibiotics should be given for suspected or confirmed injuries to the bowel and should cover coliforms and anaerobes. Suspected pancreatic injuries should be managed with serial examinations, surgical consultation, repeat CT scanning and serial lipase levels.

Refer to Chapter 15, "Genitourinary Trauma" for a discussion on renal injury.

Refer to Chapter 13, "Chest Trauma" for diaphragmatic rupture.

Specific Problems: Penetrating Abdominal Trauma

- *Background.* Penetrating abdominal trauma is usually the result of a gunshot wound (GSW) or a stab wound, but may involve any sharp object or projectile. Stab wounds are three times more common than GSWs, but the latter cause more fatalities. This is because GSWs usually have a longer trajectory through the abdominal cavity and exhibit greater kinetic energy than stab wounds. Any penetrating trauma is much more likely to involve vascular structures than blunt trauma. Due to the high-energy nature of GSW injuries, certain considerations must be taken into account. First, the wound tract can be deceptive. There is always some blast effect and the dissipation of kinetic energy can damage structures that were not in direct contact with the missile. Second, due to the force of the missile, the wound tract can actually close in on itself and lead to an inaccurate assessment of tissue damage when evaluating the path of injury. The most frequently injured organ after a GSW is the small bowel, followed by the colon and then the liver. Stab wounds of the abdomen occur most commonly in the upper quadrants, the left more than the right.
- *Clinical presentation.* A thorough examination of these patients is critical because the wounds may be small and well hidden in body recesses and under fat folds. Remember to examine all skin surfaces of the abdominal wall, back, buttocks, perineum, and axilla.

Gunshot Wounds: High Energy

- *Diagnostic testing.* In stable patients, time may be taken to obtain imaging studies. Abdominal and chest radiographs (using a radiopaque marker to indentify entry and exit wounds) may be useful to identify the location of the bullet fragment, especially if no exit wound is found on examination. Radiologic studies are also necessary to identify spinal or pelvic fractures. A CT scan with IV contrast may be useful to identify the path of the bullet and any involved organs in the hemodynamically stable patient.
- *ED Management.* As a general rule, all gunshot wounds to the anterior abdomen, thoraco-abdomen, back, and flanks require surgical exploration. Most surgeons advocate immediate surgery for all patients who have sustained penetrating abdominal trauma from a high-velocity projectile. ED management involves ABCs, thorough examination to identify all wounds, hemodynamic support, and immediate surgical consultation. Prophylactic antibiotics should be given to cover anaerobes and coliforms.

Stab Wounds: Low Velocity

- *Diagnostic studies.* A chest radiograph is indicated to evaluate for thoracic involvement (pneumo- or hemothorax) or bowel penetration. A CT scan with IV contrast is useful in the hemodynamically stable patient if examination of the wound suggests underlying organ injury, or if the wound tract cannot be fully evaluated. An ultrasound is useful to confirm free fluid (blood) in the abdominal cavity. Angiography can be used to further evaluate organ injury and has the added benefit of therapeutic embolization if active bleeding is found.

- ***ED management.*** Patients who have an abdominal stab wound, and who are hemodynamically unstable or have clinical evidence of peritonitis require immediate surgery. However, in the absence of these findings, the wound may be locally explored in the ED to assess depth and possible extension into the peritoneal cavity. Approximatily 30% of anterior abdominal stab wounds do not penetrate the abdominal cavity. Prophylactic antibiotics should be given to cover anaerobes and coliforms if there is peritoneal penetration.

Special Considerations
Pediatrics

- For the most part, all of the preceding principles apply to children and adults. However, young children have a slightly different anatomy that predisposes them to certain injuries. The anteroposterior abdominal distance is usually smaller and the rib cage is more compliant than in adults, resulting in less force being required to compress the abdominal organs against the vertebral column.
- Young children who are preverbal or very anxious and uncooperative are much more difficult to assess and examine. Early surgical consultation is advocated in this population.
- Remember that nonaccidental trauma is a common cause of abdominal trauma.

Women and Pregnancy

- The pregnant trauma patient has an additional organ that must be considered with abdominal trauma, namely the gravid uterus. The most common complication of severe blunt abdominal trauma is placental abruption. This is very common, even with a very minor mechanism of injury in the third trimester, less so in the second, and virtually absent in the first trimester. Signs of abruption include uterine tenderness, contractions, vaginal bleeding, or leakage of amniotic fluid.
- Obstetric consultation is advised for pregnant patients with abdominal trauma especially if the pregnancy is viable (after 20 weeks). An ultrasound is used to document normal fetal movement and heart rate. The Kleihauer-Betke (KB) test is used to determine the presence of fetal blood in the maternal circulation of an Rh-negative patient with significant trauma. Routine use is not indicated in the ED, and obstetrical consultation should be sought.

Teaching Points

Abdominal trauma is very common, but often missed because other injuries distract attention from the abdomen. The delay in the development of signs and symptoms further confounds the ability to identify problems. Moreover, the bulk of injuries are seen in healthy young men whose compensatory capacities are high.

An objective evaluation of the abdomen is often necessary with ultrasound or diagnostic peritoneal lavage followed by imaging studies dependent on the patient's stability.

Penetrating injuries, especially high-velocity gunshot wounds, carry an almost 98% chance of internal injury, so virtually all of these patients will require laparotomy.

Blunt injuries are harder to recognize, but can sometimes be managed with less invasive care, reserving laparotomy for patients who cannot be stabilized, who destabilize after initial resuscitation, or who reveal features of hollow viscus damage.

Suggested Readings

American College of Surgeons, Committee on Trauma. Advanced Trauma Life Support Manual. Chicago: American College of Surgeons; 1997.

Marx, JA, Isenhour J. Abdominal trauma. In: Marx JA, Hockberger RS, Walls RM (editors). Rosen's Emergency Medicine: Concepts and Clinical Practice (6th ed). Philadelphia: Mosby, 2006, pp 489–514.

Richardson JD. Changes in the management of injuries to the liver and spleen. J Am Coll Surg 2005;200:648–669.

Sikka R. Unsuspected internal organ traumatic injuries. Emerg Med Clin North Am 2004;22:1067–1080.

Todd SR. Critical concepts in abdominal injury. Crit Care Clin 2004;20:119–134.

Udeani, J. Abdominal trauma, blunt. emedicine.com, 2004. eMedicine journal. Available at *http://www.emedicine.com/med/topic2804.htm*. Accessed May 21, 2005.

CHAPTER 15

Genitourinary Trauma

Raj J. Patel ▪ Juan Reynoso ▪ Gary M. Vilke

Red Flags

Flank, abdominal, rib, back, or scrotal pain ● Unable to void spontaneously ● Hemodynamic instability (tachycardia or hypotension) ● Gross hematuria or blood at the urethral meatus or vaginal introitus ● Perineal ecchymosis ● High riding prostate ● Pelvic fracture

Overview

Most genitourinary (GU) injuries occur from blunt force. Most genitourinary trauma is not immediately life-threatening. Look for "red flags" (see Box) when assessing these patients. The exceptions include renal vein laceration or a shattered kidney. Renal artery avulsions, intimal tears, and renal venous injuries are also significant injuries. Renal pedicle injuries (these include the major renal vessels and ureter) have a low kidney salvage rate but only account for 1% to 2% of all renal injuries.

Injuries to the upper tract (kidneys and ureters) require a high degree of force. Upper tract injuries often have a more subtle presentation and are associated with other nonurologic injuries, some of which may be life-threatening. Hematuria is the most common sign of renal trauma, but its presence does not correlate directly with the degree of injury. Hematuria is not a reliable indicator for ureteral injury. Blunt injury to the renovascular pedicle or penetrating ureteral injury may not produce gross or even microscopic hematuria.

Injuries to the lower tract (bladder and urethral injury) and external genitalia result from a more localized, less forceful mechanism. Most significant lower urinary tract injuries will be accompanied by either the presence of a pelvic fracture or blood at the urethral meatus. Most patients with a bladder laceration have gross hematuria. However, gunshot wounds to the bladder often result in microscopic hematuria.

Initial Diagnostic Approach
General

- All trauma patients must initially be assessed using the basic ABC (*a*irway, *b*reathing, and *c*irculation) approach as discussed in chapter 8.
- The diagnostic evaluation is always done in a retrograde fashion by first ruling out any lower tract injuries (urethral injury before bladder injury) before upper tract injuries (ureteral or renal injury) in the stable patient. Nevertheless, there is a good correlation with where the trauma was sustained on the body (i.e., blows to the flank or upper abdomen will be associated with renal injuries, while pelvic trauma is more likely to involve the urethra or bladder).
- The secondary survey should evaluate for pelvic fracture (Chapter 16), blood at the urethral meatus, or gross hematuria that will identify all significant lower urinary tract injuries. The presence of flank, abdominal, rib, back, or scrotal pain and inability to void should be assessed. Abdominal tenderness, especially in the presence of a pelvic fracture, suggests a bladder rupture in addition to other intra-abdominal injuries. Any hematoma or ecchymosis of the penile shaft, scrotal skin, or perineum should be identified. Blood at the vaginal introitus, especially in the presence of a pelvic fracture, should be evaluated with a thorough vaginal examination to look for vaginal lacerations or possible urethral injury.
- Gross blood at the urethral meatus is diagnostic of a urethral injury and dictates the need for early retrograde urethrography, which can be performed in the operating room in situations requiring emergent surgical exploration for life-threatening injuries.
- A Foley catheter should preferably not be introduced when there is suspected urethral trauma without first evaluating urethral integrity by retrograde urethrography to avoid converting a partial urethral tear into a complete disruption.
- Unlike male urethral injuries, urethrography is not helpful in suspected female urethral injuries because of the urethra's short length. Successful passage of a Foley catheter in a patient with blood at the vaginal introitus does not exclude urethral injury. Difficulty passing the Foley catheter may be concerning for a urethral injury.
- Rectal examination evaluates sphincter tone, bowel wall integrity, and most important, the position of the prostate, which is normally palpable and well defined. A pelvic fracture may cause a large pelvic hematoma that can displace the prostate superiorly, resulting in a boggy, ill-defined mass on rectal examination. A "high riding" or "nonpalpable" prostate may be concerning for a urethral injury. However, this examination finding is often unreliable, as a result of examiner inexperience or the presence of a tense pelvic hematoma, which can blur the tissue planes and make palpation difficult (especially in young men with small prostates).

Laboratory

- Hematuria is the best indicator of traumatic injury to the urinary system. Microscopic hematuria (more than five red blood cells per high-power field), heme-positive urine dipstick, and gross hematuria are the strongest indicators of genitourinary injury. However, the degree of hematuria does not necessarily correlate with degree of injury. Furthermore, blunt injury to the renovascular pedicle or penetrating ureteral injury may not produce gross or even microscopic hematuria.

■ The best urine sample for assessment of hematuria in the trauma patient is the first voided or catheterized specimen, because a later sample can often be diluted by diuresis. Other studies include a baseline hematocrit and creatinine, as well as a urine pregnancy test in all women of reproductive age.

Radiography

■ *Retrograde urethrogram (RUG).* This study is indicated in any suspected urethral injury. The procedure should be performed at a 30-degree oblique angle from the horizontal. The contrast is retrogradely injected into the urethra using a special catheter to occlude the urethral orifice to prevent reflux of contrast. Static images are then obtained. Dynamic images using fluoroscopy are preferred.

■ *Cystogram.* This study is indicated in any suspected bladder injury. A Foley catheter can be placed directly into the bladder, the urine drained, and the bladder refilled with contrast material. It is important to fully distend the bladder to avoid missing small injuries. Images are then obtained as described under RUG.

■ *Ultrasound.* This imaging study can rapidly outline kidney parenchyma and provide evidence of intraperitoneal fluid.

■ *Computed tomography (CT scan).* The diagnostic test of choice for GU trauma is a CT scan, but only if the patient is stable enough to be able to tolerate the study.

■ *Arteriogram.* This study is needed if the mechanism suggests a renal artery injury since it can provide detailed information regarding vascular injury.

■ *Intravenous pyelogram (IVP).* This study was formerly the only means to study the upper GU tract, but today is less commonly used.

Emergency Department Management Overview
General

■ The ABCs (*a*irway, *b*reathing, and *c*irculation) should be addressed. Establish two large-bore IV lines, place the patient on a monitor, and give supplementary oxygen to any patient who is being evaluated after major trauma to maintain the oxygen saturation > 95%.

Medications

■ *Analgesia.* Pain relief is appropriate for most injuries. Morphine sulfate at a dose of 2 to 5 mg IV or 0.1 mg/kg IV is useful in most patients. Fentanyl 50 to 100 mcg IV is an alternative agent. It has less histamine release than morphine, and thus causes less hypotension. Avoid medications with anti-platelet activity potential such as nonsteroidal anti-inflammatory drugs (NSAIDS) if there is any concern for further bleeding.

■ *Antibiotics.* Use broad-spectrum coverage to include anaerobic bacteria for all cases of penetrating trauma and possible bowel injuries.

Emergency Department Interventions

■ *Urinary catheter.* To avoid complicating a urethral injury, do not place a Foley catheter in patients who have gross blood at the urethral meatus or a high-riding, nonpalpable prostate gland on rectal examination.

Disposition

■ *Consultation.* Other than for microscopic hematuria, it will be prudent to consult with a urologist for other GU tract injuries.
■ *Admission.* Most patients with significant genitourinary trauma will require hospital admission. If microscopic hematuria is the only GU finding, and this is not a case of gun shot wound penetration of the abdomen, the patient can be safely observed as an outpatient.
■ *Discharge.* Stable and reliable patients with no identifiable injury can be discharged home. Patients with microscopic hematuria should have a repeat urinalysis in 1 to 2 weeks to identify any potentially missed injury. Patients who develop gross hematuria at home after discharge, should return to the emergency department (ED) for reevaluation.

Specific Problems
Upper Tract
Blunt Renal Trauma

■ *Background.* Of renal injuries in the United States, 80% are a result of blunt trauma. Renal injuries typically are caused by a significant blunt force such as motor vehicle crashes.
■ *Clinical presentation.* Clues to suspected renal injury include abdominal pain and tenderness over the kidney, denoting significant force transfer. There may be a large flank ecchymosis, palpable mass, or hematoma. Unfortunately, it is possible to have significant injury without any physical findings.
■ *Diagnostic testing.* Obtain a urinalysis, complete blood count, and chemistry panel to assess for hematuria and a baseline hematocrit and renal function. The CT scan is the imaging study of choice because it can also evaluate for other abdominal injuries. Intravenous urography is rarely used any more; it has no role in the unstable patient; but may rarely still be useful if there are long delays in obtaining a CT scan, or the patient is already in the operating room. An US has a more limited role but can reveal fluid in the abdomen. Arteriography is most useful in showing injuries of the renal artery, although many patients are evaluated with CT scan alone. The following grading system is useful to describe renal injuries:
    ■ Grade I: Contusion or subcapsular hematoma without parenchymal laceration

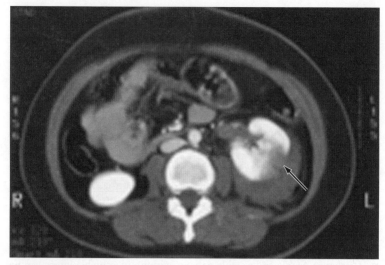

Figure 15–1. Computed tomography image revealing a grade II renal injury. There is a major tear of renal cortex (*arrow*) with perinephric hematoma. *(From Goldman SM, Sandler CM. Eur J Radiol 2004;50, p. 87.)*

- Grade II: Cortical laceration or perirenal hematoma smaller than 1cm (Figure 15–1)
- Grade III: Cortical laceration larger than 1 cm, without collecting system rupture
- Grade IV: Parenchymal laceration involving the collecting system or main renal artery or vein injury with contained hemorrhage
- Grade V: Completely shattered kidney or renal artery thrombosis or avulsion of the renal pedicle
- ***ED management.*** Tertiary care involves the trauma surgical service and urology consultation. Usually there will be nonoperative treatment of grades I through III, and operative management with possible nephrectomy for hemodynamically unstable patients with higher grade lesions.
- ***Helpful hints and pitfalls.*** Hematuria with associated hypotension (systolic blood pressure < 90 mm Hg) is associated with significant risk for renal injury.

Penetrating Renal Trauma

- ***Background.*** Of renal injuries in the United States, penetrating injuries comprise 20%, resulting in a higher renal loss than blunt injury.
- ***Clinical presentation.*** The evidence of penetrating trauma to the flank should be obvious on examination; however gunshot trajectories with known entry points not involving the flank can still involve the kidney.

- *Diagnostic testing.* Urinalysis, complete blood count, and chemistry panel to assess for hematuria and baseline hematocrit and renal function. Imaging is detailed in the section discussing blunt renal trauma. The same grading system is used. The major difference is that these patients require imaging regardless of the absence of hematuria because of the high risk of damage to the ureter as well as the kidney when there is a penetrating injury. This is especially true of gunshot wounds.
- *ED management.* There will still be a need for management by trauma surgery along with urology. Although the same nonoperative treatment of grades I to III exists, exploration of the abdomen is required for most gunshot wounds, with selective operative management for stab wounds.
- *Helpful hints and pitfalls.* Small superficial penetrating lesions can appear to be misleadingly benign. Administer antibiotics as necessary as penetrating objects are assumed to be contaminated.

Ureteral Disruption

- *Background.* The ureter is the least commonly injured part of the GU system. Eighty percent of these injuries are a result of penetrating trauma. In children, blunt injuries can occur at the ureteropelvic junction (UPJ) as increased mobility of the spine can lead to a shearing effect at this point.
- *Clinical presentation.* Think of the possibility of this injury when there is an appropriate mechanism of injury in patients with or without abdominal pain. There are no physical findings that define a ureteral injury, but the presence of signs of penetration should suggest the possibility of one.
- *Diagnostic testing.* Obtain a urinalysis to look for hematuria. When present, obtain a CT scan or an arteriogram as defined in prior sections. Penetrating ureteral injury may not produce gross or even microscopic hematuria.
- *ED management.* Obtain consultation with a trauma surgeon and urologist. Surgical repair is primarily done by direct reanastomosis or stenting and temporary diversion.
- *Helpful hints and pitfalls.* Because of the high rate of missed ureteral injuries, the possibility should be considered in trauma patients with worsening abdominal pain, fever, leukocytosis, or an unexplained fluid collection that could represent a urinoma.

Lower Tract
Bladder Injury

- *Background.* Most bladder injuries are from blunt trauma. Injuries can further be separated as extraperitoneal (80%) or intraperitoneal. Extraperitoneal rupture is almost universally associated with pelvic fractures. Intraperitoneal ruptures require a high degree of force exerted on a full bladder.
- *Clinical presentation.* Key findings on physical examination include pelvic tenderness and focal suprapubic or generalized abdominal pain.

There may be bruising and ecchymosis around the bladder and thighs, and often there is an inability to void.

- **Diagnostic testing.** The urinalysis typically shows gross hematuria. Gunshot wounds to the bladder may result in microscopic hematuria. Rupture of the bladder can be seen on screening abdominal CT scan and more accurately with a CT cystogram (Figure 15–2). CT cystography, performed with 400 mL of contrast administered in a retrograde fashion, is as accurate as a retrograde cystogram.

- **ED management.** Intraperitoneal bladder rupture requires exploratory laparotomy and repair through a layered closure whereas extraperitoneal

Contrast extends into the extraperitoneal space.

Contrast extravasation into the rectus abdominus musculature.

Air and contrast within the bladder. For CT cystogram, several hundred cc's of contrast are injected into the bladder via foley catheter prior to CT imaging. This is necessary to distend the bladder adequately. Simply scanning the bladder after routine CT is not adequate to exclude rupture.

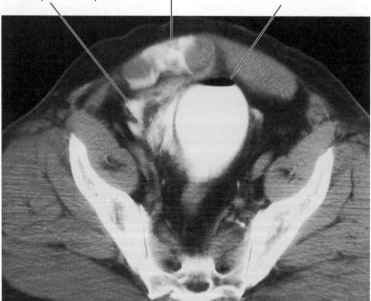

Figure 15–2. Computed tomography cystogram revealing bladder rupture. The contrast has been injected through the Foley catheter into the bladder and is extravasating into the extraperitoneal space with extension into the rectus abdominus musculature. (*From Jason Scott Stephens, M.D., The University of Texas Southwestern, Department of Radiology.*)

injuries can be managed with bladder drainage alone. Both should be managed in consultation with a trauma surgeon and urologist.

- *Helpful hints and pitfalls.* Urologic follow-up and antibiotics are needed to prevent long-term complications including strictures, fistulas, infection, and delayed healing. Remember that, like men, women can sustain bladder injuries, even though the incidence is much lower; women can also experience urethral injuries. There may not be much help in the physical examination for finding these injuries in women because there is no prostate gland, but with unstable pelvic fractures, especially straddle injuries, the urethra can be damaged as well.

Urethral Injury

- *Background.* Most injuries occur as a result of blunt trauma and occur primarily in men as the woman's urethra is short and mobile. Nevertheless, female patients do sustain this injury. Injuries are a result of high-energy impact or straddle mechanism. Look for it with any pelvic fracture. For classification of male injuries, the urethra is divided into a posterior segment (prostatic and membranous) and anterior segment (bulbous and pendulous). Posterior segment injuries are associated with pelvic ring fractures while anterior injury is a result of external blunt or straddle injuries.

- *Clinical presentation.* Blood at the urethral meatus, a high-riding prostate, pain, swelling, and ecchymosis in the penis or perineum will be found with this injury.

- *Diagnostic testing.* Gross hematuria is common. A retrograde urethrogram reveals extravasation of contrast anywhere during the course of the urethra confirms the presence of disruption. If bladder filling is noted then the lesion is considered partial, while no contrast ending up in the bladder is indicative of a complete tear.

- *ED management.* Minor injuries can be managed conservatively with passage of a catheter. Most injuries require suprapubic cystostomy and delayed repair of the urethral injury.

- *Helpful hints and pitfalls.* Evaluation of potential injury with retrograde urethrogram optimally will be undertaken before placement of a Foley catheter because the placement of a Foley catheter can convert a partial tear into a complete one. Sometimes a suprapubic cystostomy tube will have to be empirically placed because the patient cannot pass urine, but is too unstable from other injuries to allow the diagnostic study.

External Genitalia

Penile Injuries
Penile Fracture

- *Background.* This typically occurs during vigorous sexual intercourse when the penis is misdirected against the partner's pubic bone or self-inflicted by abrupt bending of the erect penis during masturbation. There is disruption of the tunica albuginea surrounding the corpora cavernosa.

- *Clinical Presentation.* The patient reports a popping sound as the tunica tears, followed by pain, swelling, and rapid detumescence. On physical examination, the penis is swollen and ecchymotic. The fracture line in the tunica is often palpable. There is associated urethral injury in up to one third of cases.

- **Diagnostic Testing.** Urinalysis will show microscopic and often gross hematuria. Retrograde urethrography should be performed to rule out urethral injury, particularly in the presence of gross hematuria, inability to void, or blood at the urethral meatus.
- **ED Management.** If suspected, a urologist should be immediately consulted. Early surgical treatment is essential to prevent complications such as deformity, impotence, erectile dysfunction, and urethral stenosis.

Penile Amputation

- **Background.** This is a very rare problem seen in the ED. It is due to self-mutilation in the hands of a psychotic patient, violent assault, or a devastating complication of circumcision.
- **ED Management.** Emergent urologic consultation is required for immediate reimplantation. Successful reimplantation has been accomplished up to 24 hours after amputation. The penis should be preserved in saline-soaked gauze and placed within a sterile plastic bag, which should be immersed over ice slush.

Testicular Trauma

- **Background.** The testicles may be injured by a direct blow, motor vehicle crashes, or sports-related activities. The right testicle, possibly because of its higher lying position, is more commonly injured than the left. Injuries include contusion, hematocele, rupture, dislocation, or traumatic torsion.
- **Clinical presentation.** Testicular pathology can be difficult to distinguish on examination alone, and imaging is required to assess the extent of the damage. Findings can include significant pain, swelling, and ecchymosis in the scrotal area.
- **Diagnostic testing.** An ultrasound study should include Doppler flow studies to assess arterial flow. Findings to suggest rupture include heterogeneous parenchyma, loss of tunica albuginea continuity, and a hematocele with extrusion of seminiferous tubules.
- **ED management.** Ice and adequate analgesia should be used while obtaining a urologic consultation.
- **Helpful hints and pitfalls.** Do not delay consultation for imaging studies if the testicle appears ruptured. Complications of testicular trauma include testicular atrophy, infection, infarction, and infertility. Ten percent of males diagnosed with testicular cancer give a history of recent trauma to the testicle.

Special Consideration
Pediatrics

- In regard to renal injuries, caution must be used in all children younger than 10 years with microscopic hematuria because this finding may be the only clue to injury.

- In adults, a relatively higher threshold of hematuria is used to determine the need for radiologic evaluation of renal injury. In children, the threshold is as low as 20 RBC/hpf; however, some experts would recommend imaging with any degree of microscopic hematuria in children.
- All perineal injuries in children should be examined under anesthesia in the operating room by the surgeon. Evaluation in the ED with or without sedation is suboptimal and prone to missed injuries and hurried repair.
- Sexual abuse is involved in a significant number of rectal and perineal injuries and a full abuse evaluation must follow.

Teaching Points

Gross hematuria always requires imaging evaluation, but microscopic hematuria should be counted by urinalysis sediment and requires clinical interpretation.

Most renal injuries can be managed nonoperatively, but this will depend on the patient's stability, degree of renal injury, and concomitant injuries to other abdominal structures.

If the traumatic forces were applied to the lower trunk and pelvis, there must be aggressive investigation to find urethral or bladder injuries, especially in the presence of straddling injuries and pelvic fractures. Women are often not considered to be at risk for these problems because there is a male predilection, but they do occur in women and should be thought of and looked for.

Urologic consultation should not be delayed for significant trauma involving the penis and testicles.

Suggested Readings

Dreitlein DA, Suner S, Balser J. Genitourinary trauma. Emerg Med Clin North Am 2001;19:569–590.

Iverson AJ, Morey AF. Radiographic evaluation of suspected bladder rupture following blunt trauma: critical review. World J Surg 2001;25:1588–1591.

Kawashima A, Sandler CM, Corl FM, West OC, Tamm EP, Fishman EK, Goldman SM. Imaging of renal trauma: a comprehensive review. Radiographics 2001;21:557–574.

Morey AF, Iverson AJ, Swan A, Harmon WJ, Spore SS, Bhayani S, Brandes SB. Bladder rupture after blunt trauma: guidelines for diagnostic imaging. J Trauma 2001;51:683–686.

Mulhall JP, Gabram SG, Jacobs LM. Emergency management of blunt testicular trauma. Acad Emerg Med 1995;2:639–643.

Palmer LS, Rosenbaum RR, Gershbaum MD, Kreutzer ER. Penetrating ureteral trauma at an urban trauma center: 10-year experience. Urology 1999;54:34–36.

Rosenstein D. McAninch JW. Urologic emergencies. Med Clin North Am 2004;88:495–518.

Samm BJ, Dmochowski RR. Urologic emergencies: trauma injuries and conditions affecting the penis, scrotum, and testicles. Postgrad Med 1996;100:187–90, 193–4, 199–200.

Velmahos GC, Degiannis E. The management of urinary tract injuries after gunshot wounds of the anterior and posterior abdomen. Injury 1997;28:535–8.

CHAPTER 16

Pelvic Trauma

CHRISTOPHER S. COURTNEY ■ ERIC A. GROSS

 Red Flags

Hemodynamic instability ● Neurologic deficit ● Abdominal pain
● Ecchymosis of the perineum ● Unstable pelvis

Overview

Pelvic fractures and dislocations often involve a significant amount
of traumatic force. Look for "red flags" (see Box) which may be
concerning for a more significant injury.

Bleeding from pelvic fractures, especially those involving posterior
structures can be life-threatening. There are four potential sources
of blood loss in these patients: fractured bone surface, pelvic venous
plexus, pelvic arterial injury, or an extrapelvic source. Persistent
hypotension in the multisystem trauma patient may indicate ongoing
bleeding from sacral vessels. Early closure of the pelvic space may
mitigate hypotension. Patients with significant pelvic fractures require
a thorough physical examination looking for associated injuries
including trauma to the urethra, rectum, and vagina.

Pelvic Anatomy
Bony and Ligamentous Anatomy

■ The bony pelvis consists of the ilium, ischium and pubis, which fuse at
the acetabulum (Figure 16–1).
■ The posterior ligaments (anterior and posterior sacroiliac, sacrotuberous,
sacrospinous, and iliolumbar) provide the bulk of mechanical support.
■ Disruption of the posterior ligaments is the dominant reason for
instability of the pelvic ring.

Related Structures

■ The lumbosacral nerve plexus is in close proximity to the sacrum.
Vertical sacral fractures and transverse fractures above S3 are associated
with neurologic injuries.

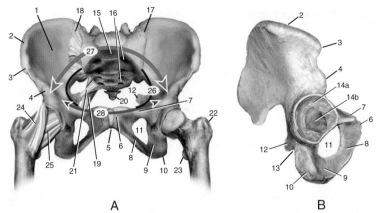

Figure 16–1. Pelvic anatomy. **A,** Anterior view of pelvis. **B,** Lateral view of right innominate bone. *1,* Iliac fossa; *2,* iliac crest; *3,* anterior superior iliac spine; *4,* anterior inferior iliac spine; *5,* symphysis pubis; *6,* body of pubis; *7,* superior ramus of pubis; *8,* inferior ramus of pubis; *9,* ramus of ischium; *10,* ischial tuberosity; *11,* obturator foramen; *12,* ischial spine; *13,* lesser sciatic notch; *14,* acetabulum (*14a,* articular surface; *14b,* fossa); *15,* sacrum; *16,* anterior sacral foramina; *17,* sacroiliac joint; *18,* anterior sacroiliac ligament; *19,* sacrotuberous ligament (sacrum to ischial tuberosity); *20,* coccyx; *21,* sacrospinous ligament; *22,* greater trochanter of femur; *23,* lesser trochanter of femur; *24,* iliofemoral ligament; *25,* pubofemoral ligament; *26,* arcuate line; *27,* posterior or femorosacral arch, through which main weight-bearing forces are transmitted; *28,* anterior arch. *(From Rosen's Emergency Medicine: Concepts and Clinical Practice (5th ed). St. Louis, MO: Mosby, 2002: p. 626)*

■ The bladder, urethra, vagina, rectum, perineum are all in close proximity to different areas of the bony pelvis.

Vessels

■ The sacral venous plexus and sacral arteries are in close proximity to the sacrum and sacroiliac joints. Bleeding will be retroperitoneal in most cases; thus, it may not be recognized by abdominal sonography or diagnostic peritoneal lavage (DPL). Hemorrhagic shock may result from uncontrolled bleeding from these structures.

■ The sacral venous plexus is more commonly responsible for hemo-dynamic instability in the setting of posterior pelvic fractures and posterior sacroiliac (SI) joint disruptions.

■ Arterial bleeds are far less common than venous bleeds, but may be amenable to embolic therapy via arteriography.

■ The superior (most commonly due to proximity to the SI joint) and inferior gluteal vessels are responsible for most arterial blood loss.

Initial Diagnostic Approach
General

- Assess the ABCs (*a*irway, *b*reathing, and *c*irculation) as discussed in Chapter 8.
- As an adjunct to the primary survey, the AP pelvic x-ray may reveal a pelvic fracture that may be the source of significant blood loss. If present, simple techniques should be promptly utilized to splint the unstable pelvic fracture.
- Evaluation of the pelvis is typically conducted as part of the secondary survey. Excessive manipulation of the pelvis should be avoided.

History

- In addition to the mechanisms of injury, inquire about risks of bleeding, previous pelvic or hip problems, and pregnancy.

Physical Examination

- Appropriate physical examination of the bony pelvis includes (a) gentle distraction and lateral compression at the iliac crests, (b) palpation of the symphysis pubis, and (c) palpation of the SI joints and sacrum. An unstable pelvis is able to rotate externally; the pelvis can be closed by pushing on the anterior superior iliac spines. Leg-length discrepancy or rotational deformity without a fracture of that extremity is another clinical clue to the presence of an unstable pelvis. One proficient examiner should check pelvic stability. Multiple manipulations should be avoided.
- Ecchymosis of the scrotum, flanks, or perineum may signify the presence of a fracture, but may also connote bladder rupture with extravasation. Obviously both may coexist. A high-riding prostate or blood at the urethral meatus may also signify fracture; either of these findings should also prompt an evaluation of the urethra (see Chapter 15).
- Cauda equina syndrome (see Chapter 21) or radiculopathies (see Chapter 46) may be present in patients with sacral fractures. Full motor, sensory (including perineal) and rectal examinations are important to exclude neurologic injury. Insertion of a Foley catheter, after appropriate evaluation of the urethra, may reveal urinary retention.
- The perineum, vagina, and rectum must be inspected for lacerations. If present, these may signify an open pelvic fracture that contributes significantly to higher morbidity and mortality. The examination must be done carefully to avoid worsening the initial injury. Likewise, the examiner must take care not to be personally injured by protruding spicules of bone.

Laboratory

- A complete blood count (CBC) is useful for obtaining a baseline hematocrit level. Serial monitoring of the hematocrit may assist in identifying ongoing blood loss; however, this is not helpful in the initial period of hemorrhage.

- Coagulation studies are needed as a large percentage of patients with pelvic-related bleeding will have or develop a coagulopathy.
- A urine pregnancy test should be performed in all females of reproductive age.
- A urinalysis should be obtained to look for hematuria.

Radiography

- An anteroposterior (AP) view of the pelvis serves as the initial screening tool for the evaluation of traumatic bony pelvic injury. This view has been routine on all blunt trauma victims for many years, but its use has decreased because abdominopelvic scans have become more frequent. It certainly should be obtained in any hypotensive trauma patient to rule-out a pelvic fracture as a source of bleeding.
- Although a CT scan of the pelvis is more accurate than plain films, and reveals much useful information, it should be obtained only in the hemodynamically stable patient.
- Special views such as the inlet, outlet, and Judet views may be helpful in detecting certain fractures. The inlet views can demonstrate fractures in the posterior arch, widening of the SI joint, and inward displacement of the anterior arch. The outlet view is helpful for sacral fractures or disruptions of the SI joint. The Judet views (internal and external oblique views) are useful for imaging the acetabulum.
- Radiographs are not necessary in the asymptomatic, alert patient who has a normal examination of the pelvis.

Special Studies

- Focused assessment with sonography for trauma (FAST) and diagnostic peritoneal lavage (DPL) should be used in the setting of hemodynamic instability preventing CT scan evaluation. Intra-abdominal gross bleeding mandates surgical exploration, but cell count–positive (no gross blood) DPL can be followed with serial studies in an attempt to avoid laparotomy. The FAST is discussed in Chapter 93. The DPL procedure is reviewed in Chapter 91.
- Angiography and embolization are sometimes beneficial although arterial bleeding is not as common as venous plexus bleeding.
- A retrograde urethrogram and cystogram should be obtained in all patients with pelvic fractures who have signs of urethral injury (see Chapter 15).

Emergency Department Management Overview
General

- The ABCs (*a*irway, *b*reathing, and *c*irculation) should be addressed. Establish two large-bore IV lines, place the patient on a monitor, and give supplementary oxygen to any patient who is being evaluated after major trauma.
- *Pelvic fracture management—stable patient.* Pelvic fractures in the hemodynamically stable patient are handled according to the type of fracture (see Tile classification system under Specific Problems).

■ *Pelvic fracture management—unstable patient.* This situation requires aggressive intravenous fluid (IVF) resuscitation, and the early use of blood products. It is useful to search for alternative causes of hypotension, or hemorrhage. An attempt should be made to approximate the disrupted pelvic space. This can be accomplished by wrapping a sheet around the pelvis, application of a pneumatic antishock garment such as the military antishock trousers or MAST suit, or external fixation in the ED or operating room. If there is persistent hypotension, angiography and embolization may be effective. Some cases require emergency laparotomy.

Disposition

■ *Consultation.* All patients with a pelvic fracture as part of a multisystem trauma should be evaluated by a trauma surgeon. All pelvic fractures require orthopedic consultation. All patients with neurologic deficits require both neurosurgical and orthopedic consultation. All patients with urethral or bladder injuries require urologic consultation.

■ *Admission.* All patients with a pelvic fracture as part of a multisystem trauma should be admitted to the hospital. Certain isolated, low-energy pelvic fractures may be managed on an outpatient basis.

Specific Problems
Classification of Pelvic Fractures

■ Several classification schemes exist for pelvic fractures.

■ *Young and Burgess classification system.* This system assesses patterns of injury and its relation to associated organ injuries, resuscitative requirements, and expected mortality rates. Injury patterns include anteroposterior compression (APC), lateral compression (LC), vertical shear (VS), and combined mechanisms. For example, patients with APC injuries mostly die as a result of pelvic bleeding and abdominal injuries.

■ *Tile classification system.* This system reflects various mechanisms of force that collectively determine treatment strategies and complications associated with the specific type of pelvic injury. Tile type A fractures are stable injuries in which the posterior arch is intact. These usually do not require operative intervention, and are treated with rest and analgesia. Tile type B and C fractures are often associated with intraperitoneal injuries, hemorrhage, and injuries to other parts of the body as a result of the large amount of forces involved. In type B injuries, there is incomplete disruption of the posterior arch. In type C injuries, the posterior arch is completely disrupted.

Acetabular Fractures

■ Fractures of the acetabulum are classified separately from the other types of pelvic fractures.

■ Acetabular fractures are intra-articular fractures of the hip joint. They are concerning because of their disruption of a major weight-bearing articular surface.

- Acetabular fractures may be missed on standard plain films. An acetabular fracture should be suspected in any patient complaining of hip pain after a traumatic injury who is unable to ambulate, especially if initial plain films appear to be negative for an acute fracture. Special plain films called Judet views (internal and external oblique views) are very useful for imaging the acetabulum. The CT scan is the best imaging modality for further delineation of these fractures.
- Many acetabular fractures are associated with hip dislocations, a true orthopedic emergency due to disruption of the blood supply to the femoral head and impending avascular necrosis.

Sacral Fractures

- Sacral fractures (Figure 16–2) commonly cause neurologic injury. The sacral foramina provide the outlet to sacral nerve roots. Fractures through the foramina or fracture fragments compressing the foramina may injure these nerve roots.
- Zone one: The fracture is lateral to the foramina. There is likely damage from an L5 nerve root impingement. Six percent of these fractures have associated neurologic injury.

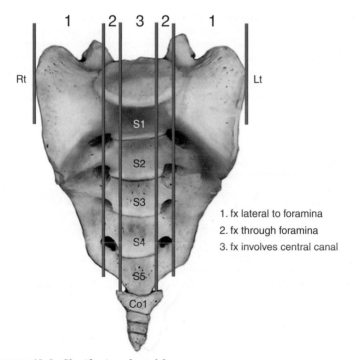

Figure 16–2. Classification of sacral fractures.

- Zone two: The fracture is through the sacral foramina. This may result in unilateral sacral anesthesia. This injury requires operative debridement of the foramina and definitive fixation.
- Zone three: This fracture is through the sacral body (medial to the foramina). These fractures have the highest association with neurologic injury and need operative intervention. Unfortunately this fracture often causes a cauda equina syndrome resulting in a neurogenic bladder.

Special Considerations
Pediatrics

- Pelvic fractures in pediatric patients are rare. Compared with the adult pelvis, the immature pediatric pelvis is more elastic and requires more force to cause a fracture. However, associated injuries are common. Visceral injuries involving the urinary tract or other intra-abdominal organs occur in up to 19% of patients.
- Control of hemorrhage may be augmented initially with a MAST suit. The high pressures required (50 mm Hg in extremity and 40 mm Hg in abdominal compartments) may intefere with ventilation resulting in the need for mechanical ventilary support.

Pregnancy

- Maternal pelvic fractures, particularly in late pregnancy, are associated with bladder injury, urethral injury, retroperitoneal bleeding, and fetal skull fracture. After 12 weeks of gestation, the maternal uterus and bladder extend outside of the pelvis and are more susceptible to direct injury.
- A supraumbilical approach for DPL is indicated when the gravid uterus is palpable above the pubis. The open or minilaparotomy technique should be used in all pregnant patients.

Teaching Points

Pelvic fractures are seen following transmission of high energy forces as with auto crashes. They are often subtle in the amount of bleeding that is occurring, and can be anticipated to require aggressive volume and blood replacement. They require pelvic stabilization as well as volume replacement. This can be commenced in the ED with the wrapping of the pelvis with a sheet, or the insertion of an external fixator device. With marked posterior displacement, there is an increased probability of an arterial bleed, and these patients may require arteriography and embolization.

Suggested Readings

Collinge C, Tornetta P. Soft tissue injuries associated with pelvic fractures. Orthop Clin North Am 2004;35:451–456.

Cwinn AA. Pelvis. In: Marx JA, Hockberger RS, Walls RM. Rosen's Emergency Medicine: Concepts and Clinical Practice (6th ed). Philadelphia: Mosby, 2006, pp 717–735.

Gonzalez RP, Fried PQ, Bukhalo M. The utility of clinical examination in screening for pelvic fractures in blunt trauma. J Am Coll Surg 2002;194;121–125.

Hak DJ. The role of pelvic angiography in evaluation and management of pelvic trauma. Orthop Clin North Am 2004;35:439–443.

Musgrave DS, Mendelson SA. Pediatric orthopedic trauma: principles in management. Crit Care Med 2002;30(11 Suppl): S431–43.

CHAPTER **17**

Extremity Trauma

COLLEEN N. ROCHE ■ DANIEL DAVIS

Overview

Extremity injuries involve more than fractures, dislocations, sprains, and strains. Injuries to nerves, vascular structures, and other soft tissues can be devastating and result in substantial morbidity. The key to successful diagnosis of neurovascular injuries is considering them in the first place, and then being willing to arrange appropriate diagnostic testing and consultation.

Patients with orthopedic injuries may arrive at the ED with isolated injuries or multisystem trauma. When evaluating a trauma patient with orthopedic injuries, the overall trauma evaluation must be completed before focusing on the orthopedic injuries. Unfortunately orthopedic injuries may distract the patient from complaining about more serious injuries, and may mislead the physician into thinking that the obvious open fracture is the patient's only, or most serious, problem.

Orthopedic injuries can lead to both long-term and short-term complications, including: compartment syndrome, infection, vascular injury, hemorrhage, neurologic injury, fat emboli, thromboembolic disease, avascular necrosis, delayed union or malunion, and arthritis.

While most extremity injuries are not life-threatening, they may indeed be limb-threatening. True extremity emergencies are listed in Table 17–1.

Table 17–1	True Extremity Emergencies Requiring Immediate Intervention
Problem	**Concern**
Open fracture	Infection
Hip dislocation	Avascular necrosis of the femoral head
Posterior sternoclavicular joint dislocation	Injuries to the subclavian artery and vein, trachea, and brachial plexus
Major pelvic fracture	Hemorrhage
Septic joint	Joint destruction
Any injury with associated neurovascular compromise	Ischemia or permanent neurologic deficit
Compartment syndrome	Ischemic contracture; myoglobinuria, renal failure
Proximal amputation or partial amputation	Ischemia or permanent neurologic deficit

Spine injuries are discussed in Chapter 12, pelvic fractures are discussed in Chapter 16, and pediatric orthopedic problems are discussed in Chapter 81. Laceration repair is discussed in Chapter 94; septic joint, tendinitis, and bursitis are covered in Chapter 42; and other soft-tissue infections and ulcerations are discussed in Chapter 54.

Initial Diagnostic Approach

- **General.** Evaluate the ABCs (*a*irway, *b*reathing, and *c*irculation), and test for major neurologic disability as in any other trauma patient. See Chapter 8. A more focused evaluation is sufficient for most individuals presenting to the ED with extreme trauma.
- **History.** The history should include the exact mechanism of injury, position of the extremity at the time of injury, the time and duration of injury, handedness, allergies, medications, illness, prior injury to the affected part, care of the stump and amputated part before arrival in the ED, occupation, avocations, and tetanus history (for open wounds).
- **Physical examination.** The extremity must be completely visualized, and the integrity of the skin must be noted. The examination needs to focus on areas of swelling and tenderness, stability of involved bones and joints, range of motion, and full assessment of adjacent joints. Look for associated neurovascular injuries with any fracture or dislocation. Pulses, capillary refill, color, warmth, sensory deficits, or ischemic pain are used to assess vascular integrity. Neurologic assessment is summarized in Table 17–2. The Allen's test is used to determine the integrity of

Table 17–2 Neurologic Assessment of Extremity Injuries

	Motor	Sensory	Comment
Brachial plexus	Impaired active range of motion in the shoulder girdle.	Usually restricted to the axillary distribution along the lateral aspect of the shoulder, but may occur in the dermatomal distribution of any affected nerve.	The brachial plexus is normally formed from the ventral rami of C5–T1 spinal nerves. This structure allows for the formation of peripheral nerves, which supply the upper extremity and shoulder girdle.
Axillary nerve	The deltoid muscle should be palpated for contraction because of the action of the supraspinatus and rotation of the scapula.	Sensation over the deltoid, but motor function is better at detecting injury.	Commonly injured by fractures or dislocations about the shoulder.
Musculocutaneous nerve	Contraction of the biceps muscle.	Sensory examination is of no great value because complete anesthesia is rare.	Most commonly is injured by penetrating injuries, anterior dislocation of the shoulder, or fractures of the humeral neck.
Radial nerve	Innervates the dorsal extrinsic muscles in the forearm, which extend the wrist and MP joints, and both abduct and extend the thumb.	Sensory over the dorsal first web space is best at detecting a deficit of the radial nerve.	Injured most often by fractures of the humeral shaft. Gunshot wounds are the second most common cause of radial nerve injury. No intrinsic muscles in the hand are innervated by the radial nerve.
Median nerve	Have the patient oppose the thumb to the index digit.	Sensory deficit is best detected over the volar tip of the index finger.	May be injured by fractures of the distal radius and by fractures and dislocations of the carpal bones.

Continued

Table 17–2   Neurologic Assessment of Extremity Injuries—*cont'd*

	Motor	Sensory	Comment
Ulnar nerve	Weakness of the interossei muscles of the hand (abduction of the fingers)	The superficial branch of the ulnar nerve supplies sensation to the ring and little fingers. The best place to test for sensation is the volar tip of the little finger.	The nerve bifurcates at the wrist into deep and superficial branches. Often is injured by dislocations of the elbow, supracondylar and condylar fractures, and injuries at the wrist.
Sciatic nerve	If complete, there is paralysis of the hamstring muscles and all muscles below the knee. With partial injury, a peroneal palsy with weakness of the extensor hallucis longus (extends big toe, dorsiflexes ankle) muscle is the most sensitive clinical sign.	There is a sensory loss below the knee and along the posterior thigh. The deep-tendon reflex at the ankle is absent or diminished.	Complete traumatic injury may result from a deep penetrating wound to the hip, thigh, or buttock. Also seen in posterior hip dislocations and fracture-dislocations.
Femoral nerve	Marked weakness of knee extension	The most reliable spot is superior and medial to the patella. The deep tendon reflex of the knee will be diminished or absent.	Rarely seen with femoral shaft fractures. The iliac and femoral arteries are commonly involved because of their anatomic proximity. Most often traumatized in penetrating trauma of the pelvis, groin, or thigh.
Peroneal Nerve	Test ankle and toe dorsiflexion (deep peroneal nerve function) and foot eversion (superficial peroneal nerve function).	Test the first dorsal web space in the foot (deep peroneal nerve) and sensation dorsal lateral foot (superficial peroneal nerve).	Commonly damaged in lower extremity injuries.
Tibial nerve	Inversion of the foot	Sole of the foot (except the medial border of the instep), the lateral surface of the heel, and the plantar surface of the toes.	Less commonly damaged than peroneal nerve.

collateral circulation between the ulnar and radial artery through the palmar arch. The ankle brachial index (ABI) is used to assess for vascular compromise to the lower extremities (see Appendix 2). Injuries involving the hand should include two-point discrimination (of the volar aspect of the finger tips, should distinguish two points at 6 mm or less), rotational deformity of the fingers (with a closed fist, all fingers should be in alignment and point toward the scaphoid), and the integrity of the flexor tendons. The flexor pollicis longus is tested by having the patient bend the tip of the thumb against resistance. The flexor digitorum profundus (FDP) is tested by having the patient flex the distal phalanx of each finger while the proximal interphalangeal joint (PIP) is stabilized in extension by the examiner. The flexor digitorum tendon superficialis (FDS) is tested individually by asking the patient to flex the PIP joint while the other fingers are held in extension to block the flexion produced by the profundus tendons.

- *Laboratory.* Patients with orthopedic injuries rarely require laboratory evaluation other than that required for preoperative management. Patients with injuries associated with vascular injury should have a hematocrit level and coagulation studies performed, and type and cross match of packed red blood cells should be obtained. Significant extremity trauma may result in muscle breakdown and rhabdomyolysis. This should be evaluated with a serum creatine phosphokinase level (CPK) and assessment for myoglobinuria. A complete blood count (CBC) and erythrocyte sedimentation rate (ESR) are ordered if there is concern for infection (see Chapter 42).
- *Arthrocentesis.* Arthrocentesis may reveal occult fracture in patients with a painful, swollen joint after a traumatic injury when radiograph findings are negative (see Chapter 91). Its diagnostic utility is primarily for inflammatory joint disease (Chapter 42).
- *Radiography.* The characteristics of both fractures and dislocations are often evident on plain radiographs. Common orthopedic terminology is listed in Table 17–3. With upper and lower extremity injuries, true posterior-anterior (PA) and lateral views, shot perpendicular to each other, are required to properly evaluate the location injured; otherwise, fractures may go undetected. Additional specialized views may add to the diagnosis and management of the patient with an orthopedic injury (see Table 17–4). Common normal plain films of bone are briefly described in Chapter 92. Computed tomography (CT scan) can be useful in detecting occult fractures, particularly in the pelvis and hip. The CT scan is often used to help delineate the extent of particular fractures, such as fractures of the calcaneous, talus, tibial plateau, and acetabulum. Magnetic resonance imaging (MRI) has a limited role in detecting acute orthopedic injuries; it is more useful in the outpatient setting in aiding the treatment plan. An arteriogram is the gold standard for excluding vascular injury.

Emergency Department Management Overview
General

- Regardless of the injury, the ABCs (*a*irway, *b*reathing, and *c*irculation) are the first priority and should be addressed. Establish two intravenous (IV)

Table 17–3 Terminology to Describe Orthopedic Injuries

Term	Comment
Anatomic location	Long bones are divided into thirds: proximal, middle, and distal. May also be described by specific anatomic part (e.g., femoral neck).
Closed (simple) vs. open (compound) fracture	In a closed fracture, the skin and soft tissue overlying the fracture site are intact. If the fracture is exposed to the outside environment in any manner, it is open.
Complete fracture	Interrupts both cortices of the bone.
Incomplete fracture	Bones of children are soft and resilient and therefore sustain a number of incomplete fractures. Examples include a torus fracture and greenstick fracture seen in the pediatric population.
Intraarticular fracture	When a fracture extends into and involves an articular surface. Frequently, the percentage of articular surface that is involved is estimated. In some cases the percentage that is involved will dictate the need to perform a surgical reduction.
Pathologic fracture	A fracture that occurs through abnormal bone. A pathologic fracture should be suspected whenever a fracture occurs from seemingly trivial trauma.
Fracture line or pattern	
Avulsion fracture	Rupture of a piece of bone at the site of insertion of a ligament or tendon.
Comminuted fracture	Greater than two fragments of bone at a fracture site.
Compression fracture	Occurs when an excessive axial load compresses the bone beyond its limits. Typically occurs in the vertebral bodies.
Depressed fracture	Due to a force that breaks and depresses one segment below the level of surrounding bone.
Impacted fracture	Opposing bony surfaces are driven together.
Oblique fracture	Fracture line is at an angle to the long axis of the bone.
Spiral fracture	Usually the result of torsion on a long bone resulting in a spiral pattern.
Transverse fracture	Fracture line is perpendicular to the long axis of the bone.

Table 17–3 Terminology to Describe Orthopedic Injuries—*cont'd*

Term	Comment
Relationship of fragments	
Angulation	The angle between the longitudinal axis of the main fracture fragments. It is described as the relationship of the bone distal to the fracture site with respect to the proximal bone. An alternative description is the direction in which the apex of the fracture points. Ulnar, radial, dorsal, and volar are terms used to describe angulation in the arm and hand. In the foot, plantar and dorsal are used. Valgus means that the distal part is angled laterally relative to the proximal part. Varus means the distal part is angled medially.
Displacement	Any deviation from normal position. The position of the distal fragment is described relative to the proximal one.
Dislocation	Complete disruption of the articulating surfaces of a joint
Rotation	Fragments that are rotated with respect to one another must be recognized and corrected. This may be noted on physical examination. The joints above and below the injury should be imaged.
Subluxation	Partial disruption of the articulating surfaces of a joint.

lines, place the patient on a monitor, and give supplementary oxygen to any patient who is being evaluated after major trauma.

Medications

- *Pain management.* Orthopedic injuries are often very painful and require aggressive and adequate pain management in the ED (see Chapter 90.1). Digital or regional nerve blocks (see Chapter 94) may help pain relief but may make neurologic evaluation by a consultant impossible.
- *Antibiotics.* Antistaphylococcus antibiotics should be used for highly contaminated wounds or open fractures.
- *Tetanus.* Prophylaxis should be given on all open extremity injuries.

Emergency Department Interventions

- *Open fractures.* When a fracture fragment violates the skin surface, there is a substantial risk for osteomyelitis to develop in the involved bone. The management of patients with open fractures includes the placement of sterile dressing over the exposed site, tetanus prophylaxis, IV administration of a first-generation cephalosporin (an aminoglycoside should be

Table 17–4   Special Plain Film Views for Orthopedic Imaging

Scaphoid view (wrist)	May help identify a scaphoid fracture. Clenched fist view with ulnar deviation.
Axillary or transcapular Y view (shoulder)	Can identify shoulder dislocations and the position of the humeral head in relation to the glenoid process. The transcapular Y view does not require abduction of the shoulder.
Inlet and outlet views (pelvis)	May reveal subtle pelvic injuries.
Judet views (pelvis)	A 45-degree oblique views of the pelvis to evaluate for an acetabular fracture.
Sunrise view (knee)	May reveal patellar fractures undetected by anteroposterior and lateral views of the knee.
Mortise view (ankle)	This is an additional, standard view when evaluating the ankle; it reveals the integrity of the articular surface of the ankle. Stress views of a joint may be obtained to reveal ligamentous instability, but should be done with caution, if at all.
Harris view (calcaneous)	Should be performed to image the calcaneal tuberosity, subtalar joint, and sustentaculotalar joints if standard plain films are unrevealing.
Stress views	Are used in some instances to evaluate the degree of ligamentous injury in certain joints. The ankle and foot are the most common examples. They are no longer indicated for acromioclavicular injuries.

added for more contaminated wounds), and emergent orthopedic consultation for operative intervention. Even an innocuously appearing break in the skin near a fracture should be concluded to be an open fracture and treated with appropriate aggression.

■ *Dislocations.* Any dislocation with neurovascular compromise must be reduced immediately. Most other dislocations can be reduced after plain films are done (Table 17–5; Figures 17–1, 17–2, 17–3, and 17–4).

■ *Arthrocentesis.* Arthrocentesis may provide substantial relief in patients with an associated hemarthrosis, since stretch on the joint capsule is quite painful. Once the hemarthrosis has been evacuated, injection with an anesthetic, such as bupivicaine, can aid in acute pain management. This approach is of particular benefit in elbow and knee injuries.

■ *Splinting.* For fractures, splint all joints with which the injured bone articulates (e.g., the joints above and below the fracture). For dislocations and sprains, place the splint so that the affected joint is immobilized in all planes of movement. The ideal splint conforms to underlying structures, which requires molding of the splint during the initial minutes of hardening. This also requires that the individual applying the splint

Table 17–5 Joint Dislocations

Joint	Anatomy	Mechanism	Diagnostic Clues	Reduction	Comment
Shoulder (glenohumeral) Figure 17–1.	Most common is anterior dislocation of humeral head; posterior and inferior less common	Anterior: forced extension or abduction external rotation. Posterior: seizures or electric shock	Anterior: prominence of the acromion and flattening of the normal shoulder contour; arm is held in abduction and external rotation Posterior: posterior fullness of shoulder and a prominence of the coracoid process. Inferior: may present with arm raised (luxatio erecta)	Milch maneuver and traction–countertraction are commonly used (Figures 17–2 and 17–3). Stimson technique: patient lies prone, 5-kg weights are attached to the arm for 20–30 min, gentle external and internal rotation of the shoulder aids reduction. Scapular manipulation: the inferior tip of the scapula is pushed medially while the superior aspect of the scapula is stabilized. Adequate relaxation is critical for most reductions.	Complications include axillary nerve injury, Hill-Sachs deformity (notch on posterior humeral head), Bankhart's lesion (fracture of anterior glenoid) in anterior dislocations. The injuries are reversed in posterior dislocations.

Continued

Table 17–5 Joint Dislocations—*cont'd*

Joint	Anatomy	Mechanism	Diagnostic Clues	Reduction	Comment
Elbow	Posterior dislocation of ulna on distal humerus is most common	Posterior: fall on the outstretched hand or wrist, with elbow extended or hyperextended.	Prominence of olecranon posteriorly	Assistant immobilizes the humerus; apply traction at the wrist. Flex the elbow as steady countertraction is applied to the anterior surface of the distal humerus. Apply long arm splint at 90 degrees of flexion at elbow.	Complications include neurovascular (ulnar > median nerve and brachial artery) injury, and associated fractures (e.g., corocoid)
Interphalangeal	Dislocation of middle phalanx on proximal phalanx is most common	Axial load ("jammed finger") or hyperextension most common	Often palpable deformity; significant swelling and immobility with misalignment at area of dislocation	Distraction and direct pressure on middle phalanx; digital block works well.	Injury to volar plate and collateral ligaments are common; finger splint; orthopedics hand follow-up important

Table 17-5 Joint Dislocations—*cont'd*

Joint	Anatomy	Mechanism	Diagnostic Clues	Reduction	Comment
Hip	Most commonly posterior from motor vehicle accident (dashboard injury)	Posterior dislocation of femoral head from acetabulum; 10% are anterior	Posterior: typically patient holds the hip flexed, adducted, and internally rotated. The extremity is shortened. Anterior: hip held in abduction, slight flexion, and external rotation. Radiograph of posterior dislocation: lesser trochanter not seen on anteroposterior view due to internal rotation, femoral head appears smaller, and Shenton's line disrupted.*	See Figure 17–4 for Stimson and Allis techniques. Axial distraction with adequate relaxation is critical.	Requires immediate reduction to prevent avascular necrosis of the femoral head. Other complications include sciatic nerve injury, acetabular chip fractures, or compression of the femoral nerve, artery, or vein. Sciatic nerve injury; high incidence of eventual avascular necrosis make this time critical; may see acetabular chip fracture.
Knee	Most commonly posterior dislocation of tibia on distal femur, but can go in any direction	Dashboard injury or hyperextension (posterior); also water-skiing or other high-energy injuries	May appear reduced upon arrival in the ED; severe instability with ecchymosis suggests this injury, swelling variable depending on capsule integrity	Usually easy to reduce with axial distraction due to disruption of ligaments	Must exclude popliteal artery injury; need angiogram if signs of vascular compromise; concurrent ligamentous injuries exist. Peroneal injury is common.

Continued

Table 17-5 Joint Dislocations—*cont'd*

Joint	Anatomy	Mechanism	Diagnostic Clues	Reduction	Comment
Patella	Lateral displacement of patella on femur	Either hyperextension with strong quadriceps contraction or direct blow to patella	Often self-reduces; otherwise, should be able to palpate patella lateral to knee	Full knee extension with relaxation of quadriceps, then apply pressure on patella pushing it medially	Often occurs in young females; tends to be recurrent; knee immobilizer with orthopedic follow-up; low concern for neurovascular injury
Ankle	Described according to the direction of displacement of the talus and foot in relation to the tibia.	Axial loading of a plantar-flexed foot; requires high energy. Dislocation of the talus without fracture is rare.	Significant ankle swelling with palpable or visible deformity; use location of calcaneus to help orient	Axial traction with ankle in plantar flexion, reduce, then place ankle in dorsiflexion for splinting	Moderate concern for neurovascular injury; usually associated with grossly unstable ankle that will require operative repair
Toe	Usually dislocation of middle on proximal phalanx	Typically axial load ("stub")	Limited mobility with pain and swelling; often palpable deformity	Axial traction and direct pressure on distal bone involved	Orthopedic referral for great toe; other toes less critical; post-op shoe appropriate

*Shenton's line: smooth curved imaginary line drawn along the superior border of the obturator foramen and medial aspect of the femoral metaphysis.
MCP, metacarpophalangeal; DIP, distal interphalyngeal joint.
(From Roberts: Clinical Procedures in Emergency Medicine (4th ed). 2004, Elsevier and Rosen P, Chan TC, Vilke GM, Stembach G. Atlas of Emergency Procedures, 2001, Mosby.

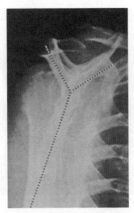

Figure 17-1. Shoulder dislocation. A posterior dislocation: Trans-scapular projection showing the dislocated humeral head, posterior in relationship to the intersecting limbs of the Y. (*From Radiology of the Emergency Patient. New York: John Wiley & Sons, 1982, p. 512.*)

needs to maintain the affected limb in the desired position for at least 10 minutes to avoid cracking or creasing during the critical period of hardening. Splints can lead to skin breakdown, especially at bony prominences. Adequate padding (e.g., Webril, cotton roll) should be placed over these sites before application of the plaster or fiberglass. The application of water to plaster or fiberglass splint material creates an exothermic reaction that can lead to thermal burns. Use cool water and adequate padding. Cooler water temperatures also extend the setting time, allowing more time for proper application and molding (see Table 17–6).

Disposition

- **Consultation.** Consultation with an orthopedic specialist should be sought for the treatment of most long-bone fractures, open fractures, flexor tendon injuries, and injuries with actual or potential neurovascular compromise. Orthopedic consultation is also required for follow-up of certain patients (e.g., severe sprains) initially treated in the ED. Vascular surgery should be consulted for vascular injuries. Emergent consultations with the reimplantation team should be done as soon as possible for patients with amputations and partial amputations who may be candidates for reimplantation.
- **Admission.** Patients requiring admission include those needing operative repair, with actual or risk for neurovascular compromise, or a social situation that prevents a safe discharge from the ED.
- **Discharge.** Most patients presenting with extremity injuries can be followed as outpatients within 5 to 7 days. The patient should be given complete instructions on care of the injured extremity and when to

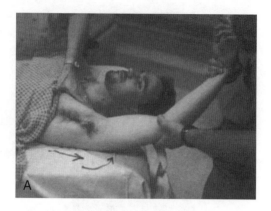

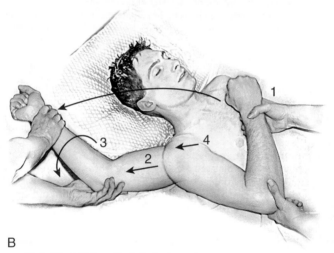

Figure 17–2. The Milch method. Reduction of an anterior shoulder dislocation includes *(1)* abduction and external rotation, and *(2)* slow and steady gentle traction. When reduced, the arm is adducted *(3)*. Pressure to the humeral head with the operator's hand during traction *(4)* may aid the reduction. *(From Clinical Procedures in Emergency Medicine, 4th ed., Philadelphia: Saunders, 2004, p. 957.)*

return to the ED. Splint care instructions include not "testing" the splint for several hours after application, strict avoidance of getting the splint (or the underlying skin) wet, adhering to non–weight-bearing instructions, and return parameters such as signs and symptoms of compartment syndrome or increasing pain at pressure points, suggesting skin breakdown.

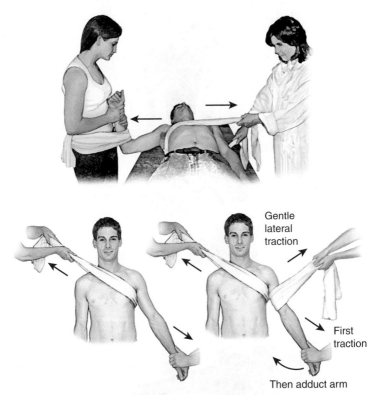

Figure 17–3. With the patient supine, a sheet or strap is wrapped around the upper chest and under the axilla of the affected shoulder. An assistant holds this sheet so as to apply the countertraction. The elbow of the affected side is flexed to 90° and a sheet or strap is wrapped around the proximal forearm and then around the operator's back, using the operator's body weight to supply the force of traction. Gentle, limited external rotation is sometimes useful to speed reduction. Applying traction to an arm that is slightly abducted from the patient's body is often successful, but some operators prefer to slowly bring the arm medial to the patient's midline while maintaining traction or to have an assistant apply a gentle lateral force to the mid-humerus to direct the humeral head laterally. *(From Respet PB. J Musculoskel Med 5:29, 1988.)*

Specific Problems
Amputation/Near-Amputation

- *Background.* The time of injury is vital when dealing with a time-sensitive ischemic limb or digit. Handedness (right or left) and occupation are sometimes used in the decision regarding reimplantation. The critical determination is whether distal perfusion has been disrupted with near amputations. Guillotine injuries are the least common but have

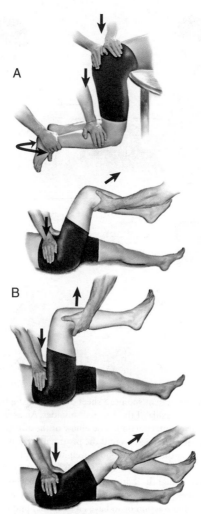

Figure 17–4. Techniques for hip reduction. **A, Stimson technique:** The patient is placed prone with the leg hanging over the bed; the hip and knees are flexed 90 degrees. The operator applies downward traction in line with the femur. The femoral head is gently rotated and the assistant pushes the greater trochanter toward the acetabulum. **B, Allis technique:** The patient is supine and the pelvis is stabilized by an assistant. With the knee flexed, the operator brings the hip slowly to 90 degrees of flexion, applying steady upward traction and gentle rotation. The assistant pushes the greater trochanter forward toward the acetabulum. *(From Rosen's Emergency Medicine: Concepts and Clinical Practice (5th ed). New York: Mosby, 2002, p. 664.)*

Table 17-6 Common Splints, Indications, and Application Techniques

Splint	Indications	Application	Illustration
Long arm posterior sling	Distal humerus or proximal radius/ulna fractures, elbow sprains/dislocations	From palmar crease along ulnar aspect of forearm to posterior humerus below axilla Thumb should point upward (neutral supination/pronation). Use arm sling with shoulder range-of-motion exercises	
Coaptation (sugar tong)	Distal radius/ulna fractures (most often Colles type), severe wrist injuries.	From palmar crease along volar forearm, around elbow to dorsal forearm ending at MCP joints. Thumb should point upward (neutral supination/pronation); wrist should be neutral for splint.	
Thumb spica	First phalangeal and metacarpal fractures/dislocations, scaphoid injuries, Gamekeeper's thumb, de Quervain's tendonitis.	From tip of thumb (remains exposed for neurovascular checks) ending distal to antecubital fossa with the wrist in neutral position. Thumb should be neutral (as if holding a soda can); thumb should be slightly adducted with gamekeeper's thumb.	

MCP, metacarpophalangeal.

Continued

Table 17-6 Common Splints, Indications, and Application Techniques—*cont'd*

Splint	Indications	Application	Illustration
Radial gutter	Second or third (index and long finger) phalangeal (severe) and metacarpal fractures, carpal fractures/dislocations.	From distal index and long fingers along radial aspect of hand ending distal to antecubital fossa. Cut large hole for thumb and thenar eminence; 90 degrees flexion at MCP with slight extension at wrist.	
Ulnar gutter	Fourth or fifth phalangeal (severe) and metacarpal fractures; carpal fractures/dislocations.	From distal ring and little fingers along ulnar aspect of hand ending distal to olecranon. Reduce boxer's fractures with splint in place; 90 degrees flexion at MCP with slight extension at wrist.	
Volar wrist	Wrist sprains; carpal tunnel syndrome; minor carpal fractures; NOT distal radius/ulna.	From palmar crease along volar aspect of hand and wrist ending at widest part of forearm flexors. Avoid excessive pressure over carpal tunnel, especially with carpal tunnel syndrome; do not immobilize thumb.

Plaster
Ace wrap
Webril
Stockinette/Webril |

Table 17-6   Common Splints, Indications, and Application Techniques—*cont'd*

Splint	Indications	Application	Illustration
Dorsal finger	Mallet finger (avulsion fracture of dorsal aspect of distal phalanx or rupture of extensor tendon).	Rigid object (splint, paper clip, popsicle stick) taped over DIP joint in full extension. Tape should be applied to both distal phalanx and middle phalanx to maintain joint in extension.	
Posterior knee splint (long leg splint)	Distal femur fractures; patellar fractures; knee injuries; proximal tibia fractures.	From distal tibia/fibula to mid-thigh (medial/lateral or posterior); may extend past ankle (tibia fractures). Use medial/lateral for MCL/LCL or meniscal injuries, posterior for ACL/PCL injuries, both for severe injuries.	
Posterior ankle	Achilles injuries; often used with stirrup splint for ankle fractures (see Bulky Jones).	From toes along plantar surface of foot behind ankle, ending just distal to popliteal fossa. Should place ankle in plantarflexion with Achilles injury; may crack at apex if used alone for ankle injuries.	

Continued

Table 17-6 Common Splints, Indications, and Application Techniques—*cont'd*

Splint	Indications	Application	Illustration
Bulky Jones	Any lower leg, ankle, or foot injury with significant swelling.	From metatarsal heads along medial and lateral aspect of lower leg; should cross ankle at malleoli. Ankle should be neutral at 90 degrees of flexion; use posterior splint for additional strength, but avoid circumferential splint. The cotton roll should be completely unrolled and split in half (with regard to thickness). It is then rerolled loosely to make application easier. After applying the stockinette, wrap the extremity loosely from toes to knee with the split cotton roll. A layer of Webril is applied to compress the cotton roll. Each Webril layer is overlaid by half of its width. The splint (posterior splint in combination with a sugar tong splint) is applied over the bulky Jones dressing and covered with an acewrap in the usual fashion.	

Table 17–7   Replantation of the Amputated Extremity
Indications
Young stable patient
Thumb
Multiple digits injured, single digits proximal to the distal interphalangeal joint
Sharp wounds with little associated damage
Upper extremity (children)
Absolute Contraindications
Associated life threats
Severe crush injuries
Inability to withstand prolonged surgery
Relative Contraindications*
Single digit, unless thumb
Avulsion injury
Prolonged warm ischemia (≥12 h)
Gross contamination
Prior injury or surgery to part
Emotionally unstable patients
Lower extremity

*If the victim is a child or if there are multiple losses, salvage reimplantations.
are attempted, and the relative contraindications are ignored.
(From Roberts JR, Hedges JR (editors). Clinical Procedures in Emergency Medicine (4th ed).
Philadelphia: Saunders, 2004: p 920.)

the best prognosis due to the limited area of destruction. Local crush injuries are the most common mechanism of injury but have a poorer prognosis due to more tissue injury. Avulsion injuries have the worst prognosis due to a significant amount of injury to vessels, nerves, tendons, and soft tissue. Power saws and lawn mowers are the most frequent causes. Indications and contraindications for reimplantation are listed in Table 17–7. The time that an amputated part can survive before reimplantation has not been determined. The success of reimplantation decreases after 6 hours but perhaps longer if the amputated part is properly cooled.

- *Clinical presentation.* Color, temperature, capillary refill, and pulses are the most common strategies for determining distal perfusion. Doppler pulsations should be determined in the digits if the hand or digits are involved. An Allen's test (Appendix 2) at the wrist may aid in determining the existence of an arterial injury. Assess the degree of hemostasis, contamination, damage to surrounding tissue, bony fragments, joint penetration, and tendon injury. Motor function should be assessed. Sensation should be assessed by pinprick and two-point discrimination tests.

- *Diagnostic testing.* Radiographs of the amputated part and proximal stump to the level of at least one joint proximal to an extremity injury should be obtained. Preoperative laboratory studies should be obtained.

- **ED management.** Any hemorrhage should be controlled with direct pressure and elevation. Vascular clamps and hemostats should not be used as they may cause more damage. A proximally placed blood pressure cuff inflated 30 mm Hg above the systolic pressure can be used to obtain hemostasis for a short period of time (<30 minutes) to control severe bleeding. Gross contamination can be removed by irrigation with normal saline. Topical antiseptic solutions should *not* be used because they will damage viable tissues. All jewelry should be removed. Emergent consultations with the reimplantation team should be obtained. Wrap the amputated part in saline-moistened gauze, place in a watertight plastic bag, and immerse the bag in a container of ice water (half water and half ice); *do not place tissue directly against ice.* Label the container with the patient's name, the amputated part, the time of the original injury, and the time that cooling began. A near-amputation with some degree of perfusion is an indication to avoid cooling; keep the wounds moist with saline-soaked gauze but do not pack in ice, as this will further compromise perfusion. If vascular compromise is present, ice packs or commercial cold packs should be applied over the dressing to cool the devascularized area. A pressure dressing and splint should be applied to the injured extremity to prevent further bleeding, injury or contamination. The extremity should be elevated to decrease edema and help control bleeding.
- **Helpful hints and pitfalls.** Amputations are usually not life-threatening injuries, and other more serious injuries must be addressed. Never discard amputated tissue until all possible uses of the severed parts are considered.

Compartment Syndrome

- **Background.** A compartment syndrome is defined as an increase in pressure within a confined osseofascial space impairing neurovascular function, causing tissue damage. It is the result of a decreased compartment volume, increased compartment content, or excessive externally applied pressure. It can develop with fractures, crush injuries, electrocution, venomous bites, or even with extreme physical exercise overuse. A circumferential splint or cast can also lead to a pseudo-compartment syndrome. The lower leg and forearm are the most frequent locations; however, gluteal, hand, foot, upper arm, thigh, and back compartment syndromes are also seen. Irreversible muscle and nerve damage may occur after 6 to 8 hours of total ischemia. Large volumes of intravascular fluid can be sequestered in the involved extremities because of increased capillary permeability. When the compression is relieved, an ischemia–reperfusion process occurs resulting in the release of toxic substances (creatine kinase, potassium, phosphate, organic acids, myoglobin, and thromboplastin) into the bloodstream with additional systemic complications causing rhabdomyolysis. Intravascular volume depletion and renal hypoperfusion, combined with myoglobinuria, can cause renal dysfunction.
- **Clinical presentation.** The first symptom is usually pain out of proportion to a given clinical situation. Pain often increases with the

passive stretching of muscles involved. There may be muscle weakness, hypesthesia, and tenseness may be palpable in the involved compartment. Paralysis may result with extensive nerve and muscle damage. *The presence or absence of arterial pulsation is not an accurate indicator of compartment syndrome*; pulses may be present in a severely compromised extremity compartment.

■ *Diagnostic testing.* Although compartment syndrome is a clinical diagnosis, measurement of compartment pressures should be obtained, especially if clinical findings are equivocal. Many methods have been described for measuring compartment pressures. The Stryker is the most commonly used commercially available device (Figure 17–5). The patient

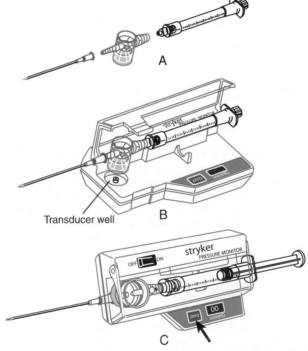

Figure 17–5. The Stryker 295 Intracompartmental Pressure Monitor System. **A,** The needle is placed firmly on the chamber stem which is then connected to the prefilled syringe; do not open and contaminate the fluid pathway. **B,** The chamber is placed in the device well. The cover is snapped close. The needle is held at approximately 45 degrees up from horizontal while fluid is slowly forced through the disposable system to purge it of air. *Caution:* Saline *MUST NOT* roll down the needle into the transducer well. **C,** The intended angle of insertion of the needle into the skin is approximated while the "zero" button is pressed. The needle is inserted into the compartment; less than 0.3 ml of saline should be slowly injected into the compartment for equilibration with interstitial fluids. The pressure is read after the display reaches equilibrium. *(From Stryker Instruments, Kalamazoo, MI.)*

should be given local anesthesia and systemic analgesia for comfort. Each compartment in the affected extremity should be tested (three in forearm, four in lower leg, Figures 17–6 and 17–7). Most compartments are superficial, and are easily accessible. Only the deep posterior compartment of the lower leg and the gluteal compartment may require a spinal needle for deeper needle placement. The needle localization and distinguishing of foot compartments is challenging because of their small size. Thus, measurement of pedal compartment pressures are usually left to an orthopedic surgeon. Normal compartment pressures range from 0 to 15 mm Hg. Compartment pressures in excess of 30 to 50 mm Hg produce clinically significant muscle ischemia. A compartment syndrome may occur at lower pressures in hypotensive patients. Myonecrosis may occur with crush injuries or a compartment syndrome. Thus, concern for rhabdomyolysis should initiate serial creatine phosphokinase levels (CPK), renal function, and electrolytes. Dark, tea-colored urine that is dipstick positive for blood despite the absence of red blood cells on microscopy is suggestive of myoglobinuria and rhabdomyolysis. A CPK level of 20,000 U/L is the threshold level for identifying those patients who are at risk and require treatment.

- ***ED management.*** It is prudent to obtain emergent orthopedic consultation for any suspicion of neurovascular injury or compartment syndrome. Vascular surgery is necessary for significant arterial injuries. Elevate the affected part to minimize pressure and edema. Remove constricting bandages and splints. A fasciotomy (opening the skin and fascia to improve blood flow) is needed for documented elevations in compartment pressure or with concerning signs or symptoms of neurovascular compromise. Patients requiring surgical intervention or serial neurovascular examinations require admission to the hospital. Vigorous fluid resuscitation is preferably started at the site of injury by prehospital personnel before reperfusion takes place. Mannitol can increase urine output and the washout of tubular myoglobin. It also has been shown to reduce intracompartmental pressure, and may be a conservative alternative to fasciotomy. Urine alkalinization with bicarbonate may decrease the toxic effects of myoglobin.

- ***Helpful hints and pitfalls.*** Left untreated, a compartment syndrome may result in permanent neurologic–muscular dysfunction and extremity deformity, or lead to shock or renal failure if myonecrosis is extensive. Mannitol should be used with caution in patients with marginal cardiac function and acute renal failure as it can cause volume overload in these patients. Intractable hyperkalemia and acidosis, refractory to volume expansion and bicarbonate administration, are the main early threats to survival in patients with rhabdomyolysis, and dialysis must be instituted promptly. The hypocalcemia that accompanies rhabdomyolysis should not be corrected unless there is danger of hyperkalemic dysrhythmias.

High-Pressure Injection

- ***Background.*** The single most important factor in the management of this injury is the type of material injected. Paint and paint thinner produce a large, early inflammatory response whereas grease causes a small

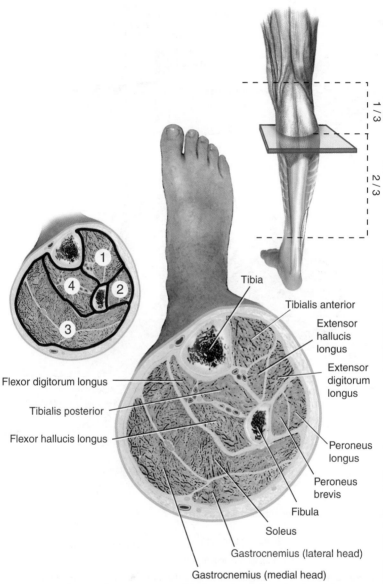

Figure 17–6. Fascial compartments of the lower leg with enclosed muscle groups. The easiest cross-sectional level for needle placement for all four compartments is approximately 3 cm on either side of a transverse line drawn at the junction of the proximal and middle thirds of the lower leg. Insert upper left: (*1*) anterior, 1 to 3 cm from anterior side; (*2*) lateral, 1 to 1.5 cm from lateral side; (*3*) superficial posterior, 2 to 4 cm from posterior side; and (*4*) deep posterior compartments, 2 to 4 cm from medial side. (*From Roberts, Clinical Procedures in Emergency Medicine (4th ed). Philadelphia: WB Saunders, 2004, p. 1066.*)

Labels in figure:

Tibia

Tibialis anterior

Extensor hallucis longus

Extensor digitorum longus

Flexor digitorum longus

Tibialis posterior

Flexor hallucis longus

Peroneus longus

Peroneus brevis

Fibula

Soleus

Gastrocnemius (lateral head)

Gastrocnemius (medial head)

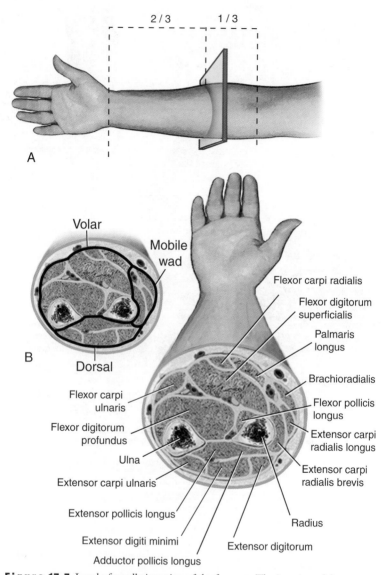

Figure 17–7. Level of needle insertion of the forearm. The junction of the proximal and middle thirds of the forearm is the cross-sectional level for needle insertion. **A,** With cross section through the upper third of the forearm **(B)** demonstrating the three forearm compartments (volar, dorsal, mobile wad). *(From Green DP [editor]. Operative Hand Surgery. New York: Churchill Livingstone, 1982.)*

inflammatory response. A large amount of material injected can cause mechanical distention with the potential for neurovascular compromise. The surface appearance is typically misleading, with much more substantial underlying tissue destruction, even with an unimpressive skin break.

■ *Clinical presentation.* The patient may have minimal symptoms and benign appearing entrance wound. Fusiform swelling of the affected digit may be present. Several hours later, the digit may become extremely painful, swollen, and pale due to vascular compromise. Performance and documentation of a detailed neurovascular examination is useful.

■ *Diagnostic testing.* Plain films are done to determine the spread of the material as many industrial paints are radio-opaque.

■ *ED management.* Initial management includes splinting, elevation, tetanus prophylaxis, analgesia, and broad-spectrum antibiotics. Digital blocks are contraindicated due to the potential for increased tissue pressure. Emergent consultation with a hand surgeon is recommended because most patients require surgical decompression and debridement.

■ *Helpful hints and pitfalls.* Do not let the innocuous appearance delay aggressive treatment. Amputation may be necessary if perfusion is significantly compromised.

Orthopedic Injuries

Common injuries are summarized in Tables 17–8 through 17–18 as follows:

■ *Hand:* See Table 17–8 for ligamentous and bone injuries and Table 17–9 and Figure 17–8 and 17–9 for simple hand infections. Hand abscesses usually require IV antibiotics and hand surgery consultation.

■ *Wrist:* See Table 17–10.

■ *Forearm and elbow:* See Table 17–11.

■ *Shoulder:* See Tables 17–12 and 17–13.

■ *Hip:* See Table 17–14.

■ *Lower extremity:* See Tables 17–15 and 17–16.

■ *Ankle and foot:* See Tables 17–17 and 17–18.

Teaching Points

Extremity injuries are common and range from minor strains and sprains to life or limb threatening injuries. Patient's must be evaluated for more subtle internal injuries, as the physician's attention may be diverted by an obvious open fracture. Any break in the skin near a fracture converts it to an open fracture, and it should be treated as such.

Radiographic images, splints, and casts should include the joint above and the joint below the injury.

Avoid circumferential casts in acute fractures because subsequent swelling can produce a compartment syndrome. Remember to be aggressive with pain management; even minor extremity problems can be very painful.

Table 17-8a   Ligamentous and Tendon Injuries of the Hand

	Definition	Mechanism	Diagnostic Clues	Treatment	Comment
Mallet finger	Detachment of extensor tendon from distal phalynx at distal interphalyngeal (DIP) joint	Forced flexion to the tip of the extended finger	Distal phalynx is flexed and cannot be fully extended actively; avulsion fracture may be present	DIP splinted in hyperextension for 6-10 wk	Improper diagnosis and treatment can lead to the development of a "swan-neck" deformity with extension at PIP and flexion at DIP
de Quervain's tendinitis	Tendonitis of the abductor pollicis longus like and extensor pollicis brevis (and sometimes extensor pollicis longus)	Thumb overuse	Finkelstein's test: thumb is held in the palm by the fingers and the wrist is deviated in the ulnar direction. Pain will occur near the radial styloid, which is also the point of tenderness.	Anti-inflammatory agents, rest, and splinting of the wrist with the thumb in 20 degrees of dorsoflexion.	Parasthesias distally or associated conditions carpal tunnel or trigger finger are not uncommon. If there is a history of trauma, treat as a possible scaphoid fracture.
Rupture of the central slip (extensor mechanism)	Disruption of the central slip of the extensor tendon hood near the PIP.	Direct blow to PIP joint or forced flexion of PIP against resistance. Dislocations of the PIP are common in athletes and are often reduced in the field.	The area of maximum tenderness is over the central slip on the dorsal aspect of the PIP. Full active extension does not assure the integrity of the central slip.	Splint PIP in extension	Boutonniere deformity develops 1-2 weeks after inciting traumatic event without proper treatment: PIP is flexed and the DIP is extended. Pain over the volar aspect of the PIP is concerning for volar plate avulsion (excessive passive PIP extension)

Table 17-8a Ligamentous and Tendon Injuries of the Hand—*cont'd*

	Definition	Mechanism	Diagnostic Clues	Treatment	Comment
Gamekeeper's thumb	Avulsion of ulnar collateral ligament	Acute forced abduction of the thumb	Pain on the medial aspect of the thumb at the MCP joint; difficulty in grasping an object between thumb and index finger; 30% have an associated fracture	Thumb spica splint	If misdiagnosed as a sprain, chronic disability may result. A "bull rider's thumb" is a torn collateral ligament on the *radial* side.

DIP, distal interphalangeal; MCP, metacarpophalangeal; PIP, proximal interphalangeal.

Table 17-8b Bony Injuries of the Hand

	Definition	Mechanism	Diagnostic Clues	Treatment	Comment
Phalyngeal fractures	Fracture to phalynx	Direct blow	Limited range of motion of finger.	Finger splint	Subungal hematomas are frequently associated
Boxer's fracture	Metacarpal neck fracture of the ring or little fingers	Direct blow; punching an object with a clenched fist	Deformity of ring or little finger knuckle. Assess for malrotation by examining the direction of the fingers in flexion. Up to 40 degrees of volar angulation is acceptable for nonoperative management.	Emergent closed reduction if angulated more than 30-40 degrees or if rotational deformities are present; ulnar gutter splint	A laceration over the MCP joint suggests a human bite (fight bite) and an open fracture unless proven otherwise. These wounds are heavily contaminated and should be aggressively managed. Less angulation is acceptable in the index and long finger metacarpals, because they are less able to compensate.
Bennett Fracture	Intrarticular fracture of the proximal thumb metacarpal with subluxation of the metacarpal joint	Axial force or striking an object with a clenched fist	Deformity and limited range of motion at thumb MCP joint	Emergent reduction and thumb spica splint	This is an unstable fracture and should be referred for consideration of surgical intervention.
Rolando fracture	Y- or T-shaped fracture involving the base of the thumb MCP joint; like a Bennett fracture but comminuted.	Axial force or striking an object with a clenched fist	Deformity and limited range of motion at thumb MCP joint	Thumb spica splint	This is an unstable fracture and should be referred for consideration of surgical intervention.

MCP, metacarpophalangeal.

Table 17–9 Infections of the Hand

	Pathophysiology	Clinical Presentation and Diagnosis	Management	Comment
Paronychia	Localized superficial infection or abscess involving the lateral nail fold due to frequent trauma or nail biting. Mostly due to *Staphylococcus aureus*, followed by streptococci.	Swelling and tenderness of soft tissue on one or both sides of the lateral nail fold. May begin as cellulitis, and then abscess.	Warm soaks, elevation, and oral anti-staphylococcal antibiotics such as dicloxicillin or cephalexin. Drain if fluctuant (see Figure 17–8)	A digital block will facilitate drainage. Soak the eponychium prior to drainage. Complications: osteomyelitis of the distal phalynx.
Felon	Infection of the pulp of the distal finger or thumb. Usually due to penetrating trauma with secondary infection with *S. aureus*	Cellulitis and inflammation in the distal pulp space causes severe pain, swelling and pressure.	Antistaphylococcal antibiotics and drainage. See Figure 17–9. The wound should be irrigated, loosely packed with gauze, and splinted. The packing is removed in 48 to 72 h, and the wound is left to close secondarily.	This differs from other abscesses due to multiple vertical septa that divide the pulp into small fascial compartments that may inhibit complete drainage. Complications: osteomyelitis and flexor tenosynovitis.

Continued

Table 17–9 Infections of the Hand—*cont'd*

	Pathophysiology	Clinical Presentation and Diagnosis	Management	Comment
Herpetic whitlow	Direct inoculation into an open wound or broken skin with herpes simplex virus.	Involves single finger; begins with pain, pruritis, and swelling, followed by clear vesicles. Systemic symptoms are absent. Vesicles coalesce to form an ulcer which may have a hemorrhagic base. A viral culture or Tzanck test of scrapings at base of unroofed vesicle (multinucleated giant cells) can confirm the diagnosis.	Prevent oral inoculation or spread. Symptomatic relief. Oral acyclovir for immunocompromised or recurrent infections.	Drainage is contraindicated and may lead to viral dissemination and secondary bacterial infection.
Flexor tenosynovitis	Acute synovial space infection. Usually due to penetrating trauma; occasionally due to hematogenous spread. S. aureus is the most common isolate.	Four cardinal signs: tenderness along the course of the flexor tendon, symmetric swelling of the finger, pain on passive extension, and a flexed posture of the finger (also called Kanavel's signs)	Consultation with hand surgeon for possible surgical drainage and IV antibiotics.	Early recognition is important as increased pressure within the tendon sheath may compromise circulation to the tendon.
Deep fascial space infections	Infection of the fascial spaces of the hand from direct penetrating trauma, infectious from contiguous site, or hematogenous seeding. Pathogens include S. aureus, streptococci, and coliforms.	Swelling and erythema. Pain with passive movement of digits or extensor tendons if on the dorsal surface of the hand.	Broad-spectrum IV antibiotics and drainage by a hand surgeon.	An infection secondary to a laceration over the MCP joint of the hand should be considered a human bite (fight bite) unless proven otherwise. These wounds are heavily contaminated and should be aggressively managed.

IV, intravenous; MCP, metacarpophalangeal.

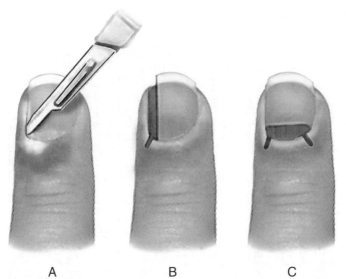

Figure 17–8. Drainage of paronychia. **A,** Eponychial fold is elevated from the nail for a simple paronychium. **B,** Lateral nail is removed if pus tracks under it. A small eponychial incision may be necessary. **C,** Proximal nail is removed if pus tracks under it. Two incisions are needed to remove the proximal nail. *(From Moran GJ, Talan DA, Emerg Med Clin North Am 11:601, 1993.)*

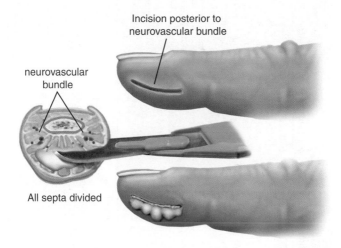

Incision posterior to neurovascular bundle

neurovascular bundle

All septa divided

Figure 17–9. Incision and drainage of felon using the unilateral longitudinal approach. The incision should be made along the ulnar aspect of digits II to IV and the radial aspects of digits I and V, avoiding pincher surfaces. The incision is begun approximately 0.5 cm distal to the distal interphalangeal joint (DIP) crease and dorsal to the neurovascular bundle of the fingertip. *(From Milford L. In: Crenshaw AH. Campbell's Operative Orthopaedics (8th ed), vol 1, St Louis, MO: Mosby, 1992.)*

Table 17–10 Bone Injuries of the Wrist

	Definition	Mechanism	Diagnostic Clues	Treatment	Comment
Scaphoid fracture	Most common carpal fracture; usually occurs in middle one third of the bone	Fall on outstretched hand	Swelling over the dorso-radial aspect of the wrist; pain in the anatomic snuff-box; up to 10% may not be radiographically evident, therefore dedicated scaphoid views may be useful	Nondisplaced fractures: thumb spica splint Displaced fractures: emergent hand referral for operative intervention within 24-48 h	The scaphoid is susceptible to development of avascular necrosis after fracture because of its proximal-to-distal blood supply
Lunate fracture	Second most common carpal fracture	Fall on outstretched hand	Swelling over the mid-dorsum of the hand; increased pain with axial loading on the third metacarpal; radiologic findings may be initially normal	Thumb spica splint	Avascular necrosis is a common complication
Lunate dislocation	Dislocation of lunate from normal anatomic position	Forceful hyperextension	Pain and swelling over the dorsum of the wrist. Deformity and swelling over volar surface of the wrist; lateral radiographs reveal the classic "spilled teacup" sign; the lunate has a triangular appearance on PA view ("piece of pie sign")	Hand surgeon consultation in the ED for reduction and stabilization.	Associated with median nerve and scaphoid injuries

Table 17–10 Bone Injuries of the Wrist—*cont'd*

	Definition	Mechanism	Diagnostic Clues	Treatment	Comment
Perilunate dislocation	Dislocation of the capitate dorsally	Fall on an outstretched hand with hyperextension	Pain and swelling over the dorsum of the wrist. Lunate remains in normal position in relation to the distal radius; the capitate is dislocated, usually in dorsal direction. PA view may show overlap of distal and proximal carpal rows.	Hand surgeon consultation in the ED for reduction and stabilization.	Associated with median nerve and scaphoid injuries
Scapholunate dislocation	Rotatory subluxation of the scaphoid	Fall on an outstretched hand with hyperextension	Pain and swelling over the dorsum of the wrist. Terry Thomas (David Letterman) sign: widening of the scapholunate joint on PA view (should be <2 mm). Signet ring sign: scaphoid seen on end with the cortex of the distal pole appearing as a ring shadow superimposed over the scaphoid on PA view.	Hand surgeon consultation in the ED for reduction and stabilization.	Standard radiographs may appear normal; need views in ulnar deviation with a clenched fist. May be associated with median nerve injury.

Continued

Table 17–10 Bone Injuries of the Wrist—*cont'd*

	Definition	Mechanism	Diagnostic Clues	Treatment	Comment
Colles' fracture	Transverse fracture of the distal radial metaphysis with *dorsal* displacement and angulation.	Fall on an outstretched hand with hyperextension	"Dinner fork" deformity	Closed reduction in the emergency department and cast. Significant displacement (greater than 20 degrees of dorsal angulation), marked dorsal comminution, or intra-articular extension require early operative repair.	Evaluate for median nerve injuries or vascular compromise. Often associated with ulnar styloid fractures. Most common wrist fracture seen in adults.
Smith's fracture	Transverse fracture of the distal radius with *volar* displacement of the fragment; also known as "Reverse Colles"	Direct blow or fall onto the dorsum of the hand or fall backward on an outstretched hand with the forearm in supination.	Distal radius fracture with volar displacement of fragment	Closed reduction in the ED and cast, OR if reduction is inadequate or the fracture is unstable.	Associated with median nerve injuries and flexor tendon injury.
Galleazzi fracture–dislocation	Fracture of the distal one third of the radius with radio-ulnar dislocation	Fall on an outstretched hand in forced pronation; direct blow to dorsolateral wrist.	Obvious deformity of the wrist. Pain with pronation or supination. The ulnar styloid may be prominent.	Operative intervention within 24 h	Rarely associated with other neurovascular injuries

Table 17–11 Bone Injuries of the Forearm and Elbow

	Definition	Mechanism	Diagnostic Clues	Treatment	Comment
Nightstick fracture	Isolated fracture to the shaft of the ulna	Direct blow to the ulna	Swelling isolated to ulnar surface of arm	Long arm cast, urgent referral within 24-48 h if displaced	Elbow film should be performed to rule out radial head dislocation (Monteggia)
Radial head fracture	Fracture of radial head	Fall on outstretched hand	Tenderness over radial head that increases with supination; fracture line may not be evident and the only radiographic clue may be the presence of an anterior or posterior fat pad	Nondisplaced fractures: sling with early range of motion Displaced fractures: posterior elbow splint and referral within 24-48 h	Associated with capitellum fractures
Monteggia fracture–dislocation	Fracture of the proximal ulna with dislocation of the radial head	Fall on an outstretched and hyperpronated hand.	The forearm may be shortened secondary to angulation; the radial head may be palpable. Elbow flexion and forearm supination is limited.	Emergent operative repair within 24 h; children may be treated with closed reduction and splinting.	Associated with radial nerve injury and recurrent subluxation of the radial head

Continued

Table 17–11   Bone Injuries of the Forearm and Elbow—*cont'd*

	Definition	Mechanism	Diagnostic Clues	Treatment	Comment
Olecranon fracture	Fracture of the olecranon process of the ulna	Direct blow or fall on an outstretched hand with elbow in flexion	May have decreased ability to extend the forearm secondary to damage to the tricep mechanism	Nondisplaced: posterior elbow splint Displacement >2 mm: splint and referral within 1-3 d	Associated with ulnar nerve neuropraxia
Condylar fracture	Fracture of either the medial or lateral condyle of the humerus at *both* the articular surface (trochlea, capitellum) *and* the nonarticular surface (mediolateral epicondyle)	Fall on outstretched hand	Decreased range of motion of elbow with swelling over either condyle	Nondisplaced: posterior elbow splint Displaced: emergent referral in the ED	

*Elbow dislocation is mentioned in Table 17–5.

Table 17–12 Soft-Tissue Injuries of the Shoulder

	Definition	Mechanism	Diagnostic Clues	Treatment	Comment
Acromioclavicular (AC) sprain	Injury to the ligamentous complex at the AC joint; ranges from minor strain of the ligaments (type I) to complete disruption of the complex (type III)	Fall on the shoulder with the arm adducted	Swelling over the distal clavicle; clavicle may appear to be displaced upward	Immobilization and early range of motion exercises	
Sternoclavicular (SC) sprain	Injury to the ligamentous complex at the SC joint; range from minor tear of the ligaments (first degree) to complete tear with displacement of the clavicle (second degree)	Fall onto the shoulder or direct force over AC joint	Swelling over medial clavicle; clavicle may appear to be displaced relative to the manubrium with third-degree sprains; Radiographs are often inadequate, and computed tomography may provide the best view	First or second degree: sling Third degree: immediate reduction	Posterior displacement of the clavicle can result in compression of mediastinal structures, and is a true emergency requiring immediate operative repair; pneumothorax, rupture of great vessels, tracheal injury and esophageal injuries may occur
Rotator cuff injuries	Tear of the tendinous insertions of the rotator cuff muscles at the greater and lesser tuberosities of the humerus	Fall onto the shoulder, heavy lifting, or forceful abduction of the arm against resistance; chronic injuries are more common	Weak, painful abduction of the arm; degenerative change or joint space narrowing may be seen on radiograph	Sling and range of motion exercise	

Table 17–13 Bone Injuries of the Shoulder Girdle

	Definition	Mechanism	Diagnostic Clues	Treatment	Key Points
Humeral shaft fracture	Usually involves middle one third of humerus	Fall on an outstretched hand or direct blow; may occur as secondary to inherent bone pathology (pathologic fracture)	Deformity of upper arm with decreased ability to move arm	Sugar-tong splint with sling and swathe	Associated with radial nerve or brachial artery injury
Proximal humerus fracture	Fractures involving the greater tuberosity, lesser tuberosity, humeral head, or proximal humeral shaft	Fall on outstretched hand or direct blow to lateral aspect of the arm	Arm is held in adduction; more common in the elderly. Neer's classification criteria**	Sling and swathe	May have associated neurovascular injuries to the brachial plexus, axillary nerve, or axillary artery. Other complications include adhesive capsulitis and avascular necrosis
Scapular fracture	Fracture of the body of the scapula and glenoid neck are most common	Direct blow to scapula/shoulder; fractures occur secondary to high energy trauma	Arm is held in adduction with posterior scapular tenderness	Sling and early range of motion exercises; glenoid fractures require referral within 1–3 d	Commonly associated with other traumatic thoracic injuries, including rib fracture, pneumothorax, and mediastinal injuries
Clavicular fracture	Occur most commonly in middle one third of clavicle	Direct force to clavicle or a force applied to the distal portion of the clavicle	Shoulder on affected side may be pulled downward secondary to lack of support; more common in children	Nondisplaced: sling. Displaced: sling and swathe	Neurovascular injuries to the brachial plexus or subclavian artery/vein or pneumothoraces may occur with displaced fractures

*Shoulder dislocation is mentioned in Table 17–5.
**An anatomic classification system for proximal humeral according to the amount of displacement of four segments: anatomic neck, surgical neck, greater tuberosity, lesser tuberosity.

Table 17-14 Bone Injuries of the Hip

	Definition	Mechanism	Diagnostic Clues	Treatment	Comment
Hip fractures	There are two types of hip fractures: **Intracapsular:** femoral head and femoral neck fractures; and **Extracapsular:** trochanteric, intertrochanteric, and subtrochanteric fractures	Falls	Lower extremity is shortened and externally rotated; most commonly seen in the elderly; Radiologic findings may initially negative; computed tomography should be ordered if concerned for this and plain films are negative	Emergent referral in the emergency department and operative repair within 1-4 d if deemed necessary	Avascular necrosis: may occur in femoral neck fractures and in patients <60 y is a surgical emergency that requires operative intervention within 24 h

Table 17–15 Bone Injuries of the Lower Extremity

	Definition	Mechanism	Diagnostic Clues	Treatment	Comment
Femoral shaft fracture	Fracture of the femoral shaft	High impact injuries; may present after minimal trauma in patients with underlying bone pathology	Painful deformity to the thigh; presence of a thigh hematoma	Hare traction splint and emergent orthopedic consultation in the ED for emergent operative intervention	High incidence of hemorrhage; large volume losses can be associated with femur fractures
Patellar fracture	Fracture to the patella; most commonly transverse	Direct blow to the patella	Pain with leg extension; limited ability extend leg; Sunrise views can pick up fractures not seen on AP/lateral radiographs	Immobilize in full extension; partial weight bearing	May be associated with patellofemoral pain (long term)
Tibial plateau fracture	Fracture of the proximal tibia; the most common fracture of the knee; often involves the articular surface	Direct axial loading; rotational stress; direct varus or valgus stress	Infrapatellar knee pain and swelling; hemarthrosis; rotational deformities may be observed if the fracture is compressed	Nondepressed: immobilization, non-weight-bearing, operative repair within 1-3 d Depressed: urgent operative intervention within 24-48 h	The popliteal and anterior tibial arteries are the most commonly injured structures. The peroneal nerve may be compromised. Also associated with concomitant ligamentous injuries and compartment syndrome.

Table 17–15 Bone Injuries of the Lower Extremity—*cont'd*

	Definition	Mechanism	Diagnostic Clues	Treatment	Comment
Maissoneuve fracture	Proximal fibular fracture that occurs in conjunction with (a) rupture of the medial deltoid ligament of the ankle OR (b) medial malleolus fracture, with disruption of the tibiofibular syndesmosis; results in an unstable ankle mortise	External rotary force applied to the ankle	Pain and swelling in both the proximal fibula and medial ankle	Urgent surgical repair within 1-3 d	May be missed without a complete physical examination and proper radiographs

Patellar and knee dislocation is mentioned in Table 17–5.

Table 17–16   Other Injuries to the Lower Extremity

	Definition	Mechanism	Diagnostic Clues	Treatment	Comment
Ligamentous injuries of the knee	Injuries involving the ACL, PCL, MCL, and LCL; most commonly affects MCL; The "unhappy triad" occurs when the MCL, ACL, medial meniscus and PCL has been disrupted	Multiple mechanisms of injury can cause ligamentous injuries to the knee; most commonly occurs secondary to valgus stress with external rotation of the flexed knee (ex: football player being clipped); mechanisms such as hyperextension or flex-and-pivot usually result in injuries to the cruciate ligament (ACL>PCL)	Hemarthrosis; tenderness along the joint line (MCL, LCL), ligamentous instability on examination; radiographs may reveal an effusion	Immobilization with knee brace; partial or non–weight-bearing depending on the extent of injury; pain control; can consider arthrocentesis for immediate relief	May be associated with chronic ligamentous instability and arthritis
Quadricep injuries	Injury to the quadriceps mechanism are secondary to one or more of the following injuries: 1. Quadricep tendon rupture 2. Patellar tendon rupture 3. Patellar fracture 4. Tibial tuberosity avulsion	Occurs when the quadriceps muscles are suddenly contracted against the body's weight (i.e., trying to prevent yourself from falling)	Knee swelling; high-riding patella (patella alta) or a low-riding patella (patella baja); limited active or passive extension of the leg; may feel a depression at the site of patellar insertion	Immobilization in full extension; early orthopedic referral within 24-48 h	Contractures and adhesions may develop, with resultant limitation of knee mobility, with delayed diagnosis or improper management

Table 17-16 Other Injuries to the Lower Extremity—*cont'd*

	Definition	Mechanism	Diagnostic Clues	Treatment	Comment
Gastrocnemius strain	Tear of the muscle or musculotendinous junction	Sudden ankle dorsiflexion in the involved leg in which the knee has been previously extended and the ankle plantar flexed.	Sudden intense pain and tenderness in the posterior medial aspect of the calf; swelling and variable loss of function. Ankle dorsiflexion elicits pain. MRI is superior to CT scans or plain films.	Rest and non–weight bearing for several days for mild cases. Splint in equinus position for 8 wk for incomplete tears. Complete tears require surgical repair.	Compartment syndrome may occur. Tenderness from a plantaris strain is located just lateral to the midline in the posterior calf.

ACL, anterior cruciate ligament; CT, computed tomography; LCL, lateral collateral ligament; MRI, magnetic resonance imaging; MCL, medial collateral ligament; PCL, posterior cruciate ligament.

Table 17–17 Bone Injuries of the Ankle and Foot

	Definition	Mechanism	Diagnostic Clues	Treatment	Comment
Malleolar fractures	**Lateral:** most commonly fractured; may be an isolated injury **Medial:** usually associated with lateral or posterior fractures; may be associated with a proximal fibular fracture (Maissoneuve fracture) **Posterior:** rarely an isolated injury **Bimalleolar:** usually lateral and medial **Trimalleolar:** all three involved	**Lateral:** inversion injury **Medial:** eversion or external rotation	The Ottawa Ankle Rules state that radiographs are needed if there is pain in the malleolar region AND one of the following: 1. Bone tenderness at the posterior edge of the distal 6 cm or tip of the lateral or medial malleolus 2. The patient is unable to walk at least four steps immediately after the injury or at the time of evaluation.	If an isolated malleolus fracture, short leg cast should be applied with orthopedic referral within 1 week; bimalleolar or trimalleolar fractures require urgent repair within 24-48 h	Associated with ligamentous injuries that can be seen as disruption of the integrity of the ankle mortise and the tibiofibular syndesmosis
Pilon fractures	Intra-articular fracture of the distal tibia; often comminuted and associated with significant soft tissue injury	Mostly high energy mechanism. The head of the talus drives itself into the tibial plafond primarily from axial compression with secondary rotation or shear forces.	Often confused with trimalleolar fractures. In pilon fractures, there is comminution of the distal tibia and fibula with the malleoli generally maintained in their usual anatomic position.	Orthopedic consultation from the ED for operative fixation.	25% are open fractures. Complications are common and include infection, malunion, and chronic pain.

Table 17–17 Bone Injuries of the Ankle and Foot—*cont'd*

	Definition	Mechanism	Diagnostic Clues	Treatment	Comment
Calcaneal fracture	Most commonly fractured tarsal bone; 10% are bilateral	Compression injury (i.e., fall from a height)	Swelling, tenderness, and ecchymosis of the hind foot; depressed fractures present when Bohler's angle is calculated to be <20 degrees on lateral radiograph A Harris view (axial) should be performed. Often requires CT scan.	Nondisplaced: posterior splint and orthopedic referral within in 1-3 d Displaced and intra-articular: emergent orthopedic consultation in the ED for repair within 24-48 h	Associated with thoracolumbar compression fractures (10%-15%) and other lower extremity fractures (25%). Also associated with compartment syndrome of the foot, which is commonly misdiagnosed
Jones fracture	Transverse fracture of the proximal diaphysis of the fifth metatarsal	Direct force to lateral foot	Swelling and pain at proximal fifth metatarsal	Nonweight-bearing short leg cast	High association with delayed union or nonunion Often misdiagnosed as a Dancer's fracture.
Pseudo-Jones fracture or Dancer's fracture	Avulsion fracture of the proximal fifth metatarsal at the insertion of the peroneus brevis	Inversion injury to plantar flexed foot	Swelling and pain at proximal fifth metatarsal	Extra-articular: compression dressing and hard-soled shoe Intra-articular: short leg cast and early orthopedic referral.	Often misdiagnosed as an ankle sprain.

Continued

Table 17-17 Bone Injuries of the Ankle and Foot—*cont'd*

	Definition	Mechanism	Diagnostic Clues	Treatment	Comment
Lisfranc fracture–dislocation	The Lisfranc joint is between the mid foot and the forefoot and is primarily stabilized by the second metatarsal and a ligamentous complex.	High-energy injury. Due to axial loads, crush injury, or rotational forces. Most are from motor vehicle collisions. One third are from trivial mechanisms.	Swelling and tenderness over tarsometatarsal joint; inability to weight-bear; radiographs can reveal: disruption of the normal alignment of the medial cuneiform with the medial aspect of the second metatarsal; fracture at the base of the second metatarsal; widening at the base of the first and second metatarsals	Emergent orthopedic consultation in the ED for surgical management within 24-48 h	Often misdiagnosed and can lead to chronic pain syndromes and long-term biomechanical dysfunction of the foot. Weight-bearing views are sometimes helpful.

Ankle dislocation is mentioned in Table 17-5.

Table 17–18 Other Injuries to the Ankle and Foot

	Definition	Mechanism	Diagnostic Clues	Treatment	Comment
Ankle sprain	Injury to the stabilizing ligaments of the ankle mortise; is usually lateral and most commonly involves the anterior talofibular ligament (>90%) and the calcaneofibular ligament (20%); medial sprains of the deltoid ligament are less common, and usually occur in conjunction with medial malleolar fractures	Medial: inversion and lateral rotation of the plantar-flexed foot Lateral: eversion and external rotation of the foot	Pain and swelling at the ankle joint, but minimal bony tenderness; high grade sprains are associated with significant functional loss, inability to bear weight, and ligamentous laxity with stress testing; avulsion fractures may be seen on radiography	Sugar-tong splint of ankle	May be associated with Maissoneuve fracture (see Table 17–15), an avulsion fracture of little toe metatarsal, peroneal tendon subluxation/ dislocation, or fracture of talar dome
Achilles tendon rupture	Tear of the Achilles tendon from its insertion at the base of the calcaneous Commonly seen in middle-aged males who participate sporadically in recreational sports	Forceful dorsiflexion of the foot with the ankle in the relaxed state, direct trauma to a taut tendon, or extra stretch applied to a taut tendon	Palpable defect at site of Achilles tendon or in gastrocnemius muscle; limited plantar flexion; positive Thompson test: place the patient in a prone position, flex the knee 90 degrees, and squeeze the calf; if plantar flexion of the foot occurs, there is no rupture; if there is an absence of plantar flexion, the tendon is ruptured)	Posterior splint in plantar flexion and orthopedic referral within 1-3 d	Often misdiagnosed because even with complete rupture, many patients retain some ability to plantar flex secondary to the actions of the tibialis posterior, toe flexors, and peroneal muscles

Suggested Readings

Dalsey WC, Luk J. Management of amputations. In: Roberts JR, Hedges JR, eds. Clinical Procedures in Emergency Medicine. Section VIII: Musculoskeletal Procedures. 4th ed. Philadelphia: Saunders, 2004:919–925.

Frankel NR, Villarin Jr LA. Compartment syndrome evaluation. In: Roberts JR, Hedges JR, eds. Clinical Procedures in Emergency Medicine. Section VIII: Musculoskeletal Procedures. 4th ed. Philadelphia: Saunders, 2004:1058–1071.

Geiderman JM. General principles of orthopedic injuries. In: Marx JA, Hockberger RS, Walls RM, eds. Rosen's Emergency Medicine: Concepts and Clinical Practice. 6th ed. Philadelphia: Mosby, 2006, pp 549–576.

Malinoski DJ, Slater MS, Mullins RJ. Crush injury and rhabdomyolysis. Crit Care Clin 2004;20:171–192.

Perron AD, Brady WJ. Evaluation and management of the high-risk orthopedic emergency. Emerg Med Clin North Am 2003;21:159–204.

Simon RR, Koenigsknecht SJ, eds. Emergency Orthopedics: The Extremities. 4th ed. McGraw-Hill, 2001.

PROBLEM-SOLVING COMMON MEDICAL COMPLAINTS

CHAPTER 18

Abdominal Pain

LYNN P. ROPPOLO ■ JEREMY SPINKS ■ CRAIG REECE BROCKMAN II

 Red Flags

Extremes of age ● Immunocompromised state ● Abnormal vital signs (high fever, ↑ heart rate, ↓ blood pressure) ● Severe pain of rapid onset Signs of dehydration ● Pallor ● Diaphoresis ● Peritoneal signs ● Other co-morbid conditions: diabetes, atherosclerosis

Overview

Look for "red flags" (see Box) and consider critical diagnoses or life-threatening problems early. The initial assessment should follow the ABCs as in any potentially life-threatening emergency (see Section II).

Abdominal pain can be visceral (vague), somatic (localized), referred, or due to extra-abdominal causes (i.e., diabetic ketoacidosis, acute myocardial infarction).

Immunocompromised, elderly, and young pediatric patients often have minimal clinical signs and symptoms despite the presence of serious abdominal conditions.

All women of reproductive age require a full obstetric and gynecologic history, pregnancy test, and pelvic examination (especially if lower abdominal pain present).

Most patients with abdominal pain should have a rectal examination.

Abdominal pain is a dynamic process requiring re-evaluation of the patient in the ED. Reassessment, including repeated abdominal examinations, is indicated after any change in the patient's status, any new or worsening condition, or after any therapeutic intervention.

Up to 50% of patients have no clear diagnosis after the ED workup is completed.

Differential Diagnosis of Abdominal Pain

■ See DDx table.
■ Based on location of pain by quadrant (Figure 18–1)
■ The source of pain for patients presenting with mid-epigastric pain may be cardiac (e.g.,myocardial ischemia), gastric (e.g., gastric reflux, peptic

DDx Priority-Based Differential Diagnosis of Abdominal Pain

	Critical Diagnoses	Emergent Diagnoses	Nonemergent Diagnoses
Cardiovascular	Abdominal aortic aneurysm Myocardial infarction (22)	Congestive heart failure with hepatomegaly (52)	
Pulmonary		Right lower lobe pneumonia (67)	
Gastrointestinal	Esophageal rupture (22) Intestinal obstruction Mesenteric ischemia Perforated viscus or solid organ rupture (i.e., spleen)	Abscess (intra-abdominal and psoas) (67) Appendicitis Biliary disease Diverticulitis Gastritis Gastroenteritis Hepatitis (41) Hernia (36) Inflammatory bowel disease (27) Pancreatitis (acute) Peptic ulcer disease Spontaneous bacterial peritonitis (67)	Constipation (23) Gastroesophageal reflux disease (GERD) Irritable bowel syndrome (27) Abdominal wall pain Nonspecific abdominal pain
Genitourinary	Ruptured ectopic pregnancy (68)	Ovarian torsion/cyst (68) Pelvic inflammatory disease (68) Ureteral colic (32)	Endometriosis (68) Mittelschmerz (68)
Other		Diabetic ketoacidosis (38) Sickle cell crisis (53)	Herpes zoster (62)

( ) Refers to the chapter in which the disease entity is discussed.

ulcer disease, gastritis), pancreatic (e.g., pancreatic), vascular (e.g., aortic dissection or ruptured abdominal aortic aneurysm), or hepatobililary (e.g., cholecystitis) source.
- Pain that is diffuse may be due to an abdominal aortic aneurysm, diabetic ketoacidosis, early appendicitis, gastroenteritis, intestinal obstruction, mesenteric ischemia, peritonitis, or systemic toxin exposure (e.g., black widow spider bite).

Right Upper Quadrant	**Gallbladder** (cholecystitis) **Heart** (myocardial ischemia) **Kidney** (renal colic) **Liver** (hepatitis, hepatomegaly) **Lung** (right lower lobe pneumonia) **Pancreas** (pancreatitis) **Skin** (herpes zoster) **Stomach** (peptic ulcer disease)	**Heart** (myocardial ischemia) **Kidney** (renal colic) **Lung** (right lower lobe pneumonia) **Pancreas** (pancreatitis) **Skin** (herpes zoster) **Spleen** (splenomegaly, rupture) **Stomach** (peptic ulcer disease)	Left Upper Quadrant
Right Lower Quadrant	**Appendix** (appendicitis) **Fallopian tube** (ectopic pregnancy, pelvic inflammatory disease) **Intestinal** (diverticulitis, enteritis, hernia) **Lymph nodes** (adenitis) **Muscles** (psoas abscess) **Ovary** (cyst, torsion, mittelshmerz) **Ureter** (ureteral stone)	**Fallopian tube** (ectopic pregnancy, pelvic inflammatory disease) **Intestinal** (diverticulitis, enteritis, hernia) **Lymph nodes** (adenitis) **Muscles** (psoas abscess) **Ovary** (cyst, torsion, mittelshmerz) **Ureter** (ureteral stone)	Left Lower Quadrant

Figure 18–1. Differential diagnosis based on location of abdominal pain. System or organ involved with example diagnoses in parentheses.

Initial Diagnostic Approach
General

- Any patient who is hemodynamically unstable or appears ill should receive immediate attention. While the physician is assessing the patient, a continuous cardiac monitor and pulse oximeter should be placed. Intravenous (IV) access should be obtained. These patients should not leave the ED until stabilized or for definitive care (i.e., operating room).
- The younger the patient, the fewer and less concerning co-morbid conditions, the better the historian, and the better the patient appears on physical examination, the fewer laboratory and imaging studies may be indicated. Immunocompromised, elderly, and young pediatric patients require a more liberal diagnostic workup.

Laboratory

- Studies may include a complete blood cell count, electrolytes and renal function, liver function tests, lipase, lactate, and urinalysis.
- Patients with upper abdominal pain that is concerning for a cardiac etiology should have cardiac enzymes checked.
- Patients whose clinical appearance suggests blood loss, anemia, an abdominal aortic aneurysm, or hemodynamic instability should have blood sent for type and cross match.

EKG

- An EKG should be ordered for patients with upper abdominal pain, cardiac risk factors, radiation to the left arm, diaphoresis, shortness of breath, or exertional symptoms especially if they are over the age of 50.

Radiography

- *Plain films.* These studies are most helpful to screen for free peritoneal air secondary to perforation of a hollow viscus, bowel obstruction, or pulmonary process. They do not help in the diagnosis of appendicitis.
- *Ultrasound.* These studies are best for biliary disease such as gallstones and common bile duct dilatation, uterine or ovarian pathology, intrauterine pregnancy, and scrotal pathology. It is useful for detecting intraperitoneal fluid and the cross-sectional diameter of abdominal aortic aneurysms. Ultrasound can also reveal hydronephrosis as an indirect indicator of an obstructing ureteral calculus.
- *Computed tomography (CT) scan.* Allows for imaging of both intraperitoneal and retroperitonal structures with a high degree of accuracy. No IV or oral contrast is used in the evaluation of nephrolithiasis.
- *Angiography.* In the setting of abdominal pain, this study is mostly indicated for the evaluation of mesenteric ischemia or severe gastrointestinal bleeding.

Emergency Department Management Overview
General

- The ABCs (*a*irway, *b*reathing, and *c*irculation) should be addressed as discussed in Section II. Supplemental oxygen should be given if the patient is in respiratory distress or if the oxygen saturation is less than 95%. Two large-bore IVs should be placed and isotonic fluids should be administered if the patient is hemodynamically unstable, or may have potentially life-threatening conditions.
- Prompt ED evaluation is prudent, and a timely surgical consultation should be obtained for patients who may have surgical disease.

Medications

- *Analgesia.* Do not delay early analgesia for patients in severe distress secondary to pain. Give morphine 2 to 5 mg IV every 5 to 10 minutes until the patient is comfortable. Nonsteroidal anti-inflammatory drugs (NSAIDs) such as ketorolac are useful in treating pain associated with nephrolithiasis and gynecologic pain (i.e., ovarian cysts) but should not be given to patients who may require immediate surgery (see Chapter 90.1).
- *Antacids.* If the patient can tolerate oral medications and has symptoms consistent with gastritis, gastroesophageal reflux disease (GERD), or peptic ulcer disease, give oral antacids such as Maalox (with or without lidocaine) and an histamine (H_2) blocker or proton pump inhibitor (see Chapter 90.4). These have therapeutic but no diagnostic value (i.e., relief of pain does not confirm the diagnosis of hiatal hernia).
- *Antibiotics.* Early administration is required for patients with the clinical appearance of perforation or abdominal infection. These infections are usually polymicrobial and the antibiotic coverage should include gram negative and anaerobic bacteria (see Chapter 90.2).

Emergency Department Interventions

- ■ *Nasogastric tube.* It is useful to insert a nasogastric tube attached to low suction for persistent vomiting, gastrointestinal bleeding, suspected bowel obstruction, or severe pancreatitis.
- ■ *Urinary catheter.* A Foley catheter should be placed to relieve bladder obstruction, for critically ill patients to ensure adequate urine output, and for patients who are incontinent or are menstruating if an accurate urinalysis is needed (can use in-and-out catheter).

Disposition

- ■ *Consultation.* Obtain a surgical consultation for any patient with surgical disease.
- ■ *Admission.* Obtain admission for patients with abnormal laboratory tests or imaging studies, patients with persistent pain requiring narcotic analgesia or vomiting, or a concerning abdominal examination. It is prudent to admit the immunocompromised, elderly, and young pediatric patients due to the higher incidence of serious pathology despite minimal clinical findings in this patient population.
- ■ *Discharge.* Patients with normal laboratory tests, imaging studies, or resolution of symptoms, as well as a normal abdominal examination upon reevaluation may be discharged home with close follow-up within 24 hours and "abdominal warnings" (i.e., return to the ED immediately for severe pain, fever, or persistent vomiting).

Specific Problems

Refer to the DDx table for reference to a discussion of problems in the differential not mentioned here.

Abdominal Aortic Aneurysm (AAA)

- ■ *Definition.* This is a localized dilatation of the abdominal aortic artery that may rupture secondary to progressive weakening of the wall of the aorta. This should not be confused with *aortic dissections*, in which blood enters the media of the aorta and splits (dissects) the aortic wall.
- ■ *Epidemiology and risk factors.* Most frequent in the elderly and in men. Risk factors include hypertension, diabetes, smoking, chronic obstructive pulmonary disease (COPD), and coronary artery disease. The operative mortality for a ruptured AAA is 50%.
- ■ *Pathophysiology.* Atherosclerosis is always present. Most AAAs involve the aorta below the renal arteries. The normal infrarenal aorta is approximately 2 cm in diameter. Most ruptured AAAs have diameters greater than 5 cm. Most AAAs are true aneurysms, which involves all three layers (intima, media, adventitia) of the vessel wall. A pseudoaneursym is contained only by the adventitia or surrounding soft tissues. An AAA may rupture into the gastrointestinal (GI) tract (aortoenteric fistula) or inferior vena cava (aortocaval fistula). An aortoenteric fistula is a rare event but occurs when the AAA erodes into the GI tract or as a complication of an AAA repair.

- *History.* The pain associated with a stable, intact aneurysm is gradual in onset and has a vague, dull quality. Sudden onset of severe abdominal pain radiating to the back, followed by syncope or signs of shock, is consistent with rupture. Pain may also radiate to the groin, testes, thigh, inguinal area, and chest. An aneurysm may be associated with nausea and vomiting. Five percent of AAA cases present with peripheral emboli to the lower extremities. Patients with aortoenteric fistulas may arrive at the hospital with hematemesis or melena.

- *Physical examination.* Many aneurysms cannot be palpated. Their presence is best confirmed by an ultrasound study. There is no risk of causing rupture by abdominal palpation. Bruits are found in only 5% to 10% of cases and are a nonspecific finding. Femoral pulses should be checked, as these may be decreased with rupture. Hypotension may be present, and is an ominous sign.

- *Diagnostic testing.* Plain films (abnormal calcifications on a lateral view) are abnormal in 75% of patients. No patient with a known or suspected AAA rupture should be considered stable. A bedside ultrasound can help confirm the diagnosis in unstable patients but will not demonstrate leakage (see Chapter 93). The accuracy of ultrasound may be limited by obesity, bowel gas, and availability, and it is operator dependent. A CT scan is 100% accurate in revealing an AAA, but the patient's instability may prevent the study from being obtained (Figure 18–2). IV contrast is used in elective studies but need not be used in emergency situations. Acute hemorrhage is well visualized without contrast. A CT scan is also better at visualizing the retroperitoneum or identifying an alternative diagnosis. Angiography has no place in the emergent evaluation of the suspected ruptured AAA. Angiography can underestimate aneurysm size if significant amounts of thrombus are present. Magnetic resonance imaging (MRI) can be used electively; acutely hemorrhaged blood can be difficult to identify.

- *ED management.* Establish two large-bore IVs, type and cross match for 10 units of blood. Surgery should be consulted for emergent operative repair. It is often impossible to fully resuscitate in the ED. Hemodynamically unstable patients should go to the OR as soon as possible. If the patient is hypertensive on admission, unlike aortic dissection, there is no evidence to support lowering the blood pressure. An asymptomatic patient with an incidental finding of an AAA should be referred for elective repair.

- *Helpful hints and pitfalls.* In the older patient, an aneurysm may be mistaken for renal colic. It is estimated that AAAs smaller than 5 cm expand at a rate of 0.4 cm/y. The classic triad of pain, hypotension, and a pulsatile abdominal mass may not be present. Blood loss from a ruptured AAA may cause diminished coronary perfusion.

Appendicitis

- *Epidemiology and risk factors.* Appendicitis is most likely to occur in adolescents and young adults.
- *Pathophysiology.* Appendiceal lumen obstruction leads to swelling, ischemia, infection, and, if not removed, perforation. A fecolith is the most common cause.

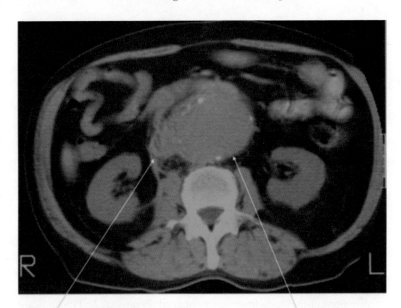

Retroperitoneal bleeding and inflammation from the leaking aneurysm.

Dilated aorta. Note the atherosclerotic calcifications in the aortic wall. An aneurysm is usually diagnosed when the aortic diameter exceeds 3 cm. Intervention is generally taken when diameter exceeds 4–5 cm or when there is rupture, leak, or increasing diameter. Slow leaking aneurysms often cause perianeurysmal fibrotic changes.

Figure 18–2. Leaking abdominal aortic aneurysm. Axial computed tomography image with no oral or intravenous contrast. *(Courtesy of Dr. Jason Scott Stephens, The University of Texas Southwestern, Department of Radiology.)*

- *History.* Vague epigastric or periumbilical pain of visceral origin is followed by anorexia, nausea, or vomiting a few hours later, and low-grade fever. Usually within a day, the pain changes to a parietal type of pain that localizes to McBurney's point in the right lower quadrant (RLQ; an area 2 cm from the anterior superior iliac spine).
- *Physical examination.* The examiner may find point tenderness, rebound, or guarding in the RLQ. Rovsing's sign (pain perceived over the RLQ when the LLQ is palpated), iliopsoas sign (pain in RLQ upon flexing thigh against resistance), and obturator sign (RLQ pain with internal and external rotation of flexed hip) also suggest appendicitis but are seen in fewer than 10% of cases. Diffuse rebound tenderness implies appendiceal rupture with consequent peritonitis.
- *Diagnostic testing.* Leukocytosis (but a normal white blood cell [WBC] count does not mean that appendicitis is absent), hematuria, or pyuria

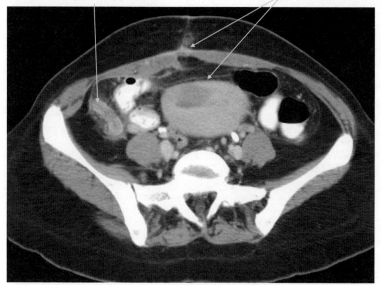

Enlarged inflamed appendix representing acute appendicitis.

Postsurgical changes in the abdominal wall and uterus from recent cesarian section.

Figure 18–3. Appendicitis. Axial computed tomography images with oral and intravenous contrast. The image shows the enlarged inflamed appendix. The patient also has postoperative changes from a caesarian delivery 3 days earlier. *(Courtesy of Dr. Jason Scott Stephens, The University of Texas Southwestern, Department of Radiology.)*

may be present. If the diagnosis is straightforward, no imaging studies are needed. Plain films are not useful. An abdominal ultrasound may reveal a noncompressible appendix and is most useful in children who are thin. A CT scan (study of choice) reveals periappendiceal fat strands. It may also visualize a distended, edematous, nonfilling appendix, fecalith, abscess, rupture, or an alternative pathology if appendicitis is not present (Figure 18–3).

- **ED management.** The patient should have nothing by mouth (NPO), IV hydration, and a surgery consult. Once the decision has been made to operate, start the administration of antibiotics to cover gram-negative and anaerobic organisms (e.g., cefotetan or cefoxitin). A nasogastric tube is often unnecessary but may be used for the patient with persistent vomiting, abdominal distention, or diffuse peritonitis.
- **Helpful hints and pitfalls.** Patients at extremes of age present atypically. Approximately 25% of women with signs suggestive of appendicitis have gynecologic disease. Thus, ancillary testing with a CT scan or ultrasound examination is usually required. The diagnosis of appendicitis during pregnancy is difficult. The rate of perforation is two to three times higher than in the general population. A normal WBC count does not indicate absence of acute appendicitis.

Biliary Tract Disease

- **Definitions.** *Cholelithiasis* is a stone in the gallbladder. *Choledocholithiasis* is a stone in common bile duct. *Biliary colic* is transient gallstone obstruction of the cystic duct causing intermittent right upper quadrant (RUQ) pain following a meal. There is no infection present. *Acute cholecystitis* is inflammation of the gallbladder caused by obstruction of the cystic duct. *Cholangitis* is due to a common duct stone and results in obstruction of the biliary tract and biliary stasis leading to bacterial infection. A *gallstone ileus* occurs when a stone erodes through the wall of the gallbladder, and into adjacent small bowel. The stone is often too large to pass, especially the ileocecal valve, and the patient presents with an episode of biliary colic that is often masked or forgotten as the patient develops a small bowel obstruction.

- **Epidemiology and risk factors.** The four F's, "A *f*at, *f*ertile (i.e., multiparous), *f*emale in her *f*orties," is classic. A gallstone ileus occurs in older patients who have had large solitary gallstones, usually present for many years. *Acalculous cholecystitis* is more common in the elderly, during recovery from non–biliary tract surgery, and in immunocompromised patients. This has a more acute and malignant course.

- **Pathophysiology.** See definitions above. Gallstones are either cholesterol stones or pigmented stones (contain calcium bilirubinate). Three simultaneous defects are typically required for the formation of cholesterol gallstones: (1) secretion of a cholesterol-supersaturated bile by the liver; (2) nucleation of cholesterol monohydrate crystals from gallbladder bile; and (3) gallbladder stasis.

- **History.** The patient will complain of RUQ abdominal pain that may radiate to the base of the scapula or shoulder and may worsen with eating. The pain may be colicky but more commonly is steady rather than intermittent. Nausea and vomiting may be present. Fever and jaundice may be present with cholecystitis, but are more common with cholangitis. *Charcot's triad* is fever, jaundice, and RUQ pain. *Reynold's pentad* includes the former three signs plus sepsis and an altered sensorium. Both are concerning for ascending cholangitis.

- **Physical examination.** The patient will have tenderness in the RUQ or epigastric region. Temperature elevation, tachycardia, and a positive Murphy's sign (inhibition of inspiration because of pain over the gallbladder), as well as a palpable tender mass in the RUQ, are often present. Sepsis is a common complication of cholangitis.

- **Diagnostic testing.** Serum aminotransferase, bilirubin, and alkaline phosphatase levels may be mildly elevated in cholecystitis but are more often within normal limits. Leukocytosis, increased bilirubin, elevated alkaline phosphatase, and moderately increased aminotransferases are common in cholangitis. Plain films show radio-opaque stones in only 10% to 15% of patients with acute cholecystis. An ultrasound in patients with cholecystitis may reveal gallstones, thickened gallbladder wall, and pericholecystic fluid (see Chapter 93). An ultrasonic Murphy's sign (inspiratory inhibition by pressure of the ultrasound probe over the gallbladder) is often present. Dilatation of the common bile duct implies presence or recent passage of a common duct stone. Ultrasonographic evidence of dilated common and intrahepatic ducts is concerning for cholangitis. Nuclear scintigraphy (hepatoiminodiacetic acid [HIDA] scan) is an excellent study for cholecystitis but is often impractical in the ED setting. A CT scan can reveal the cause of the obstruction in a gallstone ileus, since ultrasound studies are compromised by the additional bowel gas of the bowel obstruction in this setting. The diagnosis is sometimes apparent on plain films, since these solitary stones are usually highly calcified.

- **ED management.** Patients with uncomplicated biliary colic who are symptom free can be discharged with surgical follow-up for elective cholecystectomy. Antispasmodics such as glycopyrrolate and NSAIDs may relieve biliary colic pain. Patients with cholecystitis should be NPO and receive IV hydration, antiemetics, nasogastric suction (to decrease stimulus for biliary secretion and excretion), narcotic analgesia, IV antibiotics (see Chapter 90.2), surgical consultation, and hospital admission. The most serious complication is gangrene of the gallbladder, with necrosis and perforation. Patients with cholangitis are managed in a similar fashion to cholecystitis but require aggressive antibiotic therapy and hemodynamic stabilization. Early biliary tract decompression with percutaneous transhepatic cholangiography (THC), endoscopic retrograde cholangiopancreatography (ERCP) or surgery is needed. Treatment for a gallstone ileus is surgical, to relieve the small bowel obstruction, and remove the gallbladder small bowel fistula.
- **Helpful hints and pitfalls.** Immunocompromised patients (especially diabetics) are at greater risk for complications such as gangrene of the gallbladder, necrosis and perforation, emphysematous cholecystitis (gas in the gallbladder wall from gas-producing organisms), pericholecystic abscess, and fistula formation.

Diverticulitis

- **Definition.** This disease involves inflammation or local perforation of diverticulum.
- **Epidemiology and risk factors.** This is primarily a disease of the elderly. Only 2% to 4% of patients are younger than 40 years. Risk factors include low-fiber diet, chronic constipation and family history.
- **Pathophysiology.** A colonic diverticulum has become inflamed or perforated or causes local colitis. Obstruction, peritonitis, abscesses, or fistulas may result.
- **History.** Constant severe left lower quadrant (LLQ) pain with guarding. Fever, nausea, anorexia, abdominal distention, and constipation are also present. Urinary symptoms are due to inflammation of the adjacent ureters.
- **Physical examination.** LLQ tenderness, abdominal distention, diminished or normal bowel sounds, occult blood–positive stools, and fever are all possible findings. A palpable LLQ mass is rare. If perforation occurs, peritoneal signs will be present.
- **Diagnostic testing.** A leukocytosis may be present. Abdominal plain films may reveal an ileus and air-fluid levels. Even with colonic perforation, there is almost never free air. A CT scan is the imaging study of choice (Figure 18–4).

Diverticula

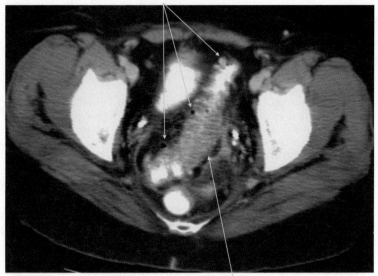

Acute diverticulitis. Note wall thickening of the sigmoid colon with extensive surrounding inflammatory changes in the pericolonic fat. A few small diverticula are seen extending from the sigmoid colon.

Figure 18–4. Diverticulitis. Single axial computed tomography image through the pelvis with oral and intravenous contrast. *(Courtesy of Dr. Jeffrey Pruitt and Dr. Jason Scott Stephens, The University of Texas Southwestern, Department of Radiology.)*

- **ED management.** This includes bowel rest, IV fluids, analgesia, and broad-spectrum antibiotics (e.g., levofloxacin and metronidazole). Diverticulitis is a surgical disease, and although many episodes can be treated conservatively without emergency surgery, many patients will require elective colonic resection. It is therefore prudent to obtain a surgical consultation even if it is decided to discharge the patient. This will expedite and produce safer follow-up care.
- **Helpful hints and pitfalls.** Colonoscopy and barium enema are avoided during active disease to prevent perforation.

Gastritis

- **Definition.** Gastritis is an inflammation of the stomach lining.
- **Epidemiology and risk factors.** The most common cause is infection with *Helicobacter pylori*, which is present in up to 50% of the adult population but most people are asymptomatic. Exposure to drugs that disrupt the protective mucosal barrier secondary to prostaglandin inhibition such

as aspirin and other NSAIDs can predispose an individual to gastritis. Other causes include hypotension, alcohol abuse, radiation, autoimmune disorders, and sarcoidosis. Erosive and hemorrhagic gastritis is seen most commonly in patients taking NSAIDs, alcoholics, and the critically ill.

- *Pathophysiology.* This demonstrates inflammation of the gastric mucosa caused by a wide variety of insults.
- *History.* The patient complains of abdominal pain mostly in the epigastric area, nausea, and vomiting. Hematemesis or coffee-ground emesis can occur, and at times frank GI bleeding.
- *Physical examination.* There may be vague abdominal tenderness in the mid-epigastric area. The abdominal examination is otherwise unremarkable. Stool is positive for occult blood in many cases even if the patient has not had hematemesis or melenic stool.
- *Diagnostic testing.* In the absence of GI bleeding, no specific diagnostic tests are necessary in the ED. If the patient is bleeding, management should be the same as for upper GI tract bleeding (see Chapter 34). *H. pylori* testing is not indicated in the ED.
- *ED management.* Treament includes the use of antacids, H_2 antagonists, or proton pump inhibitors. Most patients will do well with removal of the insult, but this is difficult to achieve in the alcoholic or chronic NSAID user. Some patients will require surgical management for a major GI bleed. Discharged patients should follow up with a primary physician.
- *Helpful hints and pitfalls.* Complications include gastric ulcer formation, possible perforation, and at times, major GI hemorrhage.

Gastrointestinal Reflux Disease

- *Definition.* Gastrointestinal reflux disease (GERD) is reflux of gastric contents into the esophagus caused by a motility disorder.
- *Epidemiology and risk factors.* About 40% of adults in the United States complain of monthly heartburn, about 20% complain of weekly heartburn, and about 7% complain of daily heartburn. Less than 1% of adults develop a Barret's esophagus, which occurs when the normal stratified squamous epithelium is replaced with metaplastic columnar epithelium. This condition can predispose a patient to adenocarcinoma of the esophagus. Risk factors include smoking, alcohol, caffeine, stress, obesity, hiatal hernia, high-fat diet, spicy foods, citrus drinks, and chocolate. Pregnancy, diabetes, and scleroderma are also associated with GERD. Calcium channel blockers, nitrates, and NSAIDs may exacerbate symptoms. It is more common in the elderly and men.
- *Pathophysiology.* Transient lower esophageal relaxation is the key motility disorder underlying most cases.
- *History.* A burning pain arises in the mid-epigastric region and radiates retrosternally to the throat, neck, or back. It is exacerbated by meals, laying down, bending over, and ingesting acidic liquids. Nausea and vomiting may be present. Dysphagia may be present in more complicated cases. The pain is relieved by ingestion of antacids, milk, or other alkaline foods. Patients may complain of bitter or acidic taste in their mouths. It is often difficult or impossible to distinguish the symptoms from those of an ischemic coronary syndrome.

- *Physical examination.* There are normal findings except for mid-epigastric tenderness. Dental erosion may be present from acid exposure.
- *Diagnostic testing.* Laboratory and radiographic studies are not indicated in most cases but should be ordered if the diagnosis is uncertain.
- *ED management.* The patients should be given antacids and be educated about social habits that may exacerbate symptoms.
- *Helpful hints and pitfalls.* Nausea and vomiting are rare in GERD. Potentially life-threatening cardiac causes for what may be considered "atypical chest pain" should be excluded. Although the history is suggestive, it will often be impossible to prove the presence of this entity without special studies that will not be available in the ED. The diagnosis should therefore be only presumptive, and the patient must have careful followup care arranged.

Intestinal Obstruction

- *Definitions.* A *closed-loop obstruction* is a segment of bowel that is obstructed at two sequential sites with a high risk of compromising blood flow. An *adynamic ileus* is when intestinal contents fail to pass through the bowel lumen due to disturbances in motility, rather than a blockage. *Intussusception* is invagination of a proximal piece of bowel into the lumen of an adjacent distal piece usually due to a lesion that serves as a lead point for invagination. A *volvulus* is an intestinal twist due to the rotation of a segment of bowel about its mesenteric axis, and is typically in the sigmoid colon or cecum.
- *Epidemiology and risk factors.* Infants and the elderly are at the highest risk for a bowel obstruction. There are multiple causes of obstruction. Large bowel obstruction (LBO) is much less common than small bowel obstruction (SBO). Carcinoma and diverticulitis are the most common causes for large bowel obstruction. Postoperative adhesions account for more than 50% of all SBOs. Other important causes of SBO are hernias and neoplasm. Sigmoid volvulus occurs in patients of all ages who have severe psychiatric or neurologic disease and in inactive elderly patients; all typically have a history of severe chronic constipation. Cecal volvulus is most common in persons 25 to 35 years of age from congenital hypofixation of bowel. In infants, look for an intussusception or congenital defects such as pyloric stenosis or duodenal atresia.
- *Pathophysiology.* Intestinal obstruction causes accumulation of fluid and air within the lumen proximal to the obstruction. Intraluminal pressures rise and may lead to compromise of first venous, and then arterial blood flow. Failure of normal intestinal motility results in bacterial overgrowth.
- *History.* Patients with an SBO complain of recurrent episodes of poorly localized, crampy abdominal pain. A change to constant severe pain may indicate complications such as intestinal ischemia or perforation. Bilious emesis, several hours of severe colicky pain, and abdominal distention are typical of a proximal obstruction. Feculent emesis is consistent with a more distal obstruction. Patients with an early or partial obstruction may continue to pass stool or flatus. Patients with complete obstruction may develop obstipation. Patients with a LBO have a more insidious onset with vomiting occurring late in the presentation. Changes in bowel

habits, especially constipation, pencil-thin stools, or small bouts of diarrhea, are especially common in LBO.

■ *Physical examination.* Depending on the stage of the disease, one may observe abdominal distention, high-pitched bowel sounds, tympany, and diffuse tenderness. Be sure to palpate for a carcinomatous mass or hernias. A rectal examination is essential to determine if there is stool in the vault or hemoccult-positive stools. Peritoneal signs raise concern for bowel strangulation or perforation.

■ *Diagnostic testing.* A significant leukocytosis may suggest strangulation. Vomiting and profound fluid loss may impair electrolytes and renal function. Serum markers of intestinal ischemia such as amylase, creatine phosphokinase (CPK), and lactate are only elevated late in the course. Plain film studies require two views, one supine and the other upright or in the lateral decubitus position. An upright chest film may be added to exclude subdiaphragmatic air. In obstruction, look for air-fluid levels and dilated loops of bowel. Small-bowel valvulae conniventes are noted in SBO (Figure 18–5). A "String of pearls" sign is also suggestive of SBO (occurs when obstructed intestine contains more fluid than gas). Loss of haustra is seen in LBO, and the bowel is dilated to a width of 6 cm or greater (Figure 18–6). A single, largely dilated loop of colon in left half of the abdomen, with both ends down and the bow positioned superiorly ("bent inner tube") is found in sigmoid volvulus. Cecal volvulus can be seen anywhere in the abdomen. Bowel gas is negligible distal to the obstruction unless the films are done early or there is a partial obstruction. In adynamic ileus, the radiologic findings involve the entire gastrointestinal tract and air-fluid levels are not so prominent as with mechanical obstruction. A CT scan is complementary to plain films, and better defines the site of obstruction or possible cause. The diagnostic test of choice for adult intussusception is a CT scan.

■ *ED management.* NPO, nasogastric tube for intestinal decompression, IV hydration, and correction of electrolyte abnormalities. Antibiotic coverage for gram-negative and anaerobic organisms is necessary when the diagnosis of bowel obstruction is entertained. Surgical consultation is prudent, and a laparotomy may be required. Up to 75% of patients with partial SBO will have complete resolution of symptoms when treated with IV hydration and bowel decompression alone.

■ *Helpful hints and pitfalls.* Plain films show SBO in 50% to 60% of cases. An abdominal CT scan can help establish the diagnosis. High fever, tachycardia, or peritoneal signs suggest strangulation, perforation, and sepsis. Respiratory compromise is another potential complication due to elevation of the diaphragm or aspiration of intestinal material.

Mesentic Ischemia (Acute)

■ *Definition.* This is caused by an acute severe reduction in intestinal blood flow.

■ *Epidemiology and risk factors.* This entity is most common in the elderly and in patients with cardiovascular disease. Arterial occlusive causes are more commonly secondary to emboli than thrombosis. Venous thrombosis and nonocclusive vascular disease are less common causes.

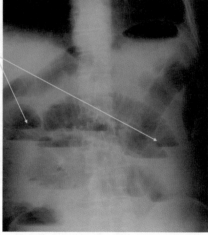

Dilated air filled loops of small bowel

Multiple dilated loops of small bowel are seen in this patient with a small bowel obstruction. No air fluid levels are seen because this is a supine film.

Small amount of air in the cecum.

Calcified bladder stone is incidentally noted in this patient with chronic obstructive uropathy.

On the upright view, multiple air fluid levels can now be seen.

Figure 18–5. Small bowel obstruction. The top image is a supine view. The bottom image is an upright view. *(Courtesy of Dr. Dan Moore and Dr. Jason Scott Stephens, The University of Texas Southwestern, Department of Radiology.)*

The mortality rate is as high as 90% once intestinal infarction has occurred.

- **Pathophysiology.** Most arterial emboli involve the superior mesenteric artery (SMA). The source of these emboli is usually the heart.
- **History.** The patient may complain of a sudden onset of severe, colicky, poorly localized abdominal pain that starts in the periumbilical region and then becomes diffuse. It is often associated with nausea, vomiting and frequent bowel movements. Patients with mesenteric arterial thrombosis may give a history of "abdominal angina" or abdominal pain after meals.

Multiple dilated loops of colon throughout the abdomen in this patient with colonic obstruction from sigmoid volvulus.

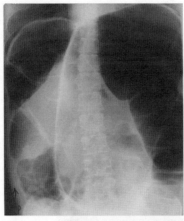

There is high risk for perforation when the diameter of the cecum exceeds 12 cm or the remainder of the colon exceeds 9 cm.

It is often difficult to distinguish large and small bowel in radiographs. The colonic semilunar folds do not extend completely across the bowel lumen whereas small bowel valvulae conniventes do. The haustra are less numerous and are more widely spaced than the small bowel folds. Location is also very helpful. The colon "frames" the abdomen while the small bowel is more centrally located.

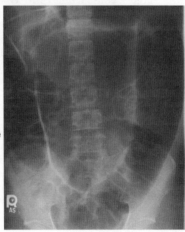

Figure 18–6. Large bowel obstruction. This figure contains two radiographs of the abdomen in a patient with colonic obstruction from sigmoid volvulus. The top image is an upright view and the bottom image is supine. *(Courtesy of Dr. Jason Scott Stephens, The University of Texas Southwestern, Department of Radiology.)*

- ■ *Physical examination.* Pain is classically out of proportion to physical findings but the most classical finding is that each patient is different. The only common thread between patients appears to be restless pain that is hard to describe or localize on physical examination. Early findings can be misleadingly benign. Hemoccult-positive stools may be present. Late in the course, a distended abdomen without bowel sounds and peritoneal signs may result.
- ■ *Diagnostic testing.* The serum lactate level is often elevated and may help in reaching this diagnosis. An increased WBC count is common but not helpful. Additional findings are hemoconcentration, metabolic

acidosis with base deficit, and hyperamylasemia. Plain films of the abdomen most often have normal findings in the acute phase but may reveal an adynamic ileus, dilated loops of bowel, and irregular bowel wall thickening (thumb printing). In the advanced stages, gas in the bowel wall (pneumatosis) or portal system may be present. A CT scan can reveal mesenteric ischemia, but angiography is a more accurate imaging modality. A CT scan may show indirect evidence of bowel ischemia such as edema of the bowel wall and mesentery, abnormal gas patterns, intramural gas, and ascites. Occasionally direct evidence of mesenteric thrombosis is seen. A large percentage of patients will have normal or nonspecific CT scan findings. Angiography remains the gold standard for diagnosis and treatment.

- ***ED management.*** Treatment includes nasogastric tube placement, IV fluids, vasopressors for severe hypotension (inotropes are preferred to alpha agonists), and antibiotics that cover bowel flora. Early utilization of angiography is helpful to improve patient outcome. It is prudent to obtain a surgery consultation early. Once the diagnosis is confirmed, infusion of papaverine directly into the SMA reduces mesenteric vasoconstriction.
- ***Helpful hints and pitfalls.*** No diagnostic strategies are available in the ED that adequately ensure the diagnosis before bowel infarction occurs. Any patient with the clinical picture of acute mesenteric ischemia requires an aggressive approach to diagnosis and management.

Pancreatitis: Acute

- ***Definition.*** Inflammatory process of the pancreas.
- ***Epidemiology and risk factors.*** Alcohol abuse and biliary tract disease are the primary causes of this disease, followed by hypertriglyceridemia, trauma, ERCP, and infection (HIV, mumps, coxsackie B), and drug induced episodes. Mortality rates are found to be 6% to 10% rising to 30% in the patients who develop acute hemorrhagic necrotizing pancreatitis.
- ***Pathophysiology.*** The pathology of acute pancreatitis is premature activation of pancreatic enzymes resulting in autodigestion of pancreatic tissue. Complications include shock from volume loss secondary to fluid sequestration or hemorrhage into necrotic pancreatic tissue, pulmonary complications (pleural effusions, hypoxia, acute respiratory distress syndrome [ARDS]), and metabolic complications (hyperglycemia, hypocalcemia). Late complications occur after the second week of illness and include abscess formation, gastric bleeds from stress ulcers, venous thrombosis, pseudoaneurysm rupture, fistula formation, and pseudocysts (develop after 4 to 6 weeks).
- ***History.*** Usually the patient will complain of an acute onset of epigastric pain radiating to the back that is partially relieved by sitting up or assuming the fetal position; pain is constant and severe, not colicky. Pain may be diffuse or described in the right or left upper quadrant. Nausea, vomiting, and low-grade fever are common.
- ***Physical examination.*** Mid-epigastric tenderness may be present. Because the pancreas is retroperitoneal, guarding and rebound are not

present unless severe destruction of the pancreas has occurred with damage to surrounding tissues (hemorrhage or pseudocyst rupture). The patient will have hypoxia and decreased breath sounds if an associated pleural effusion is present. Jaundice often accompanies an obstructing gall stone. Ileus and hypoactive bowel sounds are common. Cullen's (discoloration around umbilicus) and Grey Turner's signs (discoloration of the flank) suggest retroperitoneal bleeding as in hemorrhagic pancreatitis.

- **Diagnostic testing.** Because the lipase rises sooner, stays elevated longer, and is more specific for pancreatitis than amylase, there is no need to order both studies. The WBC count may be elevated and the hematocrit may be high or low (high due to third-space volume loss or low due to hemorrhage). Hyperglycemia is due to insulin and glucagon abnormalities. The serum calcium may be falsely low due to low albumin but may reflect a true decline as hemorrhagic pancreatitis worsens. In either event, a low serum calcium level is an ominous prognostic sign. A magnesium level should be checked in alcoholics. Elevated liver enzymes may be due to biliary pancreatitis or other hepatobiliary process such as acute fatty liver or cirrhosis, especially in the alcoholic patient. An abdominal series may show an ileus with a sentinel jejunal loop, pancreatic calcifications of chronic pancreatitis, gallstones, or pulmonary findings such as pleural effusion or atelectasis. Ultrasound is useful to rule out gallstones and common bile duct dilatation. A CT scan is performed to rule out other causes of abdominal pain or complications such as pseudocyst, hemorrhage, necrosis, or abscess. Ranson's criteria is used to predict mortality (Table 18–1).

- **ED management.** NPO, admission for IV fluids, antiemetics, and pain control should be done in the ED. Nasogastric tube suction is used for intractable vomiting or ileus. It is useful to obtain a surgical consult for complications such as abscess, pseudocyst, or acute hemorrhagic necrosis. Obtain an emergent gastroenterology consult for ERCP if secondary

Table 18–1	Ranson's Criteria
At Admission	**Within 48 H**
Age >55 y	Hematocrit drop >10%
WBC >16,000	BUN rise >5
Glucose >200 mg/dL	Ca <8
LDH >350 U/L	Po_2 <60
AST >250 U/L	Base deficit >4
	Fluid sequestration >6 L
No. Ranson's Criteria	**Mortality %**
3–4	20
5–6	40
7 or more	100

AST, aspartate aminotransferase; BUN, blood urea nitrogen; Ca, calcium; LDH, lactate dehydrogenase; WBC, white blood cell count.

to gallstones. For severe pancreatitis, use broad spectrum antibiotics to reduce sepsis and H_2 blockers for ulcer prophylaxis. All patients with acute pancreatitis should be admitted to the hospital.

- ■ *Helpful hints and pitfalls.* Chronic pancreatitis is ongoing pancreatic inflammation with subsequent ductal obstruction, mostly due to alcohol use. Pancreatic calcifications are pathognomonic and are seen on plain films in up to 50% of cases. Amylase and lipase levels may be normal. Stable patients who are not dehydrated, can tolerate oral fluids, and have adequate pain control can be managed as outpatients. Morphine is safe to use for analgesia.

Peptic Ulcer Disease (Duodenal and Gastric Ulcers)

- ■ *Definition.* Ulceration in the stomach lining or duodenum.
- ■ *Epidemiology and risk factors.* H. pylori and NSAID use are the primary etiologies. Other causes include smoking, ethanol, steroids, renal failure, and familial predisposition. Approximately 1% are caused by a gastrin-secreting tumor (Zollinger-Ellison syndrome).
- ■ *Pathophysiology.* H. pylori disrupts the gastric mucosal surface and causes inflammation and subsequent ulceration. NSAIDs cause mucosal injury directly by inhibition of prostaglandin secretion with a reduction in mucus production and indirectly by cyclo-oxygenase inhibition that also decreases the protective effect of prostaglandins. NSAIDs also cause decreased platelet aggregation that may result in more bleeding.
- ■ *History.* The patient complains of visceral (vague and midline) epigastric, burning or gnawing pain that may radiate to the chest, back, or other areas of the abdomen. Duodenal ulcers are typically relieved by eating. Pain can be relieved by antacids. The pain may awaken the patient at night as gastric acid secretion is the highest around 2 AM in most people.
- ■ *Physical examination.* There may be mild epigastric tenderness on examination and hemoccult positive stool if bleeding has occurred.
- ■ *Diagnostic testing.* Peptic ulcer disease is usually a clinical diagnosis in the ED, and most patients are treated empirically. A CBC may demonstrate anemia. Testing for *H. pylori* is not routinely part of the ED workup. A lipase should be sent to rule out pancreatitis. Abdominal plain films should be ordered if perforation is suspected.
- ■ *ED management.* The patient should stop consumption of NSAIDS and other precipitating factors. Uncomplicated cases are treated with antacids, H_2 blockers, or proton pump inhibitors before invasive studies are completed. Admit patients with pain that cannot be relieved, signs of obstruction such as gastric distention and vomiting with feeding, GI bleeding, or perforation.
- ■ *Helpful hints and pitfalls.* Antacids can relieve pain from both gastritis and peptic ulcer disease (PUD). Search for signs of complications such as hemorrhage, perforation, penetration (ulcer erodes into another organ such as the liver), and gastric outlet obstruction.

Perforated Viscus

- ■ *Definition.* Sudden rupture of a hollow organ such as the stomach or bowel.

- *Epidemiology and risk factors.* Perforation is most common in the elderly, especially those with a history of peptic ulcer disease or diverticular disease.
- *Pathophysiology.* A duodenal ulcer eroding through the serosa is the most common cause, although perforation can occur anywhere along the GI tract. Spillage of gastrointestinal contents causes peritonitis.
- *History.* Acute onset of epigastric pain is common. Nausea, vomiting, or fever may occur.
- *Physical examination.* Tachycardia is common. Shock may be present with bleeding (simultaneous GI bleeding and perforation are rare) or sepsis. Peritoneal signs with decreased bowel sounds, diffuse guarding, rebound, and a rigid abdomen may occur.
- *Diagnostic tests.* If peritonitis is present, the WBC and amylase may be elevated. Third space fluid losses may cause hemoconcentration and azotemia. An upright abdominal or lateral decubitus radiograph may show free air under the diaphragm. The CT scan is diagnostic.
- *ED management.* This includes NPO, nasogastric tube, IV fluids, antibiotics. Prompt surgical consultation is required because these patients are usually treated surgically, and do better before there is widespread contamination and spillage causing peritonitis.
- *Helpful hints and pitfalls.* Although the peritonitis caused by the perforation is initially chemical, septic complications occur early. The combination of sepsis and hypovolemia ultimately result in acidosis, shock, and death from multisystem organ failure.

Special Considerations
Pediatrics

- Refer to Chapters 77 and 78.

Elderly

- Up to one third of all elderly patients presenting with abdominal pain require surgical intervention.
- Misdiagnosis and mortality rise significantly with patients older than 50 because older patients are more likely to have catastrophic illness rarely seen in younger populations such as myocardial infarction, mesenteric ischemia, and ruptured AAA.
- Elderly patients are more likely to not have classic signs and symptoms and are more likely to have a subtle or confusing presentation.
- Common medications used by the elderly can alter their response to pain and inflammation. Examples include beta-blockers that blunt a tachycardic response to hypovolemia or anemia and steroids that can mask or cause disease.

Women and Pregnancy

- The confirmation of pregnancy is the most important initial laboratory test in all women of childbearing capacity. The primary concern is to rule out an ectopic pregnancy if the woman is pregnant and complaining of abdominal pain.

- If the woman is not pregnant, any fertility-reducing event such as ovarian torsion, pelvic inflammatory disease or a tubo-ovarian abscess must be ruled out (Chapter 68).
- Appendicitis is the most common extra-uterine cause for abdominal surgery during pregnancy, and RLQ pain is still the most common location for pain of appendicitis even though the classic teaching is that this pain migrates to the right upper quadrant as pregnancy progresses and the uterus enlarges.

Immunocompromised

- These patients are always at greater risk for complications of all abdominal pathology as mentioned repeatedly throughout this text.

Teaching Points

Abdominal pain often has no identifiable cause, and in many patients it will not be possible to establish an exact and correct etiology. It is better to consider the patient's diagnosis as "abdominal pain, etiology undefined" than to select an incorrect explanation for the pain in order to feel safe about discharging the patient.

When there is a possibility of a surgical disease, it is prudent and useful to involve the surgical consultant early.

Another common error is failure to think about rare disease entities, failure to do critical parts of the physical examination such as pelvic and rectal examinations, or failure to obtain a pregnancy test because the patient does not believe she is pregnant.

Although up to 50% these patients will never have a cause of the abdominal pain identified, complete and compulsive attention to detailed history and physical examinations, repeated assessments, and the appropriate use of imaging studies will enable accurate diagnosis and management of most serious conditions.

Finally, in the elderly or immunocompromised, as in the very young infant, history and physical examinations may be very unhelpful. It is therefore prudent to be willing to order diagnostic tests in the absence of firm findings when another explanation for the patient's pain has not been found.

Suggested Readings

Hendrickson M. Abdominal surgical emergencies in the elderly. Emerg Med Clin North Am 2003;21:937–969.

Kamin RA, Nowicki TA, Courtney DS, Powers RD. Pearls and pitfalls in the emergency department evaluation of abdominal pain. Emerg Med Clin North Am 2003;21:61–72.

King KE, Wightman JM. Abdominal pain. In: Marx JA, Hockberger RS, Walls RM (editors). Rosen's Emergency Medicine: Concepts and Clinical Practice (6th ed). Philadelphia: Mosby, 2006, pp 209–220.

Newton E, Mandavia S. Surgical complications of selected gastrointestinal emergencies: pitfalls in management of the acute abdomen. Emerg Med Clin North Am 2003;21:873–907.

Rogers RL, McCormack R. Aortic disasters. Emerg Med Clin North Am 2004;22:887–908.

Silen W. Cope's Early Diagnosis of the Acute Abdomen (19th ed). New York: Oxford University Press, 1996.

CHAPTER 19

Allergic Reactions

JEFFREY A. EVANS

 Red Flags

Vital sign abnormalities • Hoarseness or stridor • Cyanosis or hypoxia • Inability to manage oral secretions • Wheezing or diminished breath sounds

Overview

Allergic reactions range from mild and recurrent to immediately life-threatening. Look for "red flags" (see Box) that require immediate therapy. Oxygen, epinephrine, antihistamines, steroids, and intravenous (IV) fluids should be administered simultaneously to critically ill patients with allergic reactions.

Most fatalities are caused by upper respiratory tract obstruction, bronchospasm, or cardiovascular collapse. It is prudent to achieve successful intubation early in any patient with oropharyngeal swelling.

Anaphylaxis often produces signs and symptoms within minutes of exposure to an offending stimulus, but some reactions are delayed for many hours. Increased vascular permeability is a characteristic feature of anaphylaxis, and causes transfer of as much as 50% of the intravascular fluid into the extravascular space within 10 minutes. As a result, hemodynamic collapse can occur rapidly.

Most allergic reactions warrant ED observation for second phase reactions. Patients with anaphylaxis usually require hospitalization in a critical care setting.

Prevention and prophylaxis is a key component of successful allergy control. The complete care of patients with an allergic reaction will include a thorough allergy and medication history, removal of any offending drugs or allergens, and possibly discharge with an epinephrine auto-injector (Epi-Pen), a medic-alert bracelet, and referral to an allergist for hyposensitization immunotherapy.

Differential Diagnosis of an Allergic Reaction
■ See DDx table.

DDx Systems-Based Differential Diagnosis of Allergic Reactions

Respiratory	Cutaneous Diagnoses
Asthma (52)	Carcinoid syndrome (27)
COPD exacerbation (52)	Cellulitis (54)
Epiglottitis (55, 76)	Erysipelas (54)
Foreign body aspiration	Scombroid (27)
Hyperventilation syndrome*	Pheochromocytoma (39)
Pulmonary embolism (52)	Systemic mastocytosis**
Retropharyngeal abscess (64)	Viral exanthem (62)
Vocal cord dysfunction	

( ) Refers to the chapter in which the disease entity is discussed.
*Somatic diseases causing hyperventilation have been ruled out, and the somatic complaints are all related to hypocapnia.
**A rare disease characterized by an abnormal increase in mast cells in the bone marrow, liver, spleen, lymph nodes, gastrointestinal tract, and skin.

Initial Diagnostic Approach

■ Any patient who has respiratory complaints, appears ill or is hemo-dynamically unstable should receive immediate attention. A cardiac monitor and continuous pulse oximetry should be applied.

■ Anaphylactic reactions are almost always unanticipated, and can be life-threatening. Even if only mild symptoms are present initially, the potential for progression must be recognized early. Any delay in the recognition of the initial signs and symptoms of anaphylaxis can result in a fatal outcome either because of airway obstruction or vascular collapse.

■ Anaphylaxis is a clinical diagnosis, and diagnostic studies are usually not helpful.

Emergency Department Management Overview
General

■ The ABCs (*a*irway, *b*reathing, and *c*irculation) should be addressed as discussed in Section II. Give oxygen for all patients who are dyspneic, wheezing, or have vital sign abnormalities.

■ Patients with allergic reactions are exceptions to the rule that the patient who is talking has a secure airway. Hoarseness, stridor, pooling of secretions, or visible swelling may be signs of impending loss of airway. It is safer to intubate early, before progressive oropharyngeal swelling can further distort airway anatomy and interfere with successful intubation. Anticipate a difficult airway. A surgical airway may be necessary.

■ Insert a large-bore IV catheter for all patients with dyspnea, vital sign abnormalities, or oropharyngeal swelling. IV fluid resuscitation with normal saline or Ringer's lactate (2 L in adults or 20 ml/kg in children) should be given for hypotensive patients. IV access is always useful for delivery of medications even in patients who are less acutely ill. Do not delay administration of subcutaneous epinephrine while IV access is secured.

Medications

- *Epinephrine.* For mild to moderate anaphylaxis give a subcutaneous (SC) or intramuscular (IM) injection of 0.3 to 0.5 ml 1:1000 (pediatrics 1:1000 give 0.01 mL/kg/dose SC). An Epi-Pen auto-injector delivers 0.3 ml (Epi-Pen Jr., 0.15 ml). Repeat every 5 to 10 minutes for continuing or advancing signs and symptoms. For severe anaphylaxis (laryngeal edema, shock), give 10 ml 1:100,000 IV over 10 minutes. The risk of tachydysrhythmias, accelerated hypertension, and myocardial ischemia, are increased by using the IV route with epinephrine. Dilution and slow administration reduce these risks. The rate for a continuous infusion of IV epinephrine is 0.1-1.0 µg/kg/min. Inhaled epinephrine, delivered as a 2.25% solution (0.5 ml placed in a nebulizer in 2.5 mL of normal saline), may be a temporizing measure. However, epinephrine as described above is preferred.
- *H₁ blockers (Antihistamines).* Diphenhydramine (Benadryl) 25 to 50 mg by mouth (PO) or IM/IV (pediatrics 1 mg/kg) should be given. For mild urticaria or contact dermatitis, the PO route is preferred. Patients should be discharged with instructions to take diphenhydramine 25 to 50 mg PO q4-6h for 24 to 48 hours then as needed. Nonsedating antihistamines such as fexofenadine (Allegra) 180 mg PO daily or loratadine (Claritin) 10 mg PO daily are prescribed for chronic urticaria.
- *H₂ blockers.* Ranitidine (Zantac) 50 mg IV/IM or 150 mg PO, or famotidine (Pepcid) 20 mg IV/PO should be given. The pediatric dose for ranitidine is 1 mg/kg. The PO route is acceptable for mild allergic reactions. These agents speed the resolution of urticaria when used in conjunction with H₁ blockers. They should be given for all severe allergic reactions. The patient should be discharged on H₂ blockers for 24 to 48 hours.
- *Corticosteroids.* Give methylprednisolone (Solu-Medrol) 60 to 125 mg IV q6h (pediatrics 2 mg/kg per dose IV q6h) or prednisone 40 to 60 mg PO daily (pediatrics 2 mg/kg/d PO or divided twice daily). All steroids have a 4- to 6-hour onset of action. They decrease the occurrence of second-phase reactions. There is a decreased incidence and severity of urticaria when patients are discharged on a steroid burst (e.g., prednisone 60 mg PO daily for 4 days). A similar burst is recommended at discharge for all allergic reactions. Unfortunately, they may adversely affect diabetic control or worsen symptoms in patients with peptic ulcers.
- *Aerosolized β-agonists and others.* Albuterol 2.5 mg diluted with 3 ml NS may be given continuously. Levalbuterol 0.625-1.25 mg (pediatric dose 0.3-0.625 mg) diluted with 3 ml of NS may be given continuously. Ipatropium 0.5 ml (pediatric dose 0.25 mg) diluted in 3 ml NS may also be given and repeated as necessary.
- *Vasopressors.* Epinephrine, norepinephrine, or dopamine infusion can be given for hypotension unresponsive to IV fluids.
- *Glucagon.* Give one milligram IV for refractory hypotension, especially in patients taking β-blockers. This can be followed by a glucagon infusion 1 mg in 1 L D₅W IV at 5 to 15 µg/min (5-15 mL/min).

Disposition

- **Consultation.** Allergy, immunology, and hematology consultations may be indicated for patients with hereditary angioedema. Allergy and immunology referral for desensitization therapy is appropriate for patients with anaphylaxis or severe allergic reactions.
- **Admission.** Admit the following patients to a critical care setting: severe anaphylaxis, concern for upper airway obstruction, or hypotension.
- **ED observation.** A short period of ED observation is prudent hours after resolution of symptoms for most patients with allergic reactions, but is not necessary for isolated urticaria that has responded to therapy. Twenty percent of anaphylactic reactions follow a biphasic course, with a mean time to second-phase reaction reported ranging from 3 to 10 hours.
- **Discharge.** Patients with mild to moderate anaphylaxis who respond completely to initial treatment can be discharged from the ED after an observation period of 3 to 10 hours depending on the clinical situation. Patients should be discharged on an oral antihistamine (H_1) taken regularly for 48 hours, oral prednisone burst for 4 to 7 days, and possibly an oral H_2 blocker for 48 hours. All patients with a history of systemic allergic reactions (or localized oropharyngeal swelling) are at high risk for recurrence (e.g., after a bee sting) and should be discharged with an epinephrine auto-injector. Factors that define high risk include reactions that require hospitalization, asthma, reaction to trace amount of allergen, re-exposure to the allergen is likely, or there will be limited or delayed access to medical care. Prescribe the EpiPen Jr. for patients weighing 10 to 28 kg and the regular EpiPen if patients weigh above 28 kg.

Specific Problems
Anaphylaxis and Anaphylactoid Reactions

- **Definitions.** Anaphylaxis is a severe systemic allergic reaction in a previously sensitized patient. An anaphylactoid reaction is a clinically indistinguishable syndrome that occurs without sensitization. (Except for pathophysiology, anaphylaxis and anaphylactoid reactions will be discussed as one entity in this text.)
- **Epidemiology and risk factors.** No epidemiologic factors identify those at risk. No causative agent can be identified in two thirds of cases. Antibiotics (especially penicillins) and radiocontrast agents are the most common iatrogenic triggers of anaphylaxis. Hymenoptera envenomation is a common cause. Food allergy accounts for one third of cases, with peanuts and shellfish being the most common. Other important causes include latex, nonsteroidal anti-inflammatory drugs, aspirin, and exercise.
- **Pathophysiology.** Anaphylaxis is caused by an IgE antibody response in sensitized individuals. Re-exposure to a foreign protein induces the release of preformed mast cell and basophil-derived inflammatory mediators. This IgE-mediated pathway is responsible for most venom, food, and antibiotic reactions. Anaphylactoid reactions occur when the same mediators are released on first exposure to a foreign protein, independent of IgE.

- *History.* Anaphylaxis causes a wide range of cutaneous, respiratory, gastrointestinal, and cardiovascular symptoms, generally within minutes to hours of exposure to the triggering antigen. Skin changes include flushing, pruritis, and edema. Respiratory distress may be preceded by wheezing, dyspnea, chest tightness, hoarseness, dysphagia, and stridor. Gastrointestinal effects include nausea, vomiting, tenesmus, diarrhea, and abdominal pain. Palpitations, presyncope, or syncope may indicate a dysrhythmia or impending cardiovascular collapse.
- *Physical examination.* Clinical findings are variable. Patients may be anxious or unresponsive with tachypnea, tachycardia, hypotension, and hypoxia. An alternative or additional diagnosis should be considered in febrile patients. Cyanosis, flushing, urticaria, and angiodema may be present. Angioedema of the tongue or oropharynx, pooling of oral secretions, or stridor indicate impending airway obstruction. Wheezing or diminished breath sounds may accompany bronchospasm. Intestinal edema may cause diffuse abdominal tenderness.
- *Diagnostic testing.* Anaphylaxis is a clinical diagnosis, and treatment should never be delayed by diagnostic testing. Obtain an EKG, laboratory studies, and radiographic imaging to diagnose concomitant disease, especially in the elderly patient.
- *ED management.* As discussed in "Emergency Department Management Overview," IV access, supplementary oxygen, and pharmocotherapy are the mainstays of treatment. A prolonged ED observation or hospital admission is required. Second-phase reactions accompany 20% of anaphylactic reactions. Education and prevention (antigen avoidance, Epi-Pen, medic-alert bracelet, referral for immunotherapy) are important.
- *Helpful hints and pitfalls.* Even mild allergic systemic symptoms should be considered warning signs of a potentially life-threatening reaction.

Angioedema

- *Definitions.* This is caused by subdermal or submucosal plasma extravasation resulting in cutaneous and gastrointestinal edema. It is often accompanied by urticaria.
- *Epidemiology.* No epidemiologic factors identify those at risk, except for recurrent episodes in those with hereditary or acquired angioedema. The hereditary form appears in the first two decades of life, the acquired form is most often seen after the fourth decade.
- *Pathophysiology.* Angioedema is classified by etiology and includes idiopathic, allergic, C1–esterase inhibitor deficiency, hereditary, and acquired. In idiopathic angioedema, no trigger can be identified. This is the most common form. In allergic angioedema, there is IgE-mediated mast cell degranulation and release of inflammatory mediators on exposure to foreign proteins or a physical agent. Drugs (especially angiotensin-converting enzyme [ACE] inhibitors), food allergens, cold, pressure, vibration, ultraviolet radiation, and exercise have all been implicated. ACE inhibitors are thought to potentiate bradykinin release. C1-INH deficiency causes unregulated activation of the classical pathway of the complement system. Angioedema is caused by anaphylatoxins and

not by histamine release. Hereditary angioedema (HAE) occurs as an autosomal dominant disease. Twenty-five percent of cases occur from a spontaneous mutation. In acquired angioedema (AAE), there are autoantibodies against C1-INH, or there is a C1-INH deficiency associated with B-cell lymphoproliferative disorders, hepatitis, or *Helicobacter pylori* infections.

- **History.** The patient may have edema of the face, extremities, or genitalia. These are most characteristic, although any skin surface may be involved. A burning sensation is common. Pruritis is rare unless there is concurrent urticaria. Gastrointestinal submucosal swelling may cause fatal tongue and throat swelling or nausea, vomiting, diarrhea, and abdominal pain.
- **Physical examination.** Localized nonpitting edema may be present in virtually any body area. Diffuse and sometimes severe abdominal tenderness may mimic an acute abdomen. Tachypnea, hypoxia, or stridor herald airway obstruction.
- **Diagnostic testing.** Diagnostic testing is rarely helpful. A C1-INH immune assay may assist in the diagnosis of HAE or AAE but is not performed in the ED.
- **ED management.** Ensure a patent airway. It may be necessary to intubate immediately. Anticipate a difficult airway. Most angioedema is treated in a manner similar to a mild to moderate allergic reaction with antihistamines (H_1 blockers) and corticosteroids. Epinephrine is reserved for impending airway obstruction. HAE and AAE are resistant to conventional therapy, and treatment should be coordinated in consultation with an allergy specialist. Patients without oropharyngeal edema may be discharged after treatment. Hospitalization in a monitored setting is required with tongue or laryngeal swelling.
- **Helpful hints and pitfalls.** Mortality from angioedema is always a result of airway obstruction. Review all potential drug allergies and discontinue ACE inhibitors.

Contact dermatitis

- **Definitions.** This is an inflammation of the skin in response to direct chemical damage (irritant contact dermatitis) or a hypersensitivity reaction in a previously sensitized individual (allergic contact dermatitis).
- **Epidemiology.** It is extremely common overall. Atopic individuals are at higher risk of allergic contact dermatitis. This entity accounts for 90% of all work-related dermatologic complaints.
- **Pathophysiology.** Irritant contact dermatitis produces direct damage to the protective layers of the epidermis. In allergic contact dermatitis, there is a type IV hypersensitivity reaction to a foreign protein.
- **History.** The patient complains of a pruritic rash localized to skin that has come into contact with the irritant or antigen. The distribution of the lesions is the best indicator of the etiologic agent. Common irritants are soaps, detergents, and cleaning solutions; common antigens include latex, plants (e.g., poison ivy), and nickel (jewelry).

- *Physical examination.* There are papules, vesicles, or bullae over an erythematous base. Allergic contact dermatitis is frequently edematous.
- *Diagnostic testing.* Diagnostic testing is not indicated. Referral to an allergist for patch testing may identify antigens responsible for allergic contact dermatitis.
- *ED management.* This is focused on identifying and removing the irritant or antigen. Topical treatment is usually adequate and may include over-the-counter skin moisturizers, aluminum acetate (Burow's solution) compresses, and mid-potency corticosteroid creams. Systemic steroids are appropriate for severe cases. Antihistamines should be prescribed for pruritis.
- *Helpful hints and pitfalls.* The distribution of the contact dermatitis is usually the best indicator of the causative irritant or antigen.

Urticaria

- *Definition.* This condition produces pruritic, erythematous skin wheals caused by dermal edema. They arise from the same mechanism as angioedema, but produce involvement of the dermis rather than the subdermal tissue.
- *Epidemiology and risk factors.* There is a higher incidence in people with atopy. Fifty percent of cases are accompanied by angioedema. They are classified as chronic urticaria if present longer than 6 weeks.
- *Pathophysiology.* Allergic (IgE-mediated) or nonallergic release of inflammatory mediators causes dermal fluid extravasation and edema. Causes include drugs, food allergens, pollens, animal dander, viral illness, cold, exercise, heat, emotional stress, ultraviolet radiation and diseases such as systemic lupus erythematosus (SLE), viral hepatitis, tuberculosis, cryoglobulinemias, hyperthyroidism, and rheumatic fever. Fifty percent of patients with chronic urticaria have an autoimmune component.
- *History.* The patient complains of pruritic lesions that may be accompanied by angioedema.
- *Physical examination.* There may be edematous, blanchable, pink, or red wheals of variable size, often with central pallor. They are commonly accompanied by dermatographism (firm stroking of the skin produces an urticarial wheal within 30 minutes) and angioedema. Individual lesions fade in 24 hours, but new lesions may continually appear.
- *Diagnostic testing.* Diagnostic testing is not indicated. Urticaria is a clinical diagnosis.
- *ED management.* This may include observation to ensure the urticaria is not a precursor to a more severe allergic reaction. Antihistamines (H_1 blockers) are the mainstay of treatment. H_2 blockers are optional. An H_1 blocker with oral prednisone 40 mg daily for 4 days is superior to an antihistamine alone. Prescribe a nonsedating antihistamine for patients with chronic urticaria. Avoidance of the offending antigen is the only preventive measure.
- *Helpful hints and pitfalls.* All urticaria must be considered a possible precursor to a serious allergic reaction or anaphylaxis, even though most cases will not deteriorate into these more serious forms.

Teaching Points

Allergic reactions and anaphylaxis are common. They can become life-threatening with great rapidity, or take time to deteriorate because of delayed secondary reactions.

Airway obstruction is the usual pathway to mortality, and comes from an edematous upper airway obstruction. Epinephrine and early intubation are the most successful agents to prevent mortality. Steroids are useful, but have a lag time to onset.

When a cause of the anaphylaxis is identified, it may be possible to prevent recurrence by desensitization, but sometimes it is more useful for the patient to be given an EpiPen and to be taught how to use it.

Suggested Readings

Brochner BS, Lichtenstein LM. Anaphylaxis. N Engl J Med 1991;324:1785–1790.

Ellis AK, Day JH. Diagnosis and management of anaphylaxis. CMAJ 2003;169:307–312.

Frigas E, Nzeako UC. Angioedema: pathogenesis, differential diagnosis, and treatment. Clin Rev Allergy Immunol 2002;23:217–231.

Lieberman P, Kemp SF, Oppenheimer J et al. (editors). The diagnosis and management of anaphylaxis: an updated practice parameter. J Allergy Clin Immunol 2005;115(3 Suppl): S483–523.

Lin RY, Curry A, Pesola GR, et al. Improved outcomes in patients with acute allergic syndromes who are treated with combined H_1 and H_2 antagonists. Ann Emerg Med 2000;36:462–468.

Pollack CV, Romano TJ. Outpatient management of acute urticaria: the role of prednisone. Ann Emerg Med 1995;26:547–551.

Sampson HA. Anaphylaxis and emergency treatment. Pediatrics 2003;111:1601–1608.

Tran TP, Muelleman RL. Allergy, hypersensitivity, and anaphylaxis. In: Marx JA, Hockberger RS, Walls RM. Rosen's Emergency Medicine: Concepts and Clinical Practice (6th ed). Philadelphia: Mosby, 2006, pp 1818–1837.

CHAPTER 20

Altered Mental Status

DIONNE SMITH ■ JOSEPH N. MARTINEZ

 Red Flags

Extremes of age ● Immunocompromised state ● Other co-morbid
conditions: diabetes, atherosclerosis ● Acute onset of symptoms
● Overdose ● History of trauma ● Severe pain of rapid onset
● Abnormal vital signs (high fever, ↑ heart rate, ↓ blood pressure)
● Abnormal breathing pattern ● Signs of dehydration ● Focal
neurologic findings

Overview

Altered mental status (AMS) is defined as an abnormal change in
intellect, cognitive function, or behavior. There is a loss of all or a
portion of orientation to person, place, time, or situation. A patient
with AMS may be awake but confused or arrive at the ED with bizarre
behavior, somnolence, or coma.

An AMS may be found in 4% to 10% of ED patients. Multiple
etiologies exist, and are the result of either a direct central nervous
system (CNS) process (e.g., stroke, head trauma, or mass lesion) or a
secondary event affecting mental functioning (e.g., sepsis, cardiogenic
shock, or intoxication). Look for "red flags" (see Box) when evaluating
these patients.

Evaluation of a patient with AMS is challenging and often difficult.
The history is often not available, and the patient is frequently unable
to cooperate with the physical examination. The clinician must often
rely on second hand information from family members, friends, or
nursing home providers. At times, even this second hand information
is totally unavailable. The patient's baseline mental functioning may be
unknown and the etiology of the AMS may not be immediately obvious.

Normal consciousness requires both arousal and awareness. The
integrity of both cerebral hemispheres determines the state of awareness, whereas arousal is controlled by the ascending reticular activating
system (ARAS) that courses from the medulla to the thalamus. The
location of the ARAS overlaps several brain stem reflex pathways, in
particular those responsible for the pupillary light reflex and the reflex

eye movements that allow conjugate gaze. Thus, preservation of these reflexes often means that ARAS function is normal and therefore implies that the alteration in mental status is the result of deficits in both cerebral hemispheres. Conversely, pupillary asymmetry or dysconjugate gaze imply deficits in the area of the ARAS.

Definitions. *Delirium* (or acute organic brain syndrome) is an acute, reversible, organic mental disorder characterized by a reduced attention and fluctuations in level of functioning. The patient appears disoriented, fearful, agitated, and irritable, but can quickly reverse to an almost-normal state. The patient may present with hallucinations such as feeling like insects are crawling on the skin or hearing sounds or sensing smells that are not perceivable by others. This state is usually secondary to a toxic or metabolic etiology. *Dementia* is a chronic organic mental disorder characterized by a general loss of intellectual abilities. *Obtundation* is decreased alertness with limited interest in the environment. Most of the time, the patient is sleeping, but is drowsy upon awakening. In *stupor*, the patient is responsive only to vigorous stimuli and returns to an unresponsive state when left unstimulated. *Psychosis* is a mental disorder characterized by gross impairment in thinking as evidenced by coherent delusions and hallucinations.

Whatever the cause of the AMS, the initial actions to take are rapid identification and correction of reversible causes, the recognition and stabilization of any life or limb threat, and only after this can efforts be made to achieve accurate diagnosis of the patient's diseases (Table 20–1).

Differential Diagnosis of Altered Mental Status

The differential diagnosis of AMS is quite broad and diverse. The mnemonic AEIOU TIPS is found useful by some:

- **A:** Alcohol, acid-base and metabolic disorders, dysrhythmias
- **E:** Encephalopathy, endocrinopathy, electrolyte disorders
- **I:** Insulin, intestinal (e.g., intussusception or bowel obstruction)
- **O:** Opiates, oxygen (hypoxia)
- **U:** Uremia
- **T:** Trauma, thermal, tumor
- **I:** Infection, intracerebral vascular disorders
- **P:** Poisonings, psychogenic
- **S:** Seizure, shunt malfunction

Initial Diagnostic Approach
General

- Assess the ABCs (*a*irway, *b*reathing, and *c*irculation), insert an intravenous (IV) line, place a cardiac monitor, monitor pulse oximetry, and give supplementary oxygen. At this time, obtain blood for laboratory tests and perform a rapid finger-stick glucose determination.

Table 20–1   Common Problems Causing Altered Mental Status in the ED

Disease	Clinical Presentation	Management
Hypoglycemia (38)	Lethargy Slurred speech	Glucose Admit for recurrent hypoglycemia or sepsis
Meningitis (67)	Headache Neck pain Fevers Nausea and vomiting Neck muscle rigidity	IV antibiotics Admission
Electrolyte abnormality (88): hypernatremia hypocalcemia hypomagnesemia	Lethargy Tetany	Fluid and electrolyte replacement May require admission
Space-occupying lesions (35)	Headache Nausea/vomiting Weakness Neurologic deficit	Neurosurgery consult Admission
Subarachnoid hemorrhage (35)	Thunderclap headache Neurologic deficit	Neurosurgery consult Admission
Myxedema coma (63)	Hypothermia Bradycardia Areflexia or prolonged relaxation phase of deep tendon reflexes	Hydrocortisone Thyroid hormone IV fluids Admission
Seizure, postictal (51)	Tongue or cheek biting, incontinence, gradual improvement after observation period	Benzodiazepines are first-line agents. Anticonvulsants such as phenytoin
Drug overdose (72) (opioid)	Respiratory depression and pinpoint pupils	Narcan Supportive care for most

ED, emergency department; CT, computed tomography; IV, intravenous; MRI, magnetic resonance imaging; TSH, thyroid-stimulating hormone.
( ) Refers to the chapter in which the disease entity is discussed.

■ The history may narrow down the differential. Try to determine the patient's baseline mental status. Look for medical alert bracelets or medical opiate patches. If possible, establish the timeline of the events leading up to the patient's arrival and rule out trauma, overdose, pharmacologic interactions or toxic ingestions. The patient's medical history may reveal diabetes mellitus, seizures, alcoholism, or drug abuse.
■ The physical examination addresses the degree of impairment and may provide clues to the diagnosis. Once the ABCs are assessed, use the Glasgow Coma Scale (GCS) score (see Appendix 2) or AVPU scale (Alert, response to Verbal stimuli or Pain, Unresponsive state) to determine

the patient's mental status baseline at presentation so improvement or deterioration can be observed. A mini mental status examination (see Appendix 2) may be performed as time allows and the patient's condition permits. Monitor the patient's respiratory rate, looking for hypoventilation or airway compromise. The rate, depth, and rhythm of the breathing may be a reflection of nervous system pathology, particularly in patients with an altered level of consciousness. A healthy, awake patient at rest generally breathes about 12-16 times a minute with occasional deeper respirations as demanded by the levels of carbon dioxide (CO_2). When the cerebral cortex is no longer functioning, the nervous system relies on diencephalic control of breathing or *Cheyne-Stokes* respirations. Cheyne-Stokes respirations refer to a periodic breathing pattern of alternating hyperpnea and apnea. It also occurs in sleep disorders, narcotic overdose, head trauma, congestive heart failure, and uremia. It is also seen as a normal pattern in infants. Cheyne-Stokes respiration localizes the level of the neurologic lesion at or above the level of the midbrain. *Kussmaul* respiration describes the hyperventilation pattern seen in diabetics with ketoacidosis. Subtle tachypnea is often difficult to detect, but can be the solitary harbinger of serious disease. Perform as complete a neurologic examination as the patient's condition and ability to cooperate will permit. Also look for evidence of trauma, odors such as pesticide, ketones, or fetor uremia as well as signs of a possible toxidrome or any evidence of sepsis.

■ Patients with an alteration in mental status should not leave the ED unmonitored for imaging studies. They can be anticipated to worsen if left alone in the radiology department, or can harm themselves by falling or uncontrolled thrashing.

■ Use sedation for patient control when the patient is agitated. Imaging studies will not be useful if obtained in a moving, combative patient.

Laboratory

■ Immediate tests should include a rapid finger-stick glucose determination. Other tests should include a complete blood count (CBC), blood urea nitrogen (BUN), creatinine, electrolytes including calcium, magnesium, and phosphorous, and a urinalysis. A catheterized urine specimen should be obtained since urinary infections are a common cause of an acute organic brain syndrome in older patients (serious pathology must still be ruled out). Other laboratory data such as ammonia or alcohol levels, and toxicology screens should be tailored to the individual case. An arterial blood gas (ABG) may useful in the comatose patient looking for hypoxia, acidosis or CO_2 retention.

■ A lumbar puncture (LP) should be performed since sepsis, meningitis, or intracranial hemorrhage are common causes of organic brain syndrome. Nuchal rigidity may be entirely absent. Patients who are immunocompromised or at extremes of age often do not present with the classic symptoms and signs of meningitis such as headache, fever, and neck stiffness. An LP is contraindicated in unstable patients such as a hydrocephalic child who may have an obstructed shunt or a patient who is experiencing a cerebral herniation. It may be necessary to start empirical antibiotics in these patients without the information available from spinal fluid. Computed tomography (CT scan) is not a substitute for clinical assessment. It is often necessary to obtain special serologic markers for immunocompromised patients, such as for toxoplasmosis, syphilis or cryptococcosis.

EKG

■ An electrocardiogram (EKG) can reveal poor-perfusion rhythms. A wide QRS may indicate a toxidrome, especially a tricyclic antidepressant (TCA) overdose.

Radiography

■ A CT scan of the head without contrast is necessary in most patients with altered mental status. Depending on the circumstances of the individual case, it may need to be followed with a contrast scan, magnetic resonance imaging (MRI) or angiography. An MRI may be needed but is typically not performed in the ED on these patients. The contrast-enhanced cranial CT scan or MRI is invaluable in the diagnosis of a CNS abscess. MRI is also helpful in the evaluation of other infectious and noninfectious encephalitides. Although a CT scan can show hypodense lesions in the temporal lobes in patients with herpes simplex virus HSV encephalitis, an MRI scan may reveal these changes much earlier.
■ Other imaging studies should be performed as the clinical presentation indicates (i.e., a chest radiograph to evaluate for pneumonia).

Emergency Department Management Overview
General

■ The ABCs should be addressed as discussed in Section II. Give oxygen to all confused patients. A bedside glucose should be checked on any patient presenting with AMS.

Immediate Therapies

■ The acronym "DON'T" is often used to help remember immediate therapies for AMS: dextrose, oxygen, nalaxone, and thiamine.
■ Glucose: one ampule in D50W (50% dextrose in water) intravenous (IV) (pediatric dose: 2 to 4 ml/kg of D25W [25% dextrose in water]) if finger-stick glucose level is low. Patients with a mildly low glucose level who are alert and able to swallow may be given glucose orally (e.g., orange juice).
■ Thiamine 100 mg IV to the patient who appears malnourished or has a history of alcoholism.
■ Nalaxone: 0.4 mg to 2 mg IV or intramuscular (IM) (pediatric dose, 0.1 mg/kg per dose; maximum dose, 0.8 to 0.05-0.01 mg/kg/dose) to reverse adverse effects of narcotics and the patient who has AMS. The lowest dose possible should be used on patients with AMS secondary to recreational narcotic overdose to prevent significant withdrawal.

- Administer appropriate antibiotics for any patient in whom the cause of the confusion might be sepsis or meningitis.

Disposition

- Virtually all patients with an alteration in mental status will require admission. Exceptions are for those conditions that are readily reversible such as hypoglycemia or opiate overdose if the condition is easily treated and symptoms are not recurrent, or in the patient who has chronic organic brain syndrome such as a Korsakoff's psychosis, in whom a satisfactory disposition can be made. Even some of these patients may require admission if the social circumstances of discharge are unsatisfactory.

Special Considerations
Pediatrics

- The child with AMS is often described as toxic, poorly responsive, or lethargic. The differential diagnosis in children is similar to that of adults and includes infection, poisoning, hyper- or hypothermia, and metabolic abnormalities, especially hypoglycemia.
- Inborn errors of metabolism often are the cause of AMS, and whatever the individual metabolic derangement, most are symptomatic from hypoglycemia.
- It is easy to overlook uncommon pediatric causes because of the absence of history or helpful physical findings. Thus intussusception may present with lethargy rather than the more common presentation of acute severe abdominal pain. Any child with an AMS can present as a failure to feed and lethargy.

Elderly

- Elderly patients have higher rates of altered mentation; dementias and other delirious states are seen in up to 30% of elderly patients presenting to the ED.
- The easily reversible causes of AMS include hypoglycemia and hypoxia. These should be assessed during the ABCs. Elderly patients can also be affected by medication changes, chronic medications, or dosage error. A thorough medication history may be useful. A common error is to fail to appreciate the change in the elderly patient's mental status, because the patient cannot give a history and no one knows the baseline status. The patient should not be dismissed as having chronic organic brain syndrome from senility until the underlying status has been properly identified.

The Immunocompromised Patient

- In the immunocompromised patient, the differential diagnosis should be expanded to include less likely causes of encephalitis and meningitis such as fungal infections.

Teaching Points

The patient with an altered level of mental status can be in the midst of an acute or chronic change.

An acute organic brain syndrome is characterized by a waxing and waning level of awareness and brain function and can quickly change from what appears to be normal, to confusion, lethargy, and even coma. There are many causes of an acute organic brain syndrome, but the most common ones are metabolic: an acute confusional state caused by hypoglycemia; diminished function, as in the postictal patient; toxicologic as in the alcohol- or opiate-intoxicated patient; or from other pharmacologic ingestions or interactions; or finally sepsis.

It is helpful to understand the patient's level of function before the new state of activity because this may reveal the acute change and identify the cause.

A common error in the elderly patient is to assume that the loss of awareness and cerebral acumen is due to the chronic changes of Alzheimer's dementia. Another common mistake is to overlook sepsis as the cause of the confused state in the elderly; the most common source is the urinary tract.

Suggested Readings

Ferrera PC, Chan L. Initial management of the patient with altered mental status. Am Fam Physician 1997;55:1773–1780.

Flacker JM, Marcantonio ER. Delirium in the elderly: optimal management. Drugs Aging 1998;13Z:119–130.

Kanich WB, Brady WJ, Huff JS, et al. Altered mental status: evaluation and etiology in the ED. Am J Emerg Med 2002;20:67–79.

King D, Avner JR. Altered mental status. CPEM 2003;4;171–178.

O'Keefe KP, Sanson TG. Elderly patients with altered mental status. Emerg Med Clin North Am 1998;16:701–715.

Wolfe RE, Brown DFM. Coma and depressed level of consciousness. In: Marx JA, Hockberger RS, Walls RM (editors). Rosen's Emergency Medicine: Concepts and Clinical Practice (6th ed). Philadelphia: Mosby, 2006, pp 156–164.

CHAPTER 21

Back Pain

ALEC TUAN HUYNH ■ REBEKA BARTH ■ IAN R. GROVER

 Red Flags

Age >55 y • History of coronary artery or peripheral vascular disease
• Urinary retention • Bowel incontinence • Bilateral lower limb
weakness • Major trauma • History of chronic steroids or osteoporosis
• History of malignancy • Weight loss • Pain longer than 1 mo
(especially if not improved by rest) • Fever • Intravenous drug use
• Immunosuppression • Saddle anesthesia • Midline point tenderness

Overview

Back pain is one of the most common complaints of patients
presenting to the ED. Mechanical back pain is the most common cause
of back pain, but a few life-threatening and potentially debilitating
conditions must be considered. Look for the "red flags" (see Box)
concerning for emergent causes of back pain.

Search for an abdominal aortic aneurysm (AAA) in back pain
patients older than 50 with a history of hypertension. These patients
should be rapidly assessed. Immediate surgical management may be
necessary.

A brief review of spinal cord anatomy will help to understand some
common or concerning problems involving the spinal cord that may
present as back pain. The spinal cord terminates at the body of the first
or second lumbar vertebra. At its lower end the spinal cord tapers into
the conus medullaris where several segmental levels are represented
in a small area. The lumbar and sacral nerve roots form the cauda
equina as they descend caudally in the thecal sac prior to exit of the
spinal canal at the respective foramina.

A radiculopathy is a disease process that involves the nerve root.
Sciatica is a radiculopathy in the lumbosacral region and is a common
cause of back pain.

Differential Diagnosis of Back Pain

See the DDx table.

DDx Priority-Based Differential Diagnosis of Back Pain

Critical Diagnoses	Emergent Diagnoses	Nonemergent Diagnoses
Abdominal aortic aneurysm (18)	Diskitis Fracture (12)	Seronegative spondyloarthropathies (71)
Cauda equina syndrome	Malignancy	Musculoskeletal strain
Spinal cord syndrome (12)	Spinal osteomyelitis (67)	Nephrolithiasis (32) Pyelonephritis (32)
Epidural hematoma Epidural abscess	Transverse myelitis	Sciatica Spinal stenosis

( ) Refers to the chapter in which the disease entity is discussed.

Initial Diagnostic Approach
General

■ As always, the ABCs (*a*irway, *b*reathing, and *c*irculation) should be addressed immediately followed by assessing the patient for any possible neurologic dysfunction that would require immediate attention. Aggressive use of imaging studies and tertiary care consultants will preserve function in those clinical situations in which a spinal cord syndrome is developing.
■ The history and physical examination findings should suggest the need for further studies. The straight leg raise test should be performed on patients with back pain to evaluate for a radiculopathy. These patients typically present with back pain radiating to the leg. With the patient supine, the examiner raises the symptomatic leg with the knee fully extended. The test is positive if lifting that leg reproduces or worsens the pain in that leg. The pain of radiculopathy is usually worse in the leg than in the back, and almost always radiates past the knee. A positive crossover straight leg raise occurs when elevation of the asymptomatic extended leg produces radicular pain in the affected leg. This is thought to be pathognomonic for nerve root compression caused by disk herniation. If this results in pain in the normally asymptomatic leg it may indicate a central disk hernation. See Table 21–1 for clinical findings associated with lumbosacral radiculopathies.

Laboratory

■ Blood tests are only rarely necessary because most causes of back pain are mechanical.
■ If the clinical presentation suggests a leaking or ruptured AAA, the patient should have type and cross match for 6 to 10 units of blood.
■ Complete blood cell count, sedimentation rate, and C reactive protein may be helpful when searching for a spinal infection (epidural abscess, osteomyelitis, and diskitis).

Table 21–1 Radiculopathies Associated with Disk Herniation

Disk	Root	Pain Radiation	Sensory Deficit	Motor Deficit	Reflex Involved
L3-4	L4	Lateral and anterior thigh Medial calf and foot ± Great toe	Medial calf and foot ± Great toe	Quadriceps	Knee
L4-5	L5	Lateral thigh Anterior calf and dorsum of foot.	Anterior calf Medial foot First web space ± Great toe	Dorsiflexors	None
L5-S1	S1	Posterior thigh Posterior and lateral calf Heel	Posterior calf Lateral foot	Plantar flexors	Ankle

Please refer to Chapter 12, "Spinal Trauma" for loss of function in the cervical and thoracic area as well as a summary of perineal reflex assessment.

- When bony malignancy is probable, determine the serum calcium. A urinalysis should be done if there is concern for kidney stones or pyelonephritis.

Radiography

- *Plain films.* Plain films are not necessary in uncomplicated low back pain thought to be due to musculoskeletal strain or recurrent back pain that has been previously worked up. Indications for imaging include age over 50, concern for malignancy (unexplained weight loss, history of cancer especially to the breast, lung, thyroid, kidney, and prostate), pain that is worse at rest, history of trauma, neurologic deficits, pain more than 3 weeks duration, osteoporosis, history of prolonged steroid use, or intravenous (IV) drug use.
- *Ultrasound.* Ultrasound studies can be extremely useful to look for an AAA. It can show intraperitoneal fluid and measure the cross-sectional diameter of the aorta. However, computed tomography (CT scan) is necessary to demonstrate retroperitoneal leaking.
- *CT scan.* A noncontrast CT scan is the imaging modality of choice for the diagnosis of nephrolithiasis. Also, a CT scan can help clarify the extent of spinal fractures or malignancies.
- *Magnetic resonance imaging (MRI).* This study is most useful to determine a cauda equina syndrome, spinal cord compression, or an epidural abscess. An MRI can also be useful to evaluate disk herniation and malignancy.
- *Bone scan.* Bone scan may be helpful to demonstrate an infection or tumor, but is typically not performed from the ED.

Emergency Department Management Overview

General

■ Address the ABC's (*a*irway, *b*reathing, *c*irculation) on all ill-appearing patients, particularly those with presentations suggesting an AAA or a spinal cord syndrome. Any patient with an acute neurological deficit should be monitored closely for progression of symptoms.

Medications

■ *Analgesia.* NSAIDs are appropriate for most back pain due to musculo-skeletal strain. Opiates may be needed for severe pain and may be supplemented with a muscle relaxant such as a benzodiazepine (see Chapter 90.1).
■ *Muscle relaxants.* Benzodiazepines such as diazepam are useful to decrease muscle spasm in mechanical back pain. Other muscle relaxants such as cyclobenzaprine, methocarbamol, orphenadrine, and carisoprodol can also be used to decrease muscle spasm.
■ *Antibiotics.* Appropriate coverage is needed when treating infectious etiologies such as epidural abscess, osteomyelitis, diskitis, and pyelonephritis.
■ *Steroids.* Steroids may be used for tumor induced spinal cord syndromes, and may be useful in other cases of cord compression.

Emergency Department Interventions

■ A urinary catheter is necessary in patients with cauda equina or other spinal cord syndrome to relieve urinary retention, and in any patient with an AAA to monitor urinary output.

Disposition

■ *Consultation.* Emergent surgical consultation is required for suspected leaking or ruptured AAA (vascular surgery), spinal epidural abscess, cauda equina or other spinal cord syndromes (neurosurgery). Spinal fractures also require consultation with an orthopedic surgeon.
■ *Admission.* Admission is indicated for patients requiring surgery, patients with a suspected cord syndrome who require an MRI and neurosurgical consultation, patients who are unable to ambulate, as well as those who have poor pain control despite adequate analgesia.
■ *Discharge.* Most mechanical causes of back pain may be treated symptomatically and discharged if they are improved, but even if not completely symptom free. If symptoms are worsening with adequate treatment, the patient may require hospital admission to search for another etiology of the pain such as an epidural abscess that is not obvious. Patients with continued back pain and minor neurologic symptoms (e.g., paresthesias in the lower extremities) should follow up with a primary physician because they will require an MRI.

Specific Problems

Refer to the DDx table for reference to a discussion of problems in the differential not mentioned here.

Cauda Equina Syndrome

- **Definition.** A severe myelopathy in the lumber spinal cord due to mass lesion (e.g. disk herniation) that can cause permanent neurologic defects if not recognized and corrected rapidly.
- **Epidemiology and risk factors.** It is most often caused by an epidural abscess or a central disk herniations. Other causes of spinal cord cauda equina syndrome include tumors, lumbar spinal stenosis, arachnoiditis, osteomyelitis, or diskitis from infection and vertebral fractures. When the conus medullaris is solely impaired, radicular pain is less prominent.
- **Pathophysiology.** The syndrome is caused by compression of the conus medullaris or the spinal nerve roots comprising the cauda equina resulting in an acute myelopathy that can progress rapidly to permanent neurologic damage. The most commonly affected disk space is L4-5 followed by L5-S1 and L3-4.
- **History.** The patient often describes acute or chronic back pain with a rapid development of bilateral leg pain, bilateral leg weakness or numbness, saddle anesthesia, urinary retention or incontinence, constipation or fecal incontinence.
- **Physical examination.** Patients often have focal lumbar spine tenderness. Motor and sensory deficits may be present in the L4-S5 distribution, including genitals, perineum, rectum, and asymmetric paraplegia with loss of the deep tendon reflexes. Decreased rectal tone may be found on digital examination. The patient may also have a positive straight-leg raise.
- **Diagnostic testing.** Postvoid residual volume greater than 200 ml confirms urinary retention. An emergent MRI is the imaging study that is best to define compression. The MRI should include the entire spine, as it is possible to have higher spinal lesions causing similar symptoms that would be missed on a focused MRI. If there are contraindications to its use, or it is not available, a CT myelogram or myelography can be obtained.
- **ED management.** Treatment should include high-dose IV steroids and urgent neurosurgical consultation. Neurologic and orthopedic consultations are also recommended depending on the suspected etiology.
- **Helpful hints and pitfalls.** Urinary retention is the most common finding but may be preceded by increasing pain that is not relieved by adequate amounts of analgesia. Loss of rectal tone is often a late finding and is often subtle when it first appears. It is often missed because a rectal examination is not repeated as the patient's symptoms worsen.

Diskitis

- **Definition.** This is an inflammatory process involving the intervertebral disks and the end plates of the vertebral bodies.

- *Epidemiology and risk factors.* The onset may occur spontaneously, or after surgical procedures. It may also follow dental work. Spontaneous diskitis is more common in the pediatric patient population. There is an increased incidence in immunocompromised patients and in patients with systemic infections.
- *Pathophysiology.* The disease involves an infection of the nucleus pulposus, with secondary involvement of the cartilaginous end plate and vertebral body. *Staphylococcus aureus* is the most common organism, but gram-negative, fungal, and tuberculous infections have all been involved. Osteomyelitis usually starts as diskitis and then spreads to the bone.
- *History.* Fever is present in the majority of patients. Patients present with moderate to severe pain localized to the involved area that is worsened by movement. Radicular symptoms are often present. The lumbar spine is the most common site of disease.
- *Physical examination.* There is usually tenderness to palpation (focal or point tenderness) and percussion. There may be an overlying cellulitis and inflammation.
- *Diagnostic testing.* The erythrocyte sedimentation rate (ESR) and C-reactive protein level will usually be elevated. Blood cultures should be sent. Plain films may suggest an infection, but an MRI is the best imaging study to demonstrate the pathology.
- *ED management.* Start IV antibiotics, and admit the patient to the hospital. Surgical intervention is usually unnecessary.
- *Helpful hints and pitfalls.* Plain radiographs are usually not helpful until after 2 to 4 weeks.

Epidural Abscess

- *Definition.* This is caused by a focal suppurative infection located in the spinal epidural space.
- *Epidemiology and risk factors.* Risk factors include diabetes, IV drug abuse, chronic renal failure, alcoholism, and immunosuppression.
- *Pathophysiology.* Hematogenous spread to the epidural space is the most common source of infection. Skin and soft-tissue infections are the most frequently reported identified source. *Staphylococcus aureus* is cultured in more than 50% of cases. Other pathogens include aerobic and anaerobic streptococcus, *Escherichia coli*, and *Pseudomonas aeruginosa*. No organism is identified in 40% of cases.
- *History.* The patient may initially complain of a backache that becomes more severe and may be more localized. Fever, sweats, and rigors are common. Radicular symptoms may be present as the disease progresses. Later, bowel and bladder disturbance and weakness may develop. A small percentage of patients may have encephalopathy as a presenting symptom.
- *Physical examination.* Spinal tenderness is often present. Signs of myelopathy such as decreased rectal tone, paraplegia, or quadriplegia may be present.
- *Diagnostic testing.* Laboratory testing usually reveals a leukocytosis and an elevated ESR. An MRI is the best imaging study for confirming the diagnosis. Plain films are usually normal unless osteomyelitis of an adjacent vertebral body is present. A lumbar puncture is relatively

contraindicated. If MRI is contraindicated or not available, the diagnosis can sometimes be confirmed with CT scan or myelography.

- ** *ED management.*** Urgent surgical consultation for decompression is required. Intravenous antibiotics effective against the most common organisms (particularly *S. aureus*) should be started empirically.
- ***Helpful hints and pitfalls.*** The classic triad of back pain, fever, and progressive neurologic deficit is present in a minority of patients. Most often, the patients present with increasing back pain that is not relieved by adequate analgesia. A common error is to think the patient is merely drug seeking, because of a history of IV drug abuse. Irreversible paralysis and death can occur in up to 25% of patients.

Malignancy

- **Epidemiology and risk factors.** Primary bone cancer occurs primarily in children and adolescents and is rare. By contrast, secondary bone cancer due to metastasis from a primary site involving the breast, lung, prostate, kidney, and thyroid is more common. Tumors account for fewer than 1% of back pain. Risk factors include a history of malignancy and age greater than 50 or less than 20.
- **Pathophysiology.** Most of the tumor-induced skeletal destruction is mediated by osteoclasts. Malignant cells secrete factors that stimulate osteoclastic activity both directly and indirectly. Malignant cells might also stimulate bone resorption by stimulating tumor-associated immune cells to release osteoclast-activating factors.
- **History.** The patient usually has constant unrelenting pain as a presenting symptom. The pain can be worse at night, and changes in position usually do not alter the character of the pain. Patients may report an unexplained weight loss or night sweats.
- **Physical examination.** The patient usually has focal point tenderness. Lymphadenopathy and testicular or breast masses may be additional clues.
- **Diagnostic testing.** The ESR, calcium and alkaline phosphatase may all be elevated. Plain films can be useful. Metastatic bone lesions may be destructive and cause holes (lytic lesions) in the bone, or they may be bright dense white (sclerotic lesions). The CT and MRI scans are better for showing the tumors. A bone scan is a cost-effective imaging study for metastatic bone cancer. If there is concern for metastatic bone cancer but the patient has a negative ED workup and is stable enough to be discharged, a bone scan should be ordered and the patient should have close outpatient follow-up.
- **ED management.** The patient should receive adequate pain management followed by appropriate outpatient follow-up. Admission criteria include a new diagnosis of metastatic malignancy, an unstable spine from vertebral destruction, neurologic deficits, hypercalcemia, or inability to relieve the patient's symptoms.
- **Helpful hints and pitfalls.** A malignancy may be indistinguishable from infection on plain films. Many of the patient's symptoms may be due to hypercalcemia, and a common error is to conclude that nothing can be done for the patient because there is metastatic disease present.

Musculoskeletal Strain

- *Epidemiology and risk factors.* This entity accounts for 85% of patients with lower back pain. Patients with prior back strain are more likely to get recurrent flare-ups of back pain.
- *Pathophysiology.* The pain is presumed to originate from muscle spasm and ligament inflammation.
- *History.* The onset is usually preceded by repetitive movements or sudden heavy straining.
- *Physical examination.* There is often no focal point or midline tenderness. Tenderness in the paraspinous muscles may be present.
- *Diagnostic testing.* Radiographs are not indicated for this problem unless red flags are present such as elderly age, IV drug use, or a history of trauma.
- *ED management.* The best management is symptomatic treatment with nonsteroidal anti-inflammatory drugs (NSAIDs). Opioids and muscle relaxants should be used if the pain is severe or if significant muscle spasm is present.
- *Helpful hints and pitfalls.* Patients will benefit most from rapid return to normal daily activity. Avoid bed rest for longer than 24 to 48 hours, but also avoid exercise in the acute phase. Ice massages for 10 to 15 minutes will also relieve the spasm and pain, and after 48 hours, local heat or hot tub baths may provide relief.

Sciatica (Lumbar radiculopathy)

- *Definition.* This name is given to pain in the distribution of a lumbar or sacral nerve root, with or without associated neurosensory and motor deficits.
- *Epidemiology and risk factors.* Sciatica is diagnosed in only 1% of patients with back pain, but is present in almost all patients with a symptomatic herniated disk. It is more common in patients in the fourth and fifth decades of life.
- *Pathophysiology.* Herniation of the nucleus pulposus occurs in 95% to 98% of cases at the disk between the fourth and fifth lumbar vertebrae (L4-5) or between the fifth lumbar vertebra and sacrum (L5-S1), with herniation at two levels in 10% of cases.
- *History.* The patient complains of low back pain and leg pain that radiates to the foot. Motor and sensory deficits are also frequently present.
- *Physical examination.* A straight leg test to 60° should be performed with the understanding that it is 95% sensitive in patients with L4-5 and L5-S1 disc herniations (i.e., positive in most patients with the disease), but not as specific (may be positive in patients without the disease). The cross straight leg test is less sensititive but more specific. Assessment should be done for L4, L5, and S1 neurologic deficits (see Table 21–1).
- *Diagnostic testing.* Plain films are neither indicated nor helpful. An MRI can be obtained electively, if symptoms persist longer than 1 month, but should be obtained acutely if there is a significant new neurologic deficit, change in bowel or bladder function, or loss of perineal sensation (i.e., cauda equina syndrome).

- **ED management.** Usually symptomatic care will suffice with NSAIDs, opiates, and muscle relaxants. Intrathecal steroids may reduce swelling and relieve symptoms but are not typically given in the ED. An MRI and hospital admission should be arranged if neurologic deficits appear acutely, are rapidly progressive, if the patient is unable to ambulate, or if there is no relief of the pain with adequate analgesia. Some patients may require admission for sociologic reasons.
- **Helpful hints and pitfalls.** A finding of disk herniation on MRI is significant only if it correlates with the patient's level of neurologic deficits. A common error is to overlook a new neurologic deficit and assume it is chronically present because there have been prior episodes of pain.

Spinal Epidural Hematoma

- **Epidemiology and risk factors.** This is a rare condition with multiple etiologies. Predisposing factors include a coagulopathy (anticoagulation medications, thrombocytopenia, liver disease), congenital coagulation disorders (i.e., hemophilia), vascular malformations (i.e., arteriovenous malformation), arteritis, trauma, and Paget's disease of the spine. Rarely, these occur following simple lumbar or epidural puncture, or as a complication of spinal surgery. In many cases, no cause is evident.
- **Pathophysiology.** Most cases are thought to be caused by rupture of bridging veins of the cord, but no completely satisfactory explanation of the entity exists.
- **History.** The patient usually complains of a sudden onset of severe and constant back pain. There may be a radicular component. It may be noted to follow a straining episode. Neurologic deficits may progress over hours to days. Anticoagulant use or a coagulation abnormality may be present.
- **Physical examination.** Motor and sensory deficits may be present and include weakness, paresis, sensory deficits, and loss of bowel or bladder function.
- **Diagnostic testing.** An MRI is the study of choice. A coagulation profile may be abnormal. If an MRI is contraindicated, CT scan, CT myelogram, or plain myelography may confirm the diagnosis.
- **ED management.** Any coagulopathy should be corrected. Emergent neurosurgical consultation should be obtained for a decompressive laminectomy.
- **Helpful hints and pitfalls.** Up to one third of patients are on anti-coagulant therapy for another disease such as an artificial valve.

Spinal Stenosis

- **Epidemiology and risk factors.** This entity usually occurs in the sixth decade of life
- **Pathophysiology.** It is caused by a narrowing of the spinal canal at single or multiple levels. The narrowing is usually a result of degenerative changes in the spine.
- **History.** Elderly patients often present with a long history of back pain. Ninety percent of patients with spinal stenosis will have significant leg

pain with ambulation or numbness of the leg or foot. The low back pain and leg pain may be exacerbated by back extension or prolonged standing. The back and leg pain will be relieved with rest and forward flexion.

- *Physical examination.* The patient may have a normal findings on physical examination or may show sensory and motor deficits at specific nerve root levels. The physical examination is usually not helpful for determining the presence of spinal stenosis.
- *Diagnostic testing.* An MRI is optimal for showing the diameter of the stenosis and the cord compression, but it may also be demonstrated with a CT scan.
- *ED management.* Symptomatic care with NSAIDs and opiates is all that is required in the ED. If there are symptoms of an acute cord syndrome, the patient will require urgent to emergent surgical correction.
- *Helpful hints and pitfalls.* Spinal stenosis is a cause of an acute spinal cord syndrome and can occur in the cervical or lumbar regions.

Transverse Myelitis

- *Definition.* This is a focal inflammatory disorder of the spinal cord resulting in acute or subacute spinal cord dysfunction.
- *Epidemiology and risk factors.* The incidence of acute transverse myelitis has distinct peaks in adolescence, middle age, and the elderly. A viral prodrome is present in 30% of cases. It sometimes occurs in heroin addicts, with various systemic inflammatory disorders (systemic lupus erythematosus, Behçet disease, Sjögren syndrome), or may be the first symptom in patients who will be ultimately diagnosed with multiple sclerosis (see Chapter 60). Thirty percent of cases are idiopathic.
- *Pathophysiology.* The exact pathogenesis is unknown.
- *History.* The patient will have back pain, leg weakness, sensory disturbances below the level of the lesion, and sphincter dysfunction, especially urinary retention. The onset is usually acute or subacute, from a few hours to several days, but the disorder sometimes evolves over several weeks.
- *Physical examination.* Weakness is initially associated with flaccidity and hyporeflexia, but spasticity and hyperreflexia subsequently develop. A sensory level may be present over the trunk, and a band of hyperesthesia sometimes occurs just above this level. Dysautonomias may also be present from spinal cord involvement.
- *Diagnostic testing.* An emergent MRI scan should be performed to rule out any compressive lesion. The cerebrospinal fluid study findings are frequently normal but may reveal mildly elevated protein and pleocytosis.
- *ED management.* High-dose corticosteroid treatment has been used without consistent benefit. All patients should be admitted to the hospital. Neurologic consultation should be obtained.
- *Helpful hints and pitfalls.* Spinal cord compression must be ruled out.

Special Considerations

- *Pediatrics.* Children are more likely than adults to present with non-mechanical causes of back pain. These include malignancy, diskitis, severe spondylolisthesis, and scoliosis.

- **Elderly.** These patients are at a much higher risk for AAA, fracture, and malignancy.
- **Women and pregnancy.** Always consider ectopic pregnancy in women of reproductive age with back pain. Pain from placental abruption may occur in the late trimesters.
- **Immunocompromised.** These patients are at a much higher risk for epidural abscess, osteomyelitis, and diskitis.

Teaching Points

Back pain is a very common ED problem. Most cases are from mechanical causes, will not require any imaging studies, and are capable of being managed with analgesia and muscle relaxants.

Patients with a more serious etiology are likely to be immunosuppressed, elderly, posttraumatic, or IV drug abusers.

Be alert to changes in bowel or bladder function, including both incontinence and constipation. If the patient has increasing pain that does not respond to adequate analgesia, look for an acute onset of a cauda equina or spinal cord syndrome. These patients require aggressive diagnosis and management with an MRI study and rapid neurosurgical decompression if permanent loss of neurologic function is to be avoided.

Suggested Readings

Della-Giustina D. Emergency department evaluation and treatment of back pain. Emerg Med Clin North Am 1999;17:877–893.

Deyo RA, Weinstein AN. Primary care: low back pain. N Eng J Med 2001;344:363–370.

Deyo R, Rainville J, Kent D. What can the history and physical examination tell us about low back pain? JAMA 1992:286:760–765.

Freymoyer JW. Back pain and sciatica. N Engl J Med 1988;318:291–300.

Linklater DR, Pemberton L, Taylor S, Zeger W. Painful dilemmas: an evidence-based look at challenging clinical scenarios. Emerg Med Clin North Am 2005;23:367–392.

Rogers KG, Jones JB. Back pain. In: Marx JA, Hockengerger RS, Walls RN (editors). Rosen's Emergency Medicine: Concepts and Clinical Practice (6th ed). Philadelphia: Mosby, 2006, pp 260–267.

Small SA, Perron AD, Brady WJ. Orthopedic pitfalls: cauda equina syndrome. Am J Emerg Med 2005;23:159–163.

CHAPTER 22

Chest Pain

GREGORY KUTSEN ■ KURT C. KLEINSCHMIDT
■ HEATHER S. OWEN

 Red Flags

> Tachycardia, bradycardia, tachypnea, high fever ● Hypotension
> ● Hypoxia ● Cardiac risk factors: hypertension, diabetes, hyperlipidemia,
> smoking, family history, cocaine use, prior coronary artery disease
> ● Sudden onset with radiation to the back ● Associated diaphoresis,
> nausea, vomiting or difficulty breathing ● Syncope

Overview

Chest pain is a common complaint, and is seen in approximately 5% of all patients in the emergency department (ED).

Look for "red flags" (see Box) and consider critical diagnoses or life-threatening problems early.

The patient's history is the most important diagnostic tool, and will help distinguish between critical, emergent, and nonemergent causes of chest pain.

Women, elderly, and diabetic patients are more likely to present with atypical or milder symptoms of acute ischemic coronary syndrome (AICS), and thus require a more liberal diagnostic workup. An AICS occurs when the cap on an atheromatous plaque in a coronary artery tears and a clot acutely forms at the site. This occlusion results in either unstable angina, a non-ST-segment elevation myocardial infarction (NSTEMI), or an ST-elevation myocardial infarction (STEMI).

Differential Diagnosis of Chest Pain

■ See DDx table.

Initial Diagnostic Approach
General

■ Any patient who is hemodynamically unstable or appears ill should receive immediate attention. While the physician is assessing the patient,

DDX Priority-Based Differential Diagnosis of "Chest Pain"

	Critical Diagnoses	Emergent Diagnoses	Nonemergent Diagnoses
Cardiac	Acute ischemic coronary syndrome Aortic dissection Cardiac tamponade Mediastinitis	Coronary vasospasm Myocarditis Pericarditis	Aortic stenosis Dilated cardiomyopathy Hypertrophic cardiomyopathy Mitral valve prolapse
Pulmonary	Pulmonary embolus (52) Tension pneumothorax (13, 52)	Pneumonia (67) Pneumothorax (13, 52) Pulmonary edema (52)	Malignancy Pleuritis Pneumomediastinum Primary pulmonary hypertension (52)
Gastrointestinal	Esophageal rupture (Boerhaave's syndrome)	Esophageal tear (Mallory-Weiss) (34) Pancreatitis (18)	Cholecystitis (18) Esophageal spasm (28) Esophagitis (34) Gastritis (34) Gastro-esophageal reflux (18) Peptic ulcer disease (18)
Musculoskeletal			Costochondritis Fibromyalgia (71) Rib fracture (13) Herpes zoster
Neurologic			Radicular syndromes (21, 46) Thoracic outlet syndrome (46)
Other			Psychologic (somatization)

() Refers to the chapter in which the disease entity is discussed.
(From Brown JE, Hamilton GC. Chest pain. In: Marx JA, Hockberger RS, Walls RM (editors). Rosen's Emergency Medicine: Concepts and Clinical Practice (6th ed). Philadelphia: Mosby, 2006, pp 183–192.)

a continuous cardiac monitor and pulse oximeter should be placed. Intravenous (IV) access should be obtained. These patients should not leave the ED except for definitive care (i.e., catheter laboratory, intensive care unit [ICU], or operating room) unless they have had all measures to obtain stability.

■ An electrocardiogram (EKG) should be reviewed by a physician within 10 minutes of patient's presentation to the ED to determine if the patient is a candidate for early reperfusion therapy.

■ The physician should rapidly determine the likelihood of AICS. The history should include cardiac disease and risk factors. Characteristics of the pain should be elicited, and include the onset (sudden versus gradual), precipitation (with exertion, movement, food, at rest), palliation (relief by rest or self-medication), duration (prior episodes, continuous, intermittent), severity (on a 1 to 10 scale), quality (burning, tightness, pressure, pleuritic), radiation (back, neck, arms), and associated symptoms (nausea, vomiting, diaphoresis, shortness of breath). For patients with chronic chest pain, any change from the patient's usual chest pain should be assessed. Any chest pain radiating to the upper mid-back should be concerning for aortic dissection (AD). Likewise, pain that is located in the mid-epigastric area or that is reproducible on palpation, may well be cardiac in origin. Chest wall tenderness can occur in patients with pulmonary embolus, AICS, and pneumonia. A pericardial friction rub may be present in patients with an acute myocardial infarction.

Laboratory

■ Studies include cardiac enzymes (Table 22–1), complete blood count and a basic metabolic profile. Coagulation studies should be drawn prior to anticoagulation therapy. Send a type and cross match if the patient may need a blood transfusion, and a toxicology screen if a history of illicit drug (i.e., cocaine and amphetamines) use is sought.

EKG

■ A standard 12-lead EKG is the best test to identify patients with AICS but may be normal on the initial presentation.

Table 22–1   Cardiac Enzyme Kinetics

	Rises, h	Peaks, h	Remains Elevated, d
CK	4-8	12-24	3-4
CK MB	4-10	20	2
Myoglobin	2-3	4-24	1
Troponins (T and I)	6	12-18	7-14

CK, creatine kinase; CK-MB, creatine kinase MB.

Radiography

- *Plain films.* A chest radiograph should be done to look for pulmonary pathology, cardiomegaly, or a widened mediastinum.
- *CT angiogram (CTA).* This imaging study is useful to evaluate for AD and pulmonary embolus. Improper timing of the contrast bolus or too slow of an injection rate can result in a failure to fully opacify the false lumen found in AD.
- *Ultrasound.* This will not be the initial diagnostic modality for most patients with chest pain. It can be useful to evaluate a pleural effusion for the presence of loculations, or to confirm the presence of a pneumothorax. Transesophageal echocardiography (TEE) is an alternative imaging study used to diagnose AD if the patient cannot have a computed tomography (CT scan) angiogram (i.e., cannot have IV contrast or is unstable). However, it is not readily available in many institutions and requires sedation. It may reveal wall motion abnormalities in patients with an acute myocardial infarction (AMI), a pericardial effusion in patients with pericarditis, or right-sided heart flow abnormalities in patients with a pulmonary embolus.
- *Angiography.* Angiography is considered the most accurate imaging method to look for dissection, and has the added advantage that it can also study coronary artery flow, but it is not readily available. Diagnostic information from TEE or CTA is adequate, and more readily obtained. It is thought to be the most accurate imaging study for pulmonary embolus, but has more potential for complications, and is harder to obtain than a CTA.

Emergency Department Management Overview
General

- The ABCs should be addressed as discussed in Section II. Any patient with possible critical diagnoses of chest pain should be placed in a resuscitation room. These patients should receive supplemental oxygen to keep oxygen saturation above 95% and one to two large-bore IV catheters depending on the level of concern.

Medications

- Antithrombotic and adjunctive therapies for AICS are described in Chapter 90.5.
- For severe or persistent pain, give morphine 2 to 5 mg IV every 10 minutes titrated to the patient's comfort.
- Noncardiac pain control should be individualized: nonsteroidal anti-inflammatory drugs (NSAIDs) are preferred for chest pain of musculoskeletal origin, and antacids or H_1 blocking agents can be given for gastric reflux or "heartburn" pain. Relief of pain by either of these modalities does not rule out an AICS, and they have no value as a diagnostic test. They should be used for therapeutic relief of symptoms only.

Disposition

- *Consultation*. Obtain cardiac consultation for patients with AICS. Obtain a cardiothoracic surgery consultation in a patient with a valvular lesion by echocardiogram, esophageal rupture, or AD.
- *Admission*. Patients with the potential for dysrhythmias require continuous cardiac monitoring. Most patients with an AICS will be admitted to the cardiac care unit (CCU) or a monitored bed. Patients with actual or potential hemodynamic instability should be admitted to the ICU or CCU.
- *Discharge*. Patients with a low probability for life-threatening illness, resolution of pain and stable hemodynamics, normal laboratory and imaging studies, and normal or unchanged EKG findings can be discharged home.

Specific Problems

> ● ● ● Refer to the DDx table for reference to a discussion of problems in the
> ● ● ● differential not mentioned here.

Acute Ischemic Coronary Syndrome
Definitions

- See Table 22–2 for definitions of AICS.

Epidemiology and Risk Factors

- This is a leading cause of death in adults in United States.
- Hypertension, diabetes, tobacco use, family history of coronary artery disease (CAD) at an early age, male sex, hypercholesterolemia, and cocaine use are all risk factors. A positive risk factor must always be interpreted in the clinical context (e.g., a patient might have all of these risk factors and be suffering from an early community-acquired pneumonia).

Pathophysiology

- Narrowing of the coronary arteries is secondary to atherosclerotic plaques. When these plaques rupture, they cause platelet aggregation and thrombus formation at the site of rupture.
- AICS can result in death of cardiac muscle (AMI) or reversible ischemia without detectable myocardial damage (angina).
- Other rarer causes of AICS include emboli to the coronary arteries (endocarditis, prosthetic valve, mural thrombus, myxoma), vasospasm (cocaine, amphetamines, or Prinzmetal's angina), AD involving a coronary artery, vasculitis, and severe hypertension in the setting of CAD. Variant angina, or Prinzmetal's angina, is caused by coronary artery vasospasm at rest with minimal fixed coronary artery disease. The EKG

Table 22–2	Definitions of Acute Ischemic Coronary Syndromes			
	Pathology	**EKG changes**	**Biomarkers**	**Comment**
Unstable angina (UA)	Subtotal coronary thrombosis	ST depression (>1 mm) or T-ware inversion	Negative	A clinical diagnosis: new exertional chest pain, increased anginal episodes, pain at rest. Same prognosis as NSTEMI.
Non–ST segment elevation myocardial infarction (MI)	Subtotal coronary thrombosis	ST depression (>1 mm) or TW inversion	Positive	Although an incomplete ischemic event, additional myocardium is at risk for infarction.
(NSTEMI)				Same prognosis as UA, and can lead to STEMI or death
ST segment elevation MI (STEMI)	Total coronary thrombosis	ST elevations >1 mm in limb leads or >2 mm in precordial leads New LBBB Hyperacute T waves (<1 h) Q waves (>6 h) Reciprocal ST depression	Positive	Need immediate reperfusion with thrombolytics or PCI

EKG, electrocardiogram; LBBB, left bundle branch block; MI, myocardial infarction; PCI, percutaneous coronary intervention.

will reveal ST-segment elevation (STE) that is impossible to discern from AMI electrocardiographically or, at times, clinically.

History

■ Ischemic chest pain is usually described as chest pressure, heaviness, tightness, or squeezing and not typically as fleeting, sharp, or stabbing. The pain is usually substernal and in the left chest. There may be radiation to the arm (classically the left, but it can be to the right arm or shoulder), back, neck, jaw, or throat. It is a restless pain, not relieved by positional changes, and hard to describe.

■ Unfortunately, most patients do not have a classic story. Diabetic, older, and female patients often do not experience classical chest pain, but even male patients can have infarction with no or misleading types of chest pain. The patient may deny that the sensation in the chest is an actual "pain" but more of a vague feeling of discomfort. Others may describe it as indigestion or heartburn, which can also accompany ischemic chest pain, or precede it.

■ Many times an AICS will be precipitated by another disease that causes a drop in blood pressure, and those disease signs and symptoms may predominate and prevent the physician from thinking about or seeing the presence of an AICS.

Physical Examination

■ The primary purpose of the physical examination is to exclude other chest pain etiologies. There are no findings diagnostic of AICS. A S_4 gallop is common but not specific for AICS. Transient pericardial friction rubs may be auscultated in AMI, and are not helpful.

■ Virtually all other physical findings relate to low cardiac output, development of dysrhythmias, or congestive heart failure (crackles, S_3, and increased jugular venous pressure [JVP]). A new mitral regurgitation murmur in the setting of AICS represents papillary muscle dysfunction.

Diagnostic Testing

■ Serial cardiac markers (Table 22–1) only reveal death (infarction) of heart muscle (AMI). Thus absence of cardiac marker elevation does not rule out unstable angina. Evidence to support the use of a single cardiac marker are weak. Serial cardiac markers are recommended.

■ A physician should evaluate the EKG within 10 minutes of the patient's arrival in the ED. A repeated EKG should be performed at intervals to look for dynamic or reversible changes especially if the initial tracing reveals ischemic changes (i.e., T-wave inversion, ST segment depression or elevation) or the patient's chest pain changes. An attempt should be made to find an old EKG for comparison. The EKG changes give clues to the anatomic site of obstruction and infarction (Chapter 87). Fewer than 50% of patients with AMI will have ST segment elevations on the initial EKG. Nondiagnostic EKG changes are classified as *nonspecific* changes. This does not mean that they are not dangerous.

■ Patients with ST elevation in II, III, and avF (inferior wall MI) should have right-sided precordial or V leads obtained looking for right ventricle infarction. Patients with a tall R wave in V_1, or ST depression in V_1 and V_2, may have a posterior wall infarction, and should have a left scapula (V_8) lead obtained.

■ A chest radiograph may reveal cardiomegaly or congestive heart failure, and should be obtained before initiation of heparin or thrombolytic therapy as a screening test for AD unless the concern for AD is extremely low.

- An echocardiogram can detect regional wall motion abnormalities, but this is not part of routine ED evaluations.
- Exercise tolerance testing is being used at some institutions for patients with an atypical presentation, who are pain-free, have no ischemic changes on the EKG, and have negative cardiac enzymes.

ED Management

- Aspirin, nitroglycerin, morphine, and a beta-blocker should be given.

> ⠿ **Refer to Chapter 90.3, "Cardiovascular Pharmacology."**

- Anemic patients with AICS should be transfused until their hematocit level is more than 30%.
- External pacing pads should be placed for patients with symptomatic bradycardia, type II second–degree heart block, or third degree heart block.
- Each institution will have a strategy as to which patients will need percutaneous coronary intervention (PCI) or thrombolysis in the ED. In general, PCI is preferred if the facilities are available. However, reperfusion should not be delayed waiting for PCI to become available if the patient meets criteria for thrombolytic therapy (see Chapter 90.5). Each institution and cardiology service has their own preferences for the use of platelet blockers and anticoagulants. Withhold anticoagulation in those patients who are being investigated for AD or gastrointestinal bleeding.
- Patients with persistent chest pain may benefit from a nitroglycerin drip and narcotic analgesia, but some will need immediate reperfusion therapy.
- The patient with chest pain who arrives in the ED in acute pulmonary edema, but with a low blood pressure, is probably having an AMI with pump failure, and is in cardiogenic shock. These patients require immediate endotracheal intubation for respiratory failure, vasopressor therapy (e.g., dobutamine and dopamine), reperfusion therapy (e.g., thrombolysis, PCI, or cardiac bypass surgery), or cardiac surgery to replace a necrotic chorda tendinae, a ruptured ventricle, or septal necrosis. They may need an aortic pump assistance device to improve cardiac output.
- Patients with an equivocal presentation for AICS should be admitted to the hospital for observation and early stress testing. These patients can be admitted to a telemetry unit. Some hospitals have chest pain units within the ED where such patients can be observed and have early stress testing along with serial EKG and cardiac enzyme testing. Patients with an AMI are preferably admitted to a cardiac care unit. Stable patients with unstable angina can be admitted to a telemetry floor bed.

Helpful Hints and Pitfalls

- Chest pain is a somatic symptom that can easily mimic serious disease. It is often referred to as *atypical* or *noncardiac*, but while nonischemic chest pain is common, and benign, this classification should not be used to preclude further workup for AICS in patients who are at risk. It is a diagnosis of exclusion. Moreover, many patients with AICS are mistaken as chest wall pain because subtle EKG changes or cardiac enzyme elevations have not yet evolved or are unrecognized.

- Other conditions that can be associated with ischemic EKG changes: intracranial hemorrhage, pericarditis, or pulmonary embolus.
- Other conditions can cause troponin elevations: acute pericarditis, myocarditis, pulmonary embolus, acute or severe heart failure, sepsis, renal failure.
- Rule out AD before initiating thrombolytic therapy if any concern exists.

Aortic Dissection (AD)
Definitions

- AD occurs when blood pushes into the medial layers of the aorta due to an intimal tear.
- This should not be confused with an aortic aneurysm, which is a localized dilatation of the aorta caused by weakening of its wall.

Epidemiology and Risk Factors

- AD is more common in older men; hypertension is the most common risk factor.
- In younger patients, predisposing conditions include congenital heart disease (aortic coarctation), Marfan's syndrome, Ehlers-Danos syndrome, other connective tissue disease, syphilis, and pregnancy (third trimester). Traumatic AD is discussed in Chapter 13.
- Without treatment, the mortality rate is as high as 75% within 2 weeks of the initial symptoms.

Pathophysiology

- There is degeneration of the media, or muscular layer, of the aortic wall. This occurs with the normal aging process, but is augmented in the face of persistent hypertension. Dissection occurs as the blood violates the endothelial lining of the aorta and dissects through degenerating media. Once a dissecting hematoma is established in the media, extension of the dissection and of the hematoma occurs, forming a *false* lumen.
- ADs have been classified by two different systems. The Stanford system classifies ascending dissections as type A, and isolated descending dissections as type B. In the DeBakey system, class I is dissection involving the ascending aorta, the arch and the descending aorta. Class II is the ascending aorta only. Class III is the descending aorta distal to the left subclavian artery.

History

- The classic history is a sudden onset of severe, tearing chest pain, most severe at onset, radiating to the upper mid-back, but only half the patients will give this history. The chest pain may move in location as the dissection progresses. The patient may also present with vasovagal symptoms such as diaphoresis, nausea, vomiting, lightheadedness, syncope, or severe apprehension.

■ Other associated symptoms depend on the course of the dissection. Dissection involving the carotids may present as stroke; those involving the coronary arteries may manifest as an AMI; the aortic root as pericardial tamponade; and abdominal pain, lower extremity weakness, or leg numbness as the dissection progresses caudally. The patient may also present with paraplegia if the dissection has involved the anterior spinal artery.

Physical Examination

■ There are no pathognomic physical findings, however, the patient is often hyper- or normotensive and in distress. Hypotension is less common but more concerning, and is usually due to rupture through the adventitia or pericardial tamponade. Pulse deficits and blood pressure discrepancies between limbs may be seen. Dissection of the aortic root can result in pericardial effusion with tamponade (muffled heart sounds, jugular venous distention [JVD], and hypotension) or aortic regurgitation (diastolic murmur). Involvement of the carotid artery can produce an acute stroke picture.

Diagnostic Testing

■ No laboratory tests define dissection. A blood sample should be sent for type and cross match. Evidence of myocardial ischemia may be present with EKG changes and elevated enzymes and troponin levels. The EKG often demonstrates left ventricular hypertrophy from chronic hypertension.

■ Chest radiograph findings that suggest dissection include a widening of the mediastinum; an indistinct aortic knob; pleural effusion; deviation of the trachea, main stem bronchus, or nasogastric tube; and separation of the calcified aortic lining from the rest of the aortic contour. Chest radiograph findings will be normal in 10% of patients.

■ Aortography is a very good imaging study, but is not available in many institutions, and has been replaced by CTA or ultrasound.

■ CTA is also a good study. Although it provides less anatomic detail of the injury aortography, it is readily available at most institutions, but it does not show the coronary arteries well.

■ TEE is a very good imaging study, especially for unstable patients, but is not always available, requires sedation, and does not give good information about downstream vessel involvement or the coronary arteries.

■ Magnetic resonance imaging (MRI) is excellent for diagnosing dissection, but is often not readily available from the ED, and is an unsafe place to image an unstable patient.

ED Management

■ Place two large-bore IVs and transfuse blood if hypotensive. The patient may need a pericardiocentesis in the ED if tamponade is present.

- Arrange emergent cardiothoracic surgery consultation.
- Hypertension needs to be controlled. The desired endpoint depends on the individual patient. A systolic blood pressure of 120 mm Hg is the generally accepted target. The initial goal is rate control with a beta-blocker. Give esmolol 500 µg/kg bolus (ultrashort acting), then an infusion of 50 to 200 µg/kg/min or metoprolol 5 mg IV every 5 minutes for three doses followed by 2 to 5 mg/hr IV infusion. Nitroprusside (initial dose of 0.3 µg/kg/ min) can be added for further blood pressure reduction. Labetalol has both alpha- and beta-blocking activity. The usual dose is 20 mg IV every 5 to 10 minutes. Pain should be controlled with IV morphine. Nicardipine 5 to 15 mg/hr IV is a calcium channel blocker, and has also been used successfully.
- Although dissections of the ascending aorta, Stanford classification A, are usually surgically repaired, descending dissections are usually managed medically with blood pressure control and observation.

Helpful Hints and Pitfalls

- Medications with negative ionotropy (beta-blockers) should be given first before vasodilators (e.g., nitroprusside) to reduce shearing forces secondary to an increase in the rate of the arterial pulse.
- AD is suggested by CP that radiates to the back, CP combined with neurologic deficits, or CP that moves to the abdomen or visa versa.

Esophageal Rupture (Boerhaave's Syndrome)
Definition

- Boerhaave's syndrome is due to perforation of the esophagus following a rise in intraesophageal pressure.
- This should not be confused with a Mallory-Weiss tear (Chapter 34), which is a longitudinal mucosal laceration in the region of the gastro-esophageal junction as a result of retching or vomiting.

Epidemiology and Risk Factors

- The most common causes of esophageal perforation are iatrogenic (endoscopy), foreign body, caustic burn, blunt or penetrating trauma, spontaneous rupture (Boerhaave's syndrome), and postoperative breakdown of an anastomosis.
- Rupture is associated with forceful emesis, straining, cough, childbirth, blunt trauma, and seizures. Alcohol and pre-existing esophageal disease are risk factors.
- Improved resuscitative and surgical techniques have decreased mortality from this condition.

Pathophysiology

- The distal esophagus is the usual site of injury, with a longitudinal tear occurring in the left posterolateral aspect.

- This esophageal injury is associated with a poor prognosis, because the forces required to rupture the esophagus result in massive mediastinal contamination. Leakage of esophageal contents causes fulminant necrotizing mediastinitis and septic shock.

History

- There is often an acute onset of severe chest pain after an episode of forceful vomiting. However a history of vomiting may be absent.
- Pain is described as severe, unrelenting, and possibly radiating to the back, neck, and shoulders. Pain is associated with dysphagia and is exacerbated by swallowing or neck flexion.
- Dyspnea may occur once inflammation progresses.

Physical Examination

- The patient is usually ill appearing with the development of cardio-vascular collapse and sepsis. Hypotension, shock, and abdominal rigidity are late findings.
- There may be subcutaneous emphysema of the neck if the proximal esophagus is involved.
- There may be a "Hamman's crunch" sign, which is a loud clicking or crunching sound heard in synchrony with the heartbeat.

Diagnostic Testing

- There are no diagnostic laboratory studies. There often is a leukocytosis with neutrophilia. A thoracentesis may yield pleural fluid with a high amylase level, low pH, and undigested food.
- An EKG should be done to screen for acute ischemic coronary syndrome.
- An upright chest radiograph may reveal mediastinal air with and without subcutaneous emphysema, left-sided pleural effusion, empyema, pneumothorax, widened mediastinum, or another cause of chest pain. Radiographic evidence of the perforation may be absent.
- A CT scan of the chest is good at detecting mediastinal air, but will often not reveal the exact location of an esophageal tear.
- An esophagogram is often required to define the extent and location of the tear precisely. Barium is most accurate, but obscures an esophagoscopy, and contaminates the mediastinum if a tear is present. Gastrograffin is less difficult to work with, but less accurate. Esophagoscopy may extend the tear, and doesn't easily visualize the tear.

ED Management

- Address airway patency, which is threatened by the perforation and mediastinitis.
- Two large-bore IVs are needed for fluid resuscitation.
- Tube thoracostomy is needed to drain pleural effusions or for a pneumothorax.

- Broad-spectrum antibiotics should be administered, and should cover streptococci, gram-negative bacteria, and anaerobes.
- Surgery should be consulted for surgical repair.

Helpful Hints and Pitfalls

- This entity is often misdiagnosed initially. The diagnosis of esophageal rupture should be sought in any patient who has unexplained sepsis, left pleural effusion, lung abscess, empyema, pneumomediastinum, or pneumothorax.
- The mortality rate is more than 90% if appropriate management is delayed for 48 hours.

Mediastinitis
Definition

- This is a rare but serious infectious process involving the structures of the mediastinum.

Epidemiology and Risk Factors

- This is associated with a high mortality rate, from 19% to 47%.
- Most patients with mediastinitis are in their third to fifth decades of life; however, it has been documented in patients as young as 2 months and as old as the eighth decade.
- The most common cause is as a postoperative complication of cardio-thoracic surgery. The second most common cause is esophageal perforation or leakage (see Esophageal Rupture).
- It can also occur from a bacteremic or contiguous spread from foci within the head and neck, retroperitoneum, sternum, vertebrae, and lung; however, the common use of antibiotics has reduced this route significantly.

Pathophysiology

- Mediastinitis secondary to cardiothoracic surgery is primarily due to gram-positive cocci with lesser contributions by gram-negative bacilli. *Candida* is increasingly associated with mediastinitis following cardiothoracic surgery.
- Head and neck infections as well as esophageal contents may extend downward into the mediastinum, and spread from the fascial planes in the neck to gain access to the mediastinum. It is also necrotizing, as the infection is often polymicrobial and includes gas-producing organisms.

History

- Patients may complain of fever, chills, pleuritic chest pain, shortness of breath, sore throat, dysphagia, or neck swelling. Chest pain is the most prominent symptom. Retroperitoneal extension may result in acute abdominal signs.

Physical Examination

- The patient usually appears ill. Examination may reveal fever, tachycardia, crepitus, and edema of the neck, face, or chest.
- Hamman's sign, a crunching rasping sound heard over the precordium synchronous with the cardiac rhythm due to emphysema of the mediastinum, may be present in up to 50% of patients with pneumomediastinum. The heart sounds may appear distant and dull.

Diagnostic Testing

- Laboratory tests usually reveal a leukocytosis with a leftward shift evident on the differential.
- Chest radiographs are rarely helpful, but may reveal widening of the mediastinum, air fluid levels, and subcutaneous or mediastinal emphysema. The lateral chest radiograph may be useful in demonstrating superior mediastinal gas not evident on PA or AP films of the chest. A pleural effusion may be present.
- A CT scan is often helpful in cases in which the diagnosis is not evident clinically or on plain films.
- The use of MRI to confirm the diagnosis of mediastinitis is becoming more common.

ED Management

- Broad-spectrum antibiotics should be started, and surgical consultation obtained.

Helpful Hints and Pitfalls

- The early diagnosis of mediastinitis in the infant or neonate is particularly challenging. A peculiar, interrupted, staccato type of inspiration has been described.

Myocarditis
Epidemiology and Risk Factors

- This disease is rare but has a mortality rate of 20%.
- Most patients are younger than 35 years.

Pathophysiology

- The enteroviruses, such as Coxsackie B, are common causative agents. Other organisms that may cause myocarditis include adenovirus, influenza A and B, *Streptococcus*, mononucleosis, *Chlamydia*, *Mycoplasma*, parainfluenza, mumps, cytomegalovirus (CMV), rubeola, rubella, rabies, lymphocytic choriomeningitis virus, hepatitis A and B, and varicella-zoster. Bacterial infections are seen in IV drug abusers and in immunocompromised patients.
- CMV and *Toxoplasma gondii* are potential causes in cardiac transplant recipients. Half of the fatal AIDS cases have myocarditis on autopsy. Chagas disease is the leading cause worldwide.

- There are three possible mechanisms: necrosis from direct invasion of the infectious agent with replication within or near myocytes, destruction of cardiac tissue from infiltration by host cellular immune components or from the cytotoxic effect of activated host humoral defenses, or the toxic effect of toxin produced by a systemic pathogen.
- Complications include ventricular dysrhythmias, ventricular aneurysm, and cardiac failure.

History

- Typical initial symptoms are those of a viral illness: fever, fatigue, myalgias, vomiting, and diarrhea. Chest pain is present in approximately 10% of patients. Shortness of breath may be present secondary to congestive heart failure (CHF).

Physical Examination

- Fever, tachycardia, tachypnea, and uncommonly, hypotension may develop. A tachycardia disproportionate to the temperature or apparent toxicity is a clinical clue.
- Cardiac and pulmonary examinations may be normal. Unexplained CHF and dysrhythmias occur.

Diagnostic Testing

- Laboratory testing reveals elevated cardiac enzymes, leukocytosis, and an elevated erythrocyte sedimentation rate (ESR). Indium-111 antimyosin antibodies bind specifically to exposed myosin in damaged myocardial cells, thereby providing a noninvasive approach for the diagnosis of myocardial necrosis. Viral titers or viral-specific IgM titers may be helpful.
- The EKG may reveal sinus tachycardia, low electrical activity, prolonged corrected QT interval, atrioventricular (AV) block, or global ischemic cardiac abnormalities such as ST-segment depression and T-wave inversion.
- The echocardiogram can show multichamber dysfunction such as reduced left ventricular ejection fraction, global hypokinesis, and regional wall motion abnormalities. Coronary angiography findings are normal. CT scan and MRI may be diagnostic.
- Endocardial biopsy is the most accurate diagnostic test.
- Antimyosin scintigraphy reveals a diffuse, faint, heterogeneous uptake of antimyosin antibody in myocarditis but is more localized in AMI. A normal antimyosin scan excludes both AMI and myocarditis. These last three studies are not typically performed from the ED.

ED Management

- All patients require admission and continuous cardiac monitoring. Hemodynamically unstable patients require ICU admission.
- Most patients require supportive therapy only. Severe cases may require cardiac transplantation. Immunotherapy and antiviral therapy may be helpful in select patients.

Helpful Hints and Pitfalls

- This diagnosis should be sought in an otherwise healthy patient with new onset CHF and dysrhythmias.

Pericarditis
Epidemiology and Risk Factors

- Possible causes include infectious (viral, bacterial, fungal), malignancy, connective tissue disease, uremia, myxedema, postmyocardial infarction (Dressler syndrome), and drug-induced (procainamide, hydralazine, bleomycin, phenytoin, and others). Pericarditis may occur as a complication of trauma to the chest.

Pathophysiology

- This involves inflammation of the pericardium. A pericardial effusion occasionally occurs.

History

- The most common symptom is a sudden onset of sharp, retrosternal chest pain. The pain is worse with movement, inspiration, and when lying supine. The pain is often reduced by leaning forward or sitting up. Patients may report low-grade intermittent fever, dysphagia, myalgias, anorexia, and anxiety.

Physical Examination

- A transient, intermittent pericardial friction rub helps confirm the diagnosis. It is heard best at the lower left sternal border or apex, but is not commonly heard clearly.

Diagnostic Testing

- No laboratory tests confirm this diagnosis. Obtain cardiac enzymes, a basic metabolic panel, CBC and blood cultures if bacterial pericarditis seems possible, and viral titers if the subsequent course is prolonged.
- An EKG may show low voltage or electrical alternans in the presence of a large pericardial effusion. Table 22–3 shows the EKG findings. The EKG changes are best seen over time, so a single tracing is often inadequate to reveal them.
- The chest radiograph study is often normal. An echocardiogram is the best way to detect a pericardial effusion.

ED Management

- Uncomplicated cases are treated with NSAIDs for 1 to 3 weeks (Ibuprofen 800 mg by mouth three times daily or indomethacin 25-50 mg by mouth every 8 hours).

Table 22–3   Electrocardiogram Comparison: Pericarditis vs. AICS

	Acute Pericarditis*	**AICS**
ST segment	Diffuse concave ST-segment elevation in limb and precordial leads and upright T waves. ST depression in aVR.	Localized ST elevation (STEMI) or ST depression (NSTEMI or UA).
Reciprocal changes PR depression	None May be present	May be present None
T waves inversion	May be present	May be present
Q waves	None	Common
Dysrhythmia and conduction abnormalities	None	Common

If no associated heart disease present.
AICS, acute ischemic coronary syndrome; NSTEMI, non–ST-segment elevation myocardial infarction; STEMI, ST-segment elevation myocardial infarction; UA, unstable angina.

■ Admission criteria include the presence of a pericardial effusion, oral anticoagulation therapy, trauma, myo-pericarditis, high fever, or possible bacterial pericarditis. Patients experiencing renal failure with a large effusion may require emergency dialysis. Aspirin and steroids are alternatives to NSAIDs for postmyocardial infarction pericarditis.

Helpful Hints and Pitfalls

■ Anticoagulation in the setting of pericarditis can lead to hemorrhage into the pericardial space and tamponade.

Pneumomediastinum (Benign)
Epidemiology and Risk Factors

■ Spontaneous pneumomediastinum generally occurs in young healthy patients without underlying lung disease.
■ It is more common in young men.

Pathophysiology

■ Pneumomediastinum is generally a benign, self-limited condition. Excessive intra-alveolar pressures lead to rupture of perivascular alveoli. Air escapes into the perivascular connective tissue, with subsequent dissection into the mediastinum. If the mediastinal pressure rises abruptly or if decompression is not sufficient, the mediastinal parietal pleura may rupture and cause a pneumothorax (in 10%-18% of patients).

- Acute production of high intrathoracic pressures is the usual cause for benign pneumomediastinum. Asthma, smoking, athletic competition, emesis, severe cough, and mechanical ventilation can all cause a pneumomediastinum. It may also be seen after a Valsalva maneuver or forceful inhalation, and is common in heroin and marijuana users.
- Pneumomediastinum in the setting of trauma, esophageal instrumentation, or a Boerhaave's syndrome is associated with significant morbidity and mortality, but it is the underlying condition that must be managed aggressively.

History

- The most common complaint is chest pain or cough.
- The chest pain is typically substernal, radiating to the back and shoulders, and pleuritic. Patients may also complain of dyspnea, dysphagia, or neck pain.

Physical Examination

- Subcutaneous emphysema is the most common sign. Auscultation of the heart can reveal a Hamman's sign (precordial crunching noise associated with heart beats).
- If pneumomediastinum results in a pneumothorax, decreased breath sounds, tachypnea, tachycardia, hypoxia, and hypotension may be present.

Diagnostic Testing

- The chest radiograph is the best test for diagnosing pneumomediastinum and to rule out an associated pneumothorax.
- An esophogram is indicated if retching or emesis is the precipitating event, or if there is any other reason to look for an esophageal tear.

ED Management

- Patients with pneumomediastinum may need to be admitted and observed for signs of serious complications such as pneumothorax or mediastinitis.
- Stable patients who develop a pneumomediastinum after Valsalva maneuver or cocaine or marijuana inhalation and without co-morbidities can be discharged safely.
- Pain should be treated as needed. Supplemental oxygen may hasten reabsorption, but specific therapy for pneumomediastinum is rarely needed.

Helpful Hints and Pitfalls

- Patients with a history of emesis, retching, or recent esophageal instrumentation need to be evaluated for an esophageal tear.

Other Causes of Chest Pain
Cardiomyopathy

■ Cardiomyopathies are diseases of the heart in which the primary feature is involvement of the heart muscle itself. There are three types: dilated, restrictive, and hypertrophic.

■ There are many causes. Patients with cardiomyopathy can present with chest pain; however cardiomyopathies are an infrequent cause of chest pain. Refer to Table 22–4 for a comparison of the three major types of cardiomyopathy. Refer to Chapter 52 for management of acute pulmonary edema.

Chest Wall Pain

■ Pain that results from inflammation of, or trauma to, the joints, muscles, cartilages, bones, and fascia that comprise the thoracic cage is common. Herpes zoster causes pain to the chest wall in a dermatomal distribution, but it often causes pain before the diagnostic rash appears, and thus can be difficult to explain or recognize in a single ED visit.

■ Refer to Table 22–5 for a description of common causes.

■ NSAIDs are commonly used to treat chest wall pain. Treatment for herpes zoster is summarized in Chapter 62.

Pleuritis

■ *Pleuritis* is a term used to denote inflammation of the parietal pleura. This chest pain increases with breathing movements, and is commonly referred to as *pleuritic chest pain*. Pleuritic pain is usually localized to the affected region rather than being diffuse, but the patient may describe referred pain in the ipsilateral neck or shoulder. There may be an associated pleural effusion.

■ Common causes of pleuritic chest pain include infection, pulmonary embolism (see Chapter 52), pneumothorax (see Chapter 52), collagen vascular disease (see Chapter 71), and sickle cell disease (see Chapter 53). Pleural effusions are discussed in Chapter 52.

Valvular Heart Disease

■ Valvular heart disease occasionally presents as a rare cause of chest pain.

■ Refer to Table 22–6 for a comparison of the most common valvular problems. Treatment for acute pulmonary edema is discussed in Chapter 52. Antibiotic prophylaxis should be given for bacteremia prone procedures.

Special Considerations

■ *Pediatrics.* Chest pain in the pediatric age group is rarely cardiac and is unlikely to be ischemic. Younger children are likely to have an organic cause, whereas adolescents are more likely to have unknown or

Table 22–4   Types of Cardiomyopathy

	Pathophysiology	Clinical Presentation	Comment
Dilated	Characterized by dilated left and right ventricles with accompanied hypertrophy, this results in systolic pump failure Causes include myocarditis, coronary artery disease, postpartum, pregnancy, HIV, ethanol, amyloidosis, HTN, connective tissue disease	Evidence of LV failure: dyspnea on exertion, orthopnea, paroxysmal nocturnal dyspnea RV failure: ascites, lower extremity edema Severe DCM is associated with mural thrombi formation and may cause peripheral embolization	Atrial fibrillation is the most common dysrhythmia Associated with: viral infections, ethanol, heavy metals, lithium, doxorubicin, stimulant use Vasodilators can cause hypotension as restrictive cardiomyopathy is very preload sensitive.
Restrictive	Diastolic restriction of ventricular filling which results in low end diastolic ventricular volume and decreased cardiac output Causes include amyloidosis, sarcoidosis, hemochromatosis, scleroderma, neoplastic, metabolic disease	Evidence of right heart failure predominates, exercise intolerance is a common complaint	Difficult to distinguish from constrictive pericarditis Associated with amyloidosis, sarcoidosis, hemo-chromatosis
Hypertrophic	Asymmetric left ventricular hypertrophy mostly involving the septum without dilatation. Reduced ventricular cavity size, impaired diastolic relaxation and obstruction to left ventricular outflow.	Many are asymptomatic Dyspnea on exertion, ischemic chest pain, Palpitations, syncope, sudden death Murmur: loud S_4 gallop and a harsh crescendo-decrescendo midsystolic murmur that is made softer by nitrates and louder by Valsalva's maneuvers, or by standing. It becomes quieter when the patient lies down, squats, or does isometric exercises, such as those using hand grips.	More than 50% of cases are inherited via an auto somal dominant fashion. Patients should avoid competitive athletics because of the associated risk of sudden death. Ionotropes are contraindicated as they can increase outflow obstruction. Can be treated with septal myomectomy, a surgical procedure.

DCM, dilated cardiomyopathy; HIV, human immunodeficiency virus; HTN, hypertension; LV, left ventricle; RV, right ventricle.

Table 22–5   Common Problems Causing Chest Wall Pain

Costochondritis	Many patients have tenderness over the costochondral junctions (junction of bony rib and cartilage), especially when they are small and slender; but this does not mean that they have costochondritis. The latter is probably a true form of arthritis, but the label should not be applied to the patient unless there is true pain and tenderness overlying the costochondral junction.
Herpes zoster	Found exclusively in patients who have had primary varicella, severe burning pain often precedes the rash. The rash is in a dermatomal distribution, and consists of grouped vesicles on an erythematous base that progress to crusting/scabbed over lesions; when it occurs on the trunk especially before vesicular eruption, the patient might complain of chest pain.
Myositis	Rarely presents as isolated chest pain, can be rheumatologic, viral or drug induced. Common causes of toxic myopathy include: lovastatin, ethanol, steroids, TCA, colchicines, chloroquine. Laboratory data will reveal an increased CK and ESR.
Somatization	Refers to a tendency to transform psychologic distress (such as from depression) into physical symptoms in the absence of organic pathology. Patients seek medical attention because they are convinced that their symptoms reflect real physical disease. They will have seen a myriad of physicians and multiple ED evaluations. It may be helpful in getting the patient to accept referral to a psychiatrist if you have a normal EKG and chest radiograph. Many of these patients can be managed symptomatically. They do not want to be told they are all right, but rather relish being told that they have problems that cannot be solved easily. Usually after telling them exactly that, they will tell you what they need to get through the day, and to go back to a primary physician.

CK, creatine kinase; EKG, electrocardiogram; ED, emergency department; ESR, erythrocyte sedimentation rate; TCA, tricyclic antidepressants.

psychogenic etiologies. Overall, the incidence of chest pain attributable to a cardiac etiology is less than 5%.

- ***Elderly.*** Fewer than half of patients over 85 years arriving at the ED with an MI will complain of chest pain. They more commonly have vague complaints such as feeling weak or tired; misdiagnosis is very common in this group of patients. Elderly patients often have co-morbid diseases, and decreased functional reserve.
- ***Women.*** Women with AICS are more likely than men to experience atypical symptoms, such as pain at rest, during sleep, or with mental stress. The risk of pulmonary embolism is increased by pregnancy or use of birth control pills.

Table 22–6 Valvular Heart Disease

	Risk Factors	Clinical Presentation	Comment
Aortic stenosis (AS)	Congenital bicuspid valve (if <65 years old) Calcific aortic stenosis (if >65 years old) RHD	Dyspnea on exertion Exertional syncope Angina Heart failure Murmur: low-pitched, rasping systolic crescendo-decrescendo murmur heard best at the base and radiating into the carotids	Medications that decrease preload or afterload should be administered with caution. Symptomatic patients may require surgery.
Aortic regurgitation (AR)	Endocarditis, aortic dissection, trauma, RHD, congenital, Marfan's	Acute: Dyspnea, orthopnea, PND Chest pain Wide pulse pressures Water-hammer pulse Murmur: soft diastolic and a midsystolic flow murmur	If suspecting acute aortic regurgitation, obtain an emergent cardiothoracic surgery consultation for valve replacement.
Tricuspid regurgitation (TR)	Right ventricular dilatation secondary to left heart failure, primary pulmonary hypertension. Endocarditis Trauma	Fatigue Dyspnea on exertion Peripheral edema Pulsatile liver Anorexia Atrial fibrillation Murmur: high-pitched, pansystolic	Rate control for atrial fibrillation and long term anti-coagulation.
Mitral stenosis (MS)	Rheumatic heart disease in >90% of cases Congenital lesions Left atrial myxoma	Exertional dyspnea Hemoptysis Palpitations (afib) PACs Fatigue Systemic emboli Murmur: low-pitched, rumbling diastolic murmur heard best at the apex	Hemoptysis can be massive. Patient may need rate control and long-term anti-coagulation for afib.

Table 22–6   Valvular Heart Disease—*cont'd*

	Risk Factors	Clinical Presentation	Comment
Mitral regurgitation (MR)	AMI Endocarditis Trauma Rheumatic heart disease Mitral valve prolapse Connective tissue disorder	Acute: Heart failure Chest pain (AMI) Fever (endocarditis) Exertional dyspnea Fatigue Murmur: high-pitched, holosystolic, and heard best at the apex, radiating to the axilla	Atrial fibrillation is very common Afterload reduction using an intra-aortic balloon pump acutely.
Mitral valve prolapse (MVP)	5%-10% of population affected Female to male ratio 3:1 Inherited in an autosomal dominant fashion	Asymptomatic (most) Chest pain Palpitations Fatigue, Dyspnea Murmur: midsystolic click followed by a late systolic crescendo murmur	Avoiding alcohol, tobacco, and caffeine may also relieve symptoms. Patients with chest pain, palpitations, or anxiety frequently respond to beta-blockers.

AMI, acute myocardial infarction; CHF, congestive heart failure; PACs, premature atrial contractions; PND, paroxysmal nocturnal dyspnea; afib, atrial fibrillation; RHD, rheumatic heart disease

■ ***Immunocompromised.*** Immunocompromised patients with chest pain are at increased risk of infections as the cause of chest pain. Many immunosuppressive agents cause hypertension and glucose intolerance, and thus contribute to atherosclerosis.

Teaching Points

The ED complaint of chest pain has a large differential diagnosis.

Most patients who present to the ED with chest pain will not have AICS.

The patient with AMI is often easily recognized from history of classic chest pain, an EKG diagnostic of ischemia, and elevated cardiac markers. The key is to provide a rapid assessment; quickly consider the need for thrombolytics, or PCI, and administer oxygen, aspirin, nitroglycerin, beta-blockers, heparin, and morphine as needed. Students should not see these patients alone, and should ensure that the senior emergency medicine resident and attending physicians are aware of these patients' presence in the ED.

The patient with chest pain with known or suspected coronary artery disease, but who is not having an AMI is a greater problem. Try to identify the patient who has unstable or new-onset angina. Unstable angina is a clinical diagnosis for which you must arrange admission, and administer oxygen, aspirin, heparin, and perhaps antiplatelet therapy according to institutional protocols.

Diseases that are easy to confuse with AICS such as aortic dissection and pulmonary embolism are much less common, but do occur and must be looked for. If their presence is possible, then one must obtain the studies that will give a definite answer. If the clinical presentation is equally suggestive of both PE and AICS, then a simultaneous evaluation for both diseases is appropriate.

Suggested Readings

American College of Emergency Physicians Clinical Policies Committee. Clinical policy: critical issues in the evaluation and management of adults presenting with suspected pulmonary embolism. Ann Emerg Med 2003;41:257–270.

American College of Emergency Physicians Clinical Policies Committee. Clinical policy: critical issues in the evaluation and management of adult patients presenting with suspected acute myocardial infarction or unstable angina. Ann fEmerg Med 2000;35:521–525.

Brady WJ, Ferguson JD, Ullman EA, Perron AD. Myocarditis: emergency department recognition and management. Emerg Med Clin North Am 2004;22:865–885.

Brown JE, Hamilton GC. Chest pain. In: Marx JA, Hockberger RS, Walls RM (editors). Rosen's Emergency Medicine: Concepts and Clinical Practice (6th edition). Philadelphia: Mosby, 2006:183–192.

Lange RA. Hillis LD. Clinical practice: acute pericarditis. N Eng J Med 2004;351:2195–2202, 2004 Nov 18.

Pollack CV Jr. 2004 ACC/AHA guidelines for the management of patients with ST-elevation myocardial infarction implications for emergency department practice. Ann Emerg Med 2005;45:355–363.

Putukian M. Pneumothorax and pneumomediastinum. Clin Sports Med 2004;23:443–454.

Rogers RL. Aortic disasters. Emerg Med Clin North Am 2004;22:887–908.

CHAPTER 23

Constipation

LEIGH P. ANDERSON ■ MARTIN DE KORT ■ JOHN SARKO

Red Flags

Neurologic deficits ● Significant abdominal pain ● Peritoneal signs (rebound or guarding) ● Abnormal vital signs (fever, hypotension, tachycardia) ● Inability to pass flatus ● Weight loss ● Rectal bleeding ● Changes in stool caliber ● Changes in bowel habits ● Absent bowel sounds ● Vomiting ● Abdominal, pelvic, or rectal masses ● Hernias

Overview

The definition of *constipation* is a difficulty in having a bowel movement. *Obstipation* is the absence of bowel movement. However, patients complain of constipation when they have many different problems such as a painful bowel movement, difficulty in initiating a bowel movement, change in character of the stool, or when they actually have obstipation.

Most patients presenting to the ED with constipation are elderly. Look for "red flags" (see Box) when evaluating these patients. No patient should be treated symptomatically without first searching for a cause. Constipation may be a symptom of serious disease. The few acute, harmful causes of constipation must be separated and sought out from an extensive list of less harmful causes (see DDx table). Most adverse outcomes are due to missed bowel perforation or obstruction.

Most causes will not be determined. The majority of these patients will be referred to their primary care physician for further workup.

Functional constipation is diagnosed by the presence of symptoms of constipation in the absence of known causes affecting the colon or anorectum. Two subtypes of functional constipation include slow-transit constipation and disorders of rectal evacuation. In patients with normal-transit constipation, constipation is likely to be caused by perceived difficulty with evacuation or the presence of hard stools. Slow-transit constipation is characterized by prolonged delay in the transit of stool through the colon allowing increased time for absorption of fluids, which produce harder and larger stools that are more difficult to pass. Disorders of rectal evacuation are characterized by either difficulty or inability to expel stool from the anorectum. Dyssynergic or obstructive defecation is a common example. These patients may also have prolonged colonic transit. Another category may exist, and comprises patients with irritable bowel syndrome who can have either slow (constipation-prone) or accelerated (diarrhea-prone) transit times (Chapter 27).

DDx Differential Diagnoses of Constipation

System	Disorder
Neurologic	Cauda equina syndrome (21) Multiple sclerosis (60) Parkinsonism Spinal cord injury (12)
Gastrointestinal	Diverticular disease (18) Fecal impaction Gastrointestinal tract neoplasm Hirschsprung's disease (77) Intestinal obstruction (18) Intestinal adhesions Intussusception (77) Inflammatory bowel disease (27) Irritable bowel syndrome (27) Painful anal conditions: hemorrhoids, fissure, stricture (48)
Endocrine/metabolic	Diabetes (38, 63) Hypothyroid (63) Hypoadrenalism (63) Hypopituitarism (63) Metabolic electrolyte abnormalities (88)
Renal	Uremia and chronic renal failure (49)
Obstetric and gynecologic	Malignancy (68) Pregnancy (68)
Rheumatologic	Collagen vascular disorders (71)
Hematologic	Porphyria
Toxicologic	Heavy metal poisoning (72)
Psychiatric	Anorexia nervosa Depression
Other	Change from daily routine Medications Old age Poor dietary habits

Differential Diagnoses of Constipation

⚬⚬⚬ See DDx table for differential diagnosis of constipation and Table 23–1 for
⚬⚬⚬ medications causing constipation.

Initial Diagnostic Approach
General

■ The younger the patient, the fewer and less concerning co-morbid conditions, the better the historian, and the better the patient appears on

Table 23–1 Medications that Commonly Cause Constipation	
Class	**Medication**
Anticholinergics	Tricyclic antidepressants Phenothiazines Antiparkinson drugs Antispasmodics Antihistamines Dicyclomine Phenylzine Oxybutynin Tolterodine tartrate
Antihypertensives	Calcium channel blockers Clonidine Diuretics
Antacids	Aluminum and calcium-containing antacids Bismuth
Analgesics	Opioids Nonsteroidal anti-inflammatory drugs
Sympathomimetics	Ganglionic blockers Serotonin antagonists Ondansetron Sumatriptan Selective serotonin reuptake inhibitor Vinca alkaloids Ephedrine Phenylephedrine Phenylpropanolamine
Miscellaneous	Laxative abuse Iron Barium sulfate Phenytoin Phenylzine Valproic acid Sucralfate

physical examination, the fewer laboratory and imaging studies (if any) may be indicated.

- Immunocompromised, elderly, and young pediatric patients require a more liberal diagnostic workup.
- The history and physical examination are the most important components in the assessment of constipation. Be specific in questioning to determine exactly what the individual patient means by constipation. Abdominal pain is not usually associated with constipation. If a patient has abdominal pain, a complete abdominal pain workup (see Chapter 18) is needed. The physician cannot assume that the constipation is the cause of the abdominal pain. A digital rectal examination and inspection of the perineum are mandatory.

Laboratory

- Testing is only needed if a specific abnormality is suspected (e.g., hypokalemia, hypercalcemia, dehydration, hypothyroidism).
- Laxative abuse may result in hypomagnesemia and hypokalemia.

Radiography

- *Plain films.* Plain films are very accurate in detecting the amount of stool in the colon. Stool, especially in a speckled pattern, is easily seen. When this pattern is seen outside the bowel, it represents perforation and abscess formation. Upright and supine abdominal films can also detect obstruction and volvulus (Chapter 18). Plain films are not needed in most cases of constipation.
- *Computed tomography (CT scan).* Abdominal and pelvic CT scans show the presence of stool in the colon, extent of dilatation of the colon (megacolon), masses, obstruction, and volvulus. It can also reveal diverticulitis (Chapter 18). A CT scan can also evaluate vertebral lesions when spinal cord compression is suspected. A CT scan is not needed in most cases of constipation.
- Other diagnostic tests include barium or gastrograffin enema, sigmoidoscopy, colonic transit time, anorectal or colonic, manometry, or defecography. These studies are typically not performed in the ED. In the patient with a sigmoid volvulus, the sigmoidoscopy may not only be diagnostic (revealing the status of the viability of the bowel muscosa), but therapeutic since it may help the volvulus detorse.

Emergency Department Management Overview
General

- The ABCs (*a*irway, *b*reathing, and *c*irculation) should be addressed as discussed in Section II. Two large-bore intravenous (IV) lines should be placed and isotonic fluids should be administered if the patient is hemodynamically unstable or may have potentially life-threatening conditions.
- Prompt ED evaluation and early surgical consultation should be obtained for patients who may have surgical disease.

Medications and Diet Modification

- Adequate hydration is the key to treating and preventing constipation. Dehydration reduces the amount of water in stool, and can worsen constipation if laxatives are used.
- Fiber in the diet is vital as well. This increases the stool bulk. To increase dietary fiber intake, patients should be instructed to increase daily consumption of raw fruits, raw vegetables, and whole grain products such as bran and grain. Prunes do have a laxative effect, and when added to the diet may overcome constipation without requiring pharmacologic laxatives.
- If possible, stop offending drugs such as opiates (Table 23–1).
- Medications used in the treatment of constipation are listed in Table 23–2. Tailor the bowel program to the patient's needs. For instance, lubricants are helpful for patients with painful perianal lesions or hard stools. Osmotic agents (with nonabsorbable sugars) are useful for patients with chronic constipation or decreased gut motility. Irritants, for short-term use only, are useful for patients with decreased gut motility, especially secondary to medication use. Laxatives can take 6 hours or longer to cause a bowel movement. It is usually not necessary to produce a bowel movement in the ED.
- Methylnaltrexone, an opioid antagonist, has been shown to reverse opioid-induced constipation within 1 minute of the first infusion. This drug is able to retain its pain-relieving qualities without constipating effects due to its inability to cross the blood-brain barrier.

Emergency Department Interventions

- *Nasogastric (NG) tube.* Place this to low wall continuous suction for intestinal obstruction.
- *Fecal disimpaction.* Manual evacuation of the rectal vault is an uncomfortable procedure, but is necessary when a fecal impaction is present. Some patients may benefit from mineral oil enemas to soften hard-stool impactions, which will ease rectal evacuation with manual disimpaction. However, disimpaction may be necessary before the enema can be effective.
- *Enema.* Typically this works quickly, but tends to be messy, and is difficult and unpleasant for an already busy nursing staff. An enema may be most helpful when evaluating constipation associated with abdominal pain and no other cause is easily found. Its advantages include the rapidity of results, and because it is given rectally, patients can remain on nothing by mouth (NPO) status. It is dangerous however if the patient has an obstruction or perforation. In the former, it will not relieve the obstruction, and often leads to a false conclusion that the patient's problems have been relieved. It also increases the risk of perforation. If perforation has already occurred, it increases the risk for peritonitis.
- *Education.* In most cases, the only interventions necessary in the ED are reassurance and education of the patient concerning proper bowel care. Patients should be encouraged to modify their diet, exercise, and attempt bowel movements at the same time every day, usually 30 minutes after meals, straining for no more than 5 minutes at a time.

Table 23–2   Treatment of Constipation

Type of Treatment	Generic Name	Dose	Precautions
Stool softeners	Docusate calcium Docusate potassium Docusate sodium	Max 500 mg/d Max 500 mg/d Max 500 mg/d	Hepatotoxic and potentiate hepatotoxic effects of other drugs.
Bulk agents	Psyllium Methylcellulose Fiber	Max 30 g/d Max 6 g/d Ideal dose 30 g/d	Without adequate fluid intake, these can cause impaction and worsen constipation
Lubricants	Mineral oil	Max 45 ml/d	Lipid pneumonitis from aspiration. Do not use in patients with swallowing disorders
Irritants	Phenolphthalein Senna extract Bisacodyl Castor oil Danthron	Max 275 mg/d two tablets or 2 tsp per day Max 15 mg/d Max 60 ml/d Max 150 mg/d	"Cathartic" colon with chronic use, best documented with Senna.
Enemas	Tap water or saline Sodium salts Mineral oil Phosphate Sulfate	Max 200 ml/d PR Max 120 ml/d PR Max 120 ml/d PR	Use sodium salt enemas cautiously in patients with CHF. Do not use phosphate enemas with renal failure.

Osmotic agents	Magnesium:
	Hydroxide
	  Citrate
	  Sulfate
	Lactulose
	Polyethylene-glycol-saline
		
		Max 30 ml/d
		Max 200 ml/d
		Max 300 ml/d
		Max 30 ml bid
		Max 6 l/d
			Magnesium can cause diffuse cramping. Sorbitol and nonabsorbable sugars can cause abdominal bloating.

Suppositories	Bisacodyl Glycerine	Max 10 mg/d PR 3 g/d PR	Discontinue use if rectal irritation develops

CHF, congestive heart failure; Max, maximum; PR, per rectum.

Disposition

- ■ *Consultation.* Surgical consultation is prudent when a surgical etiology is found, or is being investigated. The patient's primary care physician can usually evaluate simple, uncomplicated cases of constipation. A consultation with a gastroenterologist is useful for serious gastrointestinal (GI) tract pathology.
- ■ *Admission.* Admission for constipation per se is unlikely to be required. Admit for the underlying disease given its specific indications such as a need for surgery.
- ■ *Discharge.* Most patients with constipation can be discharged after the ED evaluation is completed, and patients have been educated regarding its treatment and prevention.

Specific Problems

There are several etiologies for constipation. A few of the more common problems will be briefly discussed here.

Fecal Impaction

- ■ *Epidemiology and risk factors.* This entity is characterized by inability to defecate due to a large compacted mass of stool. It is most frequentiy encountered in patients who are elderly, bedridden, and are suffering from chronic disease.
- ■ *Pathophysiology.* Patients with chronic constipation have slow gut-transit times, allowing increased time for absorption of fluids, which produce harder and larger stools that are more difficult to pass.
- ■ *History.* The problem is heralded by a feeling of urgency to defecate, rectal distention, or tenesmus. This may be associated with an elevated temperature (but if present, other sources for fever should be investigated). Occasionally, the impaction results in obstruction and dilatation with increased fluid content proximal to the impaction. This can result in a *paradoxical diarrhea* as the fluid moves past the obstructing fecal mass.
- ■ *Physical examination.* Abdominal palpation may reveal a hard mass in the lower abdomen. A dilated rectum filled with a large amount of stool is noted upon rectal examination.
- ■ *Diagnostic testing.* An abdominal radiograph may reveal excessive stool in the colon, often with solid stool visualized all the way proximal to the cecum. Seek an alternative diagnosis if there is little stool seen on the study.
- ■ *ED management.* Due to the potentially life-threatening nature of fecal impaction, it is important to manually disimpact the bowel in the ED as already described. Sedation may be useful because of the painful nature of the procedure. Once the colon has been cleared, laxatives and suppositories should be administered to prevent future stool impaction. Fecal impaction is often relieved by the colonic lavage solution polyethylene glycol.
- ■ *Helpful hints and pitfalls.* Fecal incontinence may be caused by a fecal impaction, but this should not be the conclusion before more dangerous causes, such as cauda equina, are assessed (see Chapter 21).

Intestinal Pseudo-Obstruction

- *Epidemiology and risk factors.* Intestinal pseudo-obstruction is rare, and has multiple etiologies.
- *Pathophysiology.* This disease is characterized by intestinal immotility most commonly due to visceral myopathies or neuropathies. Patients arrive for care with signs and symptoms of bowel obstruction in the absence of any lesions occluding the gut lumen.
- *History.* These patients often have complaints of obstipation, colicky abdominal pain, nausea, and vomiting.
- *Physical examination.* Signs and symptoms associated with intestinal obstruction are present.
- *Diagnostic testing.* Abdominal radiographs should be obtained to rule out an obstructive lesion and to look specifically for a dilated colon.
- *ED management.* If this is determined to be the cause of constipation, a treatment plan should be made in consort with a surgeon, with the consideration for operative or colonoscopic decompression of a severely dilated intestine.
- *Helpful hints and pitfalls.* An abdominal CT scan is often required to evaluate for other causes of obstruction. This is not a diagnosis typically made in the ED.

Obstructive Defecation (Dyssynergic)

- *Epidemiology and risk factors.* This entity has been considered the most common cause of constipation in adults. This functional defect is also known as *pelvic floor dysfunction, anismus, outlet obstruction,* and *dyschezia.* Large, hard stools or painful perianal lesions can lead to avoidance of defecation, and thus functional fecal retention. Structural abnormalities are also causes of this defecatory disorder.
- *Pathophysiology.* This is characterized by the inability to adequately evacuate rectal contents, causing storage of fecal residue for prolonged periods in the rectum. This is believed to be due to paradoxical anal sphincter and pelvic floor contraction with a defect in coordinating expulsion of stool.
- *History.* The patient often has a sensation of incomplete defecation with significant straining. Patients often complain of the need for digital evacuation or application of perineal or vaginal pressure to allow stools to pass.
- *Physical examination.* Patients with obstructive defecation often present with rectoceles found during the rectal examination. During the rectal examination, the patient should be instructed to bear down so the puborectalis and external anal sphincter tone can be assessed.
- *Diagnostic testing.* This will rarely be necessary in this condition.
- *ED management.* These patients often have little relief with diet or laxatives, and should be referred to their primary care physician for specific treatment such as neuromuscular conditioning using biofeedback techniques.
- *Helpful hints and pitfalls.* Most likely, a history of chronic laxative abuse will also be present but may not be volunteered by the patient.

Special Considerations
Pediatrics

■ A healthy child may have a soft stool only every second or third day without difficulty. However, a hard stool passed with difficulty every third day should be treated as constipation.

■ Constipation may arise from defects in filling or in emptying the rectum. Watery content from the proximal colon may leak around hard retained stool and pass per rectum unperceived by the child. This involuntary encopresis (passage of feces into inappropriate places after a chronologic age of 4 years) may be mistaken for diarrhea. A nursing infant may have very infrequent stools of normal consistency; this is usually a normal pattern.

■ Concerning causes in this population include Hirschsprung's disease, meconium ileus, congenital atresia in infants, intussusception, and intestinal obstruction (Chapter 77). Hypothyroidism can also cause constipation.

Elderly

■ The elderly are at higher risk for constipation for several reasons. They are frequently on multiple medications, have a decreased thirst mechanism that tends to produce dehydration, are on low-fiber diets, have diseases that impair gastrointestinal motility, and have sedentary life styles.

Pregnancy

■ Constipation is physiologic during pregnancy with decreased bowel transit time, and the stool may be hardened. Iron supplementation may aggravate constipation, and patients may require stool softeners. Patients should increase water intake and increase bulk in their diet (fruit and vegetables, bran). Additional dietary fibers such as Metamucil (psyllium hydrophilic muciloid) or surface-active agents such as Colace (docusate sodium) are recommended. Laxatives are rarely necessary.

■ Hemorrhoids are common in late pregnancy, especially in a multiparous patient. When prolapsed, these hemorrhoids are often painful. Although stool softeners may help, the problem may not be resolved until after delivery.

Teaching Points

Constipation is a difficult bowel movement, whereas obstipation is an absence of bowel movement. Although a common complaint, it may be a symptom of an underlying much more serious disease.

In the absence of such underlying disease, the patient will often be elderly, will have a poor diet, and will have poor mobility.

Fecal impaction results from large bulky hard stools, which are painful to pass. The best treatment for this is manual disimpaction, with subsequent manipulation of the patient's diet and fluid consumption.

Suggested Readings

Cullen N. Constipation. In: Marx JA, Hockberger RS, Walls RM (editors). Rosen's Emergency Medicine: Concepts and Clinical Practice (6th ed). Philadelphia: Mosby, 2006. pp 237–242.

Rao SSC. Constipation: evaluation and treatment. Gastroenterol Clin North Am 2003;32:659–683.

Thompson WG, Lonstreth GF, Drossman DA, et al. Functional bowel disorders and functional abdominal pain. Gut 1999;45(Suppl II):1143–1147.

Wald A. Constipation, diarrhea, and symptomatic hemorrhoids during pregnancy. Gastroenterol Clin North Am 2003;32:309–322.

Wald A. Diagnosis of constipation in primary and secondary care. Rev Gastroenterol Dis 2004;4(Suppl 2): S28–S33.

CHAPTER **24**

Cough

CAMIE J. SORENSEN ■ MICHAEL J. NELSON ■ SEAN P. KELLY

 Red Flags

Extremes of age • Acute respiratory distress • Abnormal vital signs (heart rate >100 beats per minute, respiratory rate >24 breaths per minute, temperature >100.4° F [38° C]) • Hypoxia • Hemoptysis • Immuno-compromised state • Co-morbid conditions, especially cardiac or pulmonary. • Smoker

Overview

Cough is a common condition for which patients seek medical attention.

Cough can be categorized as acute or chronic. Acute cough is a cough that has lasted fewer than 3 weeks. Chronic cough is a continuous cough that has been present longer than 3 weeks without any period of resolution. Cough is sometimes categorized as productive versus nonproductive of sputum, but the clinical significance of this distinction is minimal.

Although most patients who have a cough have generally benign problems, a cough may be a manifestation of serious disease. Look for "red flags" when evaluating these patients. The most common causes of an acute cough include viral or bacterial upper respiratory tract infections (e.g., common cold, acute bacterial sinusitis, and pertussis), asthma, chronic obstructive pulmonary disease exacerbation, allergic rhinitis, and environmental irritants (e.g., smoke). However, an acute cough may be the presenting manifestation of potentially life-threatening illness, such as congestive heart failure, pulmonary embolism (see Chapter 52), pneumonia (see Chapter 67), and conditions that predispose to aspiration (i.e., stroke). Seventy-five percent of chronic coughs in adults with negative chest radiograph findings are caused by one of three conditions: postnasal drip, asthma (see Chapter 52), or gastroesophageal reflux (see Chapter 18).

Hemoptysis is the coughing up of blood from the respiratory tract. Massive hemoptysis accounts for only 1.5% of all cases of hemoptysis, and is defined as 600 ml per 24-hour period. Impaired oxygen transfer occurs when approximately 400 ml of blood is in the alveolar space. Hemoptysis must be differentiated from pseudohemoptysis (when blood in the sputum originates in the nasopharynx or oropharynx), and hematemesis (the vomiting of blood). Worldwide, tuberculosis is the most common cause of hemoptysis. The most common causes of blood in the sputum in industrialized countries are bronchitis, bronchiectasis, and bronchogenic carcinoma. Acute and chronic bronchitis are estimated to account for up to 50% of cases.

The patient with tuberculosis (Chapter 67) may not always have the classic presentation of a chronic cough associated with night sweats, fever, hemoptysis, or weight loss. The patient may not be from an endemic area or have human immunodeficiency virus (HIV). One must think of tuberculosis in order to find it. While the patient is being worked up for this diaginosis, it is prudent to protect hospital workers and other patients by placing a face mask on anyone actively coughing. When admitted, the patient requires respiratory isolation until the diagnosis is ruled out.

Bronchiectasis is a cause of chronic cough in a relatively small number of patients; the diagnosis is established by clinical history, chest radiograph, high-resolution computed tomography (CT scan) of the thorax, and cough disappearance with specific therapy. Cough associated with flares of the disease can be treated with a combination of chest physiotherapy, drugs to stimulate mucociliary clearance, and systemic antibiotics. Inhaled antibiotics are recommended only in patients with cystic fibrosis (CF) with bronchiectasis.

This chapter will address common causes of cough in patients without underlying co-morbidities.

Differential Diagnosis of Cough and Hemoptysis

See DDx table.

DDx Differential Diagnosis of Acute and Chronic Cough

Acute Cough (Symptoms less than 3 Weeks) Acute and Emergent Etiologies	Chronic Cough (Symptoms longer than 3 Weeks) Nonemergent Etiologies
Aspiration, foreign body (5, 76)	Postnasal drip*
Asthma, acute (52)	Gastroesophageal reflux disease*
Congestive heart failure, acute (52)	Asthma, mild* (52)
Pneumonia (67)	Pertussis (cough may be
Acute bronchitis	prolonged)
URI (upper respiratory tract infection)	Medication induced
Pertussis (in early stages)	(Angiotensin-converting enzyme
Pulmonary embolism (52)	inhibitors; angiotensin receptor
Sinusitis (35)	blockers)
	Smoking
	Environmental irritants
	Tuberculosis (67)
	Carcinoma
	Sarcoidosis
	Cystic fibrosis (pediatrics)
	Psychogenic cough
	(diagnosis of exclusion)

These three diagnoses comprise 75% of adults who present with chronic cough and negative chest radiography.
( ) Refers to the chapter in which the disease entity is discussed.

Initial Diagnostic Approach
General

■ The ABCs (*a*irway, *b*reathing, and *c*irculation) must be addressed initially as discussed in Section II. All patients with cough should have documented oxygen saturation. Intravenous (IV) access and continuous cardiac monitoring should be done on patients who appear ill, are in respiratory distress, or are hemodynamically unstable.

Laboratory

■ Laboratory testing is not essential in evaluating most patients with a cough if they have normal vital signs and otherwise appear healthy. Patients with hemoptysis or concerning infection should have a complete blood count (CBC). A coagulation panel should be ordered if a coagulopathy is suspected. Blood should be sent for type and cross match if massive hemoptysis is present. If an infectious etiology to the hemoptysis is suspected, sending a sputum sample for Gram's and acid-fast stains should be done. Arterial blood gases should be sent to assess oxygenation, ventilation, and circulatory adequacy in patients with signs of hemodynamic instability and respiratory impairment. Serum chemistries should be sent for evaluation of baseline values for sicker patients.

DDx Differential Diagnosis of Hemoptysis

Cardiovascular	Left ventricular failure Mitral stenosis Erosion of aortic aneurysm Atrioventricular fistula
Pulmonary	Bronchitis Bronchiectasis Pneumonia Pulmonary embolism Tuberculosis Fungal infection (aspergillosis, coccidioidomycosis) Goodpasture's syndrome Parasite infection (amebiasis, ascariasis) Vasculitis (Wegener's granulomatosis, Churg-Strauss syndrome, Henoch-Schönlein purpura) Cystic fibrosis Pulmonary hypertension Pulmonary hemosiderosis Pulmonary endometriosis Trauma Iatrogenic
Bioterrorism related	Pneumonic plague Tularemia T2 mycotoxin
Other	Drugs: aspirin, anticoagulants, penicillamine. Laryngeal bleeding (laryngitis, laryngeal neoplasm). Trauma Epistaxis Coagulopathy

EKG

- An electrocardiogram (EKG) is not essential in evaluating patients with cough if they have normal vital signs and otherwise appear health but is useful if the cough may have a cardiac origin.

Radiography

- *Plain films.* A chest radiograph should be used to detect pneumonia, foreign body, congestive heart failure, lung masses, granulomatous disease, pneumothorax, or other abnormalities.
- *CT scan.* A CT scan is usually unecessary in the evaluation of most patients with a cough. One condition that requires a CT scan for diagnosis is a pulmonary embolism. For patients presenting with hemoptysis, a CT scan can detect masses, alveolar consolidation, bronchiectasis, and abnormally enhancing vessels.
- *Ventilation-perfusion (VQ) scans.* This test is useful in detecting a pulmonary embolus (PE) or infarction, particularly in the presence of a normal chest radiograph.

■ *Other.* Bronchoscopy is indicated to evaluate and treat patients who present with cough secondary to foreign body aspiration, selected cases of hemoptysis, and to obtain bronchial washings to evaluate for an infectious source or malignancy. For patients with massive hemoptysis, pulmonary angiography or surgery may be required.

Emergency Department Management Overview
General

■ The ABCs should be addressed. Any patient in respiratory distress should be placed in a resuscitation room and immediately be given supplemental oxygen. Fluid boluses of normal saline or lactated Ringer's solution are given to optimize hydration, especially if the patient is hypotensive, via two large-bore peripheral IV catheters.

Medications

■ *Antitussives.* Antitussive therapy is indicated when the cough serves no useful function such as clearing the airways. Specific antitussive therapy should be directed at the etiology or mechanism causing the cough (e.g., cigarette smoking, postnasal drip, asthma). Nonspecific antitussive therapy is directed at the symptom rather than the etiology or mechanism. It is indicated when specific therapy has not had a chance to work or will not work (e.g., inoperable lung cancer). Examples include guaifenesin (100-400 mg by mouth [PO] every 4 hours), dextromethorphan (10-20 mg PO every 4 hours or 60 mg every 12 hours of sustained-action liquid preparation), benzonatate (100-200 mg PO three times daily, swallowed whole), or opiate medication such as codeine.
■ *Analgesia.* Acetaminophen or nonsteroidal anti-inflammatory drugs (NSAIDs) should be provided to patients with elevated temperature. Liquid or rectal forms of medication should be provided if the patient has a sore throat and odynophagia.
■ *Antacids.* This therapy is indicated in patients with known gastro-esophageal reflux disease (GERD) that might be causing a chronic cough. The patient's primary care physician can manage ongoing treatment of GERD (see Chapter 90.4).
■ *Bronchodilators.* These agents are indicated for patients with a history of asthma, COPD, low PFT results, or wheezing on examination. They are also useful in the treament of acute bronchitis. Albuterol or other β-agonist may be given via inhalers (with or without spacer) or nebulizer treatment (see Chapter 90.6).
■ *Antibiotics.* These drugs are used when the patient is confirmed or suspected to have a treatable infectious etiology of cough.

Disposition

■ *Consultation.* A pulmonologist should be consulted in any patient with suspected foreign body aspiration or massive hemoptysis requiring bronchoscopy. Radiologic and surgical consultation should also be obtained for patients with massive hemoptysis. An oncologist should be consulted by the admitting team or primary care provider in patients with a newly diagnosed lung mass.

- *Admission.* Any patient with abnormal vital signs that do not correct with ED treatment should be admitted. Any patient requiring supplemental oxygen should be admitted (unless it is baseline). Patients requiring respiratory isolation (e.g., tuberculosis) require admission. Patients with significant co-morbidities, extremes of age, or those with poor social support may need to be admitted as well.
- *Discharge.* Patients who are otherwise healthy and have normal vital signs may be discharged home. Arrange for primary care follow-up.

Specific Problems
Acute Bronchitis and Upper Respiratory Infection

- *Definition.* An upper respiratory infection (URI) is also known as the *common cold*, but may include a localized infection such as sinusitis (Chapter 35). Acute bronchitis often occurs with a URI, but a patient may have a URI without developing acute bronchitis. Acute bronchitis is inflammation of the bronchi. It usually presents as a cough with or without sputum production, and is frequently accompanied by symptoms of upper respiratory tract infection. Other etiologies for cough must be ruled out before diagnosing acute bronchitis.
- *Epidemiology and risk factors.* Elderly patients, infants, and immuno-compromised individuals are at highest risk. Infection is spread through respiratory droplets.
- *Pathophysiology.* Most cases of acute bronchitis and URI are viral in origin. Viruses most commonly associated with lower respiratory tract infection, and thus acute bronchitis, include respiratory syncytial virus (RSV), parainfluenza, and influenzas A and B. Viruses most commonly causing upper respiratory symptoms include coronavirus, adenovirus, and rhinovirus. Bacterial causes of acute bronchitis are less common (less than 10% in nonoutbreak settings) and include *Bordetella pertussis*, *Mycoplasma pneumoniae*, and *Chlamydia pneumoniae*. The infectious agent inoculates tracheobronchial epithelium, resulting in inflammation (leading to cough and sputum production), and airway and bronchial hyper-reactivity (leading to cough and bronchospasm).
- *History.* Patients with a URI present with symptoms typical of the common cold such as rhinorrhea, generalized malaise, low-grade fever, myalgia, and congestion. Patients with acute bronchitis have a cough lasting fewer than 3 weeks usually accompanied by symptoms of URI. Approximately 75% of patients with cough due to acute bronchitis have resolution of the cough within 14 days. If the cough is persistent (4 or more weeks), consider the diagnosis of pertussis (discussed below). Patients with influenza virus typically present with abrupt onset of high fever, diffuse myalgia, and extreme fatigue. Cough may be an associated symptom of influenza, in some cases accompanied by influenza pneumonia or secondary bacterial pneumonia. Table 24–1 compares symptoms of influenza to the common cold.
- *Physical examination.* Patients may have an elevated temperature. Head, ears, eyes, nose, and throat (HEENT) examination generally reveals

Table 24–1   Symptoms of Influenza vs. the Common Cold

Symptoms	Influenza	Cold
Onset	Sudden	Gradual
Fever	>101° F (38.3°C), lasting 3-4 d	None or <101° F (38.3°C)
Cough	Dry, sometimes severe	Hacking
Headache	Prominent	Rare
Myalgias (muscle pain)	Usual, often severe	Uncommon or mild
Fatigue and weakness	Lasting 2-3 weeks	Very mild and brief
Extreme exhaustion	Early and prominent	Never
Chest discomfort	Common	Uncommon or mild
Stuffy nose	Sometimes	Common
Sneezing	Sometimes	Typical
Sore throat	Sometimes	Common

rhinorrhea, conjunctival irritation, and congestion. The pulmonary examination may reveal wheezing, even in patients without asthma. Otherwise, the examination is unremarkable. Crackles, egophany, or tactile fremitus indicate a more serious diagnosis such as pneumonia or pulmonary effusion.

- *Diagnostic testing.* Obtain a chest radiograph on any patient with cough who has abnormal vital signs or who has crackles on pulmonary examination. Bedside spirometry is helpful in cases with bronchospasm or tachypnea, with or without a known diagnosis of asthma. Oxygen saturation can be monitored to assess for hypoxia. Diagnosis of acute bronchitis or URI is a clinical diagnosis based on patient presentation, history, and physical examination findings. Rapid tests are also available for identifying influenza A or B in clinical specimens. In an otherwise healthy patient with normal vital signs and normal physical examination, no further testing is needed.
- *ED management.* This includes antipyretic drugs to reduce fever, NSAIDs to ameliorate myalgias, antitussive medication, and β-agonist bronchodilators. Often supportive treatment is the only treatment needed. Antibiotics are indicated only if a bacterial source of cough is suspected. If the patient appears to have influenza and presents within 48 hours of symptom onset, treat with a 5-day course of antiviral medication (amantadine or rimantadine for influenza A, and the neuraminidase inhibitors zanamavir or olsetamavir for influenza A or B). These drugs have been shown to reduce symptoms in otherwise healthy patients by approximately 1 day but do not reduce complications of the disease.
- *Helpful hints and pitfalls.* Fewer than 10% of patients presenting with bronchitis have a bacterial cause, yet 70% to 90% of these patients are treated with antibiotics. This is expensive, unnecessary, and harmful

to long term antibiotic utility. Secondary infection with bacterial pneumonia is a complication of respiratory viral infections. Influenza vaccination is the primary method for preventing influenza. Target groups include the elderly, those with underlying chronic medical conditions, children, pregnant, women, health care workers, and institutionalized patients (e.g., nursing home).

Pertussis

■ *Epidemiology and risk factors.* This disease is commonly known as *whooping cough.* Pertussis usually causes bronchitis but may cause pneumonia. It is highly contagious and is spread by airborne droplets with a secondary attack rate of 80% in susceptible persons. Pertussis has potentially severe complications for infants and young children. Immunity is conferred by a series of vaccinations during childhood. Vaccination is often given in combination with diphtheria and typhoid as a whole-cell or acellular version (DTP or DTaP). There has been a marked decline in incidence with vaccine development. The vaccination provides partial immunity for up to 10 years, although the exact duration is unknown. Thus, adolescents and adults are susceptible to contracting pertussis, but do not generally present with the typical symptoms, making it difficult to diagnose. Natural immunity is life-long.

■ *Pathophysiology.* Pertussis is a communicable infection of the respiratory tract caused by the gram-negative bacteria, *Bordetella pertussis.* Milder symptoms of a similar nature can be caused by a related species, *Bordetella parapertussis.*

■ *History.* The catarrhal phase lasts 1 to 2 weeks, with symptoms similar to a URI. The paroxysmal phase lasts 1 to 6 weeks, causes staccato coughing, especially at night, typically with a large inspiratory gasp after coughing, causing a distinctive *whooping* sound. Patients may have associated posttussive emesis. The convalescent phase lasts 2 to 3 weeks, with gradual resolution of cough. Most adolescent and adult patients complain of a prolonged and persistent cough with a median duration of 10 to 12 weeks. In fact, up to 20% of adults with prolonged or persistent cough show serologic evidence of infection with *B. pertussis.* Typical symptoms of pertussis such as paroxysmal cough, inspiratory whoop, or posttussive emesis may be lacking. Presentation is often indistinguishable from viral URI or bronchitis with nonspecific symptoms including rhinorrhea, malaise, low-grade fever, conjunctival irritation, and sneezing.

■ *Physical examination.* Generally unremarkable.

■ *Diagnostic testing.* There may be leukocytosis with marked lymphocytosis. Radiography is not indicated in patients with normal vital signs. The chest radiograph may show mild peribronchial cuffing, atelectasis, perihilar infiltrates, or mild interstitial edema. Bacterial culture isolated from nasopharyngeal secretions is the gold standard for diagnosis; but the organism is difficult to isolate and requires a special medium. Other modalities exist such as polymerase chain reaction, direct fluorescent antibody, or enzyme-linked immunosorbent assay serology. Often dual testing is used to confirm the diagnosis. The clinical diagnosis is defined by the Centers for Disease Control and Prevention (CDC) and World

Health Organization (WHO) as cough illness lasting at least 2 weeks without any other apparent cause (as reported by a health professional) with either a household contact diagnosed with pertussis OR one of the following: paroxysm of cough, inspiratory whoop, or posttussive vomiting.

■ ***ED management.*** If clinically suggested, or if the patient has a household contact with a known diagnosis of pertussis, antibiotic treatment should be initiated. Do not wait for laboratory confirmation of the diagnosis to start treatment. In adults, macrolides are the optimal choice for treatment of pertussis. The treatment course is 14 days of erythromycin. Fluoroquinolones are also effective as is trimethoprim-sulfamethoxazole. Antibiotic treatment eradicates the organisms from secretions, and thus decreases communicability of disease. Clinical duration is affected only if antibiotics are initiated early in the course of illness. Close contacts younger than 7 years old who have not completed the primary vaccination series should complete it with the minimal intervals. In close contacts younger than 7 years old in whom the primary series has been completed, a booster dose of DTP or DTaP should be given if it has been more than 3 years since the last dose.

■ ***Helpful hints and pitfalls.*** Any patient diagnosed with pertussis by clinical or laboratory criteria must be reported to the public health authorities. Prophylaxis is recommended for contacts of patients with pertussis. Treatment for prophylaxis is the same as treatment for disease.

Postnasal Drip

■ ***Epidemiology and risk factors.*** This is the most common cause of chronic cough in nonsmoking, immunocompetent adults with a normal chest radiograph findings.

■ ***Pathophysiology.*** Mucopurulent material drains from the sinuses into the posterior pharynx, and irritates cough receptors.

■ ***History.*** Patients commonly complain of a sensation of postnasal drainage, and a frequent need to clear the throat.

■ ***Physical examination.*** Generally unremarkable. There may be a *cobblestone* appearance of the posterior pharynx.

■ ***Diagnostic testing.*** The diagnosis is made by a therapeutic trial of a combination of decongestants and an antihistamine agent for 2 weeks. If symptoms are typical and resolve with treatment, the diagnosis of postnasal drip can be made. Sinus radiographs are not needed in initial evaluation.

■ ***ED management.*** Outpatient treatment includes decongestants, antihistamines and primary care follow-up.

Special Considerations
Pediatrics

■ Causes of cough more prevalent in the pediatric population include foreign body aspiration, asthma, pertussis, and RSV in infants. Less common but important diagnoses include cystic fibrosis and congenital anatomic abnormalities (such as vascular rings, tracheoesophageal fistula, primary ciliary dyskinesia, and congenital heart disease). For more information, please refer to Chapter 76.

Elderly

- The predominance of community living and high incidence of co-morbidities in the elderly population lead to increased susceptibility to viral or bacterial infections causing cough. Elderly patients with viral infections can readily develop community-acquired pneumonia and other bacterial infections. Many of these patients with co-morbid conditions will require admission, and in the elderly, an aggressive early diagnosis is often life-saving.

The Immunocompromised Patient

- Immunocompromised patients are more susceptible to opportunistic infections. Measure the CD4 count on every HIV patient who presents with cough, and do a more thorough workup in those patients with a CD4 count below 200 (see Chapter 37).

Teaching Points

Cough varies from being a normal protective physiologic method of ridding the respiratory tract from contaminants to being a symptom of serious disease. It can be centrally mediated or pharmacologically induced, as with ACE inhibitor treatment of hypertension. It can be almost uncontrollable, as in the patient with the paroxysm of coughing induced by pertussis, thus the common lay title of "whooping cough." It can sound like the bark of a seal, representing the upper airway constriction of croup. It can represent the ominous onset of pulmonary edema.

Thus it becomes hard to define alone as any one problem disease or physiologic manifestation, and must be interpreted in light of vital signs, age, underlying disease, and historical clues. When the patient looks well, there is ample time to investigate the source, but when the patient looks ill, the cough will have to be ignored while the ABCs are addressed.

Suggested Readings

Center for Disease Control. Health Topic: Pertussis. *www.cdc.gov/nip/publications/pink/pert.rtf.* Accessed February 3, 2004.

Corder R. Hemoptysis. Emerg Med Clin North Am 2003;21:421–435.

Gonzales R, Sande MA. Uncomplicated bronchitis. Ann Int Med 2000:133:981–991.

Holmes RL, Fadden CT. Evaluation of the patient with chronic cough. Am Fam Physician 2004;69(9):2159–2166.

Irwin RS, Madison JM. The diagnosis and treatment of cough. N Engl J Med 2000; 343:1715–1721.

Irwin RS, Boulet LP, Cloutier MM, et al. Managing cough as a defense mechanism and as a symptom: a consensus panel report of the American College of Chest Physicians. Chest 1998;114(2[Suppl]):133S–181S.

Tintinalli JE, Kelen GD, Stapezynski S (editors). Emergency Medicine: A Comprehensive Study Guide (6th ed). New York: McGraw-Hill, 2004, pp 440–442.

Widdicombe J, Kamath S. Acute cough in the elderly: aetiology, diagnosis and therapy. Drugs Aging 2004:21(4):243–258.

CHAPTER 25

Cyanosis

HOLLYNN LARRABEE ■ ANDRA L. BLOMKALNS

 Red Flags

Tachypnea ● Tachycardia ● Oxygen saturation less than 90% ● No improvement with supplemental oxygen ● Central cyanosis ● Altered mental status or coma ● Seizure activity ● Pallor ● History of anemia ● Exposure to chemical agent or new drug ● Acute unilateral cyanosis with pain

Overview

Look for "red flags" (see Box), and consider life-threatening problems early, as cyanosis is more often a sign of impending doom than a harmless process.

Cyanosis refers to a bluish or purplish discoloration of the skin or mucous membranes. Clinically, cyanosis suggests tissue hypoxia. It is detectable when >5g/dl of deoxygenated blood is present.

Cyanosis is divided into central or peripheral forms. Central cyanosis can be seen in lips, ears, tongue, and nail beds. Peripheral cyanosis is limited to the extremities. Significant interobserver variation occurs in the detection of cyanosis. Many factors such as skin tone and thickness and room lighting can affect the ability to discern cyanosis.

Peripheral cyanosis is usually secondary to an increased oxygen extraction in the peripheral capillary beds due to slow blood flow. The most concerning cause for unilateral cyanosis to an extremity is acute arterial occlusion.

Except for the relatively uncommon causes of methemoglobinemia, sulfhemoglobinemia, and some hemoglobinopathies, central cyanosis is always accompanied by a low arterial Po_2. As a result of hypoxemia, an excess amount of hemoglobin is not saturated with oxygen. It is the quantity of unsaturated hemoglobin, not the relative lack of oxygenated hemoglobin that accounts for the bluish color of cyanosis. The greater the hemoglobin content the more readily cyanosis will appear as the oxygen saturation falls. Conversely, the lower the hemoglobin content (i.e., anemia), the more oxygen saturation has to fall before cyanosis becomes manifest.

Any patient presenting with cyanosis and completely normal oxygen saturations should raise suspicion for abnormal hemoglobins, particularly methemoglobin.

Pediatric cyanosis is most commonly due to congenital cardiac anomalies (see Chapter 75).

Differential Diagnosis of Cyanosis

See DDx table regarding the differential diagnosis of cyanosis.

DDx Central Versus Peripheral Cyanosis		
	Central	**Peripheral**
Definition	Generalized cyanosis, visible in lips, nail beds, ears.	Local cyanosis. Usually only seen in the extremities.
Cause	Unsaturated arterial blood Abnormal hemoglobin	Slowing of blood flow to area Increased extraction of oxygen from normally saturated arterial blood
Differential	**Pulmonary causes** Pneumonia (67) Asthma (52) Chronic obstructive pulmonary disease (52) Pulmonary edema (52) Pulmonary embolus (52) Interstitial lung disease (52) Hemoglobinopathy Methemoblinemia Sulfhemoglobinemia **Anatomic Shunts** Congenital cardiac disease (75) Pulmonary atrioventricular fistula **Other** High altitude (65) Drug overdoses (72) Seizures (51) Shock (7)	Cold exposure (65) Shock (7) Arterial obstruction or peripheral vascular disease Deep vein thrombosis (29) Raynaud's phenomena

( ) Refers to the chapter in which the disease entity is discussed.

Initial Diagnostic Approach
General

- As always, the ABCs (*a*irway, *b*reathing, and *c*irculation) should be assessed. Search for a history of cardiovascular, hematologic, and respiratory problems, as well as toxic ingestions or exposures to drugs, chemicals, fumes, and metals. The physical examination should include inspection of the skin with attention to the mucosal surfaces (especially the tongue and conjunctiva) and a thorough cardiopulmonary examination.
- If no cardiopulmonary source is likely and central cyanosis persists despite supplemental oxygenation, think abnormal hemoglobins!
- Pulse oximetry may overestimate total oxygen saturation with abnormal hemoglobins, and underestimate it in the presence of nail polish and hypoperfusion states. At high levels of methemoglobin, for example, the oxygen saturation by pulse oximetry approaches 85%, independent of the actual oxygen saturation.

Laboratory

- Check arterial blood gases (ABGs) in cases of central cyanosis to evaluate for hypoxia and low oxygen saturation. Peripheral cyanosis usually has a normal saturation. Abnormal hemoglobins have a normal calculated saturation (normal amount of dissolved oxygen in the blood), but a reduced measured saturation (due to decreased available oxygen binding sites).
- Co-oximetry can be used to measure the quantity of methemoglobin and carboxyhemoglobin because ABG analysis may be misleading.
- A complete blood count (CBC) is helpful to evaluate for anemia or polycythemia. Polycythemia can cause sludging in the peripheral vessels.

EKG

- All patients with central cyanosis should have an electrocardiogram (EKG) performed to evaluate for possible dysrhythmias or ischemia.

Radiography

- *Plain films.* Obtain a chest radiograph in all patients with central cyanosis to evaluate for cardiac or pulmonary pathology.
- *Echocardiogram.* This study may help in the evaluation of cardiac wall motion or valvular abnormalities, but is not typically ordered from the ED.

Emergency Department Management Overview
General

- The ABCs should be addressed as discussed in Section II.
- Give 100% oxygen via nonrebreather mask if central cyanosis is present, the patient is in respiratory distress, or the oxygen saturation is less than

95%. An intravenous (IV) line is necessary for drug administration, IV hydration, and drawing blood for laboratory tests.

Medications

- *Methylene blue.* This is the treatment for methemoglobinemia.
- Use appropriate medications to improve underlying pulmonary issues such as bronchodilators, diuretics, and steroids.

Disposition

- *Consultation.* Consult with hematology or toxicology based on the etiology of symptoms. Consult vascular surgery for arterial occlusive disease.
- *Admission.* Most patients with central cyanosis will need to be admitted.
- *Discharge.* Patients with reversible causes of cyanosis may be discharged after a period of observation.

Refer to the DDx table for reference to a discussion of problems in the differential not mentioned here.

Specific Problems: Peripheral Cyanosis
Acute arterial occlusion

- *Epidemiology and risk factors.* Approximately 50% of acute arterial occlusions are caused by arterial embolism. The other 50% are caused by in situ thrombosis.
- *Pathophysiology.* Arteriosclerosis causes decreased blood supply to tissue, which can result in local hypoxia.
- *History.* The patient may complain of leg pain, numbness, swelling, or changes in surface appearance.
- *Physical examination.* In arterial occlusion, one may find arterial bruits and decreased or absent pulses. The extremity may appear pale with loss of hair and decreased sensation. The ankle brachial index (ABI) of the involved extremity should be measured as described in Appendix 2.
- *Diagnostic testing.* An arteriogram will confirm the presence and location of arterial obstruction.
- *ED management.* ED management includes pain control and vascular surgery consultation. Acute ischemia may require bypass surgery to avoid amputation. Systemic heparinization may be started immediately in the ED in consultation with vascular surgery.
- *Helpful hints and pitfalls.* Consider this diagnosis in any patient with acute unilateral extremity paresthesias or pain.

Buerger's Disease (Thromboangiitis Obliterans)

- *Definition.* Idiopathic inflammatory occlusive disease primarily involving the medium and small arteries of the hands and feet.

- **Epidemiology and risk factors.** The typical age of onset is 40 to 45 years. It is more common in men. There are no atherosclerotic risk factors other than smoking. Raynaud's phenomenon occurs in approximately 40 percent of patients.
- **Pathophysiology.** There is segmental inflammation of the smaller arteries of the extremities. It most commonly affects the distal extremities, but more proximal arterial involvement occurs as the disease progresses. The initial arterial inflammatory event may spread to the adjacent veins and nerves resulting in venous thrombosis and fibrosis of these structures.
- **History.** The patient may complain of pain in the hands and feet that worsens with cold exposure, emotional stress, and activity (claudication).
- **Physical examination.** Dependent rubor may be present in the lower extremities. Skin ulcers and gangrene of the digits may be present. Phlebitis migrans may be present and manifests as tender, reddened, dark nodules over a peripheral artery with either a reduced or absent pulse. In the upper extremities, the digital arteries are usually more involved than the radial or ulnar arteries.
- **Diagnostic testing.** Clinical criteria should be sufficient for the ED diagnosis of Buerger's disease. Noninvasive vascular laboratory testing can confirm the diagnosis, and determine the extent of involvement. A definitive diagnosis is made when the histopathology examination identifies the acute phase lesion in a patient with a clinical history of smoking. An arteriogram is obtained to evaluate for arterial disease in the extremities. Other diagnostic studies are performed to rule out other causes. An echocardiogram may be performed to rule out a cardiac source for emboli. Laboratory studies are used to rule out an autoimmune and hypercoagulable diseases.
- **ED management.** Counsel the patient on the discontinuation of tobacco use and refer for vascular testing.
- **Helpful hints and pitfalls.** Criteria for the diagnosis include age less than 45 years, current or recent history of tobacco use, distal extremity ischemia (objectively noted on vascular testing), and exclusion of autoimmune and hypercoagulable diseases.

Raynaud's Phenomena

- **Definition.** Peripheral vasospasm of the fingers, toes, ears, and nose caused by exposure to cold or stress. It is characterized by episodic attacks lasting minutes to hours.
- **Epidemiology and risk factors.** Raynaud's most commonly affects women ages 15-40. Associated diseases include systemic lupus erythematosus, scleroderma, rheumatoid arthritis, and Buerger's disease.
- **Pathophysiology.** Vasoconstriction causes areas to become white due to lack of flow, then blue due to venous pooling, and finally red as arterioles dilate and blood flow slowly normalizes.
- **History.** Attacks may cause pain, numbness, and swelling.
- **Physical examination.** This is expected to be normal unless an episode is occurring.
- **Diagnostic testing** Anti-nuclear antibody (ANA) and erythrocyte sedimentation rate (ESR) are standard to screen for autoimmune and

connective tissue disorders. Cold stimulation test may be done on an outpatient basis.

- **■ *ED management.*** Treat the underlying cause as needed. Warm extremities with warm water. Prophylactic drug treatment, such as calcium channel blockers or vasodilators, is usually reserved for those with Raynaud's secondary to another disease process.
- **■ *Helpful hints and pitfalls.*** Advise the patient to avoid cold exposure and stop smoking.

Specific Problems: Other Causes of Cyanosis

Methemoglobinemia and Sulfhemoglobinemia

- **■ *Definition.*** Methemoglobinemia is due to abnormal hemoglobin containing an iron molecule that cannot bind oxygen. Sulfhemoglobinemia is a condition in which hemoglobin binds to sulfur.
- **■ *Epidemiology and risk factors.*** This may be acquired or congenital. It is often due to exposure to oxidizing agents. Local anesthetics, such as benzocaine, are a frequent cause. There are two genetic variations: type I and type II. Type I is known as *hemoglobin M disease*, and is an autosomal dominant condition in which hemoglobin does not reduce normally. Type II is the most common, and is due to a lack of cytochrome b5 reductase. Substances that predispose to methemoglobinemia are listed in Table 25–1. Drugs that predispose to sulfhemoglobinemia are listed in Table 25–2.
- **■ *Pathophysiology.*** Methemoglobin contains hemoglobin in which the iron component has been oxidized to the Fe^{3+} state. Lacking an electron to bind to oxygen, methemoglobin is unable to bind to or transport oxygen. The agents responsible for methemoglobin formation often have other deleterious effects. For example, vasodilators such as nitrites cause tachycardia, hypotension, and circulatory inadequacy. Oxidants can

Table 25–1	Substances that Predispose to Methemoglobinemia
Drugs	Nitrates, nitrites (including nitroglycerin, nitroprusside, amyl nitrite)
	Topical anesthetics (benzocaine, lidocaine, prilocaine)
	Dapsone
	Chloroquine, primaquine, quinines
	Sulfonamides
Chemical agents	Aniline dyes
	Arsine
	Butyl nitrite
	Chlorates
	Chlorobenzene
	Chromates
	Dimethyltoluidine
	Naphthalene
	Silver nitrate
	Well water (contains nitrites)

Table 25–2   Drugs that Predispose to Sulfhemoglobinemia
Acetanilid
Phenacetin
Nitrates
Trinitrotoluene
Metoclopramide
Sulfur compounds

cause hemolysis or sulfhemoglobinemia. In sulfhemoglobinemia, the iron remains in a reduced state ($HbFe^{2+}$). Sulfhemoglobin is inert as an oxygen carrier, and can produce deep cyanosis at a relatively low concentration. In contrast to methemoglobin, sulfhemoglobin causes a *rightward* shift of the oxygen dissociation curve, giving up its oxygen more readily at the tissue level.

■ *History.* This will include exposure to predisposing substances. Patients typically present with acute shortness of breath and cyanosis. Symptoms vary, and correspond to methemoglobin levels. Normal blood contains 1% methemoglobin. No symptoms occur with levels less than 10%. Initial symptoms include skin discoloration, mostly on the mucous membranes, anxiety, headache, and dyspnea on exertion. At levels greater than 50%, symptoms include fatigue, confusion, dizziness, and palpitations. Coma and seizures are present at levels greater than 70%.

■ *Physical examination.* Cyanosis unresponsive to oxygen, despite normal arterial oxygen tension, is the hallmark of methemoglobinemia. The patient may be tachypneic and tachycardic. In sulfhemoglobinemia, the presentation may be similar, but there is persistent cyanosis that is refractory to methylene blue. Sulfhemoglobinemia may also cause venous blood to appear slate gray color.

■ *Diagnostic testing.* At a minimum, a CBC, ABG, and methemoglobin level must be done. Serum lactate levels may help determine the level of tissue hypoxia. Pulse oximetry overestimates oxygen saturation, but also reflects the diminished response to supplemental oxygenation. An ABG will show normal calculated oxygen saturation, but a decrease in measured oxygen saturation. Cyanosis becomes apparent in the presence of 1.5 g/dl of methemoglobin, in contrast to the 5 g/dl of deoxy-hemoglobin. Tests to rule out hemolysis include a CBC, reticulocyte count, lactate dehydrogenase, indirect bilirubin, and haptoglobin. An EKG should be performed to evaluate for dysrhythmias or cardiac ischemia. Both methemoglobin and sulfhemoglobin levels should be measured using a co-oximeter capable of measuring sulfhemoglobin (many do not have this capacity). For confirmation of sulfhemoglobinemia, use gas chromatography if the diagnosis is in doubt.

■ *ED management.* Treat symptomatic patients (angina, dyspnea, dysrhythmias , hypotension or mental status changes). Supplemental oxygen should be given. The antidote for methemoglobinemia is 1% solution of methylene blue (1-2 mg/kg IV over 5 minutes). Improvement should occur in 30 to 60 minutes. Repeat the dose in 1 hour if the symptoms continue. Administration of methylene blue in patients who have glucose-6-phosphate dehydrogenase deficiency can lead to hemolytic anemia. In severe cases where methylene blue is ineffective, it is necessary to treat with exchange transfusion or hyperbaric oxygen. Sulfhemoglobinemia does not respond to methylene blue, and an exchange transfusion may be necessary. Give cimetidine (300 mg IV or by mouth every 6-8 hours) if dapsone is the causative agent. Gastrointestinal decontamination may be indicated depending on the causative agent. Admit all symptomatic patients.

- *Helpful hints and pitfalls.* Cases of iatrogenic methemoglobinemia have been reported after the use of topical anesthetic for procedures such as nasogastric tube placement and nasopharyngoscopy. Venous blood appears chocolate brown in color in methemoglobinemia. Infants with severe metabolic acidosis due to diarrhea and dehydration may develop methemoglobinemia. The exact cause is unknown. Methylene blue may be ineffective and possibly harmful in cases of glucose-6-phosphate dehydrogenase deficiency, sulfhemoglobinemia, or congenital causes of methemoglobinemia.

Pseudocyanosis

- *Definition.* This entily is a bluish discoloration to the skin and mucous membranes that is not associated with either peripheral vasoconstriction or hypoxemia.
- *Epidemiology and Risk Factors.* It is caused by metals (silver, lead, iron, gold, arsenic) or drugs (phenothiazines, amiodarone, minocycline, chloroquine, hydrochloride).
- *History.* The patient does not report any cardiopulmonary symptoms.
- *Physical examination.* This will be a normal, except for the bluish discoloration of skin that does not blanch under pressure.
- *Diagnostic testing.* Arterial blood gases and the CBC should be normal.
- *ED management.* No urgent management is needed. Arrange follow-up with a primary care physician.
- *Helpful hints and pitfalls.* The skin does not blanch under pressure in contrast to true cyanotic skin, which does blanch.

Special Considerations
Pediatrics

- Congenital heart disease occurs in 8/1000 live births. Approximately 50% of cases are diagnosed within the first week of life. Cyanotic lesions usually involve right to left shunting or impedance of left ventricular outflow (see Chapter 75).
- Acrocyanosis in newborns refers to the presence of cyanosis in the extremities. It is a normal variant in newborns. It is thought to be due to vasomotor instability to environmental cold, and can last hours to days with waxing and waning of cyanosis.
- Young infants with methemoglobinemia present with nonspecific findings such as tachycardia, poor feeding, vomiting, irritability, excessive crying, and excessive sleeping.

Teaching Points

Cyanosis is almost never due to a benign cause. Therefore the patient with cyanosis must be presumed to have a significant degree of hypoxia, and the first priority is to reverse this with oxygen administration. If this does not help, then initiate a search for abnormal hemoglobin.

Methemoglobin will usually respond to methylene blue administration, but sulfhemoglobin may require an exchange transfusion.

Most cyanotic patients will not have an easily reversible cause. Therefore, cyanosis is an indication for admission to an intensive care unit.

Suggested Readings

Lu HC, Shih RD, Marcus S, Ruck B, Jennis T. Pseudomethemoglobinemia: a case report and review of sulfhemoglobinemia. Arch Pediatr Adolesc Med 1998;152:803–805.

Martin L, Khalil H. How much reduced hemoglobin is necessary to generate central cyanosis? Chest 1990;97:182–185.

Moore TJ, Walsh CS, Cohen MR. Reported adverse cases of methemoglobinemia associated with benzocaine products. Arch Int Med 2004;164:1192–1196.

Sasidharan P. An approach to diagnosis and management of cyanosis and tachypnea in term infants. Pediatr Clin North Am 2004;51:999–1021.

Schofftall J, Bouchard M, Schick P. Methemoglobinemia. eMedicine, last updated May 10, 2002. *http://www.emedicine.com/med/topic1466.htm*.

Tintinalli JE, Kelen GD, Stapczynski JS (editors). Emergency Medicine: A Comprehensive Study Guide (6th ed). New York: McGraw-Hill, 2004, pp 212–213.

Wright RO, Lewander WJ, Woolf AD. Methemoglobinemia: etiology, pharmacology, and clinical management. Ann Emerg Med 1999;34:646–645.

CHAPTER **26**

Dehydration

CHRISTIAN ARBELAEZ ■ CAMIE J. SORENSEN ■ EDUARDO BORQUEZ

 Red Flags

- Postural lightheadedness • Tachycardia • Hypotension • Muscle cramp • Syncope • Confusion • Coma • Seizures • Dysrhythmias • Muscle weakness • Anuria • Polyuria (DKA, DI) • Tetany • Hyporeflexia

Overview

Dehydration is not completely synonymous with *volume depletion*; however, these two terms are often used interchangeably. Dehydration largely refers to intracellular water deficits due to hypertonicity, and a disturbance in water metabolism. The diagnosis of dehydration cannot be established without laboratory analysis of the serum sodium level or calculation of serum tonicity. In contrast, volume depletion describes the net loss of total body sodium, and a reduction in intravascular volume. This is often a clinical diagnosis and adjunctive data from laboratory studies may be helpful. For the purposes of this chapter, dehydration will refer to volume depletion.

Total body water (TBW) is 50% to 60% of a person's weight. Two thirds of TBW is intracellular and one third is extracellular. Three fourths of extracellular fluid (ECF) is in the interstitial space and one fourth of it is in the plasma. Volume and tonicity are largely regulated by the renin-angiotensin-aldosterone system (Figure 26–1).

True volume depletion is one in which there is reduced TBW. It occurs when the rate of salt and water intake is less than the combined rates of renal plus extrarenal volume losses. In chronic volume-contracted states, input and output may be equal.

Volume depletion is a common ED presentation, especially among children and the elderly. Worldwide, volume depletion due to diarrhea is the leading cause of infant mortality. Volume depletion in the elderly is associated with a mortality of close to 50% among hospitalized patients. Pediatric dehydration is discussed in Chapter 80.

The clinical approach in this chapter addresses the severity of volume depletion, not underlying etiology. Look for "red flags" (see Box) to identify severe signs and symptoms that indicate a need for emergent or expedited work up. Volume depletion may be a consequence of many diseases, and may be mild, moderate, or severe (Table 26–1). The goal of initial management is to begin treatment of the volume depletion first, identify the underlying etiology, and tailor definitive management accordingly. Volume, acid-base, and other electrolyte disturbances take precedence over sodium and chloride abnormalities. Hypovolemic shock is discussed in Chapter 7. Acid-base disturbances are reviewed in Chapter 83. Electrolyte abnormalities are discussed in Chapter 88.

Differential Diagnosis of Dehydration

- Volume depletion can be classified as hyponatremic, isonatremic, or hypernatremic (see DDx Table).
- Although the differential is broad, the vast majority of cases of volume depletion are due to gastrointestinal fluid losses and insensible losses without adequate repletion.

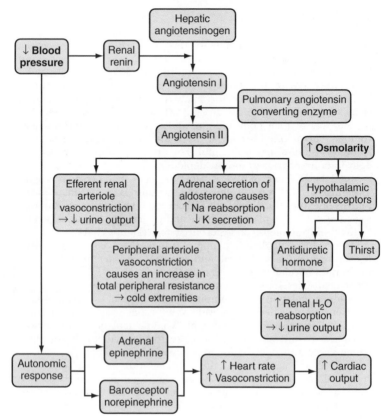

Figure 26–1. Pathophysiology of the renin-angiotensin-aldosterone system.

Initial Diagnostic Approach
General

- Any patient who is hemodynamically unstable or appears ill should receive immediate attention. While the physician is assessing the patient, a continuous cardiac monitor and pulse oximeter should be placed. Intravenous (IV) access with two large-bore catheters (16 to 18 gauge) should be obtained. See Figure 26–2 for an algorithm on the intial assessment and stabilization of these patients.
- The younger the patient, the fewer and less concerning co-morbid conditions, the better the historian, and the better the patient appears on physical examination, the fewer laboratory and imaging studies may be indicated. Immunocompromised, elderly, and young pediatric patients require a more liberal diagnostic workup. Assume a degree of dehydration

Table 26–1   Severity of Volume Depletion

	Mild <5%	Moderate 5–10%	Severe >10%
Signs and symptoms			
Level of consciousness	Alert	Lethargic	Unresponsive
Heart Rate	Normal	Increased	Markedly increased
Blood Pressure	Normal	Orthostatic	Decreased
Pulse	Normal	Thready	Faint
Urine output	Normal	Oliguria	Anuria
Mucous membranes	Normal	Dry	Cracked
Best measures in the elderly			
Speech difficulty	Clear	Rambling/ garbled	<50% understandable
Arm weakness	Normal	Moderate	Extreme weakness
Sunken eyes	Normal	Slight	Deep
Axillary sweat	Normal	Decreased	Absent
Labs			
Urine specific gravity	≤1.020	≥1.030	≥1.035
Arterial pH	7.30–7.40	7.10–7.30	<7.10
BUN	Normal	Elevated	Markedly elevated

DDx **Differential Diagnosis of Volume Depletion**

Hypo-natremic	**Iso-natremic**	**Hyper-natremic**
Concentrated fluid loss	GI fluid loss (e.g.,	Dilute fluid loss
Replacement of insensible	vomiting, diarrhea,	Heat exposure (ex:
losses with dilute fluids	obstruction)	losses through sweat,
(ex: marathoner	Diuretic overuse	heat stroke and
drinking tap water)	Plasma loss through	exhaustion)
Renal salt losses (thiazide	skin (burns,	Diabetic and alcoholic
diuretics, salt wasting	Stevens-Johnson	ketoacidosis
nephropathies)	syndrome and toxic	High metabolic rate
Hemorrhage	epidermal necrolysis)	(ex: fever,
	Adrenal insufficiency	hyperthyroidism,
		hyperventilation)
		Decreased water intake
		(pharyngitis,
		hypodipsia)
		Diabetes insipidus and
		mellitus
		Osmotic diuresis
		(mannitol, lactulose)
		Lithium salts

that is greater than the clinical appearance. Fever, for example, may increase normal insensible fluid loss by 250-500 mL per degree of fever.

■ The history will vary depending on the cause of the volume depletion. It is helpful to ascertain the acuity of the volume depletion; the amount, duration, frequency, and consistency of emesis; diarrhea, urination, drainage, or blood loss; the intake of fluids (amount and type); if there have been any ingestions; any co-morbid conditions (especially diabetes, renal disease, and heart failure); any symptoms associated with volume depletion (such as fatigue, thirst, muscle cramps, myalgias, postural lightheadedness, signs of ischemia such as chest pain, abdominal pain, delirium, and change in mental status); any symptoms associated with metabolic diseases that cause acid-base and electrolyte abnormalities (muscle weakness, polyuria, polydipsia, lethargy, confusion, and seizures); and the adequacy of the social conditions.

■ No single examination finding can be used to diagnose volume depletion or degree of volume depletion. Skin turgor and moistness of mucous membranes are unreliable in adults. The lack of physical findings does not exclude the presence of mild-to-moderate volume contraction in a given patient. Several clinical findings can be used to classify the degree of volume depletion as mild (<5%), moderate (5%-10%) or severe (10%) (Table 26–1).

■ Orthostatic vital signs are noninvasive, and easily performed at the bedside (see Chapter 2). However, in patients with acute blood loss of less than 20% of total blood volume, orthostatic vital signs lack both sensitivity and specificity.

Laboratory

■ *Bedside testing.* Evaluate for diabetic ketoacidosis (DKA) and hypoglycemia by checking a finger-stick glucose immediately, especially if the patient has altered mental status. If available, check a finger-stick hemoglobin to evaluate for blood loss, although this may be normal in acute hemorrhage.

■ *Urine sodium (UNa).* The response of the kidneys to volume depletion is to conserve sodium and water in an attempt to expand ECF volume. Except in situations in which sodium (Na^+) reabsorption is impaired (e.g., diuresis, renal disease), the urine Na^+ in hypovolemic patients should be less than 25 mEq/L. Low urine sodium is most often an indication of reduced circulating blood volume. Urinary Na^+ may also be increased in some cases of metabolic alkalosis in an attempt to excrete $HCO3^-$. The fractional excretion of Na^+ (FE_{Na}) is most useful in the differential diagnosis of acute renal failure (Chapter 49).

■ *Urine osmolality and specific gravity.* Renal retention of water in hypovolemic states is mediated by ADH, which is secreted in response to decreased tissue perfusion, resulting in relatively concentrated urine (>450 mosm/kg). However, isosmotic urine does not rule it out as the concentrating ability of the kidneys may be impaired (e.g., renal disease and diuresis). Urine specific gravity is less accurate than osmolality but a value above 1.015 is suggestive of concentrated urine as seen with hypovolemia.

- *Other urine studies.* The urinalysis is usually normal in patients with hypovolemia if the kidneys are not diseased. Proteinuria, hematuria, and myoglobinuria are present in rhabdomyolysis (e.g., from heat stroke). Urine human chorionic gonadotropin (hCG) should be measured on all females of reproductive age. Glucose level is elevated in patients with volume depletion due to hyperglycemia. Urine ketones should be checked to evaluate for DKA (Chapter 38).
- *Blood urea nitrogen (BUN) and plasma creatinine.* Both vary inversely with the glomerular filtration rate (GFR). BUN elevation can also be caused by increased urea production (e.g., gastrointestinal [GI] bleed) or tubular reabsorption. Creatinine is a more reliable estimate because it is produced at a constant rate by skeletal muscle, and is not reabsorbed. The BUN/creatinine ratio is greater than 20:1 in hypovolemia due to increased urea reabsorption. Creatinine may also increase if the hypovolemia is severe enough to lower the GFR. A normal BUN/creatinine ratio may occur in patients with hypovolemia if the urea production is reduced (e.g., decreased protein intake from vomiting).
- *Electrolytes.* Hypovolemia has variable effects on plasma Na^+ and potassium (K^+) levels. Serum Na^+ is helpful to detect hypo- and hypernatremia, which may be a clue to the etiology and can guide therapy. Volume depletion is a potent stimulus for antidiuretic hormone (ADH) and increased thirst, a combination which may cause hyponatremia in the hypovolemic patient. Na^+ may increase when water is lost in excess of solute, such as with insensible and sweat losses, diabetes insipidus, and hyperglycemia. The body's homeostatic mechanisms often prevent the development of hypernatremia. K^+ may be lost in the urine or gastrointestinal tract. It may be increased due to movement from the intracellular fluid to the extracellular fluid in metabolic acidosis, or there may be an inability to excrete it as in renal failure.
- *Acid-base balance.* Patients with vomiting or on diuretics may develop metabolic alkalosis from H+ loss and volume contraction. These patients typically have a low urinary chloride. Volume repletion with normal saline will correct both the alkalosis and volume depletion ("chloride responsive"). Loss of HCO_3^- secondary to diarrhea or reduced H^+ excretion (e.g., renal failure) can result in metabolic acidosis. A metabolic acidosis may also occur in shock states (i.e., lactic acidosis) and severe hyperglycemia (i.e., DKA).
- *Hematocrit and plasma albumin.* Both may be elevated from hemoconcentration but may appear falsely normal due to underlying anemia and hypoalbuminemia.

EKG

- Hypovolemia may cause tachycardia, ischemia and acute coronary syndrome.
- Many electrolyte abnormalities may be manifested by changes in the electrocardiogram (EKG) (see Chapter 87). For example, hypokalemia, hypomagnesemia, and hypocalcemia can all cause prolonged QT intervals.

Radiography

- An abdominal series (flat and upright abdominal film and upright chest radiograph) is useful to find bowel obstruction or perforation as causes of the dehydration.
- Abdominal computed tomography (CT scan) is most accurate in identification of intra-abdominal causes of dehydration.

Emergency Department Management Overview
General

- Address the ABCs (*a*irway, *b*reathing, and *c*irculation) as discussed in Section II. Start oxygen in any patient with hypoxia or respiratory distress.
- Two 16-gauge IVs are preferred for immediate access but may be difficult to insert in volume depleted patient. An external jugular is still considered peripheral access and should be attempted. Indications for central venous access include no peripheral IV access, need for measurement of CVP (central venous pressure), and for pressor support (usually after 2 L of isotonic fluid resuscitation). Other options include interosseous (especially in children) or a saphenous venous cutdown. Refer to Chapter 91, "Procedures".
- See Figures 26–2 and 26–3 for an algorithm on initial stabilization and fluid management.

Fluid Therapy

- Oral hydration should be given for mild dehydration in patients able to tolerate oral fluids. Indications for parenteral volume resuscitation include abnormal mental status, tachycardia at rest (>100 bpm), hypotension (<100 mm Hg systolic), any other signs of significant volume depletion or shock, or the inability to tolerate oral fluids.
- Interventions for patients with moderate to severe dehydration can be divided into three phases: resuscitation, repletion, and maintenance.
- In the *resuscitation* phase, give a fluid bolus with 20 mL/kg of 0.9% normal saline (NS) (500 ml to 2 L for adults) over 5 to 20 minutes. The patient should be reassessed after each intervention. Signs of adequate perfusion include an increase in blood pressure, improved mental status, and fuller pulses, suggesting a better cardiac output and improved peripheral perfusion. If there is no response to 2 L, consider starting pressors or giving blood (see Chapter 7). Exact volume deficits are difficult to calculate, and the patients are best monitored by response to treatment. Underresuscitation and continued losses may lead to irreversible shock. Overresuscitation may cause pulmonary edema, or adult respiratory distress syndrome.
- After perfusion is restored, in the *repletion* phase, the type of fluid given is largely dependent on the type of fluid that has been lost and any concurrent fluid and electrolyte disorders. An estimation of fluid deficit can be calculated by multiplying the patient's pre-illness weight by the clinically estimated percent of volume depletion of mild (<5%), moderate

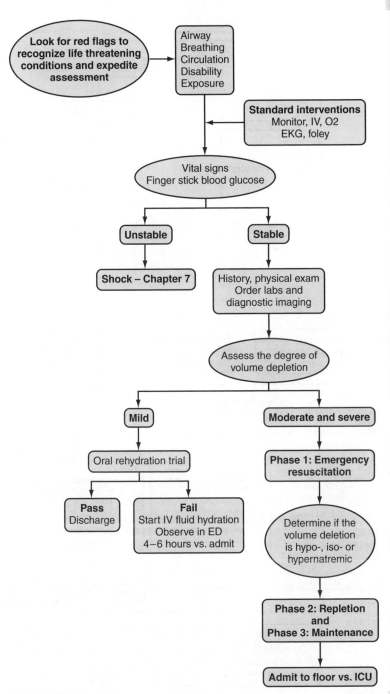

Figure 26–2. Initial assessment and stabilization.

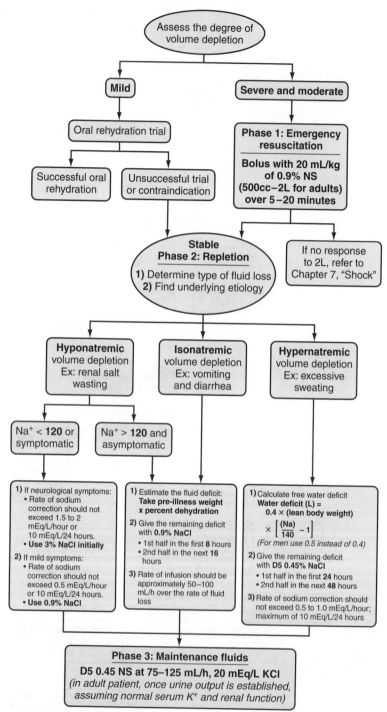

Figure 26-3. Algorithm of fluid therapy for volume depletion.

(5%-10%) and severe (10%). For patients with hypernatremia, the water deficit must be calculated (Table 26-2).

■ *Maintenance* fluids and electrolytes must be added to account for ongoing, normal losses. Average (70-kg adult) maintenance requirements are D_5 0.45% NS at 75 to 125 mL/h with 20 mEq/L KCl. Maintenance fluids should be initiated concurrently with phase 2 (repletion).

Medications

■ *Antiemetics.* Prochlorperazine 5 to 10 mg IV/IM or 25 mg per rectum (PR) is the most commonly used antiemetic agent. Others are listed in Chapter 90.4.

Emergency Department Interventions (Other)

■ *Acid-base and electrolyte replacement.* These are discussed in Chapters 83 and 88, respectively.
■ *Nasogastric tube.* For dehydration caused by surgical diseases accompanied by vomiting, gastrointestinal bleeding, bowel obstruction or severe or worsening pancreatitis.
■ *Urinary catheter.* This should be placed for moderate to severe volume depletion to monitor urinary output.

Disposition

■ *Consultation.* This will be determined by the etiology of the volume depletion.
■ *Admission.* Admission criteria are listed in Box 26–1.
■ *Discharge.* This is safe in mild cases of volume depletion that respond to oral rehydration therapy.

BOX 26–1 Admission Criteria for Patients Presenting with Dehydration

Intractable vomiting or diarrhea
Inability to tolerate PO liquids
Persistent electrolyte, acid-base or volume defect
Co-morbid illness requiring admission
Abdominal pain of unknown etiology
Gastrointestinal bleed
Persistent altered mental status
Newly diagnosed sodium > 150 or <120 mEq/L
Symptomatic or severe hypo- or hyperkalemia
Dysrhythmias
Hyperosmolar syndrome
Heat stroke

Specific Problems
Isonatremic Volume Depletion

- **Background.** This type of volume depletion results from a balanced water and salt loss. Examples include acute gastroenteritis with nausea, vomiting and diarrhea.
- **Clinical presentation.** Patients with isonatremic volume depletion will usually have symptoms and signs related to hypotension, rather than electrolyte disturbances.
- **Diagnostic testing.** Electrolytes are normal.
- **ED management.** Patients should be volume resuscitated as discussed above.
- **Helpful hints and pitfalls.** Prioritize volume, acid-base, and electrolyte disturbances over sodium and chloride abnormalities.

Hypernatremic Volume Depletion

- **Background.** This type of depletion results from water loss exceeding salt loss (dilute losses), producing a serum sodium concentration greater than 145 mEq/L. Causes include excessive sweating, fever, decreased water intake, diabetes insipidus (renal or pituitary) and mellitus, and alcoholism and lithium intoxication.
- **Clinical presentation.** Patients with hypernatremic volume depletion will have fewer volume-related symptoms than with isonatremic depletion because extracellular fluid is relatively maintained. However, neurologic symptoms include irritability, ataxia, altered mental status, seizures, coma, and intracerebral hemorrhages.
- **Diagnostic testing.** If the UNa is above 20 mEq/L or shows low urine osmolality, losses are due to renal causes (e.g., diuretic use, diabetes insipidus secondary to low or ineffective antidiuretic hormone). If the UNa is less than 10 mEq/L or there is high urine osmolality, losses are due to extrarenal sources (e.g., GI loss, skin loss).
- **ED management.** Volume resuscitation for a hemodynamically unstable patient should be accomplished with isotonic 0.9% NS. Once the patient is hemodynamically stable, IV fluids should be changed to a hypotonic 0.45% NS solution, because isotonic saline resuscitation in the absence of hemodynamic compromise may cause fluid overload while only minimally decreasing the serum sodium concentration. Although isotonic saline is given to restore volume, it also lowers the plasma osmolality because the hypernatremia patient typically has a plasma osmolality greater than 308 mEq/L (the concentration of isotonic saline). The water deficit should be calculated as described in Table 26–2. The volume used in the fluid resuscitation phase should be subtracted from this deficit. The remaining deficit must be replaced (using hypotonic 0.45% NS solution) in addition to maintenance fluid requirements from renal and extrarenal losses. When using dextrose-containing solutions, the glucose should be monitored closely, because hyperglycemia worsens hyperosmolarity and can lead to osmotic diuresis. The rate of correction in hypernatremia is important. Due to the risk of cerebral edema, the serum sodium concentration should be lowered no faster than 0.5 to 1.0 mEq/L

Table 26–2 Water Deficit Calculation in Hypernatremic Volume Depletion

	Defined	Calculation	Example
1. Normal TBW	TBW in a healthy person	60% × weight (50% for women, 70% for infants)	100 kg man 100 × 0.6 = 60 L
2. Current TBW	TBW before fluid correction. Except in rare cases, hypernatremia is due to water loss	50% × weight (40% for women, 60% for infants) Note: the percent of body water relative to weight is decreased.	100 kg man, Na+ = 170 mEq/L 100 kg x 0.5 = 50 liters
3. Ideal TBW	TBW after the administration of fluid	$\dfrac{\text{Current [Na+]} \times \text{Current TBW}}{\text{Ideal [Na+]}}$	100 kg man, Na+ = 170 mEq/L 170 mEq/L x 50 L = 61 L
4. Water deficit	Ideal TBW– Current TBW	Equation #1 – Equation #2	61L – 50L = 11 L
5. Water deficit (alternative calculation)	See above	Weight (kg) × (0.5 men, 0.4 women) × $\left(\dfrac{\text{measured [Na+]}}{140 \text{ mEq/L}} - 1\right)$	100 kg man, Na+ 170 mEq/L $100 \times 0.5 \times \left(\dfrac{170}{140} - 1\right) = 10.7\text{L}$
6. Rate of sodium correction	0.5 to 1.0 mEq/L/hour	$\dfrac{\text{Current sodium} - \text{Ideal sodium}}{\text{Rate of correction}}$	100 kg man, Na = 170 mEq/L $\dfrac{170 \text{ mEq/L} - 140 \text{ mEq/L}}{1.0 \text{ mEq/L/hour}} = 30 \text{ hours}$

TBW = total body water; 1 L water = 1 kg.

Intravenous (IVF)	Na (mEq/L)
5% dextrose in water	0
0.2% saline	34
0.45% saline	77
0.9% saline	154
3% saline	513

$$\text{Serum Na change (mEq/L) with 1 L of IVF} = \frac{\text{Na content in IVF (mEq/L)} - \text{Measured serum Na (mEq/L)}}{[\text{Correction factor} \times \text{Weight (kg)}] + 1}$$

Patient	Correction factor
Pediatric	0.6
Male, nonelderly	0.6
Female, nonelderly	0.5
Male, elderly	0.5
Female, elderly	0.45

Figure 26–4. Formula to calculate the change in serum sodium concentration with 1 L of intravenous fluids, based on the sodium content of the fluid, the current measured serum sodium concentration, a correction factor to help estimate total body water volume, and the patient's weight. This formula applies to the treatment plan for hyponatremia and hypernatremia. *(From Adrogue HJ, Madias NE. Hypernatremia. N Engl J Med 2000;342:1493–1499.)*

per hour, with a maximum decrease of 10 mEq/L per 24-hour period. No more than half of the water deficit should be replaced within the first 24 hours, with the remainder corrected over the next 1 to 2 days. See Figure 26–4 for a formula to estimate the effect of 1 L of an IV fluid on serum sodium concentration.

- **Helpful hints and pitfalls.** Most cases of hypernatremia in the ED occur over a chronic (greater than 48-hour) period of time. Lowering the plasma osmolality with hypotonic fluids too rapidly will cause an osmotic shift of water into brain cells, leading to iatrogenic cerebral edema. Eu- and hypervolemic sodium abnormalities have different etiologies and treatments (Chapter 88).

Hyponatremic Volume Depletion

- **Background.** Sodium depletion exceeds TBW volume depletion. Examples include renal (sodium-wasting nephropathy, hypoaldosteronism, or diuretic) or extrarenal (e.g., vomiting, diarrhea, severe burns) sodium losses or excessive water ingestion.
- **Clinical presentation.** Evaluation of volume status (hypo-, eu-, or hypervolemic) is critical to the evaluation of hyponatremia (Chapter 88). Neurologic symptoms and signs will predominate ranging from

headache, nausea, altered mental status, ataxia, status seizures, coma, and unresponsiveness.

■ ***Diagnostic testing.*** These patients have a low serum osmolality (less than 275 mOsm/kg), reflecting a net gain of free water. A low urinary sodium concentration (less than 20 mEq/L with a high urine osmolality) suggests extrarenal sodium and water losses, because the kidneys are reabsorbing sodium appropriately. These patients represent the most common cause for hyponatremia found in ED patients. In contrast, a high urinary sodium concentration (greater than 20 mEq/L and high urine osmolality) reflects renal sodium and water losses.

■ ***ED management.*** These patients have decreased total body sodium stores in addition to free water loss, and require either oral or intravenous sodium administration. Isotonic saline is the intravenous fluid of choice for concurrent salt and water repletion. Once the patient is euvolemic, the stimulus for ADH release is reduced, allowing excess free water to be excreted and further self-correction of hyponatremia. Thus, once hypovolemia is corrected, isotonic IV fluids should be changed to a hypotonic fluid, such as 0.45% saline, to avoid correcting the serum sodium concentration too quickly. Correction of hyponatremia too rapidly can lead to central pontine myelinolysis (CPM), recently known as osmotic demyelination syndrome (ODS). For hyponatremic patients with significant neurologic symptoms, such as seizures, severe altered mental status, or coma, aggressive therapy is necessary to avoid permanent neurologic deficits and even death from cerebral edema. In these patients, the target rate of sodium correction is 1.5 to 2 mEq/L per hour with 3% hypertonic saline (513 mEq/L sodium) for the first 3 to 4 hours, or more briefly, if symptoms improve. The maximum rise of serum sodium concentration should not exceed 10 mEq/L in the first 24 hours. Patients with mild symptoms tend to have chronic (greater than 48 hours duration) hyponatremia. In these patients, CPM very rarely develops if sodium correction is limited to 0.5 mEq/L per hour with a maximum sodium increase of 10 mEq/L over 24 hours. See Figure 26–4 for a formula to estimate the effect of 1 L of an IV fluid on serum sodium concentration. For example, a 70-kg elderly man who arrives to the ED with altered mental status and a sodium concentration of 110 mEq/L. One liter of 3% saline (513 mEq/L sodium) will increase the serum sodium concentration by approximately 11 mEq/L, as calculated by $(513 - 110)/[(0.5 \times 70) + 1]$. Thus, to increase the serum sodium concentration by 2 mEq/L in the first hour, between one fifth and one sixth of the liter (approximately 175 mL) should be given. Another simple method used to estimate the initial sodium infusion is described in Chapter 88 under the discussion of "Hyponatremia".

■ ***Helpful hints and pitfalls.*** CPM occurs 1 to 6 days after treatment. Patients develop a deteriorating mental status and progressive neurologic deficits, such as pseudobulbar palsies and spastic quadriparesis, after a transient period of improvement with fluid administration. It has a dismal prognosis and has no effective treatment. Cerebral edema may occur in the setting of hypo-osmolarity due to the osmotic movement of water into brain cells and can occur if the sodium is too low. Thus, a more rapid rate of correction is allowed in patients with neurologic symptoms.

It should be noted that a high urinary sodium and osmolality can also be seen with in euvolemic states such as SIADH (syndrome of inappropriate antidiuretic hormone), hypothyroidism, and adrenal insufficiency. In SIADH (which is usually eu- or hypervolemic), hyponatremia will *worsen* with any fluid administration because the kidney is inappropriately reabsorbing water and excreting concentrated urine.

Special Considerations
Pediatrics

See Chapter 80.

Elderly

- Several mechanisms have been proposed to explain why the elderly are especially susceptible to volume depletion. These include decreased capacity of the kidney to concentrate, decreased effectiveness of ADH, decrease in body water percentage, and decreased sensation of thirst that may be due to subclinical strokes, especially in the hypothalamus.
- Medications may also contribute to dehydration. Diuretic use is common; beta-blockers may blunt tachycardia and exacerbate hypotension; cardiac glycosides can decrease thirst.
- Management of volume depletion in the elderly is similar to management in younger adults. However, due to the higher prevalence of co-morbid conditions such as heart failure and renal insufficiency, slower infusion rates should be selected.

Teaching Points

Dehydration is a common problem that is frequently underestimated in its severity. Any illness can cause a diminished intake, and this is especially important in young infants and the elderly who cannot gain access to fluids because of motor weakness, disease, or developmental stage.

It is always prudent to assume a degree of dehydration that is greater than the clinical appearance. Fever, for example, will increase insensible fluid loss. Losses are worsened by environmental temperatures and humidity, by medications or dietary ingestions that can produce diuresis (e.g., caffeine), and by diminished ability to sense thirst, as in the elderly.

While the underlying disease will certainly contribute to continued losses, it is prudent to commence therapy with a bolus of normal saline: 20 cc/kg in the child, and 500 mL to 1 liter in the adult.

Laboratory analysis is useful in moderate to severe dehydration, but not in mild cases. Whatever the degree of dehydration, it is useful to monitor body weight, urine output, skin turgor, capillary refill, mentation, and level of activity.

Suggested Readings

Barkin RM, Ward G. Infectious diarrheal disease and dehydration. In: Marx JA, Hockberger RS, Walls RM (editors). Rosen's Emergency Medicine: Concepts and Clinical Practice (6th ed). Philadelphia: Mosby, 2006, pp 2623–2635.

Faubel S, Topf. The Fluid, Electrolyte and Acid-Base Companion. San Diego: Alert and Oriented Publishing Co., 1999, pp 145–218.

Gibbs MA, Tayal VS. Electrolyte disturbances. In: Marx JA, Hockberger RS, Walls RM (editors). Rosen's Emergency Medicine: Concepts and Clinical Practice (6th ed). Philadelphia: Mosby, 2006, pp 1933–1937.

Gross CR, Lindquist RD, Woolley AC, et al. Clinical indicators of dehydration in elderly patients. J Emer Med 1992;10:267–274.

Lavizzo-Mourey RJ. Dehydration in the elderly: a short review. J Natl Med Assoc 1987;79:1033–1038.

Lin M, Liu SJ, Lim IT. Disorders of water balance. Emerg Med Clin North Am 2005;23:749–770, ix.

McGee S, Abernethy WB, Simel D. Is this patient hypovolemic? JAMA 1999;282:1022–1029.

Rose BD, Post TW. Clinical Physiology of Acid-Base and Electrolyte Disorders (5th ed). New York: McGraw-Hill, 2001, pp 415–446.

CHAPTER **27**

Diarrhea

JENNIFER E. DELAPEÑA ■ **LEON D. SANCHEZ**

Red Flags

Severe abdominal pain ● Fever >101.5° F ● Tachycardia ● Hypotension ● Extremes of age ● Immunocompromised state ● Significant bleeding

Overview

Diarrhea, defined as an increased liquidity and frequency of stools, is a common presenting symptom in the ED. Diarrhea can be classified as infectious (85%) or noninfectious (15%). Most acute diarrhea due to an infectious etiology is self-limited. Sixty percent of these cases are viral, 20% are bacterial, and 5% are due to parasites.

Diarrhea may present with dehydration, vomiting, fever, bloody stools, and abdominal pain.

Diarrhea can be characterized as acute or chronic; acute diarrhea is defined as diarrhea present for fewer than 4 weeks. There are only a few infectious agents that cause prolonged diarrhea in immunocompetent individuals (such as *Giardia lamblia* or *Yersinia* species).

Patients with significant abdominal pain should be assessed primarily for abdominal pathology (see Chapter 18). Look for "red flags" (see Box) to identify patients with serious illness such as appendicitis, bowel obstruction, diverticulitis, mesenteric ischemia (Chapter 18), gastrointestinal bleed (Chapter 34), or organophosphate poisoning (Chapter 72).

Patients should be rapidly assessed for signs of volume depletion. Elderly and pediatric patients are more susceptible to dehydration resulting from diarrhea.

Diarrhea in the pediatric patient is discussed in Chapter 77.

Differential Diagnosis of Diarrhea

See DDx tables for the differential of acute and chronic diarrhea.

Initial Diagnostic Approach
General

- Any patient complaining of diarrhea should immediately be assessed for the severity of volume depletion, and appropriate resuscitative measures should be initiated. Any patient who is hemodynamically unstable or appears ill should receive immediate attention. While the physician is assessing this patient, a continuous cardiac monitor should be placed and large-bore intravenous (IV) catheters should be inserted.
- Important clinical history includes the onset of illness, duration of symptoms, weight loss, and any ill contacts. It is also important to quantify and characterize the stools including the presence of blood. Clues to the etiology of diarrhea can be obtained through a detailed history regarding travel to an endemic area, exposure to untreated water, medication use (particularly laxatives or recent antibiotics), and human

DDx Other Causes of Acute Diarrhea

Infectious	Noninfectious
Viral Bacterial Parasitic (protozoa and helminth)	Dietetic foods: mannitol, sorbitol, xylitol Drugs: caffeine, colchicines, hydralazine, lactulose, laxatives Constipation with overflow incontinence Food allergy Inflammatory bowel disease Irritable bowel syndrome Lactase deficiency Opiate withdrawal Initial presentation of chronic diarrhea (see below)

DDx Causes of Chronic Diarrhea

Category	Types	Definition	Examples
Watery	Osmotic	Ingestion of poorly absorbed substance	Osmotic laxative Carbohydrate malabsorption
	Secretory	Increased electrolyte secretion or reduced electrolyte absorption	Congenital syndrome Bacterial toxin Ileal bile acid malabsorption Inflammatory bowel disease Vasculitis Drugs and poisons Laxative abuse Disordererd motility and regulation Endocrine Tumors Idiopathic
Inflammatory		Diarrhea due to inflammatory or neoplastic diseases involving the gut	Inflammatory bowel disease Infectious disease Ischemic colitis Radiation colitis Neoplasia
Fatty		Defective absorption of fat in the small intestine	Malabsorption Maldigestion

immunodeficiency virus (HIV) risk factors. Patients with malabsorption may have fatty stools.

■ Because most cases of diarrhea are self-limited, diagnostic testing should be reserved for patients who are unstable, ill-appearing, immunocompromised, who are not responding to conservative management, who have persistent diarrhea or significant associated symptoms (abdominal pain, fever).

Laboratory

■ Studies may include a complete blood count (CBC) with a differential count looking for leukocytosis, hemoconcentration, and anemia. Neutropenia can occur in salmonellosis. Electrolyte levels and renal function tests can determine the extent of fluid and electrolyte depletion and its effect on renal function.

■ Stool cultures should be obtained on patients with fever, bloody diarrhea, an acute flare of inflammatory bowel disease (IBD), an immunocompromised state, recently on antibiotics, chronic diarrhea, employees involved in food handling, exposure to day care centers, and those with recent travel to endemic areas.

- Fecal leukocyte and occult blood are often present in patients with diarrhea and diffuse colonic inflammation. The presence of occult blood does not always correlate with the presence of fecal leukocytes (e.g., fissures, irritation, hemorrhoids, bowel ischemia, and malignancy). Although fecal leukocytes are associated with invasive bacterial colitis, their absence does not rule it out. The presence of fecal leukocytes does not delineate which patients will benefit from antimicrobial therapy. However, studies suggest that stool cultures are unlikely to grow pathogenic bacteria in the absence of fecal leukocytes. Fecal leukocytes are commonly absent in diarrhea due to viruses and all toxin-induced bacterial food poisoning.
- *Clostridium difficile toxin* is positive in nearly all cases of antibiotic-associated pseudomembranous colitis. Symptoms may be delayed in onset up to 10 weeks after antibiotic therapy. The most common antibiotics implicated are cephalosporins, penicillins, and clindamycin. Patients who have been treated with antibiotics in the preceding 3 months or those developing diarrhea in an institutional setting, including recent hospitalization, should be tested.
- *Escherichia coli 0157:H7 toxin* should be ordered in endemic areas and in patients with suspected hemolytic-uremic syndrome.
- Stool examination for *ova and parasites* is not routinely necessary. Patients in whom ova and parasites may be useful include those with persistent diarrhea (*Entamoeba histolytica, Cryptosporidium* species), history of travel (*Cryptosporidium, Giardia, Cyclospora* species), adults with contact with infants in day care centers (*Cryptosporidium, Giardia* species), and those with suspected HIV infection (*E. histolytica, Giardia species*).
- *Giardia antigen* may be ordered on patients at risk such as campers who drink unfiltered, mountain spring, or creek waters in the United States.
- Analysis of fecal fat is used to screen for malabsorption.

Radiography

- Abdominal radiographs should be obtained in toxic patients or patients with significant abdominal pain to look for evidence of ileus, megacolon, or other obstructive process.
- Computed tomography (CT scan) of the abdomen can reveal other serious abdominal pathology including appendicitis, diverticulitis, and mesenteric ischemia.

Emergency Department Management Overview
General

- As always, the ABCs (*a*irway, *b*reathing, and *c*irculation) should be addressed as discussed in Section II.
- Two large-bore IV catheters should be placed in any patient with hemo-dynamic instability. A single peripheral IV is usually sufficient for most patients requiring IV fluids for dehydration.

Medications

- *Analgesia.* Patients with significant abdominal pain should be assessed for serious abdominal pathology, and treated with analgesic medications such as morphine 2 to 4 mg IV every 5 to 10 minutes until the patient is comfortable.

■ *Antidiarrheal agents.* Bismuth subsalicylate (Pepto-Bismol) can be used to reduce diarrhea. Antimotility agents (loperamide) can be used in non-infectious diarrhea, but are not recommended for infectious diarrhea or patients who look seriously ill (see Chapter 90.4).

■ *Antibiotics.* Treatment with antibiotics will be discussed later in the chapter.

Emergency Department Interventions

■ Oral fluids can be used for mild dehydration. Patients with moderate or severe dehydration, vomiting, or significant electrolyte abnormalities should have IV hydration with normal saline (1-2L in young previously healthy adult patients, 250 to 500 ml in elderly individuals, and 20 ml/kg in children). The fluid should be given in boluses, the first being wide open, with reevaluation of the patient's status after each bolus.

■ *Nasogastric tube placement.* A nasogastric tube section is unnecessary unless bowel obstruction or gastrointestinal bleeding is suspected as the primary cause of diarrhea.

■ *Urinary catheter placement.* A Foley catheter should be placed in patients who are ill for careful urine output measurement.

Disposition

■ *Consultation.* A gastroenterologist should be consulted for inflammatory bowel disease. Surgery should be consulted for surgical diseases.

■ *Admission.* Patients who are hemodynamically unstable, unable to tolerate oral fluids, have significant metabolic derangements, or other serious illness, should be admitted.

■ *Discharge.* Patients who look well, have improvement in symptoms, do not have signs of volume depletion, and can tolerate oral intake can by discharged from the ED with primary care follow-up. The differential diagnosis and evaluation of chronic diarrhea is more extensive than for acute diarrhea (DDx Table). If these patients do not require admission, they should be referred for an outpatient workup.

Specific Problems: Infectious Diarrhea
Viral Diarrhea

■ Viral pathogens are the most frequent cause of acute gastroenteritis. Transmission occurs through contaminated food, person-to-person contact, raw oysters, and contaminated water. Norwalk virus and rotavirus are responsible for more than 50% of infections. Risk factors include recent travel to endemic areas and sick contacts in close environments such as schools, hospitals, and residential homes.

■ Acute viral gastroenteritis presents with diarrhea accompanied by upper gastrointestinal symptoms such as vomiting. High fever, bloody diarrhea, and abdominal pain are usually absent.

■ Overdiagnosing viral gastroenteritis is a common pitfall. It is an unlikely diagnosis in patients with an abnormal abdominal examination or if there is blood present in the stool.

Bacterial Diarrhea

- Bacterial infection is commonly caused by the ingestion of food or water contaminated with pathogenic organisms particularly in areas where people are housed together (nursing homes, daycare centers) and areas with poor hygiene. Patients with recent antibiotic use are at risk for developing pseudomembranous colitis from *C. difficile* overgrowth. Diarrhea is due to increased intestinal secretion, mucosal damage from bacterial toxins, or direct tissue invasion by the organism resulting in destruction of the mucosa (Table 27–1). Pathogens associated with inflammatory or bloody diarrhea include *Shigella*, *Campylobacter jejuni*, nontyphoidal *Salmonella*, *Vibrio parahaemolyticus*, *E. histolytica*, *C. difficile*, and enteroinvasive *Escherichia coli*.

- Fever, crampy abdominal pain, bloody or explosive diarrhea, and the passage of many stools per day are common findings. Patients with ciguatera fish poisoning often present with neurologic symptoms (see Chapter 46). Scombroid fish poisoning resembles a histamine intoxication. Patients present with facial flushing, diarrhea, severe, headache, palpitations, and abdominal cramps. Occult positive stools suggest a bacterial cause of infectious diarrhea.

- Empiric antibiotic treatment may be started on well-appearing patients with symptoms of bacterial enteritis (Table 27–1). One important exception is suspected hemorrhagic colitis from *E. coli* O157:H7 associated with the consumption of undercooked hamburger. Antibiotics are ineffective and can increase the risk of complications (hemolytic uremic syndrome). Suspected *C. difficile* infections should be treated with metronidazole or oral vancomycin.

Parasitic Infection

- *Giardia lamblia*, acquired by drinking water contaminated with *Giardia* cysts, is the most common parasitic gastroenteritis in the United States.

Table 27–1 Summary of Bacterial Pathogens

Bacteria	Food Source	Mechanism	Antibiotic*
Campylobacter jejuni	Milk	I	Macrolide
Salmonella	Raw eggs, meat, poultry	I	Quinolone
Shigella	Contaminated food	I	Quinolone
Yersinia enterocolitica	Raw milk, Pork	I	Quinolone
Eschericia coli O157:H7	Ground Beef	I	None
Vibrio parahemolyticus	Raw seafood	I & T	None
Enterotoxigenic *E. Coli* (traveler's diarrhea)	Water, vegetables, fruit peel	T	None
Staphylococcus aureus	Undercooked meat	T	None
Bacillus Cereus	Rice	T	None
Vibrio cholerae	Raw Seafood	T	Doxycycline
Scombroid	Mahi mahi, tuna, bluefish	T	None
Ciguatera	Large, predacious, coral reef fish	T	None

Invasive, I; toxin mediated, T.
Refer to Chapter 90.2 for drug dosages.

E. histolytica causes amebiasis, which predominately affects those in lower socioeconomic status in developing countries. Other parasites that are more common in patients with acquired immunodeficiency syndrome (AIDS) include *Cryptosporidium parvum*, microsporidium, and *Isospora belli* (see "Special Considerations").

- Parasites commonly cause diarrhea by causing malabsorption from the gastrointestinal (GI) tract. One exception is amebiasis, which causes an inflammatory colitis by invading the colonic epithelium. Hepatic infection may also result, causing obstruction of portal veins and hepatic necrosis. Amebiasis can cause serious extraintestinal manifestations including liver abscess, brain, peritoneal, and pericardial sac infection.
- Diarrhea of chronic duration is more likely to be parasitic than viral or bacterial in origin. Other characteristics include bloating, excessive flatulence, and profuse watery diarrhea. Parasitic infections are diagnosed by sending stool for ova and parasite examination (see "Initial Diagnostic Approach"). Parasitic disease is suggested by a high eosinophil count on the CBC differential count.
- Treatment is based on stool examination for ova and parasites. Metronidazole is effective against *Giardia* and amebiasis. Patients who look well, but have had diarrhea for 2 to 4 weeks, can be treated empirically for *Giardia*. In addition to parasitic infections, patients with chronic diarrhea should be evaluated for non-infectious causes. Most of these patients may need to be referred for a more extensive outpatient workup.

Specific Problems: Noninfectious Causes of Diarrhea
Inflammatory Bowel Disease (IBD)

- *Definition.* There is a chronic relapsing and remitting disorder characterized by gastrointestinal tract inflammation. IBD is comprised of ulcerative colitis (UC), which is limited to the colon, and Crohn's disease, which can involve the entire gastrointestinal tract.
- *Epidemiology and risk factors.* IBD is a chronic inflammatory disease of the intestine. There is a bimodal distribution in age of onset with an early peak from 15 to 30 years of age and the second peak at 55 to 60 years. There is an increased risk of colorectal cancer.
- *Pathophysiology.* The etiology of IBD is unknown but it is believed to be multifactorial involving immunologic, genetic, environmental, and psychologic factors. UC causes inflammation that is limited to the submucosa of the intestinal wall, whereas Crohn's disease results in transmural inflammation.
- *History.* IBD presents with episodic constitutional and gastrointestinal symptoms that can include low-grade fever, abdominal pain, weight loss, and chronic diarrhea. The most typical manifestation of ulcerative colitis is bloody diarrhea. Pain is uncommon but may occur. The most typical manifestations of Crohn's disease are abdominal pain and diarrhea. A careful review of systems can reveal extraintestinal manifestations (eye, skin, and musculoskeletal). A flare-up of Crohn's disease may be signaled by weight loss and the appearance of ischiorectal abscesses.
- *Physical examination.* Look for evidence of complications requiring surgical intervention (bowel obstruction, toxic megacolon, bowel

perforation, abscess). Rectal examination should be performed looking for fistulas, fissures, abscess and stool examined for gross and occult blood.

- **Diagnostic testing.** Obtain a CBC to evaluate for anemia. Electrolytes, BUN, creatinine, and stool studies should be performed. *Clostridium difficile* is not uncommon. Patients who look ill or have significant abdominal tenderness should be evaluated for serious complications of IBD with appropriate imaging.
- **ED management.** Treatment of volume depletion is similar to the treatment for infectious causes of diarrhea. Broad-spectrum antibiotics should be administered in patients who appear toxic or those with suspected perforation. Other therapy (anti-inflammatory, immunosuppressive, and steroid medications) should not be initiated unless the diagnosis of IBD is established.
- **Helpful hints and pitfalls.** IBD can cause mild symptoms that can mimic infectious diarrhea. Patients with IBD may develop axial arthritis, such as ankylosing spondylitis (Chapter 71), or a peripheral arthritis. Diseases of the eye associated with ulcerative colitis are episcleritis and iritis (Chapter 69). The major skin diseases associated with IBD are erythema nodosum (Chapter 62) and pyoderma gangrenosum. Calcium oxalate stones are the most common type of renal calculi associated with Crohn's disease. Sclerosing cholangitis is most commonly associated with ulcerative colitis. Anemia and hypercoagulopathy are common in patients with IBD. Strictures and obstructions are not uncommon in persons with Crohn's disease. Fistulae and perianal disease are not uncommon in persons with Crohn's disease. Toxic megacolon is a life-threatening complication of ulcerative colitis and requires urgent surgical intervention.

Irritable Bowel Syndrome

- **Definition.** Irritable bowel syndrome (IBS) is characterized by chronic or recurrent abdominal pain and a disturbance of defecation.
- **Epidemiology and risk factors.** It is most often seen in women younger than 40 years.
- **Pathophysiology.** This is not well understood. It is thought to involve a dysfunction in the sensory pathways of the gut resulting in hyper-responsiveness and irritability of the GI tract.
- **History.** IBS is diagnosed on the basis of history after exclusion of other serious pathology. Symptoms include chronic abdominal discomfort, alteration in stool (alternating diarrhea and constipation), bloating, dysmenorrhea, or gastroesophageal reflux. Symptoms can be triggered by dietary factors or stress.
- **Physical examination.** Usually unremarkable, including the abdominal examination. The stool should be negative for occult blood.
- **Diagnostic testing.** Studies may help to eliminate other disorders.
- **ED management.** Patients usually look well, and require little intervention in the ED. Patients can be counseled on avoidance of dietary triggers. Antispasmodic agents such as dicyclomine may be prescribed. Antidiarrheal agents can be used as well.
- **Helpful hints and pitfalls.** Patients with suspected IBS should have a thorough evaluation for other serious problems.

Special Considerations
Diarrhea in Children

- Diarrhea is the second most common pediatric complaint. It is the leading cause of death in children worldwide.
- The most common cause of acute infectious diarrhea in children is viral infection. Children, especially the very young, are extremely susceptible to severe dehydration.

Refer to Chapter 77, "Pediatric Gastrointestinal Problems," and Chapter 80, "Pediatric Dehydration"

Diarrhea in Acquired Immunodeficiency Syndrome

- Diarrhea is the most common complication, affecting half of all patients with AIDS.
- Most of these infections occur as opportunistic infections and include viral, mycobacterial, parasitic, and fungal infections (see Chapter 37).

Teaching Points

Diarrhea is a very common complaint. Most of the time it will represent a self limited viral infection, but it is not rare to see bacterial infections. Blood in the stool can help distinguish bacterial from a viral enteritis.

Any cause of diarrhea can produce significant dehydration, and any patient with moderate or severe dehydration should be treated with IV fluids. Most of these patients will require admission, whereas the ones with mild dehydration can be rehydrated, usually with oral fluids if they are not vomiting.

Unfortunately, diarrhea can also be the presenting complaint of a number of serious diseases such as mesenteric ischemic vascular bowel disease, or inflammatory bowel disease. Most of these diseases will have in common the presence of blood in the stool, additional signs which need to be investigated, and most of these patients will require admission.

Suggested Readings

Cheung O, Reguiero MD. Inflammatory bowel disease emergencies. Gastroenterol Clin North Am 2003;32:1269–1288.

Gore JI, Surawicz C. Severe acute diarrhea. Gastroenterol Clin North Am 2003;32:1249-1267.

Kroser J, Metz D. Evaluation of the adult patient with diarrhea. Gastroenterology 1996;23:629–647.

Mitra A, Hernandez CD, Hernandez CA, Siddiq Z. Management of diarrhea in HIV-infected patients. Int J STD AIDS 2001;12:630–639.

Schiller LR, Sellin JH. Diarrhea. In: Feldman M, Tschumy Jr. WO, Friedman LS, Sleisenger MH (editors). Sleisenger and Fordtran's Gastrointestinal and Liver Disease (7th ed). Philadelphia: Elsevier, 2002, pp 131–150.

Somers SC, Lembo A. Irritable bowel syndrome: evaluation and treatment. Gastroenterol Clin North Am 2003;32:507–529.

CHAPTER 28

Dysphagia

GRIFFIN L. DAVIS

Red Flags

Extremes of age • Abnormal vital signs (high fever, ↑ heart rate, ↓ blood pressure) • Signs of dehydration • Signs of respiratory compromise • Weakness • Signs of neurologic dysfunction

Overview

Look for "red flags" (see Box) first in any patient presenting with dysphagia. These patients should be rapidly assessed and evaluated. Special consideration should be given to the immunocompromised, the elderly, and very young patients.

Dysphagia is any difficulty or disruption in the swallowing process, or delay in passage of liquids or solids from the mouth to the stomach. The problem usually involves the muscles of the oropharynx, the upper esophageal sphincter, the body of the esophagus, or the lower esophageal sphincter. Patients usually complain of difficulty with food passing from the mouth to the stomach or a feeling that the food gets "stuck" somewhere in this process. It is more common among elderly patients, and affects as many as 10% of people older than 50.

Odynophagia is a term used to describe "pain" with swallowing. Any inflammatory process involving the mucosa of the oropharynx or esophagus or its muscle may cause odynophagia.

Aspiration may complicate dysphagia in as many as 75% of cases, and may lead to pneumonia.

Differential Diagnosis of Dysphagia

- The causes of dysphagia can be classified into two distinct types: oropharyngeal and esophageal (see DDx table).
- Oropharyngeal, or transfer dysphagia, results from dysfunction of the oropharyngeal swallowing mechanism or the perception that once swallowing starts, the passage of the bolus is impeded.
- Esophageal dysphagia is caused by disorders affecting the esophagus itself, and stems from one of a variety of disorders that affect the esophageal

DDx Differential Diagnosis of Dysphagia

Oropharyngeal	Neurologic and neuromuscular	Cerebrovascular accident (56) Parkinson's disease Bulbar paralysis or peripheral neuropathies: poliomyelitis, botulism (67), diphtheria (55), amyotrophic lateral sclerosis (60), brainstem tumors, diabetes (38) Tetanus (67) Multiple sclerosis (60) Myasthenia gravis (60)
	Mechanical obstruction	Anaphylaxis (19) Mass or neoplasm Zenker's diverticulum Cervical osteophyte Thyromegaly
	Skeletal muscle disorder	Polymyositis (71) Myopathy (60)
	Miscellaneous	Decreased saliva (medications, Sjögren's syndrome) Alzheimer's disease Oropharyngeal inflammation or infection: pharyngitis (55), glossitis, stomatitis, abscess Medication side effects (mucositis with chemotherapy and neuroleptic malignant syndrome) Hysteria: globus hystericus
Esophageal	Motility disorder	Achalasia Spastic motility disorder Amyloidosis Scleroderma (71) Chaga's disease
	Mechanical obstruction	Esophageal stricture Foreign body (33) Webs and rings (Schatzki) Esophageal spasm Diverticulum Neoplasm (esophageal or external compression from other lymphoma or mediastinal tumor) Aberrant subclavian artery (dysphagia lusoria) Enlarged aorta or thyroid
	Esophagitis	Gastroesophageal reflux disease (18), infection such as human immunodeficiency virus–related (37), pills, caustic ingestion, radiation

( ) Refers to the chapter in which the disease entity is discussed.

body. Both mechanical obstructing lesions and motility disorders can lead to esophageal dysphagia.

Initial Diagnostic Approach
General

- As always, the ABCs (*a*irway, *b*reathing, and *c*irculation) should be assessed. Intravenous (IV) access, pulse oximetry, and continuous cardiac monitoring should be rapidly established for any patient who is ill appearing.
- Most causes of dysphagia can be determined based solely on the history. It is important to elicit specific details of dysphagia. If an esophageal foreign body is suspected (Chapter 33), where does the patient perceive that the bolus gets stuck, and where does the patient perceive pain? Is the dysphagia intermittent or progressive? What is the duration of symptoms? Do liquids, solids or both cause the symptoms? Are there associated symptoms such as pain, neurologic deficit, difficulty breathing, or weight loss?
- During the physical examination, look for any signs of infection or airway compromise. Perform a thorough neurologic examination, including cranial nerves, to rule out a stroke or peripheral neuropathy.
- It is useful to make a clinical assessment of the degree of dehydration or malnutrition associated with the dysphagia. Patients with complete aphagia should be admitted.

Laboratory

- Laboratory testing is usually not helpful.

EKG

- An electrocardiogram (EKG) should be performed especially in the older patient whose symptoms may represent ischemic cardiac disease.

Radiography

- A barium swallow study is often the first step in evaluating dysphagia. It is very useful in identifying intrinsic and extrinsic structural lesions.
- Plain radiographs (soft-tissue lateral of the neck or chest radiograph) should be done if concerned for a mass compressing the esophagus.
- Computed tomography (CT scan) of the head should be performed if there is concern for an acute cerebrovascular event. A CT scan of the neck or chest can further delineate a mass lesion in these areas.

Other Studies (Not Typically Performed in the Emergency Department)

- Endoscopy provides the best assessment of esophageal mucosa. It is the best method for diagnostic accuracy and immediate treatment of many causes of dysphagia.
- Videofluoroscopy requires a team of a speech pathologist, otolaryngologist, and radiologist. It is best at identifying oropharyngeal swallowing difficulties.

■ Manometry assesses esophageal motor function and typically is only used if the barium swallow and endoscopy are normal.

Emergency Department Management Overview
General

■ The ABCs should be addressed as discussed in Section II.
■ Oxygen should be administered to patients with any appearance of significant illness.

Medications

■ *Analgesia.* Administer nonsteroidal anti-inflammatory drugs (NSAIDs) or narcotic medication as necessary (see Chapter 90.1).
■ *Antacids.* Proton-pump inhibitors may help dysphagia that is secondary to gastroesaphageal reflux disease or GERD (see Chapter 90.4).
■ *Muscle relaxants.* Glucagon 1 mg IV can be administered to patients who experience complete esophageal obstruction secondary to food impaction (Chapter 33). Allow at least 20 minutes for effect. It works best when the obstructing bolus is in the mid to lower esophagus because it is a smooth muscle dilator, and will not help relax striated muscle. The upper third of the esophagus is predominantly striated muscle, with a transition to smooth muscle at the level of the middle third of the esophagus.

Emergency Department Interventions

■ Maintain hydration of the patient and monitor for airway compromise.

Disposition

■ The disposition includes treatment of the underlying cause (e.g., neurologic disease or infection), or urgent referral to the specialty most appropriate for the patient's etiology of dysphagia. Most of these patients will require referral to gastroenterology for diagnostic evaluation and management. Endoscopy by a gastroenterologist may need to be performed in the ED for foreign body removal if no relief from glucagon.

Specific Problems
Esophageal Cancer

■ *Epidemiology and risk factors.* Smoking, family history, alcohol use, and GERD are the most common risk factors.
■ *Pathophysiology.* A squamous cell carcinoma is the cell type in 95% of cases worldwide, but adenocarcinoma is increasing in incidence in the United States. In GERD, there is replacement of the normal stratified squamous epithelium with metaplastic columnar epithelium in a condition known as Barrett's metaplasia. There is a strong correlation between the development of Barrett's metaplasia and adenocarcinoma of the esophagus.

- ■ *History.* This history usually reveals dysphagia that is progressive and associated with anemia and weight loss. Pain and hoarseness may be signs of advanced disease.
- ■ *Examination.* Any physical findings may represent metastasis or perforation.
- ■ *Diagnostic testing.* A barium swallow is a very accurate imaging study to detect esophageal cancer. Endoscopy allows an accurate diagnosis because a biopsy of the tumor can be performed.
- ■ *ED management.* The patient will need tertiary care referral. ED treatment is focused on hydration, pain relief, symptom control, and appropriate follow-up. Admission is indicated for complications such as perforation, mediastinitis, dehydration and cachexia, pain control, sepsis, or aphagia. Most patients will require surgery, chemotherapy, and radiation, but the 5-year survival rate remains low.
- ■ *Helpful hints and pitfalls.* Barrett's esophagus from prolonged exposure to reflux may be a precursor in cases of adenocarcinoma.

Motility Disturbance

- ■ *Definitions. Achalasia* is caused by the inability of the lower esophageal sphincter to relax causing a functional obstruction. *Diffuse esophageal spasm* is caused by an inability of the entire esophagus to relax causing obstruction.
- ■ *Epidemiology and risk factors.* These occur equally in men and women, and usually occur between 25 and 60 years of age.
- ■ *Pathophysiology.* The underlying mechanism is unknown.
- ■ *History.* The dysphagia is usually intermittent, and may be associated with heartburn and weight loss.
- ■ *Physical examination.* There are no physical findings.
- ■ *Diagnostic testing.* A barium swallow is a very useful imaging test. It shows a bird's beak appearance with a dilated proximal esophagus. Manometry is useful to demonstrate high resting lower esophageal sphincter pressures
- ■ *ED management.* Calcium channel blockers and beta-blockers help in a small percentage of cases. Appropriate tertiary care referral is necessary. Some patients will require treatment and admission for dehydration or inanition.
- ■ *Helpful hints and pitfalls.* Endoscopy is performed diagnostically to rule out other etiologies, and therapeutically to dilate the sphincter. Because many of these patients are elderly, they may have concomitant cardiac disease that is missed because they have known achalasia, and their symptoms are misinterpreted as esophageal rather than cardiac.

Special Considerations
Pediatrics

- ■ Although achalasia can occur in children, it is usually seen in infants. Remember that children explore the world with their mouths, and foreign body ingestion is always a possibility (Chapter 33).

Elderly

■ These patients represent the largest group of patients with dysphagia that may be secondary to other conditions.

The Immunocompromised Patient

■ Look for consider infectious etiologies such as esophagitis in this population.

Teaching Points

Dysphagia is a common symptom usually relating to diseases of the esophagus. It can be seen at any age, but is most common in older patients. It may signify a chronic problem with acid reflux from the stomach, but it can also be a signal that there is major disease present within the esophagus. Unfortunately, there are almost no physical signs that can help distinguish any of the esophageal diseases, and it will require an imaging study, and often an esophagoscopy.

The principle concern is that serious problems such as ischemic cardiac disease can coexist or cause identical symptoms to esophageal reflux disease. It can be difficult or impossible to distinguish the two in the ED. Dysphagia may also be one of the initial presenting symptoms of a patient with a neurologic syndrome. When in doubt, it is safest to initiate the workup and management of the patient in the ED to avoid the risk of missing a potentially life-threatening diagnosis.

Suggested Readings

Leslie P, Carding PN, Wilson, JA. Investigation and management of chronic dysphagia. BMJ 2003:326;433–436.

Lowel M. Espophagus, stomach, and duodenum. In: Marx JA, Hockberger RS, Walls RM (editors). Rosen's Emergency Medicine: Concepts and Clinical Practice (6th ed). Philadelphia: Mosby, 2006: pp 1382–1401.

Owen W. ABC of the upper gastrointestinal tract: dysphagia. BMJ 2001;323;850–853.

Siddiq MA, Sood S, Strachan D. Pharyngeal pouch (Zenker's diverticulum). Postgrad Med J 2001:77;506–511.

Spieker MR. Evaluating dysphagia. Am Fam Physician 2000:61;3639–3648.

Wong P. Esophageal webs and rings. eMedicine Journal[serial online]. Last updated June 7, 2005. Available at *http://www.emedicine.com/med/topic3413.htm.*

CHAPTER 29

Edema

JULIE A. ZELLER ■ LAURA MACNOW

 Red Flags

History of hypercoagulable state, malignancy, contraceptive use, previous DVT or PE, trauma, or recent surgery ● Severe pain ● Pain out of proportion to examination ● Dyspnea ● Chest pain ● Fever ● Tachycardia ● Tachypnea ● Hypotension ● Hypoxia ● Pulseless or cool extremity ● Hemorrhagic bullae

Overview

Edema is most often a symptom of another clinical condition. It may be generalized or focal. Edema may be the initial complaint of a patient with congestive heart failure, liver failure, renal failure, lymphedema, deep venous thrombosis, trauma, infection, allergic reaction, or vascular insufficiency.

Some of these patients can be quite ill. The emergency physician should always check for "red flags" when evaluating the patient presenting with edema (see Box).

Differential Diagnosis of Edema

See DDx table for nonfocal and focal causes of edema.

Initial Diagnostic Approach
General

- Any patient who is in respiratory distress, hemodynamically unstable, or appears ill should receive immediate attention with priority given to the ABCs (*a*irway, *b*reathing, and *c*irculation). While the physician is assessing the patient, a continuous cardiac monitor and pulse oximeter should be placed. Intravenous (IV) access should be obtained.
- Obtain a complete history, including the time of onset, history of trauma, underlying medical conditions (such as congestive heart failure [CHF] or liver failure), medications (such as angiotensin-converting enzyme [ACE] inhibitors, which may cause angioedema), and associated symptoms (such

DDx Differential Diagnosis of Edema	
Nonfocal	**Focal**
Congestive heart failure (52)	Deep venous thrombosis
Cirrhosis (41)	Superficial thrombophlebitis
Renal failure (49)	Cellulitis (54)
Nephrotic syndrome	Lymphangitis
Acute nephritic syndrome	Allergic reaction (19)
Myxedema (63)	Ruptured Baker's cyst
Pregnancy	Hematoma
Medications (vasodilators, NSAIDs)	Abscess (54)
Superior vena cava syndrome	Muscle or soft tissue injury
Idiopathic	Necrotizing fasciitis (54)
	Compartment syndrome (17)
	Venous stasis

as pain, paresthesias, fever, or shortness of breath). The characteristics of urine output (color and quantity) should also be ascertained. Women should be questioned about the possibility of pregnancy.

■ The physical examination should include characteristics and extent of edema, evidence of liver failure or congestive heart failure, and the integrity of circulation in the affected extremities.

■ When considering arterial versus venous insufficiency of an extremity, note that arterial insufficiency is usually worse with walking, and worse when the legs are elevated. Cold tends to aggravate the symptoms, whereas warmth tends to relieve them, and compression stockings usually aggravate the pain. The opposite is true in venous insufficiency. In both cases peripheral pulses may be difficult to palpate. In addition to carefully documenting pulses, ankle-brachial indices (ABIs) are helpful to evaluate the extent of vascular insufficiency from arteriosclerosis. (See Appendix 2 for ABI measurements.)

Laboratory

■ Laboratory testing should be tailored to the individual patient and history. For example, patients with signs of acute CHF should have complete blood count (CBC), electrolytes, cardiac enzymes drawn, and perhaps a brain natriuretic peptide or BNP (see Chapter 52). Patients with liver disease should have liver function tests, electrolytes, and coagulation studies sent. Blood cultures should be considered for any patient with edema associated with cellulitis and systemic signs or symptoms of infection. A CBC and coagulation studies with an international normalized ratio (INR) should be ordered in any patient who is going to be started on anticoagulation therapy.

■ D-dimer levels may be elevated in any medical condition that causes clotting of the blood. Unfortunately, the D-dimer test is positive in many conditions other than DVT. It can be elevated in trauma, recent surgery, hemorrhage, cancer, and sepsis. D-dimer levels remain elevated in DVT for about 7 days.

EKG

- An electrocardiogram (EKG) should be ordered for any patient with dyspnea in the setting of edema.

Radiography

- ***Chest radiograph.*** Any patient with dyspnea in the setting of edema, cough, or a history of CHF or other cardiac history should also have a chest radiograph.
- ***Extremity radiograph.*** Obtain a radiograph of the extremity with edema in the setting of trauma, extensive infection, or ulceration to examine for fracture, foreign body, osteomyelitis, or subcutaneous air in necrotizing fasciitis.
- ***Duplex ultrasonography.*** An ultrasound study (US) should be obtained in the evaluation of extremity edema for DVT. It may also be used in the case of a large abscess to help determine the depth of the cavity.

Emergency Department Management Overview
General

- The ABCs should be addressed as discussed in Section II.

Medications

- ***Diuretics.*** These drugs are essential therapy in patients with acute dyspnea thought to be related to CHF. Beware of worsening renal function with over diuresis.
- ***Analgesia.*** Pain management should be addressed in all patients. Avoid nonsteroidal anti-inflammatory drugs (NSAIDs) in patients with renal failure. Narcotic analgesics are indicated for patients with moderate to severe pain (see Chapter 90.1).
- ***Anticoagulation.*** If the diagnosis of DVT is confirmed, heparin (or low-molecular-weight heparin) should be started while loading oral warfarin (Coumadin) therapy.
- ***Antibiotics.*** Empiric antibiotics should be started in the ED if concerned for an infection, such as cellulitis.

Emergency Department Interventions

- Therapeutic paracentesis in a patient with cirrhosis and ascites (see Chapter 91).

Disposition

- ***Consultation.*** Consult a surgeon emergently for any patient with surgical disease such as necrotizing fasciitis or acute vascular occlusion.
- ***Admission.*** Many problems with acute edema will require admission, whereas many problems that produce chronic edema can be safely managed in the outpatient setting. Patients who are immunocompromised, elderly, noncompliant, have suspected pulmonary embolism,

other significant co-morbidities, or a poor social situation should be admitted to the hospital.

- *Discharge.* Patients who are discharged must have a clear follow-up plan in place, understand how to use their medications, and know what signs or symptoms should prompt return to the ED for evaluation.

Specific Problems: Nonfocal Edema
Nephritic Syndrome

- *Definition.* Acute glomerulonephritis (AGN) is a clinical syndrome that frequently manifests as a sudden onset of hematuria, proteinuria, and red cell casts. This clinical picture often is accompanied by hypertension, edema, and impaired renal function.
- *Epidemiology and risk factors.* Most cases occur in patients aged 5 to 15 years. Cases of acute nephritis may progress to a chronic form.
- *Pathophysiology.* Glomerular lesions in AGN are the result of glomerular deposition or in situ formation of immune complexes. There are three broad categories of AGN: postinfectious, renal (idiopathic), and systemic diseases such as lupus, Wegener's granulomatosis, and Goodpasture's syndrome. Poststreptococcal AGN is one of the most common causes and has a peak incidence between the ages of 2 and 6 years.
- *History.* Symptom onset usually is abrupt, and the patient may have nonspecific symptoms, including weakness, fever, abdominal pain, and malaise. In the setting of postinfectious acute nephritis, a latent period of up to 3 weeks occurs before onset of symptoms. The onset of nephritis within 1 to 4 days of streptococcal infection suggests preexisting renal disease. Systemic nephritis can be distinguished by other associated findings in the history. Hemoptysis occurs with a Goodpasture's syndrome or idiopathic progressive glomerulonephritis. The triad of sinusitis, pulmonary infiltrates, and nephritis defines a Wegener's granulomatosis. Skin rashes occur with hypersensitivity vasculitis, systemic lupus erythematosus (SLE), and perhaps due to the purpura that can occur in hypersensitivity vasculitis, cryoglobulinemia, and Henoch-Schönlein purpura (HSP).
- *Physical examination.* Most commonly, patients have noticeable edema, frequently including the face, specifically the periorbital area. Hypertension is found in as many as 80% of patients in all populations affected. Patients may have gross hematuria, skin rashes, and abnormal neurologic examination or an altered level of consciousness, occurring because of malignant hypertension or hypertensive encephalopathy.
- *Diagnostic testing.* Laboratory and radiologic imaging is similar to that for nephrotic syndrome.
- *ED management.* The ED treatment is etiology dependent. In poststreptococcal AGN, oral antibiotic therapy may be initiated. Penicillin is indicated in nonallergic patients. Note that early antibiotic therapy in streptococcal infections does not prevent the development of poststreptococcal glomerulonephritis. Fluids should be restricted in patients with singnificant edema. Admission is recommended for patients with anuria, oliguria, renal failure, massive proteinuria, significant hypertension, or pulmonary symptoms. Patients with severe hypertension associated with signs of cerebral dysfunction require immediate

aggressive treatment. Useful agents to treat hypertension include diuretics (if edema is present), hydralazine, nitroprusside, and labetolol. Steroids and cytotoxic agents may be indicated in nonstreptococcal glomerulonephritis secondary to hypersensitivity, HSP, lupus, Wegener's, Goodpasture's, or idiopathic AGN. Nephrology may need to be consulted immediately for dialysis of the rare oliguric patient.

- *Helpful hints and pitfalls.* Be cautious in attributing hematuria to a simple urinary tract infection, and always consider the possibility of AGN.

Nephrotic Syndrome

- *Definition.* Nephrotic syndrome is not a disease but an edematous clinical condition characterized by the triad of proteinuria (greater than 40 mg/m^2/d or urine dipstick result showing more than 2+ protein), hypoalbuminemia (usually less than 2.5 g/dl), and hypercholesterolemia.
- *Epidemiology and risk factors.* Most cases of primary nephrotic syndrome occur in children, and are due to minimal-change disease. In adults, the most common form of glomerulopathy causing nephrotic syndrome is membranous glomerulonephritis, followed by focal segmental glomerulosclerosis. In many areas, diabetic nephropathy is emerging as a major cause of nephrotic syndrome. Risk factors include infection (group A beta-hemolytic streptococcus or viral infections including varicella and Epstein-Barr virus [EBV]), underlying collagen vascular diseases (lupus and rheumatoid arthritis), sickle cell disease, diabetes, malignancy, and medications including angiotensin-converting enzyme (ACE) inhibitors, lithium, and warfarin.
- *Pathophysiology.* There is an increase in permeability of the glomerular capillary wall, which leads to massive proteinuria and hypoalbuminemia. The cause of the increased permeability is not well understood. High glomerular permeability leads to hyperalbuminuria, and, eventually, to hypoalbuminemia. In turn, hypoalbuminemia lowers the plasma colloid osmotic pressure, causing greater transcapillary filtration of water and the development of edema.
- *History.* The first sign in children is usually swelling of the face; periorbital edema is a common presentation, followed by swelling of the entire body. Adults more often have edema of dependent parts. In most cases, this includes the ankles or legs. Patients may also complain of lethargy, poor appetite, weakness, occasional abdominal pain, decreased urine output, and frothy urine.
- *Physical examination.* Edema is the predominant feature.
- *Diagnostic testing.* The amount of protein in a random urine sample usually exceeds 100 mg/dL; values as high as 1000 mg/L are common. Hematuria may be present. The serum albumin is less than 2.5 g/dL. Hyperlipidemia correlates inversely with the concentrations of serum albumin. Renal function may be normal but there may be a moderate rise of serum creatinine. The hemoglobin and hematocrit may be increased due to the contracted plasma volume. Elevated white blood cell counts are occasionally seen even in the absence of infections. Hyponatremia and reduced serum osmolality are common but are usually factitious

because of hyperlipidemia. Hypocalcemia is common but the ionized serum calcium is in the normal to low-normal range. Serum levels of complement are usually normal except in those patients with membranoproliferative glomerulonephritis (MPGN). All patients should have a chest radiograph to look for a pleural effusion or pulmonary edema.

- *ED management.* Four major problems exist in newly diagnosed patients with nephrotic syndrome: edema, relative hypovolemia, infection, and thrombotic phenomena. Although the patient is edematous, tachycardia and hypotension should be quickly treated with aggressive fluid hydration. The cornerstone of treatment of nephrotic syndrome is high-dose corticosteroid therapy (2 mg/kg/d for the first 4 to 6 weeks). However, most adults with idiopathic nephrotic syndrome do not respond to corticosteroid therapy. Contraindications include active bacterial infection or a positive result on a PPD test. Patients with a new diagnosis should be admitted to the hospital, as should any child older than 6 years or those with hypertension, hematuria, or evidence of impaired renal function.

- *Helpful hints and pitfalls.* Patients with nephrotic syndrome are at risk for thrombosis. Renal vein thrombosis should be suspected in a patient with acute flank pain, renal enlargement, hematuria, and unexplained deterioration in renal function. Hyponatremia in nephrotic syndrome should not be too aggressively corrected. Any fever or infection should be treated aggressively in these patients because they are relatively immunocompromised, even before steroid therapy is initiated.

Superior Vena Cava Syndrome

- *Definition.* Superior vena cava syndrome (SVCS) is characterized by gradual, insidious compression or obstruction of the superior vena cava (SVC).
- *Epidemiology and risk factors.* The SVCS is most commonly associated with malignancy. More than 90% of patients with a SVCS have an associated malignancy as the cause. Bronchogenic carcinoma accounts for more than 80% of cases of SVCS. Of the nonmalignant causes of SVCS, thrombosis from central venous instrumentation (catheter, pacemaker, guide wire) is an increasingly common event.
- *Pathophysiology.* The subsequent obstruction to flow causes an increased venous pressure, which results in interstitial edema and retrograde collateral flow.
- *History.* In the early clinical course, few, if any, signs or symptoms of SVCS may be manifested. Typically, symptoms accelerate as the underlying malignancy increases in size or invasiveness. Dyspnea is the most common symptom, followed by trunk or extremity swelling. Other symptoms include facial swelling, cough, orthopnea, headache, nasal congestion, and light-headedness.
- *Physical examination.* This often reveals facial or upper extremity edema. The degree of jugular venous distention is variable. Other markers of lung malignancy, such as a Horner's syndrome or paralysis of the vocal cords or phrenic nerve are rarely present.

■ *Diagnostic testing.* The diagnosis of SVCS is often made on clinical grounds alone, combining clinical presentation with a history of thoracic malignancy. A chest radiograph should be performed followed by computed tomography (CT scan) of the thorax, especially to search for thrombus formation.

■ *ED management.* Attention to the ABCs is essential. Patients should be positioned upright to help provide relief of the dyspnea. The airway should be stabilized as needed, and steroids given if airway compromise is present. Diuretics have not shown consistent benefit in the ED. Emergent consultation for radiation treatment may be necessary, depending on the acuteness of the presentation. Because most causes of SVCS are related to bronchogenic carcinoma, a pulmonary consultation is useful.

■ *Helpful hints and pitfalls.* In patients in whom the diagnosis of lung cancer is not known, the most common mistake by the care provider is not appreciating the subtle swelling (or not believing the patient's complaints of bilateral arm swelling, facial fullness, and related symptoms) as a possible SVCS.

Specific Problems: Focal Edema
Deep Vein Thrombosis

■ *Definition.* DVT refers to a blood clot in one of the major deep veins of the lower legs, thighs, or pelvis. This blockage can cause pain, swelling, or warmth in the affected leg.

■ *Epidemiology and risk factors.* Death from DVT is attributed to massive pulmonary embolism. Multiple risk factors exist and are listed in Table 29–1.

■ *Pathophysiology.* One or more elements of Virchow's triad (venous stasis, vessel wall injury, and hypercoagulable state) causes coagulation in areas of reduced blood flow. A DVT of the lower extremity usually begins in the deep veins of the calf around the valve cusps or within the soleal plexus. The vast majority of calf vein thrombi dissolve completely

Table 29–1 Risk Factors for Development of Deep Vein Thrombosis (DVT)

General	Medical	Other
Age	Cancer	Trauma including
Immobilization longer than 3 days	Previous DVT	the spinal cord or lower extremity
	Stroke	fractures
Pregnancy and the postpartum period	Acute myocardial infarction (AMI)	IV drug use
Major surgery in previous 4 weeks	Congestive heart failure (CHF)	Oral contraceptives or estrogen
	Sepsis	
Long plane or car trips (>4 h) in previous 4 weeks	Nephrotic syndrome	
	Ulcerative colitis	
	Hematologic disorders such as protein c or protein s deficiency, Factor V Leiden, antithrombin III deficiency	

without therapy. Approximately 20% propagate proximally. Propagation usually occurs before embolization.

■ *History*. Patients may complain of pain and swelling. In addition, some complain of erythema of the involved extremity. Chest pain and shortness of breath may be present if there is embolization to the lungs.

■ *Physical examination.* This may demonstrate unilateral edema, warmth, erythema, or tenderness on palpation. Massive edema with cyanosis and ischemia (phlegmasia cerulea dolens) is rare. A palpable cord may be present. The presence or absence of pain on dorsiflexion of the foot (Homan's sign) is not a reliable test to rule in or exclude DVT.

■ *Diagnostic testing.* The Well's clinical prediction guide quantifies the pretest probability of DVT. The model enables physicians to stratify a patient into high-, moderate-, or low-risk categories. Combining this with the results of objective testing simplifies the clinical workup of patients with suspected DVT. In patients with no identified risk factors, DVT is confirmed in only 11%. In patients with three risk factors, the number rises to 50% (Table 29–2). The diagnosis of DVT is established with duplex ultrasonography. The major ultrasonographic criterion for detecting venous thrombosis is inability to compress the vascular lumen, presumably because of the presence of occluding thrombus. The absence of the normal phasic Doppler signals arising from the changes to venous flow provides indirect evidence of venous occlusion. If a D-dimer is obtained, the results should be used as follows: (a) negative D-dimer result rules out DVT in the unlikely group (low-to-moderate risk of DVT); (b) all patients with a positive D-dimer result and all patients in the likely group (moderate-to-high risk of DVT) require an ultrasound study. Patients with the clinical appearance of a DVT and negative findings on the initial noninvasive study must be reassessed by their

Table 29–2   Well's Clinical Score for Deep Vein Thrombosis (DVT)*

Clinical Parameter Score	Score
Active cancer (treatment ongoing, or within 6 months or palliative)	+1
Paralysis or recent plaster immobilization of the lower extremities	+1
Recently bedridden for >3 d or major surgery <4 wk	+1
Localized tenderness along the distribution of the deep venous system	+1
Entire leg swelling	+1
Calf swelling >3 cm compared to the asymptomatic leg	+1
Pitting edema (greater in the symptomatic leg)	+1
Previous DVT documented	+1
Collateral superficial veins (nonvaricose)	+1
Alternative diagnosis (as likely or > that of DVT)	-2
Total of Above Score	
High probability	>3
Moderate probability	1 or 2
Low probability	<0

*Adapted from Anand SS, Wells PS, Hunt D, et al. Does this patient have deep vein thrombosis? JAMA. 1998 Apr 8;279:1094–9.

primary care providers or return to the ED in 24-48 hours for a repeated ultrasound study.

- **ED management.** Anticoagulation is the preferred treatment, and can prevent thrombus propagation, thus reducing the size and frequency of emboli. The initial dose for unfractionated heparin is 80 U/kg (about 7000 units for a 70-kg patient) with a maintenance infusion of 18 U/kg/h. The partial thromboplastin time (PTT) should be monitored at 6 hours after each change of therapy with a target of at least 1.5 times the control value. Low-molecular weight heparin (LMWH) should be used if possible. The dose is 1-mg/kg subcutaneous (SC) injection twice daily or 1.5 mg/kg SC injection daily. The optimal regimen for the treatment of DVT is anticoagulation with LMWH followed by full anticoagulation with oral warfarin for 3 to 6 months. Warfarin therapy 5 mg by mouth (PO) is overlapped with LMWH for 5 days until the INR is therapeutically elevated to 2 to 3 because of the initial transient hypercoagulable state induced by warfarin. Most patients with confirmed proximal vein DVT may be safely treated on an outpatient basis. Table 29–3 lists exclusion criteria for outpatient management.
- **Helpful hints and pitfalls.** Patients should have repeated noninvasive studies and reassessment in high-risk patients with negative findings on initial evaluations because the initial studies may be falsely negative in the presence of a DVT.

Lymphangitis

- **Definition.** Lymphangitis is defined as an inflammation of the lymphatic channels that occurs as a result of infection at a distal site.
- **Epidemiology and risk factors.** Although it may occur at any age, lymphangitis is much more common in children than adults. Risk factors include trauma, recent infection, or immunocompromise.
- **Pathophysiology.** Pathogenic organisms enter the lymphatic channels directly through an abrasion or wound or as a complication of infection. Once the organisms enter the channels, local inflammation and subsequent infection ensue, manifesting as red streaks on the skin. The inflammation or infection then extends proximally toward regional lymph nodes. In individuals with normal host defenses, group A beta-

Table 29–3 Exclusion Criteria for Outpatient Management of Deep Vein Thrombosis (DVT)

Suspected or proven concomitant pulmonary embolism
Significant cardiovascular or pulmonary comorbidity
Ileofemoral DVT
Contraindications to anticoagulation
Familial or inherited disorder of coagulation: ATIII, protein C or protein S deficiency, or factor V Leiden
Pregnancy
Morbid obesity
Renal failure
Inability to arrange close follow-up care

hemolytic streptococcal (GABHS) species are the most common causes of lymphangitis.

- *History.* Patients often have a history of a recent cut or abrasion that appears infected and spreading. They may complain of localized edema and erythema. Associated symptoms include fevers, chills, headache, anorexia, and malaise.
- *Physical examination.* Clinically, erythematous and irregular linear streaks extend from the primary infection site toward draining regional nodes. These streaks may be tender and warm. The primary site may be an abscess, an infected wound, or an area of cellulitis. Edema is also present. Lymph nodes associated with the infected lymphatic channels are often swollen and tender.
- *Diagnostic testing.* Any child who presents with lymphangitis should have a CBC, blood culture, and aspiration of the affected lymph node. A culture and a Gram's stain of a swab of the primary site of infection may help identify the infectious organism.
- *ED management.* Children in stable social situations who appear nontoxic, are older than 3 years, afebrile, and well hydrated may be treated initially with PO antibiotics on an outpatient basis. Analgesics can be used to control pain, and anti-inflammatory medications can help reduce inflammation and swelling. Hot, moist compresses also help reduce inflammation and pain. If possible, the affected extremity should be elevated to reduce swelling, pain, and the spread of infection.
- *Helpful hints and pitfalls.* Lymphangitis may spread within hours and bacteremia and sepsis can occur.

Ruptured Baker's Cyst

- *Definition.* A Baker's cyst, also called a *popliteal cyst*, is the most common mass in the popliteal fossa, and results from fluid distention of the gastrocnemiosemimembranosus bursa. The most common complication of a Baker's cyst is the rupture or dissection of fluid into the adjacent proximal gastrocnemius muscle belly, which results in a pseudo-thrombophlebitis syndrome mimicking symptoms of a DVT.
- *Epidemiology and risk factors.* Rupture of the cyst most often occurs spontaneously, and most patients will present with atraumatic leg pain and swelling.
- *Pathophysiology.* A Baker's cyst is a synovial cyst located posterior to the medial femoral condyle between the tendons of the medial head of the gastrocnemius and semimembranosus muscles. This usually communicates with the joint via a slitlike opening at the posteromedial aspect of the knee capsule just superior to the joint line. Idiopathic cysts usually are seen in young patients without symptoms. Cyst contents usually are viscous. Secondary or symptomatic cysts communicate freely with the knee joint and contain synovial fluid of normal viscosity. Secondary cysts are associated with underlying articular disorders including osteoarthritis, rheumatoid arthritis (RA), and psoriatic arthritis.
- *History.* The most common associated complaint is a popliteal mass or swelling (76% of patients). Other key points in the history may be posterior knee pain, swelling, or redness, or a buckling or locking sensation of the knee when trying to bear weight or walking.

- **Physical examination.** If the cyst has ruptured, the patient may have diffuse edema of the leg below the knee, pain on palpation of the calf, and difficulty walking secondary to pain.
- **Diagnostic testing.** On ultrasound, a simple Baker's cyst appears as an anechoic mass with posterior acoustic enhancement that communicates with the knee joint.
- **ED management.** Treatment of popliteal cysts is conservative, including NSAIDs, ice, and assisted weight bearing, in addition to correction of underlying intra-articular disorders as appropriate. Patients should follow up with their primary care provider, who may ultimately refer them to an orthopedist for surgical removal.
- **Helpful hints and pitfalls.** Rarely, dissection or rupture of a popliteal cyst can increase pressure within the deep posterior compartment of the leg, causing posterior compartment syndrome. It is prudent to perform a workup to diagnose or exclude a DVT, even in patients with a documented Baker's cyst.
- Venous insufficiency syndromes are caused by valvular incompetence in the high-pressure deep venous system, low-pressure superficial venous system, or both. Untreated venous insufficiency in the deep or superficial system causes a progressive syndrome involving pain, swelling, skin changes, and eventual tissue breakdown.

Teaching Points

Edema may be secondary to a focal or systemic disease process. The history is important to distinguish the underlying etiology and help define appropriate diagnosis and treatment.

Deep vein thrombosis is common but at times difficult to define. It must be distinguished from arterial disease, musculoskeletal trauma, or infection such as necrotizing fasciitis. Venous duplex ultrasonography is very helpful in confirming the diagnosis. If it is unavailable, it may be prudent to commence anticoagulation with low molecular weight heparin while the patient is transferred to a facility that has the diagnostic technology.

Suggested Readings

Anand SS, Wells PS, Hunt D, et al. Does this patient have deep vein thrombosis? JAMA 1998;279:1094–1099.

Cho S, Atwood JE. Peripheral edema. Am J Med 2002;113:580–586.

Lensing AW, Prins MH, Davidson BL, Hirsh J. Treatment of deep venous thrombosis with low-molecular-weight heparins. A meta-analysis. Arch Intern Med 1995;155:601–607.

O'Brien JG, Chennubhotla SA, Chennubhotla RV. Treatment of edema. Am Fam Physician 2005;71:2111–2117.

Wells PS, Anderson DR, Rodger M, et al. Evaluation of D-dimer in the diagnosis of suspected deep-vein thrombosis. N Engl J Med 2003;349:1227–1235.

CHAPTER 30

Facial Weakness

JAMES HWANG ■ KAMA Z. GULUMA

 Red Flags

Facial weakness that does not involve the forehead ● Altered mental status or other neurologic deficits ● Head or facial trauma ● Immunocompromised ● Fever ● Hypertension

Overview

Look for "red flags" (see Box) and consider critical diagnoses and life-threatening problems early. Upper motor neuron findings or concomitant neurologic deficits should prompt initiation of a stroke protocol.

Idiopathic peripheral facial palsy (Bell's palsy) is the most common cause of isolated facial weakness seen in the ED. Trauma is the second most common cause. Although less common, other causes of facial nerve paralysis such as infection must also be considered.

The facial nerve or cranial nerve (CN) VII originates from the pontomedullary junction of the brainstem, exits the brain stem at the cerebellopontine angle, and then enters the internal auditory canal with CN VIII (auditory nerve for hearing). CN VII has four major branches in the temporal bone: the greater and lesser petrosal nerves (through which it sends parasympathetic secretomotor fibers to the lacrimal glands), the nerve to the stapedius muscle, and the chorda tympani (through which it provides taste to the anterior two-thirds of the tongue and parasympathetic salivary stimuli to the submandibular, and sublingual glands). CN VII then exits the temporal bone at the stylomastoid foramen. Lastly, it enters the parotid gland, and divides to innervate the muscles of facial expression (frontalis, orbicularis oculi, buccinator, orbicularis oris, and platysma) and supply sensation to a part of the posterior external auditory meatus.

Bilateral facial paralysis is rare. The diseases most commonly associated with bilateral facial paralysis include Guillain-Barré, Bell's palsy, benign idiopathic hypertension, syphilis, leukemia, Lyme disease, sarcoidosis, bacterial meningitis and brainstem encephalitis.

Differential Diagnosis of Facial Weakness

- Ninety different conditions have been reported to cause facial weakness.
- Please see DDx table for a priority-based differential diagnosis list.

Initial Diagnostic Approach
General

- The approach to managing patients with facial weakness begins with a rapid assessment of the ABCs (*a*irway, *b*reathing, and *c*irculation), followed by determination of whether the etiology is upper motor neuron versus lower motor neuron in nature.
- The physical examination requires thorough ear, nose, and throat (ENT) and neurologic examinations with a specific focus on CN VII.
  - *Facial weakness with relative sparing of the forehead.* Implies a supranuclear upper motor neuron (UMN) lesion, due to the bilateral cortical innervation of the upper facial musculature.
  - *Facial weakness involving the forehead.* Implies a lower motor neuron (LMN) lesion at the facial nucleus or distally.

DDx Priority Based Differential Diagnosis of Facial Weakness

Critical Diagnoses	Emergent Diagnoses	Non-Emergent Diagnoses
Cerebrovascular event (56)	Facial or skull trauma (9, 10)	Bell's Palsy
Botulism (67)	Infectious	Hemifacial spasm
Iatrogenic during surgery	Lyme disease (67)	
	Ramsay-Hunt Syndrome	
	Otogenic infection/ mastoiditis (64)	
	Basilar meningitis (67)	
	Encephalitis (67)	
	Syphilis (67)	
	Ebstein-Barr virus	
	Cytomegalovirus	
	Kawasaki's disease (79)	
	HIV (37)	
	Autoimmune	
	Guillain-Barré (60)	
	Multiple Sclerosis (60)	
	Myasthenia Gravis (60)	
	Sarcoidosis	
	Malignancy	
	Benign intracranial hypertension (35)	
	Hyperglycemia (38)	

( ) Refers to the chapter in which the disease entily is discussed.

- *LMN weakness + hyperacusis + loss of taste, salivation, and lacrimation.* Implies a cerebellopontine angle or internal auditory meatus lesion.
- *LMN weakness + loss of taste and salivation only.* Implies a facial canal lesion.
- *LMN weakness only.* Implies a distal facial canal or mastoid lesion.
- *LMN weakness in a specific muscle group only.* Implies isolated involvement of a CN VII branch by a parotid gland or distal facial lesion.

Refer to Appendix 2 for evaluation of other cranial nerves.

Laboratory

- Studies ordered should be guided by the history and clinical examination. Patients with an infectious etiology may need Lyme titers, Monospot, rapid plasma reagin (RPR)/VDRL test, or cerebrospinal fluid (CSF) studies. Idiopathic facial weakness may require no laboratory studies at all.

Radiography

- *Plain films.* Plain skull films aid in visualization of extracranial structures only, but an air fluid level in the sphenoid sinus will indicate a basilar skull fracture that may explain the facial nerve injury. This is best seen on a lateral cervical spine study.
- *Computed tomography (CT scan).* A noncontrast enhanced brain CT scan is helpful in the evaluation of causes such as mass lesion, hemorrhage, or infarction. In cases of suspected skull base fracture, fine cuts through the temporal bones and skull base should be obtained, but are often hard to read and may reveal no more than the sphenoid air fluid level of the plain films.
- *Magnetic resonance imaging (MRI) with gadolinium.* This study can be difficult to obtain, but yields the most information regarding infectious, inflammatory, neoplastic, and ischemic causes of facial weakness. This is also the optimal study to demonstrate a cerebellopontine angle tumor.

Emergency Department Management Overview
General

- Address the ABC's for patients with a cerebrovascular accident (CVA) or head trauma, and for patients whose facial weakness represents a rapidly progressive polyneuropathy (e.g., myasthenia gravis, botulism) capable of affecting ventilatory function.

Medications

- *Antivirals.* These are often used in patients with amenable viral causes of facial weakness, such as a Ramsay-Hunt syndrome or Bell's palsy.

- **Steroids.** If the patient is seen early after the onset of the neurologic deficit, these are often used in infectious or inflammatory etiologies of facial weakness, such as Ramsay-Hunt syndrome, Bell's palsy, myasthenia gravis, and multiple sclerosis.
- **Other.** Medications such as analgesics and antibiotics should be given depending on the condition causing the paralysis.

Disposition

- **Consultation.** Consult neurology for patients with cerebral infarction or progressive neurologic syndromes, neurosurgery for patients with intracranial hemorrhage or central nervous system (CNS) tumors, head and neck surgery for penetrating injuries to the face, traumatic facial nerve injury in the ear canal, or facial tumors, and ophthalmology for patients with ocular complications.
- **Admission.** Admit patients with cerebral infarctions, intracranial bleeds, significant trauma or penetrating injuries to the face, or tumors that need prompt intervention. Admit patients who are at risk for ventilatory compromise or severe disability.
- **Discharge.** This is appropriate in stable patients with causes of weakness that are appropriately managed in the ED.

Specific Problems

Refer to the DDx table and specific problems below for reference to a discussion of problems in the differential not mentioned here. A few of these disease entities will briefly be discussed.

Autoimmune Causes of Facial Weakness (Chapter 60)

- Inflammatory demyelination and scarring of CNS corticobulbar tracts in multiple sclerosis (MS), diminution in the number of postsynaptic acetylcholine receptors at the neuromuscular junction in myasthenia gravis (MG), and autoimmune demyelination or axonal loss affecting cranial nerves in Miller-Fisher Syndrome (a descending peripheral neuropathy variant of Guillain-Barré Syndrome), may all result in a presentation with a primary symptom of facial weakness.
- The patient with MFS may have ophthalmoplegia, dyarthria, ataxia, and areflexia, with minimal if any limb weakness initially.

Cerebral Vascular Accidents (Chapter 56)

- On close examination, stroke patients with seemingly isolated facial weakness may have other concomitant neurologic deficits such as facial sensory loss, mild hemiparesis or sensory loss, dysarthria or aphasia, clumsiness, ataxia, nystagmus, or visual changes. Lesions involving the vertebrobasilar circulation are more likely to produce cranial nerve abnormalities.
- A central etiology of the facial weakness should be of concern if the forehead is intact. In contrast, Bell's palsy affects all branches of cranial nerve VII (i.e., the forehead is not spared).

Head and Face Trauma (Chapters 9 and 10)

■ After a Bell's palsy, the most common cause of facial paralysis is trauma. This includes basilar skull fractures, temporal bone fractures, and penetrating injuries to the face.
■ CN VII is the most commonly injured cranial nerve in head trauma.
■ Transection of CN VII results in an acute onset of symptoms whereas nerve edema typically presents with more of a delayed onset.
■ Findings consistent with CN VII transection require ENT consultation and possible surgical exploration.

Idiopathic Peripheral Facial Palsy (Bell's Palsy)

■ *Epidemiology and risk factors.* A Bell's palsy is the most likely cause of isolated facial weakness presenting to the ED. The prevalence is similar in men and women, and typically affects patients who are 30 to 50 years old. Bell's palsy affects the left or the right side of the face equally. About 60% of patients note a viral prodrome.
■ *Pathophysiology.* By definition, Bell's palsy is idiopathic, but there is evidence to suggest that viral infection with herpes simplex is a possible cause.
■ *History.* There is an acute onset of unilateral facial droop. Patients also complain of subjective facial numbness, tearing or dryness of the eye, ear pain or fullness, hyperacusis, or dysgeusia. Maximal deficit by 5 days is noted in almost all cases.
■ *Physical examination.* Patients will have facial weakness that involves the forehead. Patients may also have incomplete eyelid closure, drooling, or pocketing of food in the mouth. The Bell's phenomenon may also be present: an upward and outward rolling of the eye on attempted lid closure. Look for possible ocular complications (e.g., corneal abrasions or ulcers).
■ *Diagnostic testing.* No laboratory or imaging studies are indicated.
■ *ED management.* The goal of therapy is to educate the patient, and to decrease the inflammatory changes present in CN VII. Approximately 85% of patients have complete recovery. The degree of deficit correlates with the prognosis: patients with partial deficits (demyelinating injury that leads to a neurapraxia) usually have excellent results, whereas those with more severe symptoms (Wallerian degeneration in which part of the nerve dies off) have the poorest prognosis. Risk factors for poor outcomes include advanced age and slow recovery. For those with partial deficits, recovery usually begins within 2 weeks, and is usually complete at 2 to 3 months. For those with severe symptoms, recovery is slower because the nerve regenerates at a rate of 1 inch per month. Patients with axonal regeneration are at risk for aberrant reinnervation that may lead to crocodile tears and facial synkinesis (presence of both weakness and hyperkinesis). If there is to be maximum benefit from steroids, they need to be started within 24 hours of onset of symptoms. If started within 1 week of onset of symptoms, steroids may hasten recovery. Prednisone 60 mg orally may be given once a day for 5 to 7 days followed by a 5- to 7-day taper for a total of 10 to 14 days of therapy. Alternatively, prednisone 1 mg/kg/d for 7 to 10 days without a taper is also acceptable. For pediatric patients, the dose is 2 mg/kg/d. Acyclovir also needs to be started early in

the patient's course if it is going to improve functional nerve recovery. Acyclovir should be started within 3 to 7 days after symptom onset. The dose of acyclovir is 400 to 800 mg orally five times a day for 7 to 10 days. Valacyclovir (100 mg three times daily) and famciclovir (500 mg three times daily) are newer oral antiviral agents that have better oral absorption, are better tolerated, and good alternatives to acyclovir. Eye lubricants and covering are essential to prevent corneal dryness that can lead to ulceration and perforation of the globe. The goal of therapy is to keep the eye moist. Provide preservative-free artificial tears (flood the eye every hour while awake) and ointments (overnight). Patients should be referred to a neurologist for atypical or complicated cases. Refer to an ENT doctor to determine the need for additional therapy (e.g., surgical decompression). Ophthalmology referral should be done as needed.

- *Helpful hints and pitfalls.* A Bell's palsy is a diagnosis of exclusion. Immunosuppressed patients often have severe courses, and usually need to be admitted for IV antiviral treatment.

Lyme Disease (Chapter 67)

- CN VII is the most commonly affected cranial nerve and in endemic areas, up to 50% of facial weakness in children is secondary to Lyme disease (LD). Facial weakness is bilateral in up to one third of cases.
- CSF analysis in patients with isolated cranial nerve palsies usually reveals a lymphocytic pleocytosis that is similar to aseptic meningitis. Isolating the organism is often difficult, and serologic testing for antibodies is not always reliable. The diagnosis is frequently based on the history of a tick bite and characteristic clinical findings.
- Patients with cranial nerve palsies may require 3 to 4 weeks of an oral antibiotic such as doxycycline or amoxicillin.

Malignancies Resulting in Facial Weakness

- The following malignancies can cause facial weakness: facial nerve schwannomas, acoustic neuromas, meningiomas, parotid gland tumors (adenomas), metastatic lesions (from the breast, lung, ovarian, prostate, thyroid, kidney), and leukemia.
- Refer patients to the appropriate consultant depending on the type of malignancy involved. Although many tumors are benign, such as acoustic neuroma, they can become life-threatening by bulk alone, and can be very incapacitating as a result of pain and focal neurologic deficits.

Otogenic Infections and Mastoiditis (Chapter 64)

- Infectious processes affecting the auditory canal, the middle ear, and the mastoid prominence can result in damage to the facial nerve because of its anatomic proximity.
- Imaging with a contrast-enhanced CT scan or MRI will help delineate the underlying process.
- Consult ENT, because treatment of otogenic infections severe enough to cause facial weakness often requires myringotomy and IV antibiotics, as in the case of an acute suppurative process, or surgical debridement and

mastoidectomy, as in the case of a more indolent, invasive, or coalescing process.

Ramsay-Hunt Syndrome

- *Epidemiology and risk factors.* The frequency of herpes zoster in patients with facial weakness is approximately 6% to 12%. Women are affected slightly more often than men, and the overall incidence is higher in patients older than 50 years.
- *Pathophysiology.* Ramsay-Hunt Syndrome (RHS) is secondary to the activation of dormant varicella zoster virus (VZV) within the geniculate ganglion of the facial nerve. Activation of VZV leads to edema and degeneration of CNVII, which results in ipsilateral facial weakness and a ipsilateral zoster rash with characteristic vesicular lesions.
- *History.* There is often a viral prodrome, and the initial symptoms include pain in and around the ear. LMN facial weakness and herpes zoster rash typically develop approximately 7 days later. RHS can present as a cranial polyneuropathy. After CNVII, the most commonly involved cranial nerves, in order of frequency, are cranial nerves V, VIII, IX, and X. Tinnitus, hearing loss, and vertigo may also be present. The pain is almost always the first symptom, and can be intense. The correct diagnosis is usually dependant upon the appearance of the typical rash.
- *Physical examination.* The erythematous vesicular rash of RHS is typical of herpes zoster, and develops on or around the ear. The rash is classically in the ipsilateral external ear (zoster oticus), or vesicles may be seen on the hard palate. The distribution is dependent on the sensory ganglia involved. It can also involve the face, neck, shoulders, tongue, buccal mucosa, palate, and uvula.
- *ED management.* Inform the patient that the facial weakness will progress to a maximum by 10 to 20 days, and some degree of recovery will probably occur by 6 months. Complete recovery has been noted in 66% of patients with partial weakness, but in only 10% of patients with complete paralysis. In general, when compared with a Bell's palsy, the prognosis is poorer. Postherpetic neuralgia may develop, but usually not to a severe degree. Steroids, acyclovir, and eye care are used as in the treatment of a Bell's palsy.
- *Helpful hints and pitfalls.* A relatively hidden vesicular eruption in the external auditory canal may be the only evidence of rash in a patient with facial palsy due to RHS, and this location is very easy to miss. The absence of rash in the patient who presents with acute facial weakness does not rule out VZV reactivation. Furthermore the rash may appear up to 10 days after the weakness develops. Patients with HIV or immune compromise who have RHS often have a more serious course, and may require admission and IV antiviral therapy.

Special Considerations
Pediatrics

- Although meningitis and irritability are the most common neurologic complications of Kawasaki's disease, facial palsy has been reported. The paralysis is thought to be due to ischemia of the nerve secondary to arteritis.
- Management includes supportive care, including high-dose aspirin.

Pregnancy

- Bell's palsy occurs 3.3 times more frequently in pregnant women than in nonpregnant women. The pathogenesis is not completely understood. It occurs most commonly during the third trimester or immediately after delivery.
- Treatment is with prednisone, which poses minimal risk to the fetus.

HIV

- Acute facial palsy can be a direct result or secondary to an HIV infection (e.g., herpes zoster). In the later stages, facial nerve involvement may be related to immunodeficiency, resulting in cephalic herpes zoster or systemic lymphoma.
- The prognosis is similar to that of the general population.

Teaching Points

There are many different possible explanations for facial nerve weakness. The most frequent cause for a patient to present to the ED with this deficit is due to Bell's Palsy. The patient will have a peripheral nerve deficit of CNVII, flat expressionless facies on the involved side, and an inability to wrinkle the forehead on that side. If seen early on, the patient will benefit from steroids and antiviral agents. The patient is usually unable to close the eyelid completely, and this often requires special ophthalmologic management.

Immunosupressed patients will require admission for IV antiviral treatment.

The second most common cause is trauma. These nerves are less likely to be transected when the trauma is blunt, and the onset of dysfunction is delayed after the trauma.

Suggested Readings

Benecke Jr JE. Facial paralysis. Otolaryngol Clin North Am 2002;35:357–365.

Coyle PK, Schutzer SE. Neurologic aspects of Lyme disease. Med Clin North Am 2002;86:261–284.

Mattox DE. Clinical disorders of the facial nerve. In: Cummings, CW, Flint PW, Haughey BH, et al. Otolaryngology: Head and Neck Surgery (4th ed). Philadelphia: Elsevier, 2005, pp 3333–3353.

Furuta Y. Varicella-zoster virus reactivation is an important cause of acute peripheral facial paralysis in children. Pediatr Infect Dis J 2005;24:97–101.

Ho SY, Kveton JF. Acoustic neuroma: assessment and management. Otolaryngol Clin North Am 2002;35:393–404.

Pascuzzi RM. Peripheral neuropathies in clinical practice. Med Clin North Am 2003;87:697–724.

CHAPTER 31

Fever

JOSHUA M. COTT ■ DEBORAH GUTMAN

 Red Flags

Hypotension ● Extremes of age ● Headache ● Petechial rash
● Lower back pain ● Intravenous drug use ● Change in mental status
● Fever >41° C ● Weight loss ● Night sweats ● Travel ● Asplenia
● Immunocompromise ● Recent antibiotic use with question of partially
treated meningitis ● Sudden arrival of many patients with similar
complaints (bioweapons)

Overview

Fever is a common finding in patients seen in the ED. Always look
for "red flags" (see Box) and other primary complaints (DDx table) to
assist with prioritizing the diagnostic and management priorities in
these patients.

Young adults with fever usually have benign, self-limited causes. The
challenge is identifying the rare case of life-threatening infection, such
as meningococcemia or meningitis.

Elderly patients and those with chronic diseases are at a higher risk
for serious illness. Life-threatening infections are most commonly due
to sepsis, respiratory failure, or central nervous system infection.

Fever is defined as a core temperature above 38°C. Normal body
temperature can vary by as much as 0.5°C over the course of the day
in a healthy individual. The rectal temperature is the most accurate
and is usually 0.6°C higher than the oral reading, but patients with
exaggerated mouth breathing may have differences of up to 1.8°C.
Fever does not necessarily indicate infection. Evaluate for the other
causes described in this chapter.

Fever and hyperthermia are not synonymous. In a fever, the hypothalamic homeostatic set point is adjusted upward by circulating
pyrogens, and the body responds appropriately to this readjustment
by increasing temperature. In hyperthermia, the hypothalamic set
point remains normal, but the body temperature rises because of
exogenous or endogenous heat production. Hyperthermia represents
an inappropriate and uncontrolled increase in body temperature, so

the primary treatment goal must be to actively lower the patient's core temperature. It is frequently impossible to initially differentiate between fever and hyperthermia. Antipyretics reduce fever but not hyperthermia. In most adults, a temperature of greater than 41.5°C represents hyperthermia.

Fever of unknown origin (FUO) is a specific term that should be used appropriately to minimize confusion. The definition of FUO includes (a) temperature >38.3°C on several occasions; (b) duration of fever of at least 3 weeks, and (c) an uncertain diagnosis after 1 week in the hospital.

Drug fever is a term defined as a febrile response to drug administration. If recognized, the drug can be stopped, and a prolonged workup for fever can be avoided. It is only rarely possible to identify a drug fever in the ED, and so a fever workup is often necessary. Most drug fevers begin 1 to 2 weeks after initiation of therapy, but any time frame is possible. ED management consists of discontinuing the offending drug.

Pediatric fever is discussed in Chapter 79.

DDx Complaint Based List of Differential Diagnosis in Patients with Fever

Chief complaint	Disease
Headache (35)	Meningitis, encephalitis, brain abscess, intracranial hemorrhage, sinusitis, Rocky Mountain spotted fever (RMSF)
Altered mental status (20)	Meningitis, encephalitis, sepsis, urinary tract infection
Cough (24)	Pneumonia, influenza, active tuberculosis
Sore throat (55)	Peritonsillar abscess, retropharyngeal abscess, epiglottitis, mononucleosis, pharyngitis
Chest pain (22) or shortness of breath (52)	Pneumonia, pericarditis, pulmonary embolus, myocardial infarction
Back pain (21) or flank pain (32)	Epidural abscess, pyelonephritis
Abdominal (18) and pelvic pain (68)	Appendicitis, cholecystitis, diverticulitis, colitis, pancreatitis, inflammatory bowel disease, intra-abdominal abscess, peritonitis, tubo-ovarian abscess, pelvic inflammatory disease, cystitis
Joint pain (42)	Septic arthritis, disseminated gonococcemia, crystal arthritis, collagen-vascular diseases, serum sickness
Extremity pain (29,54,67)	Cellulitis, deep-tissue infections, deep venous thrombosis, osteomyelitis

DDx Complaint Based List of Differential Diagnosis in Patients with Fever—*cont'd*

Chief complaint	Disease
Rash (37, 62, 67, 79)	Meningococcemia, RMSF, measles, rubella, fifth disease, roseola , scarlet fever, Kawasaki disease, chicken pox, toxic shock syndrome, Lyme disease, erythema multiforme, erythema nodosum, secondary syphilis, shingles, rickettsia, acute HIV
Temperature >41° C and autonomic instability	Serotonin syndrome, neuroleptic malignant syndrome, malignant hyperthermia
Prolonged fever with no source (63,67,71)	Endocarditis, thyroid storm, drug induced, malignancy, sarcoid, lupus
Recent travel (67)	Brucellosis, Q fever, leptospirosis, amebic dysentery, malaria, yellow fever, dengue, viral hemorrhagic fever, typhoid fever, typhus fever, hantavirus
Tick exposure (67)	Lyme disease, ehrlichiosis, babesiosis, tularemia
Intravenous drug use (21, 67)	Endocarditis, epidural abscess
Biologic weapons (86)	Anthrax, smallpox, plague, tularemia, hemorrhagic fever viruses, Q fever, brucellosis, glanders, typhoid fever, ricin poisoning
New medication	Anticholinergic drug fever, sympathomimetic drug fever, Jarisch-Herxheimer reaction (fever after penicillin in syphilis) phlebitis (after intravenous medicines), hypersensitivity, idiosyncratic drug fever, G6PD deficiency

( ) Refers to the chapter in which each chief complaint is discussed.

Differential Diagnosis of Fever

- The DDx table provides information on chief complaint–based fevers and Table 31–1 describes clinical clues.
- Temperatures greater than 42°C (107.6°F) are most often noninfectious in origin. Causes of such dramatically elevated temperatures include neuroleptic malignant syndrome, seratonin syndrome, heatstroke, and malignant hyperthemia. See Table 31–2.

Initial Diagnostic Approach
General

- There should be an immediate assessment of the ABCs (*a*irway, *b*reathing, and *c*irculation) in any patient who appears ill, especially in the

Table 31–1   Clinical Clues for Patients Presenting with Fever

Mental status and neurologic examination	Behavioral changes may be the only presenting symptom of infection in elderly or chronically ill patients or central nervous system infections.
Head and neck	Identify focal infection of the face, neck, ears, sinuses, upper respiratory tract, and oral cavity (dentition). The funduscopic examination may reveal evidence of disseminated disease such as endocarditis (retinal hemorrhage or Roth's spots) or toxoplasmosis (cotton wool spots). The neck should be palpated for the presence of lymphadenopathy. Nuchal rigidity may not always be present in cases of meningitis.
Chest	Assess for the presence of pneumonia (rales, rhonchi, decreased resonance with percussion) or endocarditis (heart murmur), however, physical examination findings may be normal in both.
Abdominal	Assess for peritonitis or focal infection such as appendicitis, diverticulitis, and cholecystitis.
Back	Assess for costovertebral angle tenderness (pyelonephritis), tenderness over the spine (osteomyelitis, malignancy, or epidural abscess).
Perineal and perirectal	Assess for local infection, fistula, or abscess.
Pelvis	A complete pelvic examination is required for all females with fever and abdominal pain (pelvic inflammatory disease, cervicitis, tubo-ovarian abscess).
Skin and extremities	Evaluate for rash, petechiae, joint inflammation, soft-tissue infection, osteomyelitis, malignancy, decubitus ulcers.

presence of altered mental status or abnormal vital signs. These patients should have an expeditious workup and be placed on a cardiac monitor, continuous pulse oximetry, and IV access should be obtained. The use of diagnostic testing varies greatly depending on the patient population and the patient's condition (Table 31–3).

■ The history should include questions about the degree and duration of fever, travel history, potential zoonotic exposures (animals that may transmit disease to humans), intravenous (IV) drug use, recent surgeries and illnesses, history of cardiac murmurs or valve replacements, sick contacts, medications taken recently, environmental exposure, and a detailed review of systems (ROS).

Disease	Mechanism	Differentiating factor	Time course	Treatment
Neuroleptic malignant syndrome	Impaired thermoregulation in hypothalamus and basal ganglia due to relative lack of dopamine activity	Antipsychotic medication use, diaphoresis; incontinence; tremor; muscular rigidity	Gradual, progresses over several days	Stop offending medication(s) Hydration Active cooling Intravenous benzodiazepines to relax muscles and control agitation Neuromuscular blockade (nondepolarizing agents) Controversial: Bromocriptine or amantadine Dantrolene
Serotonin syndrome	Excess serotonin and dopamine levels in central nervous system	Medications that increase serotonin levels (e.g., SSRIs, MAOIs, dextromethorphan, lithium, meperidine, tramadol, tryptophan); diaphoresis; diarrhea; shivering or tremor; muscular rigidity; hyperreflexia.	Usually rapid after introduction of new medication or increase in dose; can be gradual	Stop offending medication(s) Hydration Active cooling Cyproheptadine
Heat stroke	Environmental heat stress	Environmental exposure history; sweating may be absent; muscular rigidity rare	Rapid or gradual	Hydration Active cooling
Malignant hyperthermia	Genetic instability of sarcoplasmic reticulum, causing massive calcium release after administration of triggering medication	Occurs after administration of inhalational anesthetic or succinylcholine; masseter spasm is an early sign; muscular rigidity	Sudden, provoked by administration of anesthetic	Stop anesthetic Hydration Active cooling Dantrolene

SSRIs, Selective serotonin reuptake inhibitors; MAOIs, monoamine oxidase inhibitors.

Adapted from: Winter MA, Lavonas EJ. Antipsychotics. In: In: Marx JA, Hockberger RS, Walls RM eds. Rosen's Emergency Medicine: Concepts and Clinical Practice. 6th ed. Philadelphia: Mosby: 2445–2451.

Table 31–3	**Examples of Patients Presenting with Fever and Suggested Emergency Department Evaluation**
A young, healthy patient with an obvious pharyngitis or local cellulitis	No additional tests are necessary.
Elderly, immunocompromised, or multiple co-morbidities	These patients may have an unimpressive fever, history, and physical examination, but may still be septic. In this population, the basic fever workup includes a complete blood count, blood cultures, chest radiograph, and urinalysis and culture.
Patients with any change in mental status and fever	Should have a lumbar puncture with cerebrospinal fluid analysis and culture.
Back pain and fever	If there is concern for an epidural abscess, get an erythrocyte sedimentation rate, but key test is magnetic resonance imaging.
Patients with abdominal pain	In addition to a complete blood count and metabolic panel, laboratory studies should include a urinalysis, lipase, liver function tests, and analysis of peritoneal aspirate (if ascites is present). Many of these patients will require an abdominal CT scan with oral and intravenous contrast. All female patients require a complete pelvic examination and a pregnancy test if age appropriate.
Diarrhea with fever	Check stool cultures and a fecal leukocyte count (see Chapter 27).
If there is concern for a hyperthermic syndrome due to a poisoning	Acetylsalicylic acid and acetaminophen levels should be checked. A routine toxicology screen can be performed, but may not reveal certain ingestions such as with anticholinergics and sympathomimetics. Also consider serotonin syndrome, malignant hyperthermia or neuroleptic malignant syndrome. Efforts should be made to elicit a history of possible ingestion of these agents.
Fever after travel to a tropical area	Specialized testing may not be available in the emergency department. However, blood can be sent for a thin and thick smear if malaria or babesiosis is suspected.

- A thorough physical examination is required particularly in patients without an obvious source of the fever (Table 31–1). A fever may cause mild elevations in the heart rate and respiratory rate. Bradycardia may be medication induced (i.e., beta blocker) or may be a manifestation of an infectious disease process such as typhoid fever, brucellosis, leptospirosis, rheumatic fever, Lyme disease, viral myocarditis, or endocarditis. Pay particular attention to potential sources of infection that may not be obvious (i.e., infected decubitus ulcer, perirectal or rectal abscess, odontogenic infection, otitis media, septic joint, osteomyelitis, meningitis), especially if the patient is elderly or incapable of communicating appropriately.

- There is no single fever workup that can be applied to all patients. See Table 31–3 for suggested ED evaluation for patients presenting with a fever. In the otherwise healthy patient, the workup can safely be focused on the primary complaint with a paucity of laboratory testing and imaging studies.

- Certain patient populations such as the elderly, immunocompromised, and IV drug users often present with nonspecific or atypical symptoms that make localization of the source difficult. Furthermore, the patient's mental statues may be altered or the patient may be too sick to give a helpful history. Thus, a more comprehensive investigation is warranted.

- Pediatric fevers have their own protocol and are discussed in Chapter 79.

Laboratory

- A CBC with differential, metabolic profile, coagulation panel, urinalysis with microbiology, and blood and urine cultures (before antibiotic administration) should be initially drawn on all ill appearing and immunocompromised patients. Do not delay antibiotic administration in patients with possible meningitis because a lumbar puncture (LP) has yet to be performed.

- The erythrocyte sedimentation rate (ESR) may be elevated in the presence of any inflammatory or malignant disease, and may be a clue to subtle but serious infections early in their course such as epidural abscess. The ESR does not differentiate one infectious or inflammatory process from another. C-reactive protein is comparable to ESR but increases earlier.

- Other laboratory studies will depend on the individual clinical presentations (i.e., thyroid-stimulating hormone (TSH) for suspected thyroid storm).

EKG

- An electrocardiogram (EKG) should be ordered for patients with chest pain to evaluate for dysrhythmias, ischemia, or pericarditis.

Radiography

- In general, a fever workup may include various imaging studies. These are chosen according to the possible source of fever, but in the patient who cannot localize symptoms, or manufacture signs because of age, immunosuppression, confusion, or competing concurrent diseases, it will be necessary to order studies without obvious clinical manifestations of disease. For example, in many young children and elderly adults, a chest radiograph may be a part of the fever workup even though specific respiratory findings are lacking.

Emergency Department Management Overview
General

- The ABCs should be addressed for any ill appearing patient as discussed in Section II. Two large-bore IV catheters (at least 18 gauge) should be inserted for patients with hypotension, significant tachycardia (fever can cause mild tachycardia), or concern for dehydration. Remember that insensible fluid loss is increased by about 200 ml for each degree of fever.
- Begin the initial fluid resuscitation with 250 ml of normal saline for elderly patients or those with a history of congestive heart failure or renal failure and 1 L normal saline for younger patients, then reassess.
- Supplemental oxygen by nasal cannula or face mask should be given to keep oxygen saturation >95%.

Medications

- Analgesia should be provided for severe pain (Chapter 90.1).
- Acetaminophen 500 to 1000 mg by mouth (PO) or rectum (PR) every 4 to 6 hours (maximum, 4 g over 24 hours) or ibuprofen 400 to 800 mg PO every 6 to 8 hours may reduce fever and improve patient comfort. Temperatures above 41° C should be aggressively treated to prevent neuronal damage that can occur with extremely elevated temperatures.
- Patients whose fever is probably caused by infection should be treated with empiric broad-spectrum antibiotics. The choice of antibiotics is based on the most likely cause of infection and the presence of co-existing conditions such as being immunocompromised (see Chapter 90.2).

Emergency Department Interventions

- Place a Foley catheter early in ill-appearing patients or individuals unable to void on their own to obtain an adequate specimen for urinalysis and to monitor urine output.
- Patients with hyperthermia need rapid external cooling.

Disposition

- ***Consultation.*** Consultations will be dependent upon the clinical scenario, and may not be appropriate or necessary in the ED.
- ***Admission.*** Most elderly patients, immunocompromised patients, and IV drug users with a fever will need to be admitted to the hospital. Anyone requiring IV antibiotics should be admitted. Hyperthermia of any source requires admission and observation to monitor for rhabdomyolysis.
- ***Discharge.*** Fever alone is not a reason for admission, and if the source can be identified, and the patient has good general health and adequate home and social resources, it is often possible and desirable not to admit the patient to the hospital.

Special Considerations
Pediatrics

- Pediatric fever is discussed in Chapter 79.

Elderly

■ An atypical presentation of infection is typical in elderly patients. Defining fever in the elderly is also difficult because a blunted fever response is typical in these patients. For example, 30% of bacteremic elderly patients are afebrile on arrival at the ED.

■ Because fever often causes confusion in the elderly patient, do not assume the patient is merely senile, but search for a source and treat aggressively for sepsis.

Women and Pregnancy

■ Fever during pregnancy places the pregnancy at high risk, and therefore it is prudent to have obstetrical consultation for these patients.

Immunocompromised

■ Fever in neutropenic or immunosuppressed patients may not present with classic signs and symptoms of bacterial infections.

■ Refer to Chapter 66 for neutropenic fever.

■ Patients with suspected indwelling catheter infections should be started on vancomycin.

Intravenous Drug Users

■ IV drug users are at risk for life- and limb-threatening pathology such as endocarditis and epidural abscess. No clinical or laboratory features have been identified that allow precise diagnosis in the ED, so additional studies (such as an echocardiogram and magnetic resonance imaging) are needed. Although these studies may not be readily available in the ED, empiric antibiotics should be given and the patient should be admitted.

Teaching Points

Fever is a frequent finding in ED patients. Its workup and management will need to be individualized, and will vary in depth and detail varying with age of the patient, what the cause of the fever is likely to be, and the co-morbidities.

In the immunosuppressed patient and at the extremes of age, it is not possible to rely on patient history and signs to assist in formulating the workup, and such patients will have to have empiric testing. Thus, obtain CBC, ESR, basic metabolic panel, urinalysis, and cultures of blood, spinal fluid, stool, purulence where it is found, and spinal fluid. Do not rely on the absence of nuchal rigidity to eliminate meningitis in patients who cannot develop nuchal signs because of age, immunosuppression, or confusion.

Suggested Readings

Blum, FC. Fever. In: Marx JA, Hockberger RS, Walls RM (editors). Rosen's Emergency Medicine: Concepts and Clinical Practice (6th ed). Philadelphia, PA: Mosby, 2006, pp 134-137.

Calder KK, Severyn FA. Surgical emergencies in the intravenous drug user. Emerg Med Clin North Am 2003;21:1089–1116.

Gallagher EJ, Brooks F, Gennis P. Identification of serious illness in febrile adults. Am J Emerg Med 1994;12:129–133.

Johnson DH, Cunha BA. Fever: drug fever. Infect Dis Clin North Am 1996;10:85–91.

McKinnon HD, Jr, Howard T. Evaluating the febrile patient with a rash. Am Fam Physician 2000;62:804–816.

Norman DC, Yoshikawa TT. Fever in the elderly. Infect Dis Clin North Am 1996;10:93–100.

Mourad O, Palda V, Detsky AS. A comprehensive evidence-based approach to fever of unknown origin. Arch Intern Med 2003;163:545–551.

CHAPTER **32**

Flank Pain

DANIEL C. MCGILLICUDDY ■ CARLO L. ROSEN

 Red Flags

> Abnormal vital signs • Anti-coagulation • Pregnancy • Neurological symptoms • Co-morbidities (i.e., diabetes mellitus) • Immuno-compromised • Age greater than 50

Overview

The flank refers to the area between the anterior and posterior axillary lines from the inferior costal margins to the iliac crests. Look for "red flags" (see Box), and consider critical diagnoses early. These patients should be rapidly assessed, and have an expeditious emergency department (ED) evaluation. Pain should be addressed early in the ED visit.

Elderly, immunocompromised, and pregnant patients may have minimal or atypical clinical symptoms despite the presence of serious disease. These patients will likely require a more urgent and detailed diagnostic evaluation.

All female patients require an obstetric and gynecologic history, pregnancy test, and most will need a pelvic examination.

DDx Differential Diagnosis of Flank Pain

Critical Diagnoses	Emergent Diagnoses	Non-Emergent Diagnoses
Abdominal aortic aneurysm (18)	Pyelonephritis	Herpes zoster (62)
Ectopic pregnancy (68)	Perinephric abscess Renal infarction Renal vein thrombosis	Musculoskeletal strain
Retroperitoneal hematoma Psoas abscess	Nephrolithiasis Cholecystitis (18)	

( ) Refers to the chapter in which the disease entity is discussed.

Differential Diagnosis of Flank Pain
See DDx table for the differential diagnosis of flank pain.

Initial Diagnostic Approach
General

- Any patient who is hemodynamically unstable or appears ill should receive immediate attention.
- Patients in distress with flank pain should not always be assumed to have a renal stone, especially in older patients. Life-threatening disease, such as a ruptured AAA, may also present with the same clinical picture as a renal stone.
- The timing of onset (e.g., gradual or sudden), the quality of the flank pain, the presence or absence of pain radiation, the presence of a precipitating event, the presence of dysuria or hematuria, and the presence of systemic symptoms are extremely helpful in the evaluation of flank pain.
- Patients with musculoskeletal pain usually do not require further testing.

Laboratory

- Studies may include a CBC, electrolytes, renal function, urinalysis (UA) and a pregnancy test for all women of reproductive age. Microscopic hematuria may be absent in up to 20% of patients with documented nephrolithiasis. The decision to order imaging studies should not be based on the presence or absence of hematuria, but on the overall clinical presentation.
- Patients with hemodynamic instability, presence of blood loss, ruptured AAA, or ectopic pregnancy should have blood sent for type and cross match.

EKG

- An electrocardiogram (EKG) should be performed on any patient with a suspected cardiac source of flank pain, such as in any elderly patients with unexplained left flank pain, as well as to evaluate for signs of cardiac ischemia secondary to blood loss.

Radiography

- *Plain films.* Midline spinal tenderness requires imaging, especially in the setting of trauma, history of malignancy, or if the patient is older than 55 years. With the advent of computed tomography (CT scan), intravenous pyelogram (IVP) and abdominal radiographs (kidney-ureters-bladder [KUB]) are infrequently used. The IVP is still occasionally used to evaluate the collecting system and dynamic dye excretion. A KUB may also be used to evaluate the migration of known stones or to assess the status or location of ureteral stents.
- *Ultrasound.* This is a useful test in the evaluation of hydronephrosis as an indirect indicator of obstructing ureteral stone. The abdominal ultrasound is also useful in the evaluation of intra-abdominal free fluid and an AAA. The abdominal ultrasound can show the presence of an enlarged aorta, but is unable to detect retroperitoneal rupture of an AAA. Ultrasound is the study of choice in evaluating biliary tract disease. Pelvic ultrasound is used to detect ovarian pathology, and to help diagnose an ectopic pregnancy.
- *CT scan.* A noncontrast CT scan is the study of choice in evaluating for nephrolithiasis. It is also the imaging study of choice for evaluation of stable patients with suspected AAA. The addition of IV contrast allows for further delineation of intra-abdominal pathology.

Emergency Department Management Overview

General

- The ABCs (*a*irway, *b*reathing, and *c*irculation) should be addressed as discussed in Section II.
- Patients with renal stones often have severe distress secondary to pain. They should be rapidly assessed and given analgesia as soon as possible while awaiting further diagnostic studies.

Medications

- *Analgesia.* Early administration of analgesia is important in the management of flank pain. If renal colic is suspected, IV ketorolac 30 mg (or 60 mg by intramuscular [IM] injection) is the medication of choice. Narcotic analgesia should be given for more severe pain (Chapter 90.1).
- *Antiemetics.* Nausea is a common chief complaint associated with flank pain. An antiemetic is often useful in the management of nephrolithiasis. Promethazine, metoclopramide, ondansetron, or droperidol can be given IV (see Chapter 90.4).
- *Antibiotics.* Early administration of antibiotics in patients with the clinical appearance of pyelonephritis or psoas abscess is indicated. Fluoroquinolones are often used for pyelonephritis due to their oral bioavailability; psoas abscess requires a broad-spectrum antibiotic that also covers anaerobes (see Chapter 90.2).

Emergency Department Interventions

- *Urinary catheter.* A urinary catheter may be necessary for urine retention, to obtain a sterile urine specimen, in patients in whom mobility may be restricted secondary to pain, or in critically ill patients to monitor urine output.

Disposition

- *Consultation.* Urology consultation is indicated in cases of nephrolithiasis especially if the stone is too large to pass spontaneously (>5 mm), and in the presence of co-infection or perinephric abscess. A general surgery consult is indicated for all other surgical disease.
- *Admission.* All patients with surgical disease, such as psoas abscess, perinephric abscess, or retroperitoneal hematoma, should be admitted. See "ED Management" under the pyelonephritis discussion for specific admission criteria for this particular disease.
- *Discharge.* Most patients with nephrolithiasis can be discharged. They must have stable vital signs, pain relief, the ability to tolerate oral medications, and have follow-up within 24 to 48 hours.

Specific Problems

> ● ● ● Refer to DDx table for reference to a discussion of problems in the
> ● ● ● differential not mentioned here.

Nephrolithiasis

- *Definition.* Stone formation in the genitourinary tract.
- *Epidemiology and risk factors.* They are three times more common in men than women.
- *Pathophysiology.* There are many types of renal stones (i.e., calcium oxalate, struvite, and cystine), the most common being calcium oxalate. The formation of stones is a complex process relating to hydration status, urinary sodium concentration, and occasionally associated with urinary tract infection (UTI).
- *History.* The patient will complain of acute, colicky flank pain, which radiates to the groin. The patient may also complain of dysuria, urinary urgency, hematuria, and nausea.
- *Physical examination.* These patients are frequently found writhing in pain, and are unable to get comfortable. Tachycardia is common at presentation, before pain control is adequate. Occasionally the patient will have costovertebral angle tenderness, and, very rarely, mild abdominal tenderness. The genitourinary examination is normal even though a male patient may present with testicular pain.
- *Diagnostic testing.* Hematuria will be present >80% of the time. An electrolyte panel including blood urea nitrogen and creatinine should be sent to assess renal function. For patients with suspected renal colic,

a noncontrast CT scan of the abdomen and pelvis is the study of choice (Figure 32–1), especially if this is the initial episode. If the patient has had prior stones, there is no need to obtain an imaging study in the emergency department. These patients can be treated with pain relief and analgesia, with imaging studies obtained if there is no response to therapy, or if there are signs of infection. Eighty percent of renal calculi are radiopaque. A renal ultrasound is not accurate for detecting stones. However, the bedside ultrasound can be used to reveal hydronephrosis as a secondary sign of renal stone. It may also be useful in the pregnant patient to avoid radiation exposure.

- *ED management.* The initial management of renal colic is pain control. Ketorolac IV has been shown to be the most efficacious initial analgesia. An anti-emetic is frequently needed. If an NSAID does not provide adequate pain relief, narcotic pain medications should be added. Patients should also be given IV fluids. Patients with renal stones less than 5 mm in diameter will pass the stone spontaneously more than 90% of the time. Patients with signs of obstruction and infected urine should be evaluated by a urologist; they frequently require nephrostomy tube placement to relieve the obstruction. Patients with urinary extravasation, severe volume depletion, inability to tolerate oral medications, or new renal

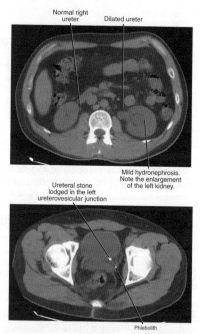

Figure 32-1. Nephrolithiasis with mild hydronephrosis. CT scan with no IV or oral contrast. The top image demonstrates mild hydronephrosis of the left kidney with dilatation of the left ureter. The bottom image shows the obstructing calculus at the left ureterovesicular junction.

insufficiency should be admitted to the hospital. Patients may be discharged if they have stable vital signs, are adequately hydrated, can tolerate oral fluids, and have adequate follow-up with a primary care physician or a urologist.

- *Helpful hints and pitfalls.* Acute flank pain in the elderly is a ruptured AAA until proven otherwise. True abdominal tenderness to palpation warrants an investigation for causes of pain other than renal colic.

Psoas Abscess

- *Definition.* An abscess of the psoas muscle in the retroperitoneal space.
- *Epidemiology and risk factors.* Risk factors for developing a psoas abscess include immunosuppression and IV drug use. It may also be seen after dental work or a ruptured appendix.
- *Pathophysiology.* This kind of abscess usually develops from hematogenous spread or from local intra-abdominal abscess extension.
- *History.* Patients frequently report a history of intermittent spiking fevers, flank and abdominal pain, hip pain or groin pain, as well as pain with ambulation.
- *Physical examination.* Flank and abdominal tenderness to palpation are often present. A limp may be evident, and flexion deformity of the hip may develop from reflex spasm, suggesting septic arthritis of the hip. The iliopsoas sign can be elicited. A tender mass may be palpated in the groin.
- *Diagnostic testing.* A CBC will frequently demonstrate a leukocytosis. A C-reactive protein (CRP) or erythrocyte sedimentation rate (ESR) will be elevated. Blood cultures should be obtained because psoas abscesses are often the result of hematogenous spread. A CT scan with IV contrast can show the psoas abscess. It will appear as a soft-tissue mass along the psoas muscle, frequently with rim enhancement, and occasionally with air-fluid levels in the abscess.
- *ED management.* A broad-spectrum antibiotic that covers gram-positive, gram-negative, and anaerobic organisms is warranted. Often double or triple antibiotic coverage is needed (i.e., ampicillin, gentamycin, and clindamycin). General surgical consultation should be obtained. Patients are often managed by percutaneous needle aspiration with drain placement. However, occasionally patients may need an open operative drainage procedure.
- *Helpful hints and pitfalls.* Psoas abscess can often be confused with appendicitis since these patients present with fever, abdominal or flank pain, and have an iliopsoas sign. It can also follow appendicitis with rupture.

Pyelonephritis

- *Definitions.* Pyelonephritis is a complicated urinary tract infection (UTI) of the renal parenchyma and collecting system manifested by the clinical syndrome of fever, chills, and flank pain. Uncomplicated urinary infections are discussed in Chapter 58.
- *Epidemiology and risk factors.* Complicated urinary tract infections are far more common in women than men until the fifth decade. Patients

with genitourinary abnormalities are at a much higher risk of developing a pyelonephritis.

- **Pathophysiology.** Pyelonephritis is the result of worsening of simple UTI that may have started as a simple cystitis.
- **History.** Patients will typically complain of dysuria, followed by fever, back pain, flank pain, nausea, vomiting, and body aches. They frequently have a history of recurrent UTIs. Other risk factors include recent genitourinary instrumentation, urinary obstruction, chronic neurologic disorders, diabetes, or pregnancy.
- **Physical examination.** Patients will frequently appear toxic. The presence of fever is common, as is the presence of costovertebral angle tenderness or suprapubic tenderness
- **Diagnostic testing.** The UA will frequently show pyuria with more than 10 white blood cells (WBCs), and may be positive for leukocyte esterase as well as nitrates. A urine culture is deemed positive if it has more than 100,000 colony forming units (CFU) or more than 1000 CFUs in males or from a catheter specimen. A CBC is nonspecific, but may show a leukocytosis with a bandemia. Typically blood cultures are not useful. A helical CT scan should be performed if there is concern for a renal stone or obstruction, in male patients, those who fail to respond to therapy, or if the diagnosis is unclear. A renal abscess should be suspected in those patients who fail antibiotic therapy. A renal ultrasound can be used in the case of pregnancy to avoid excessive radiation.
- **ED management.** This includes IV access, IV fluids, antiemetics, analgesia, and antibiotics. Many physicians will give the first dose of antibiotics IV with hydration, and try the second dose orally to see if the patient can tolerate medications by mouth. The recommended antibiotics are third-generation cephalosporins, fluoroquinolones, trimethoprim-sulfamethoxazole (TMP-SMX), or aminoglycosides. Young healthy adults without co-morbidities who can tolerate oral medications are safe for discharge with close follow-up. Patients with co-morbidities, those who are immunosuppressed, extremes of age, or patients with other genitourinary abnormalities (i.e., solitary kidney) should be admitted. Pregnant patients with pyelonephritis are usually admitted for intravenous antibiotic administration, although outpatient parenteral therapy can be effective and safe in selected patients especially in the first trimester.
- **Helpful hints and pitfalls.** A pelvic examination should be performed especially when the UA is negative to rule out pelvic inflammatory disease as an alternative diagnosis. An evaluation for genitourinary tuberculosis is mandatory for any patient with a history of tuberculosis who has back pain, dysuria, or sterile pyuria from an unidentified cause.

Renal Abscess

- **Definition.** A renal abscess is located within the body of the kidney (i.e., cortical or corticomedullary).
- **Epidemiology and risk factors.** It may occur in patients with resistant organisms causing pyelonephritis, or in noncompliant patients not completing a prescribed course of antibiotics. Common sources for cortical abscesses include skin infections, osteomyelitis, and endovascular

infections. 10% of all renal abscesses eventually rupture through the renal capsule and form a perinephric abscess.

- *Pathophysiology.* Renal cortical abscesses result from hematogenous spread of bacteria from primary infectious foci elsewhere in the body. In contrast, renal corticomedullary abscesses occur most commonly as a complication of ascending UTIs.
- *History.* Patients will typically complain of fever, flank pain, dysuria, malaise, and occasionally urinary frequency. They frequently have a history of recurrent or severe pyelonephritis that was inadequately treated, or the clinical appearance of endocarditis.
- *Physical examination.* The patient will frequently appear acutely ill. Fever is common as is costovertebral angle tenderness.
- *Diagnostic testing.* See workup for pyelonephritis. Although ultrasound is useful, abdominal and pelvic CT scan with IV contrast is the study of choice.
- *ED management.* Patients with a history consistent with a urologic source for renal abscess should have antibiotic coverage for gram-negative and anaerobic organisms. Patients in whom an infective embolic phenomena is the likely source should have broad-spectrum coverage for gram-positive organisms.
- *Helpful hints and pitfalls.* Patients with recurrent pyelonephritis or those with recurrent spiking fevers while on antibiotics are at increased risk for renal abscess.

Renal infarction

- *Definition.* This results from renal blood vessel occlusion causing necrosis of the kidney.
- *Epidemiology and risk factors.* This is a rare condition and found most commonly in patients with increased risk for thromboembolic disease.
- *Pathophysiology.* It is most commonly the result of a renal artery embolism.
- *History.* The patient may be asymptomatic but may complain of upper abdominal pain, flank pain, fever, nausea or vomiting.
- *Physical examination.* Hypertension, abdominal tenderness, and signs of extrarenal embolization may be present.
- *Diagnostic testing.* Laboratory studies may reveal gross or macroscopic hematuria, elevated WBC, increased creatinine, and a markedly elevated lactate dehydrogenase (LDH). Contrast-enhanced CT scan is the noninvasive standard of imaging for acute renal infarction in the ED.
- *ED management.* Prompt recognition and early consultation are important as thrombolysis, anticoagulation, or embolectomy may minimize the loss in renal function.
- *Helpful hints and pitfalls.* Detection is often delayed or missed, because the condition is rare and its clinical presentation is nonspecific.

Renal vein thrombosis

- *Epidemiology and risk factors.* It most commonly occurs in patients with nephrotic syndrome (Chapter 29). Malignancy and pregnancy are other risk factors.

- *Pathophysiology.* The thrombosis is the result of hypercoagulability. In nephrotic syndrome, the excess loss of urinary protein is associated with decreased antithrombin III, a relative excess of fibrinogen, and changes in other clotting factors.
- *History.* The patient may be asymptomatic, but may present with flank pain and gross hematuria.
- *Physical examination.* Signs of nephrotic syndrome may be present (e.g., edema).
- *Diagnostic testing.* Urine protein, hematuria, and loss of renal function may be present. Contrast-enhanced CT scan is currently the ED imaging study of choice.
- *ED management.* Consultation with nephrology and surgery. Treat nephrotic syndrome as described in Chapter 29. Anticoagulation is used for prophylaxis against pulmonary emboli. Surgery is rarely required. Thrombolytics or interventional radiology may be required if a vena cava filter is necessary as well as for failure of or contraindications to medical therapy.
- *Helpful hints and pitfalls.* Pulmonary emboli from RVT should be diagnosed and treated in the usual fashion.

Retroperitoneal Hematoma

- *Epidemiology and risk factors.* Retroperitoneal hematomas in the absence of significant blunt trauma are found in patients with ruptured AAA, and in patients who are anticoagulated. Patients who are on warfarin or having recently undergone percutanous angiography are at especially high risk to develop this entity.
- *Pathophysiology.* Blood tracks in the confined retroperitoneal space.
- *History.* Back pain, weakness, or symptoms of orthostasis are frequently present in patients with a retroperitoneal hematoma.
- *Physical examination.* Some findings associated with retroperitoneal hematoma include flank tenderness or paraspinal tenderness to palpation, peri-umbical ecchymosis (Cullen's sign), flank ecchymosis (Grey-Turner's sign), scrotal or perineal hematomas, or iliopsoas sign (pain with hyperextension of leg on affected side).
- *Diagnostic testing.* CT scan with IV contrast is the study of choice to make the diagnosis of retroperitoneal hematoma.
- *ED management.* Retroperitoneal hematomas are acutely life-threatening. Vitamin K and fresh frozen plasma are used to reverse the effects of warfarin, and protamine sulfate is used to reverse Heparin. Admission to the hospital is mandatory; surgery should be consulted if the patient has an AAA or if correction of the coagulopathy does not stop the blood loss.
- *Helpful hints and pitfalls.* Be cautious reversing a patient's anti-coagulation status in the presence of an artificial valve.

Special Considerations
Pediatrics

- Flank pain in children is an uncommon complaint. Children who are diagnosed with pyelonephritis need a formal urologic workup and urology consultation.

Elderly

■ Flank pain in the elderly can often by associated with a catastrophic diagnosis. Misdiagnosis of an ruptured AAA as renal colic is common.

Women and Pregnancy

■ Women with flank pain must have an ectopic pregnancy ruled out as a possible cause, and should have a pregnancy test obtained. Pregnant women with pyelonephritis are usually admitted for IV antibiotics unless they are in the first trimester, and have follow-up capability with an obstetrician.

The Immunocompromised Patient

■ The immunocompromised are at a much higher risk for complications associated with flank pain. This may include dissemination of varicella zoster virus, renal abscess, and pyelonephritis.

Teaching Points

Flank pain has many causes that range from benign musculoskeletal pain to life-threatening causes such as a ruptured AAA. Although renal stones are common, there are many other possible diseases that produce similar symptoms.

First time stone disease should always have an imaging study as well as pain and nausea relief. It is usually not necessary to obtain an imaging study if the patient has known stone disease, unless pain cannot be controlled or signs of infection appear.

Patients with pyelonephritis require an initial dose of IV antibiotics, pain relief, and reassessment in the ED to see if the patient appears non-toxic, can take oral fluids, follow instructions, and have a close follow-up plan. If there are significant comorbidities, immunosupression, extension of disease, poor social circumstances, or pregnancy, the patient should be admitted.

Flank pain may also be the presenting complaint of a ruptured abdominal aortic aneurysm or a retroperitoneal hematoma. These are very serious problems, require admission and often emergency surgery.

Suggested Readings

Gonzalez C, et al. The clinical spectrum of retroperitoneal hematoma in anticoagulated patients. Medicine 2003;82:257–262.

Hutchinson FN, Kaysen GA. Perinephric abscess: the missed diagnosis. Emerg Med Clin North Am 1988;72:993–1014.

Lee C, Henderson SO. Emergency surgical complications of genitourinary infections. Emerg Med Clin North Am 2003;21:1057–1074.

Rosen CL, et al. Ultrasonography by emergency physicians in patients with suspected ureteral colic. J Emerg Med 1998;16:865–870.

Rubenstein JN, Schaeffer AJ. Managing complicated urinary tract infections. Infect Dis Clin N Am 2003;17:333–351.

Teichman J. Acute renal colic from ureteral calculus. N Engl J Med 2004;350:684–693.

CHAPTER 33

Foreign Bodies

GARRY F. GAGNON ■ SAMUEL D. LUBER

 Red Flags

Severe wound infection or poor healing ● Drainage from any orifice
(i.e., ear, nose, vagina, rectum) ● Recurrent pneumonia in the same
location ● Unexplained rectal pain ● Injection-drug user (i.e., broken
needle parts) ● Any penetrating injury

Overview

The identification and management of foreign bodies (FB) is often
challenging and time consuming to the emergency physician. Look
for "red flags" during the evaluation of any patient with a suspected
foreign body (see Box). The consequence of a retained foreign body
may be potentially fatal (e.g., airway obstruction) or more benign (e.g.,
bug in the ear). Retained or missed FBs may serve as a nidus for
infection.

Given the vast number of potential FBs and the potential areas
of the human body that they may invade, this chapter will only briefly
review the most common foreign bodies presenting to the ED. These
include the skin, gastrointestinal tract, nose, and ears. Airway foreign
bodies are discussed in Chapter 5. Pediatric airway and gastrointestinal
FBs are discussed in Chapters 76 and 77, respectively. Environmental
foreign bodies such as sting rays and jellyfish are reviewed in Chapter
65. Foreign bodies of the eye are commonly encountered in the ED
and are discussed in Chapter 69.

Initial Diagnostic Approach

■ The history and physical examination are essential in making an accurate
diagnosis. A retained FB must be in the differential for unexplained or
non-healing wounds, even when the history does not specifically indicate
its presence. A patient may not be aware of the presence of a FB. Less
commonly, the patient may not be willing to reveal the presence of a FB
that was intentionally placed (e.g., rectal foreign body).
■ A foreign body is typically diagnosed by direct visualization, palpation, or
imaging studies. Plain films are often ordered for airway, gastrointestinal,

and soft-tissue foreign bodies. Two views such as an anteroposterior and lateral radiograph should be performed. Glass FBs larger than 2 mm or gravel larger than 1 mm are radiopaque, and thus identifiable. Organic materials such as wood are better seen by computed tomography (CT scan).

■ The presence or absence (after an appropriately thorough evaluation) of a foreign body must be carefully documented in the patient chart.

Emergency Department Management Overview

■ FBs that are not easily seen or readily palpable are often difficult to remove. Removal of a FB requires a cooperative patient. The procedure can be challenging and time consuming, especially in the intoxicated, uncooperative, mentally handicapped, or pediatric patient. Sedation and analgesia may be needed (Chapter 90.1). Although attempts should be made to remove a foreign body, patients or their guardians should be made aware that removal attempts in the ED may not be complete or may be unsuccessful.

■ If the FB is not easily removed, the appropriate specialist should be consulted. Impaled foreign bodies require surgical consultation and removal in the operating room, due to the potential for uncontrollable bleeding to occur once the foreign body is dislodged.

■ Removal of a FB in the soft tissues can be delayed up to 48 hours so that removal can be performed under optimal conditions.

■ For soft-tissue wounds, tetanus immunization should be updated (see Chapter 94). Antibiotic prophylaxis may be given.

Specific Problems

The most common foreign bodies presenting to the ED are briefly summarized in Tables 33–1 through 33–5.

Table 33–1	Gastrointestinal Foreign Bodies		
Visualization	**Medications**	**Procedures**	**Comments**
Radiograph, CT scan, indirect laryngoscopy, naso-pharyngoscopy, endoscopy	Glucagon 1-2 mg IV NGT 0.4-0.8 mg SL Nifedipine 10 mg SL Pharmacologic measures indicated in smooth FBs. These work at the lower esophageal sphincter. Most effective with food impactions.	Foley catheter: Pass distal to foreign body inflate 1-2 ml and withdraw. Endoscopy: Use for sharp objects. Forceps: Used if FB can be visualized in the oropharynx.	Glucagon: may cause nausea, vomiting, hyperglycemia. Disc batteries do not require removal if in stomach unless GI symptoms; emergent removal if in esophagus. Impacted bones do not pass.

CT, computed tomography; ENT, ear, nose, and throat or otolaryngology; GE, gastroesophageal; GI, gastroenterology; IV, intravenous; NGT, nasogastric tube; SL, sublingual.

Table 33–2   Soft-Tissue Foreign Bodies By Location or Material

Location	Imaging	Removal Technique(s)	Additional Therapy
Embedded puncture in subcutaneous tissue (e.g., nails, sewing needle, glass, metal fragments, bullets, wood)	Glass/metal usually visualized with radiograph (glass: if greater than 2 mm). Wood/vegetative matter is not seen well with radiographs; may be seen better with a CT scan. Ultrasound gaining acceptance as common method of evaluation.	Do not use blind finger to probe wound. Use local anesthetic prior to removal. Enlarge wound as necessary: linear incision above object when object perpendicular to skin; grasp object with hemostats.	Tetanus prophylaxis. Irrigation after removal of object. If noncosmetic area and small incision, may leave wound open to heal by secondary intention. If significant contamination, pack wound and close 3-5 days later. Antibiotics not routine. May use with immunocompromised or significant contamination.
Foot (e.g., nail, including pieces of shoe or sock that nail penetrated through)	If nail FB reportedly removed completely intact, may not need additional imaging unless there are additional concerns. Radiographs if suspect bony injury. If deep wound, may need to evaluate with CT scan, ultrasound.	Search for threads/rubber from puncture wound. These can serve as nidus for infection if not removed. Local wound exploration if large laceration. If infection present, probability of retained FB is high.	Tetanus prophylaxis, irrigation. Antibiotics (controversial, recommended if signs of current infection): cover for pseudomonas if rubber-soled shoe. Also cover for *Staphylococcus aureus* if diabetic.
Subungual	None, unless suspect bony damage.	Digital block for anesthesia. May need to remove part of or entire nail. Grasp with forceps or use a sterile hypodermic needle bent at the tip to hook FB.	Tetanus prophylaxis. Risk of osteomyelitis of distal phalanx. Prophylactic antibiotics may be given but are usually not necessary.

Table 33–2 Soft-Tissue Foreign Bodies By Location or Material—*cont'd*

Material	Imaging	Removal Technique(s)	Additional Therapy
Fishhooks	None	Local anesthetic. Advance hook and cut with wire cutters just proximal to barb, and then remove in retrograde fashion. Downward pressure on shaft of hook to disengage barb then traction at turn of hook to pull hook out.	Tetanus prophylaxis. Prophylactic antibiotics may be given but are usually not necessary.
Pencil lead (not actually lead, but graphite)	Ultrasound may be useful.		None
Cactus	Ultrasound or CT scan if deep foreign body is suspected	Deep wounds generally only produce granulation tissue. Superficial spines may be removed with forceps, wax, glue, duct tape.	
Rings	None	Lubrication with K-Y Jelly. May need a ring cutter.	None
Ticks	None	Early removal as soon as possible. Must remove head of tick by mechanical means.	Doxycycline 200 mg single dose to prevent Lyme disease. Provide discharge instructions with information on signs and symptoms of Lyme disease (see Chapter 67).
Zippers	None	Generous local anesthetic. Cut crossbar of the sliding portion of zipper. Often difficult to cut. May need specialized tools (check with hospital maintenance department).	Urology follow-up if penile laceration.

CT, computed tomography.

Table 33–3	Rectal Foreign Bodies		
Type	**Evaluation**	**Removal Technique**	**Disposition**
Palpable	Anoscopy, rigid sigmoidoscopy, speculum, retractor. Radiograph to obtain location and to look for sharp objects. Local anesthetic with viscous lidocaine, lubrication, and anxiolytics will likely be necessary to obtain optimal viewing and extraction.	If palpable and no signs of perforation or peritonitis, removal may be attempted. Ring forceps may be helpful for grasping some objects. Foley catheters can be used to pass balloon past object, inflate balloon, then remove with gentle traction. Some air may be passed through to relieve vacuum that may have been created by an open ended object such as a soda/beer bottle. It may be helpful to use suprapubic pressure or Valsalva to help deliver object.	Observation in ED for signs of perforation Surgical consultation if unable to remove or signs of peritonitis.
Nonpalpable	Anoscopy, radiograph to identify position/type of FB.	Do not attempt to remove in the ED.	Surgical consultation
Signs of perforation	Portable plain film radiographs to look for free air, but immediate surgical consultation is necessary.	Do not attempt to remove in the ED.	Surgery consultation

Table 33–4   Ear Foreign Bodies

Type of Object	Analgesia/Sedation	Procedure	Disposition
Nonliving: Beads, nuts, grass, button batteries	Topical lidocaine. May require conscious sedation and immobilization of the head. If object is deep or firmly embedded in canal—control pain, and ENT consult with possible removal under general anesthetic.	Irrigation: Works well with dirt, small rocks or sand. Not to be used with deeply embedded objects or vegetables as they may swell. Direct manual removal using right angle hook or alligator forceps. Small catheter with removal by inflating balloon of catheter with gentle traction. Suction catheters: works well with round objects. Dissolving agents: Acetone useful with Styrofoam.	Re-examine ear after removal. Re-examine after removal: check TM and hearing. ENT consultation in ED if infection, suspected TM rupture, severe trauma, or unable to remove FB. ENT follow-up in one day if object not able to be removed. Button batteries may lead to corrosive perforation of TM within hours. This will require emergent ENT consultation.
Living object: (cockroach is most common)	Immobilize the insect by killing with lidocaine* prior to procedure. Mineral oil has been reported to kill roaches.	Same as for nonliving foreign bodies.	Same as for nonliving FBs.

ED, emergency department; ENT, ear, nose, throat, or otolaryngology; TM, tympanic membrane.
*Lidocaine can cause vertigo in patients with TM perforation.

Table 33–5 Nasal Foreign Bodies

Anesthetic	Procedures	Disposition
Topical anesthetic achieved with bilateral nasal packing or swab after soaking in lidocaine with epinephrine; can also try oxymetazoline (Afrin). Benzocaine spray. A cooperative patient is essential. This is especially the case with children.	Visualization with speculum is necessary to identify position of object. Radiographs may be useful. If in anterior nares, then alligator forceps or a hooked probe may be able to grasp object. May use catheter with balloon insufflated past object to gently remove with traction. Apply cyanoacrylate glue to the end of a stick, then press it against the FB for 1 minute and remove. Positive pressure via bag-valve-mask or by having parents blow forcefully into mouth while maintaining pressure on opposite nares. A tight seal must be maintained over mouth. Small button batteries should be removed immediately to prevent necrosis.	Re-examine with attention to the ears as well. If unable to remove then admission for removal under general anesthesia is necessary Monitor the airway as there is a risk of aspiration if the FB is dislodged into the posterior pharynx.

Teaching Points

Retained foreign bodies are a common complication, and may result in an adverse outcome for the patient. Therefore, the practitioner should feel comfortable with removal procedures, know when specialty consultation is necessary, and as with all procedures, discuss with the patient the various treatment and removal options before proceeding with attempted removal.

A retained foreign body should be included in the differential diagnosis for complaints of local pain, infection, drainage, or respiratory irritation.

Suggested Readings

Davies PH, Benger JR. Foreign bodies in the nose and ear: a review of techniques for removal in the emergency department. J Accid Emerg Med 2000;17:91–94.

Kalan A, Tariq M. Foreign bodies in the nasal cavity: A comprehensive review of aetiology, diagnostic pointers, and therapeutic measures. Post Grad Med J 2000;76:484–487.

Lamers RL. Soft tissue foreign bodies. Ann Emerg Med 1988;17:1336.

Nagendran T. Management of foreign bodies in the emergency department. Hosp Physician 1999;35:27–40.

Roberts JR, Hedges JR (editors). Clinical Procedures in Emergency Medicine (4th ed). Philadelphia: Saunders, 2004.

CHAPTER **34**

Gastrointestinal Bleed

Scott B. Murray ■ Edward Ullman

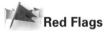
Red Flags

History of liver disease or known GI bleeding ● Frequent use of alcohol or nonsteroidal antiinflammatory agents (NSAIDs) ● Chest pain or abdominal pain ● Dyspnea or tachypnea ● Lightheadedness or syncope ● Altered mental status ● Hypotension ● Tachycardia ● Cool extremities ● Hematemesis ● Hematochezia

Overview

Look for "red flags" (see Box). Patients may initially present with the complications of anemia and hypovolemia, such as cardiac ischemia, dyspnea, weakness, lightheadedness, syncope, or altered mental status, rather than obvious bleeding. Any signs or symptoms of hypoperfusion require immediate resuscitation.

Once stability has been established, identifying the site of bleeding is critical. Using the ligament of Treitz as a boundary, anything above is an upper GI tract bleed (UGIB), anything below, a lower GI tract bleed. Clinical distinction between the two is still difficult, and at times the distinction can only be made with endoscopy or imaging studies.

A rectal examination should always be performed in these patients. Stool color does not accurately localize the bleeding site. While hematochezia (bright red blood per rectum or maroon stools) suggests a lower GI bleed (LGIB), nasogastric (NG) lavage should be performed to rule out a briskly bleeding upper source. Melena (black, tarry stool) often suggests an upper source of bleeding; however, it can be from the small bowel or ascending colon as well. Slow or occult bleeding is rarely a cause of a visit to the ED until the patient becomes symptomatic from the anemia.

Differential Diagnosis of Gastrointestinal Bleed

See DDx table.

Initial Diagnostic Approach
General

- Any patient who is hemodynamically unstable or appears ill should receive immediate attention. While the physician is assessing the patient, a continuous cardiac monitor and pulse oximeter should be placed. Two large–bore intravenous (IV) lines should be obtained, and labaratory tests should be sent, including blood for type and cross match. Unless these patients are going for definitive care (i.e., operating room, angiography, or ICU for endoscopy), they must be stabilized prior to transfer.

- *History.* Important information includes the presence and duration of hematemesis (red or coffee grounds), abdominal pain, and character of stools to help localize source of bleeding, but they are not completely reliable (Table 34–1). The probability of a variceal bleed is higher in patients with a prior history of cirrhosis. A history or presence of an AAA or its repair is helpful in making the diagnosis of aortic enteric fistula (AEF). Crampy mid-lower abdominal pain from colonic spasm induced by blood may come from LGIB or UGIB. Severe, diffuse pain and tenderness is concerning for peritonitis due to perforation or bowel ischemia. Rectal pain is most often associated with anal fissures and

DDx Differential Diagnosis of Gastrointestinal Bleeding

Upper GI Source	Lower GI Source	Non-GI Source
Peptic ulcer disease	Diverticulosis	Nasal/oropharyngeal
Gastritis	Atrioventricular	Hemoptysis (24)
Varices	malformation	Red dyes (guiac-negative
Mallory-Weiss tear	Neoplasm/polyp	red stool/vomitus)
Aortoenteric fistula	Anal fissure/	Bismuth salts, iron (guiac-
	hemorrhoid (48)	negative dark stool)
	Colitis	
	Meckel's diverticulum	

GI, gastrointestinal.
( ) refers to the chapter in which the disease entity is discused.

Table 34–1 **Presenting Signs of Upper and Lower GI Bleeding**

	Upper GI Source	Lower GI Source
Hematochezia	10%	90%
Melena	90%	10%
Hematemesis	Frank or coffee ground	Rare

GI, *gastrointestinal.*

external hemorrhoids. Ask about traumatic anal penetration. Patients may be reluctant or embarrassed to offer such information. Intake of iron or bismuth salts can produce Guiaic negative melenic stools. Epistaxis can mimic hematemesis. Ingesting red dyes can masquerade as hematochezia or hematemesis.

- **Physical examination.** Tachycardia and hypotension are warning signs of hemorrhage and inadequate volume resuscitation. Patients taking beta-blockers, calcium channel blockers, or digoxin often cannot mount a tachycardic response. Low or normal blood pressure in patients with a history of hypertension is ominous. Positive orthostatic vitals signs (pulse elevation of >20 beats per minute or severe postural dizziness) may be seen with high-volume acute blood loss, but are often not present with adult losses of less than 20%. Normal orthostatics does not mean lack of significant bleeding. See Chapter 2 for the technique used to perform orthostatic vital signs. A narrowed pulse pressure occurs with acute blood loss. This is defined as the difference between systolic and diastolic blood pressure (normal is 40 mm Hg). Alterations in mental status indicate brain hypoperfusion. Pale conjunctiva can indicate a low hematocrit. Inspect the oropharynx, sputum, and nares for alternate bleeding sources in patients with hematemesis. Epigastric tenderness indicates gastritis or peptic ulcer disease. Abdominal tenderness elsewhere indicates inflammation or infection. Diffuse peritonitis suggests perforation. Signs of liver disease (telangiectasias, ascites, fluid wave, hepatomegaly) suggest portal hypertension. Cool extremities indicate hypovolemia. Perform a rectal examination and visually inspect the stool, as the patient's historic report of the stool color may be inaccurate. Check for external and internal hemorrhoids. A painful rectal examination indicates rectal pathology (see Chapter 48). Always test stool for occult blood as red dyes can turn stool red, and black stools can result from bismuth salts or iron supplements. Inspect vomitus for blood and ensure "coffee grounds" are not succus entericus of a small bowel obstruction.

Laboratory

- Obtain a complete blood count (CBC), metabolic panel; and type and cross match for 2 units of packed red blood cells (PRBCs) if the patient is stable and at least 4 units if the patient is symptomatic or unstable. Also obtain coagulation studies especially in patients with liver disease or who are being treated with anticoagulants.

- Obtain cardiac enzymes if there are symptoms of cardiac ischemia from anemia or hypovolemia. This is of special concern in elderly patients or individuals with known coronary artery disease as they can develop demand ischemia if the hematocrit becomes too low.
- The blood urea nitrogen (BUN) level may be elevated due to digested blood in the GI tract. The creatinine may be elevated in the presence of hypovolemia and prerenal azotemia.
- The hematocrit may be normal initially until volume losses have been replaced with saline or the patient has had time to reconstitute plasma volume. Transfusion of each unit of PRBCs typically raises the hematocrit approximately 3%, unless the patient is continuing to hemorrhage.

EKG

- An electrocardiogram (EKG) should be obtained in any patient with known or suspected coronary artery disease, abnormal vital signs, or chest pain.

Nasogastric Lavage (NGL)

- Use normal saline, not free water to avoid inducing hyponatremia. Ice-water lavage does not slow bleeding, and can induce hypothermia and coagulopathy.
- NGL can be grouped into four categories: *positive* (blood present but clears with lavage), *positive* (but does not clear with lavage), *negative* (no blood, and bile is seen in lavage), or *indeterminate* (no blood but no bile seen). Lack of bile in NG aspirate suggests that there is no active bleeding in the esophagus or stomach, but offers no information about the duodenum, as the NG tube has failed to pass the pylorus and duodenal contents (bile) have not refluxed into the stomach (see Chapter 91 for NG tube placement technique).
- NGL is safe in the presence of esophageal varices and should be performed in order to monitor for an ongoing UGIB. Patients with varices also frequently bleed from a lower GI source, so NGL is useful to exclude an acute upper GI source of the hemorrhage. In a patient with esophageal varices that have recently been banded, consultation with a gastroenterologist is recommended as blind tube placement may dislodge the bands.

Anoscopy

- Anoscopy should be performed in cases of hematochezia to identify the presence of an actively bleeding hemorrhoid. It is risky to assume that hemorrhoids are the sole cause of hematochezia without visualizing an actively bleeding internal hemorrhoid. Even if a bleeding hemorrhoid is noted, there is no guarantee that it is the isolated source of GI bleeding.

Radiography

- *Radiographs.* Obtain an upright portable abdomen or chest radiograph in patients with severe pain and peritoneal signs to evaluate for free intraperitoneal air from bowel perforation, or a potential foreign body in the GI tract.

- *Ultrasound.* An aortic aneurysm may be detected, suggesting an aortoenteric fistula.
- *Computed tomography (CT scan).* An abdominal CT scan with IV contrast may be useful if the patient is stable, and there is a concern for AEF, colitis, or mass lesion.
- *Tagged red cell scan.* This test is useful for patients with slow, continual bleeding suspected to be an atriovenous malformation (AVM) that is not in the field of view of lower or upper endoscopy. Nuclear scintigraphy can detect hemorrhage at rates as low as 0.1 ml/min. It is not a test to obtain in the ED due to the time required to radiolabel blood and obtain images. It is not suitable for unstable patients.
- *Angiography.* Angiography has the potential advantages of localization and treatment in patients who have vigorous bleeding in whom a upper or lower endoscopy would be difficult. Its utility is limited because bleeding is intermittent, unpredictable, and has often stopped by the time the patient has arrived for angiogram.

Endoscopy

- This is the diagnostic and therapeutic test of choice for upper GI bleeding.

Emergency Department Management Overview
General

- The ABCs (*a*irway, *b*reathing, and *c*irculation) should be addressed as discussed in Section II. Supplemental oxygen should be given if the patient is in respiratory distress or if the oxygen saturation is less than 95%.
- Two large-bore IVs (preferably 16 gauge or larger) should be placed and isotonic fluids should be administered for all patients with a GI bleed. Initiate and repeat fluid boluses of 500 ml normal saline (NS) until vital signs normalize (250 ml NS in the elderly or in those patients with a history of congestive heart failure [CHF]).

Blood Products

- Begin transfusion of PRBCs if hypotension remains after 2 L of replacement crystalloid fluid, if there is evidence of ongoing rapid bleeding, or decreased hematocrit. Elderly patients or those with significant co-morbidities (e.g., coronary disease) should receive packed red blood cell transfusions to maintain the hematocrit above 30%. Young and otherwise healthy patients should be transfused to maintain their hematocrit above 20%.
- Transfuse fresh frozen plasma (FFP) to correct an abnormal prothrombin time or partial thromboplastin time in patients with liver disease, on warfarin, or with other coagulopathy. Subcutaneous vitamin K should be given to patients on warfarin; however, new vitamin K-dependent factors take 24 to 48 hours to synthesize. Due to this time delay, FFP should also be given in order to provide a rapid (although temporary) reversal of the warfarin effect by directly providing active vitamin K-dependent

factors. Patients who are on heparin (with elevated partial thrombo-plastin time) or low molecular weight heparin should be given IV protamine to reverse their coagulopathy. In the setting of acute bleeding, transfuse platelets to at least 50,000/μL. Any patient with hemophilia should be corrected to 100% of the missing factor. Refer to Chapter 84 for additional information.

Medications

- *Analgesia.* Pain should be treated with parenteral analgesia such as IV morphine.
- *Antacids.* Oral antacids and sucralfate should be avoided unless requested by the gastroenterologist, as these can interfere with upper endoscopy. In the setting of UGIB, proton pump inhibitors have been found to significantly reduce the rate of ulcer rebleeding, and should be administered; a finding that has not been demonstrated with histamine-2 (H_2) blockers (see Chapter 90.4).
- *Antibiotics.* Gram-negative and anaerobic coverage should be given (third generation cephalosporin or fluoroquinolone with metronidazole) for any patients with suspected perforation or with LGIB suspected to be from an infectious source (those with fever, colitis, bloody diarrhea, inflammatory bowel disease, or other systemic signs of infection). Add ampicillin to cover enterococci if perforation has occurred. The administration of erythromycin may enhance the clearance of residual blood and blood clots from the stomach and the duodenum as well as reduce the need for second-look endoscopy. Cirrhotics with GI bleeding are at risk for infection. Up to 20% of cirrhotics who are hospitalized secondary to GIB have bacterial infections, and an additional 50% develop an infection while hospitalized. The most common site for infection is the urinary tract, followed by peritoneal cavity and respiratory tract. Prophylactic antibiotics have been shown to reduce infectious complications and possibly decrease mortality in these patients (see Chapter 90.2).
- *GI Vasoconstrictor Therapy.* Somatostatin inhibits the release of vaso-dilator hormones, indirectly causing splanchnic vasoconstriction and decreased portal inflow. The initial dose for somatostatin is 250-μg bolus followed by 250-μh/h infusion. Octreotide is a long-acting analog of somatostatin. The starting dose of octreotide is 50-μg bolus followed by 50-μg/h infusion. When used with endoscopy, these medications may reduce the risk of rebleeding better than does endoscopic therapy alone. Both drugs may also reduce the risk of bleeding due to nonvariceal causes. Vasopressin 0.2-0.4 U/min is a potent splanchnic and systemic vasoconstrictor. It must be administered with nitroglycerin but is less commonly used today.

Emergency Department Interventions

- *Nasogastric tube (NGT).* Nasogastric lavage is more of a diagnostic test than a treatment for GIB. Applied alone, an NGT cannot be expected to alter outcomes in patients with confirmed GIB.

- *Urinary catheter*. Any hemodynamically unstable or incontinent patient should have a Foley catheter placed, and urinary output monitored (maintain >0.5 ml/kg/h) to assess resuscitation.

- *Esophagogastroduodenosopy (EGD)*. This procedure is rarely performed in the ED by a gastroenterologist. In severe bleeding, the airway must be secured before the EGD is performed. Endoscopy provides visualization of the esophagus, gastric mucosa, and proximal duodenum. It is both diagnostic and therapeutic. Esophageal varices can be sclerosed, banded, or injected. Gastric or duodenal ulcers may be injected and sclerosed.

- *Esophageal tamponade.* Indicated for variceal bleeding when vasoactive medications are ineffective, and endoscopy is unavailable or ineffective. Esophageal tamponade achieves short-term hemostasis in 60% to 90% of all variceal hemorrhages. Three types of balloons have been used: (1) the standard or modified Sengstaken-Blakemore tube, (2) the Minnesota tube, and (3) the Linton-Nachlas tube. Before the placement of any one of these tubes, endotracheal intubation is necessary to decrease the risk of airway compromise or aspiration. The lubricated tube is then advanced though the mouth or nose into the stomach. Once gastric intubation has been accomplished and verified by epigastric auscultation, the balloon should be inflated partially, and its position checked radiographically. After radioligic verification of placement in the stomach, the gastric balloon is fully inflated and traction applied. The esophageal balloon is then inflated.

Disposition

- *Consultation.* A gastroenterologist capable of performing endoscopy should be consulted. Endoscopy is diagnostic *and* therapeutic for UGIB. If endoscopy is not available, and the patient is to be admitted, the patient should be transferred to a hospital that can provide it. If available, interventional radiology can be diagnostic and therapeutic for LGIB. General surgical consultation should be obtained in cases of peritonitis, ongoing life-threatening bleeding, or any episode of hypotension. Indications for surgery are listed in Box 34–1. A vascular surgeon should be consulted immediately if aortoenteric fistula is a possible diagnosis.

BOX 34–1 Indications for Surgical consultation for Gastrointestinal Bleeding

Upper:
1. Inability to see source of bleeding in massively bleeding patient
2. Inability to achieve hemostasis by endoscopic means
3. Special situations: aortoduodenal fistula

Lower:
Hemodynamic instability, transfusion requirements, and persistent or recurrent hemorrhage

---

BOX 34–2 **Intensive Care Unit Admission Guidelines**

Older than 75 years
History of portal hypertension or esophageal varices
Any episode of hypotension
Ongoing bleeding
Uncorrected coagulopathy
Concurrent cardiac ischemia
Hematocrit below 20% or a more than 8-point drop from baseline
    hematocrit
Upper endoscopy shows visible vessel or overlying clot

- *Admission.* Eighty percent of patients admitted with GIB will not need an invasive intervention as an inpatient, but it is impossible to predict the 20% who will require urgent endoscopy, embolization, or surgery. Nevertheless, all patients with UGIB and LGIB will need to be admitted to the hospital for serial hematocrit checks and vital sign monitoring. Patients with LGIB who cannot be definitively indentified as having a benign rectal bleed (e.g., hemorrhoid) should be admitted. ICU admission may be required in as many as 50% of patients with UGIB. Level of care and monitoring capabilities vary between hospitals, but general guidelines for ICU admission are listed in Box 34–2.
- *Discharge.* Some stable patients with a bleeding hemorrhoid on anoscopy may be discharged home with a diagnosis of hemorrhoids, as long as they have close follow-up and have the ability to return immediately for any further significant bleeding or other complications. The bleeding must be controlled before discharge is safe. Criteria for discharging patients with UGIB are controversial, but low risk UGIB patients have been identified. See Box 34–3.

BOX 34–3 **Candidates for Outpatient Management**

Younger than 75 years
No significant co-morbid illness
Reliable patient with close follow-up, and able to return to emergency
    department
No evidence of portal hypertension or ascites
Systolic blood pressure above 100 mm Hg (>120 mm Hg in a patient with
    existing hypertension), normal heart rate, and no orthostatic changes
    during 6 hours observation
Normal coagulation function
Hematocrit above 32%

Specific Problems

Please refer to the "Overview" and "Initial Diagnostic Approach" for a more detailed discussion of historical and physical examination findings.

● ● ● Refer to the DDx Table for reference to a discussion of problems in the
● ● ● differential not mentioned here.

Upper Gastrointestinal Tract Bleeding
Aortoenteric Fistula

- *Epidemiology and risk factors.* Patients with an AAA or an abdominal aortic graft.
- *Pathophysiology.* Erosion into the duodenal wall by graft or aneurysm. Rupture of an artery causes rapid exsanguination.
- *History.* Because most of these fistulas are into the duodenum, hemorrhage usually manifests as hematemesis or melena, but there can be brisk hematochezia in conjunction with a history of an aneurysm or graft. Classically, a rapid, "herald" bleed precedes the fatal bleed. The initial bleeding episode may last several days or longer, is often minor, and results from erosion of vessels in the bowel wall. Abdominal pain, back pain, and fever may be present.
- *Physical examination.* The presence of a pulsating mass in the abdomen suggests the presence of an AAA, but the aneurysm is often not palpable, and many are not seen without ultrasound or CT studies.
- *Diagnostic testing.* Plain films may reveal calcification of the aortic wall or a paravertebral soft-tissue mass in AAA, but will not show an AEF. Bedside ultrasound can show an AAA (but may be limited by obesity and with excess bowel gas), but cannot reliably determine whether the AAA has ruptured, or if an AEF is present. If AEF is suspected, and the patient is stable, emergency upper endoscopy should be performed. If negative, CT scan with IV contrast of the abdomen may demonstrate an AEF or inflammation around the aortic anastomosis. If the diagnosis of AEF is suspected, and the patient has a negative CT scan, angiography may be pursued.
- *ED management.* These patients are typically unstable, and those with epidemiological risk factors and clinical instability warrant immediate vascular surgical consult with angiogram performed in the OR.
- *Helpful hints and pitfalls.* A minor episode of GI bleeding in these patients may represent a herald bleed, and should be aggressively evaluated.

Erosive Gastritis, Esophagitis, and Duodenitis

- *Epidemiology and risk factors.* Alcohol, nonsteroidal anti-inflammatory drugs (NSAIDs), steroids, and stress (burns, ICU admission, and severe illness) are all associated with erosive mucosal disease. Pills (tetracyclines most commonly) and infection can cause esophagitis. Duodenitis has the same risk factors as PUD.
- *Pathophysiology.* At the mucosal edge, mucous is secreted to protect the epithelial cells from caustic digestive products. NSAIDs lower

prostaglandin levels that are important in promoting mucous production. Stress results in increased acid production. Gastric reflux increases the risk of esophagitis.

- *History.* Patients most commonly describe epigastric pain, which is burning or stabbing in quality. Patients may have no pain on presentation. Typically inflammation presents as a slow, constant bleed rather than abrupt and intermittent.
- *Physical examination.* Occasionally, patients have epigastric tenderness to palpation.
- *Diagnostic testing.* The diagnosis of these problems is sometimes made clinically in the ED but an EGD is required for diagnosis.
- *ED management.* As with all upper GI bleeding, initiate therapy with a proton pump inhibitor. Any offending agent must be avoided.
- *Helpful hints and pitfalls.* Beware of the premature diagnosis of gastritis in patients with epigastric pain with nausea and vomiting.

Esophageal Varices and Portal Hypertensive Gastropathy

- *Epidemiology and risk factors.* Bleeding from varices accounts for one third of all deaths in patients with cirrhosis. Esophageal varices develop at a rate of 50% per year, and ultimately occur in up to 90% of all patients with cirrhosis. The risk of recurrent bleeding approaches 70%.
- *Pathophysiology.* Portal hypertension from liver cirrhosis results in elevated venous pressures at portal-systemic anastomoses, producing engorged venous outpouching in the esophagus, gastric, and duodenal veins.
- *History.* Patients typically describe bright red hematemesis. A history of risk factors for developing cirrhosis (hepatitis C, chronic alcohol abuse) or a known diagnosis of varices suggests variceal bleeding. There is usually minimal abdominal pain.
- *Physical examination.* Stigmata of liver disease or cirrhosis (caput medusa, spider angiomas, ascites, facial telangiectasia, palmar erythema, signs of feminization) or portal hypertension (splenomegaly and dilated periumbilical veins) may be present. Anorectal varices sometimes present as dilated veins resembling hemorrhoids.
- *Diagnostic testing.* Concurrent liver failure may result in coagulopathy that should be corrected. The serum ammonia level may be elevated contributing to altered mental status. Patients with a transjugular intrahepatic portosystemic shunt (TIPS) or portocaval shunt should have a Doppler ultrasound to assess shunt patency and flow direction. Endoscopy is diagnostic and therapeutic.
- *ED management.* Secure and manage the airway if the patient has abnormal mental status and hematemesis. The airway must also be secured if the patient has severe bleeding and requires emergent endoscopy. The Sengstaken-Blakemore tube can be used in cases of severe life-threatening bleeding. Replacing fluid and blood is essential in the orthostatic or hypotensive patient, but avoid overexpanding volume in the stabilized individual because it may increase portal pressure and accelerate hemorrhage. Somatostatin or octreotide should be started as soon as the diagnosis of variceal hemorrhage is suspected. Endoscopic therapy and somatostatin infusions are effective in arresting hemorrhage in 80% to 90% of cases. The patient should be admitted to the ICU.

- *Helpful hints and pitfalls.* Patients with variceal bleeding frequently bleed from nonvariceal sources necessitating NG lavage to distinguish upper from lower GI bleeding. The presence of varices is not a contra-indication to NG tube placement, unless recently endoscopically banded.

Mallory-Weiss Tear

- *Epidemiology and risk factors.* Hiatal hernia, alcohol consumption, and esophagitis are all risk factors for a Mallory-Weiss tear, as well as anything that causes repetitive vomiting. Bulimia is can also cause a Mallory-Weiss tear.
- *Pathophysiology.* Repetitive and forceful vomiting causes tears through the mucosa and submucosa of the stomach, although about 15% occur in the esophageal mucosa.
- *History.* Typically a patient who has had several episodes of nonbloody emesis will develop bloody emesis.
- *Physical examination.* The patient may appear dehydrated from frequent vomiting.
- *Diagnostic testing.* Obtain a chest radiograph to examine for pneumo-mediastinum indicative of esophageal rupture.
- *ED management.* In the absence of significant blood loss, this disease is usually self-limited, and treatment should include anti-emetics to remove the cause of the tear. Boerhaave's syndrome (Chapter 22) (esophageal rupture) is spontaneous rupture of the full wall of the esophagus, while Mallory-Weiss tears are limited to the mucosa. A chest radiograph should be obtained if the patient complains of chest pain or shortness of breath. Pneumomediastinum in this setting suggests esophageal rupture, requiring broad spectrum antibiotics and surgical consultation.
- *Helpful hints and pitfalls.* Search for a Boerhaave's syndrome in patients with suspected Mallory-Weiss tear who develop chest pain or who appear toxic.

Peptic Ulcer Disease

- *Epidemiology and risk factors.* Peptic ulcer disease (PUD) is more common in patients over 50 years of age, but can also be seen in children and young adults. Tobacco and alcohol are associated risk factors.
- *Pathophysiology. Helicobacter pylori* is a treatable source of many duodenal and gastric ulcers. It causes increased acid secretion and decreased protective mucous production.
- *History.* Sharp, burning pain in the epigastrium near eating suggests PUD. A change to diffuse pain is worrisome for perforation. Develop-ment of back pain suggests posterior penetration.
- *Physical examination.* Tenderness over the epigastrium may be present. Diffuse peritoneal signs indicate perforation.
- *Diagnostic testing.* Obtain an upright abdominal or chest radiograph to evaluate for free intraperitoneal air if perforation is suspected. Endoscopy is both diagnostic and therapeutic.
- *ED management.* Proton pump inhibitors should be started. Antibiotics should be given, and surgical consultation obtained if perforation is suspected.

- *Helpful hints and pitfalls.* Forty percent of all UGIB are from PUD (two thirds are duodenal and one third is gastric).

Lower Gastrointestinal Tract Bleeding

Arteriovenous Malformation

- *Epidemiology and risk factors.* Age, hypertension, and aortic stenosis are all associated risk factors. Most are located in the ascending colon and small intestine. These lesions are likely congenital, and most are seen in patients younger than 30 years.
- *Pathophysiology.* Abnormal connections of the arterial and venous system that are superficial to the bowel mucosal surface can rupture and bleed. An AVM is an interconnection of aberrant arteries and veins with thick hypertrophic walls.
- *History.* Rupture leads to sporadic, rapid, and painless bleeding.
- *Physical examination.* Patients are usually not tender to palpation, and often lack any physical examination findings other than the presence of bloody stool.
- *Diagnostic testing.* These are usually diagnosed during endoscopy.
- *ED management.* Once the diagnosis in made, surgical resection is the usual treatment. Angiography may localize the site of active bleeding, and permit embolization or infusion of vasopressin to stop the bleeding.
- *Helpful hints and pitfalls.* The terms *arteriovenous malformation*, *angiodysplasia*, *telangiectasia*, and *hemangioma* describe distinct entities but have been used interchangeably to describe the same lesion.

Diverticulosis

- *Epidemiology and risk factors.* Patients with diverticular disease, especially those older than 60 years, are at risk for diverticular bleeding.
- *Pathophysiology.* Low-fiber diets and constipation are thought to cause small invaginations in the colon wall, bringing the mucosa externis into close proximity to the arterioles in the deeper layers. Arterial bleeding into the colonic lumen occurs from minor trauma due to straining and fecal movement.
- *History.* Diverticulosis is typically painless bleeding. It can be intermittent and very rapid.
- *Physical examination.* Mild tenderness or fullness in the left lower quadrant may be present.
- *Helpful hints and pitfalls.* Diverticular disease includes diverticulosis (painless bleeding) and diverticulitis (Chapter 18). Painful GI bleeding (other than mild cramping prior to defecation produced by intraluminal blood), is not due to diverticular disease alone.

Ischemic Colitis

- *Epidemiology and risk factors.* Risk factors for ischemic colitis include age, atrial fibrillation, peripheral vascular disease, coronary artery disease, or any other cause of a hypoperfused state. Inflammatory bowel disease and infectious diarrhea are discussed in Chapter 27. Risk factors for infectious colitis include recent travel and exposure to sick contacts with similar symptoms.

- *Pathophysiology.* All types result from mucosal sloughing and bleeding into the colon. Thromboembolism in atrial fibrillation or low-flow states in mesenteric arterial stenosis cause ischemia and necrosis of the innermost colon wall.
- *History.* A history of abdominal angina (abdominal pain due to ischemia after eating), advanced age, or presence of risk factors should prompt consideration of mesenteric ischemia. Hematochezia is a late finding in mesenteric ischemia, and patients are gravely ill by that time. Fever and abdominal pain may be present.
- *Physical examination.* Tenderness and bloody diarrhea are not present until late in ischemic colitis. Initially, ischemic colitis may present as pain out of proportion to the physical examination.
- *Diagnostic testing.* An EKG is useful to diagnose atrial fibrillation. A rapid CT scan (with IV contrast only) is recommended to assess for mesenteric ischemia.
- *ED management.* Broad-spectrum antibiotics covering gram-negative and anaerobic bacteria should be administered early in the patient's course. Fluid loss may outweigh blood loss as the colon loses the ability to reabsorb fluids. Therefore, aggressive fluid resuscitation is recommended. Early surgical involvement is required for patients with suspected mesenteric ischemia.

Special Considerations

Pediatrics

- Clinically significant GIB in pediatric patients is rare, and severe bleeding is usually from varices of cirrhosis or a Meckel's diverticulum (Chapter 77).

Elderly

- There is 70% mortality during an acute GIB in the elderly that is usually due to complications of co-morbid disease, adverse effects of medication, and the aging process.
- The elderly are more likely to have mesenteric ischemia, aortoenteric fistula, diverticulosis, and AVM.
- Close attention should be paid to the pulmonary status in patients who have CHF when giving crystalloid and blood products, but do not delay resuscitation. Continuous re-evaluation of patients is critical.

Women and Pregnancy

- Perform a vaginal examination in women presenting with hematochezia to rule out a gynecologic source.

The Immunocompromised Patient

■ Common causes of HIV-related UGIB are infectious esophagitis, idiopathic esophageal ulcers, a Kaposi sarcoma, and lymphoma. Patients with AIDS may also develop CMV colitis.

■ Most LGIB cases are directly associated with HIV, and include CMV colitis, idiopathic colon ulcers, Kaposi sarcoma, and lymphoma. Hemorrhoids and anal fissures are more likely to cause significant bleeding in these patients.

Teaching Points

GI bleeding is a frightening entity whether it is upper or lower. It may be hard to distinguish the origin of the bleeding in the ED, and the priority is for stabilization and resuscitation. Although nasogastric tubes are useful to help determine the site of bleeding, and help direct further investigation, there is no evidence that their use affects the outcome. Placement of a nasogastric tube is not contraindicated by the presence of esophageal varices, especially because the cirrhotic patient also has a high incidence of bleeding from duodenal ulceration, but special precautions should be taken if the patient has been recently banded. Be aggressive in blood replacement, and obtain surgical consultation in patients who are not responding rapidly to crystalloid and packed red cell replacement.

Suggested Readings

Bono MJ. Lower gastrointestinal tract bleeding. Emerg Med Clin North Am 1996;14:547–556.

Hamoui N, Docherty SD, Crookes PF. Gastrointestinal hemorrhage: is the surgeon obsolete? Emerg Med Clin N Am 2003;21:1017–1056.

Henneman PL. Gastrointestinal bleeding. In: Marx JA, Hockberger RS, Walls RM (editors). Rosen's Emergency Medicine: Concepts and Clinical Practice (6th ed). Philadelphia: Mosby, 2006, pp 220–227.

Leung FW. The venerable nasogastric tube. Gastrointest Endosc 2004;59:255–260.

McGuirk TD, Coyle WJ. Upper gastrointestinal tract bleeding. Emerg Med Clin North Am 1996;14:523–546.

Simoens M, Rutgeerts P. Non-variceal upper gastrointestinal bleeding. Best Pract Res Clin Gastroenterol 2001;15:121–133.

Toy RM. Gastrointestinal bleeding. In: Frank LR, Jobe KA. Admission and Discharge Decisions in Emergency Medicine. Philadelphia: Hanley and Belfus, 2001, pp 65–68.

CHAPTER 35

Headache

WENLAN CHENG ■ ALAN WEIR ■ LYNN P. ROPPOLO

Red Flags

New-onset headache ● Headache brought on by exertion ● Sudden onset of severe headache ● "Worst headache of my life" ● Change in pattern of headache ● Older than 50 years ● Headache that disrupts sleep or presents on awakening ● History of chronic illness such as human immunodeficiency virus, tuberculosis, or cancer ● History of recent trauma ● History of intravenous drug abuse ● Systemic illness (i.e., fever, nausea, vomiting, severe vertigo) ● Altered level of consciousness or behavior ● Acute loss of vision ● Neck stiffness ● Abnormal neurological examination ● Abnormal vital signs especially high fever, tachycardia, hypertension.

Overview

Look for "red flags" (see Box) and consider critical diagnoses early. *Primary headaches* include migraine headaches, tension headaches, and cluster headaches, in all of which the headache itself is the illness. Ninety percent of patients arriving at the ED with a complaint of headaches will be diagnosed with one of these.

Secondary headaches represent a spectrum of diseases in which the headache is the symptom of a different underlying disease.

The diagnosis of a primary headache should be made only after all life-threatening causes have been ruled out.

Differential Diagnosis of Headaches

See DDx table for information on the differential diagnosis of headaches.

Initial Diagnostic Approach
General

■ Patients with any "red flags" require immediate attention and an expeditious ED evaluation. Indications for "no further workup" in the ED include patients with intermittent similar headaches in the past and

DDx Priority-Based Differential Diagnosis of Headache

Critical Diagnosis	Emergent Diagnosis	Nonemergent Diagnosis
Subarachnoid hemorrhage	Cerebral abscess	Migraines
Subdural hematoma (9)	Brain tumor	Tension headache
Epidural hematoma (9)	Cerebral venous thrombosis	Cluster headache
Stroke (56)	Shunt failure	Dental (61)
Carotid and vertebral artery dissection	Hypertensive emergency (39)	Cervicogenic headache
Acute angle closure glaucoma (69)	Pseudotumor cerebri	Post-lumbar puncture
Carbon monoxide poisoning (72)	Anemia (66)	Post-traumatic (9)
Temporal arteritis	Sinusitis	Hypertension (39)
Meningitis (67)		Ophthalmic zoster (69)
Encephalitis (67)		Trigeminal neuralgia Temporomandibular joint disease Medication overuse or substance withdrawal Substance use: cocaine, cannabis, alcohol (72)

( ) Refers to the chapter in which the disease entity is discussed.

a normal physical examination. This is particularly true for the non-concerning headache that resolves spontaneously in the ED or with appropriate analgesia (i.e., typical migraine pain, tension headaches, sinus headache).

■ *History.* A headache that is sudden in onset or the "worst headache of my life" should raise concerns for subarachnoid hemorrhage (SAH). A mass lesion should be considered in patients who present with a chronic headache, especially if behavioral changes are present. A headache that is unilateral may have a benign etiology such as migraine or sinus disease, but may also result from serious pathology such as a mass lesion, temporal arteritis, or glaucoma. Nausea and vomiting are nonspecific symptoms, but significant vomiting is concerning for increased intracranial pressure. The presence of fever and a headache suggests an infectious etiology such as meningitis. An acute headache and altered mental status can be associated with many critical diagnoses. Headaches that are the result of trauma are often benign (e.g., concussion), but can also be due to more serious injuries such as intracranial hemorrhage or skull fracture.

■ *Physical Examination.* Determine if there are any vital sign abnormalities, especially significantly elevated blood pressures (Chapter 39) or fever. Intra-ocular pressures and vision testing should be checked in patients with a unilateral headache and vision complaints. Funduscopy should be performed to evaluate for papilledema or retinal pathology. Nuchal rigidity is typically associated with meningitis and subarachnoid hemorrhage, but its absence does not rule out either of these diagnoses. A complete neurologic examination should be performed on any patient complaining of a headache.

Laboratory

■ Laboratory studies may include a complete blood count (CBC) to evaluate for anemia or infection, erythrocyte sedimentation rate (ESR) or C-reactive protein (CRP) if temporal arteritis is suspected, and a carbon monoxide (CO) level if there is concern for CO poisoning.

■ Coagulation studies should be performed on elderly patients, individuals with co-morbidities (e.g., cirrhosis), if there is concern for intracranial hemorrhage, and in patients who may require a lumbar puncture (LP).

■ A pregnancy test should be done on every woman of child-bearing age due to concern for pre-eclampsia.

■ Free T_4 and thyroid-stimulating hormone (TSH) levels should be ordered if concerned about hypothyroidism as a cause of the headaches.

Lumbar Puncture (LP)

■ An LP needs to be performed on patients suspected of having subarachnoid hemorrhage (SAH), meningitis, encephalitis, or idiopathic intracranial hypertension (see Chapter 91 for LP technique and Appendix 1 for CSF results).

■ Pretreatment with antibiotics for suspected meningitis will not affect cell counts if the LP is performed within a few hours of starting the antibiotic therapy.

■ A shunt tap rather than an LP should be performed if the patient has a ventriculoperitoneal (VP) shunt and fever. Neurosurgery should be consulted.

Radiography

■ *CT scan.* Abnormalities that require emergent interventions, such as bleeding, cerebral edema, herniation, depressed skull fractures, masses, and hydrocephalus, are readily seen on noncontrast CT scans. However, a noncontrast CT scan of the head may be normal in the setting of increased intracranial pressure, and can miss up to 8% of cases with SAH. Thus, an LP should follow a negative CT scan if there is concern for a subarachnoid bleed. A shunt series in addition to a noncontrast CT scan is used to evaluate VP shunt malfunction.

■ *Magnetic resonance imaging (MRI).* This imaging study is not often used acutely in the ED due to limited availability and difficulty in monitoring patients while in the magnet. It is better than a CT scan for identifying cerebral infections, metastases, and cerebral ischemia. It is also the best modality for identifying posterior fossa pathologies, since CT scan images in that area are limited by artifact and cortical structures.

- *Magnetic resonance angiography (MRA) and MRV.* MRA and MRV are noninvasive and useful for assessing vascular structures. MRA is 90% accurate for detecting aneurysms larger than 3 mm. They are not usually performed in the ED. MRA is preferred for detecting carotid or vertebral artery dissection. MRV is preferred for diagnosing cerebral venous thrombosis.

Emergency Department Management Overview
General

- Patients with abnormal vital signs or altered mental status should be rapidly assessed for airway or hemodynamic compromise (see Section II).

Medication

- *Analgesia.* Nonsteroidal anti-inflammatory drugs (NSAIDs) and acetaminophen are first-line agents for mild to moderate pain. Morphine 2 to 5 mg via intravenous (IV) route can be given for severe pain every 5 to 10 minutes (see Chapter 90.1). See Table 35–1 for migraine headache therapy.
- *Anti-emetics.* See Chapter 90.4 for common antiemetic agents, some of which are used for migraine treatment (e.g., prochlorperazine) Ondansetron 4 mg IV is given for nausea with less of a sedating effect, but is more costly than other agents.
- *Antibiotics.* Administer antibiotics early for patients with potential intracerebral abscesses or meningitis (see Chapter 67). An LP and CT scan should not delay the administration of antibiotics if intracranial infection is suspected.

Disposition

- *Consultation.* Potential surgical problems such as SAH, intracerebral abscess, or mass lesion should be referred to the neurosurgery service. Brain metastases or central nervous system (CNS) lymphoma should be referred to the medicine service with evaluation by an oncologist. Ophthalmology should be consulted for vision loss associated with headache.
- *Admission.* Admit patients with critical or emergent diagnoses, patients with persistent severe pain despite aggressive management, patients with altered mental status, patients with suspected intracranial infection, or patients with an abnormal neurologic examination. Admission is prudent in immunocompromised and elderly patients due to the higher incidence of serious pathology despite minimal clinical findings.
- *Discharge.* If there is no concern for serious disease after a careful ED evaluation, the patient may safely be discharged with appropriate analgesia and follow-up. Patients should be told to return for fever, severe persistent headache, vomiting, or neurologic changes.

Table 35–1   Migraine Pharmacotherapy

Mild Symptoms	Adult Dosage	Precautions
Acetaminophen	500 -1000 mg PO	Liver disease, no more than 4 g in 24 h
Ibuprofen	600-800 mg PO	Peptic ulcer disease, renal disease, elderly, class B in pregnancy (D in third trimester)
Naproxen	275-825 mg PO	Peptic ulcer disease, renal disease, elderly, class B in pregnancy (D in third trimester)
Ketorolac	10 mg PO, 30 mg IV, 60 mg IM	Peptic ulcer disease, renal disease, elderly, class C in pregnancy (D in third trimester)

Moderate to Severe Symptoms	Adult Dosage	Precautions
Ergot alkaloids Dihydroergotamine	1 mg SC, 0.251 mg IM/IV, max 3 mg *Medicate with an anti-emetic due to common side effect of nausea and vomiting	Pregnancy, CAD, PVD, uncontrolled HTN, sumatriptan use in last 24 h
Serotonin agonists Sumatriptan	6 mg SC, max 12 mg SC	Pregnancy, CAD, PVD, uncontrolled HTN, ergot use in last 24 h
Zolmitriptan	2.5-5 mg PO, 5 mg intranasal	Same as sumatriptan
Opioid analgesics Morphine	5-10 mg IM/IV	Allergic reactions
Hydromorphone	2-4 mg PO	Allergic reaction
Meperidine	50-100 mg IM/IV	Allergic reactions
Dopamine antagonists Metocloperamide	10 mg IV/PO	Drowsiness, dystonic reaction, class B in pregnancy
Prochlorperazine	10 mg IV/PO	Drowsiness, dystonic reaction, orthostatis hypotension, class C in pregnancy

CAD, coronary artery disease; HTN, hypertension; IM, intramuscular; IV, intravenous; PO, by mouth; PVD, peripheral vascular disease.

Specific Problems

> ●●● Refer to the DDx table for reference to a discussion of problems in the
> ●●● differential not mentioned here.
> ●●●

Brain Tumors

- *Epidemiology.* Most brain tumors are metastatic cancers from a primary tumor elsewhere in the body, the most common being lung, breast, kidney, and melanoma. Primary brain tumors are less common and are usually seen in patients younger than 50 years.
- *Pathophysiology.* The headache may be caused by involvement of pain-sensitive areas such as the meninges or cerebral blood vessels or secondary to increased intracranial pressure (ICP).
- *History.* Headaches, weakness, personality changes, and cognitive deficits are the typical symptoms. The headache may initially be present only on awakening but progressively becomes continuous. The headache often disrupts sleep and awakens the patient at night, and it may be associated with straining or bending over.
- *Physical examination.* Examination will often reveal weakness or focal deficits in two-thirds of the patients. About 25% of the patients will have cognitive deficits upon careful testing.
- *Diagnostic testing.* MRI is the preferred choice of imaging; however, a CT scan with IV contrast may be the best option in the ED.
- *ED management.* Emergent neurosurgery referral should be made for evidence of cerebral edema, mass effect, or altered level of consciousness. Dexamethasone 10 mg IV push then 4 mg every 6 hours should be initiated in the ED to treat edema. Seizures should be treated with phenytoin. Prophylactic seizure treatment is not recommended.
- *Helpful hints and pitfalls.* Look for this entity in patients with cancer complaining of new headaches or unexplained cognitive deficits in an otherwise healthy young-to-middle aged patient.

Carotid and Vertebral Artery Dissection

- *Epidemiology.* Dissections can be spontaneous or due to trauma. There have been reported cases associated with neck torsion or chiropractic manipulation. Hypertension and a history of collagen vascular disease such as Marfan syndrome are risk factors for spontaneous dissection.
- *Pathophysiology.* Dissection typically involves the extracranial segments of these vessels. It is usually caused by primary hemorrhage of the vasovasorum, or an intimal tear resulting in intramural hemorrhage and ensuing local or circumferential hematoma. This hematoma can then lead to vascular occlusion. The timing of these events is variable. There will be pain at the time of the initial tear but symptoms of cerebral ischemia may take days to years to develop.
- *History.* There is usually an abrupt onset of ipsilateral headache, neck, and face pain, but the symptoms may be of gradual onset. Vertebral

artery dissection will usually present with unilateral posterior headache, and rapid progressive neurologic deficits consistent with a brainstem or cerebellar stroke. Patients may complain of nausea and vomiting, gait disturbances, unilateral tinnitus, and vertigo. Carotid artery dissection may present with a unilateral headache, pulsatile tinnitus, and signs of cerebral or retinal ischemia such as amaurosis fugax (temporary monocular loss of vision caused by transient retinal ischemia) or weakness. Transient ischemic attacks are common. Seizures, episodic lightheadedness, and syncope have also been reported.

- **Physical examination.** An ipsilateral, partial Horner's syndrome (ipsilateral ptosis, miosis, but no anhidrosis of the face), aphasia, neglect, visual disturbances, and contralateral hemiparesis may be found with carotid artery dissection. A carotid bruit may also be noted. Ataxia, diplopia, hemiparesis, and unilateral facial weakness may be present with vertebral artery dissection.
- **Diagnostic testing.** An MRI and MRA of the neck or duplex scanning can help establish the diagnosis. If the MRA is nondiagnostic, angiography must be performed. Catheter angiography is the gold standard. Half of all vertebral artery dissections will have associated subarachnoid hemorrhage; therefore, a noncontrast head CT, may have positive findings. Usually, the CT scan will be normal in carotid artery dissection. Cerebrospinal fluid (CSF) analysis may appear similar to that of SAH.
- **ED management.** Anticoagulant and antiplatelet therapies are recommended for stroke prevention. SAH must be ruled out before starting anticoagulation. The head of the bed should be elevated to 30 degrees. Neurology and neurosurgery should be immediately consulted. The patient should be admitted to the intensive care unit (ICU).
- **Helpful hints and pitfalls.** Consider this diagnosis in young patients presenting with head or neck pain and focal neurologic findings.

Cerebral Venous Thrombosis

- **Epidemiology.** Cerebral venous thrombosis (CVT) is an extremely rare condition affecting all ages with a slight increase in incidence in young women due to the use of oral contraceptives and in pregnancy, both of which increase coagulation.
- **Pathophysiology.** The causes are divided into infectious and noninfectious etiologies. The common infectious causes include sepsis, tuberculosis, endocarditis, intracranial infections (abscess, empyema, meningitis), and regional infections (otitis, sinusitis, tonsillitis). Cavernous sinus thrombosis is the most common form of septic thrombosis, usually due to an infection of the middle third of the face or after ethmoid or frontal sinusitis. Paranasal sinusitis, most commonly the sphenoid after basilar skull fracture, accounts for 30% of cases. Common noninfectious causes include head injury, neurosurgical procedures, dural punctures, pregnancy, coagulation disorders, connective tissue disorders, and severe dehydration. The thrombotic event is the same as anywhere else in the body. Cerebral venous thrombosis classically causes bilateral hemorrhagic infarcts with prominent vasogenic edema, which is different from arterial infarcts.

- *History.* Symptoms are varied with headache being the earliest presenting complaint. It is often diffuse, progressive, and permanent. The onset is subacute, often longer than 48 hours but less than 30 days; a thunderclap-type headache is described in 15%. Seizures and focal deficits may be reported. Decreased level of consciousness is also reported, but is often a very late sign. Patients with septic cavernous sinus thrombosis present with an acute headache following a facial infection, fever, and eye complaints. There is unilateral periorbital edema that almost always spreads to the other eye, which helps distinguish it from preseptal or orbital cellulitis.
- *Physical examination.* This may reveal focal deficits and papilledema. Cavernous sinus thrombosis will usually present with decreased visual acuity, chemosis, proptosis, and ophthalmoplegia involving cranial nerves III through VI; most of these patients appear quite toxic.
- *Diagnostic testing.* MRI combined with MRV approaches the sensitivity of angiography in diagnosing CVT. A CT scan with and without contrast is an adequate initial study in the ED. Most commonly seen signs on a CT scan include small ventricles with swelling and edema, hyperdensity of a thrombosed sinus, and hemorrhage from swelling secondary to venous congestion. The D-dimer level may be elevated. Leukocytosis and abnormal CSF results are present in up to 90% of patients.
- *ED management.* The most important management strategy is to treat the causes of the thromboses. If infection is suspected, then broad-spectrum antibiotics should be started. Heparin should be initiated to prevent further clot formation and promote recanalization. Catheter-based thrombolytics should be considered in patients with a rapidly deteriorating neurologic status. Symptomatic seizure treatment is also appropriate. Prompt neurology consultation is needed.
- *Helpful hints and pitfalls.* Search for this entity in patients with an unexplained headache, especially when combined with a focal neurologic deficit, papilledema, or seizures. A noncontrast CT scan is not adequate to rule out CVT. An MRI with MRV is recommended.

Cluster Headache

- *Epidemiology.* These headaches are more common in men than women with an onset in the mid twenties. Male-to-female ratio is 6:1.
- *Pathophysiology.* The etiology is unclear but thought to be vascular- or serotonin-related.
- *History.* They often present with multiple episodes of sharp, stabbing unilateral pain over the orbital, supraorbital, or temporal area. Pain is acute in onset, and escalates rapidly. Headaches can last from minutes to many hours. Each cluster of headaches will last a few weeks. Remissions between cluster periods usually last 6 months to a year. Most sufferers have two to three cluster periods annually. They may be precipitated by alcohol, stress, or climatic changes. The patient may also have tearing and nasal congestion.
- *Physical examination.* This may reveal a partial Horner's syndrome with ptosis and miosis. Lacrimation, conjunctival injection, and nasal congestion may also be present.

- *Diagnostic testing.* None.
- *Management.* High-flow oxygen at 7 to 10 L/min for 15 minutes is effective. Another preferred abortive therapy is sumatriptan 6 mg via subcutaneous injection. Dihydroergotamines (DHEs) can also be used as an alternative therapy. Prophylactic therapy may be considered in patients with repeated attacks and includes calcium channel blockers, beta-blockers, methysergide, divalproex, and topiramate. A short course of oral prednisone may abort an attack in some patients. Intranasal valium and lidocaine has given quick relief for some patients.
- *Helpful hints and pitfalls.* Rapid treatment is recommended due the abrupt nature of this presentation.

Intracerebral Abscess

- *Epidemiology.* The age distribution varies with the predisposing condition that led to the formation of the abscess. Twenty-five percent of cases are in children, usually from an otogenic focus or in relation to cyanotic congenital heart disease. The mortality rate is in the range of 24%.
- *Pathophysiology.* The abscess usually forms from contiguous infection or hematogenous spread with the vast majority of abscesses arising from a sinus or otogenic origin. Brain abscesses that arise from hematogenous spread are usually due to a cardiac or pulmonary source, and tend to be multiple. Streptococcal species account for up to 70% of all cases, mostly the *Streptococcus milleri* group. *Staphylococcus aureus* accounts for 10% to 15% of cases, and is usually found in patients with endocarditis or cranial trauma. Anaerobes are isolated from 40% to 60% of cases. Gram-negative species can be found in patients with chronic otitis externa or in immunocompromised patients. Fungal infections are predominantly due to Candida species, and are found in patients who have central venous catheters, or who are diabetic or otherwise immunocompromised. Toxoplasmosis is a common cause in patients who have human immunodeficiency virus (HIV). Meningitis is a rare cause except in neonates. One fifth of brain abscesses are cryptogenic (unknown origin).
- *History.* The clinical presentation ranges from indolent to fulminant. Most of the symptoms are due to size and location of the lesions, not the systemic effects of the infection. Focal signs, most commonly altered mental status and hemiplegia, are seen in 50% of patients. Fewer than 50% of the patients will present with the classic triad of fever, headache, and focal neurologic deficits.
- *Physical examination.* Patients rarely appear toxic unless it is late in the course of disease. Fever may be present. The mental status may be altered and focal neurologic deficits may be present on examination. Papilledema is only seen in 25% of the cases.
- *Diagnostic testing.* A CT scan with contrast will classically show a lesion with a hypodense center and uniform, peripheral ring enhancement surrounded by another hypodense area of brain edema (Figure 35–1). An MRI is the imaging modality of choice, but is often difficult to obtain in the ED. Blood cultures should be obtained, but are positive in 10% of cases. Serologic testing for the presence of anti-*Toxoplasma* immunoglobulin G (IgG) antibody should be obtained in patients positive for

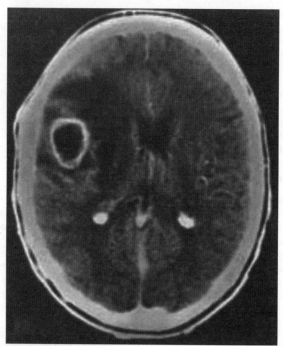

Figure 35-1. Brain abscess. Contrasted-enhanced CT scan in the coronal projection. Abscess appears as a lesion with a hypodense centre composed of necrotic debris surrounded by ring enhancement, which may in turn be surrounded by hypodense cerebral edema. *From: Cohen & Powderly: Infectious Disease, 2nd ed., Copyright © 2004 Elsevier.*

HIV. Stereotactic biopsy or aspirate of the abscess cavity yields a microbiologic diagnosis in up to 96% of cases.

- *ED management.* Administer antibiotics in the ED if the diagnosis of brain abscess is made. Empiric antibiotic choices include vancomycin, metronidazole, and a third-generation cephalosporin, such as ceftriaxone or cefotaxime. If the abscess is of otogenic origin, coverage should be expanded to include *Pseudomonas aeruginosa*. See Chapter 37 for toxoplasmosis treatment. If there is a mass effect or severe edema, steroids should be administered, and the patient should be intubated. Early neurosurgery consult should be obtained for possible excision and drainage of the abscess. A select group of patients are managed with antibiotic therapy alone.
- *Helpful hints and pitfalls.* The diagnosis should be considered in patients with a headache, fever, focal neurologic deficit or concern for elevated ICP.

Idiopathic Intracranial Hypertension (also called Pseudotumor Cerebri or Benign Intracranial Hypertension)

- *Epidemiology.* Typical patients are young obese females of childbearing age with chronic daily headaches.
- *Pathophysiology.* The exact mechanism is unknown. It has been linked to oral contraceptive use, vitamin A intoxication, anabolic steroids, obesity, and tetracycline.
- *History.* Patients will complain of a generalized daily chronic headache of nonspecific pattern. The headache may be worse with Valsalva maneuvers or bending over. Bifrontotemporal distribution is the most common involvement Transient visual loss may occur secondary to ischemia of the visual pathways, and is permanent in 10% of patients. The patient may also complain of nausea or tinnitus.
- *Physical examination.* This is typically normal except for papilledema or visual field defects. A sixth nerve palsy (inability to move affected eye laterally) may be noted.
- *Diagnostic testing.* Neuroimaging studies are normal and without mass lesions or ventricular enlargement; however, an axial CT scan may show narrow slitlike ventricles. There may be normal or low CSF protein, but the cell count will be normal. The opening pressure of the LP is greater than 200 mm H_2O.
- *ED management.* This is initially directed at pain management. Obese patients are also advised to lose weight. If the patient is asymptomatic without papilledema or visual loss, no treatment is needed. The headache may improve or resolve with an LP. If performing an LP to reduce the headache, only 5 to 10 ml of CSF should be removed at a time. The goal is to reduce ICP to less than 200 mm H_2O or until the patient is asymptomatic. If there are signs of visual disturbances, aggressive management should be pursued. Four to 6 weeks of furosemide or acetazolamide is given to reduce CSF production. Steroids have been used, but their mechanism of action is unclear. Urgent referral should be made to ophthalmology. A ventricular shunt or optic nerve sheath fenestration may be indicated for patients with impending vision loss or severe symptoms.
- *Helpful hints and pitfalls.* Opening pressure should be measured on all patients in whom an LP is performed so that this diagnosis is not missed.

Migraine Headaches

- *Epidemiology.* Migraine headaches usually start in the first three decades of life. It is more common in women than men. Classic migraine is described in association with an aura, but up to 80% of patients with vascular headaches have no associated aura. There is a relationship between migraines and menses in 15% of individuals. Most migraine sufferers have a family history of migraines. Table 35–2 describes different types of migraine headaches.
- *Pathophysiology.* This is probably due to a disorder of neurovascular regulation in the brain. The exact pathology is unknown but several theories exist. Research suggests that at least three mechanisms are

Table 35–2	Types of Migraines
Type of Migraine	**Description**
Migraine with aura	May occur with or without headache; most aura develops over 5-20 min and resolves within 1 h; please see chapter for descriptions of some of the auras.
Migraine without aura	Diagnostic requirements: Headache lasting 4-72 h; headaches with at least two of these characteristics (pulsating quality, unilateral pain, aggravated by activity, moderate to severe intensity); during the headache, at least one of these symptoms (nausea and vomiting or photophobia)
Hemiplegic migraine	Begins in childhood and stops in adulthood; sporadic and a familial form; attacks precipitated by minor head injury; hemiplegia may be part of the aura lasting an hour to being part of the headache that lasts for days.
Ophthalmoplegic migraine	Acute CN III palsy with dilated pupil and unilateral eye pain; CN IV and VI are rarely involved; the ophthalmoplegia can last from days to months; LP may be needed to rule our an infectious process if there is no prior history; MRI and MRA with contrast may show some enhancement of the oculomotor nerve.
Basilar migraine	Female predominance; severe headache preceded by visual aura and signs and symptoms of brainstem pathologies, including, ataxia, nausea and vomiting, vertigo, diplopia, nystagmus, and altered level of consciousness.

CN, cranial nerve; LP, lumbar puncture; MRA, magnetic resonance angiography; MRI, magnetic resonance imaging.

involved: alteration in cranial circulation, neurogenic inflammation, and abnormalities in pain modulation in the brainstem. Serotonin (5-HT) appears to play a role.

■ *History.* There is a history of chronic and recurrent headaches. The headache is often described as unilateral, but may be bilateral in 40% of patients. The headache is gradual in onset, pulsating in quality, moderate to severe in intensity, and associated with photophobia, nausea, or vomiting. Migraine with aura typically starts with fully reversible neurologic symptoms preceding the headache. These symptoms include scintillating scotomas (bright rim around an area of visual loss), photopsia (poorly formed brief flashes of light), blurred vision, or fortification spectrums (aerial view of a fortress or walled city). They typically develop over a short amount of time, and do not last more than 1 hour. The visual auras are the most common, but there are also others, such as hemiparesis, paresthesias, aphasia, or even ophthalmoplegia. Paresthesia is the second most common aura. Patients often describe triggers such as menstruation, certain smells, stress, or alcohol.

- *Physical examination.* A thorough neurologic examination should be performed. If the patient is suffering from an uncomplicated migraine attack, the examination will be normal. Cranial nerve palsies may be seen in opthalmoplegic migraines.
- *Diagnostic testing.* No imaging or laboratory study is needed if the history and physical examination do not reveal any "red flags", or if the patient describes the headache as a "typical" migraine.
- *ED management.* Many different options for pain control exist (Table 35–1). Narcotic analgesia should be reserved for patients who do not respond, have contraindications to other therapy, or need rescue medication. The use of steroids is controversial, but may be effective for prolonged attacks. Calcium channel blockers are useful in some patients with auras, but must be given before the headache is full blown. Some patients report that a daily aspirin tablet is effective prophylaxis. Valproic acid (Depakote®) may prevent migraine, but will not cure a headache once it is started.
- *Helpful hints and pitfalls.* Migraine sufferers with a change in pattern of the headache should have a thorough ED evaluation looking for possible SAH, or other intracranial pathology.

Post–Lumbar Puncture Headache

- *Epidemiology.* This is a common complication of an LP, occurring in up to 49% of patients. The duration is typically less than 5 days.
- *Pathophysiology.* It is most likely due to a persistent CSF leak resulting in low CSF pressures, and causing the brain to descend in the cranial vault when the patient assumes an upright position. The amount of time a patient remains in the recumbent position immediately after a lumbar puncture does not affect the incidence of this complication.
- *History.* The patient complains of a diffuse, throbbing, headache that worsens in the upright position. The patient may also complain of neck stiffness, nausea and vomiting, auditory disturbances, blurred vision, and diplopia.
- *Physical examination.* This is normal.
- *Diagnostic testing.* Studies are not indicated.
- *ED management.* Most resolve after conservative treatment of bed rest and analgesics. Oral caffeine (300 mg every 4-6 hours) or caffeine benzoate (500 mg in 1 L of IV fluid) may be effective for persistent headaches. An epidural blood patch by an anesthesiologist will relieve the headache in the majority of severe cases; and should be obtained when the patient fails to obtain relief from the above and adequate analgesia.
- *Helpful hints and pitfalls.* Smaller-diameter needles and inserting the needle with the bevel of the needle facing straight up toward the ceiling (assuming that the patient is in the lateral decubitus position) may decrease CSF leakage.

Sinusitis

- **■ *Epidemiology.*** Viral URIs and allergic rhinitis are the most common causes. Other predisposing factors include immunocompromised state, structural abnormalities, foreign bodies, and instrumentation. Allergic rhinitis is associated with allergen exposure and prior episodes. *S. pneumoniae*, nontypable *H. influenzae*, and *M. catarrhalis* are the primary pathogens responsible for acute bacterial sinusitis. Anaerobic bacteria, streptococcal species, and *S. aureus* are causes of chronic sinusitis. *P. aeruginosa* is associated with HIV infection and cystic fibrosis.

- **■ *Pathophysiology.*** Ostial obstruction, inflammation, ciliary dysfunction and increased mucous impair drainage of the sinuses. These processes lead to inflammation and bacterial overgrowth.

- **■ *History.*** Allergic sinusitis is associated with sneezing and itchy eyes. During the first 5-7 days, it is difficult to distinguish between viral and bacterial sinusitis. Bacterial disease is suggested by worsening symptoms after 5 days. Symptoms include nasal congestion, mucopurulent nasal discharge, nasal obstruction, postnasal drip and cough, malaise, fever, teeth pain, and facial pain or headache over the involved sinus. The exception to this is in cases of sphenoid sinusitis, which may present with vague headaches and focal points almost anywhere in the head.

- **■ *Physical examination.*** This may reveal fever, nasal mucosal erythema and edema, purulent nasal discharge, and tenderness over the involved sinus. Pain caused by ethmoid, sphenoid, and frontal sinusitis is exacerbated by placing the patient supine and relieved by positioning the patient's head in an upright position.

- **■ *Diagnostic testing.*** This is usually a clinical diagnosis. An axial and coronal CT scan is the imaging study of choice. Its use should be limited to questionable diagnosis, to unresponsive disease, or to search for complications. The CT scan findings suggestive of sinusitis include air-fluid levels, sinus opacification, sinus wall displacement, and 4 mm or greater mucosal thickening.

- **■ *ED management.*** Selected use of antibiotics is recommended as most cases resolve spontaneously. Ten days of amoxicillin is still the first-line agent. Alternative agents include trimethoprim-sulfamethoxazole, amoxicillin-clavulanate, second-or third-generation cephalosporins, clindamycin, macrolides, or fluoroquinolones. Topical and systemic decongestants should be prescribed. Topical agents should only be used for 3 days to avoid rebound vasodilatation and worsening congestion. Antihistamines should be prescribed for allergic sinusitis. Chronic sinusitis should be referred to an otolaryngologist. Frontal or sphenoid sinusitis with air-fluid levels require hospitalization. Multiple sinus involvement should also be admitted, as well as any patient with single sinus involvement who appears toxic.

- **■ *Helpful hints and pitfalls.*** Sinus mucosal thickening is seen in about 40% of asymptomatic patients. Complications include facial cellulitis, periorbital cellulitis, periorbital abscess, optic neuritis, blindness, orbital abscess, and intracranial infection (e.g., cavernous sinus thrombosis, brain abscess).

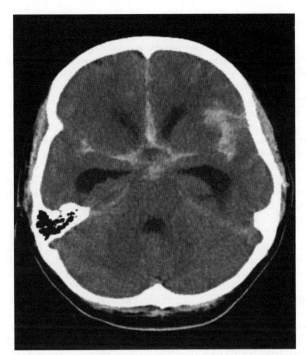

Figure 35-2. Subarachnoid hemorrhage. Noncontrast head CT scan of a subarachnoid hemorrhage with diffuse blood filling the basal cisterns in the classic star-shaped pattern. There is also some blood in the left sylvian fissure and mild ventricular enlargement. *Courtesy of Dr. Peter Panagos, Brown Medical School, Department of Emergency Medicine.*

Subarachnoid Hemorrhage

- *Epidemiology.* Hypertension, alcohol, drug use, cigarette smoking, and a family history of SAH are risk factors. Patients with fibromuscular dysplasia, polycystic kidney disease, and connective tissue diseases have a higher incidence of aneurysms. The overall occurrence is more common in women.
- *Pathophysiology.* SAH is defined as blood in the subarachnoid space of the brain. Most are caused by trauma. Of nontraumatic cases, 80% are due to ruptured intracranial aneurysms. In children and adolescents, an atrioventricular (AV) malformation is the most common cause of spontaneous SAH.
- *History.* The classic history includes sudden onset of a severe or "thunderclap" headache, usually "the worst headache of my life" accompanied by nausea and vomiting, photophobia, or meningismus. The patients may have neurologic complaints such as seizures or diplopia, a transient loss of consciousness, or a persistent altered level of

consciousness. The onset of headache may be associated with exertion, coughing, or a Valsalva maneuver. The patient may give a history of a less severe headache, which may represent a *sentinel bleed.*

- **Physical examination.** Nuchal rigidity occurs in 70% of cases. Funduscopy may reveal retinal or vitreous hemorrhage. Up to 15% of patients have a third nerve palsy that will manifest as papillary dilatation, with the same eye in the *down and out* position due to an expanding aneurysm compressing the third nerve. Twenty percent of patients have focal neurologic findings.

- **Diagnostic testing.** A noncontrast CT scan of the head can reveal most cases when performed within 24 hours of symptom onset (Figure 35–2). Still, negative findings on a CT scan do not ever rule out a SAH. There is a false-negative rate of 3% to 8% with noncontrast CT scans. The ability of a CT scan to correctly identify a SAH decreases rapidly to less than 50% after 1 week. The CT scan may also be falsely negative if the patient's hematocrit is less than 30%, or if the hemorrhage is very small. An LP should be performed on all patients in whom SAH is clinically suggested, and who have a normal noncontrast head CT scan. Xanthochromia is the yellowish pigmentation that is found in the CSF from the metabolism of hemoglobin. Xanthochromia may be absent very early (<12 hours), or very late (>2 weeks) in SAH. A traumatic LP is suggested by the presence of a clot in one of the tubes or by the clearing of the CSF and decreasing red blood cell counts from tubes, one to three. When peripheral cell counts are normal, the CSF from a traumatic lumbar puncture should contain around 1 white blood cell (WBC) per 700 red blood cells (RBCs).

- **Management.** All patients with a positive CT scan or persistently bloody or xanthrochromic CSF should undergo vascular imaging, either MRA or CT angiography. Emergent neurosurgery consultation should be obtained. Blood pressure control to maintain a mean arterial pressure of 110 mm Hg or a systolic blood pressure of less than160 mm Hg can decrease the rebleeding risk. The head of the bed should be elevated to 30 degrees. Vasospasm occurring after a ruptured aneurysm may be controlled by nimodipine, 60 mg by mouth (PO) every 6 hours. Phenytoin should be given for seizure prophylaxis. All patients should be admitted to the ICU for close monitoring.

- **Helpful hints and pitfalls.** Pain relief or normal CT scan findings do not rule out SAH.

Temporal Arteritis (also called Giant Cell Arteritis)

- **Epidemiology.** This disease is rare before the age of 50. The mean age of onset is 71. Women have a greater incidence of the disease than men. Visual loss occurs in 36% of untreated cases.

- **Pathophysiology.** The pathology reveals a granulomatous inflammation with multinucleated giant cells. The arteritis most commonly affects branches of the carotid artery but may involve any large or medium size artery.

- **History.** Headache is the most common presenting symptom, present in 80% to 90% of all patients. The headache is described as continuous or intermittent, and is worse at night or after cold exposure. Pain is localized to the frontotemporal region, and is described as sharp and throbbing. It may also be associated with jaw claudication, fatigue, weight loss, fever, night sweats, and visual disturbances such as unilateral vision loss or diplopia. Amaurosis fugax can also occur before permanent visual loss. There is also an association with polymyalgia rheumatica, with patients complaining of early-morning shoulder girdle stiffness.

- *Physical examination.* This may reveal a tender temporal artery with decreased pulsation, beading, or erythema over the surrounding skin. Funduscopy may reveal disc edema or pallor.
- *Diagnostic testing.* ESR and CRP will be elevated. The ESR is usually greater than 50 mm per hour, however, an ESR of less than 40 mm per hour has been found in 5% of people with temporal arteritis. The CBC may show a mild anemia.
- *Management.* Treatment with steroids should be started for any patient with the clinical picture of temporal arteritis. Prednisone should be started at a dosage of 1 mg/kg/d. Start oral prednisone daily, up to a maximum dose of 120 mg daily. In the rapidly deteriorating patient or a patient with one or more neurologic symptoms, IV methylprednisolone can be used, typically 1 g/d divided into two to four doses. The steroids do not change the results of the biopsy, but may prevent progression to visual loss. A temporal artery biopsy is the gold standard to clinch the diagnosis. If there are visual disturbances, ophthalmology should be consulted. Rheumatology should be consulted for complicated cases.
- *Helpful hints and pitfalls.* If the diagnosis is delayed, the most serious complication is visual loss, caused by ischemic optic neuritis. A low ESR may be found in a small percentage of patients.

Trigeminal Neuralgia (Tic Douloureux)

- *Epidemiology.* This entity is more common in women than in men, mostly between the ages of 50 and 69 years.
- *Pathophysiology.* It is an idiopathic disorder but may involve compression of the trigeminal nerve root.
- *History.* The patient experiences brief electric shocklike pains in the distribution of one or more branches of the trigeminal nerve, occurring spontaneously or elicited by minimal stimuli.
- *Physical examination.* A thorough examination should be performed to rule out other sources of pain or neurologic disease.
- *Diagnostic testing.* A CT scan or MRI is necessary to rule out any underlying mass lesion.
- *Management.* Several drugs have been found to be effective and include carbamazepine, phenytoin, baclofen, valproate sodium, lamotrigine, and gabapentin. Thirty percent of patients do not respond to medical therapy. Surgical management includes nerve blocks or microvascular decompression.
- *Helpful hints and pitfalls.* Patients with any neurologic deficit require urgent imaging studies to rule out a mass or vascular abnormality; these patients do not have trigeminal neuralgia.

Special Considerations
Pediatrics

- Most headaches in the pediatric population are benign. Most of these headaches are due to upper respiratory infections or migraines.
- Indications for imaging are similar to those for adults.

Pregnancy

- Consider the diagnosis of pre-eclampsia, which is discussed in chapter 68.

Immunocompromised

- All HIV and oncology patients with new headaches or neurologic deficits require neuroimaging. A head CT scan *with* contrast is the preferred imaging study in the ED, unless there is a concern for a subarachnoid hemorrhage.

Toxicology

- Consider carbon monoxide poisoning and alcohol withdrawal as possible etiologies.

Teaching Points

Headache is a common, usually not serious, but often troublesome problem in the ED. However, it may signify a very serious disease that may be presenting at a time when a tragic deterioration of neurologic function can be averted.

The clues for this are sudden onset, the history of "the worst headache" ever experienced by the patient, and no historical support for another diagnosis such as migraine.

Every emergency physician will see rare but dangerous causes for headache, such as brain tumor. The clue may be in a history that is not commonly part of a vascular headache picture, and subtle neurologic changes.

Do not be afraid to workup the patient who has had a history of "migraine" headaches, especially if he or she has never had a complete workup.

Do not forget to perform lumbar punctures; a CT scan will not reveal small bleeds, infection, or increased intracranial pressures.

Suggested Readings

American College of Emergency Physicians. Clinical policy: critical issues in the evaluation and management of patients presenting to the emergency department with acute headache. Ann Emerg Med 2002;39:108–122.

Edlow JA. Diagnosis of subarachnoid hemorrhage in the emergency department. Emerg Med Clin North Am 2003;21:73–87.

Heilpern KL, Lorber B. Infectious disease emergencies: focal intracranial infections. Infectious Dis Clin North Am 1996;10:879–898.

Henry GL, Russi CS. Headache. In: Marx JA, Hockberger RS, Walls RM (editors). Rosen's Emergency Medicine: Concepts and Clinical Practice (6th ed). Philadelphia: Mosby, 2006, pp 169–175.

Peters KS. Secondary headache and head pain emergencies. Prim Care Clin Office Pract 2004;31:381–393.

Qureshi F, Lewis D. Managing headache in the pediatric emergency department. Clin Ped Emerg Med 2003;4:159–170.

Schoenen J, Sándor PS. Headache with focal neurological signs or symptoms: a complicated differential diagnosis. Lancet Neurology 2004;3:237–245.

Stahmer SA, Raps EC, Mines DI. Neurologic emergencies: carotid and vertebral artery dissections. Emerg Med Clin North Am 1997;15:677–698.

Widico CR, Newman DH. Does this patient have temporal arteritis? Ann Emerg Med 2005;45:85–87.

CHAPTER **36**

Hernia

Jason N. Collins ■ Adam H. Miller

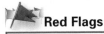
Red Flags

> Abnormal vital signs ● Peritoneal signs ● Toxic appearance ● Repeat visits to the ED ● New or acutely changed symptoms with known hernia such as the inability to reduce a previously reducible hernia ● Symptoms or signs concerning for bowel obstruction (vomiting, constipation or obstipation) ● Persistent pain after reduction → Incomplete reduction or reduction of gangrenous bowel

Overview

Hernias are common in patients arriving at the ED. While usually problematic only because of pain, they can produce both morbidity and mortality. Look for "red flags" (see Box) early in any patient presenting with a hernia.

A hernia is a protrusion of a structure or part of a structure through the tissues in which it is normally contained. The site of formation is structurally weak, either congenitally or through surgery or trauma. The contents of the hernia sac may include bowel or other organs, omentum, fat, vascular structures, or masses.

A visible or palpable mass usually accompanies the diagnosis. However, a hernia can present with vague, poorly localized pain, and must be considered in any patient presenting with abdominal pain (see Chapter 18).

Two broad categories exist—internal and external—and are further characterized by their respective specific anatomic locations (Table 36–1). An external hernia breeches the abdominal wall; an internal hernia is a protrusion of intestine through a defect within the peritoneal cavity.

The most common type is an inguinal hernia. Inguinal hernias are classified as *direct* or *indirect*. The sac of an indirect inguinal hernia passes from the internal inguinal ring obliquely toward the external inguinal ring and into the scrotum. The sac of a direct inguinal hernia protrudes outward and forward, and is medial to the internal inguinal ring and inferior epigastric vessels. It may be difficult distinguish between an indirect and a direct inguinal hernia clinically. However, this distinction is of little importance in the ED since the complications are similar, and both types require surgical repair.

If the structure can be relocated to a normal position, the hernia is *reducible*. An *incarcerated* hernia is present when the contents become irreducible. *Strangulation* implies compromise of blood flow to a component of the hernia and subsequent ischemic necrosis. The latter two cases require urgent or emergent surgical intervention.

Differential Diagnosis

■ See the DDx table for the differential diagnosis of a groin mass.

DDx Differential Diagnosis of a Groin Mass	
Genitourinary	Epididymitis (50)
	Hydrocele (50)
	Orchitis (50)
	Scrotal abscess (50)
	Scrotal edema (50)
	Spermatocele (50)
	Testicular infarction (50)
	Testicular torsion (50)
	Testicular tumor (50)
	Undescended testicle
	Varicocele (50)
Vascular	Hematoma
	Pseudoaneurysm
Skin	Epidermal inclusion cyst
	Lipoma
Infection	Groin abscess
	Hidradenitis suppurativa (62)
	Lymphogranuloma venereum (67)
Other	Lymphadenopathy
	Tumor

( ) Refers to the chapter in which the disease entity is discussed.

Table 36–1 Specific Types of Hernias

Hernia	Description	Epidemiology/Risk factors	Presentation and Complications
Inguinal	• Located in the inguinal canal; may protrude through external ring to scrotum/labia • Indirect: through deep inguinal ring • Direct: through region of the abdominal wall bound by the rectus muscle (medially), inguinal ligament (inferiorly), and inferior epigastric vessels (laterally)	• Most common site; 75% of all • Majority are indirect • More common in males and on the right side of the body • Associated with processes that increase intra-abdominal pressure	• Found incidentally on examination • Presents with a bulge or mass • The patient may report vague discomfort or pain in groin • Indirect hernias have higher risk of strangulation
Femoral	• Found inferior to inguinal ligament, medial to femoral vessels	• 3% of all hernias • More common in women	• Groin or medial thigh pain • 35% of all strangulated hernias are femoral
Incisional	• Located at site of prior incision (laparotomy and laparoscopic)	• Occur with 2-10% of abdominal surgeries • Most develop within 1 yr of surgery	• Asymptomatic bulge or pain at prior surgical site • Tend to enlarge, may progress to incarceration/strangulation • High recurrence rate after repair
Umbilical	• Located at the umbilicus	• Congenital in children; usually close spontaneously; repaired by age 4 otherwise • In adults, associated with pregnancy, obesity, ascites	• Usually asymptomatic • Peri-umbilical pain • May spontaneously rupture in persons with ascites
Spigelian	• Lateral/inferior edge of rectus muscle • Intraparietal (found deep to external oblique muscle)	• Acquired, rare • More common in middle-aged adults	• Pain at lateral edge of rectus • High risk of incarceration
Internal	• Within abdominal cavity • Form at sites of weakness/anomalous formation of mesentery or prior surgery/trauma	• Congenital or acquired • Rare, more frequent in adults	• Most are asymptomatic • Acute obstruction may progress to strangulation

Initial Diagnostic Approach
General

- As always, any patient who is hemodynamically unstable or appears ill should receive immediate attention. Patients with a history of a hernia who arrive in the ED complaining of a change in symptoms such as an inability to reduce the hernia, constipation or obstipation, fever, vomiting, and abdominal pain should have a complete and expeditious ED workup to evaluate for incarceration or strangulation.
- Vital sign abnormalities are indicators of more serious disease. The physical examination should look for asymmetry between opposite sides of the body, take note of surgical scars, auscultate bulges for bowel sounds or bruits, palpate for crepitus or fluctuance, and attempt to delineate the extent of the fascial defect surrounding a hernia sac.
- Inguinal hernias require examination in the standing and supine positions. If the patient is supine, ask the patient to flex the leg on the side being examined. Gather enough loose tissue from the base of the scrotal sac so that there will be comfortable insertion of the finger. Follow the spermatic cord as it moves up towards the inguinal canal, which is parallel and 1 cm above the inguinal ligament. If no mass is felt, ask the patient to bear down or turn his head away from the examiner and cough. A direct hernia can be felt pressing on the side of the examiner's finger. An indirect hernia can be felt pressing on the tip of the examiner's finger (see Figure 36–1). Bulges below the inguinal ligament usually represent femoral herniations.

Laboratory

- No testing is necessary or useful unless the hernia is incarcerated or strangulated.

Radiology

- *Plain films.* An upright chest film with a flat and upright abdomen may show bowel obstruction; free air represents bowel perforation but is rare even with strangulation,
- *Ultrasound.* May be useful in distinguishing a hernia from other masses.
- *Computed tomography (CT scan).* This imaging modality provides an excellent means to study the anatomy of the abdominal wall and can be useful in diagnosing internal hernias.

Emergency Department Management Overview
General

- If the patient appears ill, search for strangulation. The ABCs (*a*irway, *b*reathing, and *c*irculation) should be addressed as discussed in Section II.

Medications

- *Analgesia/sedation.* Opiates and benzodiazapines are the mainstays of treatment for patient comfort and to facilitate reduction. A combination

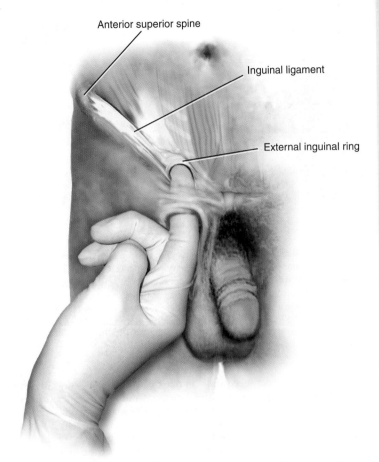

Anterior superior spine

Inguinal ligament

External inguinal ring

Figure 36–1. Technique of invagination of the scrotum to permit thorough palpation of the inguinal canal. *(From Dunphy JE, Botsford TW. Physical Examination of the Surgical Patient (4th ed). Philadelphia: WB Saunders, 1975, p 124.)*

of agents such as morphine or fentanyl plus midazolam is generally effective (see Chapter 90.1).

- *Antibiotics.* Broad-spectrum antibiotics effective against anaerobes are indicated in cases of strangulation (see Chapter 90.2).

Emergency Department Interventions

- Strangulated and incarcerated hernias in the adult patient require surgical correction, and should not be reduced in the ED.
- If the hernia is not incarcerated, reduction in the ED is appropriate. Passive treatments (e.g., sedation, analgesia, Trendelenburg position, and ice packs) are used to assist in the reduction. If the ED physician is unable

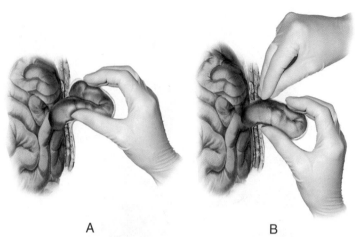

A   B

Figure 36–2. Reduction technique. Ballooning of contents. **A,** When reducing a hernia, the contents may ride up over the edge of the fascial defect. This leads to ballooning of the contents around the neck of the hernia, which hinders the reduction. **B,** By placing fingers along the edge of the hernia neck, one can direct the contents into instead of over the fascial defect. *(From Manthey DE. Abdominal hernia reduction. In: Roberts JR, Hedges JR (editors). Roberts' Clinical Procedures in Emergency Medicine (4th ed). Philadelphia: Elsevier, 2004, p 864.)*

to reduce the hernia successfully in one or two attempts, surgical consult should be obtained as multiple unsuccessful attempts can increase swelling, and prevent successful non-operative management.

- Technique for hernia reduction: identify the fascial defect with the non-reducing hand and apply gentle pressure to the neck of the hernia (Figure 36–2). This helps prevent overriding of the sac about the neck as steady pressure is applied to the hernia in a direction opposite to the line of presentation with the other hand (i.e., for inguinal hernias apply pressure from the scrotum or external inguinal ring toward the internal ring). It is important to reduce the most proximal part of the hernia first so that the apex does not block reduction of the remainder of the hernia sac. Continue applying direct, steady pressure until the entire hernia sac is reduced.

Disposition

- ***Consultation.*** Early surgical consultation is necessary for ill-appearing patients, and those who have incarceration, strangulation, or in whom reduction attempts are unsuccessful. Persistent pain after reduction suggests a partial reduction or reduction of already ischemic tissue and warrants further investigation.
- ***Admission.*** This is straightforward in cases of strangulation or incarceration, because emergent surgical correction is needed. Admission is also

necessary in patients who have peritoneal signs, evidence of obstruction, and those with intractable pain or vomiting.

- ***Discharge.*** Patients who are asymptomatic or have easily reducible hernias may be discharged to home with advice to be reevaluated in 24 to 48 hours, and are referred for elective surgical repair. Patients should be instructed to avoid activities that may predispose to reformation of the hernia (i.e., straining, heavy lifting, or other activities that increased intra-abdominal pressure). A prescription for analgesia and stool softeners may be helpful.

Special Considerations
Pediatrics

- Patients may have any of the hernias described in this chapter although there are a number of hernias specific to this age group. Congenital diaphragmatic hernias, including its variants Bochdalek's and Morgagni, are associated with a serious morbidity, and carry a significant risk of mortality. Congenital umbilical hernias are generally small, and close spontaneously between 6 months and 3 years of age. Strangulation usually does not occur, but umbilical hernias can produce a bowel obstruction even in a child.
- Inguinal hernias in infants often incarcerate, do not resolve spontaneously, and are often bilateral although they may present on a single side. They do not strangulate. They are seen in both boys and girls. In the girl, the uterus or ovary can be part of the herniation, and sometimes makes reduction impossible.

Women and Pregnancy

- The overall occurrence of a hernia is disproportionately low compared with that for men although certain types (femoral, umbilical, ventral) may be seen more often in women. The differences are likely due to a combination of hereditary and anatomical factors. A careful search must be made in the female patient when she complains of groin or pelvic pain as a visible or palpable mass is often hard to find.
- A hernia may be initially diagnosed during pregnancy as symptoms develop secondary to increased intra-abdominal pressure. Indications for surgery are similar to those listed in preceding sections.

Trauma

- Herniation secondary to trauma may be diagnosed acutely or may be seen as a late complication of the initial injury. Diaphragmatic hernias are more common after blunt trauma versus penetrating trauma to the chest or abdomen, and typically traverse the left hemidiaphragm (see Chapter 13). Diagnosis may be difficult in the acute setting. Classic findings include auscultation of bowel sounds in the chest, or nasogastric tube seen above an indistinct left hemidiaphragm on radiograph.

Teaching Points

Hernias are common problems in the ED. They most often present because of pain, but can be referred for elective surgical evaluation unless they are incarcerated or strangulated.

Pediatric hernias frequently incarcerate, but do not strangulate. Umbilical hernias in children often resolve by age three. In adults, they can incarcerate and strangulate, although this is rare in children.

Adult inguinal hernias are best reduced in the operating room when incarcerated, and should never be reduced if they are strangulated. Strangulated hernias of any type are surgical emergencies, and surgical consultation should be obtained early.

Appropriate preparation, positioning, sedation, analgesia, and manipulation are the keys to successful reduction.

All adult hernia types can progress to incarceration or strangulation. Any discharged patient should be given appropriate warnings and follow-up.

Femoral hernias are more common in women, but are easy to miss on physical examination because they are often hidden in the crura of the thigh. They have a high propensity for incarceration and strangulation.

An indirect inguinal hernia is the most common hernia, regardless of gender.

Suggested Readings

Malangoni MA, Gagliardi RJ. Hernias. In: Townsend CM, Beauchamp RD, Evers BM, Mattox KL (editors). Sabistson Textbook of Surgery (17th ed). Philadelphia: Elsevier, 2004, pp 1199–1217.

Manthey DE. Abdominal hernia reduction. In: Roberts JR, Hedges JR (editors). Roberts' Clinical Procedures in Emergency Medicine (4th ed). Philadelphia: Elsevier, 2004, pp 860–867.

McCollough M, Sharieff GQ Abdominal surgical emergencies in infants and young children. Emerg Med Clin North Am 2003;21:909–935.

CHAPTER 37

HIV

ROLAND C. MERCHANT ■ MICHELLE MCMAHON-DOWNER

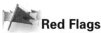 **Red Flags**

CD4+ T cell count of <200 cells/μL ● History of any AIDS defining illness ● Abnormal vital signs, especially tachycardia or hypotension ● Oxygen saturation < 95% ● Fever ● Altered mental status ● Headache ● Dehydration ● Diarrhea ● Dyspnea ● Hemoptyisis ● Diffuse rash ● Vision changes

OVERVIEW

Definition of HIV and AIDS

The *human immunodeficiency virus* (HIV) is a retrovirus that causes destruction of the immune system, particularly CD4+ T-cell lines.

The *acquired immunodeficiency syndrome* (AIDS) is the end result of an HIV infection. It is a syndrome characterized by the presence of *opportunistic* infections, and probable infection-related diseases not typically found in immune-intact humans. In the United States, AIDS is diagnosed by the presence of one or more of the 25 illnesses listed in the U.S. Centers for Disease Control and Prevention (CDC) 1993 case definition for AIDS (Table 37–1), or by the occurrence of CD4+ T cell counts below 200 cells/μL of blood in a person with an HIV infection in the absence of an AIDS-defining illness.

Epidemiologic Overview

In the United States, HIV and AIDS have predominately affected gay men and intravenous drug abusers. Recipients of blood product transfusions before 1985 in the United States were formerly at risk. Before the advent of prophylactic antiretroviral medications, perinatal transmission was a common source of HIV infection of children. Perinatal prophylaxis during pregnancy, delivery, and the neonatal period in the United States has dramatically decreased the incidence of HIV infections among children.

In most of the developing world, most persons are infected with HIV through heterosexual sex. In the United States, the number of new HIV infections transmitted through heterosexual sex is increasing. The incidence of HIV is increasing among women; women now comprise almost 50% of new HIV infections worldwide.

Natural History of HIV

HIV transmission. HIV is transmitted from exposure to the virus through contact with HIV-infected blood or body fluids containing HIV. Exposures typically occur through unprotected anal or vaginal sexual intercourse, and sharing of injecting-drug equipment. Transmission may also occur from transfusions with HIV-infected blood products, although this is rare worldwide because of screening of blood products for HIV. In the United States, HIV has been transmitted perhaps fewer than 57 times through health care worker exposures to blood or body fluids containing HIV. HIV is not transmitted through contact with saliva, sputum, urine, vomit, or feces.

HIV seroconversion and detection. After exposure and infection with HIV, HIV antibodies appear in the blood in about 3 to 6 months. HIV infections are diagnosed in most cases with assays that detect antibodies to HIV.

HIV viremia variability. HIV is at its highest levels in the blood (viral load) of an infected person within 3 to 6 weeks after an acute infection, and again near the end stage of AIDS. Persons with an HIV infection may be at their most infectious at these periods.

AIDS progression. In the United States, the median time from HIV infection to the onset of AIDS is approximately 10 years. Some patients have a more fulminant course to AIDS, and a few, termed chronic nonprogressors, remain without an AIDS-defining illness despite many years of being infected. Highly active antiretroviral therapy (HAART) has successfully delayed the onset of AIDS for many patients with HIV in the United States. Although not perfectly correlated, a patient's CD4+ T-cell count is a marker of when opportunistic infections occur (Table 37–1). The use of HAART and prophylaxis against opportunistic infections typically alter the CD4+ T-cell count at which these conditions manifest. Look for concerning signs and symptoms ("red flags"; see Box) in all HIV patients seen in the ED.

Antiretroviral Medications

In 2004 Department of Health and Human Services (DHHS) and the HIV Medicine Association/Infectious Disease Society of America (IDSA) recommended initial antiretroviral and prophylactic treatment regimens. The preferred initial antiretroviral regimens are listed in Table 37–2. Common adverse effects of antiretroviral medications are listed in Table 37–3.

Successful prophylaxis has been identified against *Pneumocystic carinii* pneumonia (PCP), toxoplasmic encephalitis, disseminated *Mycobacterium avium* complex (MAC) infection, cryptococcal meningitis, and cytomegalovirus (CMV) disease.

Table 37–1 AIDS Surveillance Case Definitions

Condition	CD4 Count
Cryptococcosis, extrapulmonary Cytomegalovirus retinitis Herpes simplex: chronic ulcers, bronchitis, pneumonitis, or esophagitis Lymphoma, brain primary Mycobacterium avium complex or M. kansasii, disseminated or extrapulmonary Toxoplasmosis of brain	<50
Candidiasis of bronchi, trachea, or lungs Cryptosporidiosis, chronic intestinal Cytomegalovirus disease other than liver, spleen, or nodes Encephalopathy, HIV-related Isosporiasis, chronic intestinal Lymphoma, Burkitt's Lymphoma, immunoblastic Pneumocystis pneumonia Pneumonia, recurrent Wasting syndrome due to HIV	<100
Coccidioidomycosis, disseminated or extrapulmonary	<250
Candidiasis, esophageal Kaposi's sarcoma Mycobacterium, other species or unidentified species, disseminated or extrapulmonary Mycobaterium tuberculosis, extrapulmonary Progressive multifocal leukoencephalopathy Salmonella septicemia, recurrent	<200
Histoplasmosis, disseminated or extrapulmonary	<150
Cervical cancer, invasive Mycobacterium tuberculosis, pulmonary or extrapulmonary	Any

Table 37–2 Infectious Disease Society of America (IDSA) and Department of Health and Human Services (DHHS)-Recommended Initial Antiretroviral Regimens

Preferred Initial Antiretroviral Regimens
NNRTI-based regimen efavirenz + (lamivudine or emtricitabine) + (zidovudine or tenofovir) *PI-based regimen* lopinavir/ritonavir + (lamivudine or emtricitabine) + zidovudine

NNRTI, *nonnucleoside reverse transcriptase inhibitors;* PI, *protease inhibitors.*

Table 37–3	HIV Medications and Common Side Effects
Nucleoside Reverse Transcriptase Inhibitors	
Abacavir	Nausea, vomiting, diarrhea, fever, chills, malaise, fatigue, headache, insomnia, loss of appetite, redistribution of body fat
Didanosine	Anxiety, headache, insomnia, irritability, restlessness, dry mouth, diarrhea, dyspepsia, flatulence, nausea, vomiting, rash
Emitricitabine	Headache, nausea, diarrhea, rash, skin discoloration of palms and soles, redistribution of body fat
Lamivudine	Splenomegaly
Stavudine	Arthralgia, myalgia, anorexia, chills, fever, rash, asthenia, gastrointestinal disturbances, headache, insomnia
Tenofovir*	Abdominal pain, anorexia, asthenia, diarrhea, dizziness, dyspnea, flatulence, headache, nausea, rash, vomiting, redistribution of body fat
Zalcitabine	Headache, fatigue, oral ulcers, stomatitis, abdominal pain, nausea, vomiting, diarrhea, constipation, rash, pruritis, urticaria
Zidovudine	Headache, insomnia, myalgia, nausea, changes in pigmentation, hyperpigmentation of nails, redistribution of body fat, malaise, anorexia
Nonnucleoside reverse transcriptase inhibitors	
Delavirdine mesylate	Rash, abdominal pain, asthenia, fatigue, fever, flu syndrome, headache, diarrhea, nausea, vomiting, anxiety, depression, insomnia, cough, bronchitis, sinusitis, pharyngitis, upper respiratory infection
Efavirenz	Euphoria, impaired concentration, insomnia, somnolence, depression, anxiety, rash, nausea, diarrhea, vomiting, dyspepsia, abdominal pain, anorexia, constipation, malabsorption, redistribution of body fat, vision changes, arthralgia, asthenia, myalgia, tinnitus
Nevirapine	Rash, fever, gastrointestinal disturbances, headache
Protease inhibitors	
Amprenavir	Abdominal pain, diarrhea, nausea, oral paresthesia, rash, vomiting, depression or other mood disorders, fatigue, peripheral paresthesia, taste perversion, redistribution of body fat, hyperglycemia
Atazanavir	Jaundice, abdominal pain, back pain, cough, depression, diarrhea, headache, redistribution of body fat, nausea, vomiting, rash, microscopic hematuria, hyperglycemia
Fosamprenavir	Rash, diarrhea, nausea, vomiting, headache, oral paresthesia, abdominal pain, depression, redistribution of body fat, hyperglycemia

*Tenofovir is a nucleoTide (not nucleoSide) reverse transcriptase.

Table 37–3   HIV Medications and Common Side Effects—*cont'd*

Indinavir sulfate	Asthenia, abdominal pain, nausea, diarrhea, vomiting, headache, insomnia, taste perversion, somnolence, hyperglycemia
Lopinavir	Redistribution of body fat, diarrhea, nausea, abdominal pain, abnormal stools, asthenia, headache, insomnia, rash, vomiting, hyperglycemia
Nelfinavir mesylate	Diarrhea, nausea, flatulence, rash, redistribution of body fat, hyperglycemia
Ritonavir	Redistribution of body fat, asthenia, nausea, diarrhea, vomiting, anorexia, abdominal pain, taste perversion, circumoral and peripheral paresthesias, fever, headache, malaise, vasodilatation, constipation, dyspepsia, flatulence, throat irritation, myalgia, insomnia, somnolence, pharyngitis, sweating hyperglycemia
Saquinavir	Abdominal pain, diarrhea, nausea, anxiety, asthenia, Buccal mucosal ulceration, constipation, depression, dyspepsia, eczema, fatigue, flatulence, headache, insomnia, musculoskeletal pain, paresthesia, rash, taste disturbance, vomiting, hyperglycemia
Fusion inhibitors	
Enfuviritide	Local injection site reactions, diarrhea, nausea, fatigue, anorexia, anxiety, asthenia, conjunctivitis, constipation, cough, depression, flu-like syndrome, insomnia, lymphadenopathy, myalgia, pruritis, taste disturbance, sinusitis, skin papilloma, abdominal pain

Initial Diagnostic Approach
General

- Any patient who is hemodynamically unstable or who appears ill should receive immediate attention. For ill patients, a continuous cardiac monitor and pulse oximeter should be placed. IV access should be obtained.
- Obtain the patient's history relevant to the chief complaint including duration, location, qualities, inciting and relieving factors, and history of related pertinent symptoms. Solicit the patient's medical history including the presence of any medical conditions, AIDS-defining illnesses, the patient's HIV history (last CD4 count and viral load, how and when HIV diagnosis made, ongoing risk factors for HIV infection such as injection-drug use and unprotected sex), recent hospitalizations, surgeries, medications (current and previous medications, especially HIV-related medications), and drug allergies. Perform a comprehensive review of systems because HIV infection may involve multiple organ systems. For the same reason most patients should receive a complete physical examination. A funduscopic examination looking for papilledema

or retinal changes should be performed on patients with visual changes or headache.

- The HIV patient must be considered to be immunosuppressed until proven otherwise. Although there may be a previously documented normal CD4, the patient's count may have changed.

- Patients with fever and HIV also need special attention. The differential diagnosis for this is lengthy, and includes a variety of infectious causes, malignancies, and drug reactions. If the absolute CD4+ lymphocyte count is less than $200/mm^3$, the likelihood of PCP or other opportunistic infections is significantly increased. A low count should prompt the physician caring for the patients to perform a diligent search for any serious pathology, such as pneumonia or meningitis. As with many other immunosuppressed patients, serious infection can be subtle, the patient may have atypical symptoms and may not have the expected physical findings. For example, headache and fever in a patient with AIDS must be assumed to be a CNS infection. A lumbar puncture should be performed even in the absence of nuchal rigidity or irritation.

Laboratory

- Obtain laboratory tests that help support or refute the putative diagnoses entertained. An arterial blood gas on room air (if possible) should be obtained on patients in respiratory distress, those who have low oxygen saturations on pulse oximetry, or if PCP is suspected.

- Obtain chemistry profiles, liver enzymes, and complete blood counts when considering adverse effects of antiretroviral medications. Obtain a serum lipase level for patients taking protease inhibitors when pancreatitis is a possible diagnosis.

- A standard or rapid HIV test, HIV viral load, and CD4+ count should be ordered on admitted patients with actual or suspected HIV. If discharged, follow-up should be coordinated with their outpatient medical providers.

Radiography

- Order imaging studies pertinent to the diagnoses being considered (e.g., chest radiograph for cardiopulmonary complaints, computed tomography [CT scan] or magnetic resonance imaging (MRI) for central nervous system (CNS) disease).

Emergency Department Management Overview
General

- The ABCs (*a*irway, *b*reathing, and *c*irculation) should be addressed as discussed in Section II. Provide oxygen to patients with hypoxia, dyspnea, and cardiopulmonary disorders to maintain SaO_2 greater than 95%.

Medications

- Provide antibiotics as quickly as possible when infections are suspected.
- Prescribe medications to relieve pain quickly, and as are appropriate to the patient's complaint and condition (Chapter 90.1).

Emergency Department Interventions

- When pulmonary tuberculosis is suspected (i.e., most patients with HIV with cough and fever), place the patient in respiratory isolation at least until pulmonary tuberculosis can be ruled out by radiography or sputum testing, as appropriate.

Disposition

- *Consultation.* Consult an HIV specialist as appropriate for HIV-infected patients whose diagnosis is unclear, or who will require further evaluation of their condition. Consult other specialists as pertinent, and required by the patient's condition.
- *Admission.* Admit patients who require further inpatient evaluation or monitoring of their condition; IV antibiotics, pain medications or fluids; transfusions; oxygen; or who are unable to adequately provide medical care for themselves.
- *Discharge.* All HIV patients discharged from the ED should be referred to their primary care or HIV specialist for follow-up.

Specific Problems
Primary HIV Infection

- *Overview.* An acute infection with HIV may become symptomatic approximately 2 to 6 weeks after an HIV exposure.
- *Pathophysiology.* A rise in viremia (viral load), and production of an immune response to HIV leads to symptoms. Recurrent symptomatic HIV infection, which results from an acute increase in viral load, may occur in patients who discontinue antiretroviral therapy.
- *History and physical examination.* Fever, lymphadenopathy, fatigue, pharyngitis, diarrhea, weight loss, rash, and myalgias may be present.
- *Diagnostic studies.* Order (or arrange follow-up to obtain) a standard or rapid HIV test, HIV viral load, and CD4+ T-cell count. The patient should be tested for mononucleosis, which may have a similar presentation.
- *ED management.* Provide symptomatic relief, HIV risk-reduction counseling, and appropriate referral for follow-up of testing.
- *Helpful hints and pitfalls.* Counsel patients on the importance of follow-up for a repeat HIV test in 3 to 6 months should the initial test be negative, and the need to reduce behaviors that may lead to infecting others with HIV. Patients are highly infectious for HIV shortly before and during the symptoms of a primary HIV infection.

HIV Complications

- See Table 37–4.

Table 37–4   HIV Complications

System	Disease	Overview	Clinical Presentation	Diagnosis	Management
Central nervous system	Crypto-coccus	*Cryptococcus neoformans*, a fungus, is transmitted via the respiratory system.	Subacute meningitis or meningoencephalitis. Fever, malaise, headache, neck stiffness, photophobia. Altered mentation. Disseminated disease and pulmonary infection.	CSF: mildly ↑ protein, ↓ slightly glucose, few lymphocytes, numerous cryptococci. Opening pressure is frequently >200 mm H_2O. Cryptococcal antigen +	Amphotericin B 0.7–1mg/kg/day with flucytosine 25mg/kg po q6h. ↑ ICP might cause clinical deterioration.
	Toxoplasmosis	*Toxoplasma gondii*, a protozoa, is acquired by humans from eating undercooked meat or ingesting oocysts shed in cat feces.	Headache, confusion, weakness, fever, focal neurologic deficits, seizures, stupor, and coma. Commonly presents as encephalitis.	CT scan or MRI of the brain reveals multiple contrast-enhancing lesions often with edema. Most patients are seropositive for anti-toxoplasma IgG antibodies. Brain biopsy for patients not improving with therapy.	Pyrimethamine 200 mg po ×1 then 75–100 mg/day plus sulfadiazine 1–1.5 gm orally q6 plus folinic acid 10–15 mg/day for six weeks. Steroids for mass effect. Anticonvulsants for seizures. IV trimethoprim 5 mg/kg/day and sulfamethoxazole 25 mg/kg/day if unable to tolerate po.
	HIV dementia	Progressive cognitive deterioration occurs in 7% of HIV-infected patients	Memory impairment, altered cognition, slow motor skills, unstable gait, seizures, stupor, coma, hyperactive deep tendon reflexes.	Neuroimaging reveals atrophy and diffuse deep matter changes. The LP and CSF results are normal. HIV dementia is a diagnosis of exclusion.	Referral for social services as needed.

Table 37–4 HIV Complications—*cont'd*

System	Disease	Overview	Clinical Presentation	Diagnosis	Management
	Neuro-syphilis	HIV-infected patients may have more rapid and severe CNS disease than other patients.	Meningitis, meningovascular disease, uveitis, optic neuritis, and deafness.	CSF: mild mononuclear pleocytosis (10-200 cells/μL), a normal or mildly ↑ protein and a reactive CSF-VDRL. The CSF may be normal in some cases.	IV penicillin G, 3-4 million units IV q 4 hours or procaine penicillin 2.4 million units IM qd plus probenecid 500 mg po qid for 10-14 days. For penicillin allergic patients, desensitization is preferred. Ceftriaxone 2 g qd IV for 10-14 days is an alternative.
	Progressive multifocal leukoencephal-opathy (PML)	This is caused by the JC polyoma virus and results in demyelination.	Insidious onset but progresses rapidly. A typical presentation includes cognitive dysfunction, dementia, seizures, ataxia, aphasia, cranial nerve deficits, paresis, and coma.	A CT scan reveals single or multiple hypodense, nonenhancing cerebral white matter lesions without mass effect. PCR for JC viral DNA in the CSF may be diagnostic. Definitive diagnosis is via brain biopsy.	Admit for definitive diagnostic evaluation as required. No antimicrobial treatment is effective.

Continued

Table 37–4 HIV Complications—*cont'd*

System	Disease	Overview	Clinical Presentation	Diagnosis	Management
	Cytomegalo-virus (CMV) retinitis	CMV causes retinal necrosis and edema that results in retinal scarring. Retinal detachment may occur in 25% of cases.	Painless, visual impairment or loss, scotomata, "floaters" or flashing lights.	Funduscopy reveals white, fluffy, lesions with hemorrhage near retinal vessels.	Valganciclovir 900 mg BID PO, ganciclovir 5mg/kg/dose BID IV, intravenous foscarnet 60 mg/kg/dose q8h IV, or cidofovir 5 mg/kg/week IV. A ganciclovir intraocular implant with oral valganciclovir may be used.
Peripheral nervous system	Myopathy	May be related to HIV infection itself, an adverse side-effect of HIV medications, or CMV myelitis in patients with CD4 counts <100/μL.	Myalgias, muscle weakness. Spastic paraparesis, bowel and bladder dysfunction, and ataxia.	CK may be elevated. If CMV myelitis is suspected, CSF should be examined for CMV DNA by PCR. Electromyography, nerve conduction studies, and muscle biopsy may be required as further evaluation.	Symptomatic treatment. Prednisone 1mg/kg/ day. Antiretroviral treatment may help or may be the source of the problem.
	Neuropathy	May be related to opportunistic illnesses, HIV infection, or HIV medications.	Many manifestations: distal symmetric polyneuropathy is most common.	Nerve conduction testing can confirm the diagnosis. Other causes of neuropathy shoul be ruled out.	Narcotics, tricyclic antidepressants, or anticonvulsants may be required in treatment of pain from neuropathy.

Table 37-4 HIV Complications—*cont'd*

System	Disease	Overview	Clinical Presentation	Diagnosis	Management
Pulmonary	PCP	*Pneumocystis carinii*, formerly popularly referred to as the cause of PCP, has been reclassified as an infector of rodents. *Pneumocystis jiroveci*, a fungus with protozoan characteristics and source of PCP in humans, is transmitted through the respiratory system.	Subacute onset of progressive exertional dyspnea, fever, nonproductive cough, and chest discomfort. Marked hypoxia. Tachypnea, tachycardia, and diffuse dry rales. Pulmonary auscultation may be normal in 50% of patients.	Chest radiograph may show a diffuse interstitial infiltrate, nodules, cavitation, bullae, pneumonthorax or no findings. A CT scan may demonstrate patchy ground-glass attenuation. Sputum may reveal the organisms. LDH is often ↑. Bronchoscopy or sputum may identify organisms.	Trimethoprim 15 to 20 mg/kg/day of trimethoprim and sulfamethoxazole 75 to 100mg/kg/day divided q 8 hr, PO or IV. Alternative therapy: trimethoprim-dapsone, clindamycin-primaquine, pentamidine, and atovaquone. If room air pO₂ <70 mm/Hg or arterial-alveolar O₂ gradient >35 mm/Hg, give prednisone 40 mg po bid with a tapering dose.

Continued

Table 37-4 HIV Complications—*cont'd*

System	Disease	Overview	Clinical Presentation	Diagnosis	Management
	Pulmonary TB (see Chapter 67)	May occur at any CD4+ count; extrapulmonary TB is more common for CD4+ T cell counts <200 cells/μL. Mycobacterium avium complex generally results in disseminated disease particularly in patients with CD4+ T cell counts <50 cells/μL.	Fever, hemoptysis, night sweats, and weight loss are common.	Chest radiograph may reveal upper lobe infiltrates, cavitary lesions, alveolar infiltrates, interstitial infiltrates, a miliary pattern, pleural effusions, intrathoracic adenopathy, or no findings. Obtain sputum (expectorated or induced) for AFB staining. Bronchoscopy may be required.	Place in respiratory isolation rooms. Begin isoniazid, rifampin or rifabutin, pyrazinamide, and either ethambutol hydrochloride or streptomycin only if TB is the known diagnosis. Consider treatment for PCP or community acquired pneumonia.
	Community Acquired Pneumonia (see Chapter 67)	Bacterial pneumonia is the most common pulmonary complication. Recurrent pneumonia is an AIDS-defining illness. Infections can occur at any CD4+ count. *Pseudomonas aeruginosa* causes a more severe pneumonia.	Chills, rigors, pleuritic chest pain, and purulent sputum that develop over a short period of time; slower developing symptoms favor PCP, TB, or fungal pneumonias. Fever, tachypnea, tachycardia, and rales or rhonchi may be present.	Chest radiograph may show a focal infiltrate whereas the atypical bacterial pneumonia and viral pneumonia may show a diffuse interstitial infiltrate. Sputum Gram's stain and culture should be obtained before antibiotics. Consider testing for PCP and TB, especially for patients with abnormal CD4+ T cell counts.	Extended spectrum cephalosporin and a macrolide or a fluoroquinolone effective against *S. pneumoniae*. Cover for *P. aeruginosa* and other gram-negative bacilli in patients with severe immunodeficiency.

Table 37–4 HIV Complications—*cont'd*

System	Disease	Overview	Clinical Presentation	Diagnosis	Management
	Histo-plasmosis	May occur in up to 27% of AIDS patients in endemic areas. *Histoplasma capsulatum*, causes disease by primary infection or reactivation of a latent infection.	Fever, fatigue, weight loss, cough, chest pain, and dyspnea. Disseminated histoplasmosis may manifest as meningitis, sepsis, skin or mucosal lesions, and diarrhea.	Chest radiograph often shows interstitial or reticulonodular infiltrates, but may also show focal infiltrates, pleural effusions, mediastinal adenopathy, calcified granulomas or no findings. Other: Wright's smear, immunoassay, histology, sputum culture.	IV amphotericin B 0.7-1 mg/kg/day. Itraconazole 200 mg qd or bid may be prescribed for patients who do not require hospitalization.
	Coccidio-mycosis	*Coccidioides immitis and Coccidioides posadasii* are fungi and cause infections from inhalation of organism and or reactivation.	Fever, cough, and chest pain in pulmonary and primary infections. Disseminated disease: meningitis, lymphadenopathy, skin nodules or ulcers, peritonitis, liver abnormalities, and less commonly with bone and joint involvement.	Chest radiograph may reveal diffuse interstitial infiltrates. Definitive diagnosis requires isolation of the fungus in respiratory fluids or histopathologic examination of involved tissue. Serology may be obtained.	IV amphotericin B 0.5-0.7 mg/kg/day. Ketoconazole, fluconazole, or itraconazole might be appropriate alternatives for patients with mild disease.

Continued

Table 37–4   HIV Complications—*cont'd*

System	Disease	Overview	Clinical Presentation	Diagnosis	Management
	Aspergillosis	*Aspergillus fumigatus* primarily causes lung disease in AIDS patients but can disseminate.	Presents as parenchymal disease (fever, cough, dyspnea, chest pain, hypoxia, or hemoptysis) or tracheobronchial disease (dyspnea, cough, stridor, or wheezing).	Chest radiograph reveals cavitary lesions, focal infiltrates, or bilateral interstitial infiltrates. Histopathologic examination confirms the diagnosis.	Voriconazole 400 mg IV or PO BID. Amphotericin B and itraconazole are alternative regimens.
Gastro-intestinal	Candidiasis	Nearly all AIDS patients have oral candidiasis (thrush) at some point during their illness; esophageal candidiasis is the AIDS-defining illness in about 14% of patients; disseminated candidiasis in AIDS is rare and is caused by *Candida albicans*, a fungus.	Oral lesions are typically painless, creamy white, plaque-like lesions of the tongue, buccal or oropharyngeal mucosa that can be scraped. Later, the lesions may appear erythematous and atrophic. In esophageal candidiasis, lesions may cause odynophagia, dysphagia, or retrosternal burning or pain.	Examine scrapings under microscopy using potassium hydroxide for the presence of fungal lesions. Refer for endoscopy, although barium swallow studies may assist in making the diagnosis. CMV and HSV should be considered as etiologies of esophagitis.	Topical therapy with clotrimazole 10 mg troches 5 times/day or nystatin suspension 4-6 ml 4 times/day or troches 4-5 times/day or oral fluconazole or ketoconazole 100-200 mg daily for 7-14 days is effective for oral candidiasis. Fluconazole 200 mg qd for 14-21 days is preferred for esophageal candidiasis; amphotericin B may be useful in refractory cases.

Table 37-4 HIV Complications—*cont'd*

System	Disease	Overview	Clinical Presentation	Diagnosis	Management
	Ulcerative oral lesions	May be due to viruses (herpes simplex, CMV, herpes zoster), bacteria, and other microorganisms (syphilis, candida); adverse side-effects of medications; cancers (Kaposi's sarcoma, non-Hodgkin's lymphoma) or aphthous ulcers.	Lesions are typically painful. HSV lesions present as multiple shallow ulcers <1 cm on the buccal mucosa or tongue while herpes zoster may appear as grouped lesions on the hard palate. CMV lesions are several small ulcers <1 cm on the buccal mucosa. Syphilitic lesions may appear as fissured ulcers. Aphthous ulcers are shallow, round or oval with a grayish ulcerative base.	HSV is diagnosed via viral culture and CMV is diagnosed by either viral culture or biopsy. Syphilis is typically diagnosed by serology. Aphthous ulcers are a diagnosis of exclusion.	HSV: oral famciclovir, valacyclovir, or acyclovir for 7 days. CMV: ganciclovir. Syphilis: depends upon the stage of the illness. Aphthous ulcers: ointments, including triamcinolone hexacetonide in Orabase, fluocinonide gel in Orabase, amlexanox 5% oral paste, thalidomide, and corticosteroids.

Continued

Table 37–4 HIV Complications—*cont'd*

System	Disease	Overview	Clinical Presentation	Diagnosis	Management
	Infectious diarrheal illness	May be the result of bacteria (e.g., *Salmonella*, *Campylobacter*, and *Shigella* species), parasites (e.g., *Cryptosporidia*, *Microsporidia*, *Isospora*), viruses (e.g., rotaviruses, Norwalk viruses), opportunistic infections (e.g., Kaposi's sarcoma, lymphoma) or an adverse-effect of medications. Cryptosporidial or Isosporal diarrhea of more than 1 month's duration are an AIDS-defining illnesses.	Nausea, vomiting, diarrhea, cramping, loss of appetite, and malaise are typical of infectious diarrheal diseases. For chronic or persistent infections, only diarrhea and weight loss may be present. Diarrhea of bloody stools or with sepsis suggests invasive disease. *Cryptosporidia* and *Isospora* cause non-bloody watery diarrhea.	Stool cultures, fecal leukocyte, and ova and parasite examinations. Colonoscopy with biopsy may be required for patients with chronic diarrhea.	Supportive therapy as needed with IV fluids, antiemetics, and antimotility agents. Begin ciprofloxacin 500 mg orally BID for empiric treatment for HIV-infected patients with fever and diarrhea. There is no effective antimicrobial agent for *Cryptosporidia*.

Table 37–4 HIV Complications—*cont'd*

System	Disease	Overview	Clinical Presentation	Diagnosis	Management
Renal	Nephro-pathy	This may be the result of adverse side-effects of medications, chronic infections, new infections, or direct infection with HIV.	Edema (particularly peripheral), fatigue, malaise may be present.	Urinalysis: proteinuria, hematuria, leukouria, and casts. Renal ultrasonography (showing large, echogenic kidneys) and renal biopsy are generally necessary to make the diagnosis.	Corticosteroids, cyclosporine, and angiotensin coverting enzyme inhibitors along with anti-retroviral medications are typically used in treatment of HIV-associated nephropathy.
Skin	Herpes simplex	90%–95% of HIV-infected patients are seropositive for HSV-1 or HSV-2. Reactivation may be due to sunlight, stress, immune dysfunction, or intercurrent illnesses.	In mucocutaneous infections, symptoms include burning or tingling followed by the eruption of grouped vesicles on an erythematous base or the formation of ulcers. Deep ulcerations may occur in severely immunocompromised.	Viral culture of lesions. Fluid from lesions may be examined in a Tzanck preparation for a more rapid diagnosis. Serology will likely not be useful.	Mild eruptions are treated with oral famciclovir 500 mg BID, valacyclovir 1 g BID, or acyclovir 400 mg TID for 7 days. Moderate-to-severe HSV lesions are best treated initially with intravenous acyclovir 5 mg/kg TID.

Continued

Table 37-4   HIV Complications—*cont'd*

System	Disease	Overview	Clinical Presentation	Diagnosis	Management
	Herpes zoster	15-25 times more common in HIV-infected patients than other patients. Herpes zoster is due to reactivation of varicella zoster virus from the sensory dorsal root ganglia.	Pain resembling a burn or muscle injury; characteristic grouped vesicles on an erythematous base in a single dermatome follow within a few days. In disseminated herpes zoster, multiple dermatomes are affected.	Lesions are typically diagnostic in herpes zoster. A viral culture of lesions may assist when the diagnosis is uncertain.	Acyclovir 800 mg 5x/day, valacyclovir 1 g TID, or famciclovir 500 mg TID PO may be initiated. If severe, begin IV acyclovir 10 mg/kg/dose TID and admit the patient. Steroids to prevent postherpetic neuralgia is not recommended in HIV.
Oncology	Lymphoma	Non-Hodgkin's lymphoma and primary CNS lymphoma are AIDS-defining illnesses, but Hodgkin's lymphoma is not.	May present with fever, chills, and weight loss, or symptoms specific to the body systems affected (typically gastrointestinal, pulmonary, hepatic, and hematopoietic). Primary CNS lymphomas may cause mental status changes, focal neuralgic deficits, headaches, or no symptoms.	A CT scan of the affected areas. Bronchoscopy, endoscopy, or colonoscopy. Definitive diagnosis is by biopsy. In brain lymphomas, tumors are more often solitary, ring-enhancing, rapid growing lesions in the cerebral hemispheres. CSF examination for Epstein-Barr virus or CSF cytology for malignant cells may assist in the diagnosis.	Symptomatic treatment, such as pain relief, related to the areas affected should be provided. Chemotherapy and antiretroviral therapy may be useful for non-Hodgkin's lymphoma. Radiation, antiretroviral therapy, and sometimes chemotherapy for CNS lymphomas. Corticosteroids for known brain lymphomas may decrease symptoms

Table 37–4 HIV Complications—*cont'd*

System	Disease	Overview	Clinical Presentation	Diagnosis	Management
	Kaposi's sarcoma	A vascular tumor that can be localized or systemic, is probably caused by human herpesvirus-8 perhaps in conjunction with HIV.	Skin and oral lesions predominate, but lesions may be present in other organ systems. Lesions are usually painless, elliptical papules of various shades from pink to purple or brown, and are more common on the lower extremities, face, and genitalia. Profound lymphedema may be present.	Diagnosis can be confirmed by biopsy.	Treatment depends upon the extent of the lesions and their manifestations. In most cases, treatment of symptoms may suffice. For localized lesions, intralesional chemotherapy, radiotherapy, laser therapy or cryotherapy may be effective. Various chemotherapeutic agents have been utilized for more extensive disease. The majority are managed on an outpatient basis.

Continued

Table 37–4   HIV Complications—cont'd

System	Disease	Overview	Clinical Presentation	Diagnosis	Management
	Invasive cervical cancer	Invasive cervical cancer is an AIDS-defining illness, and moderate to severe cervical dysplasia may be a feature of HIV infections in women. Human papilloma virus types 16 and 18 are likely causative.	Most women will have no symptoms, but some may notice abnormal bleeding, discharge, or pain with intercourse. Examination of the cervix may reveal lesions, especially with acetoacetate staining.	Papanicolaou smears, colposcopy, biopsy.	Symptomatic relief and referral for further gynecologic evaluation. Definitive treatment may involve surgery and chemotherapy.

AFB, Acid-fast bacilli; AIDS, autoimmune deficiency syndrome; CK, creatine kinase; CMV, cytomegalovirus; CNS, central nervous system; CSF, cerebrospinal fluid; CT, computed tomography; HIV, human immunodeficiency virus; HSV, herpes simplex virus; ICP, intracranial pressure; LDH, lactate dehydrogenase; LP, lumbar puncture; MRI, magnetic resonance imaging; PCR, polymerase chain reaction; TB, tuberculosis.

Teaching Points

The HIV-infected patient must be considered immunosuppressed until proven otherwise. Although the patient's last CD4+ count may have been normal, the count may not be the same on the day of the ED presentation. As with other immunosuppressed patients, sepsis and other serious conditions can be difficult to recongnize. For example, AIDS patients with fever and a headache should be assumed to have a CNS infection. A lumbar puncture should be performed on these patients even in the absence of classical signs and symptoms of meningitis.

The evaluation of HIV-infected patients relies upon knowledge of their health status. This knowledge is predicated on an assessment of their current CD4+ count, coexisting medical conditions, behavioral history (e.g., sexual habits and drug usage), and history of HIV- and AIDS-related illnesses. Some HIV-related medical problems are more likely to occur at a lower CD4+ count, such as PCP, while others are possible at any count, such as tuberculosis.

Many HIV-infected patients may require admission for conditions that, for patients with an intact immune system, would otherwise be safely managed as an outpatient. Furthermore, some AIDS patients have poor social resources, coexisting morbidities, and deleterious behaviors (e.g., injection-drug use) that limit their chances of effective outpatient treatment. Patients with established clinical providers typically have better access to resources that can help obviate hospital admission.

Laboratory and radiologic evidence of disease may lag behind clinical findings for patients with AIDS. It is prudent to evaluate the patient thoroughly for HIV- and AIDS-related conditions. Anticipation of and perhaps empirical treatment for certain conditions may be necessary.

Suggested Readings

AIDSInfo. US Department of Health and Human Services. *http://aidsinfo.nih.gov.*

amfAR Global Link. HIV/AIDS Treatment Information. American Foundation for AIDS Research (amfAR), accessed January 10, 2005, *http://web.amfar.org/treatment/index.asp.*

Centers for Disease Control and Prevention, National Institutes of Health, and the HIV Medicine Association/Infectious Disease Society of America. Treating Opportunistic Infections among HIV-infected Adults and Adolescents. *MMWR Recommed Rep.* 2004;53(RR-15):1–112.

Libman H and Makadon HJ. HIV (2nd ed). Philadelphia: American College of Physicians, 2003.

Princeton DC. Current Clinical Strategies: Manual of HIV/AIDS Therapy. Current Clinical Strategies Publishing, 2003.

Rothman RE, Marco CA, Yang S, and Kelen GD. AIDS and HIV. In: Marx JA, Hockberger RS, Walls RM (editors). Rosen's Emergency Medicine Concepts and Clinical Practice (6th ed). Philadelphia: Mosby, 2006, pp. 2071–2096.

CHAPTER 38

Hyperglycemia and Hypoglycemia

SANDRA S. YOON ■ PHILIP D. ANDERSON

 Red Flags

Altered mental status or coma ● Abnormal vital signs (hyperthermia, hypothermia, tachycardia, hypotension, tachypnea) ● Diaphoresis ● Tremulousness/Nervousness ● Focal neurologic signs ● Seizures ● Hyperventilation (Kussmaul's respiration) ● Fruity odor on breath

Overview

Look for "red flags" (see Box), and consider critical diagnosis early. These patients should be assessed rapidly, and treated for hyper- or hypoglycemia immediately with subsequent evaluation and treatment of underlying causes after stabilization.

Hyperglycemic patients not meeting criteria for diabetic ketoacidosis (DKA) or hyperglycemic hyperosmolar nonketotic coma (HHNC) can still be critically ill due to underlying problems.

A bedside finger-stick glucose level should be checked in every patient who has an altered mental status. Symptomatic hypoglycemia occurs in most adults at a blood glucose level of 40 to 60 mg/dl. Hypoglycemic patients not in coma or with only mild hypoglycemia can still be critically ill due to underlying precipitants such as sepsis, liver failure, and adrenal insufficiency.

This chapter will discuss hyperglycemia and hypoglycemia in general, focusing on the most concerning emergency department (ED) presentations of each: DKA, HHNC, and symptomatic hypoglycemia. Alcoholic ketoacidosis is also discussed. Although the blood sugar may be low or normal in this situation, its similar presentation to DKA warrants discussion.

Differential Diagnosis of Hyperglycemia and Hypoglycemia

■ See "Critical Diagnosis Table."
■ See Table 38–1 and 38–2 for causes of hyperglycemia.
■ See Table 38–3 for causes of hypoglycemia.

DDx Critical Diagnoses of Hyperglycemia and Hypoglycemia

Hyperglycemia	Hypoglycemia
Diabetic Ketoacidosis (DKA)	Hypoglycemic Coma
Alcoholic Ketoacidosis (AKA)	Symptomatic Hypoglycemia
Hyperglycemia Hyperosmolar NonKetotic Coma (HHNC)	

Table 38–1   Common Causes of Hyperglycemia

Insulin lacking (DM I and II)
Intrauterine pregnancy (or ectopic)
Insult (trauma/surgery, stress, emotional upset, burns, heat stroke)
Infection (UTI, pneumonia, etc.)
Infarction (MI, CVA, PE)
Indiscretion (Dietary noncompliance)

Table 38–2   Other Causes of Hyperglycemia

	Hyperglycemia from tissue insensitivity to insulin	Hyperglycemia from reduced insulin secretion
Hormonal tumors	Acromegaly Cushing's syndrome Glucagonoma Hyperthyroidism Pheochromacytoma	Somatostatinoma Pheochromocytoma Hyperthyroidism
Pharmacologic agents	Glucocorticoids Niacin Sympathomimetics	Thiazide diuretics Phenytoin Pentamidine

Organ disorders	Liver: cirrhosis,
	    hemochromatosis
		Pancreas: pancreatitis,
		    hemosiderosis,
		    hemochromatosis

Adipose tissue disorder	Lipodystrophy Truncal obesity	
Insulin receptor disorders	Acanthosis nigricans syndrome Leprechaunism	

Table 38–3	**Causes of Hypoglycemia**
Endocrine Deficiencies	Adrenal insufficiency (Addison's)
	Hypopituitarism
	Glucagon deficiency
	Thyroid insufficiency (Myxedema)
	Growth hormone deficiency
Drugs/Ingestions	Insulin (including factious hypoglycemia)
	Sulfonylurea
	Alcohol
	Pentamidine
	Quinine
	Salicylates
	Sulfonamides
	Propanolol
	Beta blockers
	Akee fruit
Endogenous Hyperinsulin	Insulinoma
	Ectopic insulin secretion
	Beta cell disorders
	Secretagogue (sulfonylurea)
Non Beta-cell Tumors	Mesenchymal tumors (fibrosarcoma, mesothelioma),
	Epithelial tumors (hepatic carcinoma, adrenalcortical tumors, carcinoid)
	Rhabdomyosarcoma
	Liposarcoma
	Leukemia
	Lymphoma
	Melanoma
	Teratoma
Metabolic	Liver failure
	Renal failure
Fed or Reactive	Postprandial
	Post gastric surgery (from rapid gastric emptying and increased insulin response)
	Early manifestation of DM type II
Other	Sepsis
	Starvation
	Autoimmune
	Prolonged exercise
	Alcohol

Initial Diagnostic Approach
General

■ Any patient who is hemodynamically unstable or appears ill should receive immediate attention. While the physician is assessing the patient, a continuous cardiac monitor and pulse oximeter should be placed. Intravenous (IV) access should be obtained. Bedside finger-stick glucose should be immediately obtained.

■ The history is important. Patients with hyperglycemia typically present with polydipsia, polyuria, polyphagia, visual blurring, weakness, weight loss, nausea, vomiting, and abdominal pain. Abdominal pain may occur in children. In adults, however, abdominal pain more often signifies true abdominal disease. Any precipitants of the hyper- or hypoglycemic state should be addressed. Alcohol use and nutritional intake should be assessed to determine risk for alcoholic ketoacidosis.

■ The physical examination should assess for altered sensorium, tachypnea with Kussmaul's respiration (ventilates with rapid, large tidal volumes), tachycardia, hypotension or orthostatic blood pressure changes, hydration status, odor of acetone (a fruity smell) on the breath, and evidence of infection. An elevated temperature is rarely caused by DKA itself, and suggests the presence of infection.

■ The patient should also be assessed for other conditions causing hyperglycemia (heat stroke, hyperthyroidism, seizures).

Laboratory

■ Studies include a complete blood count (CBC), electrolytes with renal function tests, lipase level, serum ketones, lactate level, cardiac enzymes (for patients at risk for cardiac ischemia as these patients may not have chest pain with acute coronary syndrome), urinalysis, blood gas, and a urine pregnancy test.

■ The finger-stick glucose may give a falsely high or low reading if the hematocrit is below 30% or above 55%.

■ Venous pH is not significantly different from arterial pH in a patient with DKA, unless the patient has decompensated to the point of respiratory failure or cardiac arrest.

■ The need for urine and blood cultures should be dictated by clinical findings.

■ An elevated urine specific gravity, blood urea nitrogen (BUN), and hematocrit suggest dehydration.

■ Hyperglycemia causes a dilutional hyponatremia (often mislabeled as *pseudohyponatremia*). The sodium level is actually low as measured, and will resolve naturally with correction of the hyperglycemia. To calculate the corrected sodium level, add 1.6 mEq/L to the measured sodium for every 100 mg/dl of glucose above 100.

■ Anion gap equals: sodium – (chloride + bicarbonate). The normal value is from 12 to 16 mEq/L, is typically elevated in DKA, and is secondary to elevated plasma levels of acetoacetate and beta-hydroxybutyrate, although lactate, free fatty acids, phosphates, volume depletion, and several medications also contribute to an increase in the anion gap condition.

■ Serum and urine tests for ketones are based on the nitroprusside test. The test may be falsely negative because it only reacts with acetone and acetoacetate, not beta-hydroxybutyrate, which accounts for the majority of circulating ketones in patients with DKA.

■ Laboratory testing should also address all suspected causes of the hypoglycemia, including ethanol or other drug ingestion. If factitious hypoglycemia is suspected, testing for insulin antibodies or low levels of C peptide may be helpful. Acute renal insufficiency may also cause hypoglycemia in patients on diabetic medications.

EKG

- An electrocardiogram (EKG) should be done to look for changes related to hyperkalemia or hypokalemia. It should also be performed on all patients at risk for CAD as hyperglycemia may be precipitated by a myocardial infarction.

Radiography

- *Plain films.* Chest radiograph should be obtained to look for infectious causes.
- *Computed tomography (CT scan).* A noncontrast head CT scan should be obtained to look for other causes of change in mental status. An abdominal CT scan with contrast may be needed to look for infection or neoplasm.

Emergency Department Management Overview
General

- The ABCs (*a*irway, *b*reathing, and *c*irculation) should be addressed as discussed in Section II. Isotonic IV fluids should be given via two large-bore IVs if the patient has tachycardia, hypotension, appears dehydrated, or has other potentially life-threatening conditions.
- The administration of IV insulin should be withheld until the potassium level is known, particularly in patients suspected to be in DKA. IV insulin decreases serum potassium, and may precipitate life-threatening dysrhythmias in a patient who is already potassium depleted.
- Normal saline restores volume and lowers glucose concentrations by hemodilution and increased urinary losses.

Medications

- *Insulin.* Lowers blood glucose levels by decreasing hepatic glucose production, increasing glucose transport into muscle and fat cells, and is needed to close the anion gap created in DKA by decreasing ketone production and increasing ketone metabolism. See Table 38–4.
- *Oral hypoglycemic agents.* There are a variety of agents with different mechanisms of action. See Table 38–4.
- *Dextrose 50% (D50).* One ampule (50 ml) contains 25 g of glucose. This is given IV for individuals with symptomatic hypoglycemia who are unable to take glucose orally.
- *Glucagon.* 1 to 2 mg intramuscular (IM) injection; should only be given if unable to establish IV access, and the patient is unable to tolerate oral intake. Glucagon stimulates adenylate cyclase to produce increased cyclic adenosine monophosphate (AMP), which promotes hepatic glycogenolysis and gluconeogenesis, raising serum glucose levels.
- *Octreotide.* 50 to 100 µg via subcutaneous (SC) injection or IV every 12 hours. Octreotide is a semisynthetic somatostatin analog, which inhibits insulin release. It is useful in hypoglycemia due to sulfonylurea and meglitinide ingestion, or insulin secreting tumors.

Table 38–4   Insulins and Oral Hypoglycemic Agents

Drug	Onset/Duration (hours)	Metabolism/ Elimination
INSULINS		
Ultra-short Acting	0.3/3-5	Hepatic and Renal
Aspart (Novolog R)	0.25/6-8	Hepatic and Renal
Lispro (Humalog R)		
Short Acting		
Regular (Novolin R)	0.5-1/8-12	Hepatic and Renal
Intermediate Acting		
Insulin Zinc Suspension (Lente)	2/18-24	Hepatic and Renal
Isophane Insulin Suspension (NPH)	2/18-24	Hepatic and Renal
Isophane Insulin Suspension and Regular Insulin Injection (Novolin R 70/30)	0.5/24	Hepatic and Renal
Long Acting		
Extended Insulin Zinc Suspension (Ultralente)	4/20-36	Hepatic and Renal
Insulin Glargine (Lantus)	2/>24	Hepatic and Renal
ORAL AGENTS		
SULFONYLUREAS – act by stimulating insulin release from pancreatic beta cells	**Duration (hours)**	
Acetohexamide (Dymelor)	12-24	Hepatic and Renal
Chlorpropamide (Diabinese)	24-72	Hepatic and Renal
Tolazamide (Tolinase)	16-24	Hepatic and Renal
Tolbutamide (Orinase)	6-12	Hepatic and Renal
Glimepride (Amaryl)	24	Hepatic and Renal
Glipizide (Glucotrol)	16-24	Hepatic and Renal
Glyburide (Micronase, Glynase, Diabeta)	18-24	Hepatic and Renal
BIGUANIDE – act by stimulating tissue glucose uptake and inhibiting gluconeogenesis	**Half Life (hours)**	
Metformin (Glucophage)	1.3-4.5	Renal
ALPHA-GLUCOSIDASE INHIBITOR - acts by inhibiting intestinal absorption of starch and disaccharides	**Half Life (hours)**	
Acarbose (Precose)	2	Renal
Miglitol	2	Renal
THIAZOLIDINEDIONE – act by increasing insulin action	**Half Life (hours)**	
Troglitazone (Rezulin)	16-34	Fecal
Rosiglitazone (Avandia)	3-4	Hepatic and Renal
Pioglitazone (Actos)	16-24	Hepatic and Renal

Continued

Oral Agent	Onset/Duration (hours)	Metabolism/ Elimination
Table 38–4 Insulins and Oral Hypoglycemic Agents—*cont'd*		
MEGLITINIDES – act by increasing insulin secretion	**Duration (hours)**	
Repaglinide (Prandin)	Up to 24 hours	Hepatic
Nateglinide (Starlix)	4 hours	Hepatic

- *Activated charcoal (AC).* 1 to 2 g/kg by mouth (PO) in cases of intentional or unintentional oral hypoglycemic agent ingestions.
- *Thiamine.* 50 to 100 mg IV simultaneous with treatment of hypoglycemia in the chronic alcoholic or otherwise malnourished patient to avoid precipitating Wernicke's encephalopathy.
- Antibiotics should be given to treat underlying infections.

Emergency Department Interventions

- Interventions include respiratory and hemodynamic stabilization of the patient, early bedside glucose monitoring, rapid correction of hyperglycemia or hypoglycemia, and initiation of appropriate treatment for the underlying medical problems.

Disposition

- *Consultation.* Consultation with an obstetrician should be obtained for any patient who is pregnant and becomes hypo- or hyperglycemic. Outpatient medication adjustments should be made in collaboration with the patient's endocrinologist or primary care provider.
- *Admission.* This is prudent for any patient with a questionable diagnosis, unresolved symptoms, unreliable follow-up, inability to tolerate oral intake, hypoglycemia secondary to sulfonylurea use, or an ill-appearance.
- *Discharge.* This is safe for mildly symptomatic patients with an identifiable cause that is corrected, and who has reliable follow-up, observation at home, and is tolerating oral intake.

Specific Problems: Hyperglycemia
Diabetes Mellitus Type I and Diabetes Mellitus Type II

- *Epidemiology and risk factors.* Diabetes mellitus type I, (DM I): younger age of onset (age <40 years), with peak between 10 and 14 years of age. DM II is more common than DM I. Patients are typically older (age >40 years). It is often diagnosed when an asymptomatic patient has elevated glucose on routine laboratory tests.
- *Pathophysiology.* **DM I:** Immune-mediated destruction of pancreatic beta cells in genetically susceptible people. This results in an absolute or near-absolute insulin deficiency leading to hyperglycemia. **DM II:** Abnormal insulin secretion and resistance to insulin action. Initially the

patient is euglycemic despite insulin resistance due to increased insulin secretion. Then insulin resistance worsens leading to postprandial hyperglycemia. Insulin levels in DM II are typically normal to high.

- *History.* Polyuria, polydypsia, and polyphagia may be present.
- *Physical examination.* Evidence of dehydration and abnormal vital signs may be present.
- *Diagnostic testing.* Well-appearing patients with normal vital signs (other than mild tachycardia from dehydration) require serum glucose, electrolytes and renal function, and urinalysis. An HbA_{1c} (an index of glucose concentration of the preceding 6 to 8 weeks) may be sent for outpatient follow-up and management. Normal values are approximately 4% to 6% of total hemoglobin.
- *ED management.* Rule out DKA and HHNC, and search for an underlying cause (infection, medication, or dietary noncompliance). Patients with normal electrolytes may be treated with IV fluid hydration alone. In reliable adult patients who are stable for discharge, an oral hypoglycemic agent such as glipizide or glyburide 10 mg daily can be initiated. Metformin is an alternative agent that is often used in obese patients, or those in whom sulfonylureas are contraindicated (e.g., sulfa allergy). If asymptomatic, prompt follow-up should be arranged. Metformin does not cause hypoglycemia but is contraindicated in patients with renal insufficiency or metabolic acidosis. It should be withheld 48 hours prior to the use of intravenous contrast agents due to the risk of acidosis.
- *Helpful hints and pitfalls.* Diabetics often present to the ED with late complications of their disease. These include accelerated atherosclerosis, nephropathy, peripheral neuropathy, retinopathy, and diabetic foot lesions. Patients with diabetes are at greater risk for infections.

Diabetic Ketoacidosis

- *Epidemiology and risk factors.* This occurs primarily in patients with DMI. It is the presenting illness in 20% to 30% of patients with newly diagnosed diabetes. DKA is associated with inadequate administration of insulin, infection, myocardial infarction (MI) or other physiologic stressor.
- *Pathophysiology.* DKA is due to a relative insufficiency of insulin and an excess of counter-regulatory or stress hormones (glucagon, growth hormone, catecholamines, cortisol). The lack of insulin causes hyperglycemia because glucose is unable to enter cells. This cellular starvation causes the release of the stress hormones that are catabolic and causes an increase in gluconeogenesis, glycogenolysis, and lipolysis. Lipolysis results in free fatty acids that are converted to ketones resulting in ketonemia.
- *History.* If the patient is able to provide a history, it may reveal the underlying precipitant (i.e., pneumonia, change or noncompliance with medications, myocardial infarction, etc.), complaints of nausea, vomiting, abdominal pain, and complaints related to dehydration.
- *Physical examination.* Abnormal vital signs (fever, hypotension, tachycardia, tachypnea), Kussmaul's respirations, dehydration, poor skin turgor, and evidence for the underlying cause may be present. The

abdominal examination is usually mild tenderness or is benign, but may resemble that of an acute abdomen in some patients.

■ *Diagnostic testing.* The defining laboratory abnormalities of DKA are hyperglycemia with an anion gap metabolic acidosis, although the degree of glucose elevation can be variable. Typical findings include a blood glucose above 300 mg/dl, pH less than 7.3, bicarbonate below 15 mEq/L, ketonemia, ketonuria, and glucosuria. A patient in DKA may have a glucose less than 300 mg/dl or a bicarbonate above 15 mEq/L. Rarely, a well-hydrated patient with DKA may have a pure hyperchloremic acidosis and no anion gap. A leukocytosis more closely reflects the degree of ketosis than the presence of infection. An increase in band neutrophils may indicate the presence of infection. Serum levels of potassium, magnesium, and phosphorus are often initially high in DKA, even in the presence of marked total body deficits. A correction for the effect of acidosis on the serum potassium determination can be made by subtracting 0.6 mEq/L from the laboratory potassium value for every 0.1 decrease in pH. Amylase (usually of salivary origin) may be increased in DKA. The falsely low sodium should be corrected by calculation (see "Initial Diagnostic Approach"), and by treating the hyperglycemia. A serum lipase can distinguish DKA alone from that caused by pancreatitis, which may also cause hyperglycemia. Other studies looking for any precipitating cause of DKA should be pursued (e.g., chest radiograph).

■ *ED management.* **IV fluids:** Patients in DKA typically have profound dehydration due to the osmotic diuretic effects of hyperglycemia. Typical fluid losses range from 3 to 6 L. Start with 2 L of IV NS over the first 2 hours. Once the patient is hemodynamically stable switch to 0.45% NS with 40 mEq KCl, as most patients with DKA have a significant potassium deficit. Switch to fluid containing dextrose when the blood glucose has been reduced to below 250 mg/dl. **Insulin:** Insulin therapy is initiated with an IV infusion of 0.1 U/kg/h of regular insulin to gradually lower the blood glucose level and close the anion gap. An initial bolus is not necessary but many clinicians will give a 0.1 U/kg bolus of regular insulin IV. Intravenous insulin must always be maintained by a continuous infusion as intermittent IV insulin boluses alone are not helpful to the patient. The blood glucose level should be monitored every hour with finger-stick glucose levels, and the infusion titrated to avoid lowering the blood glucose level by more than 100 mg/dl/h, which may increase the risk of developing cerebral edema. Continue IV insulin therapy until the anion gap is closed, at which point subcutaneous insulin can be instituted according to a sliding scale. Do not stop insulin therapy just because the blood glucose level approaches normal. **Electrolytes:** The acidemia of DKA causes intracellular potassium to shift into the extracellular space in exchange for H+. Insulin therapy causes extracellular potassium to shift back into the intracellular space, which may lead to hypokalemia. If hypokalemia is initially present, add 40 mEq KCl to IV fluids starting with the first liter. Anticipate that potassium levels will drop with IV insulin and fluid therapy, and that even if initial potassium levels are normal, supplemental potassium should be started after the second or third liter of IV fluids. Replace potassium cautiously in patients with renal insufficiency. Low magnesium levels may exacerbate hypokalemia, and therefore, should be corrected. Phosphate should also be monitored, although replacement is necessary only if the level is below 1 mg/dl. During therapy for DKA, phosphate shifts from extracellular to intracellular, and hypophosphatemia may develop 6 to 12 hours into therapy. Excessive phosphate replacement may lead to hypocalcemia. **Sodium bicarbonate:** Bicarbonate should only be used if the arterial pH is below 6.9 AND the patient displays evidence of cardiogenic shock, respiratory depression, or renal failure. If used, bicarbonate should not correct the pH above a level of 7.1. Patients with respiratory acidosis due to inadequate ventilation must be adequately ventilated. Bicarbonate therapy is not a substitute for adequate ventilation in treating respiratory acidosis. **Disposition:** All patients should be admitted except for mild cases if the hyperglycemia is corrected, the anion gap is closed, the patient is able to eat and drink, and the precipitant is found and corrected.

- *Helpful hints and pitfalls.* Insulin should NOT be discontinued in the presence of a normal blood glucose level if an anion gap still exists. Insulin should be continued with glucose added to IV fluids.

Hyperosmolar Hyperglycemic Nonketotic Coma (HHNC)

- *Epidemiology and risk factors.* HHNC is usually seen in elderly patients with DM II who are stressed by an illness or noncompliant with medications or diet. HHNC may occur in patients who are not diabetic, especially after burns, parenteral hyperalimentation, peritoneal dialysis, or hemodialysis. The mortality of HHNC is up to 25%.
- *Pathophysiology.* Insulin deficiency and resistance leads to hyperglycemia in the setting of physiologic stressors that trigger release of stress hormones, leading to glycogenolysis and gluconeogenesis. Hyperglycemia leads to hyperosmolality, osmotic diuresis, and dehydration. Residual insulin activity is adequate to suppress lipolysis and the development of ketonemia. The hallmark of the disease is severe hyperglycemia, hyperosmolality, and dehydration without ketoacidosis.
- *History.* Ten percent of these patients arrive at the ED in coma; the remainder may have an altered mental status or confusion limiting the reliability of the history from the patient. History may include polyuria, polydypsia, weight loss, weakness, drowsiness, or focal neurologic deficits. Precipitants that should be considered include pneumonia, urinary tract and other infections, gastrointestinal bleeding, pancreatitis, subdural hematoma, MI, CVA, and certain medications such as thiazide diuretics, furosemide, calcium channel blockers, phenytoin, glucocorticoids, cimetidine, propanolol, mannitol, and immunosuppressive agents.
- *Physical examination.* Findings may include dehydration, confusion, obtundation, evidence of infection (e.g., fever), and neurologic signs such as seizure or hemiparesis.
- *Diagnostic testing.* Typical laboratory abnormalities include hyperglycemia and hyperosmolarity with blood glucose above 600 mg/dl and serum osmolality above 350 mOsm/kg, pH above 7.3, lack of serum ketones, and lack of ketonuria. Although these patients do not have a ketoacidosis, they may have a metabolic acidosis secondary to some combination of lactic acidosis, starvation ketosis, and retention of inorganic acids attributable to renal hypoperfusion. The BUN and

creatinine levels are invariably elevated. These patients may have more profound electrolyte abnormalities than patients in DKA. Potassium, magnesium, and phosphorus serum levels may all be high despite a total body deficit. Sodium levels may be inaccurate due to marked hyperglycemia as mentioned in previous sections. Possible sources of acute infection or other causes for altered mental status should be pursued as indicated.

■ *ED management.* **IV fluids:** Patients with HHNC often have profound dehydration with fluid deficits of 8 to 12 L. Fluid resuscitation should be initiated with NS. Elderly patients must be monitored closely during fluid resuscitation for signs and symptoms of congestive heart failure, which can occur precipitously in patients with diminished cardiopulmonary reserve. NS 0.45 % should be used if the patient is hypertensive, hypernatremic (sodium >155 mEq/L), or if serum osmolarity is above 320 mOsm/kg. Five percent dextrose should be added when blood sugar is below 250 mg/dl. Serum glucose should be lowered at a rate no greater than 100 to 200 mg/dl/h. **Insulin:** Hyperglycemia should be treated with an IV infusion of regular insulin at 0.1 U/kg/h following initial fluid resuscitation. Insulin requirements in patients with HHNC may be less than in patients with DKA. Insulin infusion should be discontinued when serum glucose falls below 250 mg/dl. **Electrolytes:** Hypokalemia should be treated. Potassium deficits are usually greater than in DKA. Relpace potassium cautiously in patients with decreased renal function. Magnesium and phosphate should be replaced if low. **Monitoring:** Patients with HHNC should not be discharged home from the ED.

■ *Helpful hints and pitfalls.* Avoid rapid correction of glucose, as this may precipitate cerebral edema.

Special Considerations: Hyperglycemia
Pediatrics

■ Ten percent of children with new-onset DM I will have DKA.
■ Regular insulin dose is 0.05-0.1 U/kg/h. Add dextrose when glucose is below 300 mg/dl. Target rate of decrease in glucose level is 100 mg/dl/h. IV fluids should be given in 20-ml/kg bolus.
■ Cerebral edema can occur in any patient during treatment for DKA; however, this rare complication seems to occur more commonly in patients under the age of 20. The mechanism is not clearly understood, but seems to be related to a rapid fall in plasma glucose and osmolality. Symptoms usually occur 6 to 10 hours after beginning treatment, and include headache, incontinence, opththalmoplegia, and vomiting. Patients with cerebral edema should receive mannitol.
■ HHNC is rare in children.

Elderly

■ Elderly patients are at higher risk for HHNC due to more co-morbid conditions.
■ Polypharmacy, poor vision, and confusion may contribute to noncompliance or inaccurate dosing of medications.

Women and Pregnancy

- Most oral hypoglycemic agents are contraindicated in pregnancy.
- Pregnant women should be monitored for gestational diabetes, and treated with insulin accordingly. Insulin requirements may increase as the pregnancy progresses.
- DKA can occur at lower blood glucose levels in pregnancy.
- Diabetes during pregnancy increases the chance of pre-eclampsia or eclampsia, bacterial infections, macrosomic infants, hydramnios, and maternal mortality.
- Maternal hyperglycemia may be associated with increased fetal and neonatal mortality, major anomalies, preterm delivery, and hypoglycemia after birth.

Immunocompromised

- The immunocompromised may be more susceptible to infection and sepsis, hepatic and renal failure, and other co–morbid conditions that may contribute to the development of hyperglycemia.

Specific Problems: Hypoglycemia
Hypoglycemic Coma and Symptomatic Hypoglycemia

- *Epidemiology and risk factors.* This entity most commonly occurs in diabetic patients on insulin or oral hypoglycemic agents due to a mismatch between hypoglycemic medication dosing, caloric intake, and degree of physical exertion. It may also occur from intentional or unintentional overdoses, or use of other medications (Table 38–3). Symptoms usually occur when the patient's blood glucose falls below 40 to 60 mg/dl. Prolonged hypoglycemic coma can cause seizures, central nervous system (CNS) injury, and death.
- *Pathophysiology.* As the blood glucose level falls, catecholamine release is stimulated leading to many of the adrenergic symptoms of hypoglycemia (diaphoresis, anxiety, nervousness, tachycardia, hunger). The CNS is dependent on glucose for energy.
- *History.* May be unreliable due to coma or change in mental status. A history of ingestion or missed meals may be available.
- *Physical examination.* Abnormal vital signs including hypothermia may be present. Focal neurologic findings, seizures, or posturing may also be seen.
- *Diagnostic testing.* Rapid bedside glucose level should be obtained in all patients with abnormal mental status. Additional laboratory tests include a complete blood count (CBC), electrolytes and renal function, liver function tests, and a urinalysis. A noncontrast head CT should be obtained if a stroke is suspected, or symptoms do not resolve after blood glucose has normalized.
- *ED management.* Once a low blood glucose level has been identified, it should be rapidly corrected. If the patient is awake and able to tolerate oral intake, oral glucose or other high caloric liquid should be administered. If the patient has an altered mental status, IV D50 should

be administered. Continue a D5W or D10W infusion until the patient is able to tolerate oral intake. If IV access is unobtainable, glucagon 1 to 2 mg IM may be given, and repeated once. Glucagon's onset of action is 10 to 20 minutes, and it acts by releasing glucose from endogenous stores. If a patient's glycogen stores are depleted (i.e., starvation or malnutrition) glucagon will have no effect. If an agent that stimulates pancreatic insulin release (e.g., sulfanurea or meglitinide) is the source of refractory hypoglycemia, octreotide will be needed. If adrenal insufficiency is suspected, hydrocortisone should be given. Any symptomatic patient who has overdosed on a long-acting insulin or an oral hypoglycemic agent needs admission for observation and serial blood glucose checks, because the hypoglycemia will recur and persist for longer than the glucose replacement therapy will last. Patients who are unable to tolerate oral intake, or have recurrent hypoglycemia in the ED, require admission. Only those patients who have a clearly identified cause of hypoglycemia, with a normal mental status and resolution of the hypoglycemia, may be discharged if they can be observed and prompt follow-up can be arranged.

- ***Helpful hints and pitfalls.*** Hypoglycemia can mimic an acute stroke. Hypothermia related to hypoglycemia should resolve upon normalization of blood glucose. Occasionally temporizing measures such as external rewarming may be needed. Patients taking beta-blocker medications may be less able to identify the symptoms of hypoglycemia, and the hypoglycemia may persist longer than expected.

Special Considerations: Hypoglycemia
Pediatrics

- Hypoglycemic neonates can be asymptomatic or limp, and may have bradycardia, irritable, tremulousness, seizures, and poor suckling. Hypoglycemia is defined as a glucose below 20 mg/dl within the first 24 hours of life in a preterm infant, below 30 mg/dl in a newborn, and below 40 mg/dl in an infant.
- Even when asymptomatic, and euglycemic, any child who ingests a single oral hypoglycemic agent warrants admission for observation.
- Starvation, especially in children, can cause hypoglycemia.
- For therapy, give D25 2 to 4 ml/kg in children, and D10 5 ml/kg in infants.

Elderly

- Elderly patients are at greater risk for polypharmacy, medication interactions, and medication confusion.
- Worsening renal function can reduce the clearance of medications such as insulin and oral hypoglycemics and lead to hypoglycemia.

Pregnancy

- Hypoglycemia may occur late in pregnancy.
- Transient hypoglycemia is well tolerated by the fetus.
- Glucagon and D50 are safe to use in pregnancy. Try to avoid large swings in glucose when treating hypoglycemia.

- Fasting hypoglycemia and hyperinsulinemia are normal during pregnancy.
- Hypoglycemia may occur in patients with the HELLP syndrome from hepatic damage.

Immunocompromised

- These patients are more likely to have poor glycogen stores from malnutrition.

Specific Problems: Alcoholic Ketoacidosis

- *Epidemiology and risk factors.* Alcoholic ketoacidosis (AKA) is typically seen after heavy alcohol consumption for several days with little or no food intake, and may occur in alcoholics and nonalcoholics.
- *Pathophysiology.* Decreased carbohydrate intake reduces insulin levels and increases glucagon levels, which mobilizes free fatty acids causing ketosis. Alcohol may also inhibit gluconeogenesis and stimulate lipolysis. Metabolism of ethanol to acetaldehyde and then to acetic acid may further contribute to acid production. As ketosis progresses, nausea, vomiting and abdominal pains occur and limits further oral intake attempts.
- *History.* A history of alcohol consumption may be present. Nausea, vomiting, and abdominal pain are usually present for 24 to 72 hours before arrival for care.
- *Physical examination.* Tachypnea (from ketoacidosis), tachycardia (from dehydration), and abdominal pain may be present.
- *Diagnostic testing.* There is typically a high anion gap metabolic acidosis, ketonemia, and variable glucose level (low or normal). An elevated osmolar gap may be seen due to ethanol and acetone accumulation. A concomitant metabolic alkalosis due to persistent vomiting may develop, which can result in a relatively normal pH with a high anion gap. Lactate may be elevated if dehydration leading to hypoperfusion is present.
- *ED management.* IV hydration with D5 NS or D5 0.45% NS should be used. Ketoacidosis usually resolves in 12 to 18 hours. Glucose will stimulate insulin release, which in turn reduces ketoacid production. The patient must receive glucose to reconstitute hepatic glycogen, otherwise the ketoacidosis will not resolve. About 30% of alcoholics with ketoacidosis will be hypoglycemic as well. Give thiamine 100 mg IV before the administration of glucose to prevent Wernicke's encephalopathy. Hypokalemia and other electrolyte abnormalities should be corrected. Many alcoholics are profoundly hypokalemic from vomiting. A metabolic alkalosis is a sign of this, and urine pH should be monitored. At the point that it stops being paradoxically acidic, in the presence of a metabolic alkalosis, potassium losses have been replaced. Potassium should be repleted as well as magnesium, which is often low in these patients.
- *Helpful hints and pitfalls.* Serum ketones in AKA are predominantly beta-hydroxybutyrate, which is not detected by the nitroprusside test. Insulin is typically not needed in AKA, and when given can cause hypoglycemia.

See Table 38–5 for a comparison of DKA and HHNC to AKA.

Table 38–5 Comparison of HHNC vs. DKA to AKA

	HHNC	DKA	AKA
Blood glucose (mg/dL)	> 400, even > 1000	> 350, < 600	< 200
Anion gap	Not present	Present	Present
Average fluid deficit	8-12 liters	5-10 liters	Varies, use glucose containing solution
Insulin therapy	Yes	Yes	No
Acidosis	No	Yes	Yes
Serum ketones	No	Yes	Yes, but may not be detected
pH	> 7.3	< 7.3	> 7.3
Serum osmolality	> 350 mOsm/kg	< 350 mOsm/kg	

HHNC, hyperglycemic hyperosmolar non-ketotic coma; DKA, diabetic ketoacidosis; AKA, alcoholic ketoacidosis.

Teaching Points

Hypoglycemia is often hard to detect since many patients are not aware of a falling blood sugar level, and have no identifiable preliminary symptoms. A fingerstick glucose measurement should be an immediate part of any assessment of new onset confusion, coma or seizure activity, and even in known seizure disorders if the patient presents with postictal confusion or coma. The hypoglycemia secondary to ingestion of an oral hypoglycemic agent is hard to treat because the action of the drug often lasts longer than the glucose replacement therapy. Therefore these patients will often require prolonged administration of glucose solutions, and octreotide, and should therefore be admitted.

Hyperglycemia can also be hard for the patient to detect because of either slow onset, or because another disease that predominates the presentation has triggered a new onset diabetes or a deterioration of a controlled diabetes. While type I diabetes often presents with hypoglycemia, or diabetic ketoacidosis, type II is more likely to present with confusion and the dehydration of hyperosmolar coma. There are, of course, patients who will demonstrate both ketoacidosis and hyperosmolarity.

Suggested Readings

Brandenburg MA, Dire DJ. Comparison of arterial and venous blood gas values in the initial emergency department evaluation of patients with diabetic ketoacidosis. Ann Emerg Med 1998;31:459–465.

Chiasson JL, Aris-Jilwan N, Bélanger R. Diagnosis and treatment of diabetic ketoacidosis and the hyperglycemic hyperosmolar state. CMAJ 2003;168:859–866.

Cydulka RK, Pennington J. Diabetes mellitus and disorders of glucose homeostasis. In: Marx JA, Hockberger RS, Walls RM, eds. Rosen's Emergency Medicine: Concepts and Clinical Practice (6th ed). Philadelphia: Mosby, 2006, pp 1955–1975.

Hiller KM, Wolf SJ. Cerebral edema in an adult patient with diabetic ketoacidosis. Am J Emerg Med 2005;23;399–400.

Kitabchi AE, Wall BM. Diabetic ketoacidosis. Med Clin North Am 1995;79:9–37.

Marcin JP, Glaser N, Barnett P, et al. Factors associated with adverse outcomes in children with diabetic ketoacidosis-related cerebral edema. J Pediatr 2002;141:793–797.

Viallon A, Zeni F, Lafond P, et al. Does bicarbonate therapy improve the management of severe diabetic ketoacidosis? Crit Care Med 1999;27:2690–2693.

CHAPTER **39**

Hypertension

SHARI SCHABOWSKI ■ EMMIE A. CHEN

Red Flags

Severe headache ● Seizure ● Altered mental status ● Acute vision loss ● Chest pain ● Shortness of breath ● Diastolic blood pressure >120 mm Hg ● Systolic blood pressure >180 mm Hg ● Signs of volume overload ● Retinal hemorrhages on funduscopic examination ● Neurologic deficits ● Pregnancy

Overview

■ Most patients in the ED found to have very high blood pressure have no symptoms referable to hypertension, and do not have rapidly progressive end-organ disease in the short term.

■ Complications of hypertension primarily affect the heart, brain, kidneys, retina, and large arteries, referred to as the "target organs." The physician must look for "red flags" (see Box) when evaluating any patient presenting with an elevated blood pressure.

- Primary or *essential hypertension* does not have a cause that can be identified, and accounts for most cases. Secondary hypertension is the result of another disease process such as thyroid storm (see Chapter 63), catecholamine excess, or renal artery stenosis.
- A *hypertensive emergency* involves rapid and progressive decompensation with damage to these target organs caused by severely increased blood pressure. *Hypertensive urgencies* typically present with significantly elevated blood pressure, but nonspecific symptoms. This also includes patients at high risk for end-organ damage, but without evidence of new injury. Some high-risk patients have a history of target-organ disease, such as congestive heart failure, unstable angina, coronary artery disease, renal insufficiency, transient ischemic attack, or stroke. *Uncontrolled hypertension* refers to the vast majority of patients with hypertension who are often asymptomatic, and who need timely and appropriate long-term management, but who do not require acute intervention in the ED. The VA Cooperative Trial notes no adverse outcomes within the first 3 months among the 143 patients who have a diastolic blood pressure of between 115 and 130 mm Hg, regardless of whether they receive treatment or placebo. Very few asymptomatic patients with markedly increased blood pressure will experience a near-term adverse event.
- Hypertensive encephalopathy is characterized by a triad of severe hypertension, altered mental status, and (often) papilledema. The patient may present with lethargy, confusion, headache, visual disturbances, and seizures. Retinopathy may be present. The extremely elevated blood pressure overwhelms the brain's ability to autoregulate cerebral blood flow resulting in the development of cerebral edema. If not adequately treated, hypertensive encephalopathy can progress to cerebral hemorrhage, coma, and death. It is more likely to occur in previously normotensive individuals who experience a rapid increase in blood pressure such as eclampsia. The diagnosis is confirmed if the patient improves with decreasing blood pressure.
- A thorough understanding of the autoregulation of cerebral bloodflow is essential when designing a treatment plan. Cerebral vasodilatation occurs when the blood pressure decreases, and vasoconstriction results when blood pressure increases in order for cerebral perfusion pressure to remain constant despite fluctuations in mean arterial pressure (MAP). The systolic blood pressure (SBP) and diastolic blood pressure (DBP) are used to calculate the MAP. The MAP is calculated as follows: SBP–DBP/3+DBP. Normal values range from 80 to 100 mm Hg. Cerebral blood flow remains fairly constant for a MAP from approximately 60 mm Hg to up to 150 mm Hg in normal individuals. When the MAP decreases to less than the lower limits of autoregulation, cerebral hypoperfusion results. However, in chronically hypertensive individuals, the lower limit of autoregulation is increased, and autoregulation can fail at MAPs that are well tolerated in nonhypertensive individuals. Acutely, lower the MAP by no more than 20% to 25%.

- Emergent treatment of hypertension should not be based on any given number of systolic or diastolic pressure; for example, a "normal" blood pressure of 140/90 mm Hg may be a sign of hypertension urgency if it is obtained in a pregnant woman.
- At birth, a typical blood pressure is 80/50 mm Hg. Blood pressure continues to rise with age. The normal adult systolic blood pressure can be estimated by "age in years + 100".

Differential Diagnosis of Hypertension

See the DDx table describing the differential diagnosis of hypertension.

Initial Diagnostic Approach
General

- The level of blood pressure should be rechecked before any treatment is initiated. Patients with significant elevations in blood pressure should have a blood pressure measured in the other arm. To obtain an accurate measurement, a patient should be seated with the arm at the level of the heart, and the cuff bladder should cover at least 80% of the arm circumference. Blood pressure measurement with an automated cuff is often inaccurate in patients with atrial fibrillation and other heart rhythm irregularities.
- Isolated asymptomatic hypertension with no evidence of end-organ damage does not require an extensive ED workup, and can be referred for outpatient workup and care.
- Treatable causes of elevated blood pressure should be identified such as pain, hypoxia, other medications, over-the-counter preparations, or illicit drugs.
- The history should include the duration and severity of preexisting hypertension, compliance with medical therapy for hypertension, the

DDx Differential Diagnosis of Hypertension

Critical Diagnoses	Emergent Diagnoses	Nonemergent Diagnoses
Hypertensive emergency	*Hypertensive urgency*	Transient hypertension
Acute myocardial infarction	High risk but no end-organ damage	Uncontrolled hypertension (do not meet criteria for hypertensive emergency or urgency)
Unstable angina	Perioperative hypertension	
Pulmonary edema	Hypertensive pregnant patient without proteinuria or signs of preeclampsia	
Aortic dissection		
Hemorrhagic stroke		
Encephalopathy		
Acute renal failure		
Retinopathy		
Preeclampsia or eclampsia		

degree of previous success with blood pressure control and symptoms of target-organ disease.

- A complete cardiopulmonary, neurologic, and funduscopic examination should be performed on these patients. The presence of retinal hemorrhage or papilledema is evidence of end-organ damage.
- Diagnostic studies and a complete physical examination are used to diagnose or exclude acute end-organ damage caused by elevated blood pressure. The necessity of diagnostic testing is dictated by severity of hypertension, signs, symptoms and clinical risk of end-organ damage.

Laboratory

- Few studies have assessed the prognostic value of abnormal laboratory findings in patients with severe asymptomatic hypertension.
- Because renal failure is impossible to identify by history and physical examination alone, measurement of serum BUN and creatinine levels is helpful.
- A urine screen for cocaine and amphetamines might help confirm common causes of hypertension. A urinalysis is useful to evaluate for proteinuria, hematuria, and red cell casts. A urine pregnancy test should be done on all females in the reproductive age.

EKG

- New abnormalities may be seen in 22% of asymptomatic ED patients with a diastolic blood pressure greater than 115 mm Hg.

Radiography

- Imaging studies should only be performed on patients with relevant symptoms.

Emergency Department Management Overview

General

- As always, the ABCs (*a*irway, *b*reathing, and *c*irculation) should be addressed as discussed in Section II. When acute progressive end-organ damage is suspected, stabilization therapy must begin in the ED. These patients should be placed on a cardiac monitor, intravenous (IV) access should be obtained, and supplemental oxygen should be administered to maintain oxygen saturation above 95%. Most hypertensive emergencies require immediate blood pressure reduction. The important exception is cerebrovascular emergencies, in which a rapid decrease in cerebral blood flow might be harmful (see Chapter 56).
- There is no evidence to support the practice of reducing the blood pressure acutely in the ED for other patients. However some patients with no evidence of end-organ damage, but who are symptomatic from their hypertension (e.g., headache), may benefit from modest (less than 25% of MAP) blood pressure reduction in the ED.

Medications

■ An overview of the blood pressure management of the most common problems resulting from hypertensive emergencies is listed in Table 39–1. IV antihypertensive agents are listed in Table 39–2.

■ In general, beta blockers should be avoided in patients with acute heart failure or cocaine use.

■ For the treatment of newly diagnosed hypertension, there may be no need to treat in the ED, or one can start with a thiazide diuretic. The choice of therapy will depend on the patient population and co-morbidities. Commonly used oral agents for initial HTN treatment include beta-blockers, angiotensin-converting enzyme inhibitors, angiotensin receptor blockers (ARBs), and calcium channel blockers (see Table 39–3).

Disposition

■ There is no absolute level of blood pressure that mandates admission. Patients with end-organ damage or an acute underlying disease process require admission to a monitored setting.

■ Patients with no evidence of end-organ damage may be discharged from the ED. All patients with hypertension in the ED should be educated on lifestyle modification, which includes weight reduction, low-sodium diet, reduced alcohol intake, cessation of smoking, and increased physical activity. These measures should be an adjunct to all drug therapy.

Specific Problems
Coarctation of the Aorta

■ *Epidemiology and risk factors.* This is a rare lesion that is often seen in Turner's syndrome (ovarian agensis).

■ *Pathophysiology.* There is a constriction of the aorta usually located just distal to the left subclavian artery at the junction of the ligamentum arteriosum.

■ *History.* The patient will complain of headaches, exertional leg pain, and fatigue.

■ *Physical examination.* There are often prominent neck pulsations, hypertension, increased upper extremity pulses versus lower extremity pulses, prominent left ventricular impulse, aortic stenosis or insufficiency murmurs, bruit, cyanosis, and heart failure.

■ *Diagnostic testing.* A Doppler examination of the pulses may reveal flow variations. The upper limbs will have blood pressure measurements at least 10 mm Hg greater than the lower limbs. A transesophageal echo-cardiogram may show the flow variation at the level of the constriction. Magnetic resonance imaging (MRI) will show the aortic disease. A chest radiograph may show cardiomegaly and notching of the ribs as well as an abnormal aortic shadow.

■ *ED Management.* Admit for cardiac catheterization and angiography, which will show a poststenotic dilatation. Surgical correction may be required.

Table 39-1 Hypertensive Emergencies and Management

	Blood Pressure Management	Comment
Acute coronary syndrome (22)	Nitroglycerin Beta-blockers (metoprolol, labetolol, esmolol) ACI inhibitors Nitroprusside if severe	The goal is careful but rapid reduction of blood pressure to normal levels if necessary for symptom relief.
Congestive heart failure (52)	Nitroglycerin ACE inhibitors Nitroprusside (if severe) Other: furosemide morphine	The goal is careful but rapid reduction of blood pressure to normal levels if necessary for symptom relief. Beta-blockers should be avoided in acute decompensation. Diuresis should eventually be instituted but might initially exacerbate the underlying pressure natriuresis, and further stimulate the renin-angiotensin axis. Nesiritide is a vasodilator agent that may be helpful for acutely decompensated heart failure. Dobutamine is used to increase cardiac output, and is not an antihypertensive agent.
Aortic dissection (22)	Beta-blockers (esmolol) plus nitoprusside or labetolol (as monotherapy)	The goals of medical therapy are to lower the BP to a systolic level of 100 to 120 mm Hg, and to reduce the ejection force of the heart. An arterial dilator, such as nitroprusside can decrease the MAP, but may cause reflex tachycardia. Beta-blocking agents should be started before or in conjunction with vasodilator agents. Labetolol can be used as monotherapy due to both alpha and beta blocking activity. Nicardipine is not recommended as it has minimal inotropic and chronotropic effects, and may reflexively stimulate sympathetic activity.
Hypertensive encephalopathy	Nitroprusside Labetolol Nicardipine	The diagnosis is confirmed if cerebral function improves with decreasing the blood pressure. Requires careful reduction of the MAP by 25% over an hour.

Table 39–1 Hypertensive Emergencies and Management—cont'd

	Blood Pressure Management	Comment
Ischemic stroke (56)	See Chapter 56.	Reserved for those with markedly elevated blood pressures unless fibrinolytic therapy is planned or specific medical indications are present.
Hemorrhagic stroke (56) and subarachnoid bleed (35)	Esmolol or labetolol Nicardipine	Treatment should be more aggressive than for patients with ischemic strokes. The current consensus is to give parenteral agents for intracranial hemorrhage if systolic pressures higher than 160 mm Hg or diastolic pressures higher than 105 mm Hg. Nimodipine may decrease vasospasm and rebleeding after subarachnoid hemorrhages, but the drug is not recommended for blood pressure control.
Increased ICP	Beta-blockers (esmolol or labetolol) Nicardipine	Nitroprusside, nitroglycerin, and hydralazine may increase ICP.
Acute renal failure (49)	Beta-blockers (labetolol) Fenoldopam Nitroprusside	ACE inhibitor drugs definitely improve prognosis among chronic hypertensive patients with mild proteinuria, but should be used cautiously in hyperkalemic patients with acute renal uremia. ACE inhibitors can provoke acute renal failure and severe hyperkalemia in patients with bilateral renal artery stenosis.
Preeclampsia and eclampsia (68)	Hydralazine Diazoxide and Beta-blockers	Magnesium infusion is the preferred agent for seizures (eclampsia). Definitive treatment consists of delivery of the fetus.

ACE, angiotensin-converting enzyme; BP, blood pressure; ICP, intracranial pressure; MAP, mean arterial pressure (MAP=SBP-DBP/3+DBP); SBP, systolic blood pressure.
( ) Refers to the chapter in which the disease entity is discussed.

Table 39–2 Common Intravenous Antihypertensive Medications

Agent (Generic names)	Dose	Onset	Comment
Sodium nitroprusside	0.3–10 μg/kg/min IV infusion	Seconds	May cause nausea, hypotension, thiocyanate and cyanide toxicity, methemoglobinemia. Caution with high intracranial pressure or azotemia.
Nitroglycerin	5–100 μg/min IV infusion	1–5 min	Headache, nausea, tachycardia, vomiting; tolerance with prolonged use. Caution with increased intracranial pressure. Ideal agent for acute coronary syndrome and acute congestive heart failure.
Labetolol hydrochloride	20–80 mg IV bolus every 10 min up to 300 mg; 0.5–2.0 mg/min IV infusion	5–10 min	May cause, dizziness, bronchospasm, bradycardia, heart block. Do not use for acute heart failure or in patients who use cocaine.
Nicardipine	5–15 mg/h IV infusion	5–15 min	May cause hypotension, tachycardia, nausea, vomiting, flushing. For most hypertensive emergencies except acute heart failure; caution with coronary ischemia and increased intracranial pressure.
Esmolol	500 μg/kg over 1 min, IV then 50–300 μg/kg/min IV infusion	5–10 min	Hypotension, nausea.
Fenoldopam	0.1–1.6 μg/kg/min IV infusion	10–15 min	May cause reflex tachycardia, headache, flushing, hypotension. Use with caution in glaucoma. It is a peripheral dopamine-1 receptor agonist, and has been found to improve renal function acutely in patients with malignant hypertension.
Hydralazine	10–20 mg every 4–6 hr IV	10 min	May cause headaches, fluid retention, tachycardia, Lupus syndrome. Preferred agent for preeclampsia.
Enalaprilat	1.25–5 mg every 6 h IV	15 min	May cause significant hypotension, renal failure. Give this drug very slowly. May be used for acute pulmonary edema.

IV, intravenous.

Classification	Agent (Generic names)	Comment
Thiazide diuretics	Hydrochlorothiazide: 12.5-25 mg PO daily; max 50 mg/d	May cause hyperuricemia and precipitate gout. May cause potassium wasting. No significant antihypertensive effect acutely. Can reduce cardiovascular morbidity and mortality in diabetic hypertensives. First-line drug in most hypertensive patients especially in African American patients and the elderly. When combined with other antihypertensive agents, exerts a synergistic effect on blood pressure. Use loop diuretics (e.g., furosemide) for patients with chronic renal disease.
ACE Inhibitors (ACEI)	Captopril: 25 mg PO bid to tid; max 450 mg/d Fosinopril, lisinopril, and quinapril: 10 mg PO qd; max 80 mg/d	Cough (dry, hacking, nonproductive) is the most common side effect. Angioneurotic edema is an infrequent side effect. ARBS (e.g. losaritan, do not cause a cough but may cause angioneurotic edema. Serum potassium may rise with ACE inhibitor therapy particularly in the presence of diabetes or renal impairment. An increase in creatinine level (up to 30%) can occur during the first several weeks, but the drug should not be discontinued unless there is a doubling of the creatinine or significant hyperkalemia due to their benefit of long term renal protection. Avoid in renal artery stenosis and with immunosuppressive drugs.
Centrally acting anti-adrenergics	Clonidine: 0.1 mg PO bid; max 2.4 mg/d. Transdermal weekly patch: 0.1 mg/2 h, max 0.6 mg/24 h	May cause sedation, orthostatic hypotension, and large decrease in cerebral blood pressure. Avoid in congestive heart failure and with heart block. Rebound hypertension with abrupt discontinuation.
Beta-blockers	Labetolol: 100 mg PO bid; max 2400 mg/d Atenolol: 25-50 mg PO qd or divided bid; max 100 mg/d Metoprolol (immediate release): 100 mg PO qd or divided bid; max 450 mg/d	The predominant adrenergic inhibition for labetolol is at the beta-receptor site (both beta 1 and beta 2), whereas the alpha-blocker component is an ancillary effect. Atenolol and metoprolol are primarily beta-1 receptor selective. Can cause orthostatic hypotension and hepatotoxicity. Labetolol can unmask bronchospasm. Counter-regulatory responses to hypoglycemia are blunted by beta-blockers. Avoid in heart failure, heart block, bradycardia, or history of cocaine use.
Calcium channel blocker (CCB)	Amlodipine	Classified into dihydropyridines, and is a long-acting CCB. Powerful vasodilator, promotes cardiac contractility and increase atrioventricular conduction. May cause headaches, flushing, and ankle edema. Does not cause bradycardia like diltiazem and verapamil can. Ideal agent in African American and elderly.

ARBS, angiotensin receptor blockers; max, maximum; PO, by mouth; bid, twice a day; tid, three times daily.

- **Helpful hints and pitfalls.** Lowering upper extremity blood pressure may cause hypoperfusion of lower extremities. Lowering blood pressure is dangerous in pregnancy as it will reduce blood flow to the fetus.

Pheochromocytoma

- **Epidemiology and risk factors.** These are rare tumors; 10% are extra-adrenal, 10% are malignant, and 10% are familial. They are associated with multiple endocrine neoplasia (MEN) IIA and IIB, neurofibromatosis, the Von Hippel-Lindau syndrome (characterized by the formation of hemangioblastomas, cysts, and malignancies involving multiple organs and systems), tuberous sclerosis, and the Sturge-Weber syndrome (facial nevus, seizures, hemiparesis, intracranial calcifications, mental retardation).
- **Pathophysiology.** These are catecholamine-producing tumors arising from chromaffin tissues of the sympathetic nervous system with alterations in levels of circulating catecholamines.
- **History.** There are episodes of paroxysmal hypertension, headache, diaphoresis, tremors, palpitations, chest and abdominal pain. The patient may have syncopal episodes that are sometimes induced by micturition (when the tumor is in the bladder wall).
- **Physical examination.** There may be tachycardia, diaphoresis, flushing, and tremors depending on the activity of the tumor, along with hypertension. At other times there will be no physical findings and normal blood pressures.
- **Diagnostic testing.** Plasma concentrations of normetanephrines >2.5 pmol/ml or metanephrine levels >1.4 pmol/ml indicate a pheochromocytoma with 100% specificity. A 24-hour urine collection for metanephrines will also show increased levels. Although MRI is a better imaging study than abdominal CT scan for this purpose, a CT scan is 95% accurate in locating pheochromocytomas >0.5 inch in diameter.
- **ED management.** The hypertension may require alpha-blocking with phentolamine, nitroprusside, and beta-blockade. When symptomatic, the patient will need to be admitted for workup, imaging, a monitored setting, and potential surgical therapy.
- **Helpful hints and pitfalls.** Preoperative stabilization is performed using α-blockade to control hypertension followed by β-blockade with propranolol. Hypertensive crisis is controlled with phentolamine or nitroprusside used in combination with β-blockers.

Renal Artery Stenosis

- **Epidemiology and risk factors.** Five percent of hypertensive patients have this problem, which is a form of hypertension that is correctable with surgery. It is most common in older white females.
- **Pathophysiology.** There is progressive narrowing of a renal artery. The involvement is usually unilateral. This can also develop after trauma to the renal artery.
- **History.** The most common history is of asymptomatic hypertension, although there will be a history of trauma if that is the cause. The blood

pressure may have a long history of being difficult to control. Symptoms, if present, are usually a problems that are secondary to the hypertension itself, and may include vision changes (hypertensive retinopathy) or difficulty breathing (pulmonary edema).

- *Physical examination.* An abdominal bruit is present in 40% of cases. Other physical examination findings are secondary to the end-organ damage from hypertension.
- *Diagnostic testing.* This includes laboratory tests of serum electrolytes, renal function tests, and a urinalysis. Other tests may include peripheral plasma renin activity and the captopril test (stimulation of excessive renin secretion). These later studies are typically not performed in the ED. Imaging studies include a renal scan (with or without captoril), MRI, renal artery ultrasound study, or renal aortography.
- *ED management.* The therapy is to attempt blood pressure control, and surgically repair the arterial lesion (angioplasty or revascularization).
- *Helpful hints and pitfalls.* Renal failure may occur following the administration of an angiotensin-converting enzyme inhibitor.

Special Considerations
Pediatrics

- Severe hypertension in a young patient should raise the possibility of intrinsic acute renal disease, such as glomerulonephritis or coarctation. Immunoglobin A nephropathy has surpassed poststreptococcal glomerulonephritis in frequency, and, among children, Henoch-Schönlein purpura (see Chapter 77) is the most likely cause of acute glomerular disease.

Elderly

- Blood pressure increases with age. Elevations of systolic blood pressure are more common in this patient population.

Women and Pregnancy

- Hypertension is important mainly as a symptom of the underlying disorder rather than as a cause. Pre-eclampsia is important to recognize because it can progress suddenly to eclampsia, defined by the occurrence of convulsions, and can rapidly progress to coma or death. Magnesium infusion is more effective than other anticonvulsants in this setting. Definitive treatment consists of delivery of the fetus; therefore, the emergency physician usually collaborates with an obstetrician early. The mainstay of antihypertensive treatment for this population in many institutions is hydralazine followed by diazoxide and beta-blockers (see Chapter 68).

Teaching Points

Hypertensive emergencies are varied in their presentation and seriousness. The most dangerous form is hypertensive encephalopathy, but this is fortunately rare. The end-organ damage can be subtle, as with the kidney, and not noted without laboratory testing of renal function. There are no set values of blood pressure that can define any of these emergencies because other conditions, such as pregnancy, may have reset the patient's blood pressure at a low value. The hypertensive emergencies of eclampsia can then produce severe end-organ damage to mother and child at blood pressure levels that would be considered normal in a nonpregnant patient.

A hypertensive emergency is defined by signs or symptoms of end-organ damage, and should be treated in the ED. The one exception is an ischemic stroke in which lowering blood pressure may cause more damage. It is preferable to use parenteral agents with a predictable dose response curve. In the pregnant eclamptic patient, obstetrics consultation should be obtained for possible emergent delivery.

Thiazide diuretics are inexpensive first line oral agents for patients with hypertension. Other commonly used agents include ACE inhibitors, angiotensin receptor blockers, beta blockers, and calcium channel blockers. The use of these agents depends on the patient population and presence of co-morbid conditions. The decision to initiate such therapy in the ED should be coordinated with the patient's primary physician if possible, and close outpatient follow-up should be arranged.

Suggested Readings

Aggarwal M, Khan IA. Hypertensive crisis: hypertensive emergencies and urgencies. Cardiol Clin 2006;24:135–146.

Blumenfeld JD, Laragh JH. Management of hypertensive crises: the scientific basis for treatment decisions. Am J Hypertens 2001;14(11 Pt 1):1154–1167.

Chiang WK, Jamshahi B. Asymptomatic hypertension in the ED. Am J Emerg Med 1998;16:701–704.

Elliott WJ. Hypertensive emergencies. Crit Care Clinics 2001;17:435–451.

Joint National Committee on Prevention, Detection, and Treatment of High Blood Pressure. The Sixth Report of the Joint National Committee on Prevention, Detection, Evaluation, and Treatment of High Blood Pressure. Arch Intern Med 1997;157:2413–2446.

Murphy C. Hypertensive emergencies. Emerg Clin North Am 1995;13:973–1007.

Psaty BM, Smith NL, Siscovick DS, et al. Health outcomes associated with antihypertensive therapies used as first-line agents: a systematic review and meta-analysis. JAMA 1997;277:739–745.

Shayne PH, Pitts SR. Severely increased blood pressure in the emergency department. Ann Emerg Med 2003;41:513–529.

Tietjen CS, Hurn PD, Ulatowski JA, et al. Treatment modalities for hypertensive patients with intracranial pathology: options and risks. Crit Care Med 1996;24:311–322.

Veterans Administration Cooperative Study Group on Antihypertensive Agents. Effects of treatment on morbidity in hypertension. Results in patients with diastolic blood pressures averaging 115 through 129 mm Hg. JAMA 1967;202:1028–1034.

Vidt DG. Emergency room management of hypertensive urgencies and emergencies. J Clin Hypertens 2001;3:158–164.

CHAPTER 40

Intentional Trauma and Abuse

NELSSON H. BECERRA ■ THEODORE J. CORBIN

 Red Flags

Repeat ED visits ● Injury is inconsistent with clinical presentation ● Poor hygiene or malnutrition that cannot be explained ● Delay in seeking care ● Injury during pregnancy ● Multiple complaints without physical findings ● Interpersonal problems between victim and significant other ● Near strangulation by an intimate partner

Overview

Intentional trauma includes both physical and psychological injury that is not accidental, and is a consequence of the intention to harm on the part of the perpetrator. Common examples include domestic violence, child abuse, and elderly abuse. The degree of injury of some abusive acts may not be intentional, but are the result of neglect inflicted upon a helpless victim such as young children, spouse or a hard to manage elderly parent.

In many instances, the clinical presentation of nonaccidental trauma (NAT) and other forms of abuse is subtle, and often is unrecognized by inexperienced personnel. Look for "red flags" (see Box) when evaluating these patients.

Recognizing acts of abuse and intentional trauma is important. The ED is often the initial entry of many of these patients into the health care system, and may be the only cry for help by many victims. Emergency physicians can make potentially life-saving interventions by simply recognizing a victim of NAT and offering to help.

This chapter will briefly discuss three types of intentional trauma and abuse: intimate partner violence and abuse (domestic violence), sexual assault, and elderly abuse. Child abuse is discussed in Chapter 82.

Specific Problems
Intimate Partner Violence and Abuse (IPVA)

■ *Background.* This is a pattern of repetitive sexual, physical and psychological attacks that is often escalating in nature. Although women

493

are usually the victims of domestic violence, male victimization also occurs. Abused women are generally not willing to volunteer information. Screening should be performed in a nonjudgmental supportive manner in a setting in which the patient feels safe. The most dangerous period for battered women is when they attempt to leave the relationship.

- **History.** History taking should be accomplished in an area with privacy for the patient. Any significant other who accompanies the victim should be asked to leave the treatment area. There should be an attempt to obtain an accurate history of the patient's experience, assess any immediate risk, and screen for possible injuries.

- **Physical examination.** A thorough physical examination should be conducted to evaluate for signs of trauma. The definitive marker for IPVA is a nonaccidental injury presentation. Examples include bruising of different ages on the body that do not match up with the patient's history of injury. Injuries from unintentional trauma tend to be located in distal and lateral aspects of the body, and are more often unilateral. The patient should be evaluated for defensive injuries such as scratch marks and forearm injuries (e.g., nightstick fracture). The skin should also be evaluated for characteristic markings such as a hand slap, a belt, or nonaccidental burn patterns (e.g., cigarette burns, hot-water immersion injuries, iron burns). Any injury to the genital or rectal area should raise suspicion for sexual assault and abuse.

- **Diagnostic testing.** The need for radiographic studies should be dictated by that patient's complaints and findings on physical examination. A urine pregnancy test should be ordered on all women of reproductive age.

- **ED management.** All traumatic injuries should be addressed as described in Section III. Documentation should include screening questions for possible victims of domestic violence, questions to assess the patient's immediate safety, danger assessment, and any injuries noted on physical examination. The patient should be provided with referrals and resources for victims of domestic violence. Efforts should be made to ensure that the patient is returning to a safe environment. Many states have laws that require health care providers to report known or suspected cases of intimate partner violence to the police.

- **Helpful hints and pitfalls.** A particularly ominous event is an episode of near strangulation; survivors of such an episode of violence have a 30% mortality to successive violence.

Sexual Assault

- **Background.** It is estimated that only 7% of rapes are reported. One in five women will become a victim of rape at some point in her lifetime. Many of these patients will come to the ED for evaluation. Clinicians should familiarize themselves with local forms and instructions before performing an examination of a sexual assault victim. A prepackaged rape crisis kit (for evidence collection) is commonly used. Documentation of custody of all evidence obtained during examination is known as *chain of evidence*. The police officer only needs to be present in the ED, not during the examination, in order to receive the evidence from emergency personnel, and to preserve the chain of evidence. Witnessed, written, and informed consent must be obtained before beginning evaluation and treatment. Many states allow an adolescent victim of a certain age (e.g., older than 12 to 14 years) to consent to an examination for conditions related to sexually transmitted diseases (STDs), sexual assault, and pregnancy.

■ *History.* A detailed history should be obtained on all suspected victims of sexual assault (Box 40–1). History taking should always be accomplished in an area with privacy. Family members or friends should initially be asked to wait outside if they are present. Sometimes a more complete and reliable evaluation may be obtained if accompanied by a trusted friend or advocate per the patient's request. The history of the event should include only those elements necessary for the clinician to complete required forms, to perform a focused physical examination, and to collect evidence. Further questioning regarding the assault, such as the details leading up to the assault, should be left to the police investigators. The sexual assault history should assist in deciding which potential samples to collect.

■ *Physical examination.* The physical examination of the sexual assault victim differs from most other ED examinations in that there is a simultaneous medical and forensic examination occurring. In addition to documenting any traumatic injuries, the rape examination includes evaluating and obtaining specimens from the oral cavity, genital and rectal areas, fingernails, and hair (pubic hair brushings). Spermatozoa have been identified in oral smears up to 6 hours after the attack despite tooth brushing, using mouthwash, or drinking various fluids, and may show valuable evidence up to 12 hours after examination. A Wood's lamp can be used to detect semen stains on a patient's body. However, the possibility of finding seminal fluid with the Wood's lamp is negligible

---

BOX 40–1 Recommended History Taking for Sexual Assault

General medical history: acute injury or illness, chronic disease, psychiatric disorders, preexisting injuries, current medications, allergies, immunizations

Gynecologic history: gravidity and parity, last normal menstrual period, last voluntary intercourse, birth control, possibility of missed birth control pills, possible symptoms of pregnancy, recent gynecologic surgery, sexually transmitted diseases

History of the assault: date, time, and place; number and brief description of assailants; types of force and threats used; use of alcohol or drugs by victim and assailants, loss of consciousness, type of assault (fondling, oral penetration, vaginal penetration, anal penetration, foreign bodies used, ejaculation on or in the body, use of condoms, use of a lubricant)

Post assault activity: medications, alcohol or drug use, change of clothing, urination or defecation, bathing, washing, douching, eating, drinking, brushing teeth, mouthwash, tampon use

after 24 hours. Potential dried secretions may be collected with moistened swabs; the swabs are then air-dried and preserved as evidence. Toluidine dye may be used to detect smaller vulvar lacerations. For male victims, the procedures for the history, physical examination, evidence collection, and medical treatment are the same as previously described for females, allowing for male anatomic differences. If the patient reports oral copulation by the assailant, swabs from the urethral meatus, the glans, and the penile shaft should be analyzed for saliva. A digital rectal examination should be done with attention to occult or gross bleeding that indicates the need for a proctoscopic examination. A rectal swab or aspirate should be obtained for evidence of sperm or acid phosphatase. Psychological injury is always present, and the clinician needs to be sensitive to this especially during the rape examination.

- *Diagnostic testing.* The need for radiographic studies should be dictated by the patient's complaints and findings on physical examination. A urine pregnancy test should be ordered on all females of reproductive age. Gonorrhea and *Chlamydia* cultures should be sent on all patients. Blood samples are drawn for DNA testing, blood typing, and pregnancy testing. Patients started on HIV prophylaxis may require baseline liver function, renal function, and hematologic parameters as appropriate to the medications.

- *ED management.* The emphasis is placed on assessment and management of both the physical and emotional trauma to patient, the prevention of sexually transmitted disease, the prevention of pregnancy (if desired), and the appropriate documentation and collection of forensic evidence. All collected material needs to be meticulously labeled, and its collection noted and described in the chart. Prophylactic medication for the prevention of common STD and pregnancy should be offered (see Boxes 40–2 and 40–3). The risk of STDs after sexual assault are listed in Box 40-4. Factors that increase the risk of HIV transmission include type of sexual contact (anal > genital), the presence of genital or anal trauma, and exposure to ejaculate. HIV prophylaxis should be offered to patients at risk if within 72 hours of the sexual assault for those patients at high risk (Box 40–5). Three-drug regimens are recommended under the assumption of maximal viral replication suppression provided by highly active retroviral therapy (HAART); however, 2-drug regimens with 2

BOX 40–2 Current CDC Recommendation for STD Prophylaxis

Ceftriaxone 125 mg intramuscularly in a single dose, plus either **azithromycin**, 1 g orally in a single dose, or **doxycycline** 100 mg orally twice a day for 7 days.

Metronidazole, 2 g orally in a single dose, is also recommended if coverage is desired for trichomonal infections and bacterial vaginosis.

For incubating syphilis, extend doxycycline therapy to 10 days or use intramuscular benzathine penicillin.

BOX 40–3   Drug Regimens for Pregnancy Prophylaxis*

Ethinyl estradiol/levonorgestrel (Ovral, Preven Kit): two tablets taken
    twice, 12 hours apart
OR
Ethinyl estradiol/levonorgestrel (Lo/Ovral, Levelen, Tri-Levlen,
    Tri-Phasil, Nordette): four tablets taken twice, 12 hours apart

---

*Nausea is the most common side effect with these agents. Patients at risk for thromboembolic disease
should have a progestin only emergency contraceptive or an intrauterine device inserted.*

**BOX 40–4   Risk of Sexually Transmitted Disease After
                Sexual Assualt**

Disease	Risk
Gonorrhea	6-18%
Chlamydia	4-17%
Syphilis	0.5-3%
HIV	<1%

**BOX 40–5   Treatment Protocols for Postexposure HIV
                Prophylaxis**

Non-nucleoside reverse transcriptase inhibitor (NNRT) based
1. Efavirenz (Sustiva) 600 mg PO qhs
2. Lamivudine (Epivir, 3TC) 300 mg qd or emtricitabine (Emtriva, FTC)
    200 mg qd
3. Zidovudine (Retrovir AZT) 300 mg bid or tenofovir (Viread) 300 mg qd
Average total cost for 4 week supply: $1100
Protease inhibitor (PI)-based
1. Lopinavir (400 mg)/ritonavir (100 mg) (co-formulated as Kaletra) 3
    tables bid
2. Zidovudine (Retrovir, AZT) 300 mg bid
3. Lamivudine 300 mg qd or emtricitabine 200 mg qd
Average total cost for 4 week supply: $1300

Note: Common side effects of these drugs are detailed in Chapter 37.

reverse-transcriptase inhibitors may be considered when adherence and
toxicity with a 3-drug regimen is a significant concern. Give the patient
a 3-5 day starter pack or prescription and arrange follow-up with an HIV
specialist to provide additional counseling, assess medication compliance
and adverse effects, and to determine need and the patient's desire to
continue the HIV prophylaxis medications. Patients should have follow-
up HIV testing at 6 weeks, 3 months, and 6 months. The hepatitis B

vaccination should be given if the victim is unimmunized or is uncertain. Follow-up doses are given at 1-2 months and 4-6 months for a total of 3 doses. Serologic tests for syphilis should be done between 4 and 6 weeks after the assault. If the patient is stable enough for discharge, a specific follow-up plan for the patient must be generated in the ED, with liberal use of local community resources. Most states mandate that medical personnel report sexual assaults to law enforcement.

- **Helpful hints and pitfalls.** The chain of evidence must remain unbroken for evidence to be valid in legal proceedings.

Elderly Abuse

- **Background.** Of elderly patients presenting to the ED, 2.6% are victims of abuse; unfortunately only 1 in 14 are reported. The problem is defined as willful *infliction* of injury, unreasonable confinement, intimidation, or cruel punishment, resulting in physical harm, pain, or mental anguish. Also included in the definition is willful *deprivation* of goods or services that are necessary to avoid physical harm, mental anguish, or mental illness.

- **History.** When assessing a suspected victim of elder abuse, the patient's caregiver should also be interviewed, in a nonthreatening, nonjudgmental manner. The needs of both should be assessed individually. Clues to abuse include conflicting or implausible accounts of events, a history of similar suspicious episodes, the patient is not accompanied by a care giver, there is a history of "doctor shopping" or no doctor, there is a delay in seeking medical care, medication is improperly administered, or the family member is not focusing the conversation on the patient.

- **Physical examination.** Common findings of such mistreatment are bruises, sprains, abrasions, and occasionally skeletal fractures, burns, and other wounds. There may be multiple injuries in various stages of healing or unusual soft tissue injuries. Burns may have a representative shape or demarcation. The patient may present with malnutrition, dehydration, or unkept.

- **ED management.** An elderly patient who is in immediate danger should be removed from the home, usually by means of hospitalization. If there is no presence of imminent danger, the caregiver should be provided assistance by friends, family, or social service agencies. The goal to be kept in mind is preserving the family unit and avoiding institutionalization by use of in-home services. If an elderly patient is competent to make decisions and refuses interventions, this should be respected. Forty-six of the 50 states mandate emergency physicians to report cases of known or suspected elder abuse to Adult Protective Services.

- **Helpful hints and pitfalls.** Common barriers to the identification of elder abuse include difficulty interpreting subtle signs of neglect, lack of a routine for case detection and screening, inadequate social services to respond to cases, and lack of coordination between the ED and social agencies.

Teaching Points

Domestic violence and elder abuse are unfortunately common. They are hard to detect unless the problem is thought about by the physician and other personnel. Many patients cannot report their problems because of age or senility. Many domestic violence victims are afraid to report their problems, and are ambivalent about seeking help or leaving the abusive partner. A particularly ominous event is near strangulation. These women are at very high risk of being killed if they are returned to the abusive situation.

Suggested Readings

Eisenstat SA, Bancroft L. Domestic violence. N Engl J Med 1999;341:886–892.

Gremillion DH, Kanof EP. Overcoming barriers to physician involvement in identifying and referring victims of domestic violence. Ann Emerg Med 1996;27:769–773.

Lachs MS, Pillemer K. Abuse and neglect of elderly persons. N Engl J Med 1995; 332:437–443.

Martin S, Mackie L, Kupper L, Buescher P, Moracco K. Physical abuse of women before, during, and after pregnancy. JAMA 2001;285:1581–1584.

Merchant RC. Update on emerging infections: news from the Centers for Disease Control and Prevention. Antiretroviral postexposure prophylaxis after sexual, injection-drug use, or other nonoccupational exposure to HIV in the United States. Ann Emerg Med 2005;46:82–86.

Muelleman RL, Reuwer J, Sanson TG, et al. An emergency medicine approach to violence throughout the life cycle. Acad Emerg Med 1996;3:708–715.

Sachs C, Waddell. Examination of the sexual assault victim. In Roberts JR, Hedges JR. Clinical Procedures in Emergency Medicine (4th ed). Philadelphia: Elsevier, 2004, pp 1151–1167.

Waller AE, Hohenhaus SM, Shah PJ, Stern EA. Development and validation of an emergency department screening and referral protocol for victims of domestic violence. Ann Emerg Med 1997;27:754–760.

CHAPTER **41**

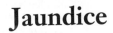

Jaundice

OREOLUWA T. OGUNJI ■ ADAM H. MILLER

 Red Flags

Immunocompromised • Elderly or young infants • Pregnancy
• Gastrointestinal bleeding • Altered mental status • Abdominal pain
• High fever • Abnormal vital signs • Pale stools • Dark urine
• Vomiting • Weight loss • Toxin exposure or overdose

Overview

Jaundice results from accumulation of bilirubin in the body tissues, including sclera, skin, and mucus membranes. It is usually noticed first in the sclera. Look for "red flags" (see Box) and consider critical diagnosis or life-threatening problems early.

Bilirubin is a product of heme metabolism formed by breakdown of the heme present in hemoglobin, myoglobin, cytochromes, catalase, peroxidase, and tryptophan pyrrolase. Eighty percent of daily bilirubin production is derived from hemoglobin, whereas the remaining 20% is from other heme-containing proteins. This unconjugated bilirubin is transported into the liver for conjugation and excretion. In the liver, unconjugated bilirubin becomes conjugated with a sugar via the enzyme glucuronosyltransferase. Once conjugated, it is soluble in bile, and can be transported into the gallbladder for storage, or into the small intestine for excretion in the stool or further metabolism and reabsorption. Jaundice can result from a malfunction in any of these processes. Jaundice can be caused by either unconjugated hyperbilirubin or conjugated hyperbilirubin depending on which stage of this process is disrupted. Clinical jaundice is usually not evident until the serum bilirubin concentration rises above 2.5 mg/dl.

In adults, jaundice alone is not an indication for admission. However, in neonates, high levels of unconjugated bilirubin can be neurotoxic and must be evaluated carefully (see Chapter 78).

Differential Diagnosis of Jaundice

See DDx table for differential diagnosis of jaundice.

Initial Diagnostic Approach
General

- Patients who appear ill, have abnormal vital signs, or altered mental status require immediate attention and an expeditious ED evaluation. A bedside glucose level should be checked on patients presenting with altered mental status due the potential for hypoglycemia in liver failure patients from diminished glycogen stores and impaired gluconeogenesis.
- The history and physical examination provide important clues regarding the etiology of jaundice. Jaundice that develops acutely with abdominal pain, vomiting, fever, and right upper quadrant pain is strongly suggestive of acute cholangitis due to obstructive disease (most commonly from choledocholithiasis). Obstructive jaundice from biliary disease or malignant neoplasms can also present with pruritus, pale stools, dark urine, and weight loss. Symptoms compatible with a viral prodrome, such as anorexia, malaise, and myalgias, make viral hepatitis a strong possibility.
- The history also may suggest that environmental hepatotoxins, ethanol, or medications are responsible for liver disease in the patient. Recent travel history may elicit exposure and risk for infectious disease that may cause hemolysis such as malaria.

DDx Priority-Based Differential Diagnosis of Jaundice

Primary Bilirubin Elevation	Critical Diagnoses	Emergent Diagnoses	Non-Emergent Diagnoses
Unconjugated		Toxin/Drugs Hemolysis (66)	Gilbert's syndrome Crigler-Najjar's syndrome
Conjugated	Ascending cholangitis (18) Fulminant hepatic failure Pregnancy related • Preeclampsia/HELLP • Acute fatty liver of pregnancy	Bile duct obstruction (18) Cirrhosis Heart failure (52) Hepatitis Infiltrative liver disease Malignancy (pancreatic, hepatocellular, metastatic) Pancreatitis (18) Primary biliary cirrhosis Primary sclerosing cholangitis Toxin/Drugs Trauma	Cholestasis of pregnancy Rotor's syndrome Dubin-Johnson

( ) Refers to the chapter in which the disease entity is discussed.
HELLP, hemolysis, elevated liver enzymes, and low platelets.
See Chapter 78 for neonatal jaundice, Reye's Syndrome, Hemolytic Uremic Syndrome.

■ Finally, a family history of jaundice or liver disease suggests the possibility of a hereditary hyperbilirubinemia or genetic liver disease. The patient should also be asked about hemoglobinopathies (i.e., sickle cell disease) or prior episodes of hemolysis.

Laboratory

■ See Figure 41–1, "Laboratory Approach to Differential Diagnosis."
■ Essential laboratory studies include serum bilirubin (total and direct fractions), alkaline phosphatase, lactate dehydrogenase (LDH) aspartate and alanine aminotransferases (AST and ALT), gamma glutamyl-transpeptidase, prothrombin time, and complete blood count (CBC). AST and ALT are markers of hepatocellular injury. Alkaline phosphatase and gamma-glutamyl transpeptidase are markers of cholestasis. Greater obstruction means greater elevation in these markers.
■ If hepatic tests other than bilirubin have normal findings, hemolysis or an isolated disorder of bilirubin metabolism should be considered. The CBC is helpful in detecting hemolysis. The blood smear may reveal schistocytes in intravascular hemolysis, spherocytes with extravascular hemolysis, sickled cells in sickle cell anemia, or Heinz bodies in cases

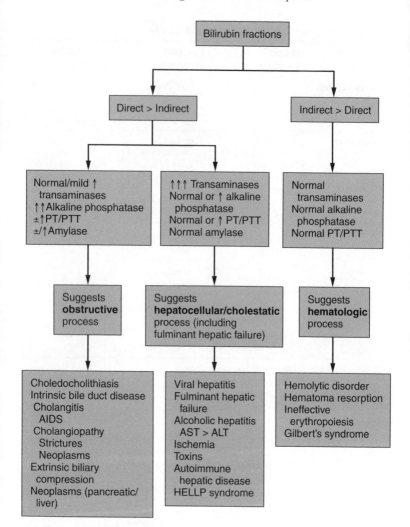

Figure 41-1. Laboratory approach to the differential diagnosis in patients with jaundice. PT/PTT, prothrombin time/partial thromboplastin time; AST, aspartate aminotransferase; ALT, alanine aminotransferase; HELLP, hemolysis, elevated liver enzymes, and low platelets. *Adapted from Heilpern KL and Quest TE. Jaundice. In: Marx JA, Hockberger RS, Walls RM, eds. Rosen's Emergency Medicine: Concepts and Clinical Practice. 6th ed. Philadelphia: Mosby, 2006:243-247.*

of glucose-6-phosphate-dehydrogenase (G6PD) deficiency. Patients with hemolysis can also have increased unconjugated bilirubin, increased lactate dehydrogenase, and decreased haptoglobin levels.

■ Further laboratory testing should be based on the most likely diagnosis determined by the history and physical examination. For example, if viral hepatitis is high on the differential, then serologic studies for viral hepatitis should be performed (see Table 41–1). If encephalopathy due to liver failure is suspected, then an ammonia level should be checked. A toxicologic screen including acetaminophen and salicylate levels should be sent on patients with altered mental status, or if an overdose is suspected. A urine pregnancy test should be sent on all women of reproductive age. Patients who are febrile should have blood cultures. Serum electrolytes, creatinine, and urinalysis should also be sent.

Radiography

■ An imaging study is chosen to confirm the presence or absence of biliary tract obstruction.

■ *Ultrasound.* An ultrasound study is the best imaging study to begin analysis of hepatobiliary disease, because it reveals intrahepatic or extrahepatic obstruction, can demonstrate cholelithiasis, show space-occupying lesions.

■ *Computed tomography (CT scan).* A CT scan of the abdomen with intravenous (IV) contrast is an alternative means of evaluating the possibility of biliary tract obstruction. A CT scan provides more information than ultrasound about liver and pancreatic parenchymal disease, reveals smaller obstructive lesions than ultrasonography, and provides technically superior images in the obese and in patients in whom the biliary tree is obscured by bowel gas. However, a CT scan is not as accurate as ultrasonography in detecting cholelithiasis because it images only calcified stones. Furthermore, it is not portable, requires use of IV contrast, and is more costly.

■ *Endoscopic retrograde cholangiopancreatography (ERCP).* This study permits direct visualization of the biliary tree as well as the pancreatic ducts, and is highly accurate in the diagnosis of biliary obstruction. In contrast to abdominal ultrasonography and CT scan, ERCP is more invasive and conscious sedation is necessary. Biopsies and brushings for cytology of lesions may be taken during the procedure. If a cause for biliary obstruction is identified (e.g., choledocholithiasis, biliary stricture), maneuvers to relieve obstruction (e.g., sphincterotomy, stone extraction, dilatation and stent placement) can be performed during the procedure. The complications associated with ERCP include respiratory depression, aspiration, bleeding, perforation, cholangitis, and pancreatitis. These rates are increased when interventional procedures are performed simultaneously. In addition, ERCP is more expensive than noninvasive imaging procedures, and is not usually performed in the ED.

■ *Percutaneous transhepatic cholangiography (PTC).* PTC complements ERCP, and is about as accurate and informative as ERCP in the assessment of biliary tract obstruction. Like ERCP, interventional procedures can be performed at the time of PTC. PTC is potentially advantageous

Table 41–1   Viral Hepatitis

Disease	Etiology/Risk Factors	Clinical Presentation	Diagnosis (Serology)	Management
Hep A	Transmitted via fecal-oral route. Most common worldwide cause of viral hepatitis. Risk factors: travel to endemic area, daycare workers, ingestion of contaminated food/water.	Common symptoms include fatigue, weakness, anorexia, nausea, vomiting, and abdominal pain; jaundice and dark urine 1-2 weeks later. Children may have asymptomatic course. Will not lead to chronic liver disease.	Acute: IgM anti-HAV. Immunity: IgG, anti-HAV. There is no chronic phase.	IV and fluid resuscitation for severe vomiting and diarrhea. The majority will have complete resolution within 2 months.
Hep B	Transmitted parenterally. Risk factors: IV drug abuse (IVDU), healthcare worker, homosexual male, hemodialysis, and perinatally. More common in adults and adolescents.	Prodrome of arthralgia or arthritis and dermatitis. Symptoms vary from asymptomatic infection to cholestatic hepatitis with jaundice, and rarely liver failure. UGI bleeding from persistent vomiting may also occur. <5% will lead to chronic liver disease.	Acute: HBsAg, IgM anti-HBc. Chronic: HBsAg, IgG anti-HBc. Immunity: IgG anti-HBc, anti-HBs	Mainly supportive care. Abnormal PT/INR or encephalopathy should raise suspicion for fulminant hepatic failure and need for admission.

Table 41–1 Viral Hepatitis—*cont'd*

Disease	Etiology/Risk Factors	Clinical Presentation	Diagnosis (Serology)	Management
Hep C	Transmitted parenterally. Risk factors: IVDU, blood transfusion, unprotected sexual intercourse, and perinatally. Major cause of chronic hepatitis, cirrhosis, and HCC and a major indication for liver transplantation worldwide.	Most do not experience clinical symptoms. If present, may have fatigue, nausea, and vomiting. Diagnosis is based mainly on exposure history. Most likely to lead to chronic liver disease (80–90%). Fulminant hepatitis is rare.	Acute/Chronic: anti-HCV, HCV RNA.	Supportive care. Refer to GI for further treatment if no signs of coagulopathy, encephalopathy.
Hep D	Transmitted parenterally. Risk factors: IV drug users, promiscuous homosexual men, and hemophiliacs.	Co-infection with HBV is more likely to cause chronic and fulminant liver disease.	Acute: IgM anti-HDV. Chronic: IgG anti-HDV.	Supportive care, admission for fulminant disease.
Hep E	Transmitted enterally. Endemic to areas such as Central America, Asia, India, Africa, and the South Pacific.	Fever, malaise, jaundice, dark urine, clay-colored stools, anorexia, nausea, vomiting, abdominal pain. Self-limited, will not lead to chronic liver disease.	Acute: IgM anti-HEV Convalescence or prior exposure: IgG anti-HEV. There is no chronic phase.	Supportive care. Pregnant women at increased risk for fulminant disease.

HCC, hepatocellular carcinoma; IVDU, intravenous drug use.

under conditions in which the level of biliary obstruction is proximal to the common hepatic duct, or in which altered anatomy precludes ERCP. PTC may be technically limited in the absence of dilatation of the intrahepatic bile ducts. The morbidity and mortality of PTC are similar to those of ERCP, and like ERCP, it is more expensive than abdominal ultrasonography or a CT scan, and is usually not performed in the ED.

- *Magnetic resonance cholangiopancreatography (MRCP).* Allows rapid evaluation of the biliary tree without the requirement of intravenous contrast agents. MRCP appears to be superior to conventional ultrasound or a CT scan for detection of biliary tract obstruction. However, the ability of MRCP to delineate smaller intrahepatic bile ducts is less clear. MRCP requires patient cooperation with breath-holding. Its expense is comparable to that of ERCP, however, it does not allow for therapeutic interventions, and is not performed in the ED.
- *Liver biopsy.* This is useful if results of serologic studies are negative, there is lack of improvement with withdrawal of suspected toxic agents, or there is no other obvious etiology for the jaundice. Liver biopsy is also useful in determining prognosis. However, there is no reason to perform this procedure in the ED.

Emergency Department Management Overview
General

- Patients with abnormal vital signs or altered mental status should be rapidly assessed for airway or hemodynamic compromise as discussed in Section II.

Medications

- *Analgesia.* IV analgesia can be given as needed to control the patient's pain. Morphine, hydromorphone, and meperidine are the drugs of choice. Despite the theoretical increase in sphincter of Oddi spasm caused by morphine, it is not clinically apparant, and morphine or meperidine are equally effective in relieving the pain of biliary disease (see Chapter 90.1). Acetaminophen at recommended dosages may be safe to use in patients with liver disease. It is safer to use than nonsteroidal anti-inflammatory drugs (NSAIDs) because it lacks gastrointestinal toxicity, renal toxicity, and inhibitory actions on platelet aggregation.
- *Antibiotics.* Patients suspected of having septic shock secondary to obstruction with infection should be promptly placed on broad-spectrum antibiotics after having blood cultures drawn. With ascending cholangitis, anaerobic coverage should be included. Antibiotics of choice are ampicillin, an aminoglycoside, and clindamycin or metronidazole for severe cases. In milder cases, second- or third-generation cephlosporins can be the initial antibiotics of choice (see Chapter 90.2).

Emergency Department Interventions

- *Nasogastric tube.* May be placed in patients who are actively vomiting if there is no response to anti-emetic agents.

■ *Urinary catheter.* Would be helpful in patients who are hemodynamically unstable, and those who require strict fluid status monitoring.

Disposition

■ *Consultation.* If extrahepatic biliary obstruction (cholecystitis or choledocholithiasis) is suspected, emergent consultation with a surgeon or gastroenterologist should be obtained. Hematology should be consulted for patients with hemolysis especially if the patient potentially requires transfusion therapy.
■ *Admission.* Patients with ascending cholangitis, intractable vomiting or pain, significant hepatic dysfunction (transaminases >1000 IU/L, bilirubin > 10 mg/dl, evidence of coagulopathy, encephalopathy), pancreatitis, cholecystitis or hemolysis requiring further evaluation or treatment require admission.
■ *Discharge.* Most patients with hepatitis or cholestatic jaundice can be discharged with close follow-up as long as they are hemodynamically stable, have normal mental status, can tolerate oral fluids, have no evidence of acute bleeding or complicating infectious process, and appropriate laboratory tests have been normal.

Specific Problems

Refer to the DDx table for reference to a discussion of problems in the differential not mentioned here.

Fulminant Hepatic Failure

■ *Definition.* Sudden illness or toxic exposure that results in hepatic necrosis. The three criteria for fulminant hepatic failure are rapid development of hepatocellular dysfunction (jaundice, coagulopathy), encephalopathy, and absence of a history of liver disease. Symptoms usually develop within 8 weeks after the onset of acute liver disease.
■ *Epidemiology and risk factors.* The most common causes are drugs (especially acetaminophen or liver toxins such as carbon tetrachloride) and viral hepatitis (Table 41–1). Other causes include Wilson's disease, poisonous mushrooms, Reye's syndrome, fatty liver of pregnancy, malignant infiltration, Budd-Chiari syndrome, and autoimmune hepatitis.
■ *Pathophysiology.* Severe injury is caused by hepatocellular necrosis or hepatocellular replacement by malignant infiltration. The injury inhibits the liver from performing its metabolic and synthetic functions.
■ *History.* The initial presentation of fulminant hepatic failure may include nonspecific complaints such as nausea, vomiting, fatigue, and malaise, but jaundice develops soon after. The patient has no history of hepatic disease, and the symptoms have developed in less than 8 weeks.
■ *Physical examination.* Patients may have moderate liver enlargement and tenderness. Patients are considered critical if they present with jaundice and any of the following: altered level of consciousness, hypotension, elevated prothrombin time, fever with abdominal pain, or active bleeding.

- **Diagnostic testing.** Laboratory studies mentioned above ("Initial Diagnostic Approach") should be part of the initial work-up. Ultrasound is preferable to a CT scan initially because it is safe, noninvasive, and can be performed at the bedside. It can be helpful to assess portal blood flow as well as evaluate for gallstones or biliary tree obstruction. A CT scan is more useful in evaluating extrabiliary causes of jaundice.
- **ED management.** In altered patients, a finger stick glucose determination is essential, as well as empiric naloxone and thiamine. Early consultation for possible liver transplantation is essential. Admit to the ICU.
- **Helpful hints and pitfalls.** Stabilize the patient before attempting to determine the cause of the liver failure. Despite aggressive management, the mortality rate of fulminant hepatic failure with severe encephalopathy can be as high as 80%.

Hepatitis and Cirrhosis

- **Definition.** Hepatitis is a generic term used to describe inflammation of the liver due to a variety of causes. This can progress to cirrhosis with the development of irreversible hepatic fibrosis and progressive hepatic failure.
- **Epidemiology and risk factors.** This impairment of hepatocellular function can be caused by a variety of disorders, including viral, auto-immune, alcoholic, or drug-induced hepatitis. It is most commonly due to viral infection (Table 41–1). Chronic hepatitis C infection and alcoholic hepatitis are the leading causes of cirrhosis. There are many other causes such as primary biliary cirrhosis, Wilson's disease (autosomal recessive disorder of copper metabolism), hemachromatosis (disorder of iron metabolism resulting in accumulation of iron in tissues), and primary sclerosing cholangitis. Between 30% and 70% of patients with hepatocellular carcinomas have underlying cirrhosis. The risk of hepatocellular carcinoma varies with the type of cirrhosis.
- **Pathophysiology.** Despite the varying etiologies, they all cause direct hepatocellular damage, inflammation of the liver, or fatty infiltration.
- **History.** The most common symptoms of hepatitis are malaise, fever, and anorexia. Patients may also present with nausea, vomiting, abdominal discomfort, and diarrhea. Cirrhotic patients may present with hematemesis (variceal or duodenal ulcer bleeding), rectal bleeding (hemorrhoids or rapid upper gastrointestinal tract bleeding), altered mental status (encephalopathy), or abdominal pain (spontaneous bacterial peritonitis [SBP] or worsening ascites).
- **Physical examination.** Fever, jaundice, right upper quadrant pain, hepatomegaly, or splenomegaly will be present. Patients who progress to cirrhosis may present with palmar erythema (alcohol abuse), spider angiomata, ecchymosis (thrombocytopenia or coagulation factor deficiency), dilated superficial periumbilical vein (caput medusae), gynecomastia, fetor hepaticus (musty odor of breath and urine found in cirrhosis with hepatic failure, small nodular liver, palpable spleen (portal hypertension), testicular atrophy, hemorrhoids, heme positive stools (if associated with GI bleeding), peripheral edema (hypoalbuminemia), ascites (portal hypertension, hypoalbuminemia), abdominal tenderness, flapping tremor, and asterixis (hepatic encephalopathy).

- *Diagnostic testing.* Patients with acute viral hepatitis typically have significant elevations (tenfold to 100-fold) of AST and ALT, with ALT being elevated in excess of AST. The bilirubin is moderately increased (5 to 10 mg/dl) but may occasionally be markedly elevated (15 to 25 mg/dl) with both fractions being elevated in equal proportions. The alkaline phosphatase and LDH may be elevated but are rarely more than 2 to 3 times normal. Elevations in the PT is a clue to hepatic dysfunction. The ammonia is elevated in encephalopathic patients but does not correlate with severity. Serum antigen and antibody levels can also be measured to determine acute or chronic infections, as well as immunized states in viral hepatitis. Imaging is usually not indicated for diagnosis. Paracentesis should be performed on patients presenting with new onset ascites for diagnostic purposes or acute abdominal pain in patients with chronic ascites to rule out SBP (see Chapter 91 for paracentesis and Appendix 1 for fluid analysis). Ultrasonography may be helpful in determining the extent of liver disease, presence of ascites, or another cause for abdominal pain and jaundice (biliary disease). A CT scan and MRI are useful for confirming the findings found with ultrasound, distinguishing benign from malignant tumors, and assessing extent of disease.
- *ED management.* Treatment of alcoholic and viral hepatitis is mainly symptomatic. IV access, fluid resuscitation, and anti-emetics should be provided for those patients showing signs of dehydration. Magnesium and thiamine replacement should be given as indicated to patients with a history of excessive alcohol ingestion. Monitor for hypoglycemia and treat accordingly. Patients with significant dehydration or electrolyte abnormalities should be admitted to the hospital. Patients who are altered or have a coagulopathy should be admitted to an ICU as well as be evaluated for fulminant hepatic failure. Toxin induced hepatitis should also be admitted. Discharged patients should have close follow-up. Cirrhotic patients should be treated according to the stage of the disease, or the presentation of its complications, and admitted for encephalopathy (lactulose 160 g/d with the goal of two to four bowel movements per day), variceal bleeding (see Chapter 34), or SBP. SBP is treated effectively with third-generation cephalosporins. Immunoprophylaxis for viral hepatitis should be provided for the patient's family members and close personal contacts.
- *Helpful hints and pitfalls.* Viral hepatitis is a reportable disease. Cirrhotic patients with altered mental status or possible gastrointestinal tract bleeding should have an expeditious ED evaluation.

Hereditary Hyperbilirubinemias

- See Table 41–2.
- Crigler-Najjar's syndrome types 1 and 2 and Gilbert's syndrome are hereditary forms of unconjugated hyperbilirubinemia that result from mutations in an enzyme that catalyzes bilirubin conjugation with glucuronic acid. In Crigler-Najjar type 1, essentially no functional enzyme activity is present, whereas patients with Crigler-Najjar type 2 have up to 10% of normal, and patients with Gilbert's syndrome have 10% to 33% of normal.

Table 41–2 Congenital Defects Causing Jaundice

Disorder	Clinical Presentation	Diagnosis	Management
Unconjugated Bilirubin (UB)			
Crigler-Najjar I	May present with poor feeding, lethargy, muscle rigidity, or seizures. Jaundice is only symptom evident in early course. Neurotoxicity, encephalopathy, and kernicterus may develop if not treated early.	Severe elevation in UB, with onset at birth. Absence of hemolysis.	If bilirubin levels >18-20 mg/dl admission and phototherapy, or exchange transfusion are needed.
Crigler-Najjar II	Similar presentation to type I, however kernicteurs is rare. Neurologic symptoms may develop during acute illness.	Levels of UB <350 umol/L, but can be higher during times of illness.	Admission usually required. Phenobarbitol as well as adjunctive phototherapy.
Gilbert's syndrome	Asymptomatic jaundice is most common complaint. Nonspecific symptoms of fatigue, malaise, weakness, and abdominal pain also common.	Mildly elevated levels of UB (50-140 umol/L). CBC, electrolytes, normal LFTs. US will show normal liver and biliary tree.	Treat acute illness. Reassurance and education are only real treatment.
Rotor's syndrome	Decreased intracellular storage and excretion of bilirubin leads to mild elevation in CB. Asymptomatic jaundice is only presentation.	Limited to elevated bilirubin about half of which is CB.	Reassurance and education are only real treatment.
Dubin-Johnson	Defective hepatic secretion leads to mild elevation in CB. Asymptomatic jaundice is most common complaint. May have vague abdominal pain. Exogenous estrogen may exacerbate the hyperbilirubin.	Limited to elevated bilirubin about half of which is CB.	Reassurance and education are only real treatment.

CB, conjugated bilirubin, UB, unconjugated bilirubin.

- Dubin-Johnson's syndrome and Rotor's syndrome, are characterized by conjugated or mixed hyperbilirubinemia with normal values for other standard liver tests.

Infiltrative Liver Disease

- Refers to other diseases in which the liver is filled with abnormal cells or substances.
- The most common disorders to produce jaundice are tuberculosis and sarcoidosis (50%-60% of cases). Others examples include *Mycobacterium avium* (particularly in an immunocompromised patient), lymphoma, drugs, α_1-antitrypsin deficiency, Wegener's granulomatosis, amyloidosis, glycogen storage diseases, Wilson's disease, hemochromatosis, or parasitic disease such as schistosomiasis.

Primary Biliary Cirrhosis (PBC)

- This is an autoimmune chronic progressive liver disease characterized by destruction of the small intrahepatic bile ducts with portal inflammation leading to fibrosis, cirrhosis, liver failure.
- Generally affects middle-aged women, and is the most common chronic cholestatic liver disease in adults in the United States. There is also a genetic predisposition.
- The diagnosis cannot be proven in the ED as a liver biopsy is required. Treatment is primarily supportive.

Primary Sclerosing Cholangitis (PSC)

- This is a chronic progressive cholestatic liver disease resulting from inflammation, fibrosis, and destruction of the bile ducts. This results in multiple areas of stricturing in the biliary tree and eventually to cirrhosis.
- This is a rare disease. There is a 2:1 male predominance. Approximately 70% of patients with PSC will have inflammatory bowel disease, more commonly ulcerative colitis than Crohn's disease.
- Many patients are asymptomatic. The most common symptom is fatigue. Other less common symptoms include pruritus, weight loss, and fever. Jaundice and hepatosplenomegaly may be present in up to 50% of patients.
- The diagnostic test of choice for PSC is cholangiography typically an endoscopic retrograde cholangiogram (ERC).
- No medical therapy has been found to be beneficial. Treatment is limited to complications that arise during the course of the disease. Consider this diagnosis in patients with inflammatory bowel disease who present with symptoms of pruritis or jaundice. Cholangiocarcinoma is a complication of this disease and has a very poor prognosis.

Special Considerations
Pediatrics

- Reye's syndrome and neonatal jaundice are two concerning causes of jaundice in the pediatric population and are covered elsewhere (see Chapter 78).

Women and Pregnancy

These problems usually present in the third trimester:

- **HELLP syndrome.** Progression of pre-eclampsia or eclampsia to hemolysis, elevated liver enzymes, and low platelets. Patients present with nausea, vomiting, right upper quadrant pain, and normal mental status. Rupture of the liver is rare. Jaundice may be present. Emergent delivery is necessary.
- **Acute fatty liver of pregnancy.** These women usually present with jaundice, fatigue, and headache, but can rapidly progress to encephalopathy, coagulopathy, seizures, and coma. Emergent delivery is necessary.
- **Cholestasis of pregnancy.** This is a benign condition. It is the most common cause of jaundice in pregnancy besides hepatitis. Patients present with generalized pruritus and mild jaundice, without fever, vomiting, or malaise. Management is by symptomatic relief with close OB follow up after other more severe causes of jaundice have been ruled out.

Teaching Points

Jaundice is perhaps the only physical finding in the ED patient that always signifies a disease. Like any other emergency problem, it is important to decide who is ill, and who has more time for accurate diagnosis and management.

While some of the causes of jaundice are oftentimes trivial, such as the minor degree that accompanies acute cholecystitis, its presence may be the first clue to a horribly serious condition such as carcinoma of the pancreas, leaving everyone to shudder at the thought of "painless jaundice."

Since jaundice may be the first sign of liver failure, it becomes critical to identify those patients who may have a reversible cause, such as bile duct stone obstruction, or pancreatitis.

Unfortunately, many of the toxicologic causes will be irreversible without liver transplantation, if they do not present before the onset of jaundice, such as acetaminophen overdose.

Chemical exposure, such as carbon tetrachloride can also lead to hepatocellular destruction, but may not destroy the entire liver as does certain mushroom ingestions, or delayed or untreated acetaminophen overdosage.

Ultrasonography has been a great boon to the bedside diagnosis of gallbladder stone disease, but is most useful for the patients who have only minor degrees of jaundice, or stone disease within the gall bladder. It may also help identify the dilated ducts of common bile duct stone, or pancreatic duct obstruction.

Infections of the liver are a common source of jaundice, with varying degrees of severity of the infection, such as hepatitis A, versus fulminant hepatitis C. Bacterial and parasitic infections can lead to jaundice as seen with schistosomiasis, malaria, and liver abscesses secondary to amebiasis (if biliary obstruction is present).

Suggested Readings

Lidofsky SD. Jaundice. In: Feldman M, Friedman LS, Sleisenger MH (editors). Sleisenger & Fordtran's Gastrointestinal and Liver Disease (7th ed). Philadelphia: Elsevier Science, 2002:249–261.

Gines P, Cardenas A, Arroyo V, Rodes J. Management of cirrhosis and ascites. N Engl J Med 2004; 350:1646–1654.

Lee WM, Acute liver failure. N Engl J Med 1993;329:1862–1872.

Heilpern KL, Quest TE. Jaundice. In: Marx JA, Hockberger RS, Walls RM (editors). Rosen's Emergency Medicine: Concepts and Clinical Practice (6th ed). Philadelphia: Mosby, 2006:243–247.

Nowicki MJ, Poley JR. The hereditary hyperbilirubinaemias. Baillieres Best Pract Res Clin Gastroenterol 1998;12:355–367.

Roche SP, Kobos R. Jaundice in the adult patient. American Family Physician 2004;69:299–304.

Tabbara IA. Hemolytic anemias: Diagnosis and management. Med Clin North Am 1992; 76: 649–668.

CHAPTER **42**

Joint Pain and Swelling

DAVID DAVIS ■ JOY MARTIN

Red Flags

Inability to bear weight • IV drug abuse • Joint prosthesis • Immunocompromised state • Elderly • Fever • Local erythema, warmth, and joint effusion • Unequal pulses, cool extremity, pale or cyanotic extremity • Open fracture • Shortened or rotated lower extremity (hip dislocation)

Overview

There is a large differential diagnosis for complaints of joint pain and swelling. The history and physical examination findings can be used to narrow the possible diagnoses into subgroups such as pediatric versus adult, traumatic versus atraumatic, and monoarticular versus polyarticular. Be aware of "red flags" (see Box) that suggest infection, vascular compromise, or other orthopedic emergencies.

When the diagnosis is unclear and an effusion is present, a joint aspiration should be performed to rule out a septic joint. Fever may not be present in septic arthritis, and the patient may still have some mobility of the involved joint.

Whenever traumatic injury is a possibility, obtain radiographs with at least two views of the affected joint.

Pediatric patients have a unique differential, and most should be imaged regardless of history of trauma (see Chapter 81 and 82). Joint trauma in adults is discussed in Chapter 17.

Differential Diagnosis of Joint Pain and Swelling

See DDx tables for information related to the differential diagnosis of joint pain and swelling based on acuity, joint involvement, and symptom duration.

Initial Diagnostic Approach
General

- Any patient who appears ill should receive immediate attention as discussed in Section II.
- The extremity examination should assess the skin, soft tissues, muscles, bones, bursae, joints (including range of motion at the involved joint), ligamentous stability, neurovascular deficits, extent of swelling, tenderness, local warmth, redness, or other abnormalities. It is also important to assess for involvement of other joints and any systemic manifestations.

Laboratory

- Studies may include a complete blood count (CBC), erythrocyte sedimentation rate (ESR), C-reactive protein (CRP), and blood cultures and synovial fluid analysis.

DDx Differential Diagnosis by Acuity*

Critical Diagnoses	Emergent Diagnoses	Nonemergent Diagnoses
Septic arthritis	Intra-articular fracture (17)	Rheumatic fever (67)
Dislocation (17)	Lyme disease (67)	Osteoarthritis
	Hemarthrosis	Gout
	Tendon rupture (17)	Sprain from ligamentous injury (17)
	Systemic vasulitic disease (71)	Tendonitis
	Reiter's syndrome (71)	Bursitis
	Rheumatoid arthritis (71)	Toxic synovitis (81)
		Systemic rheumatic disease (71)
		Viral Infection

( ) Refers to the chapter in which the disease entity is discussed.
*Pediatric orthopedics is discussed in Chapter 81.

DDX Differential Diagnosis of Arthritis by Joint Involvement and Symptom Duration

Mono-articular		Polyarticular	
Acute	Chronic or Recurrent	Acute (<6wk)	Chronic
Fracture (17)	Gout	Gonococcal arthritis	Rheumatoid arthritis (71)
Dislocation (17)	Pseudo gout	Lyme disease (67)	Osteoarthritis
Septic arthritis	Osteoarthritis	Reiter's syndrome (71)	Systemic lupus eryethematosus (71)
Hemarthosis		Rheumatic fever (67)	Scleroderma (71)
		Viral	Dermatomyositis (71)
			Ankylosing spondylitis (71)
			Psoriatic arthritis (71)

( ) Refers to the chapter in which the disease entity is discussed.

■ Joint aspiration for synovial fluid analysis is required in any patient suspected of having septic arthritis. In addition to obtaining synovial fluid for analysis, this procedure often provides pain relief by relieving pressure within the joint space (see Chapter 91 for arthrocentesis procedure and Appendix I for synovial fluid analysis).

■ Additional studies may be required for preoperative clearance if indicated.

Radiography

■ *Radiographs.* Radiographs of the joint in question should include at least two views. In children it may be advisable to get comparison views of the opposite side assuming that it is a normal joint. Whenever a traumatic injury has occurred, the physician should image the joints above and below the area in question as well.

■ *Ultrasound.* Ultrasound is a useful adjunct for arthrocentesis of certain joints, particularly pediatric hip joints.

■ *Computed tomography (CT scan).* A CT scan is useful for better delineation of fractures and suspected sacroiliac joint problems or transient synovitis, especially in children.

■ *Magnetic resonance imaging (MRI).* MRI is the study of choice in elderly patients with hip pain and no plain film evidence of fracture. Although a CT scan is more readily available in the ED, it can miss small impacted fractures or undisplaced fractures that run parallel to the axial plane. Otherwise, MRI is typically an outpatient study that is useful for evaluating ligamentous injuries.

■ *Angiography.* Angiography should be performed for joint dislocations with any evidence of altered perfusion following reduction such as posterior knee dislocations.

EKG

- An electrocardiogram (EKG) may be helpful if considering the diagnosis of rheumatic fever (prolonged PR interval) or Lyme disease (atrioventricular block).

Emergency Department Management Overview
General

- The most important ED intervention is to rule out a septic joint and treat accordingly.

Medications

- *Analgesia.* Analgesia should be provided early. Nonsteroidal anti-inflammatory drugs (NSAIDs) such as ibuprofen and ketorolac, and narcotic agents for severe pain including morphine, hydrocodone and codeine are important in controlling pain associated with most joint problems (see Chapter 90.1). Patients with rheumatoid arthritis may benefit from a prednisone taper (see Chapter 71) . Gout attacks are often acutely managed with NSAIDs, colchicine, or steroids (see "Gout and Pseudogout").
- *Antibiotics.* Antibiotics are required for all patients with documented or suspected joint infections. Empiric treatment should cover staphylococcus, streptococcus and gram-negative organisms. Recommended agents include β-lactamase resistant penicillin and aminoglycoside or a third generation cephalosporin. However if a gonococcal arthritis is suspected the preferred agents are third generation cephalosporin or fluoroquinolone (see Chapter 90.2).

Emergency Department Interventions

- *Ice and elevation.* Both act to decrease swelling, which allows for better joint assessment, facilitates joint reduction or arthrocentesis if necessary, and helps minimize pain.
- *Dislocation reduction.* This should not be delayed, especially in any patient with a hip dislocation or evidence of vascular compromise (Chapter 17).
- *Joint injection with anesthetic agent or steroid.* This can be a useful adjunct in controlling a patient's pain, particularly that associated with bursitis or tendonitis. Steroid injections have associated risks, and should not be used more than once every six weeks, and are contraindicated in patients with signs of infection and bleeding disorders.
- *Immobilization and splinting.* This limits further displacement or injury to the joint, protects surrounding soft tissue, vasculature, and nerves from further damage and decreases pain associated with continued movement of the involved joint (see Chapter 17) for splinting.

Disposition

- *Consultation.* Consult orthopedics immediately for any patient with a prosthesis dislocation or a joint dislocation that is difficult to reduce.

Orthopedics should also be consulted early for any patient in whom septic arthritis is diagnosed or suspected. If a dislocation is associated with vascular compromise, obtain vascular surgery consultation.

- ■ *Admission.* This is prudent for any patient with a joint infection, a knee dislocation, or other dislocation with suspected neurovascular injury, or intractable pain.
- ■ *Discharge.* This is appropriate for patients who have no evidence of joint infection, have pain that is controlled, are able to ambulate on their own or with the assistance of crutches, and will be able to make arrangements for the required follow-up.

Specific Problems

Refer to the DDx tables for reference to a discussion of problems in the differential not mentioned here.

Bursitis and Tendinitis

- ■ *Definition.* Bursitis is an inflammation of a bursa and is usually aseptic. *Tendinitis* refers to inflammation of the tendon only. *Tenosynovitis* refers to inflammation of the tendon and its surrounding sheath.
- ■ *Epidemiology and risk factors.* Bursitis and tendinitis result from repetitive use or trauma to certain joints.
- ■ *Pathophysiology.* Bursae are small saclike structures composed of synovial cells that act to cushion and decrease friction between joints and surrounding soft-tissue. When joints are subjected to strenuous or frequent use, polymorphonuclear (PMN) cells migrate to the site, synovial cells enlarge, and bursae can become inflamed. The same mechanism can result in inflammation of tendons and their sheaths, producing tendinitis. Pyogenic flexor tenosynovitis is an acute synovial space infection involving a flexor tendon sheath and is discussed in Chapter 17.
- ■ *History.* The chief complaint is typically joint pain that is described as mildly improving with early movement, but worsening after further exercise or use. A history of new physical activities, or increase in frequency, duration, or intensity of established work or exercise-related activities might be present.
- ■ *Physical examination.* Pain is usually localized to one area of the joint, and can be reproduced with palpation and specific movements that irritate the affected tendon or bursae. There may also be warmth, erythema, and swelling present. The strength examination may be limited due to pain.
- ■ *Diagnostic testing.* The diagnosis is made based on the history and physical examination. An ultrasound study can show bursitis or tendon thickening and surrounding inflammation.
- ■ *ED management.* Recommended treatment consists of NSAIDs and rest for several days followed by range of motion exercises. Follow-up in 1 to 2 weeks with the patient's primary physician or orthopedist is recommended.
- ■ *Helpful hints and pitfalls.* Olecranon and prepatellar bursitis can evolve to a septic bursitis, and antibiotics are often initiated. Although needle

drainage is sometimes used since it may accelerate healing, it often necessitates going through cellulitic skin resulting in an increased risk of converting the bursitis to a septic one, and may also cause a continuously draining sinus track to form. Steroid injections in patients with tendinitis or bursitis may give the patient pain relief, but can result in tendon rupture or infection.

Gout and Pseudogout

- ■ *Definition.* This is a crystal-induced arthritis in which crystals of monosodium urate (gout) or calcium pyrophosphate (pseudogout) are deposited within the joint space.
- ■ *Epidemiology and risk factors.* This typically affects men and women older than 40 years. Risk factors include obesity, alcohol consumption, hypertension, diabetes, and the use of proximal loop diuretics.
- ■ *Pathophysiology.* Gout develops when uric acid crystals are deposited in the joint space. A similar disease process, pseudogout, occurs if the crystals deposited are calcium pyrophosphate. An acute localized inflammatory response occurs as PMN cells attempt to resorb the crystals. The most commonly involved joints are those in the lower extremities, with the great toe metatarsal being affected in 75% of cases of gout, and the knee being most often affected in pseudogout. The cartilage deposition of calcium pyrophosphate is termed *chondrocalcinosis*.
- ■ *History.* Patients describe severe pain that often begins in a single joint, but may progress to involve several. Subsequent attacks often become more frequent and severe.
- ■ *Physical examination.* Affected joints may be swollen, erythematous and very tender, even with light palpation. Tophi, deposits of urate crystals in the subcutaneous tissue, may also be noted in those patients with longstanding disease. Some patients will present with fever.
- ■ *Diagnostic testing.* The white blood cell count (WBCs) and ESR may be elevated in an acute flare. Serum uric acid levels are not helpful, as they do not correlate with presence, absence, or severity of disease. Radiologic studies may show soft-tissue swelling and bony erosion. Synovial fluid analysis is the definitive diagnostic study. Patients with gout will have negatively birefringent crystals, whereas those with pseudogout have positively birefringent crystals.
- ■ *ED management.* Although gout and pseudogout are self-limited diseases, typically resolving in several weeks, appropriate treatment improves symptoms and speeds resolution of the attack. Preferred treatment for acute flares includes NSAIDs, most often indomethacin 50 mg four times daily or ibuprofen, 800 mg three times daily. In young, healthy patients with a recent onset of symptoms, colchicine can be a very effective treatment. However, its use is limited by side effects and a narrow therapeutic window. It should be avoided in patients with renal or hepatic insufficiency. Colchicine is more effective in the treatment of acute gout than pseudogout. The dose of colchicine is 0.6 to 1.2 mg orally (one to two tablets), then 0.6 mg (one tablet) every 1 to 2 hours until the attack subsides or until nausea, diarrhea, or gastrointestinal tract cramping develops. The maximum total oral dose is 4 to 6 mg. If

ineffective in 48 hours, it should not be repeated. Intravenous colchicine is also available, but is not as commonly used as in the past, due to local tissue necrosis secondary to extravasation of the drug and systemic toxicity. Prednisone 20 to 40 mg daily can be given if the patient is unable to tolerate NSAIDs or colchicine. Intra-articular steroids may be used to treat a single inflamed joint: triamcinolone hexacetonide, 5 to 20 mg, or dexamethasone phosphate, 1 to 6 mg. Do not initiate uricosuric agents (probenecid) or xanthine oxidase inhibitors (allopurinol), during an acute attack. These should not be started until the attack has resolved, but ongoing use should not be interrupted.

- *Helpful hints and pitfalls.* Always consider joint sepsis or cellulitis in the setting of a gout or pseudogout flare. There is no indication to treat asymptomatic hyperuricemia. Acute attacks of gout are occasionally associated with normal levels of uric acid.

Septic Arthritis

- *Definition.* Bacterial infection, usually of a single joint.
- *Epidemiology and risk factors.* Patients who are immunocompromised, elderly, IV drug abusers, or have prosthetic joints are at highest risk for septic arthritis. The most commonly affected joint is the knee, followed by the hip. Intravenous drug abusers are also likely to have involvement of axial skeleton joints (i.e., sacroiliac, sternoclavicular, and vertebral).
- *Pathophysiology.* Bacteria seed the joint via hematogenous spread, localized infection, and invasive procedures. The most common organism involved is *Staphylococcus aureus*. Other common organisms include streptococcus, gram-negative rods and anaerobes. Gonococcus is also a potential pathogen in sexually active patients.
- *History.* The most common presenting complaint is joint pain. Eighty percent of patients will have associated fever.
- *Physical examination.* The affected joint is typically erythematous, swollen, warm, and tender with palpation and movement. A joint effusion is usually present, however the absence of one does not rule out septic arthritis. Patients with gonococcal septic arthritis may also have painless dermatologic lesions that can be maculopapular or pustular, as well as an increased urethral or vaginal discharge.
- *Diagnostic testing.* The ESR is elevated in 90% of cases. Blood cultures will grow the organism in approximately 50% of cases. Synovial fluid analysis is the most important study. Seventy-five percent of cases will have a fluid WBC greater than 50,000 with greater than 85% PMN cells. Do not forget to request cultures of fluid as well. Radiologic studies of the joint may show evidence of soft-tissue swelling and effusion. Bony changes consistent with osteomyelitis may be noted in cases with delayed presentations.
- *ED management.* Arthrocentesis should be performed, and antibiotics initiated as quickly as possible (see "Emergency Medicine Management Overview" for initial antibiotic choices). Orthopedics should be involved early in the patient's course to help determine whether surgical drainage will be necessary. All patients with septic arthritis will require admission for IV antibiotics and pain control.

- **_Helpful hints and pitfalls._** A red, hot, swollen joint is a septic one until proven otherwise. If possible, do not aspirate a joint through an area of cellulitis as this may inoculate the joint. Do not let a history of chronic joint disease or the well appearance of patient dissuade you from pursuing a diagnosis of septic arthritis. Synovial fluid cultures have a notoriously low yield for gonococcus (<50% positive). If suspected, oropharyngeal, cervical, and urethral cultures may improve the diagnostic yield.

Spontaneous Hemarthrosis

- **_Definition._** Spontaneous joint hemorrhage.
- **_Epidemiology and risk factors._** Hemarthroses can occur secondary to joint trauma, or spontaneously, in patients with bleeding disorders. It occurs most frequently in hemophiliacs.
- **_Pathophysiology._** A spontaneous hemarthrosis in patients with hemophilia A and B occurs as a result of a deficiency of factor VIII or factor IX, respectively. The resultant abnormalities of the intrinsic coagulation pathway, and ultimately failure of hemostasis, predispose these patients to bleeding within the joint capsule.
- **_History._** The patient often gives a history of stiffness or warm sensation in the joint followed by increasing pain.
- **_Physical examination._** The earliest presenting sign of a spontaneous hemarthrosis is pain in the joint. Later findings include limited range of motion, joint held in flexion, and tense swelling of the joint space.
- **_Diagnostic testing._** Any patient with a spontaneous hemarthrosis should have coagulation studies and a platelet count sent. A patient with hemophilia VIII or IX will have elevated activated partial thromboplastin time. Factor levels are not required to manage these patients appropriately in the ED. Radiographs may reveal joint-space widening.
- **_ED management._** Any patient with hemophilia requires appropriate factor replacement. The general goal is to achieve a factor level that is 30% to 50% of normal by administering 15 to 25 U/kg of factor VIII or 30 to 50 U/kg of factor IX. Analgesia and short-term immobilization may also provide comfort. Patients should be observed to ensure cessation of bleeding. Hematology should be consulted for hemophiliacs or unexplained hemarthrosis.
- **_Helpful hints and pitfalls._** Administration of factor replacement is the most important component of treatment in diagnosed hemophiliacs.

Osteoarthritis

- **_Definition._** Joint pain due to degeneration and loss of articular cartilage.
- **_Epidemiology and risk factors._** Osteoarthritis is the most common cause of joint pain, and affects most people over the age of 65. The knee, hip, spine, and hands are most commonly involved.
- **_Pathophysiology._** The disease is symptomatic when the rate of cartilage breakdown exceeds the rate of regeneration. Primary osteoarthritis has no known cause. Secondary osteoarthritis is a consequence of a number of disorders including trauma, metabolic conditions, and other forms of arthritis.

- *History.* The most common symptoms are asymmetric joint pain and stiffness in the morning, which result in limited function at the affected joints. Patients will typically describe a gradual onset of these symptoms, and note that pain improves with rest and is exacerbated by activity. In contrast to rheumatoid arthritis there are no systemic manifestations.
- *Physical examination.* The findings include joint enlargement or deformity, and painful or limited range of motion. When cartilage destruction causes surface irregularities, crepitus may be noted during joint examination. Joint erythema and warmth are not typical findings of osteoarthritis. Distal interphalangeal (DIP) joint involvement may lead to the development of nodular swellings called Heberden's nodes. Proximal interphalangeal (PIP) joint involvement can cause nodular swellings called Bouchard's nodes.
- *Diagnostic testing.* Radiographs will demonstrate degenerative changes, including osteophytes and joint-space narrowing. Laboratory and synovial fluid examination are normal.
- *ED management.* Initiate pain control with NSAIDs and low-impact exercise, to preserve range of motion and strengthen muscles. These are recommended for initial management. Some patients with severe symptoms may require brief periods of immobilization, but this is not advised for everyone. Patients should be referred to a primary care physician for further management, which may involve referral to a physical therapist or intra-articular corticosteroid injections.
- *Helpful hints and pitfalls.* If the joint is warm or red, osteoarthritis is unlikely to be the diagnosis.

Special Considerations
Pediatrics

- Presenting pain can often be referred from another joint. Consider the hip as a source of knee pain.
- It is always prudent to look for septic arthritis (especially of the hip and sacroiliac joints) even if the patient is afebrile.
- Always consider nonaccidental trauma (see Chapter 82).

Elderly

- There is a high incidence for fractures and dislocations in this population, especially osteoporotic elderly women. There may be no history or trauma, or only a very minor episode.
- These patents have a higher risk for septic arthritis.
- NSAIDs should be used with caution in the elderly as the incidence of peptic ulcer disease, gastritis, renal insufficiency, and fluid retention are all increased in this patient population.

Women and Pregnancy

- These women have a higher risk for sacroiliac joint instability.

Immunocompromised

- These patients have a higher risk for septic arthritis.

Teaching Points

There are many forms of arthritis, but the one thing they have in common is the ability to produce acute or chronic discomfort as well as incapacitation of many common functions.

It is easy to miss an early septic joint, and to not think of the possibility in patients with chronic arthritis, but this is a true emergency because of the rapid destruction of the joint and the deterioration into septicemia. Gonorrhea is often not thought of when it presents as arthritis, and it should be sought in the sexually active patient.

Suggested Readings

Garcia-De La Torre I, Ignacio. Advances in the management of septic arthritis. Rheum Dis Clin North Am 2003;29:61–75.

Lowery DW. Arthritis. In: Marx JA, Hockberger RS, Walls RM (editors). Rosen's Emergency Medicine: Concepts and Clinical Practice (6th ed). Philadelphia: Mosby, 2006, pp 1776–1792.

Manek NJ, Lane NE. Osteoarthritis: current concepts in diagnosis and management. Am Fam Physician 2000;61:1795–1804.

Pay S. Calcium pyrophosphate dihydrate and hydroxyapatite crystal deposition in the joint: new developments relevant to the clinician. Curr Rheumatol 2003;5:235–243.

Siva C, Velazquez C, Mody A, Brasington R. Diagnosing acute monoarthritis in adults: a practical approach for the family physician. Am Fam Physician 2003;68:83–90.

CHAPTER 43

Lightheaded and Dizzy

WAME N. WAGGENSPACK, JR. ■ LYNN P. ROPPOLO

Red Flags

> Advanced age (>60 years) ● Other co-morbid conditions: diabetes, cardiovascular disease, structural heart disease ● Abnormal vital signs (high fever, ↑ or ↓ heart rate, ↓ blood pressure) ● Hypoxia or shortness of breath ● Altered mental status ● Fever ● Signs of dehydration ● Pallor ● Diaphoresis ● Severe pain (headache, chest pain, abdominal pain) ● Neurologic deficit ● Vomiting ● Blood loss

Overview

Dizziness and *lightheadedness* are common patient complaints in the ED, but can mean many different things to different people. Some patients may use these terms interchangeably. Look for "red flags" (see Box), and assess for serious pathology. Any patient presenting with these symptoms usually falls into one of four categories: presyncopal lightheadedness, vertigo, dysequilibrium, or a nonspecific dizziness that is often difficult to describe (see DDx table). Patients presenting with dizziness or lightheadedness may also describe a general feeling of weakness (see Chapter 60).

Differential Diagnosis

See the DDx table of Dizziness.

> ●●● Refer to Chapter 57 "Syncope" and Chapter 59 "Vertigo" for a more
> ●●● detailed discussion of patients presenting with presyncopal and vertiginous
> ●●● symptoms, respectively.

Initial Diagnostic Approach
General

- As always, the ABCs (*a*irway, *b*reathing, and *c*irculation) should be addressed (see Section II). Any ill-appearing patient and those with

DDx Dizziness

	Definition	Example
Presyncopal lightheadedness	A feeling that fainting (presyncope) may occur in the next few moments, and usually occurs when a person gets up quickly. It is usually due to decreased blood flow or decreased availability of vital nutrients (glucose and oxygen) to the brain.	• Decreased cardiac output (dysrhythmia, valvular disease, cardiomyopathy, pulmonary embolism) • Hypovolemia (anemia, gastrointestinal bleed) • Hypoxia (pulmonary embolism, carbon monoxide poisoning) • Orthostatic hypotension • Vasovagal • Metabolic (hypoglycemia)
Vertigo	A sensation of spinning or rotation of oneself in relation to the environment that is caused by a vestibular disorder (inner ear or brain).	• Benign positional vertigo • Meniere's disease • Acute labyrinthitis • Vertebrobasilar insufficiency • Brainstem stroke
Dysequilibrium	A feeling that one is going to fall characterized by unsteadiness or imbalance only when upright. It is usually due to a disruption in the integration between sensory input and motor output.	• Somatosensory disturbance from peripheral neuropathy • Vestibular loss • Multiple co-existing neurosensory impairments (medication side effects, neuropathy, vision impairment)
Nonspecific	Symptoms that are too vague, often difficult to describe, and are not identified within the other categories.	• Hyperventilation from anxiety • Postconcussive after head trauma

abnormal vital signs such as tachycardia, bradycardia, hypotension, or hypoxia should prompt a thorough evaluation for serious causes of lightheadedness and dizziness. The patient should be placed on a cardiac monitor and pulse oximeter and intravenous (IV) access should be obtained.

■ A thorough and accurate history should be obtained and is the most important part of the initial evaluation. Because these are subjective complaints, probably the most important clue to the diagnosis is to understand exactly what the patient is experiencing. Open-ended questions are encouraged. Identify true vertigo, associated symptoms, or any change of symptoms with position (movement of the head or upon standing), cardiac complaints such as chest pain or palpitations, abdominal pain, blood or volume loss, co-morbidities such as diabetes, and environmental exposures such as excessive heat, and medications use. Falls are common with the elderly patients. Any history of trauma should be ascertained.

■ The physical examination should focus especially on *eyes* (nystagmus, visual field deficits), *ears* (hearing loss, tinnitus or ringing in the ears, middle ear abnormalities), *cardiovascular* (tachycardia, murmurs, rhythm, central and peripheral pulses), and *neurologic* examination. Assess for orthostatic hypotension (see Chapter 2). Orthostatic vital signs should NOT be performed on patients who are already tachycardic or hypotensive.

■ Fever should prompt a complete evaluation for an infectious source. Focus on clues from the history and physical examination to guide the workup as chief complaints of lightheadedness and dizziness are rarely isolated symptoms (this is more common in the elderly and immuno-compromised patients).

EKG

■ Any patient in whom a cardiac cause is suspected should have an electrocardiogram (EKG) to evaluate for signs of cardiac ischemia, dysrhythmias, or conduction abnormalities.

Laboratory

■ Laboratory testing is rarely helpful and should be limited to evaluating specific causes based on history and physical examination.
■ Studies may include complete blood cell count, basic metabolic profile, cardiac enzymes, and urinalysis.

Radiography

■ A chest radiograph should be obtained in all patients with cardiac symptoms, shortness of breath, or hypoxia (SaO_2 <95%).
■ Computed tomography (CT scan) of the head should be reserved for patients with altered mental status, neurologic impairment, a concerning headache, or a history of head trauma.
■ Magnetic resonance imaging (MRI)/magnetic resonance angiogram (MRA) is the preferred study for imaging the posterior fossa and

brainstem. It is the study of choice for vertebrobasilar insufficiency, but may not be immediately available in the ED.

Emergency Department Management Overview
General

- The ABCs are always the first priority as discussed in Section II. Supplemental oxygen should be given to patients who are hemodynamically unstable, have potentially life-threatening conditions, or have an oxygen saturation below 95%.
- Two large-bore IV catheters (at least 18 gauge) should be inserted in all patients with hemodynamic instability. Fluid boluses of normal saline or lactated ringers should be given to hypotensive or dehydrated patients. Blood should be sent for type and cross match if there is concern for acute blood loss or severe anemia.

Medications

- Aspirin should be given if there is concern for an acute ischemic coronary syndrome.
- Vestibular suppressants such as meclizine 25 mg by mouth (PO) (antihistamine) and diazepam 5 mg PO (benzodiazepine) may be given for peripheral vertigo if the diagnosis is not in doubt.

Disposition

- ***Consultation.*** Prompt neurologic consultation is appropriate when a central neurologic cause of symptoms is suspected. Cardiology consultation is necessary for symptoms secondary to cardiac pathology such as acute coronary syndrome (ACS) or dysrhythmias.
- ***Admission***. Patients who have unstable or abnormal vital signs, hypoxia, gastrointestinal bleeding or symptomatic anemia from other causes, concern for central neurologic sources such as stroke or posterior circulation compromise, or presyncopal symptoms from possible cardiac disease should be admitted. Patients who are dehydrated and unable to tolerate oral fluids should also be admitted.
- ***Discharge***. Patients with a clear diagnosis of a benign condition, normal vital signs, normal ED evaluation, and no co-morbidities may be safely discharged home. Ensure that the patient is able to tolerate oral fluids and has outpatient follow-up.

Special Considerations
Pediatric

- Dizziness is an uncommon complaint in children.

Elderly

- Dizziness affects more than 50% of the elderly, and is the most common complaint of patients older than 75 years.

BOX 43.1 Drugs Associated With Dizziness

Cardiovascular
Alpha-blockers
Beta-blockers
Calcium channel blockers
Diuretics
Direct vasodilators
Anticholinergic
Antihistamines
Tricyclic antidepressants

Neurologic
Anticonvulsants
Lithium
Alcohol

Ototoxic
Aminoglycosides
Aspirin
Cisplatin

Other
NSAIDs
Benzodiazepines
Psychotropic drugs

■ Problems with balance are common in elderly patients. With the normal aging process, gradual deterioration in the sensory systems, the central and peripheral nervous systems, and in muscles and joints affects the functions necessary for balance. Many medications commonly prescribed for hypertension have side effects of dizziness or imbalance symptoms (Box 43–1). Vascular diseases represent the most common non-vestibular cause of dizziness and balance loss in the elderly.

■ A major concern is the increased fall risk and the morbidity associated with subsequent injury.

Teaching Points

Dizziness is a complaint that often leads the emergency physician to believe that the patient has somatizing complaints. Although this may be true in younger patients, the older the patient, the more likely the complaint is to represent serious disease.

It is often a very incapacitating complaint, and at the very least, one can improve patient comfort by ruling out serious causes, and in some cases, giving symptomatic relief.

Suggested Readings

Derebery MJ. The diagnosis and treatment of dizziness. Med Clin North Am 1999;83:163–177.
Drachman DA, Hart CW. An approach to the dizzy patient. Neurology 1972;22:323–334.
Drachman DA. A 69-year-old man with chronic dizziness. JAMA 1998;280:2111–2118.
Eaton DA, Roland PS. Dizziness in the older adult, II: Treatments for causes of the four most common symptoms. Geriatrics 2003;58:46:49–52.
Olshaker JS. Dizziness and Vertigo. In: Marx JA, Hockberger RS, Walls RM (editors). Rosen's Emergency Medicine: Concepts and Clinical Practice (6th ed). Philadelphia: Mosby, 2006, pp 142–149.

Tusa RJ. Dizziness. Med Clin North Am 2003;87:609–641.
Walker JS, Barnes SB. Dizziness. Emerg Med Clin North Am 1998;16:845–875, vii.
Wasay M, Dubey N, Bakshi R. Dizziness and yield of emergency head CT scan: is it cost effective? Emerg Med J 2005;22:312.
Weinstein BE, Devons CA. The dizzy patient: stepwise workup of a common complaint. Geriatrics 1995;50:42–46, 49.

CHAPTER **44**

Nausea and Vomiting

LARA K. KULCHYCKI ■ JASON IMPERATO

 Red Flags

Extremes of age ● Immunocompromised state ● Cardiac risk factors ● Diabetes ● Toxic ingestion ● Abnormal vital signs (high fever, ↑ heart rate, ↓ blood pressure) ● Signs of dehydration ● Severe pain of rapid onset ● Altered mental status ● Chest pain ● Abdominal pain ● Inability to pass gas ● Obstipation ● Hematemesis ● Vision loss

Overview

The symptoms of nausea and vomiting have a wide differential diagnosis that encompasses nearly every organ system. Look for "red flags" (see Box), and consider critical diagnoses first. Most of these diagnoses are discussed in detail in other chapters of this text. A careful history of the present illness and physical examination are critical in narrowing the diagnostic possibilities and selecting confirmatory testing. Vomiting must be differentiated from regurgitation. Vomiting may occur without nausea, suggesting the possibility of central nervous system (CNS) pathology. Ascertain the frequency and timing of emesis, as well as the presence of bloody, bilious, or feculent vomitus.

Complaints of nausea and vomiting are nonspecific, but not benign; they cause considerable suffering, and are often harbingers of medical or surgical emergencies.

Laboratory and imaging tests as well as treatment modalities must be directed toward identifying not only the source of symptoms, but also the presence of complications. Vomiting can result in dehydration (see Chapter 26), electrolyte depletion (see Chapter 88), acid-base abnormalities (see Chapter 83), malnutrition, aspiration, Mallory-Weiss tears (see Chapter 34), and even esophageal rupture, termed *Boerhaave's syndrome* (see Chapter 22). All women of childbearing age must be questioned regarding recent menstrual history and tested for pregnancy.

Differential Diagnosis of Nausea and Vomiting

See DDx table for information pertaining to the differential diagnosis of nausea and vomiting.

Initial Diagnostic Approach
General

- Any patient who is hemodynamically unstable or appears ill should receive immediate attention. While the physician is assessing the patient, a continuous cardiac monitor and pulse oximeter should be placed. Intravenous (IV) access should be obtained. These patients should not leave the ED except for definitive care unless they have had all measures to obtain stability.

Laboratory

- Many patients with nausea and vomiting will not require any laboratory studies. The astute clinician will use a directed history and physical examination to determine which tests, if any, are required to direct therapy. The only study that should always be obtained is a pregnancy test in women of childbearing age.
- A complete blood count (CBC) with differential may be indicated in patients with suspected infection or blood loss.
- Electrolytes and renal function panels can be useful in assessing the etiology and complications of vomiting. Electrolyte derangements, uremia, and acid-base abnormalities can be the cause or the result of persistent emesis. A properly interpreted chemistry panel can direct electrolyte repletion, and aid in the selection of appropriate IV fluids. Use the anion gap as a diagnostic aid in patients with acidosis. All patients with clinical evidence of significant dehydration, known diabetes, or suspected toxic insults should have a chemistry panel performed.
- Liver function tests (LFTs) can be useful in patients with suspected abdominal pathology such as hepatitis, biliary disease, or pancreatitis. Septic patients should also have LFTs performed both to look for the source of infection as well as to identify end organ effects of poor perfusion.
- A urinalysis (UA) is helpful in suspected cases of urinary tract infection (UTI), pyelonephritis, renal calculi, and urosepsis. In addition, the presence of urine ketones can be a useful marker of dehydration.
- Cerebrospinal fluid (CSF) analysis should be performed with suspected subarachnoid hemorrhage, meningitis, or encephalitis.

DDx Differential Diagnosis of Nausea and Vomiting

	Critical	Emergent	Nonemergent
Neurologic	Central nervous system neoplasm Head trauma (9) Hydrocephalus Meningitis/encephalitis (67) Posterior circulation stroke (56) Subarachnoid hemorrhage (9, 35)	Acoustic neuroma (59) Pseudotumor cerebri (35)	Labyrinthitis (59) Meniere's disease (59) Migraine (35) Postconcussive syndrome (9)
Ophthalmologic	Acute angle-closure glaucoma (69)		
Cardiac	Acute myocardial infarction (22) Aortic dissection (22) Ruptured abdominal aortic aneurysm (18)		
Gastrointestinal	Appendicitis (18) Cholecystitis (18) Hollow viscus perforation (18) Intestinal obstruction (18) Pancreatitis (18) Peritonitis (67)	Fatty liver of pregnancy Gastritis (18) Hepatitis (41) Inflammatory bowel disease (27) Peptic ulcer disease (18)	Irritable bowel syndrome (27) Gastroesophageal reflux disease (18) Gastroparesis Gastroenteritis (27)
Genitourinary		Renal calculi (32) Pyelonephritis (32)	
Obstetric or gynecologic	Ectopic pregnancy (68) Ovarian/testicular torsion (68)	Hyperemesis gravidarum (68) Pelvic inflammatory disease (68)	Morning sickness
Metabolic	Diabetic ketoacidosis (38) Hyponatremia (88)	Hypercalcemia (88) Uremia (49) Adrenal insufficiency (63) Hypothyroidism (63)	
Toxic	Toxins (72)	Drug withdrawal	Alcohol intoxication
Other	Sepsis (67)		Cyclical vomiting Bulimia Medication related

- Other tests can be used depending on the clinical scenario, including cardiac enzymes, lactate, medication levels, and toxicology screens. Any patient with an acute blood loss or a surgical problem should have a type and screen as well as coagulation studies sent.

EKG

- An electrocardiogram (EKG) is essential in any patient with suspected cardiac ischemia. Nausea may be the sole warning symptom of a heart attack, particularly in patients who are elderly, female, or diabetic. The EKG may also reveal characteristic abnormalities in severe electrolyte depletion, such as prominent U waves in hypokalemia.

Radiography

- An upright chest radiograph should be ordered to look for cardio-pulmonary disease in patients with suspected ischemia or sub-diaphragmatic free air in patients with suspected viscus perforation. Abdominal plain films, although often unremarkable, can reveal characteristic signs of bowel pathology in patients with bowel obstruction (see Chapter 18), volvulus, intussusception (see Chapter 77), or duodenal atresia.
- Ultrasound (US) examinations can be useful to detect hepatobiliary disease as well as evidence of genitourinary pathology, including ectopic pregnancy and ovarian or testicular torsion.
- Vomiting patients with clinical evidence of intracranial pathology will likely need noncontrast head computed tomography (CT scan), which may reveal evidence of trauma, mass, obstructive hydrocephalus, or cerebellar stroke. An abdominal CT scan may be performed with or without oral and IV contrast, depending on the differential diagnosis, the patient's allergies, and renal function. Use gastrograffin contrast if there is particular concern for bowel perforation.
- Magnetic resonance imaging (MRI) and magnetic resonance angio-graphy (MRA) may have a role in the evaluation of vomiting patients. MRI/MRA of the brain and neck may reveal ischemic strokes and evidence of aneurysms or cervical dissection. MRI of the abdomen is increasingly used to evaluate the appendix in pregnant women with abdominal pain, and to offer a non-invasive alternative to endoscopic retrograde cholangiopancreatography (ERCP) in patients with biliary disease.
- Additional studies, such as upper gastrointestinal contrast studies, may be useful in children with persistent bilious vomiting because they can evaluate for bowel malrotation and other congenital malformations such as webs and strictures.

Procedures

- A complete slit lamp examination and evaluation of intraocular pressure (IOP) is performed for suspected acute angle closure glaucoma (Chapter 69).

- A lumbar puncture (LP) is performed in patients with suspected meningitis, encephalitis, or subarachnoid bleeding. An opening pressure should be obtained; this measurement is particularly important if pseudotumor cerebri is suspected (see Chapter 91 for procedure and Appendix I for CSF analysis).

Emergency Department Management Overview
General

- The ABCs (*a*irway, *b*reathing, and *c*irculation) should be addressed as discussed in Section II. Patients with evidence of active bleeding or hemodynamic instability should have two large-bore IVs.

Medications

- Antiemetic agents should be administered for symptomatic relief. Prokinetic agents, such as metoclopramide, are useful for vomiting from gastroparesis, but should be avoided if there is any question of bowel obstruction. The 5-HT3 receptor antagonists, such as ondansetron, may be particularly useful in patients with head injury because many other antiemetics cause sleepiness that may interfere with serial examinations (see Chapter 90.4).
- All patients in pain should receive prompt treatment with analgesics (see Chapter 90.1).
- The rapid administration of antibiotics is particularly important in suspected CNS infections and sepsis.
- Patients with electrolyte abnormalities should have appropriate electrolyte repletion.

Emergency Department Interventions

- Patients who are ill-appearing, have suffered a significant trauma, or may require surgery should have nothing by mouth (NPO) until their evaluation is complete.
- A nasogastric (NG) tube may be needed for patients with pancreatitis or bowel obstruction. Patients unable to tolerate oral contrast for the CT scan may also benefit from an NG tube.
- Urinary catheterization is very important when urinary output must be monitored, such as in patients with sepsis or bowel obstruction.

Disposition

- Consultation with various medical and surgical subspecialties may be necessary depending on the working diagnosis.
- Patients with emergent diagnoses that require surgical intervention, IV fluids, or close monitoring will require admission. It is often prudent to admit the pediatric, elderly, pregnant, and immunocompromised patients.
- Well-appearing patients with adequate hydration and repleted electrolytes may be discharged if they are able to tolerate oral fluids and have appropriate outpatient follow-up.

Special Considerations
Pediatrics

■ Bilious emesis in young children is worrisome, and should prompt an evaluation for surgical disease. In particular, clinicians must rule out bowel obstruction and malrotation in infants with bilious emesis (see Chapter 77).
■ A history of any ingestion, either inadvertent or deliberate, should be elicited. Toxicology screens and medication assays should be sent as needed (see Chapter 72).

Elderly

■ Evaluating geriatric patients with nausea and vomiting can be challenging because elderly patients often present with serious illness masked by atypical presentations. The elderly often present with vague chief complaints, such as confusion or increased falls, and relatively few focal symptoms.
■ Vital signs can be misleading in this population. Elderly patients have a blunted fever response; patients with florid sepsis may be normothermic or even hypothermic. Patients with significant hypovolemia from vomiting may not mount a tachycardia due to inherent limitations in the cardiovascular system or secondary to beta blockade. A blood pressure considered normal in a younger patient may represent significant hypotension in the elderly.
■ Physical examination findings are less reliable in the elderly. For example, many healthy elderly people have nuchal rigidity from other medical conditions, such as osteoarthritis and Parkinson's disease. Ill elderly patients are also less likely to display classic physical examination findings, such as meningeal and peritoneal signs.
■ Given the higher morbidity and mortality associated with most geriatric emergencies, it is prudent to more readily obtain laboratory work, imaging, surgical consultations, and admission.

Women and Pregnancy

■ Vomiting in pregnant women cannot be dismissed as nausea and vomiting of pregnancy (NVP) without a careful history, physical examination, and appropriate laboratory investigations. Pregnant women fall prey to the same medical and surgical diseases as other women. Vomiting that begins in the third month of pregnancy is not NVP, and another source of symptoms must be sought.
■ Not all pregnancy-related vomiting is benign. Clinicians must distinguish simple morning sickness from more serious conditions, such as hyperemesis gravidarum (Chapter 68) and fatty liver of pregnancy.
■ All pregnant women with nausea and vomiting should have a urinalysis, because UTI is more common in this population.
■ Any medicine, including antibiotics and antiemetics, must be carefully selected for the safety of the fetus.
■ Never avoid a critical test due to concerns surrounding radiation exposure. Discuss the risks and benefits of any imaging with the patient

and, if necessary, with her obstetrician. Safer alternatives may exist, such as admitting a patient with suspected appendicitis for serial examinations, or imaging with MRI (see Chapter 92).

Teaching Points

Nausea and vomiting are extremely common and do not reveal a specific diagnosis or the seriousness of the disease causing them. They are a source of significant distress to the patient, and relief of them is as important as the relief of pain.

Because they are so common, it is a frequent error to underestimate their importance as a clue to serious underlying disease.

Suggested Readings

Allan SG. Antiemetics. Gastroenterol Clin North Am 1992;21:597–611.
Godbole P, Stringer MD. Bilious vomiting in the newborn: how often is it pathologic? J Pediatr Surg 2002;37:909–911.
Hanson JS, McCallum RW. The diagnosis and management of nausea and vomiting: a review. Am J Gastroenterol 1985;80:210–218.
Koch KL, Frissora CL. Nausea and vomiting during pregnancy. Gastroenterol Clin North Am 2003;32:201–234, vi.
Quigley EM, Hasler WL, Parkman HP. AGA technical review on nausea and vomiting. Gastroenterology 2001;120:263–286.
Sadow KB, et al. Bilious emesis in the pediatric emergency department: etiology and outcome. Clin Pediatr 2002;41:475–479.

CHAPTER **45**

Palpitations

PURVI SHAH ■ JEFF BEESON ■ LYNN P. ROPPOLO

 Red Flags

Extremes of age • Co-morbid conditions: coronary artery disease, history of dysrhythmia, diabetes, atherosclerosis • Abnormal vital signs (heart rate <60 or >100 beats per minute, low blood pressure) • Associated chest pain • Syncope or presyncope • Diaphoresis • Dyspnea • Hypoxia

Overview

Palpitations are described as an unpleasant awareness of a rapid or forceful beating of the heart. Patients often sense a racing, fluttering, or flip-flopping of the heart within the body.

A variety of disorders involving changes in cardiac rhythm or rate can cause palpitations. Although most cases are benign, palpitations could be a sign of serious cardiac dysrhythmia. Look for "red flags" (see Box) when evaluating these patients. Palpitations are most often caused by cardiac dysrhythmias or anxiety. Most patients with dysrhythmias do not complain of palpitations. Symptoms of a panic disorder are often described as feelings of overwhelming panic or terror accompanied by a racing heartbeat, shortness of breath or dizziness. Although panic disorder may be a likely cause of a patient's symptoms, the presence of significant dysrhythmias may still need to be ruled out as the catecholamine increase during times of stress may trigger their appearance.

An electrocardiogram (EKG) should always be obtained. Most patients will have resolved symptoms at the time of presentation. Although most patients have benign causes, serious etiologies exist such as myocardial ischemia, thyrotoxicosis, anemia, and dysrhythmias. Palpitations associated with dizziness, syncope or near-syncope, chest pain, shortness of breath, or ischemic heart disease are more concerning and generally require hospitalization. A definitive diagnosis on initial presentation is often not possible in ED.

Refer to Chapter 6, "ACLS" for algorithms used in the management of concerning dysrhythmias.

Differential Diagnosis of Palpitations

See DDx table describing the differential diagnosis of palpitations.

Initial Diagnostic Approach
General

- Any patient who is hemodynamically unstable or appears ill should receive immediate attention as described in Section II. While the physician is assessing the patient, a continuous cardiac monitor and pulse oximeter should be placed. Intravenous (IV) access should be obtained. These patients should not leave the ED except for definitive care unless they have had all measures to obtain stability.
- All patients with palpitations should have an EKG. See Box 45–1 for types of dysrhythmias causing palpitations. See Chapter 87 for EKG interpretation.
- The history should focus on the following: time of initial onset, precipitating factors, associated symptoms, characteristics of palpitations

DDx Differential Diagnosis of Palpitations

Cardiac	Dysrhythmia (87), valvular heart disease (22), pacemaker (87), atrial myxoma, cardiomyopathy (22), congenital heart disease (75) , congestive heart failure (52), pericarditis (22)
Psychiatric disorders	Panic attack/disorder, generalized anxiety disorder, somatization, depression (70)
Medications	Sympathomimetic agents, vasodilators, anticholinergic drugs, beta blocker withdrawal, beta agonists, digitalis, phenothiazine, theophylline
Habits	Cocaine (72), amphetamines (72), caffeine, nicotine
Metabolic disorders	Electrolyte imbalance (88), hypoglycemia (38), thyrotoxicosis (63)
High-output states	Anemia (66), pregnancy (68), fever (31), Paget's disease
Catecholamine excess	Stress, exercise, pheochromocytoma (39)
Other	Hypovolemia (26), pulmonary disease (52), vasovagal syndrome (57), mastocytosis, scombroid food poisoning (27)

( ) Refers to the chapter in which the disease entity is discussed.

BOX 45-1   Types of Arrhythmias Causing Palpitations

Atrial fibrillation or flutter
Atrioventricular block
Bradycardia
Bradycardia-tachycardia syndrome (sick sinus syndrome)
Multifocal atrial tachycardia
Premature ventricular contractions
Sinus tachycardia or arrhythmia
Ventricular tachycardia
Wolff-Parkinson-White Syndrome (WPW)

---

including rate and regularity, past cardiac disease, social habits, and medications. See Table 45–1 for a list of some historical clues to the diagnosis. A history of dizziness, presyncope, or syncope with palpitations may be due to ventricular tachycardia or severe bradycardia and may be an ominous prognostic sign.

■ The physical examination is rarely helpful, especially if the symptoms have resolved. Focus on the pulse (normal, slow, fast, regularity), rhythm abnormalities (regular or irregular), murmurs or extra heart sounds, cardiac enlargement, signs of heart failure (rales, gallops, peripheral

Table 45–1 Historical Clues for Determining the Cause of Palpitations

Slow heart rate	Atrioventricular block or sinus node disease
Begins and ends abruptly	Paroxysmal tachycardia such as paroxysmal atrial or junctional tachycardia, atrial flutter, or atrial fibrillation
Gradual onset and cessation	Sinus tachycardia or an anxiety state
Chaotic, rapid heart action	Atrial fibrillation
Fleeting and repetitive	Multiple ectopic beats
Multiple paroxysms of tachycardia with effort or excitement	Paroxysmal atrial fibrillation
During mild exertion	Heart failure, atrial fibrillation, anemia, or thyrotoxicosis or that the individual is severely deconditioned
Relieved suddenly by stooping, breath-holding, or induced gagging or vomiting (i.e., vagal maneuvers)	Paroxysmal supraventricular tachycardia

edema, jugular venous distention [JVD]), or conditions causing a high-output state (anemia-pale conjunctiva, delayed capillary refill, high body temperature, and signs of thyrotoxicosis). Mitral valve prolapse, which is commonly associated with palpitations, is suggested by a mid systolic click.

Laboratory

- If a young, previously healthy patient with palpitations arrives at the ED with resolved symptoms and remains asymptomatic, no further testing in the ED is needed other than an EKG. For other patients, studies may include a complete blood cell count (CBC; to evaluate for anemia), electrolytes (including calcium, magnesium, and phosphate), and thyroid function studies. Patients with chest pain that is concerning for a cardiac etiology should have cardiac enzymes checked, and be ruled out for an ischemic coronary syndrome. Patients often do not offer a history of cocaine or amphetamine ingestion; if their use is suspected, a toxicology screen should be obtained.

EKG

- Obtain a tracing in all patients with palpitations. Evaluate for rate abnormalities, rhythm abnormalities, ischemic changes or evidence of previous myocardial infarction, pre-excitation (Wolf-Parkinson-White [WPW] syndrome), conduction blocks, prolonged QT interval, and premature contractions, (see Chapter 87).

- Abnormal changes on the EKG require further cardiac investigation. These include evidence of ischemic disease, atrial or ventricular enlargement, atrial ventricular block, prolonged QT interval, short PR interval, and delta waves (WPW syndrome).
- The finding of isolated premature ventricular contractions or premature atrial contractions may require further testing depending on the clinical scenario.

Radiography

- If there is a probability of heart failure, pulmonary edema, or pulmonary infection, a chest radiograph should be obtained.

Other

- *Exercise stress testing.* This study should be performed in patients who have palpitations with physical exertion or suspected ischemic coronary artery disease.
- *Echocardiogram.* This test should be performed if concerned about structural abnormalities of the heart and to evaluate ventricular function.
- *Outpatient cardiac monitoring.* This type of testing can be safely arranged for stable patients on an outpatient basis. These devices essentially record all cardiac activity for the duration they are worn, allowing correlation of the patient's symptoms with the cardiac rhythm at that time symptoms are present. Patients with daily palpitations need outpatient Holter monitors (which are worn for 24-48 hours), whereas patients with occasional symptoms should undergo continue loop-event recordings (generally monitored for 2 weeks). Loop-event monitors are less expensive than Holter monitoring, and have a higher diagnostic yield.
- *Electrophysiologic testing.* A cardiology specialist performs this study if there is concern for a serious dysrhythmia (e.g., ventricular tachycardia). This study is not performed from the ED.

Emergency Department Management Overview
General

- The ABCs (*a*irway, *b*reathing, and *c*irculation) should be addressed as discussed in Section II. Patients who are ill-appearing, hemodynamically unstable, or have concerning dysrhythmias (i.e., second-degree type II, or third-degree heart block, symptomatic bradycardia, ventricular tachycardia, atrial fibrillation with a rapid ventricular response, or other significant tachycardic rhythm) should be placed in a resuscitation room.

Medications

- *Anti-anxiety medications.* If the patient appears to be anxious or having a panic attack, a low dose benzodiazepine (e.g., Valium 5 mg) should be given.

■ *Antidysrhythmic medications.* If the EKG shows an abnormal rhythm, treat accordingly (see Chapter 6).

Emergency Department Interventions

■ Any intervention is dependent on the etiology, type, and duration of symptoms. However, patients all need to be stabilized hemodynamically, if possible in the ED, before disposition.

Disposition

■ *Consultation.* Consultation with cardiology may be warranted for a patient with chest pain, an abnormal EKG, or dysrhythmia.
■ *Admission.* This should be arranged for patients with concern for life-threatening cardiac rhythms, hypoxia, possible acute ischemic coronary syndrome, pulmonary edema, and hemodynamic instability. Patients who present with concerning symptoms, require admission. This is especially true for elderly and patients with underlying cardiac disease.
■ *Discharge.* Patients with normal laboratory studies, EKG tracings, radiologic imaging, or resolution of symptoms may be discharged home with close follow-up, and warnings of what to watch for and when to return (i.e., return to the ED immediately for chest pain, dyspnea, syncope, dizziness). Outpatient cardiac monitoring should be arranged if indicated.

Special Considerations
Pediatrics

■ Refer to Chapters 74 and 75.

Elderly

■ The elderly gave a lower threshold for further evaluation and admission, as these patients are at greater risk for serious dysrhythmias and ischemic coronary disease.

Teaching Points

Palpitations are "chest thumps" or heart beat irregularities sensed by the patient. For the most part they are often gone by the time the patient is seen in the ED and are usually benign. However, they can represent dysrhythmias that accompany more serious disease. Thus, an EKG is required on all patients.

Although most cases are benign, studies are often prudent. Many discharged patients should have outpatient cardiac monitoring and close follow-up arranged. Patients with concerning symptoms or risk factors for ischemic cardiac disease should be admitted to the hospital.

Suggested Readings

Abbott AV. Diagnostic approach to palpitations. Am Fam Physician 2005;71:743–750.

Brawnwald E. Examination of the patient: the history. In: Heart Disease: A Textbook of Cardiovascular Medicine (7th ed). Philadelphia: WB Saunders, 2005, pp 63–76.

Kennedy HL, Whitlock JA, Sprague MK et al. Long-term follow-up of asymptomatic healthy subjects with frequent and complex ventricular ectopy. N Engl J Med 1985;312:193–197.

Kinlay S, Leitch JW, Neil A et al. Cardiac event recorders yield more diagnoses and are more cost-effective than 48-hour Holter monitoring in patients with palpitations: a controlled clinical trial. Ann Intern Med 1996;124:16–20.

Lessmeier TJ, Gamperling D, Johnson-Liddon V, et al. Unrecognized paroxysmal supra-ventricular tachycardia. Potential for misdiagnosis as panic disorder. Arch Intern Med 1997;157:537–543.

Weber BE, Kapoor WN. Evaluation and outcomes of patients with palpitations. Am J Med 1996;100:138–148.

Zimetbaum P, Josephson ME. Evaluation of patients with palpitations. N Engl J Med 1998;338:1369–1373.

CHAPTER **46**

Paresthesias

KULLENI GEBREYES

Red Flags

Abnormal vital signs • Asymmetry in weakness or pulses • Progressive weakness or neurological deficit • Difficulty breathing • Difficult ambulation

Overview

Patients presenting with paresthesias should be assessed for focal or progressive muscle weakness that may place the patient at risk for respiratory or neurologic compromise. Look for "red flags" (see Box) when evaluating these patients.

The central nervous system (CNS) involves the brain and spinal cord. *Paresthesias* are sometimes early symptoms associated with serious pathology in the CNS such as stroke (see Chapter 56) or a spinal cord injury (see Chapter 12). *Myelopathies* are processes involving the spinal cord. The most common cause of a complete cord injury is trauma. Other causes include infarction, hemorrhages, and entities causing extrinsic compression (see Chapter 21). Compression of the spinal cord above T-12 results in upper motor neuron (UMN) or long track signs such as spasticity, hyperreflexia, urinary retention with overflow incontinence, and fecal retention. Compression of the spinal cord below T-12, especially below the conus medullaris, results in lower motor neuron (LMN) or nerve root signs, and includes diminished reflexes and flaccidity.

Problems in the peripheral nervous system (PNS) may also present with potentially serious pathology such as Guillain-Barré's syndrome (GBS; see Chapter 60). The PNS consists of the 12 pairs of cranial nerves and the 31 pairs of spinal nerves and their associated ganglia. Each spinal nerve is connected to the spinal cord by two roots, the anterior (ventral) root and posterior (dorsal) root. The anterior root consists of nerve fibers (efferent motor fibers) that carry impulses to skeletal muscle. The posterior nerve root consists of afferent sensory fibers that conduct sensory information to the CNS. At each inter-vertebral foramen, the anterior and posterior nerve roots combine to form a spinal nerve, which is a mixture of motor and sensory fibers. The spinal nerve divides into the anterior and posterior ramus after emerging from the intervertebral foramen. The anterior ramus supplies all of the peripheral nerves for the upper and lower extremities via the brachial and lumbosacral plexus.

Ganglionopathies refer to involvement of dorsal root ganglia neurons with pronounced sensory loss, with or without distal nerve fiber involvement.

Radiculopathies involve the nerve roots as they leave the spinal cord. The spinal nerve roots may be injured directly by trauma or com-pressed by lesions such as tumors or herniated discs (see Chapter 21). Differentiation of these syndromes from peripheral nerve or plexus lesions thus depends on the distribution of the motor and sensory signs, and whether the signs conform to those produced by a particular myotome (anterior spinal root) or dermatome (posterior spinal root). A reduction or loss of a reflex is very helpful in localizing the root involved.

Plexopathies (brachial and lumbosacral plexus) should be suspected when the lesion is not confined to a single nerve or nerve root distribution, but to several anatomically related nerves. Thoracic outlet syndrome with compression of the brachial plexus is one example.

Neuropathies involve the peripheral nerves. This chapter will primarily focus on disorders involving peripheral nerves. Peripheral nerve disorders resulting in significant weakness, such as GBS, are discussed in detail in Chapter 60.

Differential Diagnosis of Paresthesias

- The differential diagnosis may be expanded to include not only primarily neurologic disorders, but also other diseases originating outside the nervous system. These are divided into critical, emergent, and non-emergent diagnosis (see DDx table). Most of these diseases are covered

DDx Differential Diagnosis Based on Critical, Emergent, or Nonemergent Disorders

System	Critical	Emergent	Nonemergent
Neurologic	Transient ischemic attack or stroke (56) Guillain-Barré syndrome (60) Spinal cord compression (21) Transverse myelitis (21)	Multiple sclerosis (60)	Bell's palsy (30) Carpal tunnel syndrome Migraine aura (35) Thoracic outlet syndrome Radiculopathy (21)
Cardiovascular	Arterial occlusion (25)	Deep vein thrombosis (29)	
Metabolic		Hypothyroidism (63) Electrolyte abnormalities (↑ or ↓ potassium ↓ calcium, ↑ phosphorus) (88)	Nutritional deficiency (vitamin B_1, B_6, or B_{12}) Diabetes (38)
Traumatic	Compartment syndrome (17)		Disc herniation (21) Radial nerve palsy Traumatic peripheral nerve injury
Toxicologic		Arsenic, lead, mercury	Alcohol
Infectious		Diptheria (55) Lyme disease (67)	Ciguatera fish poisoning Herpes zoster (22, 62) Human immunodeficiency virus (37)
Other		Bile from a scorpion or coral snake (65) Frostbite	Drug induced Hyperventilation (low carbon dioxide) Radiation

( ) *Refers to the chapter in which the disease entity is discussed.*

elsewhere in this book, and the reference chapter is located in parenthesis adjacent to each problem identified.

- If associated with extremity pain or swelling, the diagnoses may include a radiculopathy (see Chapter 21), deep vein thrombosis (see Chapter 29), compartment syndrome (see Chapter 17), thromboangiitis obliterans (Buerger's disease) or Raynaud's phenomena (Chapter 25), or thoracic outlet syndrome.
- The etiology for paresthesias can be categorized based on the predominance of sensory or motor symptoms, symmetry, and location of sensorimotor symptoms (see Table 46–1).
- Paresthesias may also be drug induced, and cause a distal sensorimotor polyneuropathy secondary to therapeutic agents (Table 46–2).

Table 46–1 Classification of Peripheral Neuropathies Based on Location, Symmetry, and Predominance of Sensory or Motor Symptoms

Classification	Distribution of Sensorimotor Findings	Example
Demyelinating	Symmetric, distal progressing to proximal weakness, variable sensory findings	Guillain-Barré
Distal symmetrical axonopathy	Stocking glove pattern of sensory abnormalities, symmetric. Motor findings follow sensory findings, and are in the same distribution	Diabetic Arsenic
Involvement of nerve root or plexus	Asymmetric, proximal and distal, motor and sensory involvement	Radiculopathy Thoracic outlet syndrome
Compression, entrapment, or injury to isolated nerve (mono-neuropathy)	Asymmetric, sensorimotor, usually distal	Carpal tunnel syndrome Radial and ulnar nerve
Involvement of multiple isolated nerves (mono-neuropathy multiplex)	Asymmetric, sensorimotor, usually distal	Lyme disease Vasculitis
Motor neuron disease	Purely motor findings, asymmetric, mostly distal	Amyotrophic lateral sclerosis
Ganglionopathy	Pure sensory syndrome, especially proprioception, asymmetric, initially distal	HIV Paraneoplastic

From Gallegher EJ. Peripheral nerve disorders. In: Marx JA, Hockberger RS, Walls RM (editors). Rosen's Emergency Medicine: Concepts and Clinical Practice (6th ed). Philadelphia: Mosby, 2006 pp 1687–1702.

Table 46–2 **Therapeutic Agents Associated with Peripheral Neuropathy**

Class	Drug	Relative Toxicity
Antibiotic	Chloramphenicol	S>M
	Chloroquine	S
	Colistin	S
	Ethionamide	S
	Isoniazid	S>M
	Metronidazole	S
	Nitrofurantoin	SM
Antiretroviral	Didanosine	S
	Stavudine	S
Antineoplastic	Cisplatin	S
	Vincristine	SM
	Procarbazine	SM
	Cytosine arabinoside	S
Antidysrhythmic	Amiodarone	M>S

S, sensory; M, motor.

Table 46–3 **Common Peripheral Nerve Injuries**

Peripheral Nerve	Sensory Deficit	Motor Deficit
Radial nerve palsy	First dorsal interosseous muscle	Wrist and finger drop
Ulnar mononeuropathy	Fifth finger and split fourth finger	Weak hand grip
Sciatic neuropathy	Lateral aspect of leg, dorsum or plantar aspect of foot	Knee flexion, foot dorsiflexion, toe extension
Brachial plexus	Deltoid and lateral forearm and hand	Shoulder abduction, pronation and supination of forearm, and active bicep flexion
Axillary nerve	+/– deltoid muscle	Shoulder abduction

- Physical examination findings can often identify the location of the peripheral nerve insult (Table 46–3).

Initial Diagnostic Approach
General

- Address the ABCs as discussed in section II, followed by an assessment of muscle weakness.

■ Determine the neurologic and vascular status of the affected area. Any potentially life-threatening or limb-threatening should be identified quickly.

Laboratory

■ Studies may include a complete blood count; arterial blood gas (specifically P_{CO_2}); electrolytes including calcium, potassium, magnesium, and phosphate; glucose, erythrocyte sedimentation rate, and drug and alcohol screening.
■ A lumbar puncture may reveal increased protein (e.g., with GBS).
■ Other studies include thyroid function tests, folate and vitamin B_{12} levels for nutritional deficiencies and antibodies to specific infectious agents (human immunodeficiency virus [HIV], and Lyme titer). Results for the latter tests will not be available in the ED.

EKG

■ Order an electrocardiogram (EKG) for all patients with metabolic abnormalities or evidence of vascular insufficiency (to evaluate for emboli due to atrial fibrillation).

Radiography

■ *Plain films.* These are indicated in the setting of trauma.
■ *Ultrasound.* Doppler ultrasound is helpful in assessing vascular insufficiency secondary to arterial or venous occlusion. However, angiography is the preferred study for evaluating arterial occlusion.
■ *CT scan.* A head CT scan is helpful in evaluating patients with suspected cerebrovascular insufficiency.
■ *MRI.* Patients with suspected spinal cord compression require an emergent MRI.
■ *Nerve conduction studies (NCS) and electromyography (EMG).* NCS and EMG can be performed to identify the pathological site of the motor unit as a dysfunction arising from the neural, muscle, or junctional component. In neuropathic diseases, the pattern of affected muscles also permits a lesion to be localized to the spinal cord, nerve roots, limb plexuses, or peripheral nerves. Both studies are also used determine the presence and extent of a peripheral neuropathy, distinguishing between a polyneuropathy and mononeuropathy multiplex. NCS also suggests the type of underlying pathology and, in particular, whether this is primarily axonal loss or segmental demyelination. These tests are not performed in the ED.

Emergency Department Management Overview
General

■ Address ABCs as discussed in Section II, "Life-Threatening Emergencies."

Medications

- *Analgesia.* Use the appropriate level of pain control with careful consideration of etiology. Severe pain should alert you to vascular compromise (Chapter 25), compartment syndrome (Chapter 17), or a spinal cord syndrome (Chapters 12 and 21). Neuropathic pain is described usually as burning, tingling, or numbing, and can be associated with allodynia (pain with non-noxious stimulation of normal skin) and hyperalgesia (excessive sensitivity to pain). Medications that modulate sodium channels have been found to have a beneficial effect in neuropathic pain, and include anticonvulsants (carbamazepine, gabapentin, lamotrigine, valproate), antidepressants (tricyclic antidepressants, selective serotonin reuptake inhibitor, serotonin-norepinephrine reuptake inhibitor), a 5% lidocaine patch, tramadol, and opioid analgesics. The patient can be referred as an outpatient to a specialist for nonpharmacologic treatment of neuropathic pain such as transcutaneous electrical nerve stimulation (TENS), physical therapy, and occupational therapy.

Emergency Department Interventions

- *Urinary catheter.* Place a catheter to relieve urinary retention or incontinence.

Disposition

- *Consultation.* Early consultation with neurology for neurologic deficits, neurosurgery for spinal cord compression, toxicology for toxic exposures, and vascular surgery for vascular insufficiency.
- *Admission.* Hospital admission is based on the specific diagnosis and includes all patients at risk for respiratory compromise, neurologic deficits, or other life-threatening or limb-threatening problem.
- *Discharge.* Clinically stable patients with resolving or nonprogressive symptoms may be discharged from the ED. Most patients with peripheral nerve disorders can be discharged if there are no acute active issues.

Specific Problems

> ● ● ● Refer to the DDx table for reference to a discussion of problems in the
> ● ● ● differential not mentioned here. Several specific problems will be briefly
> ● ● ● mentioned here.

Ciguatera Fish Poisoning

- *Definition.* Gastrointestinal and neurologic dysfunction secondary to ingestion of a neurotoxin called ciguatoxin.
- *Epidemiology and risk factors.* It is most common in the spring and summer months. It is endemic in fish caught around Hawaii and Florida. The most common carriers include red snapper, grouper, amberjack, barracuda, sea bass, sturgeon, jack tuna, king mackerel, and moray eels.

- *Pathophysiology.* Ingestion of ciguatoxin results in prolonged activation of sodium channels followed by inhibition of calcium regulation. It has anticholinesterase and cholinergic properties. The toxin is not deactivated nor removed by cooking, freezing, or a variety of processing techniques.
- *History.* Symptoms generally follow a meal unremarkable in taste and smell, and are exacerbated by alcohol consumption. Onset occurs within minutes or more typically within 2 to 6 hours after the meal. Acute abdominal cramps, nausea, vomiting, and diarrhea are followed by neurologic symptoms such as pruritus, perioral and peripheral paresthesias, and sensory reversal dysesthesia (cold objects are perceived as warm and visa versa). CNS changes such as ataxia, weakness, vertigo, and confusion may occur.
- *Physical examination.* Sensory reversal of hot and cold sensation may be evident. Patients may also display autonomic instability with tachycardia and hypertension or severe bradycardia and hypotension.
- *ED management.* Management focuses on supportive treatment with IV fluid replacement, anti-emetics, H_1 antagonists, and pressor support as indicated. Bradycardia, secondary to anticholinesterase activity, may be treated with atropine. Recent studies have shown that mannitol is effective for CNS manifestations. Amitriptyline 25 mg twice daily may help reduce pruritis and dysesthesias.
- *Helpful hints and pitfalls.* This is not a likely diagnosis if symptoms start 24 hours after ingestion of fish. Neurologic symptoms (especially dysesthesias and paresthesias) begin later and last longer, up to several weeks in most cases but can last years.

Distal Symmetrical Axonopathy

- *Definition.* A polyneuropathy with involvement of both sensory and motor nerves.
- *Epidemiology and risk factors.* Most commonly seen in patients with diabetes mellitus, chronic alcohol use, and exposure to toxic agents. It may also be the presentation of heavy metal poisonings such as arsenic, lead, or thallium.
- *Pathophysiology.* There is progressive injury to large and small sensory nerve fibers, motor axon dysfunction, and autonomic axon dysfunction secondary to neurotoxic effects of chronic hyperglycemia, alcohol, and other toxic agents.
- *History.* Numbness, paresthesias, and pain begins distally in the plantar surfaces of both feet and gradually spreads proximally. Symptoms progress and eventually involve bilateral hands, trunk, and scalp and face. Weakness of the feet and difficulty walking occur late in the process.
- *Physical examination.* Initial symptoms include dysesthesias with gradual progression to complete sensory loss. Motor neuropathy begins with weak dorsiflexion of the big toe and is followed by weak foot dorsiflexion, foot drop, loss of ankle reflexes, muscle atrophy, hammer toes, and abnormal gait. With heavy metal poisoning such as arsenic, there are often transverse white lines under the fingernails (Mee's lines).
- *Diagnostic testing.* NCS and EMG can assess the extent and distribution of nerve involvement.

- **ED management.** The most critical aspect of managing diabetic neuropathy is adequate blood sugar control. Neuropathic pain should be treated as mentioned above (see "Emergency Department Management Overview").
- **Helpful hints and pitfalls.** Patients are predisposed to unidentified trauma and infection of the extremities. Aggressive wound management is needed to prevent progression to gangrene and limb loss.

Median Mononeuropathy or Carpal Tunnel Syndrome

- **Definition.** Carpal tunnel syndrome (CTS) is a sensorimotor neuropathy that results from compression of the median nerve within the carpal tunnel.
- **Epidemiology and risk factors.** It is often seen between the ages of 30 and 60 years with a five-fold predominance in women. Risk factors include obesity, repetitive hand motions, pregnancy, diabetes mellitus, thyroid dysfunction, amyloid, acromegaly, and renal failure.
- **Pathophysiology.** CTS is precipitated by any condition that crowds or reduces the volume of the carpal tunnel.
- **History.** Symptoms include tingling and numbness in the median nerve distribution (thumb, index, long, radial side of ring finger) and deep aching pain that occurs in the hand and radiates up the forearm. The pain is often worse at night and may be associated with clumsiness.
- **Physical examination.** Often there is abnormal sensation of the distal palmar tip of the index finger and positive provocative testing. Tinel's sign (percussion of the median nerve at the wrist) and Phalen's test (acute flexion of the wrist for one minute) may be positive. Inflation of a blood pressure cuff on the affected arm may also exacerbate symptoms.
- **Diagnostic testing.** Refer to orthopedics for electrodiagnostic testing. Ultrasound examination of the wrist is also helpful.
- **ED management.** Conservative treatment includes splinting the affected wrist. Injection of steroids or surgical repair can be performed by orthopedics if there is no improvement with conservative therapy.
- **Helpful hints and pitfalls.** Other possible causes of the symptoms are nerve compression caused by a cervical disc herniation or thoracic outlet structures.

Radial Neuropathy

- **Pathophysiology.** This is most commonly due to prolonged compression of the radial nerve at the spiral groove of the radius, and is also known as Saturday *night palsy*. At this site, the radial nerve lies juxtaposed to the humerus, making it prone to compression, especially following prolonged immobilization such as a person falls into a deep sleep with their arm draped over a chair or bench, while intoxicated. The prolonged immobilization leads to compression and demyelination of the radial nerve at the spiral groove. Radial neuropathies with resultant wrist drop can be caused by compression at other sites, such as the axilla as in patients who use crutches incorrectly. Less commonly, radial neuropathy at the spiral groove occurs secondary to a humeral fracture, nerve infarction, or strenuous muscular effort.

- *History.* The patient typically experiences acute onset of a marked wrist and finger drop. The patient should be asked about situations causing compression of the radial nerve.
- *Physical examination.* A complete wrist and finger drop, with numbness in the lateral dorsal aspect of the hand, is most consistent with proximal radial neuropathy. There may be mild weakness of supination and elbow flexion from involvement of the supinator and brachioradialis muscles, respectively. Elbow extension remains strong, because the branch to the triceps muscle comes off proximal to the spiral groove. Median and ulnar innervated muscles are also normal. There is altered sensation over the lateral dorsal hand and dorsal aspects of the thumb through the ring digits, in the distribution of the superficial radial sensory nerve.
- *Diagnostic test.* NCS and EMG are required to make the diagnosis but they are not usually performed from the ED.
- *ED management.* A wrist splint is used to keep the wrist and fingers extended, and NSAIDs are prescribed. Any offending factors should be eliminated. The patient should be referred to a neurologist or orthopedic specialist for outpatient testing and possible surgical exploration if conservative treatment fails.
- *Helpful hints and pitfalls.* The history and physical examination should lead to this diagnosis. The length of recovery depends on whether the compression results in demyelination or axonal loss. Demyelinative lesions usually recover well after several weeks, while axonal lesions may take several months to over a year. There are other problems that can affect radial nerve function. For example, reports of lead toxicity have described a pure motor neuropathy affecting the upper more than the lower extremities, and may present as a symmetric or asymmetric wrist drop. Abdominal pain, constipation, and a microcytic, hypochromic anemia are characteristically present in lead poisoning, and serve as clinical clues to this diagnosis of lead toxicity.

Traumatic Peripheral Nerve Injury

- These produce loss or abnormal pain perception with or without loss of motor function secondary to mechanical trauma resulting in direct nerve injury (Table 46–3).
- The injuries are classified by degree of anatomical disruption and corresponding deficit and prognosis. Neuropraxia is a minor contusion with myelin sheath edema, but axonal preservation that often results in full recovery. Axonotmesis is the breakdown of the myelin sheath and axon that results in functional recovery. Neurotmesis is complete or extensive nerve injury with disruption of endoneurial tubes, and has the least favorable prognosis.

Thoracic Outlet Syndrome (TOS)

- *Definition.* A syndrome due to compression of the neurovascular structures at the superior aperture of the thorax.
- *Epidemiology and risk factors.* The brachial plexus (95%), subclavian vein (4%), and subclavian artery (1%) are affected.

- ***Pathophysiology.*** The patients develop an anatomic abnormality that predisposes them to symptoms under certain conditions. The 3 major causes are anatomic (e.g., cervical rib), trauma or repetitive activities, and neurovascular entrapment at the costoclavicular space.
- ***History.*** Almost all patients present with pain. The majority of patients have neurologic symptoms in the distribution of the nerve roots involved. The lower 2 nerve roots of the brachial plexus, C8 and T1, are most commonly involved, producing symptoms in the ulnar nerve distribution. The second most common anatomic pattern involves the upper 3 nerve roots of the brachial plexus, C5,C6, and C7, with symptoms referred to the neck, ear, upper chest, upper back, and outer arm in the radial nerve distribution. Patients with venous compression may present with swelling of the extremity due to thrombosis.
- ***Physical examination.*** This is normal in the majority of patients. The elevated arm stress test (EAST) is the most reliable screening test, and evaluates all 3 types. To perform this test, the patient sits with the arms abducted 90 degrees from the thorax and the elbows flexed 90 degrees. The patient then opens and closes the hands for 3 minutes. Patients with TOS cannot continue this for 3 minutes because of reproduction of symptoms.
- ***Diagnostic testing.*** Additional studies may include cervical spine and chest radiographs, cervical CT scan, or MRI to evaluate for areas of compression. Arteriography is performed for arterial compression.
- ***ED management.*** Patients with brachial plexus involvement should be referred for physiotherapy and shoulder girdle exercises. These patients should be referred to neurology, orthopedics, or both depending on the level of impairment. These patients rarely require surgery. Vascular surgery should be consulted for patients with arterial occlusion. Patients with a venous thrombosis should be heparinized, and are eventually treated with surgical thrombectomy or fibrinolytic therapy.
- ***Helpful hints and pitfalls.*** Most presentations to the ED are nonemergent, and require only symptomatic treatment and referral.

Teaching Points

There are many different causes of paresthesias. The history and physical examination should help identify most serious causes. Paresthesias can accompany serious problems such as spinal cord compression syndromes, stroke, or vascular insufficiency. They also may be the presenting signs of a serious poisoning such as arsenic.

More benign causes include peripheral neuropathy from traumatic compression of a nerve as in the "Saturday night" palsy of a radial nerve or minor contusion of a nerve from trauma. However, it could be a sign of a serious underlying but not recognized disease, such as a foot drop as the presenting sign of diabetes mellitus.

Most patients will be able to be managed and evaluated as outpatients, but some will require admission. Spinal cord compression syndromes, for example, need emergent relief or reversal to prevent permanent paralysis.

Suggested Readings

Dworkin RH, Backonja M, Rowbotham MC. Advances in neuropathic pain: diagnosis, mechanisms, and treatment recommendations. Arch Neurol 2003;60:1524–1534.
Gallagher EJ. Peripheral nerve disorders. In: Marx JA, Hockberger RS, Walls RM (editors). Rosen's Emergency Medicine: Concepts and Clinical Practice (6th ed). Philadelphia: Mosby, 2006, pp 1687–1702.
Grogan PM, Katz JS. Toxic neuropathies. Neurol Clin 2005;23:377–396.
Pascuzzi RM. Peripheral neuropathies in clinical practice. Med Clin N Am 2003;697–724.
Shapiro BE, Preston DC. Entrapment and compressive neuropathies. Med Clin N Am 2003;87:663–696.
Wein TH, Albers JW. Electrodiagnostic approach to the patient with suspected peripheral neuropathy. Neuro Clin N Am 2002;20:503–526.

CHAPTER **47**

Penile Complaints

CHRISTOPHER M. MCCARTHY ■ EDWARD P. CURCIO III

Red Flags

Comorbid conditions: diabetes, sickle cell disease, immunocompromise
• Acute onset of symptoms • History of trauma • Severe pain of rapid onset • Unable to urinate • Abnormal vital signs

Overview

This chapter will cover the most common ED problems involving the penis. The initial section covers complaints that are anatomic and mechanical in nature, whereas the second section covers infectious penile complaints, including sexually transmitted diseases. Pathology of the remaining male genital tract, including the scrotum and its contents, are covered elsewhere in this text.

The expanded distal end of the penis is called the glans penis. The prepuce, or foreskin, is a hoodlike fold of skin that covers the glans. The interior body of the penis is composed of three cylinders of erectile tissue: two dorsally placed corpora cavernosa, which form the main bulk of the penis, and one smaller corpus spongiosum, which lies on the ventral surface of the penis and encases the urethra (Figure 47–1). The tunica albuginea is a dense fibrous envelope that surrounds the corpus spongiosum and each corpus cavernosum. Blood is supplied through arteries lying in each of the three erectile masses and two dorsal penile arteries. A single dorsal vein drains most of the penis.

Patients may delay seeking care for many penile complaints until the pathology is at an advanced stage. Any penile problem may be accompanied by considerable anxiety on the part of the patient. Look for any "red flags" (see Box) indicative of more concerning pathology.

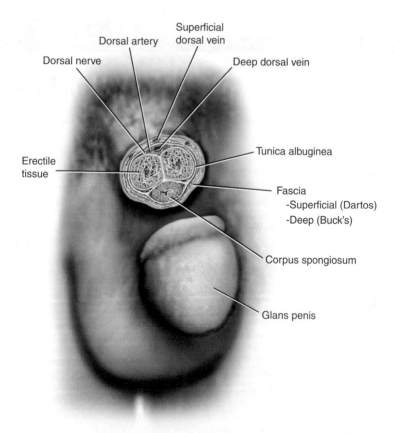

Figure 47–1. Penile anatomy. *(From Schneider RE. Genitourinary system. In: Marx JA, Hockberger RS, Walls RM (editors). Rosen's Emergency Medicine: Concepts and Clinical Practice (6th ed). Philadelphia: Mosby, 2006, p 532.)*

Differential Diagnosis

See DDx table describing differential diagnosis for penile complaints.

Initial Diagnostic Approach
General

■ Most patients with penile complaints are not toxic appearing, and do not have generalized symptoms.

Laboratory

■ Penile complaints are clinical diagnoses, made primarily by history and physical examination. In cases where infection is suspected, urine microanalysis and urethral culture (or urine polymerase chain reaction [PCR]) are indicated. Renal function should be checked if there is urinary obstruction (Chapter 47).

Radiography

■ Imaging studies are not routinely indicated in the setting of isolated penile complaints. Certain presentations may require imaging such as ultrasound, endoscopy, or retrograde urethrogram. These studies will be discussed under the headings of the individual complaints.

Emergency Department Management Overview
General

■ Noninfectious penile complaints may require surgical management by the emergency physician or consulting urologist. Infectious penile complaints are managed by empiric antibiotic therapy started in the ED, which are altered based on the availability of culture results.
■ Patients who are unable to void on their own should have a urinary catheter placed (Chapter 91).

Medications

■ Oral or parenteral analgesia may be given for pain (see Chapter 90.1).

DDx Differential Diagnoses of Penile Complaints		
Mechanical	**Infectious**	**Other**
Paraphimosis	Sexually transmitted disease (67)	Penile tumor
Phimosis	Urethritis (58)	
Penile fracture (15)	Balanoposthitis	
Urethral foreign body		
Zipper entrapment (33)		

( ) Refers to the chapter in which the disease entity is discussed.

- In certain circumstances, local or regional anesthesia may be used to control discomfort during painful procedures involving the penis. Two common regional blocks are used: the ring block and the dorsal nerve block. A ring block is performed by injecting 0.25% bupivacaine *without epinephrine* circumferentially around the base of the penis. To perform a dorsal nerve block of the penis, a 27-gauge needle is inserted into the root of the penis distal to 1 cm above the symphysis pubis. The needle is advanced 1 cm after it pierces the penile fascia. After aspiration, 2 ml of 0.25% bupivacaine *without epinephrine* is injected slowly. The needle is then withdrawn and directed to the 2 o'clock position. Two to 3 ml more of bupivacaine is injected. The needle is again withdrawn and then directed to the 10 o'clock position. Two to 3 ml of local anesthetic solution is injected. See position of dorsal nerves in Figure 47–1.

Disposition

- ***Consultation.*** Obtain a consult with a urologist for any patient with conditions requiring interventions that the emergency physician is not trained to do, or unable to successfully perform. Examples include urethral obstruction or priapism that cannot be resolved, penile abscess, or penile fracture.
- ***Admission.*** Few patients with penile complaints require admission. The decision to admit is usually made in conjunction with the urology service. Patients with urologic complications of medical disease such as sickle cell anemia and priapism or an uncontrolled diabetic with balanoposthitis may be admitted to the medicine service with urology consultation.
- ***Discharge.*** Patients with resolution of the acute problem, no surgical disease, or uncomplicated penile infection may be discharged home. Close follow-up should be arranged with either urology or a primary care physician as indicated.

Specific Problems
Balanoposthitis

- ***Definitions.*** Balanitis refers to inflammation of the glans penis. Posthitis refers to inflammation of the foreskin.
- ***Epidemiology and risk factors.*** Balanoposthitis is most often seen in uncircumcised males with poor penile hygiene. Diabetes is a major risk factor.
- ***Pathophysiology.*** The most commonly implicated organism is *Candida albicans*, followed by bacterial pathogens including group B streptococci, *Gardnerella*, and anaerobes. Various sexually transmitted diseases (STD) causing cutaneous genital lesions (see Chapter 67) may present similarly if located under the foreskin. Allergic dermatitis or premalignant skin lesions may have a similar presentation.
- ***Physical examination.*** On retraction of the foreskin, the glans and corona will be erythematous and tender, and may be purulent and malodorous. Cheesy white discharge with underlying ulceration and satellite lesions will be present in candidal infection. Diagnostic lesions may be present with selected additional organisms (human papilloma virus [HPV], herpes simplex virus [HSV], etc.).

- *Diagnostic testing.* Laboratory testing, including cultures, should be tailored to the patient's clinical presentation to help establish definitive diagnosis. Blood glucose should be tested in all patients.
- *ED management.* Meticulous hygiene is the most important step in managing balanoposthitis, and the glans and prepuce should be gently but thoroughly cleaned and dried. Fungal infection should be treated with topical nystatin or clotrimazole cream. Other bacterial infections should be treated with first or second generation cephalosporins with the addition of metronidazole if anaerobes or *Gardnerella* is suspected (Chapter 90.2). All patients with balanoposthitis should be referred to the primary care provider.
- *Helpful hints and pitfalls.* In the case of balanoposthitis that is recurrent or resistant to antibiotic therapy, biopsy with dermatologic follow-up should be considered to evaluate for malignancy.

Paraphimosis

- *Definition.* The proximal (or retracted) foreskin is unable to be reduced over the glans penis causing distal venous congestion.
- *Epidemiology and risk factors.* Uncircumcised males are at risk for paraphimosis. Other risk factors include infection, masturbation, trauma, hair or clothing tourniquets, or iatrogenic (failure to reduce the foreskin after a medical examination).
- *Pathophysiology.* Paraphimosis threatens the venous return of the glans, which causes progressive edema of both the foreskin and the glans. This can ultimately lead to arterial compromise, penile necrosis and gangrene.
- *History.* Paraphimosis will be accompanied by a history of foreskin retraction. A patient's ability to urinate should be assessed.
- *Physical examination.* The foreskin of the penis is edematous and tightly constricts the corona of the glans. The glans is erythematous and edematous. Cellulitis of the foreskin may be present.
- *Diagnostic testing.* Paraphimosis is a clinical diagnosis.
- *ED management.* Paraphimosis is a true emergency, as the viability of the glans is threatened. Local anesthesia is achieved with a ring block or local infiltration of the constricting foreskin with 1% lidocaine without epinephrine. Place an ice pack over the glans and foreskin to help decrease edema. Then direct manual pressure is applied on the glans for 5 minutes to reduce the edema enough to allow the foreskin to be replaced. Another method is to puncture the edematous foreskin with an 18- or 21-gauge needle followed by squeezing the glans penis to further facilitate drainage. If these measures are unsuccessful, a dorsal slit in the constricting foreskin band is indicated (Figure 47-2). This is a sterile bedside procedure that can be performed with light sedation and local anesthesia. Elective circumcision rather than dorsal slit of the foreskin is the definitive procedure of choice in nonemergent situations.
- *Helpful hints and pitfalls.* Although both conditions can result in painful, edematous, and erythematous glans, paraphimosis is an important diagnosis that must never be confused with balanoposthitis. In young boys, paraphimosis may be easily confused with "hair tourniquet" syndrome in which a hair encircles and constricts the penis, causing edema and impairing perfusion. Treatment is removal of the hair,

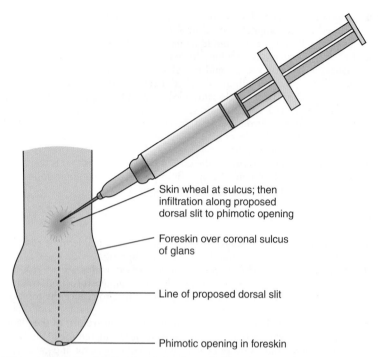

Skin wheal at sulcus; then
infiltration along proposed
dorsal slit to phimotic opening

Foreskin over coronal sulcus
of glans

Line of proposed dorsal slit

Phimotic opening in foreskin

Figure 47–2. Dorsal slit. Provide local anesthesia using 1% plain lidocaine *without* epinephrine into the dorsal midline (in proximity to the constricting band) and continue to the tip of the foreskin. A dorsal nerve block may be needed if the inner foreskin is not anesthetized. A straight hemostat is placed along the line of the proposed dorsal slit in order to crush the interposed anesthetized foreskin for 3-5 minutes. Straight scissors are then used to cut the foreskin along this line. Following the dorsal slit the foreskin swelling promptly comes down and becomes easy to fully reduce the paraphimosis. Absorbable sutures are used if hemostasis is unable to be obtained. *(From Schneider RE. Urologic procedures. In: Roberts JR, Hedges JR. Clinical Procedures in Emergency Medicine (4th ed). Philadelphia: Saunders, 2004, pp 1076.)*

followed by a retrograde urethrogram and penile Doppler ultrasound to ensure urethral and penile artery integrity.

Penile Cancer

- Carcinoma of the penis is rare and seldom found in those circumcised during infancy. The lesions are generally squamous in cell type, and are easily palpable. Infection is usually found, and must be vigorously treated before definitive therapy.
- Surgical treatment depends on the extent and location of the disease. It may consist of circumcision or partial or total penectomy, and it may include inguinal lymphadenectomy.

Penile Fracture

■ See Chapter 15.

Phimosis

■ *Definition.* Phimosis occurs when the foreskin of the uncircumcised penis cannot be retracted proximally over the glans.
■ *Epidemiology and risk factors.* Risk factors for phimosis include poor penile hygiene in uncircumcised males, chronic or repeated penile infections, previous injury to the prepuce with resultant scarring, or a complication of circumcision.
■ *Pathophysiology.* Although this condition is often initially asymptomatic, it can lead to painful erections and urinary retention.
■ *History.* Important historical details to elicit from the patient include whether the patient is able to urinate, has pain on erection, or has purulent discharge from the preputial ostium.
■ *Physical examination.* The examiner should assess for the presence of erythema, edema, and purulent discharge suggestive of *balanoposthitis*. Differentiate purulent discharge from *smegma*, the gray–white matter made up of glandular secretions and sloughed epithelial cells that is normal and does not indicate infection.
■ *Diagnostic testing.* Phimosis is a clinical diagnosis.
■ *ED management.* When phimosis is asymptomatic, no ED treatment aside from reassurance is indicated. However, when phimosis causes urinary retention, pain on erection, or inability to insert a urinary catheter, emergent treatment is needed. Initial treatment consists of local analgesia in the form of a ring block. The preputial ostium may then be enlarged with a hemostat to allow for the passage of urine or the insertion of a catheter. If these measures are unsuccessful, a dorsal slit may be required as previously described. Follow-up with a urologist is indicated as circumcision is the traditional definitive treatment modality.
■ *Helpful hints and pitfalls.* Discharge instructions for these patients should include good hygiene, and to not forcefully retract the foreskin especially in infants or young children. Asymptomatic people require no treatment.

Priapism

■ *Definition.* Sustained, often painful erection of the corpora cavernosa in the absence of sexual stimulation; although sometimes occurring after prolonged intercourse.
■ *Epidemiology and risk factors.* The most common cause in adults is medication, particularly intracarvernosally injected vasoactive therapies for impotence. Illicit substances including cocaine and ethanol have been implicated. Other common agents linked with priapism include antipsychotics and antidepressants (trazodone, chlorpromazine, etc.) as well as certain antihypertensives (prazosin). In boys, the most common cause of priapism is an underlying hematologic pathology that impairs flow, such as sickle-cell anemia or leukemia. It may occur after the use of

erection-enhancing medications such as Viagra (sildenafil citrate). Many cases are also idiopathic.

- *Pathophysiology.* Priapism is caused when the physiologic balance of blood flow into and out of the corpora cavernosa is interrupted. This causes erection of the cavernosal bodies without corresponding erection of the corpus spongiosum or glans. The more common form is *low-flow* priapism, caused by impaired outflow from the corpora cavernosa. This leads to penile ischemia and is painful. Even rarer is *high-flow* priapism, caused by the traumatic formation of an arteriovenous fistula from the penile arteries to the cavernosa. This condition is nonischemic and painless.
- *History.* A thorough medical history, including medication history and history of illicit drug use, is important. Include the time of onset of erection as well as any past episodes of priapism.
- *Physical examination.* A complete physical examination should be performed to evaluate for system manifestations of the underlying problem such as pallor, jaundice, lymphadenopathy, or signs of a toxidrome (Chapter 72). The penile examination should evaluate for the presence of a foreign body or prosthesis.
- *Diagnostic testing.* Color Doppler ultrasound of the penis may help distinguish high-flow from low-flow priapism.
- *ED management.* Priapism is a true urologic emergency, and urologic consultation is indicated. The emergency physician should attempt to identify reversible causes for low-flow priapism such as sickle cell disease, which may respond to noninvasive standard antisickling measures (see Chapter 53). Initial ED management consists of analgesia with parenteral opioids and benzodiazepines. Empiric treatment for low-flow priapism begins with terbutaline 0.25 to 0.5 mg via subcutaneous (SC) injection in the deltoid, repeated every 20 to 30 minutes or 5 mg by mouth, and repeated 15 minutes later. If no resolution occurs within 30 minutes, injection therapy is required, which consists of corporal aspiration of 30 to 60 ml of blood, followed by observation. If no improvement, an equal volume (to the amount that was aspirated) of α-agonist is injected (e.g., phenylephrine 10 mg in 500 ml of normal saline). Intracavernous injection of an α-adrenergic agonist can reverse the vascular effects of phentolamine or papaverine rapidly. Phenylephrine is the most selective and potent $α_1$-adrenergic vasoconstrictor with a rapid onset of action. High-flow priapism is treated via endovascular embolization. Oral pseudoephedrine (60-120 mg) has been shown to be effective in early onset priapism (<4 hours from onset).
- *Helpful hints and pitfalls.* Delay in treatment of priapism can lead to penile ischemia and infertility.

Sexually Transmitted Disease

- See Chapter 67.

Urethral Foreign Body

- *Epidemiology and risk factors.* Entrapment of foreign bodies in the urethra may be the result of sexual experimentation, innocent exploration by young children, or a manifestation of sexual abuse.

- *History.* Patients often complain of penile pain with dysuria, hesitancy, and hematuria.
- *Physical examination.* Indirect signs of a urethral foreign body may be present if the foreign body itself cannot be visualized. Look for trauma or evidence of infection.
- *Diagnostic testing.* Urinalysis and culture should be sent to assess for accompanying infection. Abdominal and penile plain films should be obtained to assess for radio-opaque foreign bodies. After removal (in the ED or operating room), a retrograde urethrogram must always be obtained to confirm urethral patency.
- *ED management.* If palpable and tolerated by the patient, gentle milking of the proximal end of a urethral foreign body may expose the foreign body tip and allow an attempt at manual removal. Otherwise, urologic consultation is indicated to allow for removal via endoscopy or open cystotomy.
- *Helpful hints and pitfalls.* An accurate history may not be readily obtained, because many of these foreign bodies are placed by patients themselves.

Urethritis

- See Chapter 58.

Zipper Entrapment

- See Chapter 33.

Teaching Points

Penile problems are common, and are a source of anxiety to the patient. Many lesions relate to problems of the foreskin, and it may be necessary to perform a dorsal slit of the foreskin to relieve urethral obstruction and urinary retention.

Many penile problems accompany sexually transmitted disease, and the most common pathogens are *Chlamydia* and *Gonococcus*. Herpes is another very common genital problem. In all sexually transmitted diseases, remember to arrange treatment for contacts, and look for other more subtle diseases such as syphilis.

Priapism is often a difficult problem and may require penile injection of an adrenergic agent.

Suggested Readings

Choe JM. Paraphimosis: current treatment options. Am Fam Phys 2000;62:2623–2626, 2628.

Lee C, Henderson SO. Emergent surgical complications of genitourinary infections. Emerg Med Clin North Am 2003;21:1057–1074.

Molitierno JA Jr., Carson CC III. Urologic manifestions of hematologic disease: sickle cell, leukemia, and thromboembolic disease 2003;3:49–61.

Rosenstein D, McAninch JW. Urologic emergencies. Med Clin North Am 2004;88:495–518.

Schneider RE. Urologic procedures. In: Roberts JR, Hedges JR (editors). Clinical Procedures in Emergency Medicine (4th edition). Philadelphia: Saunders, 2004, pp. 1075–1114.

Vilke G. Emergency evaluation and treatment of priapism. J Emerg Med 2004;26:325–329.

Waugh MA. Balanitis. Dermatol Clin 1998;16:757–762.

CHAPTER **48**

Rectal Complaints

JULIE A. ZELLER ■ BARBARA A. MASSER

 Red Flags

Abnormal vital signs (high fever, ↑ heart rate, ↓ blood pressure) ● Severe pain of rapid onset ● Brisk bleeding from the rectum ● Peritoneal signs ● Other co-morbid conditions: diabetes, HIV, immunocompromise ● Foreign body

Overview

Most causes of rectal pain are non-emergent. Look for "red flags" (see Box) that alter the ED course, and raise concerns for a possible emergent issue.

The goals of evaluation for rectal pain should include management of the patient's pain, determining the etiology, implementing successful treatment, and establishing appropriate specialty care or follow-up.

Differential Diagnosis of Rectal Pain

See DDx table for information on the differential diagnosis of rectal pain.

DDx Priority-Based Differential Diagnosis of Rectal Pain

Critical Diagnoses	Emergent Diagnoses	Nonemergent Diagnoses
Rectal foreign body (33)	Anorectal fistula Perianal abscess Perirectal abscess Proctitis Rectal cancer	Anal fissure Hemorrhoids Pruritis ani

( ) Refer to chapter in which the disease entity is discussed.

Initial Diagnostic Approach
General

■ Any patient who is hemodynamically unstable or appears ill should receive immediate attention.

■ When obtaining the history, quickly determine if the rectal pain is an isolated complaint, or a symptom associated with other findings (i.e., abdominal pain, constipation, nausea and vomiting) or co-morbid conditions (human immunodeficiency virus [HIV], ulcerative colitis, or Crohn's disease) to focus the physical examination.

■ Determine the quantity, color, and timing of any rectal bleeding; the character, duration, and timing of the pain; and aggravating or alleviating factors. Any pruritus or anal discharge should be noted.

■ To facilitate the examination and promote patient comfort, the patient should be examined in the left lateral decubitus position with knees drawn up toward chest. Perform an external and internal rectal examination using an anoscopy. Examine the abdomen for absent bowel sounds, rigidity, or peritoneal signs which may indicate possible perforation and peritonitis. If a foreign body is suspected, especially if large or in a high-lying position, it can occasionally be palpated during the abdominal examination (Chapter 33).

Laboratory

■ A hematocrit, platelet count, and coagulation study should be obtained if bleeding is present. Obtain a white blood cell (WBC) count with differential in cases of suspected infection.

Radiography

■ Plain films should be ordered for patients with diffuse abdominal pain or possible rectal foreign body.

Emergency Department Management Overview
General

■ For the vast majority of patients, ED management will focus on pain relief, controlling bleeding, and treating infection. Rectal foreign bodies are discussed in Chapter 33.

Medications

- ■ *Analgesia.* Oral analgesics are appropriate for most patients, but IV analgesia may be used if adequate pain control cannot be obtained by oral medications, or if there is potentially a need for sedation or surgery (see Chapter 90.1).
- ■ *Antibiotics.* Broad-spectrum antibiotics should be administered to patients with the clinical appearance of a perforation, systemic infection, or concerning localized infection. These infections are usually polymicrobial, and often involve bowel anaerobic bacteria (see Chapter 90.2).

Disposition

- ■ *Consultation.* Surgical consultation is necessary in any patient with an acute abdomen, most foreign bodies, perirectal abscess, or fistulas. A surgeon should be consulted on any patient with rectal prolapse even if reduction of the prolapse is easy.
- ■ *Admission.* Admission is necessary for patients undergoing surgery, patients with persistent pain or vomiting, with an abnormal abdominal examination suggesting perforation or peritonitis, or abnormal laboratory or imaging studies that require further evaluation and treatment. Immunocompromised patients, elderly, and pediatric patients should be admitted due to the higher incidence of serious pathology (despite minimal clinical findings) in these patient populations, unless the patient has mild symptoms and a benign cause for rectal pain is found (e.g., anal fissure or hemorrhoid).
- ■ *Discharge.* Patients should always have a follow-up plan in place with specific instructions and warning signs that describe when to return to the emergency department (ED) or obtain follow-up care.

Specific Problems
Anal Fissures

- ■ *Definition.* A superficial linear tear in the anoderm most commonly caused by passage of a large, hard stool.
- ■ *Epidemiology and risk factors.* The most common cause for a sudden onset of intensely painful rectal bleeding. It is most common in 30- to 50-year-old patients, but is also the most commonly encountered anorectal problem in pediatric patients, especially infants.
- ■ *Pathophysiology.* The dentate (pectinate) line is located in the mid-anal canal. Distal to the dentate line, the tissue is squamous epithelium, and is densely innervated. It is commonly referred to as anoderm. Lesions below the dentate line can be exquisitely painful. Above the dentate line, pain sensation is negligible. A superficial tear in the anoderm results when a hard piece of feces is forced through the anus, usually in patients who are constipated. About 90% of anal fissures occur in the posterior midline where skeletal muscle fibers that circle the anus are weakest.
- ■ *History.* Patients complain of rectal pain, usually described as burning, cutting, or tearing, worsened with bowel movements, and accompanied

by bright-red blood on the surface of stools or on the toilet paper after wiping. Mucous discharge and pruritus may also be present.

- **Physical examination.** Most fissures are visible externally when the patient bears down as if having a bowel movement. Note the depth of the fissure and its orientation to the midline. The digital rectal examination is generally difficult to tolerate because of sphincter spasm and pain. Acute fissures are erythematous and bleed easily. With chronic fissures, the classic fissure triad may be seen: deep ulcer, sentinel pile, and enlarged anal papillae. A sentinel pile forms when the base of the fissure becomes edematous and hypertrophic. This can later form a permanent skin tag, and may be associated with a fistulous tract.

- **ED management.** Use the "WASH" regimen in the treatment of anal fissures, which includes *W*arm water, shower, or sitz bath after bowel movements; *A*nalgesics, *S*tool softener, and a *H*igh-fiber diet. Most uncomplicated fissures resolve in 2 to 4 weeks with supportive care. Chronic anal fissures frequently require surgical treatment. Consult a gastroenterologist if inflammatory bowel disease is suspected.

- **Helpful hints and pitfalls.** Anal fissures found in other locations may be concerning for diseases such as leukemia, Crohn's disease, HIV infection, tuberculosis (TB), or syphilis.

Anorectal Abscesses

- **Definition.** A perianal abscess is located in the superficial subcutaneous tissue just adjacent to the anus. Perirectal abscesses are located in the fatty tissue between the rectum and ischial tuberosity. Perirectal abscesses produce tenderness and bulging, with shiny skin lateral to the anus. An ischiorectal abscess extends across the external sphincter into the ischiorectal space below the levator ani. They may be difficult to diagnose if extending superiorly because they produce little change in the anorectal skin area.

- **Epidemiology.** Abscesses can occur in all age groups, from infants to elderly patients. Men are affected more frequently than women. Approximately 30% of patients with anorectal abscesses report a previous history of similar abscesses that either resolved spontaneously or required surgical intervention. Risk factors include immunosuppression, diabetes, Crohn's disease, ulcerative colitis, anal intercourse, and pregnancy.

- **Pathophysiology.** The classic locations of anorectal abscesses listed in order of decreasing frequency are as follows: perianal, 60%, and perirectal, which is subdivided into ischiorectal, 20%; intersphincteric, 5%; and supralevator, 4% (Figure 48–1). Abscesses arise from infection of the mucus-secreting anal glands, which drain into the anal crypts. Blockage of the duct is believed to be the initiating cause of the infection that may then spread into other spaces in the area, including the intersphincteric, ischiorectal, and supralevator spaces. Perirectal abscesses are usually caused by polymicrobial aerobic and anaerobic infections. *Bacteroides fragilis* is the predominant anaerobe. Other common bacteria include *Escherichia coli* and those of the genera *Proteus*, *Bacteroides*, and *Streptococcus*. Sources of the bacteria are the skin, bowel, and, rarely, the vagina.

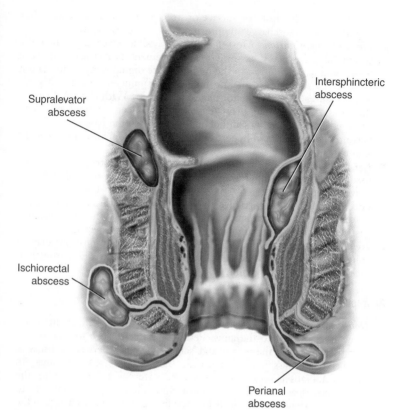

Figure 48–1. Location of common anorectal abscesses. *(From Coates W. Anorectum. In: Marx JA, Hockberger RS, Walls RM (editors) Rosen's Emergency Medicine: Concepts and Clinical Practice (6th ed). Philadelphia, MO: Mosby, 2006, p 1514.)*

■ *History.* The clinical presentation depends on the anatomical location of the abscess. Patients with perianal abscesses typically complain of dull perianal discomfort and pruritus. Movement and increased perineal pressure from sitting or defecation often exacerbate their perianal pain. These patients are usually nontoxic in appearance. In contrast, patients with ischiorectal abscesses often present with systemic fevers, chills, and severe perirectal pain and fullness consistent with the more advanced nature of this process.

■ *Physical examination.* For perianal abscesses, there is a small, erythematous, well-defined, fluctuant, subcutaneous mass near the anal orifice. External signs are minimal in patients with an ischiorectal abscess but may include erythema, induration, or fluctuance. On digital rectal examination (DRE), a fluctuant, indurated mass may be encountered. Optimal physical assessment of an ischiorectal abscess may require anesthesia to alleviate patient discomfort that would otherwise limit the extent of the examination. Patients with intersphincteric abscesses present with rectal pain, and exhibit localized tenderness on DRE. Physical examination may fail to identify an intersphincteric abscess. Though rare, supralevator abscesses present a similar diagnostic challenge. As a result, clinical presentation of pain without identifiable cause may require imaging by computed tomography (CT scan), magnetic resonance imaging (MRI), or anal ultrasonography.

- **Diagnostic testing.** A complete blood count may show leukocytosis but is unnecessary to obtain because the diagnosis is clinical. Blood cultures are indicated only in immunocompromised patients, and those who appear septicemic. Radiologic studies are rarely helpful, and should not be ordered barring exploration for some complication of the abscess, or to search for another cause of pain or fever when the diagnosis is in doubt. Endoanal, transperineal, and transvaginal ultrasonography may be used presurgically to determine the existence, extent, location, and type of abscess. Ultrasound is an accurate, painless, and cost-effective method for documenting perirectal and perianal fluid collections, fistulas, or sinus tracts. A CT scan and MRI may be used to determine the anatomy of a perirectal abscess before surgery, but are not needed for the diagnosis.

- **ED management.** Distinguish a perianal from a perirectal abscess. Perianal abscesses may be effectively treated in the ED with a single linear incision over the most fluctuant portion of the abscess in a manner described for other cutaneous abscesses (see Chapter 91). Indications for inpatient drainage are failure to obtain adequate anesthesia, systemic toxicity, extension of the abscess beyond a localized area, or recurrence of a recent perianal abscess. The patient may begin sitz baths at home 24 hours after surgery. Packing is replaced at 48-hour intervals until the infection has cleared and granulation tissue has appeared. This usually occurs within 4 to 6 days. Perirectal abscesses require a surgical consult, and must be treated in the operating suite, where optimal anesthesia can be achieved, and the abscess and any fistula or other complication may be treated definitively. The *point* of a deep abscess must not be mistaken for a superficial perianal abscess. Inadequate ED debridement of perirectal abscesses may result in increased morbidity and even mortality. Antibiotics should be given in immunocompromised patients or those with serious underlying comorbid conditions or surrounding cellulitis. Patients with perirectal abscesses should be admitted to the surgical service unless other medical conditions (elderly, obese, febrile, hypotensive, or immunocompromised), or complications from the perirectal abscess necessitate a primary medical admission, with the surgeon acting as a consultant.

- **Helpful hints and pitfalls.** The most severe pitfall would be lack of recognition of a deeper process and premature discharge from the ED.

Hemorrhoids

- **Definition.** Hemorrhoids are not varicosities but are clusters of vascular tissue, smooth muscle, and connective tissue lined by the normal epithelium of the anal canal.

- **Epidemiology and risk factors.** Familial predisposition, history of constipation or diarrhea, diet, pregnancy, and history of prolonged sitting or heavy lifting are all relevant. Ulcerative colitis and Crohn's disease may be associated with hemorrhoids.

- **Pathophysiology.** It is generally believed that this disorder arises from a history of straining with defecation, and as part of the aging process. The supportive connective tissue gives way with constant straining resulting in prolapse of the hemorrhoid cushion. Once the hemorrhoid complex begins to prolapse, venous return is impaired, resulting in engorgement, irritation, and inflammation. Erosion of the inflamed epithelium results in bleeding. Hemorrhoids are categorized into internal and external hemorrhoids which are anatomically separated by the dentate (pectinate) line. Internal hemorrhoids develop above the dentate line, are covered by anal mucosa, and lack sensory innervation. External hemorrhoids arise below the dentate line, and are covered by stratified squamous epithelium with innervation by the inferior rectal nerve. Mixed hemorrhoids are confluent internal and external hemorrhoids.

- **History.** Ask about the patient's hemorrhoid history, presence of constipation, rectal pain, or bleeding.

- **Physical examination.** Perform an inspection of the rectum, digital rectal examination, and anoscopy. The preferred patient position is the left lateral decubitus; (i.e., jack-knife position). The clinician may apply 20% benzocaine or 5% lidocaine ointment to the anal area to minimize discomfort during the examination. A prolapsed hemorrhoid appears as a bluish, tender perianal mass. During the digital examination, note any masses, tenderness, mucoid discharge, or blood. Internal hemorrhoids may not be palpable unless thrombosed. Anoscopy allows the physician to see internal hemorrhoids, and by having the patient strain, the physician may assess the grade of the hemorrhoid. Internal hemorrhoids are classified by the degree of tissue prolapse into the anal canal. Grade I hemorrhoids may present with minimal bleeding, or may be asymptomatic, but do not prolapse. Grade II hemorrhoids protrude beyond the anal verge (prolapse) with straining or defecating, and reduce spontaneously when straining ceases. Grade III hemorrhoids prolapse spontaneously or with straining, and require manual reduction. Grade IV hemorrhoids chronically prolapse, and, if reduced, fall out again. Others prolapse out of the anus and are irreducible (strangulated). Prolapsing internal hemorrhoids can cause perianal pain by spasm of the sphincter complex. A thrombosed external hemorrhoid may present with complaints of an acutely painful mass at the rectum (Figure 48–2). The pain usually peaks 48 to 72 hours after the hemorrhoid develops, and the symptoms improve by the fourth day, as the thrombus organizes. The hemorrhoid usually heals by the tenth day.

- **ED management.** Incision and drainage of the thrombosed external hemorrhoid produces faster relief of symptoms. External hemorrhoids may be excised surgically if the patient presents with a thrombosed hemorrhoid within the first 48 to 72 hours after onset of symptoms. Infiltrate under and around the hemorrhoid area with a local anesthetic, such as bupivacaine or lidocaine with epinephrine. Make an elliptical incision and excise the thrombosed hemorrhoid with the overlying skin.

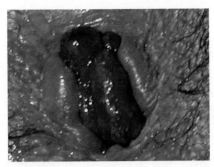

Figure 48–2. Thrombosed hemorrhoid. *(Courtesy of Gershon Effron, MD, Sinai Hospital of Baltimore. In: Seidel HM, et al: Mosby's Guide to Physical Examination, 4th ed. St. Louis, Mosby, 1999.)*

Take care not to extend the incision beyond the cutaneous layer or the anal verge. Apply a dressing, which the patient can remove after several hours. The defect heals by tertiary intention. After excision of a thrombosed external hemorrhoid, discharge home with instructions that include bed rest for several hours, sitz baths three times a day, stool softeners, and topical or systemic analgesia. Patients who have hemorrhoids excised should return for a wound check in 24 to 48 hours. If the patient presents after 72 hours from the start of symptoms, the physician can prescribe conservative medical therapy consisting of sitz baths (two to three times daily), topical and systemic analgesics, stool softeners, proper anal hygiene, and a high-fiber diet with adequate fluid intake, known as the *WASH regimen*, described under anal fissures. Internal hemorrhoids are treated according to their classification. If a patient presents with a prolapsed internal hemorrhoid, the ED physician should attempt reduction and call for a surgical consult if the hemorrhoid is grade IV. Most prolapsed hemorrhoids can be reduced, and the patient sent home for outpatient management. Treatment may be surgical or nonsurgical. Symptoms of irritation and pruritus can usually be managed with hydrocortisone suppositories, in addition to analgesic creams and warm sitz baths. Analgesic creams and hydrocortisone topical therapy should not be used for longer than 7 to 10 days because side effects such as contact dermatitis or mucosal atrophy can occur.
- *Helpful hints and pitfalls.* It is a mistake to try to incise and drain a prolapsed internal hemorrhoid. There may be some distal clot removed, but subsequently, the patient will have massive bleeding from the hemorrhoidal vessel.

Proctitis

- *Definition.* Inflammation of the mucous membrane of the rectum, often extending to the anus.

- *Epidemiology and risk factors.* There are multiple etiologies and include inflammatory bowel disease (ulcerative colitis and Crohn's disease), radiation, infectious colitis (e.g., *Salmonella, Shigella*), and idiopathic. Radiation proctosigmoiditis occurs most commonly with radiation therapy for cancers of the testes, prostate, urinary bladder, cervix, and uterus.
- *Pathophysiology.* Usually due to an inflammatory process affecting the rectum and anus.
- *History.* The patient may complain of rectal bleeding that tends to be bright red and persistent, but rarely severe. A change in bowel habits tends to occur, usually with a decrease in volume and an increase in mucoid contents. The patient may report tenesmus or fecal urgency. Diarrhea may be present but constipation is uncommon. Abdominal cramping, due to the proctitis.
- *Physical examination.* Anoscopy should be performed to evaluate the rectal mucosa.
- *ED management.* Treatment depends on the etiology. For irritable bowel disease and infectious diarrhea causing colitis, refer to Chapter 27. Conservative treatment for radiation proctosigmoiditis includes steroid enemas, sulfasalazine, and 5-ASA products given orally or as a rectal enema. Some benefit has been noted in combining oral sulfasalazine with steroid enemas or in using sucralfate enemas alone. Patients with severe rectal bleeding should be treated as a lower gastrointestinal bleed with blood transfusions as needed, and consultation with surgery and gastroenterology.
- *Helpful hints and pitfalls.* A thorough history can help determine the etiology of this problem. Although the treatment is medical in most cases, surgical intervention is sometimes indicated.

Rectal Foreign Body

- See Chapter 33.

Other Problems
Anorectal Fistula

- A fistula is a connection between two epithelium-lined surfaces. Anorectal fistulas develop in 50% to 67% of patients with ischiorectal abscesses. Other causes include Crohn's disease, trauma, foreign body reactions, TB, and cancer.
- Patients may complain of recurrent or persistent perianal discharge that becomes painful when one of the openings becomes occluded.
- Probing of fistulous tracts is not recommended, because of the danger of creating a new tract.
- Surgery should be consulted if a fistula is identified or suspected.

Pruritis Ani

- Rectal pain may due to excoriation of the anal region second to intense scratching.

- There are multiple causes, but the most common is poor hygiene and the presence of fecal material in the anal region.

Rectal Cancer

- Anal pain may occur when a low rectal cancer invades the anal canal. Other symptoms include rectal bleeding, change in bowel habits, rectal fullness, and tenesmus.
- The liver is the most frequent site of distant spread, followed by lung, retroperitoneum, ovary, and peritoneal cavity.
- The patient should be referred for staging, surgical removal, and possible chemoradiation therapy.

Rectal Prolapse (Procidentia)

- This is a disease that occurs in the very young and elderly.
- Adult patients complain of an anal mass during defecation, coughing, or sneezing. The patient may complain of incontinence, bloody or mucoid discharge, and a foul odor. Reduction should be attempted and, if successful, the patient can be discharged with agents to relieve constipation. Surgical repair is often necessary.
- In children, rectal prolapse occurs during the first 2 years of life, and may herald the presence of malnutrition or cystic fibrosis. Reduction should be attempted with sedation if necessary. The disease is usually self-limited, and does not require surgery.

Special Considerations
Pediatrics

- Anal fissures are the most common proctologic disorder occurring during infancy and childhood. Most occur in infants younger than 1 year old.
- An examination of the rectum should be included in the physical examination of any inconsolable infant.

Immunocompromised

- Immunosuppression is a risk factor for anorectal abscesses. The rectal examination may be unrevealing. Diagnostic imaging such as a CT scan of the abdomen and pelvis may be required to determine the presence of a deep seated rectal infection that is may not be appreciated on physical examination.

Teaching Points

A number of causes of rectal pain may or may not be accompanied by rectal bleeding. In the infant, the most common cause is anal fissure. In the adult, ischiorectal disease is common, and may be an indication of a more serious underlying problem such as regional enteritis (Crohn's disease).

Continued

Teaching Points—cont'd

Some patients will have only severe rectal pain for several days before the other more visible signs of an ischiorectal abscess. These abscesses will require drainage in the operating room to obtain adequate anesthesia and exposure. Perianal abscesses are also common, and are safe to drain in the ED.

Hemorrhoids are common problems, and most can be safely managed in the ED.

Foreign bodies can be difficult to locate, and even more difficult to remove, and may require removal in the operating room.

Suggested Readings

Bartolo DC. Rectal prolapse. Br J Surg 1996;83:3–5.

Coates W. Anorectum. In: Marx JA, Hockberger RS, Walls RM (editors). Rosen's Emergency Medicine: Concepts and Clinical Practice (6th ed). Philadelphia, MO: Mosby, 2006, pp 1507–1524.

Corman ML. Hemorrhoids. In: Corman ML (editor). Colon and Rectal Surgery. Philadelphia: Lippincott-Raven, 1998, pp 154–156.

Gopal DV. Diseases of the rectum and anus: a clinical approach to common disorders. Clin Cornerstone 2002;4:34–48.

Guerrero P. Hemorroids. *http://www.emedicine.com/emerg/topic242.htm*. Last updated January 14, 2005.

Hellinger MD. Anal trauma and foreign bodies. Surg Clin North Am 2002;82:1253–1260.

Janicke DM, Pundt MR. Anorectal disorders. Emerg Med Clin North Am 1996;14:757–788.

Siafakas C, Vottler TP, Andersen JM. Rectal prolapse in pediatrics. Clin Pediatr (Phila) 1999;38:63–72.

Stack LB, Munter DW. Foreign bodies in the gastrointestinal tract. Emerg Med Clin North Am 1996;14:493–521.

Thomas SH, Brown DFM. Foreign bodies. In: Marx JA, Hockberger RS, Walls RM (editors). eds. Rosen's Emergency Medicine: Concepts and Clinical Practice (6th ed). Philadelphia, MO: Mosby, 2006, pp 859–881.

CHAPTER 49

Renal Failure

DANIEL E. SURDAM ■ LYNN P. ROPPOLO

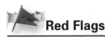
Red Flags

Elderly or immunocompromised state • Altered mental status • Chest pain • Shortness of breath • Decreased urine output • Dialysis patient who missed scheduled dialysis • Signs of dehydration or volume overload • Abnormal vital signs (fever, tachycardia, hypotension or severe hypertension) • Oxygen saturation less than 95%

Overview

Renal failure is classically divided into two categories: acute renal failure (ARF) and chronic renal failure (CRF). The time course is often arbitrary, but renal failure that arises in days to weeks is thought of as acute, whereas evidence that the process has been extending for months to years is considered chronic. Look for "red flags" (see Box), and determine whether life-threatening complications exist. These problems should be addressed while simultaneously attempting to determine the cause of renal failure so potentially reversible etiologies may be corrected.

Assessment of renal function is often done by estimation of the glomerular filtration rate (GFR) using the plasma creatinine concentration. Unfortunately, serum creatinine is very insensitive to even substantial declines in GFR. The GFR measured may be reduced by up to 50% before serum creatinine becomes elevated. Variations in creatinine production occur due to differences in muscle mass, which frequently leads to misinterpretation of serum creatinine levels. For example, a serum creatinine value in a young, healthy individual must be interpreted differently from a thin elderly individual because of a comparably smaller muscle mass.

Creatinine clearance (CrCl), which usually parallels GFR closely, is calculated using a 24-hour urine collection, a procedure not performed in the ED. GFR is more commonly estimated from the serum creatinine. One equation used to calculate the CrCl is the Cockcroft-Gault equation (Box 49–1). However, it has been found to underestimate creatinine clearance at high levels of renal function and to overestimate creatinine clearance at low levels of renal function. If the GFR is halved under steady-state conditions, the serum creatinine will double. If glomerular filtration suddenly stops, the serum creatinine will rise by 1 to 2 mg/dl/day. Rhabdomyolysis releases creatine into the plasma, and may cause the serum creatinine to increase by more than 2 mg/dl/day. Normal GFR is approximately 120 ml/min, and decreases 1% per year after age 40. The normal range of the serum creatinine level ranges from 0.5 mg/dl in thin persons to 1.5 mg/dl in muscular individuals.

Renal failure is denoted by either acute or chronic falls in GFR leading to accumulation of nitrogenous waste products and decreased ability to maintain electrolyte and fluid homeostasis. *Azotemia* is a term describing the accumulation of nitrogenous waste products (serum creatinine and urea), and *uremia* refers to a syndrome created from adverse affects of urea on different organ systems (Table 49–1).

Decreased urine output may occasionally be seen with acute renal failure. A patient with nonoliguric renal failure will have a urine output more than 400 ml/24-hour period; an oliguric patient's urine output will be less than 400 ml/24-hour period; and anuric patients have <100 ml/24-hour period of urinary output. There is greater morbidity and mortality with oliguric or anuric patients compared to their nonoliguric counterparts.

BOX 49–1   Cockcroft-Gault Equation for Calculating Creatinine Clearance

$$\text{Creatinine Clearance (mL/min)} = \frac{(140 - \text{age}) \times \text{lean body wt (kg)}}{\text{PCr (mg/dL)} \times 72}$$

PCr, plasma creatinine
In women the value must be multiplied by 0.85

Table 49–1   Common Systemic Manifestations of Uremia

Cardiovascular	Pericarditis
Nervous system	Seizures, somnolence, coma
Gastrointestinal	Nausea, vomiting, ileus
Hematologic	Anemia, platelet dysfunction, coagulopathy
Immunologic	Impaired immune system

DDx Differential Diagnoses of Renal Failure	
Prerenal	Decreased blood volume, altered vascular permeability, peripheral vasodilatation, impaired autoregulation
Renal	Tubular disease, interstitial disease, glomerular disease, vascular disease
Postrenal	Urethral obstruction, ureteral obstruction, neurogenic bladder
Chronic	Diabetic nephropathy, hypertensive nephrosclerosis, glomerulonephritis, interstitial nephritis, polycystic kidney disease

Differential Diagnosis of Renal Failure

- Etiologies of acute or chronic renal failure are traditionally classified by the area of renal anatomy being affected.
- See DDx table describing the different causes of renal failure based on this classification.

Initial Diagnostic Approach
General

- Any patient who is hemodynamically unstable or appears ill should receive immediate attention. While the physician is assessing the patient, a continuous cardiac monitor and pulse oximeter should be placed. Intravenous (IV) access should be obtained.
- No pathognomonic signs or symptoms exist for renal failure, and the clinical presentation can be varied and nonspecific often related to the underlying disorder causing the renal failure and the chronicity of the disease.
- Patients may be asymptomatic or can be critically ill. The symptoms are nonspecific, including fatigue, nausea, vomiting, shortness of breath, edema, and confusion, and often do not appear until severe uremia has developed.
- Life-threatening complications include hyperkalemia, pulmonary edema, hypertension, acidosis, encephalopathy, and uremic pericarditis. The primary responsibility of the ED physician is to treat life-threatening conditions, and to protect against those susceptible to iatrogenic-induced renal injury. A history coupled with a few simple laboratory tests often reveals the cause of renal impairment.

Laboratory

- Initial blood tests should include a complete blood count, electrolytes, glucose, calcium, phosphorus, blood urea nitrogen (BUN) and creatinine. Elevated serum potassium level is the most immediate life-threatening complication, and should be obtained quickly. In many hospitals this will be faster to obtain from the blood gas laboratory.

- Serum creatinine allows an estimation of the GFR, and the BUN allows a further characterization of the type of renal failure, and correlates with uremic symptoms better than serum creatinine.
- The BUN/plasma creatinine ratio can be normal in many forms of ARF, ranging from 10 to 15:1, but is usually greater than 20:1 in prerenal disease as urea is passively absorbed with the transport of sodium and water. The BUN will rise also in states of increased urea production such as gastrointestinal bleeding. Normal BUN and creatinine levels do not rule out ARF. Patients with a low muscle mass or vegetarians may have decreased creatinine levels, and in the setting of ARF, may result in a falsely increased creatinine clearance masking the decreased GFR.
- Other important serum markers can include creatinine kinase levels and an osmolal gap.
- Examination of the urine is inexpensive, readily available, and is a routine screening test for patients with renal failure. In addition to routine urinalysis and microscopy, urine sodium and creatinine should also be obtained if the cause of renal failure is not postrenal. Characteristic findings on renal function studies and urinalysis with microscopy can be invaluable in classifying ARF (Table 49–2). Heme-positive urine lacking erythrocytes on microscopy suggests the presence of myoglobin or hemoglobin, which would support a clinical diagnosis of rhabdomyolysis or a transfusion reaction. Examining casts can also aid in differentiating etiologies of ARF. Also looking at the specific indices, and calculating the fractional excretion of sodium and urine/plasma creatinine ratio can aid in differentiating the types of acute renal failure. The GFR by definition is very low in patients with renal failure, but urine output will be variable. Urine output is not only determined by the GFR, but also by the rate of tubular reabsorption. In the acute setting, urine output can aid in the diagnosis, with acute renal failure classified as oliguric or nonoliguric. It has been found that patients with nonoliguric acute renal failure have a better prognosis.

EKG

- An electrocardiogram (EKG) should be obtained to evaluate for hyperkalemia. This is often the most rapid means for screening for hyperkalemia, but the tracing is not abnormal until the serum potassium is greater than 6.0 mEq/ml. Changes progress as serum levels increase initially with peaked T waves, progressing to widening of the QRS complex, and eventually sine waves (see Chapter 88).

Radiography

- ***Chest radiograph.*** This will help evaluate for volume status, effusions, and infiltrates.
- ***Renal ultrasound.*** This is a rapid, safe, and effective tool to evaluate the patient with renal failure. Ultrasound images allow one to look for obstruction (markedly distended bladder or hydronephrosis), and evaluate kidney size to estimate chronicity of renal failure. A Doppler study to evaluate renal blood flow can be used. Limitations include poor

Table 49-2 Diagnostic Results in Renal Failure

	Prerenal	Intrarenal Tubular Injury	Intrarenal AIN	Intrarenal AGN	Post Renal	Chronic
Urine Dipstick	Trace or no proteinuria	Mild-moderate proteinuria	Mild-mod proteinuria; Hemoglobin; leukocytes	Mod-severe proteinuria; hemoglobin	Trace or no proteinuria; can see hemoglobin or leukocytes	Variable with trace to moderate proteinuria
Sediment	Normal or hyaline casts	Pigmented granular casts	WBC/Eosinophils and casts of each; RBC's	RBC's and RBC casts	Crystals, WBC, RBC	Variable
BUN/PCr	>20	<20	<20	<20	<20	<20
FENa*	<1	>1	>1	<1**	>1	Variable
UNa (mEq/L)	<20	>20	>40	>40	>40	>20 to 40
UCr/SCr***	>40	<20	<20	<20	<20	Variable

AIN, acute interstitial nephritis; AGN, acute glomerulonephritis; U_{Na}, urine sodium

*FENa=fractional excretion of sodium=$(U_{Na}/P_{Na})/(U_{Cr}/P_{Cr})$ P_{Na}=plasma sodium U_{Cr}=urine creatinine P_{Cr}= plasma creatinine

**When AGN is associated with tubulointerstitial abnormalities, Urine osmolality is <350, and FENa<1.

***The urine creatinine to plasma creatinine concentration is another way to estimate tubular water reabsorption.

Initially urine and plasma creatinine are equal, but the urine level gradually rises as water but not creatinine is reabsorbed.

visualization of the ureter and difficulty obtaining quality images in obese patients, and in the acute setting an undilated collecting system can occur even in the presence of obstruction.

- *Computed tomography (CT scan).* If the obstruction is not visualized on ultrasound, or is inconclusive, a noncontrast CT scan is useful to demonstrate hydronephrosis, and often better defines the level and cause of the obstruction. The CT scan also allows visualization of the renal parenchyma, collecting system, ureters, and bladder, as well as surrounding extrarenal structures. A CT scan often can better define renal masses and cysts noted on ultrasound. IV contrast should be avoided in patients with renal insufficiency or failure, and alternative imaging modalities such as magnetic resonance imaging should be utilized. If the patient is already on chronic dialysis and IV contrast is necessary, administration is safe as long as the patient will be dialyzed in the near future (ideally within 24 hours).

Emergency Department Management Overview
General

- Always address the ABCs (*a*irway, *b*reathing, and *c*irculation) first as discussed in Section II. Fluid overload and hyperkalemia are the most common cause of death in the acute setting. Place the patient on a cardiac monitor, provide supplemental oxygen to keep oxygen saturation >95%, and obtain IV access.
- If the patient's airway needs to be definitively secured, orotracheal intubation using rapid sequence intubation is the preferred method in the emergency room. Remember that succinylcholine can transiently increase serum potassium an average of 0.5 mEq/L, thus in patients in renal failure, a nondepolarizing neuromuscular blocking agent should be utilized.
- Patients who have initiated dialysis will either have a native fistula or artificial graft usually located in their arms, or a tunnel-cuffed catheter (Hickman, Quinton) usually in the right internal jugular or subclavian vein. One should avoid using these sites for blood drawing or IV access unless access elsewhere is unobtainable and emergent IV access becomes necessary. If you have to use the dialysis access for venous access, careful skin cleansing and sterile technique is a must. If withdrawal is from the fistula site, tourniquets are contraindicated and unnecessary. After obtaining blood, gentle pressure should be applied for at least 5 to 10 minutes. If the Hickman or Quinton catheter is used, aspirate 10 ml of blood (which contains heparin) before obtaining blood specimens or administering drugs. After use, the port should be flushed with 5000 units of heparin in 1 ml of saline to prevent intracatheter clot formation.

Medications

- *Hyperkalemia.* The treatment is determined by the potassium level and the EKG findings; modalities of treatment may be combined depending on the level (see Chapter 87).
- *Hypertension.* Severe hypertension associated with ARF, although rare, is a hypertensive emergency, and should be treated aggressively with IV

nitrates or sodium nitroprusside. Hypertension associated with CRF is much more common, and has a multifactorial etiology that often requires several antihypertensive agents for management. In patients with end-stage renal disease (ESRD), initial management should begin with controlling the blood volume. The rate at which the blood pressure needs to be reduced is dependent on the severity of the symptoms as with all hypertension syndromes (see Chapter 39). Oral medications that have a relatively rapid onset of action include labetolol, beta-blockers, hydralazine, α_2-agonists (i.e., clonidine), and calcium channel blockers. Angiotensin-converting enzyme (ACE) inhibitors can be used in patients with chronic renal failure, but caution should be used in patients with hyperkalemia and acute uremia. ACE inhibitors can worsen renal failure if used in patients with bilateral renal artery stenosis.

- *Pulmonary edema.* Pulmonary edema in patients with renal failure should be managed in a manner similar to that of nonrenal failure patients (see Chapter 52). Cornerstones of therapy include oxygen, nitrates, ACE inhibitors, and morphine. Diuretics such as furosemide are effective even in oliguric/anuric patients because of the pulmonary vasodilatation properties and thus increased oxygenation.
- *Hypervolemia.* Dialysis is the definitive treatment for volume overload; however, several temporizing measures should be used (see above under "Pulmonary edema").
- *Dopamine.* Low-dose dopamine (1-5 µg/kg/min) has been used to prevent and treat ARF. Dopamine at this dose dilates renal arterioles and increases the GFR and urine output.
- *Mannitol.* Mannitol provides no benefit in patients with ARF. Despite this, mannitol is routinely recommended along with large-volume crystalloid administration and sodium bicarbonate in patients with pigment nephropathy.
- *Medications to avoid.* The dosing of medications that are eliminated by the kidney or dialysis should be adjusted, and nephrotoxic agents should be carefully tailored or avoided in patients with renal insufficiency or failure (Table 49–3).

Table 49–3	**Nephrotoxic Drugs**
Mechanism	**Drugs**
Decreased Renal Perfusion	ACE-inhibitors, NSAIDs, cyclosporine, tacrolimus, amphotericin B, radiocontrast agents, Propofol
Tubular Toxicity	Aminoglycosides, radiocontrast agents, methotrexate, cyclosporine, amphotericin B, lovastatin
Tubular Obstruction	Acyclovir, trimethoprim-sulfamethoxazole, methotrexate
Allergic Interstitial Nephritis	Penicillin, loop/thiazide diuretics, cimetidine, phenytoin, allopurinol, rifampin, ciprofloxacin, NSAIDs

NSAID: nonsteroidal anti-inflammatory drugs; ACE: angiotensin converting enzyme

Emergency Department Interventions

- *IV fluids.* Determination of the patient's volume status needs to be done, and if it seems the cause of renal insufficiency appears to be prerenal, intravascular volume should be replaced by using crystalloids or blood depending on the etiology of hypovolemia. A patient with renal failure who is also hypotensive needs to be volume resuscitated, but one needs to be judicious with fluid replacement as life-threatening fluid overload can develop quickly.
- *Foley catheter.* A Foley catheter should be placed in all patients suspected of having acute renal failure. Not only will it help to rule out bladder outlet obstruction, but will enable more accurate measurement of urine output.
- *Dialysis.* Life-threatening fluid and electrolyte complications of ARF or long-term management of ESRD require renal replacement therapy (RRT), more commonly known as dialysis. RRT can be accomplished by intermittent hemodialysis (HD), continuous venovenous hemofiltration (CVVH), and peritoneal dialysis (PD). Indications for emergent dialysis are listed in Table 49–4. If no permanent access has been established, central venous access with a large-bore catheter is necessary, which is usually placed with a tunneled catheter in the right internal jugular vein. Patients undergoing RRT may have problems directly related to their vascular access or as a direct result of RRT (Box 49–2). Remember to always place the blood pressure cuff on the opposite arm from that of the HD access, and to always auscultate for a bruit and palpate a thrill that signal nonoccluded access. Although HD is the most widely used form of RRT because of its availability and efficiency, often times the critically ill cannot tolerate the hypotension and large osmotic shifts, which can exacerbate the ischemic insult to the kidneys. In this situation, CVVH, if available, is more appropriate because it allows for a tighter control of volume avoiding hypotension and has more effective clearance of urea and solutes.

Disposition

- *Consultation.* Although many aspects of the initial presentation of renal failure may be managed in the ED, early consultation with the appropriate

Table 49–4	Indications for Emergent Dialysis (AEIOU mneumonic)
Acidosis	If severe
Electrolyte abnormalities	Hyperkalemia of >6.5 or rising levels; dysnatremia Na <115 or >165 mEq/L
Ingestions	Ethylene glycol, methanol, lithium, theophylline, aspirin
Overload of fluid	Severe hypertension, pulmonary edema
Uremia	Pericarditis, encephalopathy, dyscrasia, nausea/vomiting, pruritis

---

BOX 49–2   Dialysis Related Problems

Access related (hemorrhage, thrombosis, infection, aneurysm, high-output heart failure)

Peritoneal dialysis related problems-peritonitis, tunnel catheter infection, obstruction of catheter

Hypotension

Disequilibrium syndrome

Dialysis dementia

Electrolyte abnormalities

Bleeding disorders secondary to dysfunctional platelets and transient anticoagulation

Anemia (decreased erythropoietin, decreased RBC survival times, and blood loss during dialysis)

Dialysis-related ascites

RBC: red blood cells

specialist is important for the long-term care of these patients. Consultation with urology should be done promptly in all patients with postrenal ARF. In all other patients with renal failure, consultation with a nephrologist should also be initiated early, especially if the patient will require dialysis. If dialysis is not available at your institution, the patient should be transferred to a facility with RRT capabilities.

■ *Admission.* Most patients with ARF should be admitted to the hospital. Hospitalization of patients with CRF is frequent due to the multiple co-morbid conditions and complications of dialysis in addition to the renal failure. The patients who have acute problems not easily resolved with temporizing agents in the ED or with poor follow-up should be admitted as well.

■ *Discharge.* Patients with easily correctable causes (diarrhea, overdiuresis or prerenal azotemia) may be discharged home with close follow-up if the creatinine improves to almost baseline levels with treatment. Patients with CRF who do not require dialysis or prolonged care may be discharged home with close follow-up with their nephrologist or dialysis nurse. Patients with uncomplicated urethral obstructions that have been relieved may be discharged to be followed by a urologist.

Specific Problems: Acute Renal Failure
Prerenal Causes of Acute Renal Failure

■ *Epidemiology.* Prerenal azotemia is the most common form of ARF presenting to the ED in both children and adults. Because most of the community-acquired cases of ARF are a result of volume depletion, it can be rapidly reversible if the underlying cause is corrected. About 90% of cases in the ED have a reversible cause.

■ *Pathophysiology.* Prerenal azotemia is secondary to a reduction in renal blood flow decreasing the GFR. Although the renal blood flow is reduced, it is still able to provide enough flow to sustain the viability of the kidney with intact tubular function. The decrease in the GFR is usually due to a reduction in effective arterial blood volume (EABV), which is the part of the extracellular fluid (ECF) that is contained within the arterial system and is sensed by the baroreceptors. There are three major causes of reduced EABV: hypovolemia, congestive heart failure, and systemic vasodilatation (sepsis, cirrhosis, medications).

- *History.* A history of risk factors for prerenal azotemia should be sought and include vomiting, diarrhea, fever, poor fluid intake, co-morbid illnesses (cirrhosis, pancreatitis, sepsis, heart failure), recent surgeries or hospitalizations, medications, hemorrhage, or sweating. Nonspecific symptoms such as increased thirst, decreased urination, or lightheadedness may point toward volume depletion and prerenal azotemia.
- *Physical examination.* The patient's volume status should be assessed by examining the mucous membranes and skin turgor. Vital signs, including orthostatics (Chapter 2), should be assessed, looking for signs of hypovolemia. Peripheral edema, rales, JVD, and hypertension can be signs of volume overload.
- *Diagnostic testing.* Several studies will help differentiate prerenal from intrinsic disease. Looking at the BUN-to-creatinine ratio, urine electrolytes, and urine microscopy will add invaluable information as described in the preceding paragraphs.
- *ED management.* Once life-threatening emergencies have been ruled out, treatment is guided by the underlying cause of prerenal azotemia. If the patient is hypovolemic, fluid infusion using intravenous crystalloid or blood is often all that is required.
- *Helpful hints and pitfalls.* Diuretics in a hypovolemic oliguric patient will decrease renal perfusion, and exacerbate the renal failure. Be very cautious with nephrotoxic drugs in patients predisposed to ARF (elderly, dehydrated, congestive heart failure, diabetic, CRF).

Intrinsic Renal Disease Causing Acute Renal Failure

- *Epidemiology.* Intrinsic ARF is less common in the community setting, but is the most common cause of hospital acquired ARF, of which acute tubular necrosis (ATN) accounts for up to 85% in adults. In the community setting, drugs and infection are responsible for most cases of intrinsic disease. Ischemia and toxins cause most cases in the hospital.
- *Pathophysiology.* Intrinsic renal failure may be anatomically grouped according to the site of primary injury: vasculature, interstitium, glomerulus, and tubules. If not expeditiously corrected, prerenal failure will eventually lead to ischemic tubular necrosis (ITN) resulting in the inability of the tubules to concentrate urine and reabsorb sodium. After ischemia, toxins such as aminoglycosides, IV radiocontrast, cisplatin, and myeloma light chains are frequently cited as contributors to tubular disease. Heme pigments resulting from massive hemolysis or rhabdomyolysis are concentrated in the tubules, and have obstructing and direct toxic affects on the renal tubules causing tubular necrosis. Acute interstitial nephritis (AIN) is usually caused by an allergic reaction to a medication, and is responsible for approximately 10% of cases of intrinsic renal failure in adults. Other causes of AIN include

autoimmune, infiltrative (sarcoid, lymphoma), or infectious (hanta virus, Legionnaire) diseases. Numerous disorders produce glomerular disease, but two general patterns can be used to classify the disease. A *nephritic pattern* is associated with inflammation of the glomeruli. This disease exhibits active urine sediment with red cells, white cells, casts, and a variable degree of proteinuria. A *nephrotic pattern* is not associated with inflammation, has inactive sediment, and is associated with a large amount of proteinuria (see Chapter 29). Vascular diseases causing intrinsic renal failure are most likely due to a vasculitis (e.g., Wegener's granulomatosis). Malignant hypertension, hemolytic uremic syndrome or thrombotic thrombocytopenic purpura, polyarteritis nodosa, and thromboembolic disease are other causes of vascular diseases affecting the kidney.

- *History.* The history is often helpful in identification of intrinsic disease. Patients with prolonged periods of hypotension after cardiopulmonary arrest or during surgery, imaging studies, recent hospitalizations, or exposure to nephrotoxic drugs produce a tubular disease pattern. Recent trauma, blood transfusions, substance abuse, seizures, and prolonged immobilization would make one consider pigment-induced nephropathy affecting the tubules as well. A history of a rash can be seen with allergic interstitial nephritis. Nonspecific signs and symptoms such as a rash, fever, and malaise can be seen in AIN and acute glomerulonephritis.
- *Physical examination.* Findings on physical examination depend on the underlying etiology as described above.
- *Diagnostic testing.* BUN and creatinine levels, urinalysis, urine electrolytes, and sediment are often able alone to differentiate IRF from other types of ARF. To make a definitive diagnosis and tailor therapy, a renal biopsy is often needed, which is not performed in the ED.
- *ED management.* Treatment is tailored to the underlying disorder. Many cases are readily reversible once the underlying cause is corrected. Much of the management is to remove the offending agent and give supportive care with monitoring of electrolyte and fluid balance.
- *Helpful hints and pitfalls.* Patients with preexisting renal insufficiency are predisposed to acute renal failure due to the nephrotoxins listed in Table 49–3.

Postrenal Causes of Acute Renal Failure

- *Epidemiology.* Patients at risk for developing postrenal failure are those at both extremes of age, history of malignancy, nephrolithiasis, retroperitoneal disease, and the male gender. It accounts for approximately 10% of all ARF cases.
- *Pathophysiology.* Renal failure is due to an obstruction of the renal collecting system at the level of the ureters (for failure to occur, the obstruction must be bilateral or the patient has only a single functioning kidney), in the bladder, or urethra.
- *History.* Patients may have anuria, oliguria, or normal urine output. Alternating polyuria and oliguria is strongly suggestive of obstructive uropathy. Patients may be in severe discomfort from the distended bladder.

- **Physical examination.** Look for prostatic hypertrophy, rectal or pelvic masses, and a distended bladder.
- **Diagnostic testing.** A postvoid residual should be obtained by placing a catheter after the patient attempts to void. If no urine is obtained, flush the Foley, and investigate for proper placement and the bladder size via ultrasound. If a large postvoid residual is obtained (>125 ml), the obstruction is most likely below the bladder. Urinalysis with microscopy, urine culture, BUN, creatinine, and electrolytes should be obtained.
- **ED management.** Relief of the obstruction can provide instantaneous relief, and prevent further renal damage. Depending upon the location of the obstruction, the only treatment necessary may be passing a Foley catheter, but could be as complex as placing a percutaneous nephrostomy tube. If the Foley will not pass, or the obstruction is not relieved, consultation with a urologist and urologic imaging are indicated. There is often a large postobstruction diuresis after the obstruction is relieved. It is unnecessary to periodically clamp the Foley catheter to avoid hypotension and hematuria; however, recognize large fluid losses that will need to be replaced. Admit patients with a persistent diuresis of greater than 250 ml/h for more than 2 hours.
- **Helpful hints and pitfalls.** Remember to place a Foley catheter even in someone who has normal urine output. Remember to perform a prostate examination in men, and a pelvic examination in women. When trying to pass a Foley catheter past a urethral obstruction, instill lidocaine jelly in the urethra. It is helpful to start with a Coude catheter that has a special curved tip that facilitates passage over an enlarged prostate gland. If you are still unable to pass the catheter consult urology.

Specific Problems: Chronic Renal Failure

- **Epidemiology.** The true incidence of chronic renal failure is not known. It is estimated that 6.2 million Americans have chronic renal impairment, defined by a serum creatinine level above 1.5 mg/dl. Patients older than 65 years comprise 37% of patients with ESRD, and represent 48% of new cases annually. In the United States there is an increased incidence among blacks and Native Americans. Both genders are affected. Diabetes mellitus is the most common disease responsible for ESRD, followed by hypertension. Patients with CRF undergo numerous hospitalizations secondary to underlying co-morbidities and complications from renal failure and dialysis itself. The 5-year survival rate is approximately 35%, which decreases to 20% if complicated by diabetes. Cardiac disease is the leading cause of death in patients with ESRD.
- **Pathophysiology.** This is due to a progressive destruction of nephrons over a period of months to years depending on the etiology. With progressive destruction, the kidney adapts with hyperfiltration from the remaining healthy nephrons. Over time, glomerular hypertension increases secondary to the hypertrophy of the nephrons leading to progressive renal failure. Chronic renal insufficiency (CRI) is defined as mild to moderate renal impairment, with a GFR of 30 to 70 ml/min. CRF is usually seen with a GFR below 30 ml/min. ESRD is usually seen as the GFR falls below 10 ml/min and the patient develops symptoms of uremia.

- *History.* Patients with CRF can have a wide variety of complaints and complications from their disease, such as infection (decreased immunity), weakness (anemia, uremia, neurologic effects), cardiac complaints (congestive heart failure, pericarditis), anorexia, nausea, vomiting, pruritis (uremia), and bleeding (platelet dysfunction). If they have not yet started dialysis, these complaints can be vague and nonspecific including fatigue, poor appetite, and confusion.
- *Physical examination.* This may reveal findings of underlying disease (lupus, hypertension, diabetes mellitus, atherosclerotic disease) or complications of CRF (anemia, bleeding, pericarditis, volume overload). Evaluation of the vascular access used in dialysis patients should be performed.
- *Diagnostic testing.* Obtain diagnostic studies as described above in the laboratory section.
- *ED management.* After life-threatening abnormalities have been ruled out, management of the patient in the ED consists of treating potentially reversible factors (obstruction/volume depletion) or other complications.
- *Helpful hints and pitfalls.* Avoid causing iatrogenic injury through administration of inappropriately dosed medications, nephrotoxic agents (for CRI), or too much fluid administration (especially in ESRD). Avoid inappropriate use of patient's dialysis vascular access. Look for hyperkalemia.

Special Considerations
Pregnancy

- The physiologic changes that occur during pregnancy can often mask underlying disease. The increase in vascular and interstitial volume in the kidneys during pregnancy increases creatinine clearance, making increasing levels of creatinine difficult to appreciate early on. Examples of problems causing ARF in pregnancy include hyperemesis gravidarum, severe pre-eclampsia, hemorrhage, and pyelonephritis.

The Immunocompromised Patient

- These patients are often at risk for renal disease, as they are at an increased risk of infection, drug nephrotoxicity, and prerenal azotemia. These patients have a lessened ability to show the signs of an acute disease, and therefore require earlier consideration for admission.

Elderly

- Elderly patients are susceptible to renal failure due to decreased functional reserve and inability to sustain an acute ischemic insult, propensity for hypovolemia, and increased renal-artery atherosclerotic disease.

Pediatrics

- Pediatric renal failure has a higher incidence of intrinsic renal causes for ARF secondary to diseases such as glomerulonephritis and hemolytic uremic syndrome (HUS). Many cases of renal failure in pediatrics stem from complications from congenital heart disease, solid organ transplantation, and sepsis. Continuous renal replacement therapy is preferred in children, with peritoneal dialysis for long-term management.

- Hemolytic uremic syndrome is one of the most common causes of acute renal failure in children. The most common offending agent is the verotoxin produced by *Escherichia coli* serotype 0157:H7. After the prodromal gastroenteritis (including bloody stools), patients develop sudden onset of hemolytic anemia, thrombocytopenia, and acute renal insufficiency, with possible progression to renal failure (see Chapter 78).
- Poststreptococcal glomerulonephritis (PSGN) is one of the sequelae of streptococcus pharyngitis. Treatment, however, of streptococcus pharyngitis with antibiotics has not been shown to decrease the incidence of PSGN. Renal failure is found in 2% of patients.

Teaching Points

Renal failure is a common ED problem. The majority of cases are prerenal, for which the cause must be identified and hopefully removed, while the initial treatment of volume replacement is being initiated. Chronic renal failure is more likely to be due to intrinsic renal disease, and is often identifiable by the history of prior problems. Nevertheless, the treatment of acute renal failure must be diligent and aggressive.

Hyperkalemia is the most relevant component of acute renal failure, and must be treated quickly with bicarbonate, insulin, dextrose, and calcium. If the patient has already begun dialysis, an emergent dialysis must be arranged. It is best to know the treatment capacity of your own institution as the patient may have to be transferred quickly to obtain dialysis.

Other problems common to the patient with chronic renal failure that are often overlooked are severe anemia, uremic pericarditis, or congestive failure from volume overload.

It is prudent to involve the nephrologists early in the care of these patients, but to initiate life-saving therapy rather than awaiting their physical presence to consult.

Suggested Readings

Abernethy V, Lieberthal W. Acute renal failure in the critically ill patient. Crit Care Clin 2002;18:203–222.

Conger JD. Interventions in clinical acute renal failure: what are the data? Am J Kid Dis 1995;26:565–576.

Dember LM. Critical care issues in the patient with chronic renal failure. Crit Care Clin 2002;18:421–440.

Ifudu O. Care of patients undergoing hemodialysis. N Eng J Med 1998;339:1054–1062.

Moghal NE, Brocklebank JT, Meadow SR. A review of acute renal failure in children: incidence, etiology, and outcome. Clin Nephrol 1998;49:91–95.

Thadhani R, Pascual M, Bonventre JV. Acute renal failure. N Eng J Med 1996;334:1448–1460.

Wolfson AB, Singer I. Hemodialysis-related emergencies, I. J Emerg Med 1987;5:533–543.

Wolfson AB, Singer I. Hemodialysis-related emergencies, II. J Emerg Med 1998;6:61–70.

CHAPTER 50

Scrotal/Testicular Pain and Swelling

DEEPTA S. ATRE ■ JAIME T. SNARSKI ■ TRACI THOUREEN

Red Flags

Extremes of age • Immunocompromised state • Other co-morbid conditions: diabetes, hypertension • Severe pain of rapid onset • Abdominal pain or back pain • Presyncope or syncope • Abnormal vital signs (high fever, tachycardia, low blood pressure) • Peritoneal signs

Overview

Acute scrotal pain requires immediate attention to evaluate for life-threatening (e.g., ruptured abdominal aortic aneurysm [AAA]) and fertility-compromising (e.g., testicular torsion) conditions.

Look for "red flags" (see Box), and consider critical diagnosis or life-threatening problems early. These patients should be rapidly assessed and have an expeditious ED evaluation.

The normal scrotum is relatively symmetric, with both testicles of equal mass and volume. The left testicle sits lower than the right due to the drainage of the left testicular vein into the left renal vein, while the right drains into the vena cava itself. The normal testis is found in the vertical axis with a slight forward tilt, and the epididymis is above the superior pole in the posterolateral position. The primary functions of the epididymis are sperm transit, sperm storage, sperm fertility, and motility maturation. Spermatogenesis occurs in the millions of seminiferous tubules that make up the bulk of the testicular parenchyma. The vas deferens emerges from the tail of the epididymis to become part of the spermatic cord that passes through the inguinal canal to and from the testes. The testes are enclosed in a tough capsule composed of the tunica vaginalis, tunica albuginea, with collagenous and smooth muscle elements, and the tunica vasculosa (Figure 50–1).

Differential Diagnosis of Acute Scrotal Pain

■ See DDx table.

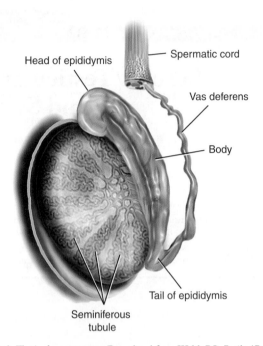

Figure 50–1. Testicular anatomy. *(Reproduced from Walsh PC, Retik AB, Vaughan ED, Wein AJ, Kavoussi LR, Novick AC, et al (editors): Campbell's Urology (8th ed). Philadelphia: WB Saunders, 2002.)*

DDx Differential Diagnosis of Acute Scrotal Pain

Critical diagnosis	Emergent diagnosis	Nonemergent diagnosis
Abdominal aortic aneurysm* (18)	Epididymitis	Hydrocele
Testicular torsion	Orchitis (mumps)	Varicocele
Fournier's gangrene (54)	Henoch-Schönlein purpura (77)	Testicular cancer (neoplasm, leukemia)
Incarcerated inguinal hernia (36)	Idiopathic testicular infarction	Retroperitoneal tumor*
Retrocecal appendicitis* (18)	Scrotal abscess	Torsion of testicular appendix
		Inguinal hernia (36)
		Nephrolithiasis* (32)
		Lower lumbar or sacral nerve root impingement* (21)
		Postvasectomy
		Postherniorrhaphy pain*

*Referred pain.
( ) Refers to the chapter in which the disease entity is discussed.

Initial Diagnostic Approach

General

- Any patient who is hemodynamically unstable or appears ill should receive immediate attention.
- Although testicular torsion is the least common cause of the acute scrotum, it should be high in the differential diagnosis because testicular salvage rates correlate inversely with time to exploration. Surgical consultation for surgical disease (e.g., testicular torsion) should not be delayed for diagnostic studies.
- Along with ultrasonography, the history and physical examination are most useful in determining the diagnosis of patients with pain localized to the scrotum and testes. The circumstances and onset of the pain are of particular interest. Isolated testicular pain of sudden onset should raise concern for testicular torsion. Ask about associated symptoms, such as nausea, vomiting, abdominal pain, back pain, dysuria, urgency, and frequency. Predisposing factors such as trauma and sexual history should be elicited.
- All patients with scrotal and testicular pain require examination of the sides, abdomen, and bilateral inguinal areas. Pay particular attention to tenderness to palpation, mass lesions, discrepancies in size, loss of testicular landmarks, scrotal edema, erythema or other skin discoloration, urethral discharge, rashes, and inguinal fullness (presence of an inguinal hernia). A thickened spermatic cord may represent a knot where the cord has twisted on itself. The *cremasteric reflex* is an essential part of the scrotal examination. It is elicited by stroking or pinching the inner thigh and observing an elevation of more than 0.5 cm of the ipsilateral testicle. Note that this reflex may be altered in certain conditions such as cryptorchidism and myelomeningocoele. Loss of the cremasteric reflex is strongly associated with torsion. The presence of the cremasteric reflex virtually excludes the diagnosis, although rare cases have been reported. *Prehn's sign* (relief of pain with scrotal elevation and support) may provide relief in epididymitis but is not reliable. The pathognomonic *blue dot sign* may be visible through the scrotal skin, representing the torsed and necrotic appendix testis. Perform a rectal examination to check for prostatitis.

Laboratory

- Patients with acute scrotal pain should have a midstream urinalysis, urine Gram's stain, and urine culture. A complete blood cell (CBC) count, electrolytes and renal function should also be evaluated in select patients (i.e., the presence of co-morbidities such as diabetes or an extratesticular source of pain). Patients with suspected torsion do not require laboratory studies but an emergent ultrasound and urologic consultation. Patients with concern for blood loss, anemia, abdominal aortic aneurysm, or hemodynamic instability should have blood sent for type and cross match and coagulation studies.

Radiography

- *Plain films.* These imaging studies are not useful, but can be obtained in a search for metastatic disease of a testicular tumor.
- *Ultrasound.* Color Doppler ultrasound is the test of choice for scrotal pathology to detect or rule out surgical emergencies. Note that ultrasound can be repeated in 30 to 60 minutes if a definitive diagnosis is not established, to make sure that blood flow is not decreasing; however, practically this is not often done. If testicular torsion is not believed to be adequately ruled out and there is still concern, a urologist should be consulted for possible surgical exploration. Ultrasound is also useful for detecting intraperitoneal fluid and the cross-sectional diameter of AAAs. It can show hydronephrosis as an indirect indicator of an obstructing ureteral calculus that may be the cause of referred pain to the scrotum.
- *Computed tomography (CT scan).* A CT scan allows for imaging of both intraperitoneal and retroperitoneal pathology. It is used in the setting of acute scrotal pain when cryptorchidism (undescended testes) is suspected.
- *Magnetic resonance imaging (MRI).* MRI is used to differentiate benign from malignant testicular lesions. For instance, MRI is superior in detecting the nodal metastases of seminoma and embryonal cell carcinoma compared to a CT scan.
- *Nuclear scan.* Nuclear scan is useful if the ultrasound is not definitive in determining testicular torsion.

Emergency Department Management Overview
General

- The ABCs (*a*irway, *b*reathing, and *c*irculation) should be addressed as discussed in Section II.
- Prompt ED evaluation and early surgical consultation should be done for patients who may have surgical disease.

Medications

- *Analgesia.* Administer analgesia for patients in severe distress secondary to pain. Administer narcotics, like IV morphine 2 to 5 mg IV every 5 to 10 minutes, until the patient is comfortable. Nonsteroidal anti-inflammatory drugs (NSAIDs) can also be used as an adjunct, but should not be given to patients who may require immediate surgery due to platelet aggregation effects (i.e., testicular torsion, incarcerated inguinal hernia, AAA; see Chapter 90.1).
- *Antibiotics.* There should be prompt administration of antibiotics in patients with the clinical appearance of an infection. These infections are usually polymicrobial: gram-positive, gram-negative, and anaerobes. Make sure to test and treat for sexually transmitted diseases (Chapter 67).

Emergency Department Intervention

- In the case of testicular torsion, manual reduction may be attempted (see discussion of "testicular torsion"), especially if surgical consultation is delayed. Even if manual reduction is successful, however, the patient should still proceed to surgery for definitive fixation.

■ *Urinary catheter.* This should be inserted to relieve bladder obstruction, for hemodynamically unstable or critically ill patients to ensure adequate urine output, for patients who are incontinent, or if an accurate urinalysis is needed (may use in-and-out catheter).

Disposition

■ *Consultation.* Consult with surgery or urology for any patient with surgical disease. Obtain a consultation early in the patient's course for Fournier's gangrene (Chapter 54), testicular torsion, suspected or actual perforation (i.e., retrocecal appendicitis), incarcerated inguinal hernia (Chapter 36), AAA (Chapter 18), or other hemodynamically unstable patients with scrotal pain.

■ *Admission.* Admit any patient with systemic signs of toxicity (fever, chills, nausea, vomiting), with abnormal laboratory tests or imaging studies, with persistent pain, or with an abnormal scrotal examination not ruling out critical or emergent causes of scrotal pain.

■ *Discharge.* Patients with normal laboratory tests, imaging studies, or improvement in symptoms after treatment in the ED, and a normal scrotal examination at reevaluation (after a short period of observation) may be discharged home with close follow-up within 24 hours and *scrotal warnings* (i.e., return to the ED immediately for severe pain, fever, increased swelling, difficulty urinating, or persistent vomiting). Most stable patients with isolated scrotal pathology such as epididymitis or varicocele may be discharged home with close follow-up. Make sure that the patient has urology follow-up with-in 2 weeks. Recommend bed rest, scrotal elevation, sitz baths, or ice packs as appropriate depending on the final diagnosis.

Specific Problems
Epididymitis

■ *Epidemiology and risk factors.* This is the most common inflammatory disease of the scrotum. The average age of the patient is 25 years. It may be sexually transmitted, associated with previous urinary tract infection, an anatomic abnormality, or the result of prior urinary tract instrumentation. A chemical epidymitis is also commonly seen in young athletes with track events such as running, jumping, hurdling etc.

■ *Pathophysiology.* There is an inflammation of the epididymis that results from retrograde ascent of bacterial pathogens, or rarely from hemato-genous spread, or from the retrograde flow of urine during intense exercise. The inflammation begins in the vas deferens and lower pole of the epididymis, spreading to the rest of the epididymis and testis. The epididymis becomes swollen and indurated, the spermatic cord thickens, and edema develops in the testis. If the process is bilateral, the end result may be sterility. In patients younger than 35 years, the most common causes are the sexually transmitted pathogens (*C. trachomatis*, accounting for two thirds of cases, and *N. gonorrhoeae*). In those older than age 40 and in prepubertal boys, suspect urinary pathogens such as *E. coli*, *Klebsiella*, and *Pseudomonas*. Epididymal abscesses are an uncommon complication of epididymitis.

- **History.** The pain is gradual in onset and may be associated with nausea, vomiting, micturition symptoms and lower abdominal or inguinal canal pain. Fever is present in 95% of patients. A urethral discharge may also be present.

- **Physical examination.** The scrotum is erythematous and edematous. The cremasteric reflex is usually intact. Swelling of the scrotum to twice its size may occur over 3 to 4 hours, and the scrotal skin will be warm. Due to congestion, the epididymis may be indistinguishable from the testis. Prehn's sign (relief of pain with scrotal elevation and support) may provide pain relief but is not reliable.

- **Diagnostic testing.** Pyuria may be seen on urinalysis in 50% of patients. A culture, Gram's stain, or DNA probe of any discharge that is present may be useful in the patients who do not respond to treatment. A CBC may reveal leukocytosis. Color-flow duplex Doppler ultrasonography or radionuclide scintigraphy can help distinguish from torsion. Blood flow in epididymitis will be preserved or increased. Be cautious as mentioned above in those patients who have spontaneously detorsed, since their blood flow will also be increased, and the torsion may be confused with epididymitis.

- **ED management.** Most cases can be treated as outpatients. Only those who are toxic in appearance requiring admission. Treatment includes antibiotics, pain management with nonsteroidal anti-inflammatory drugs or narcotics, scrotal elevation and application of ice packs. Pain relief can also be achieved by injecting the spermatic cord with 1/4% bivipucaine (Marcaine) without epinephrine. Those younger than age 35 years are assumed to have a sexually transmitted pathogen (*Chlamydia* or *Gonorrhoeae*, see Chapter 67, "Infectious Disease") should be treated appropriately, remembering to treat sexual partners as well. Those older than 35 years are assumed to have infection with gram-negative bacilli and should be treated with trimethoprim/sulfamethoxazole or a fluoroquinolone for fourteen days. Patients should be referred to a urologist for follow-up.

- **Helpful hints and pitfalls.** Mistaking testicular torsion for epididymitis could be disastrous, and lead to sterility. When in doubt get an ultrasound, and in some cases, the surgeon will need to explore the scrotum to resolve the problem!

Hydrocele

- A hydrocele is a fluid collection in the tunica vaginalis. They are most common in infancy, and present as painless testicular swelling that may be palpable or transilluminated.
- Surgical repair may be necessary if it persists beyond 2 years of age.

Orchitis

- **Epidemiology and risk factors.** It is found in 20% to 30% of post pubertal males with mumps. It may result from epididymitis; consider sexual history as a risk factor.

- *Pathophysiology.* This is usually an acute infection involving the testis, usually with an inciting epididymitis. Infection is most commonly viral or bacterial. Viral orchitis is usually caused by mumps (*Paramyxovirus*), although Epstein-Barr virus, coxsackie, varicella, and echovirus may also be implicated. Bacterial orchitis is most commonly caused by *Escherichia coli*, *Klebsiella*, and *Pseudomonas*, but may also include *Staphylococcus* and *Streptococcus species.*
- *History.* This is seen 4 to 6 days after parotitis with paramyxovirus. In 70% of cases, swelling and testicular pain begins unilaterally before spreading bilaterally in 1 to 9 days. Bacterial orchitis may cause fever, swelling, and tenderness.
- *Physical examination.* The testis is edematous and tender, and may be discolored. Prostate examination is important to do as prostatitis is often seen in association with epididymo-orchitis.
- *Diagnostic testing.* History and physical examination are usually adequate for diagnosis. A urinalysis and urine, urethral, and blood cultures are rarely helpful or necessary.
- *ED management.* Provide supportive care with analgesia and antiemetics. Mumps orchitis resolves in 4 to 5 days, and may be treated symptomatically with analgesics, ice packs, scrotal elevation, and bed rest. Bacterial orchitis mandates antibiotic treatment aimed at gram-negative coverage for sexually transmitted diseases (see Chapter 67). Follow-up with a urologist is recommended.
- *Helpful hints and pitfalls.* Doppler ultrasonongraphy is recommended to rule out more serious pathology, such as torsion, which requires emergent urology consultation. A large reactive hydrocele may require drainage by urology. Untreated orchitis may result in testicular atrophy.

Scrotal Abscess

- *Epidemiology and risk factors.* Intratesticular abscess or pyocele may be complications of epididymo-orchitis, trauma, or pelvic abscess. Diabetes is a predisposing risk factor. Superficial scrotal abscesses typically arise from an infected hair follicle.
- *Pathophysiology.* There is an infected fluid collection located within the tunica vaginalis. Epididymo-orchitis causes pyocele by compromising the testicular blood supply, leading to an infected testicular infarction that ruptures through the tunica albuginea to form the pyocele. Trauma causes pyocele when bacteria are introduced through breaks in the skin into a sterile hydrocele. After intra-abdominal infection, the mechanism of pyocele formation is thought to be tracking of bacteria from the abdomen via a patent processes vaginalis into the scrotum.
- *History.* This may elicit a history consistent with recent untreated epididymitis or orchitis, complication of ruptured appendicitis, post operative complication of circumcision or vasectomy, or Crohn's disease. The patient will complain of pain and may have fever. The patient may also note drainage or testicular mass.
- *Physical examination.* There will be a swollen, tender, erythematous scrotum that may be fluctuant.
- *Diagnostic testing.* Pyocele can have several sonographic features that distinguishes it from a simple hydrocele, including internal echoes

representing cellular debris, septae or loculations, fluid levels representing a hydrocele/pyocele interface, and even gas in the case of gas-forming organisms. A CT scan may also be useful in seeing the extent of the abscess.

- ***ED management.*** Obtain prompt urologic consultation for surgical drainage, and consideration of orchiectomy accompanied by appropriate antimicrobial agents for intratesticular abscess. A superficial scrotal abscess may be managed by incision and drainage in the ED (see Chapter 91).
- ***Helpful hints and pitfalls.*** Consider scrotal abscess in a patient with scrotal swelling and Crohn's disease.

Scrotal Edema

- This edema may be found in older men secondary to co-morbidities such as cardiac, hepatic, and renal failure. Trauma, dermatitis, human or insect bites, thrombosis of the spermatic vein, and fungal infection may also cause scrotal edema. Scrotal edema may also be secondary to pathology involving other parts of the male genitalia such as the testes, epididymis, and spermatic cord. Children aged 3 to 9 years may have idiopathic scrotal edema.
- On ultrasound, the wall of the scrotum is thickened, there is increased peritesticular blood flow, and there may be a reactive hydrocele.

Spermatocele

- A spermatocele is a cystic lesion that contains sperm.
- It is attached to the upper pole of the sexually mature testis.
- These are usually painless and incidental findings on physical examination.
- Enlargement of the spermatocele or pain is an indication for removal.

Testicular Infarction

- ***Epidemiology and risk factors.*** Segmental testicular infarction is rare whereas global infarction is the more common variant. Those with vascular disease are at higher risk for infarction.
- ***Pathophysiology.*** Global infarction is usually the result of trauma, repetitive injury (such as jack hammer use), spermatic cord torsion, severe epididymo-orchitis, or may be idiopathic. Most segmental infarctions are idiopathic, however, predisposing factors may include sickle cell disease, polycythemia, intimal fibroplasia of the spermatic artery, hypersensitivity angiitis, and trauma.
- ***History.*** The patient will complain of a painful scrotum.
- ***Physical examination.*** The scrotum typically is edematous and tender to palpation.
- ***Diagnostic testing.*** Doppler ultrasound can differentiate between testicular tumor and infarction. Infarction will be characterized by poor or absent flow on color Doppler.
- ***ED management.*** Immediate urologic consultation should be sought, as orchiectomy may be necessary.

■ *Helpful hints and pitfalls.* Remember there are many other causes of testicular infarction other than torsion.

Testicular Malignancy

■ *Epidemiology and risk factors.* This is the most common form of cancer in men between the ages of 20 and 35, with an average age of 32. The incidence is 4/100,000 making up 1% of all cancers in men. Risk factors include previous history of cryptorchidism.

■ *Pathophysiology.* Most testicular cancers are of germ cell origin, with seminomas being the most common. Other types include teratomas, embryonal carcinomas, yolk sac, choriocarcinomas, and Sertoli or Leydig cell tumors. Lymphoma and leukemia may metastasize to the testicle.

■ *History.* Usually patients will complain of a painless mass or heaviness. Sudden pain is usually the result of hemorrhage into the tumor. Minor trauma that results in severe swelling and pain may be the first sign of tumor.

■ *Physical examination.* The testicle may be firm and indurated. Some cases may present with diffuse swelling. A reactive hydrocele is present in 25% of cases. The mass may be smooth or nodular and will not transilluminate. A complete examination with attention to lymphadenopathy, abdominal masses, and hepatosplenomegaly should be performed.

■ *Diagnostic testing.* The key to diagnosis is the identification of a distinct intratesticular mass. Scrotal ultrasound is useful for identification. Chest radiograph and abdominal CT scan are obtained for staging. Tumor markers such as alpha-fetoprotein (AFP) and the beta-subunit of human chorionic gonadotropin (β-hCG) are helpful in the diagnosis, staging, and management of malignant testicular tumors, but have no role in the emergency management of these patients.

■ *ED management.* Obtain urologic and oncologic referral for biopsy. Hospitalization to expedite orchiectomy maybe necessary. Patients with seminomas will also benefit from radiation.

■ *Helpful hints and pitfalls.* The painless testicular mass is carcinoma until proven otherwise! Testicular carcinoma is most commonly misdiagnosed as epididymitis.

Testicular Torsion

■ *Epidemiology and risk factors.* The two peaks of occurrence are the first year of life and at puberty. The most common patient is a 12- to 18–year-old male, although torsion can occur at any age. Note that testicular torsion is 10 times more likely in an undescended testis (cryptorchidism). The testicular salvage rate depends on the degree of torsion and the duration of ischemia.

■ *Pathophysiology.* Testicular torsion causes venous engorgement that results in edema, hemorrhage, and subsequent arterial compromise, which results in testicular ischemia. Most patients with testicular torsion have an underlying anatomic deformity, called a *bell clapper* deformity of testicle in which the tunica vaginalis attaches above the epididymis allowing increased rotation that predisposes patients to torsion. This occurs bilaterally in 80% of patients.

- *History.* Patients usually complain of acute-onset, severe testicular swelling and pain that may radiate to the lower abdomen. This is often followed by nausea, vomiting, and a low-grade fever. Testicular torsion often occurs after exertion or during sleep. There is a lack of urinary symptoms.
- *Physical examination.* There is an exquisitely tender and swollen elevated testicle that lies horizontally. There is an ipsilateral loss of the cremasteric reflex and a negative Prehn's sign. Neither of these signs reliably exclude the diagnosis. Examination of the contralateral testicle is useful, but will not reveal the bell clapper deformity.
- *Diagnostic testing.* Color-flow duplex ultrasound to assess flow to the testicle is crucial. Torsion may be intermittent, however, and if the patient has spontaneously detorsed, there may be *increased* flow to the involved testicle, which can suggest epididymitis. Some patients will have to have this puzzle resolved by scrotal exploration, so it is always prudent to have a urologist consult for the patient when there is any confusion over the diagnosis. Radioisotope scans have a similar sensitivity and specificity to ultrasound, but take more time and are less practical.
- *ED management.* Immediate urology consultation is necessary as time is critical for survival of the ischemic testicle. Manual detorsion alleviates acute symptoms, and may obviate emergent exploration but is not a definitive treatment. Testes usually torse in an inward or medial direction, with an anteromedial rotation of the spermatic cord. Manual detorsion should proceed with one lateral or outward (viewing the scrotum from the feet) rotation (similar to opening a book). Doppler pulse evaluation may suggest successful detorsion if distal pulses return; however, the physician usually notes release and elongation of the cord followed by a marked diminution in symptoms. Successful manual reduction should be followed by elective orchidopexy.
- *Helpful hints and pitfalls.* Continuous pain more than 24 hours' duration is associated with an infarcted testicle. Nearly 41% of patients report a history of *similar* pain that resolved spontaneously.

Torsion of Testicular Appendages

- *Epidemiology and risk factors.* Usually seen in prepubertal males aged 7 to 13 years.
- *Pathophysiology.* Four embryologic remnants without function may become torsed: the appendix testis, appendix epididymis, paradidymis, and vas aberrans. The appendix testis and appendix epididymis account for 99% of appendage torsion. The appendix testis, a Müllerian duct remnant, is located at the superior pole of the testis and is the most common torsed appendage. The appendix epididymis, a Wolffian duct remnant, is located in the head of the epididymis. The appendage undergoing torsion will become ischemic and eventually infarct.
- *History.* The patient may have gradual onset of unilateral scrotal pain usually at the superior aspect of the testicle. Swelling may be apparent in later presentations. Systemic complaints such as nausea, vomiting and abdominal pain are rare.

■ *Physical examination.* This will reveal a tender nodule high in the testis or epididymis that may be palpated. The body of the testicle and epididymis will be nontender with a normal lie. Bilateral cremasteric reflex will be present. A small dark or blue dot may be present when the affected appendage is brought against the scrotal skin and transilluminated.

■ *Diagnostic testing.* Testing is usually unnecessary. If there is swelling and testicular torsion cannot be ruled out, testicular ultrasound should be performed.

■ *ED management.* Pain management, rest and scrotal elevation is all that is required. Most swelling and pain should resolve in 1 week. The torsed appendages will degenerate or calcify within 2 weeks. Urologic consultation may be necessary to rule out testicular torsion, or if there is chronic pain from a torsed appendage, which may be surgically excised.

■ *Helpful hints and pitfalls.* Always be sure to rule out torsion of the testicles! The blue dot sign is pathognomonic for torsion of the appendages. The sign is only present in 21% of cases, however.

Varicocele

■ *Epidemiology and risk factors.* This is usually seen in adolescent males. Secondary causes may result from increased pressure on the spermatic vein by diseases such as cirrhosis, hydronephrosis, or abdominal neoplasm.

■ *Pathophysiology.* There is a collection of venous varicosities of the spermatic veins from incomplete drainage of the papiniform plexus. Most varicoceles are left-sided; however, they may be bilateral up to 22% of the time. Renal cell carcinoma may present with an acute onset of left-sided varicocele due to obstruction of the left renal vein. Right-sided varicoceles are caused by inferior vena cava (IVC) thrombosis or compression from a tumor.

■ *History.* The patient may complain of a painless mass of dilated veins superior and posterior to the testis. The mass may increase upon Valsalva maneuver.

■ *Physical examination.* The patient should be examined in both supine and standing positions. Varicoceles will be more pronounced in the standing position and may be tender on palpation. They can be palpated superior and posterior to the testis. The appearance and palpation is described as a "bag of worms."

■ *Diagnostic testing.* Ultrasound should be used to rule out other sources of testicular masses if the physical examination is unclear.

■ *ED management.* Obtain urology consultation for all painful, large or bilateral varicoceles for surgical intervention. Outpatient referral for young patients is appropriate. Testicular atrophy may occur if untreated. A search for abdominal or pelvic pathology should be undertaken in the case of new varicocele in men older than 40 years or any right-sided varicocele. Uncomplicated varicoceles do not require surgery.

■ *Helpful hints and pitfalls.* An abdominal mass should always be suspected in men older than 40 years presenting with a new varicocele.

Special Considerations
Pediatrics

- Young patients may have minimal clinical signs and symptoms despite the presence of serious or surgical scrotal conditions. For instance, both the cremasteric reflex (often absent in testicular torsion) and Prehn's sign (scrotal elevation usually relieves pain in epididymitis but not torsion) are less reliable in children. Also, particular care must be taken to elicit complete histories (in private) especially in the adolescent population due to embarrassment about giving accurate sexual histories especially in the presence of parents or female health care workers. These adolescent patients often seek health care later than others.

- Testicular involvement occurs in up to 35% of patients with Henoch-Schönlein purpura (HSP). They may present with scrotal edema that resembles acute, testicular torsion (see Chapter 77).

Elderly

- Misdiagnosis and mortality rise significantly with patients older than 50 years because older patients are more likely to have catastrophic illness, such as a ruptured AAA, rarely seen in younger populations.

The Immunocompromised/Diabetic Patient

- These patients are always at greater risk for complications of scrotal pathology, specifically those involving infection, as mentioned repeatedly throughout this text. In this population orchitis may be caused by mycobacterium, Cryptococcus, toxoplasmosis, and *Candida* species as well as anaerobic bacteria.

Teaching Points

One life-threatening condition that may cause referred pain to the scrotal area is a ruptured abdominal aortic aneurysm. Acute scrotal pain has only two other entities that are true emergencies: testicular torsion and incarcerated hernia. There will be patients in whom you are sure that there is epididymitis rather than torsion, and the distinction between the two often can only be made by scrotal exploration. It is always prudent to consult with a urologist where the possibility of torsion exists.

Suggested Readings

Dogra V. Acute painful scrotum. Radiol Clin North Am 2004;42:349–363.

Escobar JI, Eastman ER, Harwood-Nuss AL. Selected urologic problems. In: Marx JA, Hockberger RS, Walls RM (editors). Rosen's Emergency Medicine: Concepts and Clinical Practice (6th ed). Philadelphia: Mosby, 2006.

Galejs L. Diagnosis and treatment of the acute scrotum. Am Fam Phys 1999;59:817–824.

Marcozzi D, Sumer S. The nontraumatic acute scrotum. Emerg Med Clin North Am 2001;19:547–567.

Rosenstein D, McAninch JW. Urologic emergencies. Med Clin N Am 2004;88:495–518.

CHAPTER 51

Seizures

MICHAEL M. WOODRUFF ■ CARLO L. ROSEN

 Red Flags

Headache, especially if severe, sudden, or unusual ● Focal neurologic deficit ● Altered mental status ● Fever ● Neck or back stiffness ● Rash, particularly petechiae ● Immunocompromised state, especially human immunodeficiency virus ● History or signs of alcohol abuse ● Change in seizure pattern, especially multiple seizures

Overview

A seizure is an episode of neurologic dysfunction (usually transient) caused by abnormal neuronal activity. Seizures may be the consequence of a potentially life-threatening condition.

An aura is the sensory (often olfactory or visual) or emotional disturbance that may precede a seizure.

Primary seizures are those that occur without a clear provoking factor. Recurring primary seizures are termed *epileptic seizures*. Secondary (reactive) seizures occur in response to a specific pathophysiologic stress. A diagnosis of epilepsy requires two or more separate seizures without identifiable cause or precipitating factor (primary or idiopathic seizures).

The postictal (post-seizure) period can involve persistent confusion, headache, or neurologic deficits that slowly resolve over minutes to hours. Todd's paralysis is any motor deficit immediately following a seizure that may persist for up to 24 hours. Status epilepticus is a life-threatening condition defined as a single seizure lasting 5-30 minutes or longer, or two or more seizures without return to normal consciousness between them. Status epilepticus is a life-threatening condition that requires emergent intervention.

Eclampsia may present with a seizure up to 8 weeks postpartum (chapter 68).

Pseudoseizures, or psychogenic seizures, are functional events that may mimic seizures but there is no abnormal CNS activity.

The ED workup should be much more aggressive in immunocompromised patients, especially those with human immunodeficiency virus (HIV) infection. All seizure patients should have a blood glucose level performed immediately. The care of epileptic patients is complicated by the lifelong presence of the disease that leads to much noncompliance.

DDx Priority-Based Differential Diagnosis of Seizures

Critical Diagnoses	Emergent Diagnoses	Nonemergent Diagnoses
Central nervous system infections (35, 67)	Cerebral neoplasm (35)	Idiopathic
Stroke (56)	Vascular abnormality (cerebral aneurysm) (35)	Congenital abnormalities
Hypoglycemia/ hyperglycemia (38)	Electrolyte abnormalities (88)	
Hypoxia (5)	• Hypernatremia	
Eclampsia (68)	• Hyponatremia	
	• Hypocalcemia	
	• Hypomagnesemia	
	Toxins (72)	
	Alcohol withdrawal (72)	
	Head trauma (9)	
	Metabolic abnormalities	
	• Uremia (49)	
	• Hepatic failure (41)	
	Hypertensive encephalopathy (39)	
	Subtherapeutic anti-epileptic medication	
	Febrile seizure (79)	

( ) Refers to the chapter in which the disease entity is discussed.

Differential Diagnosis of Seizure

- See DDx table for conditions causing seizures.
- See Table 51–1 for classification of primary seizures.

Initial Diagnostic Approach
General

- As always, the ABCs (*a*irway, *b*reathing, and *c*irculation) should be assessed. Intravenous (IV) access should be obtained, and a finger-stick glucose level should be performed. Whether the patient is having a *true* seizure should be determined.
- Family, friends, health care providers, and prehospital personnel can be valuable sources of information regarding new or recently terminated medications, or ingestion of drugs or herbal substances that might provoke seizures, and characterization of the seizure activity itself.
- Most patients with a history of seizures only require a minimal diagnostic evaluation in the ED (i.e., determination of anticonvulsant levels) if they have a normal physical examination, have one isolated seizure similar to previous episodes, have returned to baseline with no abnormalities on physical examination, and there is no concern for another cause of the patient's seizures.
- All patients who are having a first time alcohol withdrawal seizure (see Chapter 72) should have a formal seizure workup because this is a patient

Table 51–1   Classification of Primary Seizures

Type	Description
Generalized seizure	A generalized seizure consists of abnormal electrical activity involving both cerebral hemispheres and accompanied by a loss of consciousness. Secondary seizures are more likely to be generalized. Generalized seizures may be convulsive or nonconvulsive; nonconvulsive seizures result in loss of consciousness without muscular activity.
Tonic–clonic (grand mal) seizure	There is a loss of consciousness, apnea, rigidity of trunk and extremities (tonic phase), followed by rhythmic jerking (clonic) movements. They are often accompanied by urinary incontinence. The usual duration is 60 to 90 seconds. Muscle contraction may be forceful enough to cause shoulder dislocation, vertebral compression fractures, or significant oral or tongue injuries. They are frequently presaged by an involuntary yell by the patient.
Absence (petit mal) seizure	A brief loss of consciousness without loss of postural tone. These typically occur in school-aged children. Patients may appear dazed or distracted as though they are "staring off into space." There is usually no postictal period.
Tonic seizure (Myoclonic)	There is stiffening and rigidity of the trunk and extremities. There is no loss of consciousness. When the entire body is involved, the patient falls ("drop attack").
Atonic	There is a sudden loss of tone in the extremities or trunk.
Partial seizure	Abnormal electrical activity is limited to one hemisphere or area of the brain, and consciousness may be preserved. This manifests as seizure activity on one side of the body or one extremity. It may spread to involve the entire cortex, causing a generalized seizure (secondary generalization). This is also known as a Jacksonian seizure, and often connotes an underlying space occupying lesion such as a brain tumor.
Simple partial seizure	One area of the cortex is involved, and symptoms relate to the specific location in the brain. Unilateral (often focal) tonic–clonic activity, sensory symptoms, deviation of head and eyes, or isolated sensory phenomena may occur. There is no loss of consciousness.
Complex partial seizure	Involvement is localized to one region of the brain (often the temporal lobe), but involves alteration of consciousness—often with changes in thinking or behavior related to temporal lobe dysfunction. Because they often trigger complex motor actions such as lip smacking or fiddling with objects, these seizures are frequently misdiagnosed as psychiatric problems.

Continued

Table 51–1	Seizure Classification—*cont'd*
Type	**Description**
Status epilepticus	Unremitting seizure activity: two or more seizures without return to normal neurologic function in between, or a single seizure lasting more than 30 minutes. Because there is evidence that even brief periods of uncontrolled neuronal discharge can lead to cell death, some authorities advocate for a 5-minute time limit. Status epilepticus may involve generalized, complex partial, or simple partial seizures. Status epilepticus can also occur in the absence of motor activity; this is called *nonconvulsive status*, and is a difficult diagnosis to make in the unconscious patient. Status epilepticus can lead to morbidity from the metabolic stress of repeated muscle contractions, excess catecholamines, and excessive neuronal activity. Neuronal cell death (excitotoxicity) is thought to be mediated by excess glutamate release and subsequent accumulation of intracellular calcium. Rhabdomyolysis, lactic acidosis, aspiration pneumonitis, neurogenic pulmonary edema, and respiratory failure may also complicate status epilepticus.

population that has a high incidence of concomitant disease such as cerebral infection or traumatic injury.

■ Patients who have a first seizure caused by certain drug ingestions such as cocaine or amphetamine ingestion may not require an extensive workup. Nevertheless, tricyclic antidepressant overdose is a potentially life-threatening ingestion that causes seizures. Once identified, these patients should be promptly treated (see Chapter 72).

Laboratory

■ In the patient with a first seizure who has returned to normal baseline after a seizure, blood glucose determination, serum electrolytes, and toxicology screens are recommended. Further investigation is needed in patients with suspected infection, trauma, medication toxicity, or other metabolic derangement, as well as in patients with altered mental status. Women of childbearing age should have a pregnancy test performed.

■ Hyponatremia is the most common electrolyte abnormality in patients presenting with a seizure, but a patient can seize from hypernatremia as well. This is observed in patients with diabetes insipidus, as well as in the pediatric infant who has received the wrong formula (i.e., substitution of salt for sugar). Hypocalcemia is a rare cause of seizures. A history of thyroid or parathyroid surgery, pancreatitis, renal failure, or paresthesias around the mouth and fingertips should suggest this diagnosis. Hypomagnesemia can also cause seizures, and is found most often in the alcoholic patient or in the patient with an eating disorder such as anorexia nervosa. Signs and symptoms are identical to those of hypocalcemia.

EKG

- An electrocardiogram (EKG) may aid in the diagnosis of tricyclic antidepressant or other overdose, and should be performed if there is any concern for a dysrhythmia such as complete heart block, or concern for cardiac ischemic disease.

Lumbar Puncture

- A lumbar puncture (LP) to detect central nervous system (CNS) infection is recommended in the febrile adult with a seizure, and in any immunocompromised patient with a new seizure (even if afebrile). Patients who have papilledema, focal neurologic deficits, a history of malignancy, or altered mental status should undergo computed tomography (CT scan) of the head before the LP. Patients with a cerebrospinal fluid shunt should have spinal fluid obtained from the shunt itself. An LP may also be indicated after a CT scan in patients with a history suggestive of subarachnoid hemorrhage (SAH) if the CT scan is negative for abnormal findings (see Chapter 35).

Neuroimaging

- Patients with new focal deficits, persistent altered mental status, papilledema, new seizure pattern or seizure type, age above 60 years, history of a mass lesion, immunocompromise, trauma, presence of intra-cranial shunt, or other risk factors for a structural lesion should undergo imaging studies.
- HIV and other immunocompromised patients may need a contrast-enhanced head CT scan or magnetic resonance imaging (MRI) to detect a small mass lesion or an intracerebral abscess.
- It may be possible and is reasonable to arrange deferred outpatient imaging studies in a minority of patients who are young (<40 years), healthy, have a normal neurologic examination, and have no history of head trauma, malignancy, immunocompromise, fever, headache, or anti-coagulation. This is especially true if the likely precipitant of the seizure was a medication (e.g., an antidepressant) or substance abuse (especially cocaine or amphetamines). Although an MRI is often the preferred outpatient imaging modality, a noncontrast CT scan is more readily available, and is sufficient to exclude most cases of hemorrhage, mass lesion, or large stroke. If available, an MRI is more sensitive for cortical abnormalities and small masses that may act as seizure foci.
- Neurocysticercosis is the most common cause of secondary seizures in the developing world, and is a very common cause of first seizure in the Hispanic population.

EEG

- Increasingly, it has been recognized that generalized convulsive status epilepticus may evolve into a more subtle nonconvulsive status epilepticus, with ongoing abnormal electrical activity that may lead to neuronal injury and death. Although emergent electroencephalogram (EEG) may be difficult to obtain in most emergency departments, EEG should be considered for status epilepticus patients with persistent altered mental status, or those requiring long-acting paralytics or pharmacologic coma. In a stable patient with an isolated first time seizure with no clear etiology (normal head CT scan and physical examination, not related to drug use), an EEG can be deferred for outpatient acquisition with outpatient follow-up by neurology.

Emergency Department Management Overview
General

- The ABCs should be addressed as discussed in Section II.
- Most seizures are brief, self-limited events that require very little active management. For the uncomplicated seizure, intravenous medications are seldom indicated, and may lead to complications or a prolonged ED stay from unnecessary sedation.
- In any seizure, airway protection is the first priority; the patient should be placed in the left lateral decubitus position to reduce the chance of aspiration. A nasopharyngeal airway is a useful adjunct to temporarily maintain a patent airway; bite blocks can be difficult and even dangerous to place due to forceful contractions of the masseter muscles. Fingers should never be placed in the mouth of a seizing patient. In the setting of prolonged apnea, frank aspiration of gastric contents, need for gastro-intestinal decontamination, or unremitting seizures (status epilepticus), endotracheal intubation should be carried out. Short-acting paralytics should be chosen for intubation, to facilitate the detection of ongoing seizures.
- All actively seizing patients should have cardiac monitoring, pulse oximetry, supplemental oxygen, and suction available.
- While gaining IV access in an actively seizing patient is important, it can be difficult and even dangerous for both the patient and staff. Most seizures will terminate without treatment in a very short period of time; if needed, benzodiazepines and phosphenytoin can be given via the intramuscular (IM) route. Benzodiazepines may also be administered rectally in the seizing patient.
- The patient who is seizing or who may have another seizure should be protected from secondary injury by eliminating the possibility of a fall, and providing adequate protective padding so that extremities are not injured on nearby hard surfaces such as bedrails.

Medications

- Medications used to treat seizures are listed in Table 51–2.
- Seizures may be triggered by alcohol ingestion (alcohol-related seizure), or by withdrawal from chronic alcohol ingestion (more common).

Table 51–2	Medications Used to Treat Seizures		
Drug	**Adult Dose**	**Pediatric Dose**	**Comments**
Diazepam	0.2 mg/kg IV at 2 mg/min up to 20 mg	0.2-0.5 mg/kg IV/IO/ET up to 20 mg 0.5-1.0 mg/kg PR up to 20 mg	Lorazepam is equal in efficiency to diazepam but has a longer duration of action. Midazolam is the most potent.
Lorazepam	0.1 mg/kg IV at 1-2 mg/min up to 10 mg	0.05-0.1 mg/kg IV	
Midazolam*	2.5-15 mg IV 0.2 mg/kg IM	0.15 mg/kg IV then 2-10 µg/kg/min	
Phenytoin	20 mg/kg IV at ≤50 mg/min	20 mg/kg IV at 1 mg/kg/min	Use continuous cardiac and blood pressure monitoring due to risk of hypotension and cardiac dysrhythmias with rapid infusion. Do not give in dextrose solution.
Fosphenytoin	20 PE/kg at 150 mg PE/min; may be given IM	10 to 20 mg of PE/kg at a rate of 3 mg/kg/min to a maximum of 150 mg/min	When compared to phenytoin, can be given more rapidly, has few side effects, can be given IM, and can be given in dextrose solution.
Valproate	20 mg/kg PR		Absorbed slowly.
Phenobarbital	20 mg/kg IV at 60-100 mg/min	Same	May be given as IM loading dose. May cause significant sedation and hypotension.
Pentobarbital*	5 mg/kg IV at 25 mg/min, then titrate to EEG	10-15 mg/kg over 1 hour; 0.5-1 mg/kg/hr	Intubation, ventilation, and pressor support are required
Propofol*	1-3 mg/kg IV, then 1-15 mg/kg/hr	Same	Critical care monitoring needed

ET, endotracheal; IM, intramuscular; IO, intraosseous; PE, phenytoin sodium equivalents; PR, per rectum.

*If seizures persist, these medications may be used for deeper sedation and general anesthesia; the patient's airway should be protected and continuous EEG monitoring should be performed.

Prolonged alcohol-withdrawal seizures respond to benzodiazepines, but do not respond to phenytoin. Benzodiazepines also treat symptoms of acute withdrawal, and help prevent complications such as delirium tremens. A single alcohol withdrawal seizure can be managed in the ED with brief observation and appropriate detoxification referral once acute withdrawal issues are addressed.

- In patients with severe traumatic brain injury (TBI), phenytoin and carbamazepine appear to reduce the incidence of seizures in the early posttraumatic period (0-7 days), but do not reduce the incidence of late seizures. Antiseizure prophylaxis does not appear to improve overall outcomes after severe TBI. Antiseizure prophylaxis is recommended for certain high-risk situations after severe TBI: Glasgow Coma Scale below 10, cortical contusion, depressed skull fracture, subdural hematoma, epidural hematoma, intracerebral hemorrhage, penetrating head wound, and seizure within 24 hours of injury.

- In patients with cerebral edema secondary to a mass lesion, dexamethasone may be used to reduce peritumor edema, in addition to anticonvulsant therapy.

- *Glucose.* Hypoglycemia (blood glucose concentration of less than 50/60 mg/dl in adults and less than 40 mg/dl in children) may cause acute seizures. If needed, 25 to 50 g of dextrose IV should be administered to adults. The pediatric dose is 0.5-1 g/kg, or 2 to 4 ml/kg of D25W, 5-10 ml/kg of D10W (neonates). The 50% dextrose is very toxic to tissues, and care should be taken not to infiltrate this solution into soft tissues. If the patient is awake after the seizure and there is no easy IV access, glucose can be administered orally. Another option is glucagon (1mg in adults), which can be given intravenously, subcutaneously, or intramuscularly.

- *Benzodiazepines.* These medications limit seizure activity by enhancing GABA (the major inhibitory neurotransmitter) receptor activity, and are the first-line therapy for status epilepticus. Lorazepam (4-8 mg IV) is equal in efficacy to diazepam (10-20 mg IV). Diazepam has a faster onset, however, lorazepam is considered first-line therapy because of its longer duration of action. Major side effects are respiratory depression and hypotension. Valium is available in a rectal preparation ("Diastat") for pre-hospital use.

- *Phenytoin/phosphenytoin.* If seizures continue despite the administration of benzodiazepines, phenytoin 18 to 20 mg/kg IV or phosphenytoin 15 to 20 mg/kg phenytoin equivalents IV or IM should be administered. Major side effects of IV phenytoin include hypotension, cardiac dysrhythmias, and infusion-site reactions. Phenytoin should not be mixed with glucose-containing solutions. Phosphenytoin has fewer infusion-site reactions, and can be infused at a faster rate. It can also be given IM, which is an advantage when there is no easy IV access. Unfortunately it is much more expensive than phenytoin. If seizures persist after the loading dose of phenytoin or phosphenytoin, an additional 5- to 10-mg/kg dose (up to 30 mg/kg total dose) may be given.

- *Barbiturates.* IV Phenobarbital (up to 20 mg/kg) is the third-line agent for status-epilepticus. Drawbacks include profound respiratory depression and hypotension resulting from vasodilatation and cardiac depression. If this drug becomes necessary, the patient will likely need endotracheal intubation and ventilator management if this has not already been instituted.

- *Refractory status epilepticus-general anesthesia.* Continuous infusions of propofol, midazolam, and pentobarbital have been used with some success in patients who continue to seize despite the administration of benzodiazepines, phenytoin, and phenobarbital. The use of IV valproate has also been reported.
- *Thiamine/magnesium.* Thiamine 100 mg IV and magnesium 1 to 2 g IV should be used in alcoholic or malnourished patients.
- *INH overdose:* If the clinical history suggests the patient is being treated for tuberculosis, vitamin B_6 (pyridoxine) should be empirically given because the patient may have taken an overdose of isoniazid (INH), which causes intractable seizures unless treated with pyridoxine. The correct dosage will vary with the patient, but probably requires much larger amounts than may readily be available in a single hospital pharmacy. Consult poison control center for dosage recommendations, and as a source of extra supplies.

Disposition

- *Consultation.* First-time seizure patients who are being discharged should be referred to a neurologist. Patients being admitted to the hospital should have an inpatient neurologic consult, except in the case of alcohol-withdrawal seizures.
- *Admission.* The decision regarding whether the patient should be admitted to the hospital is based on the disease process identified during the initial workup. If the patient has returned to baseline function and is neurologically intact, the patient may be a candidate for discharge with outpatient follow-up. Patients with alcohol-related seizures can be safely discharged once intoxication, withdrawal, and social issues have been addressed.
- *Discharge.* The most important part of the discharge plan for a first-time seizure is close follow-up. Healthy patients with a normal neurologic examination and no structural brain lesion have a low risk of seizure recurrence, and can be discharged from the hospital without antiepileptic medications. They should be warned, however, of the risk of recurrent seizure, and should be cautioned not to engage in driving, swimming, or other dangerous activities until seen in follow-up. The physician should be aware of specific requirements of state regulatory agencies (e.g., in California, it is a legal mandate to report any new seizure activity in a driving-age patient to the motor vehicle bureau). Patients with recurrent seizures can be discharged home if they have returned to baseline, and have no new neurologic deficit. If antiepileptic levels are low, a loading dose may be required before discharge. The IV route is preferred if the patient is unable to tolerate oral medications. It is not possible to check levels of some of the newer antiepileptic medications. It is prudent to discuss additional dosing of these medications with a neurologist before discharge.
- The patient should have a ride home, and follow-up should be arranged before discharge, if possible, with the patient's primary care provider.

Specific Problems

> ● ● ●   Refer to the DDx table for reference to a discussion of problems that may
> ● ● ●   cause seizure activity.
> ● ● ●

Special Considerations
Pediatrics

- A pediatric febrile seizure is defined as a seizure accompanied by fever without CNS infection in a child between 6 months and 5 years of age (see Chapter 79).
- Children who have a first time seizure in whom the clinical presentation suggests nonaccidental trauma (NAT), should have a CT scan, and, when possible, an MRI because there is a high incidence of skull fracture, cerebral extra-axial bleed, and intracerebral bleeding in these children. The MRI is a better imaging study to reveal the sometimes subtle injuries associated with the shaken child syndrome.

Women and Pregnancy

- Management of seizures during pregnancy should be undertaken with the consultation of an obstetrician and a neurologist. Specific concerns include reducing the risk to the fetus from antiepileptic medications and diagnostic tests. Beyond 20 weeks of gestation, eclampsia should be ruled out with careful blood pressure measurement and urinalysis (see Chapter 68). Eclampsia can occur up to 8 weeks postpartum. The first-line therapy for eclamptic seizures is magnesium sulfate (4-6 g IV, then 1-2 g/h drip). The definitive therapy is delivery of the fetus. The patient should be monitored closely for magnesium toxicity (e.g., hyporeflexia).
- Stroke should be included in the differential diagnosis of seizures during pregnancy and other hypercoagulable states, but in the pregnant patient, seizures late in pregnancy are probably from eclampsia.

Immunocompromised Patients

- Infections and mass lesions may be the source of a new seizure among immunocompromised patients, particularly those with HIV (see Chapter 37). Toxoplasmosis and lymphoma are common causes of mass lesions in this population. Cryptococcal, bacterial, or viral meningitis or encephalitis can also cause seizures, as can HIV encephalopathy, PML (progressive multifocal leukoencephalopathy), CNS tuberculosis, and neurosyphilis. All immunocompromised patients should have neuroimaging prior to lumbar puncture, and virtually all of these patients will require admission.

Teaching Points

A seizure is a frightening experience for most witnesses, and is potentially life-threatening to the patient (e.g., seizure occurring in the bathtub, while driving, or while performing a risky sport such as skiing). The ABCs and a bedside glucose level should be rapidly assessed in any seizing patient. The remainder of the evaluation in patients with a first-time seizure is dictated by the history and presentation. A healthy patient who has a normal physical examination, no fever, no meningismus or headache, and whose mental status returns rapidly to normal requires an expeditious intracranial imaging study (a cranial CT scan or an MRI) and an EEG at some point. A detailed alcohol and drug use history should be obtained. A urine toxicologic analysis for drugs of abuse such as cocaine or amphetamine may be helpful.

Pediatric febrile seizures also often require no workup, and the need for LP should be determined by the appropriate management of the febrile illness rather than dictated by the seizure.

In the patient with known seizure disorder, recurrent seizure is most likely due to poor compliance with antiseizure medication. Give a dose of benzodiazepine if the patient is still seizing or having frequent seizures, and check levels of any anticonvulsant medications. The patient should receive a loading dose of appropriate medications in the ED.

Suggested Readings

Catlett C. Seizures and status epilepticus in adults. In: Ma OJ, Cline DM, Tintinalli JE, et al (editors). Emergency Medicine. McGraw-Hill, 2004, pp 1409–1417

ACEP Clinical Policies Committee. Clinical policy: critical issues in the evaluation and management of adult patients presenting to the emergency department with seizures. Ann Emerg Med 2004;43:605–625.

American College of Emergency Physicians, American Academy of Neurology, American Association of Neurological Surgeons, American Society of Neuroradiology. Practice Parameter: Neuroimaging in the emergency patient presenting with seizure. Ann Emerg Med 1996;28:114–118.

American Academy of Pediatrics Provisional Committee on Quality Improvement. The neurodiagnostic evaluation of the child with a first simple febrile seizure. Pediatrics 1996;97:769–772.

Lowenstein DH, Alldredge BK. Status epilepticus. N Engl J Med 1998;338:970–976.

Management and Prognosis of Severe Traumatic Brain Injury. The Brain Trauma Foundation and the American Association of Neurological Surgeons Joint Section on Neurotrauma and Critical Care, 2000. *http://www.braintrauma.org/guidelines/*.

CHAPTER 52

Shortness of Breath

DAVID P. BRYANT ■ TREVOR J. MILLS

 Red Flags

Rapid onset ● Extremes of age ● Immunocompromised state
● Speaking in broken words or unable to speak ● Cyanosis ● Stridor
● Altered mental status ● Absent or abnormal breath sounds
● Accessory muscle breathing ● Look and feelings of impending doom
(pale, diaphoretic, poor respiratory effort) ● Abnormal vital signs (high
fever, ↑↓ heart rate, ↑↓ blood pressure, ↑↓ respiratory rate) ● Diaphoresis
● Low oxygen saturation by pulse-oximetry

Overview

Shortness of breath, or *dyspnea,* is the uncomfortable sensation of
difficulty in breathing, or not being able to get enough air.

The evaluation of such patients follows the basic tenets of emergency medicine. First check the ABCs (*a*irway, *b*reathing, and *c*irculation) as described in Section II. Look for "red flags" (see Box) at the
time of patient presentation, indicating patients who require immediate
attention.

The problem may be primarily due to a process directly affecting
the breathing apparatus (airway or lungs), or it may be secondary to
another pathologic process affecting breathing such as cardiac failure,
anemia, or severe acidosis.

Multiple problems may present that trigger exacerbations of each
other, such as congestive heart failure (CHF) and chronic obstructive
pulmonary disease (COPD), or the problem may be multifactorial
(i.e., diabetic ketoacidosis co-existing with pneumonia).

Dyspneic patients require constant re-evaluation in the ED to determine response to treatment or need for more aggressive interventions.

Differential Diagnoses

See DDx table describing priority-based diagnosis.

DDx Priority-Based Differential Diagnosis of Shortness of Breath

	Critical Diagnoses	Emergent Diagnoses	Nonemergent Dagnoses
Pulmonary	Airway obstruction (5) Pulmonary embolus Noncardiogenic edema Anaphylaxis (19)	Spontaneous pneumothorax Asthma or COPD exacerbation Cor pulmonale Pneumonia (67)	Pleural effusion Lung neoplasm Bronchitis (24)
Cardiac	Myocardial infarction (22) Cardiac tamponade (22)	Pericarditis (22) Pulmonary edema	Stable congenital, valvular heart disease, or cardiomyopathy
Abdominal		Hypotension or sepsis from ruptured viscus, bowel obstruction, inflammatory/ infectious process (18)	Pregnancy Ascites Obesity
Psychogenic			Hyperventilation syndrome Somatization disorder Panic attack
Toxic/ metabolic/ endocrine	Toxic exposure (72) DKA (38)	Renal failure (49) Electrolyte abnormalities (88) Metabolic acidosis (83)	Thyroid disease (63)
Traumatic	Tension pneumothorax (13) Cardiac tamponade (13) Flail chest (13)	Simple pneumothorax, hemothorax (13) Diaphragmatic rupture (13)	
Hematologic	Carbon monoxide poisoning (73)	Anemia (66)	Porphyria (66)
Neuromuscular	CVA (56) Guillain-Barré syndrome (60)	Multiple sclerosis (60)	ALS (60)

ALS, amyotrophic lateral sclerosis; COPD, chronic obstructive pulmonary disease; CVA, cerebrovascular accident; DKA, diabetic ketoacidosis.

( ) Refers to the chapter in which the disease entity is discussed.

From Braithwaite S, Perina D. Dyspnea. In: Marx JA, Hockberger RS, Walls RM (editors). Rosen's Emergency Medicine: Concepts and Clinical Practice (6th ed). Philadelphia: Mosby, 2006, p 156.

Initial Diagnostic Approach
General

- Any patient presenting with dyspnea should be immediately evaluated to determine the degree of respiratory impairment. All patients in respiratory distress or who have oxygen saturation less than 95% should be placed on supplemental oxygen. Conditions resulting in hypoxia are listed in Table 52–1. If the patient is without respiratiory distress and remains resistant to oxygen therapy, cardiac shunting or an abnormal hemoglobin should be considered. These patients also should have a cardiac monitor, pulse oximetry, and intravenous (IV) access.
- Clinical clues from the initial assessment of the patient should aid in the diagnostic evaluation of the patient (Table 52–2).

Pulse Oximetry

- Pulse oximetry quickly assesses arterial oxygen saturation (SaO_2), the amount of oxygen carried by hemoglobin. The partial pressure of oxygen (PaO_2) measures the relatively small amount of oxygen dissolved in the plasma. The SaO_2 at sea level is normally between 97% and 100%. When the SaO_2 falls below 95%, hypoxia is present. For the hypoxic patient, small changes in SaO_2 represent large changes in the PaO_2.
- Limitations to pulse oximetry include severe vasoconstriction (e.g., shock), excessive movement, acrylic nails, nail polish, severe anemia, or the presence of abnormal hemoglobins (carboxyhemoglobin and methemoglobin, see Chapters 72 and 25, respectively). Normal oxygen saturation does not ensure adequate ventilation, and does not rule out serious pathology such as pulmonary embolism (PE).

EKG

- An electrocardiogram (EKG) is useful to determine the presence cardiac dysrhythmias, ischemia or patterns consistent with pulmonary disease.

Table 52–1 Causes of Hypoxia

	Description	Example
Hypoventilation	Poor ventilation drive Neuromuscular disorder	Narcotic overdose Guillain-Barré syndrome
Ventilation–perfusion imbalance	Parenchymal disease Pulmonary circulation occlusion	Pneumonia Pulmonary embolism
Inadequate transport mechanism	Abnormal hemoglobin Circulatory insufficiency Right-to-left shunt	Methemoglobinemia Shock Ventricular septal defect
Inadequate tissue oxygenation	Poisoned enzymes Abnormal tissue demand	Cyanide poisoning Hyperthyroidism

Table 52–2   Clinical Clues in Patients Presenting with Shortness of Breath

History	Diagnoses to Consider
Onset	Sudden onset is concerning for pulmonary embolism, flash pulmonary edema, spontaneous pneumothorax, or anaphylaxis. Dyspnea worsening over days may be due to congestive heart failure, COPD, pleural effusion, malignancy, infection, or neuromuscular disease.
Duration	Chronic progressive dyspnea may be due to congestive heart failure, COPD, or pulmonary hypertension. An acute episode of dyspnea may be due to an asthma exacerbation, infection, or psychogenic causes.
Exacerbating and relieving factors	Exertional dyspnea may be caused by cardiac ischemia, poor cardiac reserve, or COPD. Orthopnea (worsening with supine position) is concerning for left heart failure, COPD, and neuromuscular disorders (diaphragmatic weakness). Paroxysmal nocturnal dyspnea (occurs at night when the patient is supine) is typical of left-sided heart failure but may also be found in COPD.
Fever	May be due to an infectious process. However, noninfectious causes such as pulmonary embolism can cause a fever.
Chest pain	Associated chest pain is concerning for cardiac ischemia, pulmonary embolism, pneumonia, pleuritis, or pneumothorax. It can also be of musculoskeletal origin especially if the pain worsens with movement.
Surrounding events	Any history of trauma should be concerning for pneumothorax, hemothorax, rib fracture, pericardial effusion, or cardiac tamponade. Any patients with a history of immobilization or leg pain is concerning for pulmonary embolism.

Physical Examination	Diagnoses to Consider
Skin	Central cyanosis or diaphoresis indicates severe distress.
Neck	*JVD:* cor pulmonale, congestive heart failure, tension pneumothorax, pericardial tamponade, constrictive pericarditis, pulmonary hypertension. *Stridor:* upper airway obstruction
Lungs	*Wheezes:* pulmonary edema, asthma, anaphylaxis, COPD, pulmonary embolism, pneumonia *Rales:* pulmonary edema, pneumonia, pulmonary embolism, interstitial lung disease *Unilateral decrease:* pneumothorax, pleural effusion, consolidation, atelectasis, pulmonary contusion. *Pleural friction rub:* pleuritis, pulmonary embolism
Heart	*Muffled heart sounds:* cardiac tamponade. S_3 *gallop (early diastolic impulse):* congestive heart failure, pulmonary embolism S_4 *gallop (presystolic impulse):* suggests left ventricular dysfunction or ischemia, pulmonary embolism

Continued

Table 52–2	Clinical Clues in Patients Presenting with Shortness of Breath—*cont'd*
Physical Examination	**Diagnoses to Consider**
Heart	*Loud P₂:* may be heard in patients with pulmonary hypertension or cor pulmonale.
	Murmurs: valve abnormality (see Chapter 22)
	Friction rub: pericarditis
Extremities	*Calf tenderness, Homan's sign:* pulmonary embolism
	Edema: congestive heart failure
Neurologic	*Focal deficit:* stroke
	Symmetrical deficit: neuromuscular
	General weakness: anemia, electrolyte abnormality, toxic exposure

COPD, chronic obstructive pulmonary disease; JVD, jugulovenous distention.

Pulmonary Function Testing

■ In the ED, pulmonary function tests (PFTs) are used most commonly in patients with asthma and COPD in order to obtain objective data on pulmonary status and to assess response to therapy. They are more useful in asthma, where there is a significant reversible component of airway obstruction.

■ Neuromuscular diseases affecting ventilatory function, such as the Guillain-Barré syndrome (see Chapter 60), require screening of pulmonary function for both initial and ongoing assessment.

■ ED pulmonary function testing includes the peak expiratory flow rate (PEFR) or the forced expiratory volume in 1 second (FEV_1). The PEFR is the maximum flow rate of expired air starting with fully inflated lungs in liters per second. The FEV_1 is the volume of gas expelled during the first second of the forced expiration. Both measurements require patient cooperation for maximal effort. PEFR measures obstruction in the larger airways. FEV_1 is better for determining the severity of overall airway obstruction and ventilation. It is less dependent on patient effort than the PEFR; however, the PEFR is easier to obtain in the ED.

■ Forced vital capacity (FVC) is the sum of all the air that can be forcibly exhaled after a maximal inspiratory effort. The FVC is most often used as a measure of functional impairment in restrictive respiratory disorders such as pulmonary fibrosis or neuromuscular disease.

■ In adults, initially low-flow rates (PEFR <100 L/min) and spirometry values (FEV_1 <1 L) identify sick patients with the potential need for admission or close re-evaluation. See Table 52–3 for normal values. Although absolute values can be used, percent predicted values are preferred because they are derived from variables that include age, height, and sex. Patients with PEFR or FEV_1 values of <40% of predicted normal values after bronchodilator therapy often require admission. The percent of the patient's personal best effort is ideal.

Table 52–3   Approximate Values for Pulmonary Function Testing

Degree of Obstruction	FEV$_1$ (L)	Peak Flow (L/min)
Normal	4.0-6.0	550-650 (males) 400-500 (females)
Mild	3.0	300-400
Moderate	1.6	200-300
Severe	0.6	100

FEV$_1$, forced expiratory volume at 1 second.
From Roberts: Clinical Procedures in Emergency Medicine (4th ed). New York: Elsevier, 2004.

■ Abnormalities of maximal inspiratory pressure (MIP) and maximal expiratory pressure (MEP) are useful tests for respiratory muscle weakness (Chapter 60). A MIP less than 15 to 20 cm H_2O is often incompatible with adequate ventilation. The MEP is generated by those muscles that can be recruited for active expiration and cough. An MEP less than 40 cm H_2O is associated with a weak cough and clearance of respiratory secretions. An FVC of less than 30 ml/kg predisposes to atelectasis; values less than 10 ml/kg, or approximately 1 L, are associated with inadequate ventilation.

Laboratory

■ Studies will depend on the clinical concerns. B-type natriuretic peptide (BNP) has been demonstrated to predict acute congestive heart failure especially when levels exceed 500 pg/m. A quantitative d-dimer assay may be useful test in the evaluation of PE in the low-risk patient. Both the BNP and d-dimer assay require clinical interpretation and should be used with caution. Cardiac enzymes should be sent if concerned for cardiac ischemia.

■ Arterial blood gases (ABGs) are useful in determining the degree of hypoxia, carbon dioxide (CO_2) retention, and the presence of a metabolic versus respiratory acidosis (see Chapter 83). The alveolar-arterial oxygen gradient (A-a gradient) can be calculated from an ABG. It is the difference between the partial pressure of oxygen in the alveolar air (PaO_2) and the arterial blood (PaO_2). The A-a gradient is used primarily to differentiate between hypoxia due to hypoventilation (in which the A-a gradient is normal) and hypoxia due to ventilation–perfusion mismatch (in which the A-a gradient is abnormal). Conditions that cause abnormal oxygen exchange between the alveoli and the arterial blood result in an increase in the A-a gradient. The equation to calculate the A-a gradient on room air at sea level is $[150 - (PCO_2/0.8)] - PaO_2$.

■ A normal gradient should be less than 10 mm Hg in young persons and less than 20 mm Hg in older persons, and may be calculated as (age ÷ 4) + 4. The gradient will increase 5 mm Hg for every 10% increase in FiO_2 (fraction of the inspired air that is oxygen). The FiO_2 on room air is 21%.

Radiography

- Patients who are in respiratory distress, hypoxic, or are hemodynamically unstable should have a portable chest radiograph, and should not leave the resuscitation area. When possible, a good quality posteroanterior and lateral chest radiograph should be obtained.
- Bedside ultrasound can show pericardial tamponade, hemothorax, pneumothorax, effusions, and the quality of myocardial contraction.
- A computed tomography (CT scan) is useful for improved visualization of intrathoracic anatomy and pathology. CT pulmonary angiography using helical CT scanners and intravenous (IV) contrast delineate thoracic vasculature, and can show segmental pulmonary emboli.
- A ventilation-perfusion (V/Q) scan is a nuclear medicine study used to detect ventilation/perfusion defects in the lung, in the evaluation of suspected PE. A chest radiograph is useful in the interpretation of a scan. However, if the chest xray is abnormal, a CT angiogram is the preferred study in the evaluation of a PE.
- Angiography is considered the most accurate study for the diagnosis of PE, but is almost always performed after other diagnostic tests. Its use has been widely replaced by the use of CT angiography.

Emergency Department Management Overview
General

- The ABCs should be addressed as discussed above and in section II. If the patient in respiratory distress does not respond immediately to oxygen administration, endotracheal intubation should be performed. The decision to intubate is based on the failure to respond to therapy, not the individual diagnosis, and should never be delayed to await the numerical results of a study such as an arterial blood gas (ABG). Moreover, an ABG should never be obtained on room air in a patient in respiratory distress. Patients with high resistance failure (high blood pressure and fluid and salt overload) can often be managed without endotracheal intubation. Patients in pump failure (low blood pressure from and acute myocardial infarction) will need to be intubated early in their course.
- The decision to intubate is most often based on a failure to respond quickly to therapy. Noninvasive positive pressure ventilation (NIPPV) may be useful for some patients with asthma, COPD, and CHF to delay or avoid intubation allowing time for pharmacological measures to take effect. It is also helpful for patients with obstructive sleep apnea. NIPPV requires an alert patient who is able to cooperate. Airway management is discussed in Chapter 5.
- Emergent ED interventions include needle decompression and tube thoracostomy to relieve a tension pneumothorax or pericardiocentesis to relieve a pericardial tamponade (see Chapter 91).

Medications

- Medications given immediately to patients presenting with acute shortness of breath include bronchodilators and steroids for patients with allergic reactions (Chapter 19), asthma, or COPD exacerbations. Epinephrine or terbutaline may be given subcutaneously or IV in some cases (see Chapters 19 and 90.6).

■ Pulmonary edema may also present with severe respiratory distress. Diuretics (IV furosemide) and preload reduction (nitroglycerin) are part of the therapy (see Chapter 90.3).

■ When indicated, antibiotics should be started as quickly as possible. Once septic shock is present, mortality increases. In pneumonia, the goal is to start antibiotics within 4 hours of arrival in the hospital (see Chapter 67).

■ Anticoagulation with unfractionated heparin or low molecular weight heparin should be administered for PE. Thrombolytics may be indicated in a select number of patients (see Chapter 90.5).

Disposition

■ All dyspneic patients need frequent evaluation to observe response to therapy or disease progression.

■ Disposition will be based on the severity of the patient's symptoms and response to treatment, ability to ventilate and oxygenate, ability to take oral fluids and medications, degree of comfort, and fever control. All patients with persistent hypoxia should be admitted. Patients with multiple co-morbidities, immunocompromised status, and extremes of age are at higher risk for poor outcome, and probably require admission. Sociologic concerns may also force an admission decision (e.g., the homeless patient with a community-acquired pneumonia, will not be able to be treated as an outpatient).

Specific Problems

Acute Respiratory Distress Syndrome

Epidemiology and Risk Factors

■ Acute respiratory distress syndrome (ARDS) is a consequence of direct injury to the lungs or indirectly from circulating inflammatory mediators in response to a variety of insults. Examples of direct injury to the lungs include aspiration, inhalation injury, pneumonia, and pulmonary contusion. Indirect injury may be due to sepsis (most common), multi-system trauma, multiple transfusions, pancreatitis, high altitude (see Chapter 65), and drug overdose (e.g., aspirin and heroin, see Chapter 72). Acute lung injury (ALI) is the milder form of disease and has a PaO_2/FiO_2 ratio of less than or equal to 300 mm Hg.

■ The overall mortality rate varies between 35% and 60%.

Pathophysiology

■ ARDS is also known as noncardiogenic pulmonary edema, and is due to permeability changes in the pulmonary capillary membrane. In contrast, cardiogenic pulmonary edema primarily results from increased pulmonary hydrostatic pressure, which causes plasma ultrafiltrate to cross the pulmonary capillary membrane into the interstitium.

- Injury causes a release of cytokines that produce inflammation, increased permeability of the alveolar–capillary membrane, accumulation of protein-rich fluid in the alveolar air sacs, and fibrotic changes in the lungs. Protein-rich edema collects in dependent portions of the lung, which leads to shunting, decreased compliance, and hypoxemia.

History

- After the initial insult, symptoms of shortness of breath usually occur in 12 to 24 hours.

Physical Examination

- Tachypnea, tachycardia, and increased work of breathing. Fever may be present if an infectious source is present.
- Course rales may be present; however, initial auscultatory findings may be normal.
- Other findings include altered mental status (especially in the elderly) and cyanosis.
- Findings consistent with a cardiogenic source, such as peripheral edema, jugular venous distention, and ventricular gallop, are not present.

Diagnostic Testing

- Arterial blood gases, chest radiograph, and physical examination are used to diagnose ARDS. ARDS is defined as an acute presentation of lung injury that is characterized by a partial pressure of arterial oxygen to fractional inspired oxygen concentration ratio (PaO_2/FiO_2) that is less than 200 mm Hg (regardless of positive end-expiratory pressure or PEEP), bilateral infiltrates on chest radiograph, pulmonary artery wedge pressure less than 18 mm Hg (not relevant in the ED), or no clinical evidence of left atrial hypertension. Other studies should be directed to the underlying disease.
- Signs and symptoms of ARDS may precede chest radiograph findings. The classic findings of ARDS on chest radiograph include bilateral patchy infiltrates and normal heart size.

ED Management

- Treatment is primarily supportive, and is aimed at optimizing oxygenation and ventilation. Noninvasive ventilation techniques may be helpful particularly in ALI.
- Mechanical ventilation is often necessary for adequate gas exchange. Due to decreased lung compliance and high airway pressures, positive end-expiratory pressure (PEEP) (up to 15 cm H_2O) is frequently necessary. To minimize the risk of barotrauma, a small degree of respiratory acidosis and hypercapnia is acceptable (*permissive hypercapnea*). Tidal volumes of 6 ml/kg are recommended. Plateau pressures should be maintained at less than 30 cm H_2O to prevent barotrauma. High ventilatory rates of

more than 20 to 25 breaths per minute are often necessary in patients with ARDS because of increased physiologic dead space and smaller lung volume. Oxygen delivery (FiO_2) should be initially set at 100% until a lower value (preferably <60%) can be used to achieve adequate oxygenation. Goals of oxygen therapy include maintaining a PaO_2 of more than 58 to 60 mm Hg or oxygen saturation above 90%.

- The use of nitric oxide for ALI/ARDS should be limited to rescue therapy in patients with life-threatening hypoxemia not responding to traditional measures.
- Other ventilation therapies not routinely performed in the ED include inverse ratio ventilation (inspiratory to expiratory ratio is prolonged to 1:1 or greater) and prone positioning. Both may improve oxygenation and should be considered as a rescue therapy for patients with severe ARDS.
- Glucocorticoids in high doses have been the mainstay of treatment in severe noncardiogenic pulmonary edema because of their anti-inflammatory properties. However, they do not seem beneficial in the early phases on the disease.
- Although the pulmonary edema is not due to fluid overload, an increase in circulating blood volume can worsen alveolar fluid collection and deoxygenation. Fluid restriction should occur, but not to the degree to produce hypotension or decrease perfusion to end organs. Giving small doses of diuretics can produce significant reductions in extracellular alveolar edema, enhancing ventilatory function and oxygenation. Excessive or rapid diuresis may be harmful.

Helpful Hints and Pitfalls

- Although rarely seen in the ED, this diagnosis should be considered in individuals with rapid onset of respiratory failure and no evidence of heart failure.
- Partially treated intravascular volume overload and flash pulmonary edema can have the hemodynamic features similar to ARDS (pulmonary edema, a high cardiac output, and a low pulmonary artery wedge pressure).
- Increasing the PEEP will also increase intrathoracic pressure, and may lead to decreased cardiac output.

Asthma Exacerbation
Epidemiology and Risk Factors

- Asthma or reactive airway disease usually has an onset early in life. Adolescents and young adults are the most likely age groups to visit the ED for treatment. Acute episodic exacerbations are due to triggers such as a viral cold (most common), environmental allergens, irritants, and weather changes. Morbidity and mortality associated with asthma are due to an unperceived worsening of asthma attack frequency in a patient with moderately severe asthma, an acute unexpected external trigger, inadequate chronic management (such as no inhaled steroids), insufficient inhalation therapy, overreliance on over-the-counter medications, failure to perceive the patient's degree of increasing respiratory fatigue, or the development of a complication such as a pneumothorax.

Pathophysiology

- An attack is characterized by inflammation and reversible airflow obstruction from increased bronchial smooth muscle tone. The result is increased vascular permeability, mucus secretion, airway narrowing, limitation of airflow, bronchospasm, wheezing, lung hyperinflation, and ventilation–perfusion mismatching.
- Status asthmaticus is defined as severe bronchospasm that does not respond to aggressive therapy within 30 to 60 minutes.

History

- If the patient is able to communicate, it is helpful to know the patient's medication regimen, history of intubations or ICU admissions, last ED visit, frequency of rescue inhaler use, smoking history, presence of gastroesophageal reflux disease (GERD), cough, or postnasal drip.
- Typical complaints include coughing, wheezing, and dyspnea. The patient may also complain of chest tightness.

Physical Examination

- Diffuse wheezing is typically present. Exhalation is prolonged over inhalation. In the early stages, wheezing is expiratory. Accessory muscle use, retractions, and paradoxical abdominal movements are seen in severe cases. A chest that is quiet is an ominous sign because the patient is becoming fatigued and is unable to move enough air to cause wheezing.
- Pulsus paradoxus (see Appendix 2) greater than 20 mm Hg is often seen in asthma, but there is no absolute level of a pulsus paradoxus that determines the degree of asthmatic attack severity.

Diagnostic Testing

- An ABG is indicated for an attack that is worsening, doesn't respond to therapy, or if the patient has mental status changes. If the P_{CO_2} is normal or rising, it indicates that the patient is fatiguing, and beginning to ventilate inadequately. This patient will need endotracheal intubation and active airway management. It is preferable to avoid intubation in an asthmatic since the act itself worsens bronchoconstriction, does not overcome the airway block, and does not help the patient exhale trapped air. Nevertheless, if the patient fatigues and retains CO_2, it may be necessary. If intubation needs to be performed in the ED, use ketamine sedation because it also serves as a bronchodilator.
- Radiographs are not indicated in simple exacerbations, but should be obtained when there is concern for complications such as pneumonia or pneumothorax, or if the clinical diagnosis is uncertain.
- Serial peak flow measurements to follow improvements and degree from baseline are recommended.

ED Management

- Oxygen should always be given when the patient is hypoxic. In patients who present with a severe attack, IV access should be obtained, and the patient given gentle IV hydration.
- Inhaled β-agonists and steroids are indicated. Anticholinergic agents such as ipratropium bromide are indicated in the ED treatment of children and adults with severe acute asthma. IV magnesium has been suggested as an additional smooth muscle relaxant, and should be given in severe exacerbations. Parenteral administration of sympathomimetics (e.g., subcutaneous [SC] epinephrine) should be given for severe exacerbations and should be accompanied by electrocardiographic monitoring. Aminophylline is rarely used routinely any more, but there are some patients who seem to selectively respond to it. Leukotriene modifiers, such as nedocromil and cromolyn sodium, may benefit selected patients. Cromolyn sodium is most useful for exercise-induced asthma, but works best to prevent attacks, and will not provide therapeutic relief of an exacerbation. Steroids can often be given orally. For severe exacerbations, IV steroids should be given. A burst of steroids can be given over a 5-day period, and does not require a taper. It should be accompanied by the commencement or persistent use of inhaled steroids. Steroids take up to 8 hours to have effect if new-onset usage, but may work more quickly if the patient has taken a burst within the prior few months.
- Positive pressure ventilation with inline nebulized medications may prevent the need for intubation. PEEP can be increased to prevent small airway collapse and lessen work of breathing, but increases the risk of pneumothorax.
- If the patient is intubated, decreased tidal volumes, rapid flow rates, and decreased frequency with a prolonged expiratory phase help prevent barotrauma. Intubated asthmatic patients are prone to developing auto-PEEP and elevated intrathoracic pressure that may compromise cardiac output.
- Heliox may be considered for use in severely obstructed patients or patients with respiratory acidosis failing conventional treatment. It decreases airway resistance and respiratory work.
- The admission decision is based on a failure to improve, persistent hypoxia, CO_2 retention, multiple relapses over a short period of time, or inadequate social circumstances.
- All patients stable for discharge should receive a short burst of steroids, inhalers of bronchodilators, and instructions on appropriate use with spacers. They also require close and early follow-up. Dosing for common medications used in the treatment of asthma is listed in Chapter 90.6.

Helpful Hints and Pitfalls

- A normal range $PaCO_2$ in a tachypneic patient is an ominous finding suggesting fatigue and impending respiratory failure.
- Asthma can be precipitated by the use of beta-blocker medications or nonsteroidal anti-inflammatory drugs (NSAIDs).

Chronic Obstructive Pulmonary Disease Exacerbation
Definition

- COPD refers to a spectrum of pulmonary disorders that have the common feature of airway obstruction. The two major disorders recognized as part of the spectrum of COPD are emphysema and chronic bronchitis.
- Chronic bronchitis is defined functionally as a disease characterized by cough and mucus hypersecretion for at least 3 months of the year, for two consecutive years, with airway obstruction as defined by spirometry.
- Emphysema is the result of abnormal, permanent enlargement of the air spaces distal to the terminal bronchioles, with destruction of their walls but without obvious fibrosis.
- Chronic bronchitis and emphysema should not be considered isolated disorders, since most patients with COPD have clinical features of coexistent chronic bronchitis and emphysema.

Epidemiology and Risk Factors

- Slowly progressive airway obstruction in middle-aged and elderly patients.
- Both chronic bronchitis and emphysema are typically the result of the same etiologic factors (i.e., exposure to cigarette smoke).

Pathophysiology

- There are progressive inflammatory changes in the lung due to noxious stimuli that result in restriction of airflow. The changes are not fully reversible.
- The end results of the process include gas diffusion abnormalities, over-production of mucous, pulmonary hypertension, cor pulmonale (enlargement of the right ventricle caused by pulmonary hypertension), and reduced ability of the cilia to clear secretions.

History

- Acute exacerbations are defined clinically by a combination of increased dyspnea, sputum production, and sputum volume compared with baseline.

Physical Examination

- Dyspnea and tachypnea will be present. Course upper airway sounds or wheezes may be heard. Patients often exhibit pursed-lip respirations to ease work of breathing by maintaining a positive end expiratory pressure.

Diagnostic Testing

- Spirometry after a bronchodilator demonstrating a FEV_1 of less than 30% and a FEV_1-to-FVC ratio of less than 0.7 confirms the diagnosis.

- A chest radiograph usually demonstrates hyperinflation with flattened diaphragm, tenting of the diaphragm at the rib insertions, and increased retrosternal air space. Decreased vascular markings and bullae may be evident in patients with emphysema.

ED Management

- Aerosolized β-agonists, anticholinergic bronchodilators, and steroids are the mainstay of therapy (Chapter 90.6).
- Low-flow oxygen is indicated in all hypoxemic patients presenting with COPD exacerbation to maintain oxygen saturation levels of at least 90% to 92%. High-flow oxygen may lead to hypoxic arrest in a patient who has become insensitive to high or rising CO_2, and whose ventilation is driven by hypoxia. However, high-flow oxygen should not be withheld in the patient with severe respiratory distress and hypoxia who may require intubation. Bilevel positive airway pressure (BiPAP) or continuous positive airway pressure (CPAP) are non invasive positive pressure ventilations, and their use may decrease the need for intubation in certain patients.
- Many patients can be managed without intubation. Their status is dependent upon their level of consciousness, their ability to cough, and their level of CO_2.
- Patients with persistent hypoxemia, failure to improve, respiratory acidosis, or multiple co-morbidities are at high risk for poor outcome, and should be admitted for continued treatment.
- If discharged, patients should receive continued steroids for 3 to 14 days, bronchodilators in combination (β-agonist plus anticholinergic bronchodilators), and an antibiotic such as a macrolide, fluoroquinolone, or amoxicillin-clavulanate (Chapter 90.2). Guaifenesin can improve cough symptoms and mucous clearance, thereby lessening the duration of acute exacerbations of chronic obstructive bronchitis.
- Patients with a PaO_2 less than 55 mm Hg or pulse oximetry below 90% should be set up with home oxygen.

Helpful Hints and Pitfalls

- Many patients have concomitant COPD and heart failure, and are difficult to diagnose when short of breath. BNP levels can be elevated in patients with cor pulmonale secondary to COPD; therefore, elevated levels should be interpreted with caution and are not pathognomonic for CHF.
- Patients with chronic bronchitis present with a chronic and constant wet cough. They are usually heavy, broad-chested patients as opposed to the wasted muscular atrophic appearance of the classic patient with COPD. They often have cor pulmonale with right ventricular enlargement on EKG and severe peripheral edema. They often benefit from treatment for bronchitis with steroids, bronchodilators, and antibiotics, but also often need bed rest, diuresis, and withdrawal from tobacco. Due to overcrowding of hospitals, they often cannot be admitted, and thus do not have an opportunity to diurese and clear their bronchitis, which means recurrent visits to the ED.

Interstitial Lung Disease

- A group of disorders involving the lung interstitium and characterized by inflammation of the alveolar structures and progressive parenchymal fibrosis.
- The most common presenting complaint of patients with interstitial lung disease is gradual but progressive dyspnea. It may initially be present only with exertion, but may occur at rest as the disease progresses.
- The physical examination, including auscultation of the chest, may be entirely normal early in the disease process. Basilar crackles (Velcro rales) signal the presence of interstitial pulmonary fibrosis. However, the absence of crackles does not exclude the diagnosis.
- Cyanosis and finger clubbing may develop. With advanced disease, cardiac involvement is common as a consequence of pulmonary hypertension and right-sided heart failure. With the exception of sarcoidosis and the collagen vascular diseases, the physical findings are generally limited to the chest.
- The chest radiograph may be abnormal in the absence of significant symptoms or normal in a symptomatic patient. Early in the disease process, radiographic changes may be limited to an increase in interstitial markings, more prominent in the lower lung fields. Bilateral hilar adenopathy is suggestive of sarcoidosis. A high-resolution CT scan of the lung can reveal minimal interstitial disease not evident on conventional chest radiographs.
- Steroids are beneficial. Patients who are not acutely hypoxic and are nontoxic-appearing can be discharged. The patient should be referred to a pulmonologist for further evaluation and management.

Pleural Effusion
Definitions

- A pleural effusion is the presence of an abnormally large amount of fluid in the pleural space. A parapneumonic effusion is a pleural effusion associated with bacterial pneumonia, bronchiectasis, or lung abscess. Empyema (or pus in the pleural space) is present when there is bacteria on Gram's stain of the pleural fluid. A hemothorax is blood in the pleural space, and a chylothorax results from rupture of the thoracic duct.

Epidemiology and Risk Factors

- The most common cause in Western countries is congestive heart failure, followed by malignancy, bacterial pneumonia, and PE. The leading cause in developing countries is tuberculosis.
- Other conditions include trauma, pancreatitis, myxedema, viral infections of the lung parenchyma or pleura, cirrhosis, uremia, nephrotic syndrome, collagen vascular diseases (e.g., systemic lupus erythematosus, rheumatoid arthritis), and intra-abdominal processes (e.g., acute pancreatitis, subphrenic abscess, ascites). Esophageal perforation is a rare but serious cause of a pleural effusion.

Table 52–4	Conditions Causing Pleural Effusion
Transudate	**Exudate**
Congestive heart failure	Bacterial pneumonia
Cirrhosis with ascites	Bronchiectasis
Nephrotic syndrome	Lung abscess
Hypoalbuminemia	Tuberculosis
Myxedema	Malignancy
Renal failure	Connective tissue disease (e.g., systemic
Superior vena cava syndrome	lupus erythematosus)
Pulmonary embolism	Gastrointestinal disorders (e.g.,
	pancreatitis, esophageal rupture)
	Uremia
	Drug reaction
	Cylothorax
	Pulmonary embolism

Pathophysiology

- Fluid collects in the pleural space, and compresses the lung leading to impaired ventilation.
- Pleural fluid is classified into two categories: transudates or exudates (Table 52–4). A transudate is essentially an ultrafiltrate of plasma that contains very little protein, and develops when there is an increase in the hydrostatic pressure or decrease in the oncotic pressure within pleural microvessels. The most common cause is congestive heart failure. Exudates contain relatively high amounts of protein, reflecting an abnormality of the pleura itself, and are the result of increased membrane permeability or defective lymphatic drainage. Parapneumonic effusion and malignancy are the most common conditions associated with an exudative effusion. The pleural fluid in association with a pulmonary embolus can be transudative or exudative and can be found in up to 50% of patients.

History

- Other than when due to trauma or thoracic aortic rupture, the symptoms are slowly progressive. Symptoms include shortness of breath, dyspnea on exertion, orthopnea, cough, and pleuritic chest pain.

Physical Examination

- Tachypnea, dullness to percussion over the affected lung, or absence of breath sounds may be found on physical examination.

Diagnostic Testing

- A thoracentesis may be performed to determine if the effusion is a transudate or an exudate (see Chapter 91 for procedure and Appendix for pleural fluid analysis). The study is both diagnostic and therapeutic. Send samples for Gram's stain and culture, amylase, cell count, protein, glucose, lactate dehydrogenase (LDH), protein, and pH. Patients with bilateral pleural effusions and a reasonable explanation for the effusion (e.g., volume overload from congestive heart failure) do not require a thoracentesis in the ED, but instead should be treated for the underlying cause of the effusion (i.e., diuresis).

- Any other laboratory studies should be directed to the suspected underlying cause. It is helpful to obtain coagulation studies before attempting an invasive procedure.
- An upright chest radiograph may demonstrate blunting of the costophrenic angle (minimal amount to be seen on radiograph is approximately 150 ml) or complete opacification. Lateral decubitus views should be obtained to determine if the effusion will layer to 1 cm thick (another indication for thoracentesis).
- A CT scan is superior for demonstrating intrathoracic pathology, and may lead to a diagnosis of the underlying problem.

ED Management

- Depends on the underlying cause. A tube thoracostomy is indicated for an empyema.
- Re-expansion pulmonary edema may develop if too much fluid (usually >1.5 L) is withdrawn during the thoracentesis.

Helpful Hints and Pitfalls

- Pleuradesis may be required in recurrent effusions.
- Obtain a postthoracentesis chest radiograph to evaluate for pneumothorax.

Pneumothorax (Spontaneous)
Epidemiology and Risk Factors

- Primary spontaneous pneumothorax occurs in individuals without underlying lung disease. It is more common in tall, thin males. Smoking, substance abuse (heroine, ecstasy, marijuana, speed, and cocaine), and changes in ambient atmospheric pressure are risk factors.
- Secondary spontaneous pneumothorax is a consequence of an underlying pulmonary disease process. Individuals with Marfan's syndrome are at risk due to connective tissue defects resulting in apical pleural blebs, which then rupture. Other examples include COPD, lung cancer, cystic fibrosis, *Pneumocystis carinii* pneumonia (PCP), tuberculosis, and lung abscess.

Pathophysiology

- The visceral and parietal pleura are in close apposition to each other, with only a "potential" space between them. The negative pressure in the intrapleural space helps to keep the lungs expanded. The alveolar walls and visceral pleura form a barrier that separates this potential space from the intra-alveolar spaces, and help maintain the pressure gradient. Inspired air escapes from a defect in this barrier into the pleural space, becomes trapped, and destroys the negative intrapleural pressure. As pressure builds and ultimately becomes higher than atmospheric pressure, the lung will be unable to expand, the trachea and mediastinum will shift to the opposite side, relaxation of the heart will be impaired, pressure on the vena cava will compromise cardiac venous return, and blood pressure will drop. This is known as a *tension* pneumothorax and is a life-threatening event.

History

- There is usually a rapid onset of shortness of breath proceeded by pleuritic (made worse with deep inspiration) chest pain.
- Cough is present in a minority of individuals.

Physical Examination

- There will be a unilateral absence of breath sounds and hyperresonance to percussion. Subcutaneous emphysema (crepitus to palpation) may be present if the parietal pleura is disrupted.
- In tension pneumothorax, the patient will appear ill, and present with tachycardia, tachypnea, dyspnea, and hypotension. Jugulovenous distention (JVD) may be present. Tracheal deviation and hypotension are late findings. Hypoxemia is early and profound, but therapy should not be delayed to obtain a chest radiograph or ABG.

Diagnostic Testing

- Tension pneumothorax is a clinical diagnosis requiring immediate intervention. A chest radiograph study is useful prior and after insertion of the chest tube for a simple pneumothorax in the stable patient; expiratory films are preferred. A chest CT scan is much more accurate than a plain chest radiograph for small pneumothorax, anterior pneumothorax, and confusing diseases such as pulmonary blebs. An ultrasound study can differentiate between a pneumothorax and a large bleb.

ED Management

- Interventions for a pneumothorax are similar to those described in Chapter 13.
- For a primary pneumothorax in a stable patient, a small catheter tube thoracostomy may be performed, and attached to a Heimlich valve. The patient can be evaluated daily, and treated as an outpatient if social circumstances permit.
- If the spontaneous pneumothorax is recurrent, or if there is evidence of pulmonary blebs, a thoracic surgeon should be consulted since it may be prudent to take the patient to surgery for removal of the bleb and pleurodesis. The patient should be advised to avoid air travel and diving.

Helpful Hints and Pitfalls

- Quantifying the amount of pneumothorax is inaccurate with plain films. A CT scan may show unexpected multiple pneumothoraces or pulmonary blebs.
- Positive pressure ventilation may cause or worsen an existing pneumothorax leading to a tension pneumothorax.
- The average reabsorption rate is in the range of 1% to 2% a day and can be increased by a factor of 4 with the administration of 100% oxygen.
- Reexpansion pulmonary edema and reexpansion hypotension are rare occurrences after rapid evacuation of a large pneumothorax, and relate to how long the pneumothorax was present before re-expansion (>3 days).

Pulmonary Edema
Epidemiology and Risk Factors

- Pulmonary edema is clinically differentiated into cardiogenic and non-cardiogenic. Most people who present to the ED have cardiogenic pulmonary edema, which is mainly due to elevated pulmonary capillary hydrostatic pressure, and occurs with acute coronary syndrome, cardiomyopathy, valvular heart disease, and hypertensive emergencies.
- Noncardiogenic pulmonary edema results from an alteration in the permeability characteristics of the pulmonary capillary membrane. There are multiple causes which include drowning, high altitude, sepsis, inhalation injury, drugs or toxins, aspiration, neurogenic causes, and adult respiratory distress syndrome (discussed earlier).

Pathophysiology

- The underlying etiology can be simplified into acutely elevated afterload (high resistance failure), acute pump failure, and acute changes in hydrostatic forces. However, elements of all three underlying mechanisms may be present concomitantly.
- In elevated afterload, the peripheral resistance that the heart must pump against is pathologically higher than the pressure that the heart is able to generate. In pump failure, the left ventricle is unable to create cardiac output to circulate blood from the pulmonary vessels. Hydrostatic forces can push or pull fluid into the alveoli. Noncardiogenic pulmonary edema generally results from an alteration in the permeability characteristics of the pulmonary capillary membrane. The result, regardless of the mechanism, is fluid collection within the alveoli that decreases gas diffusion and leads to hypoxemia.

History

- Patients typically complain of shortness of breath and cough with white or pink sputum. Chest pain may be present in valvular rupture or myocardial infarction. Dyspnea on exertion is one of the earliest complaints. Orthopnea is common due to the increased venous return in the supine position. Paroxysmal nocturnal dyspnea may be present for the same reason.

■ Medications, illicit drug use, and recent procedures should be reviewed. Determine medication compliance and dietary indiscretions.

Physical Examination

■ Tachypnea, crackles, wheezing, and labored breathing are findings. Edema may be present. A systolic cardiac murmur suggests mitral regurgitation or aortic stenosis. A diastolic murmur indicates mitral stenosis or aortic regurgitation.

■ Evaluate for signs of hypoperfusion such as clammy skin, a thready pulse, or delayed capillary refill.

Diagnostic Testing

■ The EKG should be evaluated for patterns of strain or ischemia.

■ Laboratory studies include chemistry, renal function, CBC, coagulation studies, cardiac enzymes, and a urine toxicology screen (if indicated). Beta-natriuretic peptide (BNP) may help identify CHF as the origin of acute dyspnea. Levels of BNP < 100 pg/mL are unlikely to be from CHF. Levels 100-500 pg/mL may be CHF, and levels >500 pg/mL are most consistent with CHF. Other conditions that increase right filling pressures may also increase BNP levels (e.g., pulmonary embolus, cirrhosis, end stage renal failure).

■ An upright chest radiograph may reveal diffuse patchy alveolar infiltrates; cardiomegaly is usually seen with high resistance and pump failure, whereas normal heart size is seen with noncardiogenic pulmonary edema. In the early stages of CHF, minimal cardiomegaly and redistribution of the pulmonary vascularity may be seen. As CHF worsens, fluid may be seen in the interlobular septa at the lateral basal aspects of the lung (mean capillary wedge pressures of 25 to 30 mm Hg). These are referred to as Kerley B lines, are always located just inside the ribs, and are horizontal in orientation. As CHF becomes more pronounced, vessels near the hila become indistinct because of fluid accumulating in the interstitium. Pleural effusions may be present. With pronounced CHF, fluid accumulates in the alveolar spaces, and is seen as bilateral, predominantly basilar and perihilar alveolar infiltrates (>30 mm Hg) (Figure 52–1).

■ Echocardiography is helpful to gauge cardiac contractility, volume status and the presence of valvular dysfunction.

ED Management

■ Give supplemental oxygen and position the patient for comfort (e.g., head of bed elevated, feet dangling over the side of the bed).

■ Hypertensive emergencies (Chapter 39) leading to pulmonary edema require rapid reduction of the patient's afterload. Nitroprusside, labetolol, esmolol, and nesiritide are commonly used afterload reducers. Hydralazine is indicated during pregnancy.

■ If the patient is hemodynamically stable, therapy begins with diuresis (e.g., furosemide) and nitrate therapy (IV or SL nitroglycerin). Nitroglycerin decreases preload and dilates coronary vessels; it reduces afterload

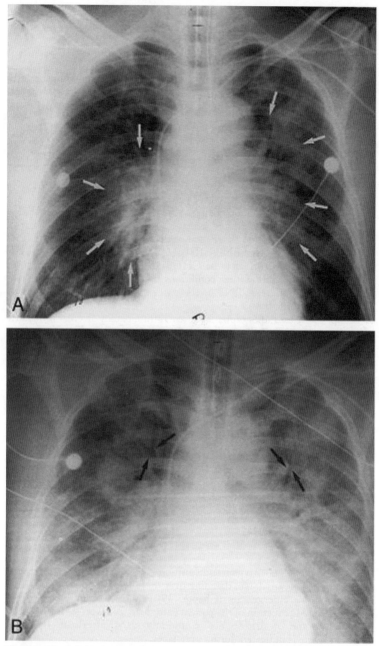

Figure 52–1. Pulmonary edema, or fluid overload, can be manifested by indistinctness of the pulmonary vessels as they radiate from the hilum **(A)**. This is sometimes termed a *bat wing* infiltrate. As pulmonary edema worsens **(B)**, fluid fills the alveoli, and air bronchograms (*arrows*) become apparent. *(From Mettler F. Essentials of Radiology (2nd ed). New York: Elsevier, 2005, p 98.)*

at higher doses. Angiotensin-converting enzyme inhibitors (ACES) are used to reduce afterload. Nesiritide may be a useful alternative to nitroglycerin. It causes venodilatation and diuresis with less hypotension.

- Patients in true cardiogenic shock often require inotropic and vasopessor therapy, intra-aortic balloon counter pulsation, and assisted ventilation. Some of these patients may require a small fluid challenge (250 ml NS) to correct hypovolemia. Dobutamine may increase cardiac contractility. Dopamine may also be needed to maintain a reasonable perfusion pressure.
- Pulmonary edema due to changes in hydrostatic forces requires supportive care. Diuretics may be required if the patient is fluid overloaded. The treatment for HAPE is discussed in Chapter 65.
- See Chapter 90.3 for Cardiovascular Pharmacology. Patients in cardiogenic shock often require endotracheal intubation. All should have hemodynamic monitoring in the critical care setting.

Helpful Hints and Pitfalls

- Failure to consider the underlying pathologic mechanism is detrimental to the patient because treatments are different.
- Heart failure is a diagnosis based on the overall clinical impression. Laboratory tests (i.e., BNP), if obtained, should only be used for confirmation, as levels can be elevated in any condition that causes ventricular dilatation.

Pulmonary Embolism
Epidemiology and Risk Factors

- Pulmonary embolism (PE) is often a difficult diagnosis to make and is often missed. One must consider the diagnosis to search for it, and the initial presentation can be misleadingly benign.
- Risk factors form the pretest probability. The Well's criteria are tools for calculating pretest probability (Table 52–5).

Table 52–5 Pretest Probability for PE	
PE is most likely diagnosis	3
Presence of a DVT	3
Heart rate over 100	1.5
Immobilized	1.5
Recent surgery	1.5
History of a VTE	1.5
Hemoptysis	1
Malignancy	1
High probability	**over 6**
Moderate probability	**2–6**
Low probability	**less than 2**

DVT, deep venous thrombosis; PE, pulmonary embolism; VTE, venous thromboembolism.
From Wells PS, et al. Excluding pulmonary embolism at the bedside without diagnostic imaging: management of patients with suspected pulmonary embolism presenting to the emergency department by using a simple clinical model and d-dimer. Ann Intern Med 2001;135:98–107.

Pathophysiology

- Virchow described a triad of stasis (prolonged bed rest or travel), vascular injury (trauma or postsurgical), and hypercoagulability as risk factors for the development of a venous thromboembolism (VTE). A PE is a VTE that dislodges and travels into the pulmonary circulation creating a ventilation–perfusion mismatch.
- Hypercoagulation may be due to genetic problems, smoking, pregnancy, obesity, hormone replacement, contraception, or malignancy.
- Most PEs are thought to originate from lower extremity due to a deep vein thrombosis. The mortality from a PE has been estimated between 5% and 10%.

History

- Shortness of breath is the most common symptom. Other patients may have pleuritic chest pain, syncope, or hemoptysis.
- Syncope may also be the initial presentation.

Physical Examination

- Tachycardia is the most common finding. Lung sounds are nonspecific.
- With massive PE, hypotension, diaphoresis, JVD, respiratory arrest, or cardiac arrest may be initial findings.
- The extremity examination may reveal unilateral pain and swelling.

Diagnostic Testing

- The EKG is nondiagnostic, and may only demonstrate nonspecific sinus tachycardia. Right axis deviation or a prominent $S_1Q_3T_3$ pattern may be seen, but is not reliably seen often enough to confirm the diagnosis.
- There are no laboratory tests diagnostic for PE. With low-probability pretest screening, some quantitative d-dimer assays have an excellent negative predictive value and preclude further workup. If elevated, the d-dimer is neither helpful nor diagnostic. The test has no value in patients with an intermediate or high pretest probability. An ABG is not diagnostic, and many patients with a normal blood gas levels have a PE. Small PEs do not impair pulmonary gas exchange, and many types of pulmonary pathology can affect the A-a gradient. A large PE often causes an increased A-a gradient, however, a normal arterial blood gas can be seen in up to 23% of patients with symptomatic PE. When a PE is present, studies such as factor V Leiden, protein C and S, antithrombin III, and antiphospholipid studies are ordered to determine if the patient has a hypercoagulable state.
- A chest radiograph should be obtained to look for other diseases and rarely can be read as a PE. An elevated right hemidiaphragm and atelectasis are common findings. A Hampton's hump (a wedge-shaped consolidation at the lung periphery is suggestive of pulmonary infarction) or a Westermark's sign (decreased pulmonary vascular markings) are rarely seen.

- Echocardiography may demonstrate right ventricular dilatation or pulmonary hypertension.
- Ventilation/perfusion (V/Q) scan requires a stable patient and often a normal chest radiograph findings. Results are reported as normal, low probability, intermediated probability, or high probability (Table 52–6). There is high likelihood of a PE in a positive scan with high pretest probability. There is low likelihood of a PE in a patient with a normal scan and low pre-test probability (approximately 1%). Many V/Q scans are nondiagnostic and the patient requires further investigation. The V/Q scan is a safe test for a pregnant patient.
- A spiral CT angiogram (CTA) can demonstrate PE down to the sub-segments of the pulmonary arterial system (Figure 52–2), but is not able to detect a subsegmental PE, which is of unknown clinical significance. A CTA must be combined with clinical pretest probability to determine disposition. It is also useful to demonstrate alternative diagnoses.
- Pulmonary angiography has been considered the most accurate diagnostic imaging study to reveal PE, but it is an invasive study, and may also miss subsegmental emboli (approximately 1%). Most interventional radiologists request a prior imaging study before proceeding to angiogram such as V/Q scan or CTA.
- Ultrasound can be used to diagnose lower extremity deep venous thrombosis in patients who have a nondiagnostic study, or are unable to have a diagnostic study. Although a positive study in a patient with chest symptoms clinches the diagnosis, it does not have a great enough frequency to be of value, even though most PE originate in the leg veins.
- An MRI is useful in pregnant patients but has not been extensively studied.

Table 52–6	**Ventilation–Perfusion Scan Interpretation for Pulmonary Embolism**
Result	**Interpretation**
Normal	No perfusion defects are seen. At least 2% of patients with PE have this pattern, and 4% of patients with this pattern have PE.
Low probability	14 % have PE overall; 40% in high clinical suspicion group, 16% in moderate suspicion, 4% in low suspicion group.
Intermediate probability	Any V/Q abnormality not otherwise classified. Approximately 40% of patients with PE fall into this category and 30% of all patients with this pattern have PE.
High probability	41% of patients with PE have this pattern and 87% of patients with this pattern have PE. In most clinical settings, a high-probability scan pattern may be considered positive for PE.

PE, *pulmonary embolism; V/Q, ventilation–perfusion scan.*

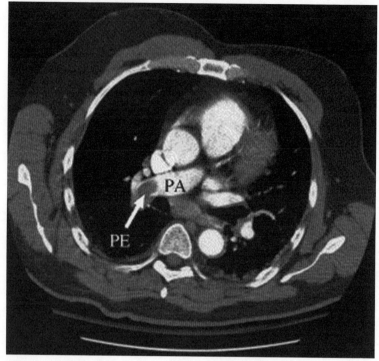

Figure 52–2. Pulmonary embolus (PE) located in the proximal pulmonary artery (PA) as seen on CT angiogram. (*From Laack TA, Goyal DG. Pulmonary embolism: an unsuspected killer. Emerg Med Clin North Am 2004;22:961–883.*)

Emergency Department Management

- Disposition will depend on pretest probability combined with the results from the chosen diagnostic study. An algorithm for a general approach to a patient with a suspected PE is described in Figure 52–3.
- For massive PE with hemodynamic instability, thrombolytics are indicated (see Chapter 90.5).
- All patients with an intermediate pretest probability should undergo further diagnostic studies. If the clinical picture is strongly consistent with PE, it may be prudent to anticoagulate with heparin (preferentially low-molecular-heparin heparin), admit the patient, and obtain further studies after admission to the hospital.
- All patients with confirmed PE should be admitted for anticoagulation, monitoring, and further evaluation.
- Patients who cannot undergo anticoagulation, or who have a recurrent PE while anticoagulated, will require an inferior vena cava filter.

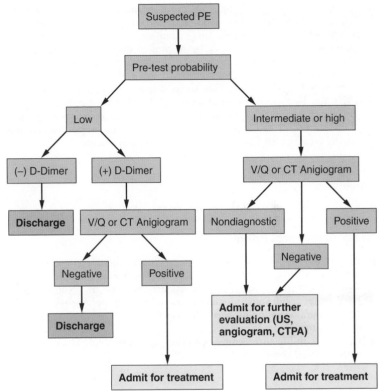

Figure 52–3. Algorithm for approach to patient with a pulmonary embolism.

Helpful Hints and Pitfalls

- Pitfalls include failure to consider the diagnosis and failure to know the type of d-dimer study available.
- Other types of emboli include air, amniotic fluid, and foreign bodies but these are not treated with anticoagulation.
- Consider PE in any patient with unexplained shortness of breath or tachycardia.

Pulmonary Hypertension

- Decreased left ventricular compliance, lung parenchymal disease (such as COPD), or decreased pulmonary artery compliance leads to increased pulmonary artery resistance. Obesity, COPD, valvular heart disease, and chronic pulmonary emboli are risk factors. Increased right ventricular pressures lead to dilatation and ultimately right heart failure (cor pulmonale).

- Patients present with dyspnea on exertion and evidence of right heart failure (peripheral edema, JVD and hepatojugular reflux). Tricuspid regurgitation may be present. Lung sounds are clear.
- Pulmonary function tests may be helpful to diagnose underlying lung disease. A chest radiograph may demonstrate pulmonary artery enlargement. An echocardiogram may detect right ventricular dilatation or tricuspid regurgitation. Due to stretch in the right ventricle, BNP levels may be elevated in the absence of left-sided heart failure.
- Treatment is supportive and admission may be required for management of cor pulmonale and hypoxia. Pulmonary and cardiology consultation is usually required for further evaluation and management.

Special Considerations
Pediatrics

- Refer to Chapter 76, "Pediatric Respiratory Problems."

Immunocompromised Patient

- Respiratory complaints in these patients are commonly encountered in the ED. Although infectious processes may come to mind initially, significant noninfectious conditions also may occur. Noninfectious pulmonary conditions include therapy-induced pulmonary toxicity, thromboembolism, pulmonary hemorrhage, and pulmonary progression of the primary disease process.
- Patients with life-threatening conditions may have fever alone or vague constitutional complaints.

Teaching Points

The dyspneic patient is immediately recognizable at the triage desk. Although there are myriad causes of dyspnea, all of these patients are seriously ill. They should be triaged quickly, and placed on oxygen, a cardiac monitor, and pulse oximetry, and have IV access.

It is useful to attempt to immediately separate cardiac from pulmonary causes, but unfortunately, many patients with chronic lung disease can develop cor pulmonale, and have a cardiac contribution to the dyspnea.

If the primary cause is cardiac, quickly distinguish between high-resistance pulmonary edema, and pump failure cardiac edema. The former will have a high blood pressure, and is unlikely to be having an acute heart attack. The latter will be in shock, and is likely to be having a myocardial infarction that involves more than 30% of the left ventricle. The former will respond to lowering the high resistance, with diuretics, morphine, oxygen, and nitrates, and will probably not have to be intubated. The latter is more consistent with cardiogenic shock, and the patient will require immediate intubation, pressor therapy, and

Teaching Points—cont'd

possibly an intra-aortic balloon pump. Dyspnea may also be the "chest pain" equivalent in some patients such as diabetics who may not develop chest pain during an acute cardiac ischemic event.

If the cause is respiratory, it is useful to separate infectious from chronic lung disease. This is accomplished by the presence of fever, chest pain, and often chest radiograph findings.

The common causes of chronic lung disease are best divided into reactive airway disease (asthma), emphysema, and chronic bronchitis. There is clearly some overlap between all of these entities since they can all have an element of bronchoconstriction and hypersecretion. Asthmatics are generally younger, have a known history of the disease, are usually taking some asthmatic medications, and have expiratory prolongation and increased secretions that are often thick and green. Emphysematous patients often have a prolonged smoking history, have severe muscle wasting, expanded anteroposterior chest diameter, and chronic respiratory failure. Patients with chronic bronchitis are usually plethoric, beefy, wide-chested patients with a chronic wet cough. They also are heavy cigarette smokers. They often have severe right-sided heart failure.

Treatment for all chronic lung disease includes bronchodilatation, steroid administration, and attempts to improve oxygenation; therapy often is successful without the admission of the patient. Patients who fail to respond to vigorous treatment may require endotracheal intubation and all require admission.

Suggested Readings

Belleza WG, Browne B. Pulmonary considerations in the immunocompromised patient. Emerg Med Clin North Am 2003;21:499–531, x–xi.

Braithwaite S, Perina D. Dyspnea. In: Marx JA, Hockberger RS, Walls RM (editors). Rosen's Emergency Medicine: Concepts and Clinical Practice (6th ed). Philadelphia: Mosby, 2006, pp 175–181.

Edlow JA. Emergency department management of pulmonary embolism. Emerg Med Clin North Am 2001;19:9995–1011.

Kosowsky JM. Pleural disease. In: Marx JA, Hockberger RS, Walls RM (editors). Rosen's Emergency Medicine: Concepts and Clinical Practice (6th ed). St. Louis, MO: Mosby, 2006;1143–1154.

Laack TA, MD, Goyal DG. Pulmonary embolism: an unsuspected killer. Emerg Med Clin North Am 2004;22:961–983.

McCrory DC, Brown C, Gelfand SE, et al. Management of acute exacerbations of COPD: a summary and appraisal of published evidence. Chest 2001;119:1190–1209.

Michelson E, Hollrah S. Evaluation of the patient with shortness of breath: an evidenced based approach. Emerg Med Clin North Am 1999;17:221–237.

Perina D. Noncardiogenic pulmonary edema. Emerg Med Clin North Am 2003;21:385–393.

Raghu G, Brown KK. Interstitial lung disease: clinical evaluation and keys to an accurate diagnosis. Clin Chest Med 2004;25:409–419, v.

CHAPTER 53

Sickle Cell Disease

PILAR GUERRERO

Red Flags

Very young • Chest pain or shortness of breath • Sepsis • Sudden drop in hematocrit • Priapism longer than 12 hours • New neurologic deficit • Fever • Tachycardia • Tachyprea • Hypotension • Hypoxia

Overview

Sickle cell disease (SCD) is a hereditary hemoglobinopathy that affects many organ systems. The result is a chronic hemolytic anemia resulting in complications that are due to vaso-occlusive disease, worsening anemia, and infection. Look for "red flags" (see Box), and identify critical patients early.

A *vaso-occlusive crisis* occurs when sickled RBCs cause obstruction in the microcirculation leading to end-organ ischemia. Pain is the most frequent complaint. Vaso-occlusive crisis can involve the bones, joints, soft tissue, abdominal organs, lungs (i.e., acute chest syndrome), central nervous system (e.g., stroke), retina (i.e., retinal hemorrhages), and penis (i.e., priapism). A *hematologic crisis* is when there is a sudden exacerbation of anemia. This may be due to acute splenic sequestration in which sickled cells block splenic outflow, leading to the pooling of peripheral blood in the engorged spleen (seen in young patients with functioning spleens), or it can occur when the bone marrow stops producing new RBCs (aplastic crisis). An *infectious crisis* is the result of the functional asplenia that is common to most adults with SCD, which predisposes them to infections with encapsulated organisms such as *Haemophilus* influenzae or *Streptococcus* pneumoniae.

In the United States approximately 1:500 African American births and 1:1000-1400 Hispanic American births are affected with SCD. Sickle cell trait (heterozygous condition) is seen in approximately 1:12 African Americans. Under normal circumstances, no clinical signs of disease or hematologic abnormalities are present. However, acidosis or hypoxia may cause sickling and vascular complications.

The responsible mutation is transferred in an autosomal recessive manner. The primary contributing factor is the substitution of valine for glutamic acid in the β-chain gene of hemoglobin A. There are several sickle genotypes. The homozygous genotype has the most severe phenotype (HbSS). When this abnormal hemoglobin is deoxygenated, it forms polymers, then a gel, and finally a crystal. This results in a less deformable, sickle structure of the erythrocyte.

The sickle cells get trapped in the venule side of the micro-circulation, causing vaso-occlusion hypoxia, and resulting in an increase in HbS polymer formation, and then the cycle continues.

Chronic anemia in SCD is caused by red cell sequestration and destruction by the spleen and liver. The life span of a normal RBC is 120 days versus a sickle cell that ranges from 4 to 20 days.

System-based complications found in SCD are listed in Table 53–1.

Table 53–1 System-Based Complications in Sickle Cell Disease*

System	Complication
Pulmonary	Infection, infarct, embolism, acute chest syndrome, pulmonary HTN
Cardiac	Congestive heart failure
CNS	Cerebrovascular accident
Vascular	Occlusion at any site
Spleen	Acute sequestration
Liver	Hepatitis, infarct
Renal	Hematuria, hyposthesuria, end-stage renal failure
Gallbladder	Gallstones
Erythrocytes	Chronic hemolysis, aplastic crisis
Leukocytes	Immunodeficiency, sepsis, meningitis
Skeletal	Infarcts, aseptic necrosis, osteomyelitis
Skin	Ulcers
Eye	Retinopathy, retinal hemorrhage
Placenta	Insufficiency, fetal demise
Genital	Priapism, impotence, decreased fertility

Common acute manifestations are in bold.

Initial Diagnostic Approach
General

- The vast majority of patients presenting to the ED have known SCD, and present with complications of the disease.
- A thorough history is most helpful. Pain that is familiar to the patient and typical for the patient's usual symptoms can be reassuring. Beware of conditions mimicking a sickle cell painful process. Patients with abdominal pain can still have appendicitis or cholelithiasis. Osteomyelitis and septic arthritis are serious causes of bone pain. Chest pain may be the result of an acute coronary syndrome, pulmonary embolism, pneumonia, or pleuritis.

Laboratory

- A peripheral smear will reveal sickle cells in each of the major sickle cell disease syndromes: sickle cell anemia (Hb SS), Hb SC disease (Hb SC), and sickle cell-β-thalassemia (Hb S-β-thal). The smear is normal in sickle cell trait. The chronic hemolytic anemia of sickle cell disease usually is associated with mildly to moderately low packed cell volume (PCV), low hemoglobin and red cell levels, reticulocytosis with reticulocyte percentages of approximately 3% to 15% (accounting for high or high-normal mean corpuscular hemoglobin), unconjugated hyperbilirubinemia, and elevated lactate dehydrogenase and low haptoglobin levels. If there is a drop of more than 2 g/dL, look at the reticulocyte count. Suspect splenic sequestration for persistent reticulocytosis, especially in the setting of a large spleen and hypovolemia. If it is low, consider aplastic crisis. Leukocytosis is expected in all patients with sickle cell anemia. Major elevation in the WBC count (i.e., >20,000 per mm^3) with a left shift raises suspicion for infection. The platelet count is often elevated. Unfortunately, no test is available that detects whether a patient is in a crisis.
- Although not available in the ED, hemoglobin electrophoresis differentiates patients who are homozygous from those who are heterozygous. The homozygous patient will have HbSS (80-90%), HbF (2-20%), and HbA$_2$ (2-4%). The heterozygous patient will have HbSS (35-40%) and the normal HbA (60-65%).

EKG

- An EKG should be ordered in the patient with chest pain to evaluate for ischemic cardiac disease.

Radiographic studies

- Studies may include a chest x-ray for patients with respiratory symptoms or chest pain. Radiographic findings may be normal in patients with acute chest syndrome. Bone films should be ordered for patients with bone tenderness; however, osteomyelitis may not appear for 8-10 days. A bone scan or MRI is better for osteomyelitis in the early stages. A head CT scan or MRI is used for patients with neurologic deficits.

Emergency Department Management Overview
General

■ The ABCs (*a*irway, *b*reathing, and *c*irculation) should be addressed as discussed in Section II. Supplemental oxygen should be given if the patient is in respiratory distress or if the oxygen saturation is less than 95%. An IV should be placed for hydration and for analgesic medication. Provide oral hydration if the patient is having a minor episode, and is not vomiting.

Medications

■ If the patient is in pain, give analgesics including narcotics and non-narcotics. Meperidine is contraindicated in patients with renal dysfunction or CNS disease because its metabolite, normeperidine (which is excreted by the kidneys), can cause seizures. A common error is to conclude the patient is *drug seeking* because of many ED visits, but in fact multiple episodes of painful crisis are the norm. See Chapter 90.1 for drug dosages.

■ Re-evaluation of pain is essential; this can be done using a pain scale or patient's self report. If there is no relief after acetaminophen with codeine or ketorolac, the drug of choice is morphine. Hydromorphone is an alternative agent. After 4 to 5 hours of treatment, if the patient is still requiring parental analgesics, or the vaso-occlusive crisis is complicated with an infection, hypoxia, or other acute event, admit the patient to the hospital.

■ Look for a precipitating factor to the crisis. Differentiate a *typical* vaso-occlusive painful process from a complicated one (ACS, splenic sequestration), or a different underlying process that may be presenting as a painful *crisis* (i.e., osteomyelitis, septic arthritis, surgical abdomen). Patients may be on long-term hydroxyurea. It promotes HbF synthesis and decreases HbS polymerization. Oral hydroxyurea has been shown to decrease painful crisis by as much as 50%.

■ Antibiotics are only used if the presentation is complicated by an infection (see Chapter 90.2).

Emergency Department Interventions

■ Exchange transfusions consist of replacing the patient's RBCs by normal donor RBCs, decreasing HbSS to less than 30%. When considering an exchange transfusion for acute chest syndrome, splenic sequestration, or cerebrovascular accident (CVA), consult hematology. Table 53–2 lists indications for transfusion therapy in SCD.

Table 53–2   Acute Indications for Exchange Transfusion in Sickle Cell Disease

Splenic sequestration	Acute multiple organ failure syndrome
Severe aplastic crisis	Preoperative preparation for major surgery
Acute stroke	Severe anemia from malaria
Acute chest syndrome	Prolonged priapism

- A simple blood transfusion is indicated for aplastic crisis and acute sequestration crisis.

Disposition

- ***Consultation.*** Hematology should be consulted for complicated cases, and for patients requiring transfusion. Consult ophthalmology for visual complaints. Consult urology for unresolved priapism. Orthopedic consultation should be done for a vascular necrosis of the hip or suspected osteomyelitis.
- ***Admission.*** Admit if there has been an inadequate response to analgesics, sepsis, acute chest syndrome, splenic sequestration, CVA, unresolved priapism, aplastic crisis, other co-morbidities, or poor social circumstances.
- ***Discharge.*** If stable, discharge the patient with appropriate follow-up, adequate analgesics, and antibiotics, when appropriate.

Specific Problems

Acute Chest Syndrome

- ***Epidemiology and risk factors.*** Criteria for diagnosing acute chest syndrome (ACS) are the presence of a new infiltrate involving at least one lung segment, and other lower respiratory symptoms (i.e., cough, dyspnea, hypoxemia, and chest pain). It is a leading cause of death among young adults with SCD, accounting for 25% of premature deaths associated with the disease. It is the second most common cause of hospitalization in this population. ACS may be precipitated by several events such as hypoventilation from a vaso-occlusive painful episode, narcotics used to treat the episode, fat emboli from bone marrow infarction, pulmonary emboli, or infection. An infection with parvovirus B19 can lead to marrow necrosis and severe ACS. An increased baseline leukocyte count has been found to be an independent risk factor for ACS. Patients older than 20 years do worse than younger patients.
- ***Pathophysiology.*** ACS arises from vaso-occlusion of lung vasculature and infarction of pulmonary parenchyma. It may also occur as a result of an acute lung injury from an infection or embolus. Hypoxia and vasoconstriction lead to an increase in polymer formation, slowing of red blood cell (RBC) transit time, and an increase in endothelial release of adhesive and pro-inflammatory molecules. Repeated episodes predispose the patient to chronic pulmonary disease and pulmonary hypertension. There is a decrease in nitric oxide (NO) during an ACS episode. NO can inhibit the erythrocyte–endothelial adhesion, and therefore reduce lung injury.
- ***History.*** ACS may be the presenting diagnosis for a patient with SCD, but equally as often, develops while the patient has a vaso-occlusive crisis, bacterial infection, or after surgery. The classic presentation is that of a young child with tachypnea and hypoxemia. Typical symptoms include chest pain, fever, wheezing, shortness of breath, and cough.

- *Physical examination.* The patient may have fever, wheezing, hypoxia, and tachypnea.
- *Diagnostic testing.* Obtain a complete blood count (CBC), arterial blood gas (ABG), sputum, blood cultures, and nasopharyngeal viral cultures. There will be a decrease in Hb and platelets. A chest radiograph may reveal new infiltrate or hazy opacity, which usually progresses rapidly (over the course of hours to several days) to involve multiple lobes. The radiologic findings may lag behind the clinical symptoms. Pulse-oximetry and ABG analysis reveals hypoxemia with a widened alveolar arterial oxygen gradient. Echocardiography may show right ventricular dysfunction, septal bowing to the left, and tricuspid regurgitation as a result of elevated pulmonary arterial pressure, as well as a hyperkinetic, dilated left ventricle. The patient may appear to have a simple pneumonia or adult respiratory distress syndrome (ARDS).
- *ED management.* The most important steps in the management of ACS are rapid recognition and treatment of any identified underlying causes of hypoxemia. Supportive care includes careful rehydration with hypotonic saline solutions to maintain euvolemia, control of infection and pain, oxygen supplementation, and simple or partial exchange transfusion as indicated. Supplemental oxygen should be provided to keep saturation above 95%. The patient may require assisted ventilation. Keep the patient well hydrated and give adequate analgesics. Incentive spirometry, bronchodilators, and analgesia are useful. Broad-spectrum antibiotics (macrolides or cephalosporins) are empirically given, and should include coverage for encapsulated organisms as well as atypical bacteria. If the severity of the syndrome is moderate, the patient may require a simple blood transfusion. However, if the patient's symptoms are more severe or the patient clinically deteriorates, becomes hypoxic, sustains a pulmonary embolus or infarction, or experiences a systemic fat embolus, an exchange transfusion may be necessary and lifesaving. A simple transfusion may still be helpful, particularly with low starting hemoglobin values, in order to decrease the fraction of sickle cells in the circulation. Hematology should be consulted. The following are associated with a more severe manifestation of ACS: a drop in the baseline hemoglobin (Hb), a platelet count of less than 200,000/uL, neurologic symptoms, confusion, or rib or sternal pain. These patients should be admitted to an intensive care unit.
- *Helpful hints and pitfalls.* The syndrome can rapidly progress to pulmonary failure, cardiovascular collapse, and death. There may be concurrent pulmonary embolism, pulmonary fat embolism, pulmonary infarction, infection, congestive heart failure (CHF), or ARDS. Almost half of the patients with ACS are admitted to the hospital suffering from another disease, and develop a superimposed ACS during their hospital stay.

Aplastic Crisis

- *Epidemiology and risk factors.* RBC production temporarily ceases. Most patients recover within a few days, but some may deteriorate into a more severe crisis that may lead to death from severe anemia, cardiac decompensation, or overwhelming sepsis.

- **Pathophysiology.** It is due to a temporary suppression of bone marrow erythropoiesis activity, usually triggered by an infection, though it can also be triggered by a folate deficiency. Most cases are precipitated by an infection with the human parvovirus B19, which can result in cytotoxicity of erythroid precursors. Patients deficient in folic acid are also at risk. Because the RBCs containing HbS only have a lifespan of 10 to 12 days, severe anemia can develop.
- **History.** Patients have a profound anemia and complain of fatigue and dyspnea. They are more prone to infections from encapsulated organisms, and may have pneumonia.
- **Physical examination.** They may have pallor, and be tachycardic.
- **Diagnostic testing.** Compare the CBC and reticulocyte count to baseline levels. A drop in baseline Hb of 2g/dl or more is significant, but the reticulocyte count is usually less than 1%. Send a parvovirus B19 IgM level, and look for Howell-jelly bodies (RBC nucleus), which confirm the absence of a spleen. Blood cultures should be obtained. An increase in reticulocyte count may indicate marrow recovery, and may spare the patient a blood transfusion. A chest radiograph may be necessary to rule out pneumonia or ACS.
- **ED management.** In many patients, bone marrow activity may be re-established within a few days; these patients will require only supportive treatment. If there is a prolonged course, the patient is febrile, or very young, broad-spectrum antibiotics, erythropoietin, and IV immuno-globulin are usually required. If the hematocrit is more than 20% below baseline, a transfusion should be given. If the aplastic crisis is known to be due to a folate deficiency, folate supplements are indicated. These patients should be admitted, and kept in reverse isolation.
- **Helpful hints and pitfalls.** This severe anemia may lead to cardiac decompensation and death. Because of the shortened half-life of sickled RBCs, these patients cannot tolerate even a brief suppression of bone marrow activity.

Gallbladder Disease

- Due to chronic hemolysis, the patient has an increased risk of developing pigmented gallbladder stones. The prevalence increases with age. Cholelithiasis may begin as early as age 4. By age 18, about 30% of patients with SCD have gallstones. Gallbladder disease is typically due to an increase in bilirubin from hemolysis.
- Symptoms, physical examination, diagnostic testing, and treatment are similar to that for the non–sickle cell patient (see Chapter 18).

Priapism

- A sustained painful unwanted erection is seen in nearly 90% of males with SCD prior to age 20. The mean age for these episodes is 12 years.
- See Chapter 47.

Splenic Sequestration

■ *Epidemiology and risk factors.* Patients with SCD (HbSS) may eventually autoinfarct their spleens, and therefore present with a splenic sequestration syndrome, usually before the age of five. Approximately 10% of children with SCD have one episode of splenic sequestration before two years of age. However even those children with sickle cell trait have splenomegaly, and are at risk for splenic sequestration into adulthood. A high concentration of HbF is protective. The recurrence rate nears 50%.

■ *Pathophysiology.* Erythrocytes become entrapped in the spleen. This gives rise to an enlarged spleen, a sudden drop in hemoglobin and hematocrit, and an increase in reticulocyte count. There is a wide spectrum of severity and presentation of splenic sequestration.

■ *History.* The patient may present with complaints of left upper quadrant pain, fatigue, decreased exercise tolerance, or shock.

■ *Physical examination.* The enlarged spleen is palpable, and there is left upper quadrant tenderness, marked anemia, and pallor. The patient may have all the signs of shock.

■ *Diagnostic testing.* Obtain a CBC, reticulocyte count, and if febrile, obtain blood and urine cultures, as well as a urinalysis. There will be a drop in erythrocytes, hemoglobin and hematocrit; thrombocytopenia and reticulocytosis will also be present.

■ *ED management.* Restore systemic perfusion with intravenous hydration until blood is available, but be cautious not to overload the patient and cause congestive heart failure. Exchange transfusion is the treatment of choice. Splenectomy shortly after an acute episode may be considered for children older than 3 years, or electively in older patients. Some patients, especially if younger than 2 years, may be on a chronic transfusion program, until a splenectomy can be performed. These patients should be admitted to a monitored setting. Any patient with fever and leukocytosis above 20,000/mm should be given IV antibiotics, and a source of infection should be sought.

■ *Helpful hints and pitfalls.* Impaired splenic function leads to an increased risk of sepsis due to inadequate clearance of bacteria from the circulation. These patients are more prone to infections with encapsulated organisms such as *Streptococcus pneumonia*, *Hemophilus influenzae*, and *Mycoplasma pneumoniae*.

Stroke

■ In patients with SCD, the prevalence of a cerebrovascular accident is nearly 10%. Many times it occurs in childhood, and it is usually caused by an infarction.

■ The presentation is similar to stroke in the general population (see Chapter 56).

■ Because a simple transfusion would increase viscosity, an exchange transfusion is indicated in the acute stage of an ischemic stroke. The aim is to reduce the HbS to less than 30%. If intractable to other treatment, a bone marrow transplant may stabilize the vasculopathy.

Special Considerations
Pediatrics

■ Dactylitis or hand-foot syndrome is commonly the earliest presentation of SCD in infants. It is characterized by painful swelling of hands and feet from vaso-occlusion of the metacarpal and metatarsal bones. It usually affects children younger than 3 years. The earlier the presentation, the worse is the prognosis. One may see signs of avascular necrosis on the radiograph.

■ Due to an increased susceptibility for infections, children should be up to date with immunizations, and should receive pneumococcal, parvovirus B19, and influenza vaccines. The patients are also treated with folic acid and penicillin prophylactically.

Women and Pregnancy

■ Prophylactic transfusion may be needed in pregnancy. These patients are prone to placental insufficiency and fetal demise.

Teaching Points

Sickle cell disease is a congenital abnormality of hemoglobin structure that leads to organ dysfunction that is widespread, and ultimately to death. There will be many episodes of acute pain defined as *crises*; and although these often respond to hydration, oxygenation, and adequate analgesia, it is too often the case that analgesia is not adequate. The patient needs to be treated in conjunction with a primary care physician so that pain management as an outpatient can be achieved.

Unfortunately, at some point these patients will develop serious complications of their disease that may cause acute worsening of the anemia, co-morbities such as sepsis, renal failure, and pulmonary failure. They may require exchange transfusions, and certainly require admission to an intensive care unit.

Suggested Readings

Hamilton GC, Janz TG. In: Anemia, polycythemia, and white blood cell disorders. Marx JA, Hockberger RS, Walls RM (editors). Rosen's Emergency Medicine: Concepts and Clinical Practice (6th ed). Philadelphia: Mosby, 2006, pp 1867–1891.

Sadowitz PD, Amanullah S, Souid AK. Hematologic emergencies in the pediatric emergency room. Emerg Med Clin North Am 2002;20:177–198.

Stuart MJ, Nagel RL. Sickle cell disease. Lancet 2004;364:1343–1360.

Tahir A, Kazzi Z. Anemia, sickle cell. eMedicine. http://www.emedicine.com/EMERG/topic26.htm Updated April 3, 2006. Accessed May 3, 2006.

Wilson RE, Krishnamurti L, Kamat D, Management of sickle cell disease in primary care. Clin Pediatr 2003;42:753–761.

CHAPTER 54

Soft Tissue Infections and Ulcerations

E. GREGORY MARCHAND

 Red Flags

Diabetes or immunocompromised status • Intravenous drug use
• Immobility • Peripheral vascular disease • Abnormal vital signs:
fever, unexplained tachycardia, hypotension (may be a late finding)
• Hemorrhagic bullae • Crepitus • Pain out of proportion to external
examination

Overview

Infections of the soft tissues are those that involve the skin (including
the subcutaneous tissue), the fascia, and, in severe cases, the muscles.
They may be superficial, but easily treated with oral or topical
antibiotics. Others may be extensive, deep, or life- or limb-threatening
infections requiring emergency debridement.

Look for "red flags" (see Box) in any patient with infection to the
soft tissues. Accurate and early diagnosis of severe infections and
prompt intervention are key to a good outcome.

Differential Diagnosis

See DDx table.

Initial Diagnostic Approach
General

- The primary diagnostic tools when evaluating patients with soft-tissue
  infections are the history and physical examination.
- The vital signs are important. Fever and a tachycardia are both concerning. A rapid respiratory rate may indicate an underlying acidosis.
  Patients with gangrene may be septicemic and hypotensive upon
  presentation.

DDx Differential Diagnosis of Soft-Tissue Infections

Classification	Example	Brief Description
Pustular lesions	Impetigo	Superficial infection of the skin limited to the dermis.
	Folliculitis	Inflammation of hair follicle caused by infection, physical injury or chemical irritation.
Abscesses	Furuncle (boil, subcutaneous abscess)	Walled off collection of pus forming a fluctuant mass. There is more inflammation than in folliculitis.
	Carbuncle Hydradenitis suppurativa	A collection of furuncles. Recurrent abscess formation of the apocrine sweat glands.
Cellulitis	Cellulitis (general)	Skin infection that extends into the subcutaneous tissues; margins are ill defined
	Erysipelas	Skin infection that involves the superficial layers of the skin and cutaneous lymphatics; well demarcated with raised borders.
Necrotizing infections	Necrotizing fasciitis	Infections involving subcutaneous tissue and fascia
	Fournier's gangrene	Soft tissue infection with widespread fascial necrosis
	Myonecrosis	Infection involving the muscle
Extremity ulcerations	Diabetic foot ulcer	Infected diabetic foot ulcer usually a consequence of uncontrolled diabetes and peripheral neuropathy.
	Venous stasis ulcers	Infected lower extremity ulcer resulting from chronic venous stasis.

- The findings of crepitus and hemorrhagic bullae are ominous indicators of serious disease (e.g., necrotizing infection), even in nontoxic appearing patients.
- Younger patients with less concerning co-morbid conditions, normal vital signs, and focal examination findings usually require no other diagnostic workup.

Laboratory

- Most patients do not require laboratory studies. Patients who appear ill, who are immunocompromised, or who have diabetes warrant basic laboratory tests, including complete blood count (CBC) and chemistry panel (especially in diabetics).

Radiology

- Imaging is useful in patients in whom there is a concern for a deeper infection.
- Plain films may show deposits of gas in the deep tissues, indicative of gangrene caused by *Clostridia* species. Other anaerobic infections may also produce gas. These include *Streptococcus* (necrotizing skin infections), *Coliforms*, anaerobic *Bacteroides*, and *Aerobacter* aerogenes.
- Computed tomography (CT scan) is often useful in determining extent and depth of infection.

Emergency Department Management Overview
General

- The ABCs (*a*irway, *b*reathing, and *c*irculation) should be addressed as discussed in Section II.

Medications

- *Antibiotics.* Early administration of appropriate parenteral antibiotics is essential in orbital cellulitis, necrotizing fasciitis, gangrene, and diabetic foot infections. Use broad-spectrum antibiotics for diabetics, as the infections tend to be polymicrobial. See Table 54–1 for antibiotics used to treat complicated soft-tissue infections. Details on specific antibiotics are located in Chapter 90.2.
- *Analgesia.* Do not fail to relieve pain, especially in addicts whose abscesses are caused in the process of substance abuse. Extensive infections are painful, and the patient may cooperate better with both further examination and treatment if good analgesia is provided.

Emergency Department Interventions

- The procedure to perform incision and drainage of an abscess is reviewed in Chapter 91.

Disposition

- *Consultation.* Consult with a surgeon for any patient with surgical disease such as debridement of necrotizing infection, deep-space infection, or an abscess unable to be drained in the ED (e.g., one that is overlying vital structures, or if it is impossible to obtain adequate analgesia).
- *Admission.* Patients with significant co-morbidities (diabetes, human immunodeficiency virus [HIV]), elderly patients, or those with prosthetic implants should be admitted. Patients can be discharged with close follow-up if they are well-appearing, and have a minor localized infection. Patients unable to take oral medication, have a deep-space infection, or demonstrate signs of systemic toxicity should also be admitted.

Table 54–1 Antibiotic Treatment in Complicated Soft-Tissue Infections

Risk Factor	Organism	Recommended Antibiotics
Human bite	Aerobes include *Eikenella corrodens*, *Streptococcus*, *Staphylococcus aureus*. Anaerobes include *Bacteroides* and *Peptostreptococcus* species	Amoxicillin-sulbactam, cefoxitin, and ticarcillin-clavulanate. Penicillin allergic patients may receive clindamycin plus trimethoprim-sulfamethoxazole or clindamycin plus a fluoroquinolone.
Dog or cat bite	*Pasteurella multicida*	Most β-lactam antimicrobials especially ampicillin-clavulanate and ampicillin-sulbactam; second- and-third generation cephalosporin; tetracycline; quinolones; trimethoprim-sulfamethoxazole. Resistant to vancomycin, clindamycin, dicloxacillin, nafcillin; borderline susceptibility to aminoglycosides. Oral first-generation cephalosporins and erythromycin may not be effective. Check need for rabies prophylaxis (Chapter 94).
Fresh-water lakes, rivers, and streams	*Aeromonas hydrophila*	Aminoglycosides, fluoroquinolones, chloramphenicol, trimethoprim-sulfamethoxazole (cotrimoxazole) and third-generation cephalosporins, but this organism is resistant to ampicillin
Aquariums or following injuries in swimming pools.	*Mycobacterium marinum*	Rifampin (rifampicin) plus ethambutol, tetracycline or trimethoprim-sulfamethoxazole.
Stepping on a nail	*Pseudomonas aeruginosa*	Aminoglycosides, third-generation cephalosporins such as ceftazidime, semisynthetic penicillins such as ticarcillin and piperacillin, or fluoroquinolones.

Table 54-1 Antibiotic Treatment in Complicated Soft-Tissue Infections—*cont'd*

Intravenous drug user	Mostly polymicrobial, mostly staphylococci and streptococci; high prevalence of oropharyngeal flora; rare gram-negative enteric bacilli; anaerobes.	Penicillinase-resistant penicillins and first-generation cephalosporins directed primarily against *S. aureus* and *Streptococcus* species. Vancomycin for possible methicillin-resistant *Staphylococcus aureus* (MRSA).
Chronic lower extremity ulcers	*S. aureus* and *P. aeruginosa.* Suspect MRSA. Diabetic foot ulcers are often polymicrobial.	A broad-spectrum antibiotic with gram-positive and gram-negative organisms until sensitivities return and appropriate antibiotic choices are made. Clindamycin, cotrimoxazole, fluoroquinolones, or minocycline may be considered in some cases of non–life-threatening infections of MRSA; vancomycin or linezolid for more serious MRSA infections. Rifampin may be added to improve outcomes for MRSA but should not be the sole agent. Fluoroquinolones are currently the only oral agents presently available to treat pseudomonal infection. More serious infections require intravenous antibiotics with aminoglycosides, third-generation cephalosporins such as ceftazidime, semisynthetic penicillins such as ticarcillin and piperacillin, or fluoroquinolones.
Hospitalized, immuno-compromised	Gram-negative, including *P. aeruginosa*; *Stenotrophomonas maltophilia.* Suspect MRSA.	Antibiotics for MRSA *P. aeruginosa* as mentioned above. Trimethoprim-sulfamethoxazole and ticarcillin-clavulanate are active in vitro against *S. maltophilia.*

*The incidence of community acquired MRSA is increasing.

- **Discharge.** Patients with localized minor infection, no systemic signs of toxicity, and no significant co-morbid disease can be discharged from the hospital.

Specific Problems

Cellulitis

Cellulitis and Erysipelas

- **Epidemiology and risk factors.** Cellulitis occurs in all age groups. The lower extremities are the most common site (>70%). Erysipelas is a disease of the young or old, in patients with impaired lymphatic or venous drainage (mastectomy, saphenous vein harvesting), and in immunocompromised patients. Recurrence is relatively common. It occurs predominantly on the lower extremities (70%-80%), but occasionally involves the face (5%-10%). Recurrent streptococcal cellulitis of the lower extremities may be caused by group A, C, or G streptococci in association with skin lesions such as chronic venous stasis, chronic lymphedema, or healed burns, especially if the skin is colonized by dermatophyte fungi. Recurrent staphylococcal cutaneous infections occur in individuals who have eosinophilia and elevated serum levels of immunoglobulin E (Job's syndrome), and among chronic nasal carriers of staphylococci.
- **Pathophysiology.** Cellulitis extends into the subcutaneous tissues; erysipelas involves the superficial layers of the skin and cutaneous lymphatics and is usually caused by group A β-hemolytic streptococci. In adults and older children, the most common organisms are group A streptococci and *S. aureus*. In children under the age of 3 years, *Haemophilus influenzae* type B was common, but with immunization, is now rarely seen. In patients with underlying co-morbidities, cellulitis is often caused by organisms other than *S. aureus* or group A streptococcus, such as *Acinetobacter, Clostridium septicum, Enterobacter, Escherichia coli, H. influenzae, Pasteurella multocida, Proteus mirabilis, P. aeruginosa,* and group B streptococci. Cellulitis associated with cat bites, and, to a lesser degree, dog bites is commonly caused by *P. multocida*.
- **History.** Symptoms may occur acutely. Associated fevers are common, but not always present. In elderly or immunocompromised patients, systemic illness and malaise may be present or even precede the development of the skin lesion.
- **Physical examination.** Classic findings of cellulitis *(rubor, color, and dolor)* are red, warm, and painful. The margins are ill-defined and not raised. Induration is often present, but fluctuance is rare until an abscess forms. Crepitus is an ominous finding (see Necrotizing Fasciitis). Bullae may be present, and are also indicative of a deeper infection. In erysipelas, the lesions are tender, hot, and red with a sharply demarcated raised border. It differs from other types of cellulitis in that lymphatic involvement *(streaking)* is prominent.
- **Diagnostic testing.** Isolation of the etiologic agent is difficult, and is usually not attempted nor necessary. Fever, mild leukocytosis with a left

shift, and a mildly increased sedimentation rate may be present. Blood cultures are positive only about 5% of the time, and should only be drawn if systemic signs are present. They typically do not guide therapy especially in an otherwise healthy adult patient. If there is a concern for a deeper infection, radiologic studies, a CT scan, or MRI may reveal the extent of the soft-tissue infection, or may reveal associated cellulitis.

■ *ED management.* Previously healthy adults and children who have reliable follow-up and are not ill-appearing, may be treated as outpatients. Empiric treatment with antibiotics aimed at staphylococcal and streptococcal organisms is appropriate in adults. Initial antibiotic therapy includes nafcillin, oxacillin, first-generation cephalosporin, erythromycin, and ampicillin-clavulanate. If methicillin-resistant staphylococci are endemic, use vancomycin or clindamycin. Gram-negative coverage should be included for patients at risk (e.g., amino-glycoside). *P. multocida* should be treated with a β-lactam antimicrobial such as amoxicillin combined with a β-lactam inhibitor. This organism is resistant to some commonly used cephalosporins such as cephalexin. Ampicillin-clavulanate, ampicillin-sulbactam, or cefoxitin are good choices for treating animal or human bite infections. Patients should be rechecked in 24 to 48 hours to ensure that the infection is not spreading. Admit patients at higher risk for complications such as diabetics, patients with peripheral vascular disease, immunocompromised patients, IV drug users, and young (<3 years old) children. Indications for admission include any toxic-appearing patient, infection that is circumferential or involves more than 30% of a limb, questionable ability to follow-up or to comply with treatment, and failure to respond to outpatient treatment. Most patients may be safely treated with oral antibiotics, and discharged from the ED. Pain can be relieved with cool Burrow's compresses and oral analgesia. Elevation of the leg hastens recovery for lower leg infections.

■ *Helpful hints and pitfalls.* Diabetics with cellulitis of the legs often have polymicrobial infections, and require broad-spectrum antibiotics. Outbreaks of epidemic furunculosis and severe invasive pediatric infections should raise suspicion for community-acquired methicillin-resistant *S. aureus* (MRSA) infection. Empirical therapy with vancomycin should also be considered for serious infections in patients with a history of MRSA colonization, IV drug use, and other risk factors (recent hospitalization, recent antibiotics, or chronic illness).

Periorbital and Orbital Cellulitis

■ See Chapter 69.

Pustular infections
Abscesses

A brief discussion on the most common abscesses are listed in Table 54–2.

■ *Epidemiology and risk factors.* Patients who are immunocompromised, afflicted with diabetes, undergoing hemodialysis, or who are IV drug abusers are at increased risk of developing abscesses.

Table 54–2 Common Abscesses

Type of Abscess	Description	Management
Furuncle	Walled-off collection of pus, involving the hair follicle. There is more inflammation than a folliculitis that extends from the follicle into the surrounding dermis.	Warm compresses, incision and drainage. Antibiotics to cover *Staphylococcus aureus* and *Streptococcus* species are indicated in the presence of recurrent infection, cellulitis, septicemia, diabetes, or immunocompromise.
Carbuncle hidradenitis suppurativa	A collection of furuncles Recurrent abscess formation of apocrine sweat glands of the groin and axilla. Occluded apocrine ducts are infected with strains of *Staphylococcus, Streptococcus, Escherichia coli,* or *Proteus species*.	Same as furuncle Better perianal hygiene, warm compresses, and broad-spectrum antibiotics. Incision and drainage of isolated lesions but the recurrence rate approaches 40%. Referral to a surgeon for wide excision of advanced chronic disease may be necessary.
Bartholin cyst abscess	An infected Bartholin gland or duct cyst. Mixed infections are typical. Common pathogens include *Neisseria gonorrhoeae, Chlamydia trachomatis, E. coli,* and *Proteus mirabilis*.	Usually requires drainage and antibiotics for concurrent vaginal, cervical or urethral infection. The incision is made on the mucosal surface of the vestibule just lateral to the hymenal ring, or A Word catheter (or Iodoform gauze, Penrose drain) is placed for 24 h to promote drainage. A Word catheter is a 10-French, 5-cm-long latex catheter with a 5-ml balloon that is inflated with water. Sitz baths promote continued drainage.
Pilonidal abscess	Pus and a wall of edematous fat, resulting from rupture of an infected follicle into fat, most commonly found in the intergluteal fold.	Incision and drainage. Antibiotics are generally not indicated unless the patient has a medical condition such as rheumatic heart disease, or is immunosuppressed. Surgery referral to obtain definitive treatment to prevent recurrence.

Felon and paronychia are discussed in Chapter 17; epidural abscess is discussed in Chapter 21; perianal and perirectal abscesses are discussed in Chapter 48; and scrotal abscess is discussed in Chapter 50; peritonsillar and retropharyngeal abscess are discussed in Chapter 64.

- *Pathophysiology.* An abscess is a walled off collection of infection that ultimately accumulates pus. It is surrounded by an area of cellulitis. They are painful and tender before they become fluctuant. Most are caused by bacteria, although occasionally they may be a sterile inflammatory response to a foreign body or a chemical necrosis. The infection is usually localized, but in some patients it may disseminate to become a systemic infection.

- *History.* The pain of the abscess is what commonly leads patients to seek assistance. There may be some remembered trauma, but more often a "boil" that continues to grow and become more painful is reported.

- *Physical examination.* A tender fluctuant warm mass is the classic description of an abscess. If the collection is in deep tissues, the fluctuance may not be appreciable, but there is typically erythema, and the pain elicited by palpitation is often greater than that expected in a simple cellulitis. Fluctuance is also absent early on when the induration and cellulitis predominate. There is usually no fever, until late in the development, and even then, low-grade fever only is common.

- *Diagnostic testing.* In healthy, nontoxic-appearing patients, laboratory testing is of no benefit.

- *ED management.* Simple cutaneous abscesses are best treated by incision and drainage. See Chapter 91 for a more detailed discussion of this.

- *Helpful hints and pitfalls.* Most abscesses are easily managed by the emergency physician.

Folliculitis

- *Epidemiology and risk factors.* A moist environment, maceration, poor hygiene, and drainage from adjacent wounds and abscesses can be provocative factors.

- *Pathophysiology.* There is inflammation of the hair follicle secondary to infection, physical injury or chemical irritation. It is usually caused by *S. aureus.* Gram-negative folliculitis with *Pseudomonas aeruginosa* occurs with infected hot tubs and swimming pools, or in individuals taking antibiotics for acne.

- *History.* The patient complains of local pain, erythema, and swelling in affected areas.

- *Physical examination.* This reveals a pustule with a central hair. The lesions are usually on the buttocks and thighs, occasionally in the beard or scalp, and may cause mild discomfort.

- *Diagnostic testing.* Gram's stain of the lesions is diagnostic.

- *ED management.* Antiseptic cleanser such as povidone-iodine or chlorhexidine every day or every other day for several weeks is usually adequate. For patients with extensive involvement, treat with a 10-day course of a penicillinase-resistant systemic antibiotic, such as cephalexin, dicloxacillin, or cloxacillin. In chronic recurrent folliculitis, daily application of a benzoyl peroxide lotion or gel can facilitate resolution.

- *Helpful hints and pitfalls.* Include instructions to improve hygiene to prevent recurrent disease.

Impetigo

- **Epidemiology and risk factors.** Impetigo is seen predominantly in children. The peak incidence is in summer, especially in regions with high humidity. This is a highly contagious skin infection. Poor health and hygiene, malnutrition, and atopic dermatitis are risk factors.
- **Pathophysiology.** Impetigo is a superficial infection of the skin limited to the epidermis. Colonization of skin usually occurs about 10 days before the appearance of the infection, which results from some minor trauma to the skin. Two forms of the disease are seen. Bullous disease is rare (<10%), and typically found in infants. Nonbullous disease is the most common form. *Staphylococcus aureus* is the most common pathogen, followed by Group A *Streptococcus*.
- **History.** Lesions begin as small, painless pustules. They are often described as pruritic. Fever is rare.
- **Physical examination.** Patients do not appear toxic. If the pustules have ruptured, the pus forms a classic golden-yellow "honey" crust over the skin around the lesions.
- **Diagnostic testing.** This is a clinical diagnosis.
- **ED management.** Educate the patient and family on infection control measures. Treatment with the topical antibiotic mupirocin 2% ointment (Bactroban) is effective in up to 90% of cases. Cephalosporins or macrolides for 5 to 7 days are also effective. Oral penicillinase-resistant semisynthetic penicillin such as dicloxacillin is effective in treating bullous disease, although minor lesions can be treated with mupirocin.
- **Helpful hints and pitfalls.** Poststreptococcal glomerulonephritis may occur after infection with streptococci. Antibiotic treatment is not preventative of the glomerulonephritis. Ecthyma is similar to impetigo, and is characterized by dry crusted lesions of the skin, and may be caused by the same organisms. Unlike impetigo, this lesion extends into the dermis, and may therefore lead to posttreatment scarring.

Soft-Tissue Necrotizing Infections

- These are a spectrum of diseases often caused by a polymicrobial infection of the subcutaneous tissues. They are seen predominantly in adults, may be elusive in diagnosis, and are rapidly progressive in nature. Ludwig's angina is discussed in Chapter 64.

Fournier's Gangrene

- **Epidemiology and risk factors.** This is most commonly seen in older men (average age of 50) and diabetics (up to 70% of cases). Other risk factors include cancers of the pelvic floor and immunosuppression.
- **Pathophysiology.** This is a polymicrobial necrotizing infection of the skin and soft tissues of the perineum, often resulting from perianal infection (up to 50% of cases). Other sources include genitourinary infection and perineal or genital skin trauma.
- **History.** Fever and malaise are common complaints. Nonspecific perineal or abdominal discomfort is often reported initially. A history of recent

perianal surgery is suggestive, as is a history of hemorrhoids. Later in the course, the patient will complain of pain and swelling in the perineum and genitalia. The progression of symptoms is rapid.

- *Physical examination.* Fever is often present. Erythema, marked tenderness of the perineum, edema, and (occasionally) crepitus are indicators of Fournier's gangrene. Dermal necrosis is a late finding.
- *Diagnostic testing.* Laboratory findings are similar to those seen in necrotizing fasciitis. A CT scan is useful in early cases, both to diagnose and to plan surgical treatment. If the patient is toxic, surgical treatment should not be delayed to obtain a CT scan.
- *ED management.* As with necrotizing fasciitis, patients with Fournier's gangrene require aggressive volume resuscitation, and prompt administration of broad-spectrum antibiotics. Definitive treatment is surgical, and thus urology and surgery should be consulted as early as possible.
- *Helpful hints and pitfalls.* Do not be fooled by an apparently benign physical examination. Extensive disease may be present in patients with few external cutaneous findings.

Myonecrosis or Myositis (Gas Gangrene)

- *Epidemiology and risk factors.* This is most often seen in postoperative patients, but may also result from trauma. As with other soft-tissue necrotizing infections, the risk is increased in patients who are diabetic, immunocompromised, or suffering from a malignancy.
- *Pathophysiology.* The infection is caused by a member of the clostridium species, most commonly *C. perfringes*. These are spore-forming anaerobic gram-positive bacilli that produce a toxin. Nonclostridial myonecrosis is caused by anaerobes such as *B. fragilis* along with grampositive aerobes such as *Staphylococcus*. Healthy muscle is not involved. It results from superinfection of previously traumatized or necrotic tissue.
- *History.* There is a history of recent surgery or trauma.
- *Physical examination.* Patients typically appear toxic. Fever and tachycardia are expected findings. The examination is remarkable for crepitus, bullae with foul-smelling dark drainage, and ischemic changes of the skin that develop over a short time. Pain in excess of physical findings is often the initial sign of this infection.
- *Diagnostic testing.* The same as already described for other necrotizing infections. Plain radiographic studies will occasionally show gas, but normal radiologic findings do not rule out gas gangrene, especially if the patient is early in the course of the disease.
- *ED management.* The best prognosis is achieved with early recognition and aggressive surgical treatment. Parenteral antibiotics should cover anaerobes and enterics. Hyperbaric oxygen may be helpful early in the disease.
- *Helpful hints and pitfalls.* Do not rely on radiographic studies in isolation to establish the diagnosis.

Necrotizing Fasciitis

- *Epidemiology and risk factors.* Although not common (500 to 1500 cases per year), necrotizing fasciitis is a disease with significant morbidity and mortality (up to 50%). Risk factors include age over 50, diabetes (present in up to 60% of patients with a necrotizing soft-tissue infection), immunocompromise, peripheral vascular disease, recent surgery, chronic alcoholism, and skin popping of illicit drugs.

- *Pathophysiology.* This is an aggressive infection of the subcutaneous tissues extending along the fascial planes. It is typically polymicrobial, with about half being a mix of aerobic and anaerobic species. If a single organism is the pathogen, the most common is group A beta-hemolytic streptococci. The organisms are not always gas producing.

- *History.* Patients typically have complaints similar to those with simple cellulitis, but often have severe pain greater than can be accounted for by the physical findings before the diagnosis is recognizable. Since many of these patients are abusing illicit drugs, a common mistake is to not think of the possibility of necrotizing fasciitis, and erroneously conclude the patient is merely seeking pain pills. The symptoms rapidly progress and are not ameliorated with oral antibiotics. An inciting trauma is a rare cause.

- *Physical examination.* The early symptoms may mimic simple cellulitis. Clues of a deeper infection being present include: pain out of proportion to the physical examination findings, edema extending beyond the erythema noted on surface examination, and tachycardia not explained by fever. Later presenting signs include hemorrhagic bullae, crepitus, and systemic signs of shock.

- *Diagnostic testing.* A leukocytosis with a bandemia is frequently present, although leukopenia may also be seen. Hyponatremia and hypocalcemia have been reported as probable indicators of the presence of a necrotizing infection. Later findings include a severe lactic acidosis and evidence of multiorgan system failure. A Gram's stain of a punch biopsy of the involved tissue is often helpful and diagnostic. Several sites should be sampled to ensure that the diagnosis is not missed. Plain films may show gas in the soft tissues. A CT scan is more accurate, and an MRI even more so. Imaging studies should be reserved for stable patients in whom the diagnosis is a possibility.

- *ED management.* Early diagnosis and treatment are key to decreased morbidity and mortality. Patients with presumed necrotizing fasciitis will require aggressive volume resuscitation. Consult surgery for early and aggressive surgical debridement. Administer broad-spectrum antibiotics (to cover gram-positive and gram-negative organisms as well as anaerobic pathogens).

- *Helpful hints and pitfalls.* If the diagnosis of necrotizing fasciitis is probable, do not delay surgical consultation pending laboratory or radiologic test results. The diagnosis is a clinical one. Patients who have early, quick, and aggressive care have the best prognosis.

Ulcerations
Diabetic Foot Ulcers

- *Epidemiology and risk factors.* About 12% of diabetics will develop foot ulcers. Approximately 82,000 limb amputations are performed each year on patients with diabetes.

- **Pathophysiology.** Precipitating factors commonly seen in patients with long-standing diabetes include: autonomic neuropathy and small-vessel arterial vascular disease. The former renders the patient insensate in the feet, and thus often unaware of trauma or small sores on the feet. The latter results in poor oxygen delivery to the tissue and delayed and impaired healing.
- **History.** Typically the patient does not initially note the ulcer, or it is a chronic wound that has been slow to heal. The inciting factor to seeking ED care is often the fact that the patient or a caretaker notices a foul-smelling discharge coming from the wound, or that the affected leg has begun to swell. Fever may be absent.
- **Physical examination.** Assess the foot for signs of infection. Superficial infections cause some induration and erythema. Evidence of deeper infection includes the presence of fluctuance and crepitus. Pain is often not elicited on examination. Tachycardia, especially in the absence of fever, may be a sign of systemic infection.
- **Diagnostic testing.** A leukocytosis may be present. Infections commonly precipitate an episode of diabetic ketoacidosis. Laboratory studies should evaluate for this. Radiographic studies will help screen for osteomyelitis.
- **ED management.** Early identification of serious infection is important. If the laboratory results are unremarkable and the patient looks well, management is safe as an outpatient. Antibiotics should have broad-spectrum coverage. Refer the patient to surgical or orthopedic wound clinic for follow-up care. Any patient with signs of systemic infection, concerning infection requiring debridement, or whose diabetes is poorly controlled should be admitted for parenteral antibiotics and surgical debridement of the wound.
- **Helpful hints and pitfalls.** Remember that the absence of a fever does not make the presence of serious systemic infection less likely.

Venous Stasis Ulcers

- **Epidemiology and risk factors.** In the United States, up to 2.5 million people each year are affected by venous stasis ulcers. Venous reflux from incompetent perforator vein valves is recognized as the primary precipitating factor.
- **Pathophysiology.** The exact pathogenesis of venous stasis ulcers is not well understood. Due to sludging of the blood and inadequate return to the heart, tissue oxygenation becomes impaired, and easily breaks down to form an ulcer. As a result of the impaired superficial microcirculation, the wound does not heal.
- **History.** The patient has chronic, nonhealing ulcers that may be secondarily infected.
- **Physical examination.** A chronic-appearing ulcer, often with incomplete granulation of the base is seen. Typically a serous (clear) drainage is seen. The surrounding skin shows features of chronic stasis dermatitis such as decreased hair on a brawny, erythematous, shiny, indurated base with patches of overlying scale. Evidence of a superimposed infection includes fever, increased pain, foul odor, cloudy or purulent drainage, redness, and warmth of the surrounding skin.

- **Diagnostic testing.** Venous duplex imaging may be of help to rule out deep vein thrombosis, but may also identify specific points of venous reflux. Arterial insufficiency should be ruled out as compression stockings used for venous stasis may impede arterial flow if arterial insufficiency is present. An ankle-brachial index (ABI) less than 0.8 indicates moderate arterial insufficiency, in which case compression stockings may further impede arterial inflow. If infection is present, plain films of the leg should be performed as an initial screening test for osteomyelitis. If wound cultures are to be taken, they should only be obtained after the wound is thoroughly debrided and irrigated due to the presence of colonizing bacteria.

- **ED management.** Venous stasis ulcers are chronic diseases, and are often difficult to manage. The patients need education in elevating their limbs to promote drainage, to cover the wound with a compressive medicated dressing (such as an Unna boot), and to be referred to a wound clinic for follow-up. Patients sometimes have an element of phlebitis that complicates the wound, and may benefit from anticoagulation. Surgery should be consulted for infected wounds that need debridement. Broad-spectrum antimicrobial therapy and admission is required for significant infections. Topical antibiotics can be used for minor superficial infections. Silver sulfadiazine (Silvadene) provides gram-positive and gram-negative coverage. Mupirocin (Bactroban) covers gram-positive infections, including MRSA, although resistance is emerging. Polymyxin B sulfate provides gram-negative coverage, including *Pseudomonas* species. Metronidazole (MetroGel) provides coverage for anaerobic infections. Triple-antibiotic ointment should be avoided because it contains neomycin and bacitracin; either of these may cause contact allergy sensitization in this population.

- **Helpful hints and pitfalls.** The ulcer is sometimes accompanied by deep vein thrombosis, and since the limb is chronically swollen and painful, this may be missed if not sought with venous duplex ultrasound imaging studies. Simultaneous arterial vascular disease can also complicate the picture, and may require arteriography. ABIs should be assessed in the ED.

Teaching Points

Soft-tissue infections are very common problems presenting to the ED. Abscesses are best treated with incision and drainage when they have become fluctuant. Most of these patients can be safely treated as outpatients. However, patients with high-risk co-morbidities, a history of intravenous drug use, severe pain, abnormal vital signs, a toxic appearance, or extensive infection require a more expeditious ED evaluation, prompt initiation of intravenous antibiotics, and consultation with a surgical specialist. Certain diseases such as necrotizing fasciitis are rapidly fatal if immediate treatment is not initiated.

Suggested Readings

Bhumbra NA, McCullough SG. Skin and subcutaneous infections. Prim Care Clin Office Pract 2003;30:1–24.

Brem H, Kirsner RS, Falanga V. Protocol for the successful treatment of venous ulcers. Am J Surg 2004:188(1A Suppl):1–8.

Brem H, Sheehan P, Boulton AJM. Protocol for treatment of diabetic foot ulcers. Am J Surg 2004;187(Suppl);1S–10S.

Ebright JR, Pieper B. Skin and soft tissue infections in injection drug users. Infect Dis Clin N Am 2002;16:697–712.

Kuncir EJ, Tillou A, St Hill CR, et al. Necrotizing soft-tissue infections. Emer Med Clin N Am 2003;21:1075–1087.

Stevens DL. Cellulitis, pyoderma, abscesses and other skin and subcutaneous infections. In: Cohen J, Powderly WG, Berkely SF (editors). Infectious Diseases (2nd ed). St. Louis, MO: Mosby, 2004, pp 138–141.

Valeriano-Marcet J, Carter JD, Vasey FB. Soft tissue disease. Rheum Dis Clin N Am 2003; 29:77–88.

CHAPTER **55**

Sore Throat

GERARD M. TOSO ■ **ANDREW SUCOV**

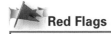

Red Flags

Extremes of age ● Co-morbidities: human immunodeficiency virus, diabetes ● Abrupt onset or presence more than 3 weeks ● Drooling ● Muffled voice ● Neck stiffness ● Abnormal vital signs: tachycardia or hypotension ● Dyspnea or stridor

Overview

Sore throat is a common symptom that ranges in severity from mild discomfort to severe pain. Always assess the airway, and look for "red flags" (see Box) that may indicate more concerning diagnoses.

Viruses or bacteria cause most sore throats. Local irritation is another common cause. Although often associated with pharyngitis, throat pain may also herald a variety of other underlying disorders, both common and uncommon. These disorders range from local to systemic diseases, and include infectious as well as noninfectious etiologies.

Deep infections of the neck may present as sore throat. The neck spaces are interconnected with each other, and also connect with the mediastinum so that infection can easily spread to a variety of these areas. Examples include retropharyngeal abscess, parapharyngeal abscess, as well as infection of the sublingual and submental space, including Ludwig's angina (Chapter 64).

Differential Diagnosis of Sore Throat

See DDx table describing the differential diagnosis of sore throat.

Initial Diagnostic Approach
General

- Although most patients complaining of a sore throat are nontoxic appearing, airway compromise should be the first diagnostic consideration in all patients. Airway assessment (e.g., swelling, obstruction, dyspnea, stridor) should be evaluated during the initial evaluation of any patient presenting with a sore throat. The airway should be secured prior to any other diagnostic testing or interventions (see Chapter 5).
- *History.* Important historical considerations should include the age of the patient, onset and duration, co-morbidities, recent trauma, ill contacts, immunization status, and cancer risk factors (i.e., smoking and alcohol). Although retropharyngeal abscess is most common in children, peritonsillar abscess and infectious mononucleosis are mostly seen in teenagers and young adults. Ludwig's angina is mostly seen in young and middle-aged men. The administration of a vaccine also affects the population in which certain infections are found. Diphtheria and epiglottitis

DDx Priority-Based Differential Diagnosis of Sore Throat

Critical Diagnoses	Emergent Diagnoses	Nonemergent Diagnoses
• Epiglottitis (76) • Retropharyngeal abscess (64) • Acute myocardial infarction (22) • Foreign body, airway (5)	• Angioedema (19) • Peritonsillar abscess (64) • Ludwig's angina (64) • Smoke inhalation • Foreign body GI (33) • Chemical ingestions	• Pharyngitis • Pertussis (24) • Laryngitis • Uvulitis • Gastroesophageal reflux (18) • Malignancy (critical diagnosis if causing airway impingement or massive bleeding)

GI, *gastrointestinal*
( ) Refers to the chapter in which the disease entity is discussed.

are not found in the vaccinated pediatric population of the United States. Diphtheria is usually found in unvaccinated travelers or adults with inadequate vaccination. Adults are more susceptible to epiglottitis by different pathogens than are children. A patient's family history, medical history, and allergies might be helpful in making the diagnosis of angioedema. Assess for associated symptoms such as the presence of fever, discomfort, pain, malaise, malodorous breath, nasal congestion, cough, dysphagia, odynophagia, reflux, and ear pain.

- ■ *Physical examination.* Examination of the ears, nose, pharynx, and neck are most helpful. The abdomen should be examined for the presence of splenomegaly that may be present in infectious mononucleosis, which should be suspected in the presence of fever, tonsillar exudates, and generalized tender lymphadenopathy (typically posterior cervical). The epitrochlear nodes (at the elbow) are rarely enlarged by any disease other than infectious mononucleosis, or very rarely, lymphoma.
- ■ The U.S. Centers for Disease Control and Prevention (CDC) criteria, which comprise four physical findings, greatly help in making the diagnosis of a group A beta hemolytic streptococcus (GABHS) pharyngitis. These criteria include a history of fever, tonsillar exudates, absence of cough, and tender cervical lymphadenopathy.
- ■ The season of the year might indicate which pharyngitis is most likely to be of bacterial origin. GABHS pharyngitis usually occurs in the winter and early spring months.

Laboratory

- ■ In the case of pharyngitis, a rapid antigen test (RAT) is performed only to diagnose GABHS. Properly performed, a RAT is almost as accurate as a throat culture. The swab must be obtained from the surface of both tonsils and the posterior pharyngeal wall. This is done on patients with two, or more of the CDC criteria. Patients with a negative RAT should get a throat swab culture (if the diagnosis is still thought to be bacterial in origin). The culture's final reading is taken 24 to 48 hours later. However, the culture's results will not be available during the emergency department (ED) visit, and thus cannot easily alter treatment plans. Throat cultures need to be obtained when cases of diphtheria, gonococcal pharyngitis, and GABHS outbreaks are suspected.
- ■ Most clinical laboratories use some form of latex agglutination method, such as the monospot test, to evaluate for infectious mononucleosis. This heterophile antibody is usually present at the time of infection. The monospot test may be negative early in the course of illness, and is unreliable in children younger than 4.
- ■ In the case of peritonsillar abscesses, an aspirate can be obtained, and sent for Gram's stain and culture. If the patient is septic, a complete blood count (CBC) and blood cultures should be performed.

Radiography

- ■ *Plain films.* Obtain a lateral soft-tissue neck study for concerns of epiglottitis or retropharyngeal abscess. The airway must be secured before any diagnostic study. If any concern for a parapharyngeal space infection spreading to the mediastinum exists, a chest x-ray should be obtained to rule out mediastinitis. Plain films of the chest may reveal mediastinal widening, air-fluid levels, and subcutaneous or mediastinal emphysema in mediastinitis. The lateral chest radiograph may be useful in demonstrating superior mediastinal gas not evident on upright films.

- *Computed tomography (CT scan).* This study is helpful to determine the extent of an abscess or other mass in the parapharyngeal spaces.
- *Other.* Direct and indirect laryngoscopy evaluates the epiglottis and vocal cords. This is performed when the concern for epiglottitis is still present despite normal findings on a lateral soft-tissue neck film. Preparations for emergency airway management should be available at the bedside.

Emergency Department Management Overview
General

- Address the ABCs (*a*irway, breathing, and *c*irculation) as discussed in Section II. Intravenous (IV) fluids should be given when the patient is dehydrated, or unable to take oral fluids.
- When respiratory distress is present, supplemental oxygen is started while definitive airway control is secured.

Medications

- *Analgesia.* Parental or liquid forms of analgesia are often required in patients with sore throat. Ketorolac 30 mg IV or 60 mg via intramuscular (IM) injection is currently the only nonsteroidal anti-inflammatory drug (NSAID) available in parental form. Opioid analgesia can be given for severe pain (see Chapter 90.1). Topical anesthetics may provide temporary relief.
- *Antibiotics.* If certain infections are suspected, antibiotics can be instituted before their confirmation. This is the case when all four CDC criteria for GABHBS pharyngitis are present, or if concerned for diphtheria, gonococcal pharyngitis, cellulitis, or abscess (see Chapter 90.2).
- *Antihistamines.* Histamine blockers are used to treat angioedema (Chapter 19), but success is variable especially in chronic angioedema.
- *Steroids.* Steroids are also used in angioedema (Chapter 19), but also provide varied effects. Steroids are also considered useful for epiglottitis, croup, and bacterial tracheitis (Chapter 76). They also appear to shorten the course of symptoms for severe pharyngitis, and may be used in selected cases of infectious mononucleosis.
- *Epinephrine.* It may provide some benefit for angioedema, and for the edema of anaphylaxis, and is useful in croup, but probably has no benefit for epiglottitis, although many physicians still use it in severe cases. In no case is it a substitute for active airway management. See Chapter 19 for dosing.

Emergency Department Interventions

- *Airway control.* See Chapter 5.

■ *Abscess drainage.* The incision and drainage of a peritonsillar abscess can be achieved with needle aspiration and good suction (see Chapter 64).

Disposition

■ *Consultation.* Consult an ear, nose, and throat (ENT) specialist for surgical disease involving the pharynx or possible airway compomise.
■ *Admission.* Patients who are septic, dehydrated, or unable to tolerate oral intake need to be admitted for IV antibiotics and fluids. Patients in respiratory distress must be admitted to an intensive care unit (ICU) after their airway has been actively controlled. Some patients with abscesses will be taken to the operating room for drainage and airway control before the ICU admission.
■ *Discharge.* Patients with no signs of airway distress and stable vital signs who are able to tolerate oral intake can be discharged home. They should receive instructions to return if symptoms worsen and to follow-up with their primary care physician.

Specific Problems

> ● ● ● Refer to the DDx table for reference to a discussion of problems in the
> ● ● ● differential not mentioned here.

Diphtheria

■ *Epidemiology and risk factors.* Diphtheria is highly contagious, and transmitted by direct contact or aerosolized pathogens. Adolescents and adults with decreased vaccine induced immunity, and immigrants with inadequate vaccination are susceptible.
■ *Pathophysiology. Corynebacterium diphtheriae* causes tissue necrosis in the upper respiratory tract. This leads to an ulcerated pharynx, and the production of a gray pseudomembrane, which can cause bleeding when dislodged. The bacteria also produces an exotoxin that causes systemic effects, hepatitis, nephritis, bulbar and peripheral paralysis, neuropathy, myocarditis, atrioventricular block, or endocarditis
■ *History.* Fever, sore throat, pain with swallowing, change in voice, loss of appetite, muscle weakness, and difficult breathing are present.
■ *Physical examination.* Pharyngeal erythema with a gray pseudo-membrane, tender cervical lymphadenopathy, and fetid breath are common findings. Airway obstruction can result from progression of the pseudomembrane. Evaluate the patient for systemic manifestations of the disease.
■ *Diagnostic testing.* The diagnosis can initially be made clinically. Cultures need to be obtained from underneath the membrane. The culture medium must contain tellurite. CBC, electrolytes, blood urea nitrogen (BUN), creatinine, liver transaminases levels and an electrocardiogram (EKG) should be obtained to evaluate systemic effects of the exotoxin.
■ *ED management.* IV fluids, antibiotics (erythromycin), and an antitoxin are required. Penicillin is an alternate antibiotic choice. Antibiotics

should be given for 14 days. ICU admission with respiratory precautions is mandatory for airway monitoring. A diphtheria booster is recommended for all diphtheria contacts. Nonimmune contacts should also receive prophylactic antibiotics.

- *Helpful hints and pitfalls.* Dysphonia occurs early on, as the palate muscles are the first ones to become paralyzed. Paralysis of the intrinsic and extrinsic muscles of the eye causes strabismus and ptosis. Diphtheria cases must be reported to local public health officials. Infected patients must be isolated, and all soiled articles properly disposed.

Laryngitis

- *Epidemiology and risk factors.* Laryngitis can occur at any age.
- *Pathophysiology.* Edema of the vocal cords due to an infection, overuse, or local trauma results in acute laryngitis. A viral upper respiratory infection is the most common etiology. Some of the frequent pathogens include adenovirus, rhinovirus, parainfluenza, coronavirus, measles, and mumps. A bacterial superinfection of the cords caused by *H. influenza* or *S. aureus* can produce thick secretions. Shouting or singing can result in submucosal vocal cord hemorrhage and edema.
- *History.* Cough, runny nose, sore throat, and hoarseness can be present depending on the etiology.
- *Physical examination.* The larynx typically has diffuse erythema, edema, vascular engorgement of the vocal folds, and occasionally mucosal ulceration but this is typically not appreciated during a typical physical examination in the ED.
- *Diagnostic testing.* Diagnosis is made on the basis of history and physical examination. Laryngitis due to trauma requires examination by flexible fiber-optic laryngoscopy to evaluate for possible edema or hematoma.
- *ED management.* Acute viral laryngitis requires symptomatic treatment. Mucolytics may be helpful. Antibiotics are needed only when there is a bacterial superinfection. If laryngitis is the result of vocal cord overuse, patients are advised to rest their voices for several days. There is no need for admission, unless there is airway compromise.
- *Helpful hints and pitfalls.* Epiglottitis is always a possibility (see Chapter 76). If hoarseness lasts longer than 3 weeks, follow-up with the ear, nose, and throat (ENT) service is recommended. Other possible causes include recurrent laryngeal nerve damage, laryngeal tumors, or vocal cord nodules.

Oropharyngeal Cancer

- *Epidemiology and risk factors.* Tobacco products and alcohol are the most common etiologic factors associated with squamous cell carcinoma (SCC) of the upper aerodigestive tract.
- *Pathophysiology.* Tumors of the upper aerodigestive tract can grow rapidly, with tumor doubling rates of less than 6 weeks. SCC accounts for more than 90% of all malignant oropharyngeal neoplasms.
- *History.* Patients complain of throat irritation, a burning sensation with acidic food, neck lump, and odynophagia. Referred unilateral otalgia is common. Hemoptysis or oral bleeding can occur with tonsillar cancers.

Late symptoms include dysphagia, dysarthria, or hot potato voice, trismus, obstructive airway symptoms, serous otitis media secondary to eustachian tube obstruction, weight loss, and inanition.

- *Physical examination.* These patients require a thorough head and neck examination to evaluate for a mass lesion.
- *Diagnosis.* The diagnosis is often delayed. A CT scan with contrast is the preferred imaging study in the ED.
- *ED management.* Stable patients with no concern for airway impingement who can tolerate oral fluids can be referred to ENT for a diagnostic evaluation, which will also include direct inspection of oropharyngeal lesions with a flexible nasopharyngoscope.
- *Helpful hints and pitfalls.* Be cautious in treating empirically with antimicrobial and topical anesthetic agents without first performing a thorough head and neck examination. Early referral to a specialist can often establish an early diagnosis, and thus result in improved prognosis of oropharyngeal cancer.

Pharyngitis: Bacterial

- *Epidemiology and risk factors.* It affects 30% of children between the ages of 5 and 15 years and 5% to 15% of adults. It is often seen in winter and early spring.
- *Pathophysiology.* It is an inflammation of the oropharynx mucous membranes. GABHS is the pathogen of concern. *Neisseria gonorrhea*, *Mycoplasma pneumoniae*, *S. aureus*, and other streptococci can cause pharyngitis, but with a lesser frequency.
- *History.* Patients usually complain of sore throat. Patients with bacterial pharyngitis do not usually have cough or rhinorrhea, and are likely to have fever. Headache, nausea, and mild abdominal pain may be present.
- *Physical examination.* Tender anterior cervical lymphadenopathy and exudative tonsillitis.
- *Diagnostic testing.* Refer to previous discussion under "Initial Diagnostic Approach". Clinical criteria to make a clinical diagnosis of GABHS pharyngitis include a history of fever, tonsillar exudates, absence of cough, and tender cervical lymphadenopathy.
- *ED management.* Patients with pharyngitis thought to be due to GABHS should receive a 10-day course of penicillin or equivalent antibiotic if they are allergic (see Chapter 90.2). Macrolides (preferably erythromycin) as well as first and second generation cephalosporins are alternative agents in the penicillin allergic patient.
- *Helpful hints and pitfalls.* Gonococcal pharyngitis is always a possibility. in patients engaging in orogenital sex. Rheumatic fever can be prevented if GABHS is treated with antibiotics within 9 days of infection, whereas glomerulonephritis cannot be prevented.

Pharyngitis: Viral (and Infectious Mononucleosis)

- *Epidemiology and risk factors.* It is the most frequent type of pharyngitis. It can occur at any age. Epstein-Barr virus (EBV) is a widely disseminated herpes virus that manifests clinically as infectious mononucleosis (IMn).

Humans are the major reservoir, and it is transmitted via saliva. It mostly affects patients between the ages of 10 and 25 years. Fewer than 10% of children develop a clinical infection despite a high rate of exposure to EBV. There is a decline of infectious mononucleosis after the age of 35 to 40 years. EBV can be present in the oropharynx for up to 18 months following resolution of symptoms.

- *Pathophysiology.* There is inflammation of the mucous membranes of the oropharynx. Other common viral pathogens include adenovirus, rhinovirus, parainfluenza virus, influenza virus, and enterovirus. EBV infects B cells in the oropharynx, and these cells spread the infection throughout the entire lymphoreticular system. The incubation period is from 30 to 50 days. This infection induces the production of antibodies against viral antigens and other unrelated antigens found in sheep and horse red cells. These latter antibodies are of the IgM type and are called heterophile antibodies. Rarely, antibodies against neutrophils, erythrocytes, and platelets are produced. Atypical lymphocytes are activated T cells that appear between one and three weeks from the onset of symptoms. Infectious mononucleosis is not caused by EBV in 10% of the cases. Cytomegalovirus, toxoplasmosis, human herpes virus and primary HIV infection can cause this EBV-negative mononucleosis.
- *History.* Gradual onset of low-grade fever, sore throat, cough, nasal congestion, and myalgias are typical complaints. Patients with infectious mononucleosis can also complain of severe fatigue, abdominal pain, nausea, and left shoulder pain. Acute symptoms resolve in 1 to 2 weeks. However, fatigue can persist for months.
- *Physical examination.* Most patients have a mildly inflamed oropharynx and tender anterior cervical lymphadenopathy. The triad of fever, exudative tonsillar pharyngitis, and generalized tender lymphadenopathy characterizes infectious mononucleosis. This lymphadenopathy is symmetric, and involves the posterior cervical chain, axillary, and inguinal nodes. It may also enlarge the epitrochlear nodes at the elbow, which is almost pathognomonic for this diagnosis. Petechiae of the soft palate are occasionally seen. Splenomegaly is found in 50% to 60% of patients. Splenic rupture is a rare occurrence, but it tends to be spontaneous in over half of the cases.
- *Diagnostic testing.* If the clinical presentation suggests infectious mononucleosis, a monospot heterophile agglutination test may be obtained. These antibodies appear within 1 week from the onset of symptoms, and last up to a year. A negative test can occur early on the illness. Therefore, a repeated heterophile test is warranted if early in the patient's course of disease. A CBC may demonstrate leukocytosis, and more than 10% atypical lymphocytes. Atypical lymphocytes are not specific to EBV. There is no need to test for all other etiologies of viral pharyngitis, but it is important to distinguish GABHS from a viral pharyngitis.
- *ED management.* Most cases of viral pharyngitis are self-limited and require supportive treatment. IV fluids are indicated for dehydration. Patients unable to tolerate oral intake require admission. Patients with IMn should be informed that symptoms can last for several weeks, and that contact sports need to be avoided (due to splenomegaly). They must

return to the ED with worsening abdominal pain or difficulty breathing. A primary care physician follow-up is indicated before returning to normal activities. The use of steroids is suggested in patients who have severe thrombocytopenia or hemolytic anemia, or potential for airway obstruction as a result of enlarged tonsils.

■ *Helpful hints and pitfalls.* Splenic rupture can be spontaneous or result from direct abdominal trauma. Contact sports should be avoided while IMn symptoms persist. A maculopapular or petechial rash develops in 70% to 90% of patients with infectious mononucleosis when ampicillin or amoxicillin is given. Rare complications of infectious mononucleosis include Guillain-Barré's syndrome, cranial nerve palsies, transverse myelitis, optic neuritis, encephalomyelitis, hemolytic anemia, aplastic anemia, thrombocytopenia, thrombotic thrombocytopenic purpura, hemolytic uremic syndrome, disseminated intravascular coagulation, acute renal failure, and malignancy.

Uvulitis

■ *Epidemiology and risk factors.* There is no specific age distribution. Medication, IV dye contrast, bee stings, or food allergies can result on angioedema of the uvula.

■ *Pathophysiology.* The two etiologies include infectious and angioedema (Chapter 19). Infection of the uvula results from the progression of local infections, such as pharyngitis, tonsillitis, odontogenic, or epiglottitis. The infectious pathogens include *H. influenzae*, streptococcus, *Candida albicans*, and viruses.

■ *History.* Patients usually complain of sore throat, gagging, and the sensation of a foreign body in the back of the throat. Patients with angioedema of the uvula can also present with pruritis, urticaria, or edema of the face and tongue. Fever, headache, facial pain, trismus, odynophagia, and neck pain can be present with infectious uvulitis.

■ *Physical examination.* The uvula is red, firm, swollen, and tender with infectious uvulitis. In cases of angioedema, the uvula appears pale, boggy, and edematous. A uvula with angioedema resembles a grape. Airway compromise can occur.

■ *Diagnostic testing.* This is a clinical diagnosis.

■ *ED management.* Antibiotics are necessary in the case of infectious uvulitis. Angioedematous uvulitis is treated with corticosteroids, epinephrine, and antihistamines. Admit if there is airway compromise, a complicated infection, or inability to tolerate oral fluids.

■ *Helpful hints and pitfalls.* The hypopharynx must be evaluated in cases of airway distress to rule out epiglottitis. Angioedematous uvulitis can lead to airway compromise and must be admitted.

Special Considerations
Pediatrics

■ See Chapter 76 for a discussion of croup, bacterial tracheitis, and epiglottitis.

■ See Chapter 64 for retropharyngeal abscess.

Immunocompromised Patient

- Diabetes, HIV, chemotherapy, or chronic steroid use can result in an immune-suppressed state. These patients are susceptible to fungal pharyngitis.
- *C. albicans* is the most common pathogen. A white removable plaque on an erythematous base characterizes this infection. It is treated with nystatin swish and swallow or oral fluconazole.

Teaching Points

Sore throat is a very common cause for ED visits. Although usually representing the start of a viral upper respiratory infection, it can also be the presenting complaint for more serious disease. The clue to all of these serious etiologies is the complaint of pain that exceeds the findings on physical examination. If you see such a patient, that is the time to look for peritonsillar abscess, Ludwig's angina, retropharyngeal or paratracheal abscess, or epiglottitis.

Most patients do not need extensive workup but will benefit from symptomatic treatment and early relief of the odynophagia that is the principle reason for seeking medical attention. This can often be achieved with a short burst of oral steroids.

Although most patients are not life- or limb-threatened, remember that cardiac pain can radiate to the throat, and an acute coronary ischemic syndrome may be another cause of pain out of proportion to the pharyngeal physical findings.

Suggested Readings

Cooper RJ, Hoffman JR, et al. Principles of appropriate antibiotic use for acute pharyngitis in adults. Ann Emerg Med 2001;37:711–719.

Marvez-Valls E, Ernst A, Gray J, et al. The role of bexamethasone in the treatment of acute exudative pharyngitis. Academ Emerg Med 1998;5:567–572.

Bisno AL, Gwaltney JM, Schwartz RH. Diagnosis and management of group A streptococcal pharyngitis: a practice guideline. Clin Infect Dis 1997;25:574–583.

Aldrete, JS. Spontaneous rupture of the spleen in patients with infectious mononucleosis. Mayo Clin Proc 1992;67:910.

CHAPTER 56

Stroke

Kerlen Chee ■ Peter D. Panagos

Red Flags

Presentation within 3 hours of symptom onset ● Sudden onset of severe headache ● Vomiting ● Unable to speak ● Profound unilateral motor weakness ● Altered level of consciousness ● Unable to handle secretions or protect airway ● Low oxygen saturation on pulse oximetry ● Significantly elevated blood pressure or bradycardia

Overview

Stroke is an acute disruption in the blood supply to the brain causing neurologic deficits. Eighty-eight percent of strokes are ischemic caused by obstruction to blood flow, 9% are due to intracerebral hemorrhage (ICH), and 3% are from subarachnoid hemorrhage (SAH). The first priority is to address the ABCs (*a*irway, *b*reathing, and *c*irculation). Any "red flags" should be identified (see Box).

Transient ischemic attack (TIA) is an abrupt onset of a neurologic deficit traditionally lasting < 24 hours attributed to focal cerebral ischemia without evidence of acute infarction. The proposed re-definition of TIA, based on new imaging techniques, is for symptom resolution in less than one hour. Following a TIA, 5% of patients sustain a stroke within 2 days.

All patients with suspected stroke should have a noncontrast head computed tomography (CT scan) immediately.

Reperfusion is time constrained and limited for the most part to patients who are within a three hour window from the time of perfusion.

Differential Diagnosis of Stroke

See DDx table describing differential diagnosis.

DDx Priority-Based Differential Diagnosis of Stroke		
Critical	**Emergent**	**Nonemergent**
Ischemic stroke	Drug toxicity	Complicated
Hemorrhagic stroke	Hypoglycemia (38)	migraine (35)
Hypertensive	Diabetic ketoacidosis (38)	Neoplasm
encephalopathy (39)	Hyperosmotic coma (38)	Multiple
Epidural hematoma (9)	Encephalitis (67)	sclerosis (60)
Subdural hematoma (9)	Meningitis (67)	Bell's palsy (30)
Subarachnoid	Todd's paralysis (51)	Meniere's disease (59)
hemorrhage (35)	Uremia (49)	Psychiatric
Carotid or vertebral	Hyponatremia (88)	
artery dissection (35)	Wernicke's encephalopathy*	

*Wernicke's encephalopathy: oculomotor disturbances (usually nystagmus and ocular palsies), abnormal
    mentation (usually confusion), and ataxia resulting in part from thiamine deficiency.
( ) Refers to the chapter in which the disease entity is discussed.

Initial Diagnostic Approach
General

- The patient with a possible acute stroke should be placed in a resuscitation area, and should receive immediate attention. The ABCs should be assessed as discussed in Section II. Intravenous (IV) access, cardiac monitoring, pulse oximetry measurement, and confirmation of blood glucose are done while obtaining an accurate and focused history. Administer supplemental oxygen. Determining the exact time of onset of the stroke symptoms is an important determinant of candidacy for thrombolytic therapy.
- See Figure 56–1 for a general approach to the stroke patient.
- A standardized assessment of severity of neurologic dysfunction is the National Institutes of Health Stroke Scale (NIHSS), which grades level of consciousness, visual function, motor function, cerebellar function, sensation and neglect, and language (Table 56–1). The NIHSS is very useful because it may help predict outcome and risk for bleeding in the setting of thrombolysis.
- A noncontrast CT scan of the head is the most important study done early in the course as most treatment algorithms for acute stroke hinge on the presence or absence of intracranial blood on a brain CT study.

Laboratory

- A finger-stick blood glucose should be obtained immediately to rule out hypoglycemia that can mimic stroke, and to evaluate for hyperglycemia. Electrolytes and renal function studies may show abnormalities that can also cause neurologic dysfunction mimicking stroke.
- Other tests to check include the following: complete blood count (CBC) to look for polycythemia or thrombocytosis, which are risk factors for stroke, and to look for thrombocytopenia, which is a contraindication to thrombolytic therapy; coagulation studies to determine if the

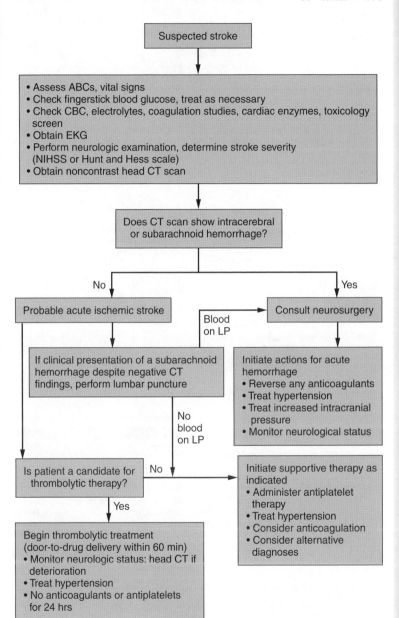

Figure 56–1. Algorithm for a general approach to the stroke patient. *Adapted from American Heart Association. Part 7: The Era of Reperfusion, Section 2: Acute Stroke. Resuscitation 46(2000):239-252.*

Table 56–1 The National Institutes of Health Stroke Scale

Category	Response	Score
1a. Level of consciousness	Alert	0
	Drowsy	1
	Stuporous	2
	Comatose	3
1b. Ask age and current month	Both correct	0
	One correct	1
	Both incorrect	2
1c. Ask patient to close eyes and make a fist	Both correct	0
	One correct	1
	Both incorrect	2
2. Best gaze	Normal	0
	Partial gaze palsy	1
	Forced deviation of eyes	2
3. Visual fields	Normal	0
	Partial hemianopia	1
	Complete hemianopia	2
	Bilateral hemianopia	3
4. Facial weakness	Normal	0
	Minor weakness	1
	Partial weakness	2
	Complete weakness	3
5-8. Motor function (test all four limbs while supine)	No drift	0
– raise arms to 45° and hold 10 sec	Drift	1
	Some effort against gravity	2
	No effort against gravity	3
– raise legs to 30° and hold 5 sec	No movement	4
	Not testable	9
9. Limb ataxia	Absent	0
	Present in one limb	1
	Present in two limbs	2
10. Sensory	Normal	0
	Partial loss	1
	Complete loss	2
11. Best language	No aphasia	0
	Mild to moderate aphasia	1
	Severe aphasia	2
	Mute	3
12. Dysarthria	Normal articulation	0
	Mild to moderate dysarthria	1
	Unintelligible	2
	Untestable	X
13. Neglect	None	0
	Partial neglect	1
	Complete neglect	2
Total		0-42

1b. Aphasic or stuporous patients are scored 2.

5-8. Patients with amputation or joint fusion are scored 9 and should be explained.

10. Only sensory loss due to stroke is scored (sensory loss from neuropathy is not evaluated).

11. Comatose and intubated patients are scored 3.

12. Comatose and intubated patients are marked X and should be explained.

prothrombin time (PT)/international normalized ratio (INR) meets eligibility criteria for thrombolytic therapy. A toxicology screen (cocaine and amphetamine ingestion) and cardiac enzymes should be ordered as appropriate. A urine pregnancy test should be sent on all women of childbearing age.

- If no common risk factors are identified, screening for hypercoagulable disorders should be considered, especially in patients younger than 50 years. Such tests include proteins C and S, antiphospholipid antibody, antithrombin III, antinuclear antibody, activated protein C resistance, and factor V Leiden, but are typically not ordered from the ED.

EKG

- An electrocardiogram (EKG) should be obtained on all patients to look for dysrhythmias or cardiac ischemia. Atrial fibrillation and acute myocardial infarction (MI) are associated with up to 60% of all cardioembolic strokes. T wave inversions can occur in up to 75% of acute stroke patients.

Radiography

- An emergent noncontrast head CT scan is the imaging modality of choice. This will allow for differentiation of ischemic versus hemorrhagic stroke.
- A chest radiograph may be obtained to rule out any acute cardiopulmonary processes such as aortic dissection. Proximal aortic arch dissections may be associated with stroke.
- An MRI is being used more frequently in the evaluation of an acute stroke but is not typically performed from the ED.
- An MRA will be obtained if there is question of a subarachnoid hemorrhage, especially from intracranial aneurysm.

Emergency Department Management Overview
General

- The ABCs should be addressed as discussed in Section II. Supplemental oxygen should be given to hypoxic patients (SaO_2 <95%).
- Patients should not leave the department for a head CT scan unless the airway is secured. Patients with a significant reduction in level of consciousness should be intubated early on for airway protection. See Chapter 5.

Medications

- *Glucose control.* Patients who are hypoglycemic should be given dextrose, and hyperglycemia should be corrected with IV hydration and insulin.
- *Anticonvulsants.* Treat seizures with benzodiazepines (lorazepam 1-4 mg IV over 2-10 minutes). Phenytoin may prevent recurrent seizures but prophylactic administration is not indicated in ischemic strokes.
- *Antihypertensive therapy.* Treatment is reserved for patients with markedly elevated blood pressures in the setting of end-organ damage

or potential fibrinolytic therapy. Treatment of hypertension in patients with intracranial hemorrhage (ICH) or subarachnoid hemorrhage (SAH) is more aggressive than for patients with ischemic stroke. The current consensus for ICH is to give parenteral agents for systolic pressures higher than 160 mm Hg or diastolic pressures higher than 105 mm Hg. Sublingual nifedipine is not recommended because it can produce a precipitous drop in blood pressure. Nitroprusside and nitroglycerin are cerebral venodilators, and should be used with caution because they may cause intracranial pressure to increase. Alternative agents include labetlol and the calcium antagonist nicardipine. See Table 56–2.

- *Reversal of anticoagulation.* This should be carried out in some patients with an intracerebral hemorrhage. Protamine sulfate is used to reverse heparin (1 mg of protamine sulfate per 100 units of heparin) but should not be used in patients who are allergic to fish. Vitamin K and fresh frozen plasma (FFP) are used to reverse warfarin (10 mg of vitamin K and 10-20 ml/kg of FFP). Cryoprecipitate, FFP, and e-aminocaproic acid are used to reverse thrombolytic agents in the setting hemorrhage such as ICH. The dose is 6 to 10 units of cryoprecipitate and 5 g of e-aminocaproic acid infused over 60 minutes for continued bleeding.
- *Heparin or low-molecular-weight heparin (LMWH).* No definitive data confirm a significant improvement in clinical outcome in patients with acute ischemic stroke treated with either unfractionated heparin or LMWHs.
- *IV thrombolytic therapy.* This may be administered to patients with ischemic strokes who meet the eligibility criteria (see Chapter 90.5).

Emergency Department Interventions

- *Aspiration precautions.* Because patients may present with a decreased level of consciousness or neurologic deficits may impair swallowing, patients should be maintained on nothing by mouth (NPO) until swallowing ability has been appropriately assessed. The airway should be secured (see Chapter 5).
- *IV fluids.* Overhydration and the administration of hypotonic solutions should be avoided to prevent cerebral edema. Dextrose-containing solutions should be avoided in normoglycemic patients suspected of having a stroke because elevated blood glucose levels may worsen an ischemic deficit.
- *Temperature regulation.* Hyperthermia should be controlled in all ischemic stroke patients, as an elevated core temperature is known to be harmful in the setting of stroke.
- *Increased intracranial pressure.* See Table 56–3.

Disposition

- *Consultation.* A consultation with neurology should be sought for any patient with a stroke, and with neurosurgery for any hemorrhagic stroke or cerebellar infarction that has potential for herniation.
- *Admission.* All patients with acute ischemic stroke, ICH, or SAH are admitted to the hospital, often to an intensive care unit (ICU). Most

Table 56–2 Antihypertensive Therapy in Stroke

Blood Pressure	Treatment
PATIENTS INELIGIBLE FOR THROMBOLYTICS	
1. DBP > 140 mm Hg	Sodium nitroprusside (0.5 µg/kg/min)
2. SBP > 220, DBP 121-140 mm Hg	Labetalol 10-20 mg over 1-2 min. May repeat or double dose every 10 min to max dose of 300 mg OR Nicardipine 5 mg/hr. May titrate by increasing 2.5 mg/hr every 5 min to max dose of 15 mg/hr
3. SBP < 220, DBP < 120 mm Hg	May use labetalol. Defer treatment in the absence of aortic dissection, MI, CHF, or hypertensive encephalopathy.
PATIENTS ELIGIBLE FOR THROMBOLYTICS	
Pretreatment	
SBP > 185, DBP > 110 mm Hg	1-2 in of nitropaste or 1-2 doses of labetalol 10-20 mg. If BP not <185/110 in 1 hr, do not administer rt-PA
During and after treatment	Check BP every 15 min × 2 hrs then every 30 min × 6 hrs then every 1 hr x 16 hrs.
1. DBP > 140 mm Hg	Sodium nitroprusside (0.5 µg/kg/min)
2. SBP > 230, DBP 121-140 mm Hg	Labetalol 10 mg over 1-2 min. May repeat or double dose every 10 min to max dose of 300 mg, or bolus and start drip at 2-8 mg/min OR Nicardipine 5 mg/hr. May titrate by increasing 2.5 mg/hr every 5 min to max dose of 15 mg/hr If BP not controlled, consider sodium nitroprusside.
3. SBP 180-230, DBP 105-120 mm Hg	Labetalol 10 mg over 1-2 min. May repeat or double dose every 10-20 min to max dose of 300 mg, or bolus and start drip at 2-8 mg/min.

Reproduced from Adams et al. Guidelines for the Early Management of Patients with Ischemic Stroke: A Scientific Statement from the Stroke Council of the American Stroke Association. Stroke 2003;34:1056-1083.

patients with a TIA are admitted. The decision to admit or not is presently institution or physician dependent.

■ *Discharge.* Candidates for discharge include patients with TIAs who are not operative candidates for high-grade carotid stenosis to prevent future stroke, those who have been seen by a neurologist and completed

Table 56–3	**Management of Increased ICP**
Positioning	Keep the head of bed elevated 20-30 degrees.
Hyperosmolar therapy and diuresis	Mannitol load 0.5-1.0 g/kg IV with maintenance dose 0.25-0.5 g/kg q6 hr titrated to serum osm 300-310 mOsm/kg H_2O Lasix and acetazolamide may be added.
Hyperventilation	Goal pCO_2 30-35 mm Hg Increase ventilation rate at constant tidal volume of 12-14 mL/kg. Hyperventilation can also lower ICP because hypocarbia causes cerebral vasoconstriction, but its effect is usually short-lived (only about 12 hours), and may result in a rebound increase in ICP. Overaggressive hyperventilation will lower cerebral blood flow.
Sedation	Propofol or ativan drip
Paralysis	Vecuronium or pancuronium in combination with sedation. Pretreatment for rapid sequence intubation should include lidocaine IV.
Barbiturate coma	Thiopental 1-5 mg/kg titrated to EEG activity
Ventriculostomy	Placement of a ventriculostomy tube through a burr hole, esp. if hydrocephalus
Surgical decompression	Neurosurgical intervention to evacuate hematoma

testing, or those who will have immediate follow-up with a neurologist. Testing may include a cardiac echocardiogram and carotid duplex ultrasonography. An MRI will probably be obtained, but is not needed acutely.

Specific Problems
Cerebellar Hemorrhage or Ischemic Infarct

- *Epidemiology and risk factors.* Increased age, black race, and all stroke risk factors (hypertension, smoking, diabetes, and vascular disease) increase risk of hemorrhagic and ischemic infarct.
- *Pathophysiology.* Hypertension or presence of a neoplasm predisposes to bleeding. Ischemic infarcts are caused by thrombosis or dissection of a vessel, or emboli from other sites.
- *History.* Patients typically have sudden onset of severe headache, severe vertigo, ataxia, and vomiting. Brainstem symptoms such as diplopia, dysphagia, dysarthria, and facial weakness may also be present.
- *Physical examination.* It may be difficult to perform a neurologic examination due to the severity of the patient's vertigo and its association with vomiting. Findings include ataxia, poor coordination, and unsteady gait. The patient may fall to the side of the lesion or may be unable to walk.

- *Diagnostic testing.* A CT scan may not visualize the posterior fossa well, but it is sufficient to detect major bleeding, and is rapidly and easily obtained from the ED. An MRI has better imaging of the posterior fossa but the acquisition process is too dangerous for unstable patients. An angiography/MRA is used to evaluate for an aneurysm or to identify a bleeding vessel. In patients with hemorrhage, coagulation parameters should be obtained, and corrected immediately if abnormal. Type and screen may be required if significant blood loss is suspected, or if the patient is going immediately to the operating room.
- *ED management.* Unlike patients who have profound coma after hemispheric infarction, patients who have coma secondary to cerebellar infarction might make useful recoveries after prompt decompression. Thus, when the CT scan findings suggest a posterior fossa mass effect in a severely comatose patient, neurosurgical consultation should be sought even in the absence of hemorrhage. If cerebellar hemorrhage is found, urgent neurosurgery consultation is warranted. The patient must be observed for signs of increased ICP, and treated as indicated to avert impending herniation (Table 56–3).
- *Helpful hints and pitfalls.* The acuity and severity of this presentation may mimic peripheral causes of vertigo. The age of the patient, risk factors, presence of truncal ataxia, or cranial nerve deficits all favor this diagnosis.

Hemorrhagic Stroke: Spontaneous Intracerebral Hemorrhage

- *Epidemiology and risk factors.* The prognosis for ICH is often poor, with a mortality rate of 30% to 50% within 30 days. Chronic hypertension is the most prevalent risk factor for ICH. Other risk factors include excessive alcohol consumption, tobacco use, illicit drug use, anticoagulation or antiplatelet therapy, cerebral amyloid angiopathy, intracranial aneurysms or tumors, arteriovenous malformations, prior stroke, male gender, Asian or black race, and advanced age. Eclampsia accounts for more than 40% of ICHs in pregnancy, and is a common cause of death from eclampsia.
- *Pathophysiology.* ICH occurs when blood leaks into the brain parenchyma due to the rupture of a vessel wall. A vessel may be prone to rupture because of chronic degeneration of the vessel wall from hypertension, amyloid accumulation, or because of a bleeding diathesis. A hemorrhage may also be due to a spontaneous rupture of an aneurysm or vascular malformation. Regardless of the cause, the common pathway is the formation of a hematoma with the release of vasoactive factors that promote the development of surrounding edema. Neurotoxic proteins are also released from the hematoma, leading to necrosis of neurons. Increasing cerebral edema within the enclosed space of the skull can disrupt the brain's autoregulatory mechanisms, and rapidly increase the intracranial pressure (ICP), resulting in herniation syndromes. In addition, compression of the cerebrospinal fluid (CSF) outflow tracts from the edema can lead to the development of hydrocephalus, which if left untreated can be fatal.
- *History.* The presentation of ICH can vary from headache and vomiting to a gradual decline in consciousness hours after the onset of initial

Location	Signs and symptoms
Table 56–4 Anatomic Location of Intracerebral Hemorrhage (ICH)	
Frontal lobe	Frontal headache, contralateral arm>leg weakness, behavioral disinhibition
Parietal lobe	Parietal headache, contralateral sensory deficits, neglect in nondominant hemisphere, visual field deficits
Temporal lobe	Temporal headache, aphasia in dominant hemisphere, visual field deficits
Occipital lobe	Ipsilateral periorbital headache, visual field loss
Putamen	Contralateral weakness/sensory deficit, aphasia in dominant hemisphere, neglect in nondominant hemisphere
Thalamus	Contralateral sensory deficit>weakness, gaze deviations
Cerebellum	Vomiting, ataxia, decreased level of consciousness
Pontine	Coma, quadriplegia, posturing, pinpoint pupils

Adapted from Panagos PD, Jauch EC, Broderick JP. Intracerebral hemorrhage. Emerg Med Clin North Am 2002;20:631-655.

symptoms to a sudden loss of consciousness, all symptoms of increased ICP. Neurologic deficits vary according to the location of the hemorrhage. Patients may report weakness, sensory deficits, visual field deficits, or difficulty ambulating. Family members may note that the patient appears confused, and does not answer questions appropriately, indicating underlying aphasia. Although ICH may not always be distinguishable from ischemic stroke, complaints of headache and vomiting or loss of consciousness are more common with hemorrhage. Other valuable information includes any incidence of recent trauma or seizure activity.

■ *Physical examination.* The focus should be on ABCs and a complete neurologic evaluation. Cushing's reflex occurs with increasing ICP and the loss of cerebral blood flow (CBF) regulation. Clinical signs include increased systemic blood pressure and bradycardia secondary to increased vagal tone. The presence of a dilated or "blown" pupil suggests compression of the oculomotor nerve due to mass effect and a herniation syndrome. Information gathered from the history and physical examination combined can help to identify the anatomic location of the hemorrhage (Table 56–4).

■ *Diagnostic testing.* A noncontrast head CT scan is the most reliable method for diagnosing ICH. Blood appears hyperdense in comparison with the normal brain parenchyma (Figure 56–2). Angiography may be indicated in those patients whose ICH can be attributed to an aneurysm or arteriovenous malformation. There is no clear role for an MRI in ICH because of its lower sensitivity for detecting hemorrhage. However, MRA is a noninvasive test that may be used to visualize the cerebral vasculature to identify any aneurysms or vascular malformations that may require repair.

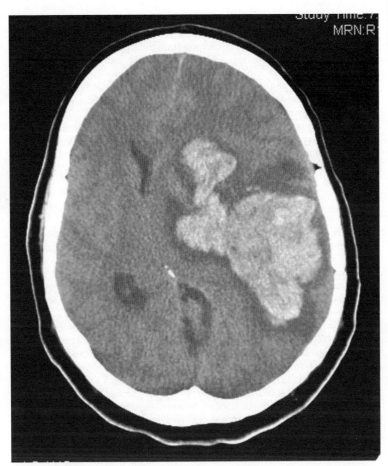

Figure 56-2. Noncontrast head CT scan of an acute intracerebral hemorrhage in the left temporal lobe in a patient found unresponsive with a history significant for an intracranial mass and deep venous thromboses requiring anticoagulation with warfarin. There is significant midline shift to the right. *Courtesy of Dr. Jerrold L. Boxerman, Department of Radiology, Rhode Island Hospital.*

- ■ *ED management.* Treatment is centered on airway protection (Chapter 5), management of increased ICP (Table 56–3) and control of blood pressure (Table 56–2). Anticoagulation should be reversed as mentioned above under "Emergency Department Management Overview". Lowering the blood pressure can reduce additional bleeding from the ruptured vessel. However, aggressively treating the hypertension may reduce cerebral perfusion, and exacerbate neuronal injury. Antihypertensive therapy in ICH is similar to that in ischemic stroke. Nitroprusside should be used with caution due to its potential to increase ICP. Labetolol or nicardipine may be preferred. Patients with ICH can also present with hypotension, which should be treated with intravenous fluid hydration and vasopressor agents if hypotension persists despite fluid therapy. Neurosurgery should be consulted early to evaluate candidates for hematoma evacuation. Surgical candidates include patients with cerebellar hemorrhages with hydrocephalus and neurologic deterioration, patients with aneurysms or vascular malformations amenable to repair, and patients younger than 50 years old with large lobar hemorrhages.

- *Helpful hints and pitfalls.* ICH is most commonly the result of long-standing hypertension, and typically begins abruptly and worsens over a few minutes to hours. Severe headache, vomiting, and decreased level of consciousness may help to differentiate from ischemic stroke before imaging.

Ischemic Stroke

- *Epidemiology and risk factors.* Stroke is the third leading cause of death and the leading cause of disability in the United States. Stroke can occur in all ages, but the risk of stroke increases with age, with 75% occurring in patients older than 65 years. Causes of ischemic stroke include atherosclerotic disease, atrial fibrillation, recent MI, valvular heart disease, cardiomyopathies, cardiac shunts such as a patent foramen ovale, hypercoagulable disorders, hyperviscosity syndromes, arterial dissection, vasculitis, and infections (such as meningitis and tuberculosis). Modifiable risk factors include hypertension, tobacco use, diabetes, excessive consumption of alcohol, illicit drug use, hyperlipidemia, carotid stenosis, dysrhythmias, heart disease, hypercoagulable states, physical inactivity, and obesity. A TIA is a significant warning, requires a complete workup, and may lead to anticoagulation or surgical repair of stenotic lesions that will prevent a subsequent stroke (discussed separately).
- *Pathophysiology.* Acute arterial occlusion may occur due to thrombosis or embolism. Thrombotic strokes are frequently caused by atherosclerotic lesions. Embolic strokes are caused by emboli from arterial sources, such as emboli from atherosclerotic plaques in vessels, or from cardiac sources, including atrial fibrillation, recent myocardial infarction, cardiomyopathies, mural thrombus, and valvular heart disease. Once vascular occlusion occurs, the hypoperfused neural tissue is deprived of oxygen and glucose. The central core of this ischemic tissue is characterized by irreversible neuronal injury due to anaerobic metabolism with resultant necrosis within minutes. The area surrounding the core, the ischemic penumbra, which has reduced blood flow with ongoing aerobic metabolism, contains neurons with potentially reversible injury. Therefore, therapy for ischemic strokes is directed at quickly restoring blood flow to the penumbra before necrosis ensues.
- *History.* Delineating the exact time of onset of symptoms is crucial in determining eligibility for thrombolytic treatment. Patients may present with a variety of symptoms according to the distribution of the ischemia. Patients may report weakness, numbness, slurred speech, visual deficits, vertigo, or difficulty ambulating. Other relevant information to elicit includes presence of associated symptoms, such as headaches or loss of

Table 56–5 Ischemic Stroke Syndromes

Occluded Artery	Signs and Symptoms
Anterior cerebral artery	Contralateral leg>arm weakness/numbness, dyspraxia
Middle cerebral artery	Contralateral face+arm>leg weakness/numbness, dysarthria, aphasia in dominant hemisphere, neglect in nondominant hemisphere
Posterior cerebral artery	Contralateral visual-field cut
Basilar artery	Quadriplegia, locked-in syndrome
Vertebrobasilar syndrome	Dizziness, vertigo, diplopia, ataxia
Penetrating arteries	"lacunar infarcts," pure motor or sensory deficits

Adapted from Kasner SE, Morgenstern LB. Neurology: Cerebrovascular Disorders. ACP Medicine 2004; 1-16.

consciousness, medical history that may indicate risk factors for stroke, and details surrounding the event, such as seizure activity or recent trauma. It is always useful to find out from a relative or care taker when the patient was last observed without symptoms or signs.

■ *Physical examination.* After the ABCs are addressed, a thorough physical examination should be performed with special attention to the neurological examination. Neurologic findings can help to determine the location and size of the ischemic insult (Table 56–5). The patient should be examined for any signs of trauma. Carotid and vertebral auscultation may reveal bruits, suggesting carotid or basivertebral stenosis. The cardiac examination may reveal dysrhythmias such as atrial fibrillation or the presence of murmurs, which may suggest underlying valvular disease. Unequal pulses in the extremities may indicate aortic dissection.

■ *Diagnostic testing.* Most ischemic strokes will not be detected by a noncontrast CT scan in the first 6 hours. If present, early findings may be subtle, and can include loss of gray–white matter interface and loss of sulci. There may be hypodensity with or without surrounding cerebral edema causing mass effect and midline shift (Figure 56–3). MR imaging (MRI) of the brain is not routinely utilized in the emergent diagnosis of stroke because it is more time-consuming than a CT scan, it has limited availability, and it is contraindicated in patients with pacemakers or metal fragments in the body. However, MRI is more sensitive in detecting acute ischemic lesions, and may identify some missed by CT. Diffusion- and perfusion-weighted MRI can also outline the core and penumbra regions and identify the extent of tissue with reversible injury. MRA is a noninvasive test that allows visualization of the cerebral vessels, and can help identify possible candidates for intra-arterial thrombolytic treatment. However, its use is also limited as it possesses the same disadvantages as MRI. Cerebral angiography is the

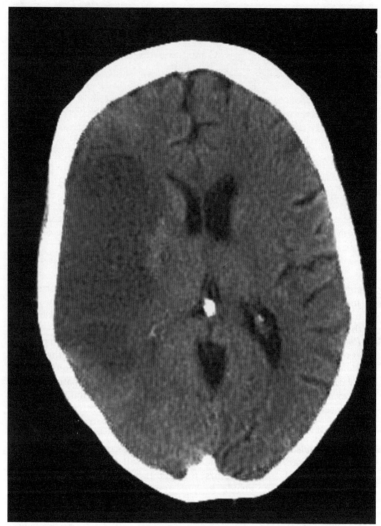

Figure 56–3. Noncontrast head CT scan of an ischemic stroke. This image demonstrates an infarct (hypodense area) evolving in the right middle cerebral artery territory. There is partial effacement of the right lateral ventricle due to edema. *Courtesy of Dr. Jerrold L. Boxerman, Department of Radiology, Rhode Island Hospital.*

gold standard for evaluating the vasculature. It will demonstrate any arterial occlusions, and also allows such interventions as direct delivery of intra-arterial thrombolytics to a culprit lesion. However, the procedure itself carries the risk of inducing a stroke and is not available at all hospitals. Transcranial Doppler (TCD) and carotid ultrasound studies are imaging studies that may be obtained once the patient is admitted to evaluate for any occlusive lesions in the intracranial arteries, and in the vessels in the neck that may be amenable to intra-arterial thrombolytic therapy or to carotid endarterectomy. In addition, an echocardiogram is a part of the nonemergent workup to be done as an inpatient to help identify the etiology of the stroke. Echocardiography is helpful in revealing ventricular wall hypokinesis in the setting of a recent or acute myocardial infarction, mural thrombus, valvular disease or endocarditis.

- *ED management.* Aspirin therapy produces a significant benefit in prevention of recurrent strokes; 50 to 325 mg of daily aspirin should be initiated within 48 hours of stroke onset, but should be withheld for 24 hours after thrombolytic therapy. No studies to date support the use of heparin and LMWH in ischemic stroke given the risk of intracerebral hemorrhage. They may be started in patients with atrial fibrillation or cardioembolic strokes because these patients will require long-term anticoagulation with warfarin; however, anticoagulation should be withheld for the first 3 to 4 days. Thrombolytic therapy (see Chapter 90.5) is given within 3 hours of symptom onset according to strict guidelines, and results in a significant reduction in morbidity. The dose of tPA for stroke is different than the dose for myocardial infarction. The patient's neurologic status must be closely monitored for signs of ICH. Any deterioration or complaints of headache, nausea, or vomiting warrants stopping the infusion, obtaining a head CT scan immediately, and administering cryoprecipitate in the event of an ICH. Rapid lowering of blood pressure will reduce cerebral blood flow and exacerbate the ischemia. Aim for 10% to 20% reduction in blood pressure (Table 56–2).
- *Helpful hints and pitfalls.* Increased intracranial pressure secondary to edema is rare early on in acute ischemic strokes, except in cerebellar infarctions, which can compress the brainstem and cause hydrocephalus.

Transient Ischemic Attack

- *Epidemiology and risk factors.* The risk factors for TIA are the same as those for stroke. TIAs carry a substantial short-term risk for stroke, hospitalization for cardiovascular events, and death. TIAs are often described as a warning sign for stroke, because 10% of patients will develop a stroke in the subsequent 90 days, half of these over the first 48 hours.
- *Pathophysiology.* This is similar to acute ischemic strokes. TIAs are caused by a reduction in blood flow due to thrombosis or embolism. However, the insult is transient, and does not cause permanent neuronal injury and cell death.
- *History.* A detailed history including time of onset and duration of symptoms must be obtained. Patients may present with a variety of symptoms according to the distribution of the ischemia. Patients may report weakness, numbness, slurred speech, visual deficits, or difficulty ambulating. Such fleeting symptoms may be subtle and typically last less than 15 minutes. Some patients may present only with transient monocular blindness (amaurosis fugax), characterized as a "shade coming down over the eye." It is caused by retinal ischemia that will typically resolve after a few minutes. If a patient has a history of multiple TIAs,

it is important to determine how often the symptoms are occurring, as crescendo TIAs warrant admission and urgent intervention to prevent the stroke from completing. Other relevant information to elicit would include presence of associated symptoms, medical history, and details surrounding the event, such as seizure activity or recent trauma.

- **Physical examination.** A general physical examination and thorough neurologic examination should be performed in a similar fashion as described for acute ischemic stroke. Most patients will have a normal neurologic examination by the time of arrival in the ED.
- **Diagnostic testing.** A noncontrast head CT scan will generally yield few or no findings, but it should nevertheless be obtained, as it could reveal an unsuspected ischemic stroke, an intracranial mass, or a subdural hematoma. As with an acute ischemic stroke, imaging of the carotid arteries and cerebral vessels and of the heart can be done on a nonemergent basis to evaluate for potential causes for the TIA.
- **EM management.** Because aspirin reduces the long-term risk of stroke after a TIA, 50 to 325 mg of daily aspirin should be initiated. If a patient has a TIA despite daily aspirin therapy, daily clopidogrel 75 mg or dipyridamole 200 mg can be added, or the patient can be switched to an aspirin-dipyridamole combination (Aggrenox) or ticlodipine 250 mg twice daily. Heparin anticoagulation can be initiated in patients with atrial fibrillation or cardioembolic sources as a bridge to lifelong anti-coagulation with warfarin. Although risk reduction is not an ED treat-ment , the patient can be advised of the importance of smoking cessation, exercise, weight loss, and limiting excessive alcohol consumption. If the patient has undergone the necessary diagnostic testing for possible causes of the TIA, and these are negative, the patient is a candidate for discharge. Discharge medications should include lipid-lowering agents if hyperlipidemia is present, and antihypertensive medications, such as angiotensin-receptor blocks or beta-blockers, if there is a history significant for hypertension. The decision to admit or not is institution or physician dependent.
- **Helpful hints and pitfalls.** Patients eligible for discharge from the ED include patients with high-grade carotid stenosis (>70%) who are not operative candidates for a carotid endarterectomy (CEA), are already on antiplatelet therapy, patients who have completed the TIA workup (laboratory test, EKG, and imaging studies), or will complete the workup within 24 hours and in whom high-grade carotid stenosis has been ruled out. Yet, most patients should be admitted to the hospital for observation, and to facilitate an expedited risk factor evaluation. The short-term risk for stroke alone is 10% at 90 days.

Vertebrobasilar Insufficiency (VBI)

- **Epidemiology and risk factors.** All risk factors for stroke and athero-sclerosis apply.
- **Pathophysiology.** This is a transient ischemic attack affecting the vertebrobasilar system. The usual cause is atherosclerotic disease. It may also be caused by dissection.

- *History.* Patients have abrupt onset of vertigo, usually lasting several minutes. It is almost always associated with other posterior circulation neurologic deficits such as ataxia, diplopia, dysarthria, dysphagia, and facial numbness or weakness.
- *Physical examination.* The symptoms are temporary, so patients may have a normal neurologic examination at the time of presentation.
- *Diagnostic testing.* A noncontrast CT scan may be used to look for infarction, but does not visualize the posterior fossa or brainstem well. An MRI is also used to look for infarction or hemorrhage. It is time-consuming, often difficult to obtain in the ED, and not a prudent study in an unstable patient. MRA and CT angiography are definitive studies to look for occlusion or atherosclerosis of the vertebrobasilar system.
- *ED management.* Neurology and vascular surgeons should be consulted. Antiplatelet agents should be administered. For severe, progressive symptoms, full anticoagulation should be considered.
- *Helpful hints and pitfalls.* Older patients with vascular risk factors may only have intermittent symptoms. A normal examination on presentation does not exclude VBI.

Special Considerations
Pediatrics

- Cerebrovascular disorders are among the top 10 causes of death in children, with rates highest within the first year.
- Causes include sickle cell disease, congenital heart diseases, hereditary hypercoagulable disorders, and infections (e.g., meningitis, tonsillitis, cat scratch disease).
- Children with sickle cell disease have a 10% per year risk of stroke making this the most important cause of ischemic stroke among black children. Prophylactic exchange transfusion to maintain hemoglobin S under 30%, adequate hydration, and oxygenation are recommended therapies.
- Child abuse (nonaccidental trauma) and substance abuse must always be considered in the differential diagnosis of hemorrhagic stroke.
- In infants, irritability and a full fontanelle may be the only signs of stroke. The presence of murmurs may direct attention toward a congenital heart disease. Diminished femoral pulses are suggestive of coarctation of the aorta.
- Thrombolytic therapy has not been widely approved for the use in children with ischemic stroke though many tertiary centers have experience using it safely and effectively.

Pregnancy

- Risk factors for stroke in the pregnancy and postpartum periods are the same for any patient and include eclampsia, postpartum cerebral angiopathy, peripartum cardiomyopathy, choriocarcinoma, and amniotic fluid embolism.
- SAH is the third most common nonobstetric cause of maternal death.

- Pregnant patients with embolic strokes will require anticoagulation with heparin. Warfarin is contraindicated because it can cross the placenta, is teratogenic in the first trimester, and is unsafe near delivery because of fetal and maternal bleeding complications. Low-dose aspirin (150 mg/d) during the second and third trimesters is safe.

Teaching Points

Thrombolytics have been proven to be safe and effective in the treatment of acute ischemic stroke. Failure to strictly adhere to the inclusion/exclusion criteria governing the use of intravenous thrombolytics may lead to an increased risk of intracerebral hemorrhage.

The most common problem in the management of patients with stroke is to be too skeptical about the ability to help these patients. It is certainly true that only a few patients will meet the 3 hour requirement for reperfusion, but it should be sought vigorously especially in the younger patient. While it is true that the mortality for reperfusion is probably higher because of induced hemorrhage, it is also true that neurologic outcome, when the hemorrhagic complication has not occurred, is better. This becomes a choice for the patient and family, and should not be missed because you are personally unwilling to risk a cerebral hemorrhage.

The place where you can do the most good is in the patient with a TIA. This is the patient in whom finding a carotid or basivertebral bruit may enable stroke preventive medical or surgical therapy. TIAs are ominous predictors of future morbidity and mortality, carrying a substantial short-term risk for stroke, hospitalization for cardiovascular events, and death.

Similarly, in the young patient with a warning bleed from an aneurysm, the time to discover this is before the aneurysm bursts with terrible destruction of neural tissue.

There are also a small group of patients with posterior bleeds who will do very well with timely neurosurgical intervention, but to find them means being fastidious about testing gait in all patients, and not putting this off because of difficulties perceived in mobilizing an elderly sick patient. Cerebellar hemorrhage or infarction can rapidly produce critical brainstem compression, and threaten the life of the patient. Immediate neurosurgical consultation is recommended.

Elevated blood pressure in the setting of an acute ischemic stroke is common, and may be adaptive to maintain cerebral blood flow. Aggressive lowering of blood pressure is not recommended and may actually worsen neurological injury. Finally, it will be possible to effect great change in neurologic function when the deficit is being caused by an acute metabolic disturbance or an acute toxicologic state. Hypoglycemia is common, and may mimic a focal neurological deficit. Rapid identification and correction will normally lead to symptom resolution.

Suggested Readings

Adams, Jr. HP, Adams RJ, Brott T, et al. Guidelines for the early management of patients with ischemic stroke: A Scientific Statement from the Stroke Council of the American Stroke Association. Stroke 2003;34:1056–1083.

American Heart Association. Heart Disease and Stroke Statistics—2005 Update. Dallas,TX: American Heart Association, 2005.

Broderick JP, Adams HP, Barsan W, et al. Guidelines for the management of spontaneous intracerebral hemorrhage: a statement for healthcare professionals from a special writing group of the Stroke Council, American Heart Association. Stroke 1999;30:905–915.

Ingall TJ, O'Fallon WM, Asplund K, et al. Findings from the Reanalysis of the NINDS Tissue Plasminogen Activator for Acute Ischemic Stroke Treatment Trial. Stroke 2004;35:2418–2424.

Johnston SC. Transient ischemic attack. N Engl J Med 2002;347:1687–1691.

Lewandowski C, Barsan W. Treatment of acute ischemic stroke. Ann Emerg Med 2001; 37:202–216.

Manno EM. Subarachnoid hemorrhage. Neurol Clin 2004;22:347–366.

Panagos PD, Jauch EC, Broderick JP. Intracerebral hemorrhage. Emerg Med Clin North Am 2002;20:631–655.

CHAPTER **57**

Syncope

COLLEEN JOHNSON ■ H. GENE HERN, JR.

 Red Flags

Elderly ● History of coronary artery disease or risk factors, peripheral vascular disease, gastrointestinal bleeding ● Polypharmacy ● Abrupt onset ● Duration more than a few seconds ● Repeated episodes of syncope ● Occurrence while sitting or supine ● Shortness of breath ● Chest pain ● Severe headache ● Abdominal pain ● Back pain ● Abnormal vital signs: tachycardia, bradycardia, hypotension, hypertension ● Pallor ● Gastrointestinal bleeding ● Focal neurologic signs

Overview

Although there is no qualitative difference between syncope and presyncope with respect to differential diagnosis, the latter differs from the former in that there is no actual loss of consciousness.

Syncope is an abrupt transient loss of consciousness associated with inability to maintain postural tone, followed by a rapid complete return to baseline neurologic function. The episode is usually due to hypoperfusion to the cerebral cortex and the cerebral reticular activating system. Both of these structures depend on cerebral metabolism and the delivery of oxygen and glucose for proper function.

Syncope is a transient event of decreased blood flow to the brain and not a specific disease. It is most often benign and self-limiting, but may cause other associated traumatic injuries. However, syncope can be a warning sign of sudden cardiac death, especially in patients with structural heart disease.

The cause of syncope is not often obvious. The evaluation, management, and treatment approach is to detect the patient at highest risk for a poor outcome including sudden death. Look for "red flags" (see Box) in the evaluation of these patients. Although most causes of syncope are not serious, search for the serious causes in the elderly patient (>60 years). Syncope may also be the presenting complaint of a leaking aortic aneurysm or pulmonary embolus.

Syncope is extremely common, accounting for up to 6% of medical admissions and 1% to 3% of ED visits. The highest incidence of syncope and increased risk for morbidity is seen in the elderly. There is 6% annual incidence in those over 75 years old, while 12% to 40% of adults younger than 40 years will experience syncope at some point. Several decision rules describe patients at risk for poor outcome. Increased death is seen with the presence of an abnormal electrocardiogram (EKG), history of ventricular dysrhythmia, congestive heart failure, and age more than 45 years. Another syncope decision rule describes increased risk of serious outcomes within 7 days for patients with abnormal EKG findings, history of congestive heart failure (CHF) or dyspnea, a hematocrit of less than 30%, or hypotension.

Prognosis is related to the underlying etiology, not the symptoms. Cardiac causes of syncope are associated with higher mortality rates than noncardiovascular causes. Any disease that decreases cardiac output may cause syncope such as valve obstruction, pump failure, dysrhythmias, or conduction defects.

Differential Diagnosis of Syncope

- The differential diagnosis is broad and includes benign and life-threatening causes (see the DDx table).

Initial Diagnostic Approach
General

- Any patient who is hemodynamically unstable or appears ill should receive immediate attention. While the physician is assessing the patient, a continuous cardiac monitor and pulse oximeter should be placed. Supplemental oxygen should be given especially if the patient is elderly,

DDx Differential Diagnoses of Syncope

Cardiac, 23%
- Obstruction to flow (22)
- Dysrhythmias (45,87)
- Vascular disease: pulmonary embolism (52), aortic dissection (22), abdominal aortic aneurysm (18), myocardial infarction or ischemia (22).

Noncardiac, 77%
- Neurologic: head trauma (9), migraine (35), seizure (51), stroke or transient ischemic attack (56)
- Vasovagal
- Orthostatic
- Medications
- Pregnancy
- Psychogenic
- Unexplained

( ) Refers to the chapter in which the disease entity is discussed.

has respiratory symptoms or has an oxygen saturation less than 95%. Intravenous (IV) access should be obtained. These patients should not leave the ED until stabilized or for definitive care (i.e., operating room). The younger the patient, the fewer and less concerning co-morbid conditions, the better the historian, and the better the patient appears on physical examination, the fewer laboratory and imaging studies may be indicated.

■ *History.* A careful history and physical examination will identify the cause of syncope in more than half of the patients in whom a diagnosis can be determined. Because syncope is transient, most patients will be asymptomatic on presentation. Witnesses of the event should be sought as they can often provide additional information. Both critical and benign causes of syncope are suggested with information regarding prodromal signs, current symptoms, medication list, past medical history and family history. A family history of syncope or sudden death may suggest a cardiac dysrhythmia or a prolonged QT syndrome. Obtain a detailed description of associated symptoms or preceding events, the patient's position, environmental stimuli, activity or exercise before the event and duration of symptoms. Syncope occurring after prolonged exposure to heat suggests orthostasis. Syncope occurring after an emotional event or pain is more likely the result of a vasovagal episode. Complaints of diaphoresis, light-headedness, graying of vision (tunnel vision) may suggest orthostasis or a vasovagal response; however, serious causes of syncope cannot be excluded. Syncope that occurs in the supine position is more concerning for a cardiac etiology. Syncope during exertion should be concerning for cardiac outflow obstruction. Anything causing a Valsalva maneuver (i.e., straining, coughing) may result in syncope. Syncope associated with shaving the neck or head turning is classically associated with carotid sinus hypersensitivity. Critical symptoms that may precede or follow an episode of syncope include: chest pain (myocardial infarction, aortic dissection, pulmonary embolism, aortic stenosis), shortness of breath (myocardial infarction, pulmonary embolism, congestive heart failure), headache (subarachnoid hemorrhage), abdominal pain or back pain (leaking aortic aneurysm, ruptured ectopic pregnancy). Seizures, although not a true syncopal event, may be preceded by an aura. These "red flag" symptoms should be specifically asked about in every patient with syncope.

■ *Physical examination.* A thorough physical examination should be completed on all patients with syncope, and may aid in determining some of the causes of syncope. Abnormal pulse and blood pressure measurements may indicate a critical cause of syncope. Tachycardia may suggest pulmonary embolism, hypovolemia, or tachydysrhythmia. Bradycardia may be a sign of a cardiac conduction defect, or an acute coronary syndrome causing syncope, but it is also seen in vasovagal fainting. Specific testing for orthostatic hypotension can be suggestive, but is frequently unreliable. The reproduction of syncopal or near-syncopal symptoms is far more helpful than any arbitrary change in blood pressure or heart rate. See discussion of orthostatic hypotension under "Specific Problems". Heart auscultation may reveal a murmur due to valve stenosis or insufficiency. Significantly unequal blood pressure measurements in both arms (>20 mm Hg change) is suggestive of an aortic coarctation dissection, or a subclavian steal syndrome. Tachypnea may suggest pulmonary embolism or congestive heart failure. Focal neurological findings may be due to a cerebral vascular accident. A rectal examination should be performed on any patient with concern for gastrointestinal bleeding.

EKG

■ A 12-lead electrocardiogram (EKG) should be ordered for all patients with syncope regardless of age. Cardiac causes of syncope are associated with higher morbidity and mortality. The EKG is of greatest importance in patients with cardiac risk factors, including coronary artery disease, congestive heart failure, diabetes, shortness of breath, or any family history of sudden cardiac death. Evaluate for acute ischemia, heart block, and dysrhythmia. Dysrhythmias associated with syncope are listed in Table 57–1. An EKG showing right-sided ventricular strain pattern may suggest pulmonary embolus, whereas diffuse ST elevation or electrical alternans will help diagnose pericarditis associated with pericardial tamponade. The presence of an abnormal EKG is not proof of a cardiac cause for syncope, but places the patient in a higher risk category (see Chapter 87).

Laboratory

■ Because syncope is an event with many various causes, there are only a few routine laboratory tests.

■ *Glucose.* This should be checked by rapid finger-stick test on all patients with syncope. Loss of consciousness due to hypoglycemia is not likely to spontaneously resolve. Despite its low yield, hypoglycemia should not be missed in the evaluation of any patient.

Table 57–1	Dysrhythmias That May Cause Syncope
Bradyarrhythmias	• Sick sinus syndrome • Second- and third-degree atrioventricular block • Atrial fibrillation with slow conduction • Pacemaker malfunction
Tachydysrhythmias	• Ventricular fibrillation • Ventricular tachycardia • Torsades de pointes • Superventricular • Atrial fibrillation with fast conduction • Brugada syndrome • Wolff-Parkinson-White syndrome

- **Stool guaiac.** This should be performed in all adult patients with syncope if concerned for occult bleeding.
- **Hemoglobin and hematocrit.** A low hematocrit has been shown to be an indicator of poor outcome in some risk stratification schemes. Selective use is recommended in orthostatic hypotension, patients with heme-positive stool, and most patients with any cardiac risk factors for syncope.
- **Serum electrolytes and renal function.** Empiric use of these tests has a low diagnostic yield in syncope. A history of diuretic use warrants evaluation of electrolytes as does the suggestion of profound dehydration. Any patient with altered mental status or suspicion of seizure activity should have electrolytes checked.
- **Cardiac enzymes.** This is indicated in any patient with a history of chest pain or shortness of breath preceding the syncope. It should also be considered in any patient with cardiac risk factors.
- **Arterial blood gases.** This is used to evaluate for hypoxemia or hyperventilation.
- **Urine pregnancy test.** Obtain this in all reproductive age women.
- **Drug screen and ethanol level.** These studies should be ordered if intoxication is suspected.

Radiography

- **Chest radiograph.** This may be helpful in patients with any cardiac or respiratory symptoms.
- **Computed tomography (CT scan).** The noncontrast head CT scan is frequently of low diagnostic yield, but is indicated if the patient has new neurologic deficits, new-onset or focal seizure, or head trauma secondary to a syncope-associated fall. A chest and abdominal CT should be ordered on stable patients with concern for aortic dissection or abdominal aortic aneurysm. Patients with a possibility for a pulmonary embolism should have a CT angiogram (or ventilation-perfusion scan).
- **Echocardiography.** Echocardiography is recommended in patients with syncope when concerned for outflow obstruction, tamponade, or thoracic aortic dissection. An echocardiogram is frequently only suggestive of a

diagnosis but may be prognostic if left ventricular dysfunction is present. It can specifically establish the diagnosis if severe aortic stenosis or an atrial myxoma is seen.

■ ***Ultrasound.*** Ultrasound can be performed at the bedside, and may be useful in patients in whom a ruptured abdominal aortic aneurysm or ectopic pregnancy is suspected.

■ ***Outpatient studies.*** Transient dysrhythmias can be detected with either Holter or loop EKG long-term monitoring. In selected patients, stress-testing (myocardial ischemia) or electrophysiologic studies (dysrhythmia) may be indicated in consultation with cardiology. Carotid ultrasound can be ordered to evaluate for stroke or transient ischemic attack (TIA), but is more often being done as an inpatient. Magnetic resonance imaging (MRI) is sometimes ordered to evaluate for seizures or stroke (but is rarely performed on an outpatient basis for stroke). Electroencephalography should be ordered if an undiagnosed seizure is suspected. Tilt table testing may have diagnostic value in elderly patients and children in whom chronic orthostatic hypotension is suspected.

Emergency Department Management Overview
General

■ The ABCs (*a*irway, *b*reathing, and *c*irculation) should be addressed as discussed in Section II.

Emergency Department Interventions

■ Syncope is a symptom of various disease states. There are no medications or interventions that apply to all causes of syncope. Treatment is based on the underlying cause, and is frequently directed at preventing recurrence or injury.

Disposition

■ ***Consultation.*** Specialty consultation is dictated by the suspected etiology of syncope. Cardiology consultation is warranted for any patient with acute ischemia, other abnormal EKG findings, or signs of structural heart disease. Early surgical or vascular consultation should be obtained for any unstable patient with abdominal pain or chest pain and evidence of aortic dissection or ruptured abdominal aortic aneurysm. Consultation with neurology is helpful for patients showing sign of stroke, or when seizure is a possible explanation for the patient's loss of consciousness. Psychiatric evaluation is recommended when symptoms suggest psychogenic disorder, or there is a previous known psychiatric disorder and other causes of syncope have been ruled out.

■ ***Admission.*** Admission is warranted in elderly (>60 years) patients with a suspicion of cardiac or neurologic syncope. Criteria for hospital admission are listed in Box 57–1. Hospitalization alone does not always determine the cause of syncope or prevent future episodes of syncope. Syncope from cardiogenic causes has a much higher 1-year mortality rate than noncardiogenic causes. Mortality is high in patients with advanced

> **BOX 57–1 Admission Criteria for Patients with Syncope**
>
> - Shortness of breath as a chief complaint
> - Chest pain or findings of cardiac ischemia
> - Abnormal electrocardiogram (new ischemic changes, dysrhythmia, or bundle branch block)
> - Hematocrit <30%
> - Systolic blood pressure <90 mm Hg
> - Congestive heart failure
> - Evidence of valvular heart disease
> - Stroke or focal neurologic symptoms

heart failure who also have syncope of any etiology. In patients with congestive heart failure, the 1-year risk of sudden death is 45% versus 12% in those without syncope.

- **Discharge.** As many as 50% of ED patients will have no diagnosis at discharge. Most patients without concern for cardiac or neurologic syncope may be safely discharged from the ED. All patients with syncope should follow-up with a primary care physician. Education on preventing recurrence is very important for orthostatic and situational syncope. Patients with recurrent syncope are at risk for severe trauma from falls, and should be counseled on avoiding high-risk situations like climbing ladders and driving. Definitive recommendations for return to any high-risk activities like driving or operating heavy machinery can be deferred to the patient's primary care physician. It is helpful to know the pertinent state laws concerning mandatory reporting of syncope to the Motor Vehicle Bureau. Some discharged patients may require further evaluation as an outpatient, which might include a holter or continuous EKG monitoring device, an EEG, or an electrophysiology study, depending on the suspected etiology.

Specific Problems

> ° ° ° Refer to the DDx table for reference to a discussion of problems in the
> ° ° ° differential not mentioned here.

Cardiovascular Causes of Syncope
Cardiac Outflow Obstruction

- **Epidemiology and risk factors.** There are many causes of outflow obstruction (Box 57–2). Aortic stenosis is a disease primarily of the elderly, and is the most common structural abnormality causing syncope. In young people, hypertrophic cardiomyopathy may lead to outflow obstruction.
- **Pathophysiology.** Diseases of the heart valves, muscle structure, or pericardium can cause obstruction to forward flow. This leads to a decrease in cardiac output, and may precipitate a syncopal episode.

BOX 57–2 Causes of Cardiac Outflow Obstruction

- Aortic or subaortic valve stenosis
- Mitral valve stenosis
- Pulmonary valve stenosis
- Hypertrophic cardiomyopathy
- Restrictive cardiomyopathy
- Pulmonary embolus
- Pericardial tamponade
- Atrial myxoma

- *History.* Syncope from cardiac outflow obstruction may occur suddenly without prodromal symptoms. Cough or dyspnea may suggest a pulmonary embolism or other obstructive cause. Obstructive syncope occurs often in the setting of physical exertion, or in the setting of vasodilatation from medications or a hot environment.
- *Physical examination.* Hypertrophic cardiomyopathy may reveal a loud S_4 heart sound or a harsh systolic crescendo/decrescendo murmur loudest at the left sternal border. Aortic stenosis has a diamond-shaped, midsystolic murmur that often radiates to the neck. Neck vein distention can be seen with a variety of cardiopulmonary diseases.
- *Diagnostic testing.* Obtain a 12-lead EKG. Intraventricular conduction delays (QRS > 0.12 seconds), atrial enlargement, and left ventricular enlargement are all signs of heart disease. An echocardiogram is helpful in evaluating patients with possible structural heart disease.
- *ED management.* Cardiac diseases that obstruct the outflow of blood frequently require surgical correction, and appropriate cardiology consultation is helpful. Treatment is directed at the underlying problem. Admission of these patients is frequently warranted.
- *Helpful hints and pitfalls.* Avoid vasodilators such as nitrates as this may worsen the condition by decreasing preload. Patients with structural heart diseases are predisposed to ventricular dysrhythmias and ischemia that may be the underlying cause of syncope and sudden death.

Dysrhythmias

- Dysrhythmias are more likely to occur in patients with underlying heart disease. The elderly are particularly at risk. Consider this in any patient with underlying cardiac disease. Syncope due to dysrhythmias may also occur in less common diseases like prolonged QT syndrome or Brugada syndrome, which is an autosomal dominant inherited disease occurring in the structurally normal heart, and is characterized by ST segment elevation in the right precordial leads (V_1 to V_3), right bundle branch block, and increased susceptibility to ventricular tachydysrhythmias.
- Bradyarrhythmias or tachydysrhythmias interfere with cardiac output, and may lead to syncope. Tachydysrhythmias do not allow enough time for diastolic filling. Bradycardiac syncope occurs when the heart rate is to slow for adequate cerebral perfusion. See Table 57–1.

Subclavian Steal Syndrome

- ***Epidemiology and risk factors.*** This is a rare cause of syncope. Risk factors are the same as those for atherosclerotic disease.
- ***Pathophysiology.*** There is occlusion or severe stenosis of the proximal subclavian artery typically due to atherosclerosis. This leads to decreased antegrade or retrograde flow in the ipsilateral vertebral artery. When the ipsilateral extremity exercises, the vessels dilate to provide adequate tissue perfusion to ischemic limbs and blood that was destined to the vertebral artery flows retrograde into the arm and out of the cerebral perfusion. This lack of cerebral perfusion occasionally causes syncope or other neurologic symptoms referable to the posterior circulation.
- ***History.*** Patients are usually asymptomatic. The patient may complain of upper extremity ischemic symptoms such as fatigue, exercise-related aching, coolness or numbness. Neurologic symptoms include vertigo, diplopia, decreased vision, or unsteady gait.
- ***Physical examination.*** The most common physical finding is the significant difference in systolic pressures between the two arms. The affected arm will have an average of a 40 mm Hg lower systolic pressure. The pulse is delayed and of smaller volume on the affected side. There may be a supraclavicular bruit.
- ***Diagnostic testing.*** Duplex ultrasonography is the test of choice for subclavian steal. It is rapid and non-invasive, and demonstrates not only anatomy, but can document retrograde flow in the vertebral artery. Other imaging studies include noninvasive upper extremity arterial flow studies and arteriography.
- ***ED management.*** The disease is benign in most patients, and requires atherosclerosis risk factor modification and aspirin. The only significant treatment option is surgical.

Neural Reflex–Mediated Causes of Syncope
Vasovagal

- ***Epidemiology and risk factors.*** Vasovagal syncope is the most common cause of syncope in young patients, but may occur at any age, and is not typically life threatening. Often preceded by a painful, emotional, or stressful stimulus, this type of syncope frequently occurs in a standing or sitting position, and thus may be associated with traumatic injuries.
- ***Pathophysiology.*** Abnormal vasodepressor reflexes or inappropriate withdrawal of the sympathetic excitation to the heart and peripheral vascular system causes an increased vagal tone, vasodilatation, and bradycardia.
- ***History.*** A history of identifiable prodromal symptoms is common. Most patients with vasovagal syncope will have warning symptoms for seconds to minutes before the event. The symptoms are varied, but may include dizziness, pallor, nausea, diaphoresis, or blurred (tunnel) vision. Vasovagal syncope rarely occurs without warning, and this diagnosis should not be made without the prodromal symptoms described above.
- ***Physical examination.*** Frequently, no physical abnormalities are identified, but a careful search for signs of trauma is warranted.

- **Diagnostic testing.** Laboratory tests are of little diagnostic yield in vasovagal syncope, but should be sent if the cause of syncope is unclear, and the clinical presentation suggests suspicion of underlying hemorrhage or electrolyte abnormality exists. An EKG should be obtained to rule out any underlying dysrhythmia.
- **ED management.** The patient should be reassured, and referred to a primary care physician. Treatment is aimed at preventing conditions that contribute to or trigger syncope.
- **Helpful hints and pitfalls.** Do not make this diagnosis in a patient without the typical warning signs and symptoms of vasovagal syncope. Patients with obvious stressors may still have a cardiac cause of syncope. Keep your differential broad.

Situational

- A physical stimulus that causes syncope may be associated with another underlying disease process. For example, prostatic hypertrophy with micturition syncope, esophageal stricture in swallow syncope, or a tight necktie in carotid mediated syncope.
- The mechanism is similar to vasovagal, except it is associated with a specific activity. It is an abnormal or hypersensitive autonomic reflex response to a specific physical stimulus such as coughing, micturition, defecation, swallowing, or shaving that leads to transient cerebral hypoxia.
- Most patients report warning symptoms before the syncopal event. This is a diagnosis of exclusion. Patients should be counseled on avoiding situations that may cause syncope.

Carotid Sinus Hypersensitivity

- **Epidemiology and risk factors.** This is more common in men, the elderly, and those with ischemic heart disease, vascular disease, hypertension, and head or neck malignancies. This should be considered in all elderly patients with recurrent syncope and a negative cardiac evaluation.
- **Pathophysiology.** The carotid body is a pressure sensitive organ, and stimulation may lead to bradycardia and asystole or decreased blood pressure.
- **History.** Historical features suggestive of carotid sensitivity such as syncope after turning head rapidly or accidental carotid massage (shaving, tightening a necktie).
- **Physical examination.** No physical signs may be present.
- **Diagnostic testing.** Careful carotid massage may be used to diagnose carotid sinus hypersensitivity. It should be done with continuous cardiac and blood pressure monitoring. Massage each carotid body separately for 5 to 10 seconds. Do not massage if bruits are present, or the patient has had a recent stroke. Carotid sinus massage may precipitate an embolic stoke in patients with carotid vascular disease. The test is considered positive if there is an asystolic pause of 3 or more seconds. Carotid massage during tilt-table testing has been used to increase the accuracy of this test.

- **ED management.** Cardiology consultation should be obtained for further evaluation, and possible pacemaker placement. Instruct not to wear tight collars, and to maintain good hydration.
- **Helpful hints and pitfalls.** This is a difficult diagnosis to make. Only 5% to 20% of patients with carotid hypersensitivity on testing have a true carotid sinus syndrome with spontaneous symptoms.

Neurologic Causes of Syncope

- The most common neurologic reasons for a patient to have syncope include seizure, stroke or transient ischemic attacks, migraines, and Arnold-Chiari's malformations (malformations of the posterior fossa, characterized by a displacement of the cerebellum). Neurologic causes account for fewer than 10% of all cases of syncope. Most of these patients are later found to have had a seizure rather than true syncope.
- It should be briefly noted that seizure is the most common event mistaken as syncope. Seizures are a probable cause of 5% to 15% of apparent syncopal episodes. Consider this in making the diagnosis of syncope. The history is very important in differentiating seizure from syncope. Tonic movements of the extremities and urinary incontinence may be seen in both. Postictal confusion is a very reliable feature that differentiates seizure related causes of loss of consciousness from syncope. Seizure patients rarely have a fast and complete recovery. A tongue or cheek laceration or contusion supports the diagnosis of seizure, but the absence of them does not exclude a seizure. For more information on diagnosing and treating seizures, please refer to Chapter 51.
- Transient ischemic attacks or strokes are a rare cause of syncope but must be considered in any patient with neurologic signs or symptoms. For syncope to occur with a cerebral vascular event, either both hemispheres or the vertebrobasilar circulation must be involved. Posterior circulation ischemia leads to decreased blood flow to the reticular activation system, and a sudden loss of consciousness. These patients often have associated symptoms such as diplopia, vertigo, nausea and vomiting, difficulty talking or ataxia. For more information about strokes and transient ischemic attacks, please refer to Chapter 56.
- A history of a severe headache may point to a subarachnoid bleed as a cause of syncope. Any history of head trauma (recent or remote) may suggest a subdural or epidural hematoma. For more information about intracranial bleeding please refer to Chapters 9 and 35.

Orthostatic Related Causes of Syncope
Orthostatic Hypotension

- **Epidemiology and risk factors.** The elderly are most susceptible to orthostatic hypotension. Many cases in the elderly are caused by medication effects that blunt normal autonomic responses. Other common causes of orthostatic syncope are conditions that lead to volume depletion including bleeding, diuretic use, or gastrointestinal losses. Orthostatic hypotension may also be due to primary autonomic dysfunction, spinal cord injury, or other neurologic diseases.

- **Pathophysiology.** Normally when a person stands, 500 to 800 ml of blood is displaced to the abdomen and lower extremities, resulting in a decrease in cardiac output, and stimulation of aortic, carotid, and cardio-pulmonary baroreceptors that trigger a reflex increase in sympathetic outflow. In orthostatic hypotension, there is an abnormal autonomic or sympathetic response to positional changes. Dehydration and decreased intravascular volume contribute to orthostasis. In the absence of volume depletion, orthostatic syncope is most commonly caused by autonomic neuropathy or medications. Insufficient response in heart rate, peripheral vascular resistance, cardiac output and blood pressure causes decreased cerebral perfusion and syncope.

- **History.** Symptom onset is usually within the first several minutes after being in an upright position. This may be delayed in some patients. Symptoms include dizziness, blurred vision, or tunnel vision. The patient's medications must be reviewed carefully for any drugs associated with orthostatic hypotension (Box 57–3).

- **Physical examination.** The physical examination is frequently normal. Always assess for occult trauma from falling.

- **Diagnostic testing.** A 20–mm Hg drop in systolic blood pressure or a 10–mm Hg drop in diastolic blood pressure within 3 minutes of standing is considered positive for orthostatic hypotension. Measurements are taken after lying supine for 5 minutes, and after standing for 1 to 3 minutes. Laboratory testing should include hemoglobin and hematocrit to evaluate for anemia. In acute blood loss, the hematocrit value, when determined soon after the onset of bleeding, will not reflect blood loss accurately. Because equilibration with extravascular fluid and subsequent hemodilution requires several hours, a single hematocrit level may not reflect the degree of bleeding. A basic metabolic panel with electrolytes is prudent if anemia or hypovolemia are considered as a likely cause for syncope or in patients taking diuretics.

- **ED management.** Correct anemia and hypovolemia if diagnosed. If the patient requires a blood transfusion, the target to which the hematocrit

---

BOX 57–3   Common Medications Associated with Orthostatic Hypotension

- Anti-dysrhythmics
- Beta-blockers
- Calcium channel blockers
- Anti-anginal/nitrates
- Alpha-blockers
- Anti-hypertensives
- Diuretics
- Antidepressants/antipsychotics
- Sedatives
- Benzodiazepines
- Opiates
- Erectile dysfunction medications

should be raised varies; in elderly patients it should be 30%, whereas in younger, otherwise healthy patients, hematocrit values in the 20% to 25% range may be satisfactory; in those with portal hypertension, it should not be above 27% to 28%. Discharge instructions for patients who do not require admission include avoidance of volume depletion when taking medications that block sympathetic responses; changing positions slowly, in stages, to full standing; and wearing support stockings to minimize venous pooling. Arrange follow-up with a primary care physician to discuss discontinuation of any unnecessary medications, and for further evaluation of other causes of orthostatic hypotension.

- *Helpful hints and pitfalls.* Use caution in making this diagnosis. Five percent to 55% of patients with other causes of syncope will also have orthostatic hypotension on testing. Patient must have a recurrence of symptoms while testing to make this diagnosis. All patients with orthostatic hypotension should be referred to a primary care physician for further evaluation upon discharge. In general, patients with orthostatic syncope have an excellent prognosis.

Psychiatric

- This is seen in younger patients with multiple somatic symptoms associated with the syncopal event. In one study of syncope patients, up to 20% met diagnostic criteria for a psychiatric disorder or substance abuse problem. Women are more likely than men to present with a psychiatric etiology of syncope.
- Young patients found to have no structural heart disease and multiple episodes of syncope (>5 in preceding year) are less likely to have a dysrhythmia and are more likely to have psychiatric illnesses.
- Causes of syncope in this population are various. Hyperventilation in patients with panic disorders may lead to syncope by hypocarbia and cerebral vasoconstriction. In other patients an acute stress may lead to a vasovagal response. Occasionally a patient may be fully conscious, and attempt to mimic syncope for secondary gain, or others may be in a dissociative or conversion state with no control over their behavior.
- Patients should be referred for psychiatric evaluation. Although compliance is low, psychiatric therapy has been found to be successful in reducing the frequency of syncope in these patients.

Special Considerations
Pregnancy

- Syncope is a common presenting symptom of early pregnancy, and may occur before the patient is aware of being pregnant. It probably relates to the volume changes occuring with pregnancy, but may be a clue to a pregancy induced anemia.

Pediatric

- As many as 15% of children have at least one syncopal event before the end of adolescence.

- Most causes are benign, but rarely may be due to significant cardiac, neurologic, or metabolic pathology. A thorough history and physical examination is required to evaluate for risk of sudden death, dysrhythmias, congenital heart disease, seizures, or metabolic disorders.

Teaching Points

Syncope is a common entity. Although it may be the signal of an underlying critical condition such as a leaking abdominal aortic aneurysm, or the presenting sign of a pulmonary embolus, it is usually far less serious. Over the age of 60 years, it is far more likely to represent a serious cardiac or neurologic pathology, and unless a trivial cause can be proven, it will be prudent to admit these patients for observation and an extensive workup.

Under the age of 60, it is far more likely to have a benign cause. The patient can undergo expeditious workup with a good history and physical examination, a finger-stick glucose test, an electrocardiogram, and a complete blood count. If all are normal, the patient can be safely discharged. Although often no specific diagnosis can be established in the emergency department, it is usually not necessary.

Vasovagal syncope is very common and can usually be determined by history, the finding of a precipitating cause such as pain, pregnancy, or confining positions (e.g., the fainting Buckingham Palace guard) and needs little workup or concern.

Suggested Readings

American College of Emergency Physicians. Clinical Policy: critical issues in the evaluation and management of patients presenting with syncope. Ann Emerg Med 2001;37:771–776.

Brignole M, Alboni P, Benditt D, et al. Task Force on Syncope, European Society of Cardiology. Guidelines on Management (Diagnosis and Treatment) of Syncope. Eur Heart J 2001; 22:1256–306.

Calkins H, Zipes DP. Hypotension and syncope. In: Zipes DP, Libby P, Bonow RO, Braunwald E (editors). Braunwald's Heart Disease: A Textbook of Cardiovascular Medicine (7th ed). Philadelphia: Elsevier, 2005, pp 909–919.

De Lorenzo RA. Syncope. In: Marx JA, Hockberger RS, Walls RM (editors). Rosen's Emergency Medicine: Concepts and Clinical Practice (6th ed). Philadelphia: Elsevier, 2006, pp 193–199.

Martin TP, Hanusa BH, Kapoor WN. Risk stratification of patients with syncope. Ann Emerg Med 1997;29:459–466.

Massin MM, Bourguignont A, Coremans C, et al. Syncope in pediatric patients presenting to the emergency department. J Pediatr 2004;145:223–228.

Quinn JV, Stiell IG, McDermott DA, et al. Derivation of the San Francisco syncope rule to predict patients with short-term serious outcomes. Ann Emerg Med 2004;43:224–232.

CHAPTER 58

Urinary Complaints

ANNA I. CHEH ■ BARBARA A. MASSER

 Red Flags

Elderly • Comorbidities (especially diabetes) • Trauma associated wtih urinary complaints • Pregnancy • Abdominal pain or back pain • Fever • Abnormal vital signs (e.g., tachycardia, hypotension) • Decreased urine output • Hematuria • Concern for urethral foreign body

Overview

Many patients with urinary complaints have minor illnesses that can be effectively diagnosed and treated, and the patient can be discharged from the ED. An example is an uncomplicated urinary tract infection (UTI).

There are a smaller number of critical cases for which therapy should be initiated quickly. Look for "red flags" (see Box). These patients may need admission and emergent urological consultation.

Patients who present with urinary incontinence should be evaluated for potentially serious underlying pathology, particularly neurologic conditions such as a spinal cord lesion (Chapters 12 and 21). Incontinence may also indicate a seizure that was unrecognized by the patient. Other causes of incontinence are stress incontinence (common in women), infection, and overflow from urinary retention. Urinary retention is more common in men and is most often due to obstruction due to an enlarged prostate. Medications are the next most common cause of urinary retention.

This chapter will discuss a general approach to a patient with urinary complaints, giving special attention to patients presenting with dysuria and hematuria.

Differential Diagnosis of Urinary Complaints

■ See DDx tables for dysuria and hematuria.

701

DDx Differential Diagnosis of Dysuria

Critical	Emergent	Nonemergent

Urosepsis
Obstructing calculi (32)
Major trauma (15)
	Urinary tract infection
	• Cystitis/urethritis/
	  prostatitis
	• Pyelonephritis (32)
	Sexually transmitted
	  diseases (67)
	Foreign body (47)
		External irritation/
		  trauma (minor)

( ) Refers to the chapter in which the disease entity is discussed.

DDx Differential Diagnosis of Hematuria

Critical	Emergent	Nonemergent

Leaking aortic abdominal
  aneurysm (18)
Urinary tract
  obstruction
Urinary tract trauma (15)
Endocarditis (67)
Malignant hypertension
  (39)
Renal vein thrombosis (32)
Renal infarction (32)
	Prostatic enlargement
	Kidney stone (32)
	Urinary tract infection
	Kidney diseases
	• Glomerulonephritis
	  (49)
	• Goodpasture's disease
	  (71)
	• Polycystic kidney
	  disease
	Coagulopathy
	Foreign body (47)
	Vascular disorders
	• Atrioventricular
	  malformation
	• Vasculitis (71)
		Transient hematuria
		Excessive exercise
		Genitourinary
		  carcinoma
		Benign bladder
		  polyps
		Medications
		Diet (e.g., beets
		  or rhubarb)
		Systemic diseases
		• IgA nephropathy
		• Sickle cell disease
		  (53)

( ) Refers to the chapter in which the disease entity is discussed.

Initial Diagnostic Approach
General

- Most patients with urinary complaints are typically stable with no respiratory or hemodynamic compromise. Any patient who appears ill or has significantly abnormal vital signs requires immediate attention.
- A thorough history and physical examination are essential to direct the initial workup, and establish the underlying pathology of urinary complaints. Many patients with sexually transmitted diseases (STDs) or pelvic pathology have urinary complaints. A common error is failure to perform a pelvic examination, and to mistakenly diagnose an uncomplicated UTI when an STD or other pelvic pathology is present.

Laboratory

- A urinalysis (UA) should be obtained in all patients with urinary complaints. There is no absolute consensus for what constitutes a positive UA, so results must be interpreted in the context of the clinical signs and symptoms. In general, leukocyte esterase on the initial dip indicates the presence of inflammation and often infection. Likewise, positive nitrites indicate the presence of nitrite-producing bacteria. Many gram-negative and some gram-positive organisms are capable of this conversion, and a positive dipstick nitrite test indicates that these organisms are present in significant numbers (i.e., more than 10,000/ml). Thus, a positive result is helpful, but a negative result does not rule out UTI. A urine cell count can be obtained to confirm the diagnosis suggested by elevated white blood cell (WBC) counts with no epithelial cells (indicating a "clean catch"). Men normally have fewer than two WBCs per high-power field (HPF); women normally have fewer than five WBCs per HPF. Casts in the urinary sediment may be used to localize disease to a specific location in the genitourinary tract. Hyaline and WBC casts may be present in patients with pyelonephritis. Red blood cell casts may be found in glomerulonephritis, but may also be found in individuals who play contact sports.
- A culture should be sent in those with a history of resistant or frequent urinary tract infections (more than three in 1 year), those currently on antibiotics, significant co-morbidities like an immunocompromised state, abnormal urinary anatomy, acute or subclinical pyelonephritis, hospitalized patients, patients with a chronic indwelling catheter, and all pregnant women, children, and adult men. Organisms such as *Chlamydia* and *Ureaplasma urealyticum* should be considered in patients with pyuria and negative cultures. Other causes of sterile pyuria include balanitis, urethritis, tuberculosis, bladder tumors, viral infections, nephrolithiasis, foreign bodies, exercise, glomerulonephritis, and corticosteroid and cyclophosphamide (Cytoxan) use.
- A urinary pregnancy test should be performed on all women of reproductive age.
- Complete blood cell count (CBC), electrolytes, renal function tests, and coagulation studies may be warranted in the ill-appearing patient.

Radiography

- *Plain films.* Plain films can be ordered to verify the proper placement of urethral stents if present. Although plain films may sometimes reveal renal stones (see Chapter 32), this modality has been replaced by noncontrast computed tomography (CT scan) at many institutions.
- *Intravenous pyelography (IVP).* An IVP study was formerly used to visualize the upper and lower urinary tracts, but it has now been largely supplanted by other modalities. Findings on an IVP are often nonspecific in comparison to the CT scan. As the cost of a CT scan has approached that of an IVP, it has become more common to use a CT scan due to its increased accuracy and ability to diagnose other pathologies outside of the GU tract.

- **Ultrasound.** An ultrasound examination can be used in cases of urinary incontinence or retention to determine the level of postvoid residual but is not routinely performed for this purpose in the ED. It can also be used for detecting kidney stone, hydroureter, or hydronephrosis in patients for whom a CT scan may be less desirable (such as in pregnancy).
- **CT scan.** The noncontrast CT scan allows visualization of stones, masses, and obstruction. Contrast is not used in evaluating for nephrolithiasis; however, intravenous (IV) contrast can subsequently be given to evaluate for other pathology, and to assess the drainage of the collecting system if no stone is seen.
- **Magnetic resonance imaging (MRI).** MRI is the optimal imaging study for the investigation of spinal cord syndromes such as cauda equina (see Chapter 21).

Emergency Department Management Overview
General

- IV access should be obtained in any patient who is ill-appearing, dehydrated, in significant pain, or who is having nausea and vomiting. IV hydration, antiemetics, and analgesics can then be given as needed.

Medications

- **Analgesia.** Pain should be quickly addressed and alleviated. Nephrolithiasis can be extremely painful, and narcotics should not be withheld. Ketorolac (15-30 mg via IV or intramuscular [IM] injection) is often effectively used for pain relief in nephrolithiasis, and should be tried before giving opiates that may themselves cause nausea, vomiting, and urinary retention (see Chapter 90.1). Phenazopyridine (100-200 mg by mouth three times daily for 2 days) may be added for patients with dysuria or spasm.
- **Antibiotics.** Antibiotics should be administered to any febrile or ill-appearing patient with signs or symptoms of an infection. They are also warranted in any patient with evidence of a UTI (see Chapter 90.2).

Emergency Department Interventions

- **Urinary catheter.** A urinary catheter should be placed immediately for both diagnostic and therapeutic purposes in any patient with urinary retention (>200 ml postvoid residual is considered positive). A catheter should also be placed in the setting of renal failure, sepsis, or other disorders requiring close monitoring of urinary output. An in-and-out catheterization should be performed if a sterile specimen is difficult to obtain (for example, in a female patient during menstruation or in an altered patient). See Chapter 91 for techniques of bladder catheterization.

Disposition

- **Consultation.** Emergent consultation is required for a UTI or renal failure in the presence of acute obstruction, deep tissue infection such as Fournier's gangrene (Chapter 54), traumatic urologic injury, or complications of urologic surgery. Patients with incontinence secondary to urethral obstruction due to more chronic conditions such as BPH may be referred for close outpatient follow-up after any urinary retention is relieved with a Foley catheter. However, the inability to place a Foley catheter to relieve urinary obstruction by ED staff requires emergent urologic consultation.

- *Admission.* Patients with intractable nausea, vomiting, or pain often require admission. Hemodynamic instability and emergent surgical findings are less common, but clear indications for admission. Hematuria in a patient with significant coagulopathy warrants inpatient reversal. Postobstructive diuresis (defined as >200 ml/h over 2 hours) can lead to electrolyte abnormalities, and should also prompt inpatient admission for 24 to 48 hours. Patients who do not respond to an initial IV dose of antibiotics, fluid replenishment, and pain relief also require admission. Patients in the second and third trimesters of pregnancy who have a complicated UTI (formerly called pyelonephritis) should be admitted.

- *Discharge.* A patient with a simple (uncomplicated) UTI or nephrolithiasis may be treated as an outpatient. Being able to establish adequate pain control with oral medications is crucial. A patient must also be able to void before discharge. Proper referral to an urologist should be arranged for patients discharged with an indwelling urinary catheter for retention. Prophylactic antibiotic treatment is not needed. Follow-up should be within 24 to 48 hours, and it will be necessary to arrange this with the urologist before the patient is discharged from the ED.

Specific Problems: Urine Infections
Asymptomatic Bacteriuria

- *Definition.* The isolation of 100,000 colony forming units (CFUs) of a single organism per milliliter from a clean-catch specimen, or the presence of more than 10,000 colonies of a single bacterial species in two successive cultures from an asymptomatic patient.

- *Epidemiology and risk factors.* Prevalence among the general female population is 5% to 9%, but can be up to 40% in elderly female nursing home residents. Although the rate is similar in pregnant and non-pregnant women, about 20% to 40% of pregnant women (a rate about three to four times higher) will develop a complicated infection (pyelonephritis.) Appropriate antibiotic therapy will reduce this rate down to just 3%. Urethral catheters remaining in situ for over 30 days are considered chronic indwelling catheters. Bacteriuria is universal in patients with chronic urethral catheters and urethral stents. There is a greater number of species and higher quantitative count of bacteria isolated in urine collected through a catheter in place for several days than a simultaneous urine specimen collected through a freshly placed catheter.

- *ED management.* There are multiple antibiotic treatment options. Nitrofurantoin remains a popular choice due to its high concentrations in the urinary tract while maintaining a low gram-negative resistance rate. Longer courses (2 weeks) might be warranted for bacteriuria that originates in the kidney as indicated by the finding of WBC casts or granular casts in the UA. Some pregnant women will be started on nitrofurantoin or cephalexin suppressive therapy for persistent bacteriuria (more than two positive cultures). Patients with chronic indwelling catheters should have the catheter changed before the urinary specimen is obtained. Treatment should be given if the bacteriuria is thought to be contributing to the patient's problem.

- *Helpful hints and pitfalls.* Treatment of bacteriuria in patients with a chronic indwelling catheter or urethral stent is not always beneficial, and may be harmful.

Prostatitis

- *Epidemiology and risk factors.* There is a bimodal distribution of cases occurring in young men who are sexually active (from STD pathogens) and elderly men with a recent UTI or genitourinary infection, indwelling bladder catheters, recent urethral instrumentation, or chronic co-morbidities.
- *Pathophysiology.* This disorder is caused by acute or chronic inflammation or infection of the prostate gland. Most are nonbacterial in origin, but an ED visit is more likely in a patient with an acute bacterial etiology.
- *History.* Patients complain of fevers and chills, urinary frequency and urgency, dysuria, and groin, perineal, or back pain. Varying degrees of bladder outlet obstruction and retention may be present. Patients often have constitutional symptoms of arthralgia, myalgia, and malaise.
- *Physical examination.* The patient is often febrile, with a tender, warm and firm prostate on rectal examination along with exquisite perineal tenderness.
- *Diagnostic testing.* The UA is often positive for leukocytes, and there is often an elevated WBC count.
- *ED management.* If the patient appears nontoxic, he can be discharged on a 4 to 6 week course of bactrim or fluoroquinolone. If the patient appears acutely ill, the patient should be admitted to the hospital for further treatment and evaluation. Parenteral antibiotics include ciprofloxacin or ceftriaxone with or without an aminoglycoside. The patient needs close follow-up with the primary care provider or urologist because these infections can worsen even with recommended therapy and good patient compliance. If urinary retention is present, urology should be consulted for suprapubic drainage. Transurethral bladder catheterization should be avoided in the acute presentation to avoid possible hematogenous spread.
- *Helpful hints and pitfalls.* When acute bacterial prostatitis is suspected, prostate massage should be avoided because of the risk of causing bacteremia. Prostatitis requires a longer antibiotic course than an uncomplicated UTI. *Chlamydia* and *Neisseria gonorrhoeae* cultures should be obtained as well as a regular bacterial culture in any male patient with dysuria. Do not ignore a possible STD in an elderly patient. The hallmark of chronic prostatitis is relapsing UTI with the same organism.

Urethritis

Sexually transmitted diseases are discussed in Chapter 67.

- ***Epidemiology and risk factors.*** Ureaplasma is the most common non-STD pathogenic cause of urethritis in men. *Chlamydia* species and *Mycoplasma hominis* are other causes of nongonoccocal urethritis.
- ***Pathophysiology.*** The urethra becomes inflamed from infection.
- ***History.*** Symptoms are often identical to cystitis in women. In men, the main complaint is usually dysuria with or without penile discharge.
- ***Physical examination.*** The examination is largely benign and should include a scrotal and testicular examination.
- ***Diagnostic testing.*** A UA should be obtained to evaluate for infection.
- ***ED management.*** Most patients will be well enough to be discharged home on oral antibiotics. Doxycycline or azithromycin are good choices for nongonococcal urethritis. Ceftriaxone, cefixime, ciprofloxacin, or ofloxacin can be used if gonococcal urethritis is suspected. Patients should be treated for both.
- ***Helpful hints and pitfalls.*** The most common cause of urethritis in men is an STD. Always treat for STDs in men with urethritis, unless this diagnosis is ruled out by culture or immunofluorescence studies. Men are also subject to a chemical urethritis from reflux caused by heavy physical exercise.

Urinary Tract Infection (Uncomplicated)

- ***Epidemiology and risk factors.*** A greater prevalence exists in women than men. Repetitive sexual intercourse is a key risk factor. This may represent a blunt traumatic cystitis rather than true infection, and the urinalysis often shows mostly hematuria. Pregnant women are particularly susceptible.
- ***Pathophysiology.*** The infection arises from pathologic colonization of the urogenital tract. *E. coli* is the causative pathogen in over 80% of cases.
- ***History.*** Dysuria is usually the primary complaint, often accompanied by suprapubic pain, urinary frequency, urgency, or hematuria. The severity of symptoms can vary greatly. Elderly patients in particular may present atypically, with symptoms of malaise, fatigue, lethargy, or generalized weakness.
- ***Physical examination.*** A bimanual or speculum pelvic examination should be performed especially if lower abdominal pain or vaginal discharge are present. A thorough external examination should be performed to look for irritative external causes of dysuria. Many patients will have suprapubic tenderness. The patient should also be assessed for costovertebral tenderness to screen for more complicated infection. Complicated UTIs (pyelonephritis) are discussed in Chapter 32.
- ***Diagnostic testing.*** A urinalysis and urinary culture should be obtained according to the guidelines listed in "General Diagnostic Approach." All women of childbearing age should have a pregnancy status established. STD testing should be performed on all patients with pelvic or penile symptoms. Renal function should be checked if there is concern for obstruction or higher tract infection and in a toxic-appearing patient.
- ***ED management.*** Antibiotics should be started empirically for any high-risk patient with signs or symptoms of a UTI, or evidence of infection on the urinalysis. Antibiotic selection will depend on local resistance patterns as well as the individual patient. Generally, in areas without

significant resistance, Bactrim DS is recommended as first line therapy in a healthy young adult with simple cystitis. Fluoroquinolones such as ciprofloxacin should be reserved for cases of documented resistance or in complicated infections. Phenazopyridine (pyridium x 1-2 days) should also be added for relief of dysuria and spasm.

■ *Helpful hints and pitfalls.* Always consider sexually transmitted etiologies for dysuria in women with pelvic symptoms or lower abdominal pain. Urology should be consulted for any patient with a UTI and hydronephrosis, perinephric abscess or underlying anatomic abnormality.

Urosepsis

■ Urosepsis is a life-threatening condition caused by dissemination of bacteria, most commonly gram-negative, from the urine in a patient with bacteriuria.
■ Antibiotics such as a third-generation cephalosporin, imipenem, or ampicillin with gentamycin should be given as soon as possible. A urinary catheter should be placed for precise monitoring of urinary output.
■ See Chapter 67 for a brief discussion of sepsis.

Specific Problems: Hematuria
Hematuria

■ *Definitions. Microscopic hematuria* is defined as three or more red blood cells (RBCs) per HPF on microscopic evaluation of two of three properly collected specimens. *Gross hematuria* is overtly bloody, smoky or tea colored with RBCs too numerous to count on microscopic analysis. This is a common complaint in the ED. *Pseudohematuria* is a reddish discoloration of urine without RBCs on microscopic analysis.
■ *Epidemiology and risk factors.* Urinary tract infections, tumors, kidney stones, systemic disorders, and medications such as anticoagulants or nephrotoxins can all cause hematuria. The most common reason for hematuria in a man 50 years of age or older is benign prostatic hypertrophy. Voiding problems, trauma, and excessive exercise (*jogger's hematuria*) may also cause blood in the urine. Hematuria of renal origin can be divided into glomerular and nonglomerular categories. IgA nephropathy, Berger's disease, is the most common cause of glomerular hematuria. Nonglomerular causes include pyelonephritis, polycystic kidney disease, granulomatous disease (tuberculosis), interstitial nephritis, and renal cell carcinoma.
■ *Pathophysiology.* The etiology and pathophysiology of hematuria are extremely varied. The amount of bleeding can be variable, but as little as 1 ml (0.03 oz) of blood will turn the urine red.
■ *History.* Inquire about any recent dietary or medication changes. Other important historical clues are risk factors for significant underlying diseases such as smoking, chemical or dye occupational exposure, known urologic disease, cancer, irritative voiding symptoms, UTI, pelvic surgery, or radiation. Travel or recent immigration from Africa or the Middle East should raise concern for *Schistosomias haematobium*, a common cause of bladder cancer in developing nations.

- *Physical examination.* Try to rule out trauma or other lesions. A more complete physical examination is indicated if there are any other systemic symptoms or illnesses.
- *Diagnostic testing.* UA and pregnancy status must be obtained. If a patient is menstruating, debilitated, or has altered mental status, a catheterized sample is necessary to obtain an uncontaminated sample. The presence of RBC casts or proteinuria in the UA suggests glomerular disease. The presence of bacteriuria, nitrites, or leukocytes confirms an infectious etiology. CBC and coagulation studies are rarely helpful unless the patient is anticoagulated or has a known bleeding disorder. Imaging (such as a CT scan) is rarely indicated emergently unless there is concern for obstruction, stone, perinephric abscess, or trauma.
- *ED management.* In more than half of the presentations, a cause is easily identifiable, and treatment of the underlying cause should be initiated if possible. Treatment is specific to the identified disease process. In general, for gross hematuria, a larger-caliber urinary catheter (26 French) should be placed for irrigation and clot evacuation. If bleeding does not clear, urology should be consulted after a three-way Foley catheter is placed. An exception is in the setting of blunt or penetrating trauma. An aggressive workup for the source must be initiated in the ED before Foley catheter insertion (see Chapter 15). Otherwise, gross hematuria can be worked up on an outpatient basis if the patient is hemo-dynamically stable, has minimal symptoms, is able to void, and can tolerate oral fluids. Patients may also be discharged with a catheter and urology follow-up if the source is a benign obstructive process like benign prostatic hypertrophy or bladder cancer screening.
- *Helpful hints and pitfalls.* Never put a patient on continuous irrigation with an infusion pump as this may result in bladder rupture if there is outflow tract obstruction.

Special Considerations

Pediatrics

- Painless hematuria is due to a glomerular lesion until proven otherwise.
- A urine sample should be obtained in all febrile infants younger than 2 months, febrile boys younger than 6 months, and febrile girls younger than 2 years without a known source of infection. Urine culture should be obtained in all children.
- Look for sexual abuse as an etiology for UTIs in children.
- Urologic referral should be arranged for boys of any age and girls younger than 5 years for work up of underlying anatomic abnormalities.
- Admission is recommended for those younger than 1 year.
- Longer antibiotic courses (7-10 days) should be prescribed for pediatric outpatient therapy.

Elderly

- UTI presentations may be atypical, often presenting with altered mental status as the only complaint.

Women and Pregnancy

■ Twenty percent to 40% of pregnant women with asymptomatic bacteriuria will develop complicated UTI if not properly treated. Treatment duration of asymptomatic bacteriuria is the same as that for simple cystitis.

■ Fluoroquinolones should be avoided during pregnancy as should sulfa medications during the third trimester. Aminoglycosides have a higher rate of transient renal dysfunction in pregnancy.

■ Any indication of preterm contractions or cervical changes necessitates an obstetric consultation, and admission for fetal monitoring.

■ Complicated UTI (i.e., pyelonephritis) may be treated as an outpatient in the first trimester following the same guidelines as for the nonpregnant patient (see Chapter 32), but all women with complicated UTI in the second and third trimester should be admitted.

Immunocompromised Patient

■ Immunocompromised patients are at a higher risk for complications and more emergent presentations of any genitourinary pathology.

Teaching Points

Urinary tract infections were formerly thought to be benign if they were in the lower urinary tract, and serious if in the upper tract. It has proved to be confusing to try to distinguish, so the modern and more useful classification is between *complicated* (formerly called pyelonephritis) and *uncomplicated* (cystitis). It is safe to treat patients with a complicated urinary tract infection as an outpatient if there are no criteria for admission; if the patient responds to an initial ED dose of intravenous antibiotics, pain relief, and symptom relief; and if the patient is able to take oral fluids and medications.

The criteria for admission are immunosupression, male gender, extremes of age, diabetes, recurrent infection already on antibiotic treatment, and the second and third trimesters of pregnancy.

Suggested Readings

Gupta K, Hooten TM, Stamm WE. Increasing antimicrobial resistance and the management of uncomplicated community-acquired urinary tract infections. Ann Intern Med 2001;135:41–50.

Fantl JA, Newman DK, Colling J, et al. Urinary Incontinence in Adults: Acute and Chronic Management. Clinical Practice Guideline No. 2, 1996 Update. Rockville, MD: U.S. Department of Health and Human Services. Public Health Service, Agency for Health Care Policy and Research. AHCPR Publication No. 96-0682. March 1996.

Nicolle LE. Asymptomatic bacteriuria: when to screen and when to treat. Infect Dis Clin North Am 2003;17:367–394.

Rubenstein JN, Schaeffer AJ. Managing complicated urinary tract infections: the urologic review. Infect Dis Clin North Am 2003;17:333–351.

Simerville JA, Maxted WC, Pahira JJ. Urinalysis: a comprehensive review. Am Fam Physician 2005;71:1153–1162.

Yun EJ, Meng MV, Carroll PR. Evaluation of the patient with hematuria. Med Clin North Am 2004;88:329–343.

CHAPTER 59

Vertigo

JENNIFER C. SMITH ■ WILLIAM A. WITTLAKE

 Red Flags

Any focal neurologic deficit or finding ● Elderly patient ● Vascular risk factors: diabetes, smoking, atherosclerotic heart disease, stroke ● Insidious onset and lengthy duration ● No ear or hearing complaint ● New onset of altered mental status ● Vertical nystagmus ● Abnormal vital signs especially elevated blood pressure or fever

Overview

Vertigo is the false perception of movement of the patient or the environment, and is associated with a sense of disorientation in space.

Most patients will have associated autonomic symptoms such as nausea, vomiting, diaphoresis, and malaise.

Many patients present with a chief complaint of dizziness, and the physician must determine whether this is true vertigo rather than presyncope, light-headedness, or dysequilibrium (see Chapter 43). The history is key in making this distinction.

Vertigo has central causes (disorders of the cerebral cortex, cerebellum, and brainstem), peripheral causes (disorders of the eighth cranial nerve or vestibular apparatus), and systemic causes (such as cardiovascular or metabolic disorders).

The history combined with a thorough physical examination should guide the acquisition of indicated imaging studies.

Look for "red flags" (see Box) that may signify more critical diagnoses requiring an expedited workup and treatment.

Differential Diagnosis of Vertigo

See DDx table describing the differential diagnosis of vertigo.

Initial Diagnostic Approach
General

■ As always, the ABCs (*a*irway, *b*reathing, and *c*irculation) should be addressed as described in Section II.

DDx Priority-Based Differential Diagnosis of Vertigo

Critical Diagnoses	Emergent Diagnoses	Nonemergent Diagnoses
Cerebellar hemorrhage/ Infarct (56)	Suppurative labyrinthitis	Benign paroxysmal positional vertigo
Central nervous system infection (67)	Toxic labyrinthitis	Meniere's disease
Vertebrobasilar insufficiency (56)	Subclavian steal (57)	Vestibular neuronitis
	Alcohol intoxication	Acoustic neuroma
	Hypoglycemia (38)	Basilar artery migraine (35)
	Central nervous system tumor	Foreign body in ear canal (33)
		Multiple sclerosis (60)
		Posttraumatic syndromes

( ) Refers to the chapter in which the disease entity is discussed.

- The history and physical examination should help the clinician determine whether the vertigo is due to a peripheral lesion (e.g., involving the inner ear) or a central process, such as cerebrovascular disease or a neoplasm. Assess for nystagmus, ear problems, hearing deficits, or abnormalities on the neurologic examination, with close attention to cerebellar function (see Appendix 2). All patients with concern for a central source of vertigo should be promptly evaluated. This is particular true for patients with a cerebellar hemorrhage or infarction. These patients can rapidly develop critical brainstem compression and threaten the life of the patient (see Chapter 56).
- A comparison of clinical findings in central verses peripheral vertigo is listed in Table 59–1.

Laboratory

- Laboratory studies are rarely indicated. A serum glucose measurement should be checked. A complete blood count (CBC) and cultures are indicated for ill-appearing patients in whom an infectious source is suspected. Other tests may include electrolytes for protracted vomiting and coagulation studies for an acute stroke.

Radiography

- *Computed tomography (CT scan) and magnetic resonance imaging (MRI).* If the patient has any focal neurologic deficit, a noncontrast head CT scan should be performed to search for a mass lesion or hemorrhage. An MRI is a superior study for visualizing cerebellar lesions, but is often not readily available to the ED, and is inappropriate for unstable patients. An MRI (with gadolinium) is also used to look for acoustic neuroma.
- *Angiography/MR angiography.* These studies are used when vertebrobasilar insufficiency or other vascular abnormalities are suspected.

Table 59–1 Characteristics of Central and Peripheral Vertigo

Characteristic	Central	Peripheral
Onset	Usually gradual	Usually sudden
Duration	Weeks to months (constant)	Seconds to days (intermittent)
Nausea/vomiting	Mild to severe	Often severe
Nystagmus	May be vertical, does not improve with visual fixation, not fatigable.	Horizontal or rotatory but never vertical, improves with visual fixation, fatigues
Symptoms related to position	Not usually	Usually
Neurologic findings	Usually have focal findings	No focal findings
Hearing loss/tinnitus	Absent	May be present
Severity	Initially mild	Often severe

Provocative Maneuvers

■ *Dix-Hallpike maneuver (also called the Nylèn-Barany maneuver).* This may be used to help distinguish between central and peripheral vertigo and to diagnose benign paroxysmal positional vertigo (BPPV). It is described in detail in Box 59–1.

Emergency Department Management Overview
General

■ The ABCs are always the first priority as discussed in Section II.
■ Patients with severe or protracted vomiting may require IV fluids for rehydration as well as IV antiemetics.

Medications

■ *Vestibular suppressants.* There are several classes of medications that suppress the vestibular system. Antihistamines such as meclizine (25-50 mg by mouth [PO] every 6 hours) and diphenhydramine (50 mg PO/IV every 4 to 6 hours) are effective. Benzodiazepines such as diazepam (2.5-5 mg PO or intramuscular [IM] injection or IV q8h) or clonezepam (0.5 mg PO every 8 hours) are also used. Vestibular suppressants may interfere with central habituation; therefore, they should not be used for more than a few days in peripheral causes.
■ *Antiemetics.* All except the mildest cases of vertigo, whether peripheral or central, are associated with nausea and vomiting. Antiemetics such as prochlorperazine can be administered. Odansetron 4 mg IV may have less of a sedating effect but is more costly than other agents (see Chapter 90.4).

BOX 59–1   Dix-Hallpike Maneuver

- The patient sits upright on the bed, and should be positioned so that when lying flat, the head will extend beyond the edge of the bed.
- The examiner stands at the head of the bed, and helps the patient to rapidly move from sitting to lying flat.
- The patient's head should be held with 30 degrees of neck extension just beyond the edge of the bed, and turned rapidly 45 degrees to one side. This will sometimes cause vomiting.
- The examiner then observes the patient in this position, and watches for the development of nystagmus as well as asking whether the patent is experiencing vertigo.
- Peripheral vertigo is associated with horizontal or rotatory nystagmus with a latent period of around 5 seconds. The symptoms will decrease upon repeated testing. Lack of fatigability, no latency, and vertical nystagmus are signs of a central etiology.
- If no symptoms are elicited, the maneuver is repeated, this time with the examiner turning the patient's head to the opposite side. The symptoms will usually occur when the affected side is toward the floor.
- Pretreatment with a benzodiazepine will prevent vomiting, which is preferable for the patient and the physician.

- *Antibiotics.* These are required for any patient in whom infection is suspected. Patients with suppurative labyrinthitis or any type of central nervous system (CNS) infection will require admission for IV antibiotics.
- *Diuretics.* Diuretics such as acetazolamide (250-500 mg PO twice daily [BID] for 3-12 months) and a low-salt diet are frequently used in the treatment of Meniere's disease.
- *Analgesics.* Analgesia may be necessary for patients with associated headache. Standard analgesics such as nonsteroidal anti-inflammatory drugs and opiates may be used (see Chapter 90.1), but for basilar artery migraine, specific antimigraine medications may be more effective. These include sumatriptan and ergotamine (see Chapter 35).

Disposition

- *Consultation.* Consult neurology for most central lesions that cause vertigo (transient ischemic attack), neurosurgery for mass lesions (small acoustic schwannoma), or vascular surgery (subclavian steal). Otolaryngology (ear, nose, and throat [ENT]) consultation or confirmed follow-up is necessary for conditions involving the inner ear, or if a foreign body is present, and cannot be removed in the ED.
- *Admission.* Many central causes of vertigo will require admission to neurosurgery (intracranial hemorrhage, brain abscess, tumor), medicine or neurology (meningitis, encephalitis, ischemic stroke), or vascular surgery (subclavian steal), depending on the cause.
- *Discharge.* Most patients with peripheral causes of vertigo may be discharged home with symptomatic therapy and follow-up if they

ambulate in their usual fashion and tolerate fluids. They should not drive themselves home even if their symptoms have resolved without drug therapy.

Specific Problems
Acoustic Neuroma (also called Vestibular Schwannoma)

- *Epidemiology and risk factors.* This is most common in the fourth through sixth decades with a 5:1 predilection for women. Most cases are sporadic, but they are occasionally related to cranial radiation or to familial syndromes such as neurofibromatosis type 1 or 2. Acoustic neuromas account for 80% of all cerebellopontine angle tumors.
- *Pathophysiology.* This is an extra-axial, slow growing, benign tumor of the schwann cells of the eighth cranial nerve. These start as a peripheral cause of vertigo, but as they enlarge, may become a central cause. They can cause neurologic damage via direct compression on the eighth cranial nerve. Continued growth of the tumor may result in compression of structures in the cerebellopontine angle, where the facial and trigeminal nerves may be compressed and damaged. Larger tumors may further encroach upon the brainstem, and if large enough may compress the fourth ventricle, ultimately resulting in signs of increased intracranial pressure (ICP).
- *History.* These patients complain of slowly progressive but continuous vertigo associated with unilateral sensorineural hearing loss and tinnitus. The tumors may also cause imbalance, headache, fullness in the ear, and otalgia. At later stages, other cranial nerve complaints may develop, such as facial weakness.
- *Physical examination.* Unilateral hearing loss will be present. Truncal ataxia and cranial nerve deficits develop as the tumor enlarges. Many patients have an absent or diminished corneal reflex.
- *Diagnostic testing.* An MRI with gadolinium and eighth cranial nerve views is the imaging study of choice. An audiogram is normal in 15% of patients.
- *ED management.* Appropriate referral for an audiogram, and for otolaryngology or neurosurgery follow-up because most patients are treated surgically.
- *Helpful hints and pitfalls.* Acoustic neuroma is likely to be missed on the first or second presentation. Patients with asymmetric hearing loss or unilateral tinnitus should be evaluated to rule out acoustic neuroma. A careful neurological examination is helpful in patients who appear to have had peripheral vertigo for a long time. If the diagnosis is not considered, an MRI will never be obtained that will reveal the tumor.

Benign Paroxysmal Positional Vertigo (BPPV)

- *Epidemiology and risk factors.* This most commonly begins in the fifth to seventh decades, with a slight predominance in women. In younger or posttraumatic patients, this predominance does not exist. Most cases are primary or idiopathic. Secondary causes include Meniere's disease, trauma (may cause bilateral BPPV), and inner ear surgery. There is also some association with migraine headache.

- *Pathophysiology.* This syndrome may be caused by a variety of inner ear diseases. The most common theory postulates that particles (otoconia) are dislodged and float through the endolymph of the semicircular canals, activating hair cells, and causing them to discharge. This creates a false sense of motion. In certain secondary causes, other factors such as inner ear vessel spasm (migraine) or hydropic damage to the cupula (Meniere's disease) are suspected.
- *History.* Patients complain of sudden, severe episodes of vertigo triggered by head motion. Common triggers include extending the neck to look up or rolling over in bed. The symptoms usually last less than 30 seconds, but the patient may have a residual sense of dysequilibrium.
- *Physical examination.* The Dix-Hallpike maneuver (Box 59–1) can confirm the diagnosis. The vertigo and nystagmus should have about 5 seconds of latency, and should fatigue. It should reverse direction when the patient sits back up. The neurologic examination should otherwise be normal.
- *Diagnostic testing.* The Dix-Hallpike maneuver is the primary diagnostic test. Further imaging or laboratory work is unnecessary unless other causes are suspected.
- *ED management.* Once the diagnosis is made, the patient should be reassured of the benign nature of the disease. The Epley maneuvers are otolith-repositioning maneuvers. They involve sequential movement of the head into four positions, staying in each position for approximately 30 seconds. Few emergency physicians have experience with these maneuvers (see Box 59–2 for technique). Most patients improve spontaneously over weeks to months, due to otolith repositioning or central habituation. Symptomatic therapy with vestibular suppressants or antiemetics is helpful. The patient can follow-up with an ear, nose, and throat (ENT) specialist.
- *Helpful hints and pitfalls.* If the patient has the classic history of BPPV but no nystagmus or concern for any other etiology of vertigo, the patient can be treated symptomatically or with the Epley maneuver.

BOX 59–2   Epley Maneuvers

- Contraindications include ongoing CNS disease, unstable heart disease, and severe neck disease.
- Have the patient sit upright on the gurney with the head turned 45° to the affected side (the side that has a positive Dix Hallpike).
- Guide the patient down with the head dependent (head hanging) or place in Trendelenburg if unable to tolerate. Maintain position until nystagmus disappears, or for at least 30 seconds. Do this for each remaining position.
- Rotate the head 90° to the opposite side.
- Ask the patient to roll on his or her side, and rotate the head so that it is facing downward.
- Raise the patient to a sitting position while maintaining the head rotation and have the legs hang over the edge of the gurney.
- Simultaneously rotate the head to a central position, and move it 45° forward.

Labyrinthitis (Acute Suppurative)

- *Epidemiology and risk factors.* This entity develops in patients with an acute or chronic infection of the tissues surrounding the labyrinth. This includes otitis media (OM), mastoiditis, cholesteatoma, and meningitis. It has become rare since the introduction of antibiotics.
- *Pathophysiology.* Caused by bacterial invasion of the inner ear. Prompt diagnosis and treatment with parenteral antibiotics are needed to prevent spreading of the infection to the temporal bone and intracranial structures, leading to meningitis or brain abscess. If allowed to progress, acute suppurative labyrinthitis leads to profound loss of hearing and vestibular function, and patients may be left with permanent sequelae.
- *History.* In addition to vertigo, patients with known ear infection may have fever, mastoid or ear pain, and headache despite previous antibiotic therapy.
- *Physical examination.* Focal neurologic deficits are a late finding, and indicate intracranial extension of infection. Patients may develop seventh cranial nerve paresis with mastoiditis. There may be erythema and tenderness in the peri-auricular region and mastoid. The tympanic membranes may show evidence of OM with dullness, bulging, and decreased motion.
- *Diagnostic testing.* The diagnosis is clinical, but a CT scan may be used to look for intracranial extension of infection. Obtain a CBC and cultures when serious infection is suggested by the clinical appearance of the patient.
- *ED management.* Antibiotics should not be delayed while obtaining other studies. If meningitis is a possible etiology, lumbar puncture (if increased ICP is not suspected) should be performed.
- *Helpful hints and pitfalls.* Patients who are obviously worse despite prolonged antibiotic therapy and immunocompromised patients should be considered at higher risk for this unusual entity. A non-infectious labyrinthitis can be due to a variety of ototoxic drugs such as aminoglycosides, cisplatin, loop diuretics, or salicylates.

Meniere's Disease

- *Epidemiology and risk factors.* This may be sporadic, familial, post-traumatic or postinfectious.
- *Pathophysiology.* Although the precise mechanism is not clear, it is commonly thought to be caused by endolymphatic hypertension (hydrops) distending the endolymphatic system and damaging hair cells.
- *History.* Patients complain of sudden attacks of severe vertigo (often strong enough to cause the patient to fall to the ground). The vertigo is associated with hearing loss or tinnitus, and a sense of aural fullness. Symptoms are recurrent, last for several hours, and may occur in clusters. Clusters are often separated by long symptom-free intervals. Between attacks, function may be normal early in the progression of the disease. Persistent sense of disequilibrium may be present for days after an acute episode. Later, permanent hearing loss may develop.
- *Physical examination.* During attacks patients will have nonpositional vertigo, nystagmus, and hearing loss. No other focal neurologic deficits should be present.

- *Diagnostic testing.* A Dix-Hallpike test can be used to evaluate for BPPV. An MRI may be needed to rule out acoustic neuroma. Definitive testing is performed by an otolaryngologyist.
- *ED management.* This is achieved by symptomatic therapy with vestibular suppressants. Diuretics (e.g., acetazolamide), and a low-salt diet may be instituted.
- *Helpful hints and pitfalls.* This is not a diagnosis to be made quickly in the ED. Because of the potential for chronicity, careful discussion with the patient about establishing follow-up care is important.

Posttraumatic

- Head and neck trauma can lead to vertigo through a variety of mechanisms. Basilar skull or temporal bone fractures may cause a labyrinthine concussion or a perilymphatic fistula (communication between the perilymphatic and middle ear spaces), leading to temporarily altered function of the labyrinth. Head trauma may also displace otoconia, causing BPPV (often bilateral). Neck trauma or whiplash injuries may also lead to vertigo.
- Episodes last seconds to minutes, and are associated with turning the head. Symptoms are usually self-limited, but may last weeks to months. A head CT scan should be performed to rule out fractures or mass effect.

Vestibular Neuronitis (Neurolabyrinthitis)

- *Epidemiology and risk factors.* The highest incidence is seen between the third and fifth decades. The entity may be preceded by viral infection or toxic exposure.
- *Pathophysiology.* This is due to inflammation or viral infection of the vestibular nerve or labyrinth.
- *History.* There is a sudden onset of severe vertigo, increasing over hours, and then subsiding over days. Mild positional symptoms may persist for weeks to months. Hearing loss is present in some cases. Many will report a flulike illness within the preceding 2 weeks.
- *Physical examination.* The rapid segment of nystagmus will be toward the diseased ear. No focal neurologic deficits are present. Hearing loss may or may not be present.
- *Diagnostic testing.* No imaging or laboratory work is needed unless more serious causes are suspected (infection or mass lesion).
- *ED management.* Reassurance and symptomatic therapy with vestibular suppressants and antiemetics. Some recommend steroids and antiviral medications, but conclusive evidence is lacking for their ability to decrease symptom duration.
- *Helpful hints and pitfalls.* This is a very common cause of vertigo in the younger population without vascular risk factors. Substantial recovery occurs even if vestibular damage is present because the brain compensates by rebalancing tone at the level of the vestibular nuclei. Most young patients can return to work in a few weeks. Older patients may have a more protracted course.

Special Considerations
Pediatrics

- Young children are unable to give a clear history. Vertigo may cause crying, inattention, or falling, and may be attributed to behavioral issues or being uncoordinated.
- Always assess for presence of foreign body in the ear canal.
- The most common causes of vertigo in children are infectious (OM, meningitis), BPPV, and migraine.

Women and Pregnancy

- Always consider pregnancy in a dizzy or nauseated woman of childbearing age.
- Basilar artery migraine is more common in women and adolescents.

Elderly

- The elderly are at increased risk for vascular and central causes of vertigo.
- The incidence of BPPV increases with age, but so do more serious causes.
- A careful medication history is important. Many of the elderly are on multiple drugs and ototoxic drugs are more common in this population.

Immunocompromised Patient

- These patients are at higher risk for infectious and malignant causes of vertigo.
- Immunocompromised patients are more likely to have been exposed to potentially vestibulotoxic medications.

Teaching Points

Vertigo is an entity that intimidates many emergency physicians. It is possible to simplify it to a degree: Is the vertigo central or peripheral? Is it related to the middle ear or to the brain itself?

Fortunately, many patients have a benign positional variety. It is easy to test this with the Dix-Hallpike positional diagnostic test and with the Epley head-turning positional maneuvers. It also responds well to antiemetics, especially antihistamines and benzodiazepines.

Probably the next most common cause is an excess of alcohol. This is usually not subtle, and is often self-limited until the alcohol has been metabolized, but some patients will develop a form of benign positional vertigo for a couple of days after the acute intoxication, and will benefit from treatment with benzodiazepines.

In the elderly, central causes of vertigo are much more common. These patients require immediate attention to prevent life-threatening or neurologic devastation.

Suggested Readings

Baloh RW. Dizziness: neurologic emergencies. Neurol Clin 1998;2:305–321.

Baloh RW. Vertigo. Lancet 1998;5:1841–1846.

Parnes LS, Agrawal SK, Atlas J. Diagnosis and management of benign paroxysmal positional vertigo. CMAJ 2003;169:681–693.

Olshaker JS. Dizziness and vertigo. In Marx JA, Hockberger RS, Walls RM (editors). Rosen's Emergency Medicine: Concepts and Clinical Practice (6th ed). Philadelphia: Mosby, 2006, pp 142–149.

Rubin AM, Zafar SS. The assessment and management of the dizzy patient. Otolaryngol Clin N Am 2002;35:255–273.

Tusa RJ. Dizziness. Med Clin N Am 2003;7:609–641.

CHAPTER 60

Weakness

WAME N. WAGGENSPACK, JR. ■ LYNN P. ROPPOLO

 Red Flags

> Advanced age • Other co-morbid conditions: diabetes, cardiovascular disease, structural heart disease, history of cerebrovascular accident or transient ischemic attack • Altered mental status • Respiratory distress
> • Abnormal vital signs (↓ or ↑heart rate, ↓ or ↑blood pressure)
> • Abnormal pulmonary function tests: forced vital capacity <20 ml/kg
> • Signs of dehydration

Overview

Weakness may be the presenting complaint for a variety of conditions, both benign or life-threatening, and acute or chronic. Patients with "red flags" (see Box) should be assessed rapidly, and have an aggressive evaluation. Watch for signs of impending cardiovascular or respiratory collapse.

The terms *malaise* and *weakness* are often used interchangeably, but deserve clarification. Strictly speaking, *malaise* is a generalized feeling of discomfort, illness or lack of well-being that can be associated with a disease state. It can be accompanied by a sensation of exhaustion or inadequate energy to accomplish usual activities. *Weakness* refers to motor strength. Patients presenting complaining of "weakness" may also describe a feeling of "lightheadedness" or "dizziness" (see Chapter 43).

This chapter will discuss the approach to patients with weakness with a more detailed discussion of problems due to defects in neuromuscular transmission, demyelinating disorders, myelopathy, and myopathy.

Differential Diagnosis

- See Box 60–1 for life-theatening causes of weakness.
- See DDX table for conditions that may present as weakness.
- See Table 60–1 for conditions causing weakness based on anatomic location.

Initial Diagnostic Approach
General

- As always, the ABCs (*a*irway, *b*reathing, and *c*irculation) should be addressed first as discussed in Section II. Any ill-appearing patient and those with abnormal vital signs (bradycardia, hypotension, or hypoxia) or any neurologic deficit should prompt a thorough evaluation for serious causes of weakness.
- The diagnostic workup begins with differentiating true weakness from fatigue or lack of energy (asthenia), and focal from generalized weakness. Generalized complaints of weakness with no neurologic findings should begin with evaluation for anemia, electrolyte abnormalities, or endocrine abnormalities such as decreased thyroid function or diabetes.
- Fever should prompt an evaluation for sepsis (see Chapter 67).
- Clinical evaluation of acute neuromuscular weakness should focus on airway and respiratory compromise. Assess ability to handle secretions and speech. Rapid, shallow breathing is the hallmark of neuromuscular respiratory failure. Due to the intact respiratory drive, oxygen saturation and PCO_2 levels on arterial blood gas measurement may remain normal until sudden respiratory collapse. Therefore, any patient suspected of having an acute, progressive neuromuscular disorder should undergo selected pulmonary function testing (see Chapter 52).

BOX 60–1   Life-Threatening Causes

- Myasthenia gravis
- Guillain-Barré syndrome
- Botulism
- Adrenal insufficiency
- Acute myopathy
- Hypokalemia

DDx Differential Diagnosis of Weakness

Cardiopulmonary	Hypoxemia Hypercapnia Hypotension Bradycardia Impaired cardiac output (cardiac insufficiency, pericardial effusion) Dysrhythmias (45, 87) Myocardial infarction (22)
Hematologic	Anemia (66) Porphyria (66)
Rheumatologic	Systemic lupus erythematosus (SLE) (71) Polymyositis (71) Polymyalgia rheumatica (71)
Infectious	Botulism (67) Diphtheria (55) Tetanus (67) Tick paralysis (67) Human immunodeficiency virus myopathy, neuropathy (37) Acute viral illness (influenza, mononucleosis) (24, 55) Acute hepatitis (41)
Toxicologic/ drug-induced	Carbon monoxide (CO) (72) Lithium (72) Neuropathy (isonizide, nitrofurantoin, organophosphates, heavy metals) Myopathy (steroids, hydrocarbons, cocaine, statins) Any drug associated with bradycardia, vasodilation, and diuresis
Metabolic/endocrine	Alterations in serum sodium, potassium, calcium, phosphorus (88) Hyper- or hypoglycemia (38) Familial periodic paralysis Adrenal insufficiency (63) Uremia (49) Hypothyroidism (63) Hyperthyroidism (63) Vitamin B_{12} deficiency
Neurologic	Cerebrovascular accident/transient ischemic attack (56) Myopathy Neuropathy (Guillian-Barré syndrome, Eaton-Lambert syndrome) Myelopathy (12, 21) Myasthenia gravis Multiple sclerosis
Other	Chronic fatigue syndrome Malignancy Fibromyalgia (71) Deconditioning

( ) Refers to the chapter in which the disease entity is discussed.

Table 60–1 Examples of Conditions Causing Weakness Based on Anatomic Location

	Location	Characteristic Location of Weakness	Examples
Upper motor neuron	Cortex	Contralateral hemiparesis	Stroke
	Brainstem	Ipsilateral cranial nerve palsy, contralateral hemiparesis	Stroke
	Spinal cord (myelopathy)	Symmetrical paresis below lesion	Trauma Transverse myelitis
Lower motor neuron	Radiculopathy	Dermatomal weakness and sensory loss	Herniated disc
	Peripheral mono-neuropathy	Weakness in distribution of single peripheral nerve	Radial nerve palsy
	Acute inflammatory demyelinating polyneuropathy	Progressive ascending weakness; eventually may involve respiratory muscles	Guillain-Barré
	Chronic inflammatory demyelinating polyneuropathy	Distal, symmetric weakness	Diabetes
Combined upper and lower motor neuron	Motor neuron	Asymmetric, primarily distal, pure motor neuropathy with weakness only	Amyotrophic lateral sclerosis (ALS)
Neuromuscular transmission	Neuromuscular junction	Weakness of ocular, facial, bulbar muscles; proximal weakness, respiratory compromise	Myasthenia gravis Botulism
	Presynaptic cholinergic cell	Weakness of limbs Dysphagia	Lambert-Eaton syndrome
Myopathy	Muscle	Bilateral symmetric, proximal weakness	Polymyositis Muscular dystrophy Drug induced

■ Elderly patients may complain of weakness rather than chest pain when they are having a myocardial infarction.

EKG

■ Any patient in whom a cardiac cause is suspected should have an electro-cardiogram (EKG). Weakness may be the chief complaint in cardiac ischemia, dysrhythmias, or other conduction abnormalities, especially in the elderly.

Laboratory

■ Extensive laboratory testing is rarely helpful, and should be limited to evaluating specific causes of symptoms based on history and physical examination. Common studies include complete blood cell count (evaluate for anemia), basic metabolic profile (evaluate for electrolyte or renal abnormalities), cardiac enzymes, and urinalysis.
■ Patients with suspected rheumatologic etiologies may have studies such as erythrocyte sedimentation rate (ESR), antibodies to double-stranded DNA (anti-DS-DNA), and rheumatoid factor (RF) sent to be followed up by the consultant (Chapter 71). A creatine phosphokinase (CPK) level should be sent if concerned for a myopathy.
■ All women of reproductive age should have a urine pregnancy test.
■ Blood should be sent for type and cross match if there is concern for acute blood loss or severe anemia (hematocrit <30% in elderly patients; <20% in younger adult patients).

Radiography

■ A chest radiograph should be obtained in all patients with cardiac symptoms, shortness of breath, or hypoxia (SaO$_2$ <95%).
■ Computed tomography (CT scan) of the head should be reserved for patients with altered mental status or neurologic deficits.
■ Except in acute hemorrhagic stroke, an MRI is better than a CT scan for the diagnosis of an acute cerebrovascular accident (CVA), but may not be as readily available in the ED. An MRI should be performed emergently for suspected spinal cord compression.

Other Studies

■ Other studies may be used by a neurologist for diagnostic purposes, although these are not normally done in the ED.
■ Somatosensory evoked potentials (SEPs) aid in finding and localizing lesions of the somatosensory pathways within the central nervous system (CNS). SEPs are accomplished by stimulation of a mixed nerve or its sensory branch, and recording the response more proximal and distal as well as over the spine and scalp. They are particularly useful in detection of subclinical multiple sclerosis lesions for diagnostic purposes.
■ An electromyogram (EMG) is a recording of the electrical activity from muscle, and, in diseases of the motor units, permits localization of the

pathology to the neural, muscle, or junctional component. They may be used in myasthenia gravis, myopathies, amyotrophic lateral sclerosis (ALS), and other neuromuscular disorders. EMG results are often not pathognomonic of a specific disease process, and must be used with the clinical picture for diagnostic purposes.

■ Nerve conduction studies are often done in conjunction with EMG, and are used to detect dysfunction of peripheral nerves. Clinically, they are used to differentiate weakness due to peripheral nerve pathology from pathology of other parts of the motor unit.

Emergency Department Management Overview
General

■ The ABCs are always the first priority as discussed in Section II.

Disposition

■ *Consultation.* Should be prompted by the clinically most likely etiology.
■ *Admission.* Patients who present with unstable or abnormal vital signs, autonomic instability, hypoxia or signs of respiratory distress or failure should be admitted. Patients in whom the diagnosis of a Guillain-Barré syndrome is suspected should be admitted to a monitored setting with close attention to their respiratory status. In patients with stable but serious conditions (i.e., lupus, multiple sclerosis), disposition should be made with the appropriate specialist.
■ *Discharge.* Patients with a clear diagnosis of a benign condition, normal vital signs, normal examination, and no co-morbidities may be safely discharged home with close follow-up.

Specific Problems

> ● ● ●   Refer to the DDx table for reference to a discussion of problems in the
> ● ● ●
> ● ● ●   differential not mentioned here.

Amytrophic Lateral Sclerosis (ALS)

■ *Background.* This is an uncommon (incidence approximately 5/100,000) disease of unknown etiology characterized by slowly progressive upper and lower motor neuron degeneration. ALS is eventually fatal secondary to respiratory muscle weakness. It is commonly known as Lou Gehrig's disease. Age of onset is usually 40-60 years. Median survival is 3-5 years.
■ *Pathophysiology.* There is no known etiology at this time. ALS eventually progresses to a diffuse disease, but the onset of symptoms is often focal, and may involve only upper or lower motor neuron signs.
■ *History.* It is of utmost importance to distinguish ALS from an acute CVA, and a careful and complete history of chronic symptoms will allow the distinction. Common presenting symptoms include slurred speech or swallowing difficulty, clumsiness, and difficulty ambulating.

- *Physical examination.* The hallmarks of ALS are asymmetric, distal, pure motor neuropathy; lower motor neuron signs of atrophy, fasciculations, and hyporeflexia combined with upper motor neuron signs of spasticity and hyperreflexia in affected limbs. Dysarthria, dysphagia, and respiratory compromise may be present. Pain and paresthesias are almost always absent. Muscular weakness is the most common initial complaint, and most patients have noticeable muscular atrophy and weight loss by the time they seek medical care.
- *Diagnostic testing.* The diagnosis should be made from the clinical picture, and there is no definitive test for ALS available in the ED. However, all patients coming to the ED in whom this diagnosis is suspected should be referred for electrophysiologic confirmation against standardized criteria.
- *ED management.* This should focus on supportive care and treatment of complications related to the disease such as infections. Referral for neurologic evaluation is indicated in patients without prior diagnosis. Patients presenting with respiratory compromise should be treated as needed, and according to their desires.
- *Helpful hints and pitfalls.* Although this is a rare disease entity, consider this diagnosis in the patients with both upper and lower motor neuron findings in the absence of any sensory findings.

Lambert-Eaton Syndrome (LE)

- *Background.* Cancer, usually small cell lung cancer (SCLC), is found in 40% of patients. This syndrome is very rare in children; the usual age of diagnosis is late adulthood.
- *Pathophysiology.* The disorder is characterized by auto-antibodies to the voltage-gated calcium channels (VGCCS) of the presynaptic terminal at the neuromuscular junction. Symptoms result from impaired release of acetylcholine (ACh) at the pre-synaptic terminal that inhibits cholinergic nerve conduction to striated (skeletal) muscle.
- *History.* The symptoms usually progress slowly and insidiously, and most patients have symptoms for months or even years before the diagnosis is made. In patients with cancer, the symptoms of LE syndrome will often precede the diagnosis of cancer. Common complaints include relative lower extremity weakness involving proximal muscles. There may be mild involvement of the bulbar muscles, but respiratory difficulties are uncommon. Patients may complain of a dry mouth or metallic taste. LE syndrome is occasionally diagnosed in patients with prolonged paralysis after neuromuscular blockade. As with myasthenia gravis, multiple common medications (beta-blockers, calcium channel blockers, macrolides, flouroquinolones, etc.) may worsen symptoms. Inquire about long-term smoking, as this obviously increases risk of lung cancer.
- *Physical examination.* As with myasthenia gravis, patients with LE syndrome may come to the ED with a wide variety of complaints. A waddling gait is due to proximal lower extremity muscle weakness. Patients may have a dry mouth and mild ptosis. Tensilon testing can improve symptoms but not so dramatically as in myasthenia gravis.
- *Diagnostic testing.* Laboratory testing will not be available in the ED. In the undiagnosed patient, the clinical picture is the only evidence available to suggest the diagnosis.

- **ED management.** As with myasthenia gravis, focus on the airway and respiratory compromise, though respiratory failure is uncommon in this disorder. Consult with a neurologist. Admission is indicated in cases of unclear or unknown diagnosis, or profound weakness with respiratory involvement. Patients with a confirmed diagnosis of LE syndrome will need a diagnostic search for malignancy.
- **Helpful hints and pitfalls.** Signs and symptoms may be similar to myasthenia gravis, but respiratory symptoms are rare and the symptoms are often slowly progressive.

Guillain-Barré Syndrome (GBS)

- **Background.** This is the most common acute neuromuscular paralytic syndrome (incidence 1-2/100,000).
- **Pathophysiology.** Demyelination of peripheral nerve fibers and spinal roots by an autoimmune attack is most commonly implicated in GBS, which markedly impairs nerve conduction. Involvement of cranial nerves is seen in more than half of cases. Less than half of patients have permanent neurologic sequelae.
- **History.** Patients often complain initially of paresthesias in the lower extremities, but those presenting later in the disease course may have progressed to overt weakness or paralysis. A history of an antecedent viral illness, especially gastroenteritis, is common, and is associated with *Campylobacter jejuni* infection. Symptoms are usually at a maximum 2 weeks after onset. Cranial nerve involvement predominates in the Miller-Fisher's variant.
- **Physical examination.** The hallmark of GBS is weakness with severely diminished or absent deep tendon reflexes. Despite patient complaints of paresthesias, the sensory examination is often normal. Autonomic dysfunction, reflected by fluctuating heart rate, blood pressure, and temperature, may be present, and along with respiratory symptoms, is a sign of serious illness.
- **Diagnostic testing.** Cerebrospinal fluid (CSF) testing usually reveals a normal cell count and glucose with elevated protein, but a mild pleocytosis (<100 lymphocytes) may be present. Pulmonary function testing should be performed on all patients suspected of having GBS (see Chapter 52).
- **ED management.** This should focus on airway and respiratory management as respiratory failure is common, seen in about one quarter of cases. Factors associated with progression to respiratory failure include a vital capacity less than 20 ml/kg, maximal inspiratory pressure below 30 cm H_2O, or maximal expiratory pressure less than 40 cm H_2O. Patients exhibiting these levels of dysfunction should be intubated. Patients who are intubated electively (versus emergently) have better outcomes. The negative inspiratory force (NIF) is measured by having the patient inhale against resistance. A value of less than −20 cm H_2O is also indication for intubation. In addition, patients with severe GBS may exhibit marked autonomic instability. Hypotension usually responds to IV fluids, and hypertension should be treated with short-term parenteral agents. Atropine is indicated for bradycardia, and temporary pacing may be needed for those patients who develop high grade atrioventricular

blockade. All patients with autonomic instability or respiratory compromise should be admitted to an intensive care unit. Obtain consultation with a neurologist.

- ■ *Helpful hints and pitfalls.* Avoid succhinylcholine in patients requiring intubation due to the risk of fatal hyperkalemia. The dose for nondepolarizing paralytic agents may need to be reduced.

Multiple Sclerosis (MS)

- ■ *Background.* The most common debilitating illness of young adults (incidence approximately 100/100,000), MS is an inflammatory demyelinating disease of the central nervous system (CNS).
- ■ *Pathophysiology.* MS is an autoimmune disease, and the hallmark of this illness is multicentric and multiphasic CNS inflammation and demyelination. Areas most commonly involved include optic nerves and periventricular white matter of the cerebellum, brain stem, basal ganglia, and spinal cord.
- ■ *History.* Patients may have a multitude of symptoms. Paresthesias are a common early complaint, as are visual disturbances. Patients may complain of muscle cramping from spasticity. Patients with a known diagnosis may also come to the ED during flare-ups. Flare-ups may be precipitated by exposure to heat, such as from a sauna or hot tub. Infection is a known precipitant of MS flare-ups. Urinary tract infections are very common. Multifocal plaque formation due to CNS inflammation manifests in a wide variety of neurologic disorders that include those in Table 60–2.
- ■ *Physical examination.* The funduscopic examination may be normal in 50% of patients with optic neuritis due to retrobulbar involvement. Anterior involvement causes papillitis. An afferent papillary defect is present, and vision is impaired. The classic finding is bilateral internuclear ophthalmoplegia, which produces incomplete or slow adduction of the eye ipsilateral to the lesion, and nystagmus of the contralateral eye during abduction. A complete neurologic examination should identify spinal cord involvement (e.g., spasticity, paralysis, hyperreflexia, decreased joint position and vibration sense) or cerebellar findings (e.g., ataxia). Lhermitte's sign may be present. It is an electric shock wave in the torso or extremities during neck flexion. Encephalitis presents with altered mental status, neurological impairment, and meningismus.
- ■ *Diagnostic testing.* A lumbar puncture is indicated in acute disease if the diagnosis is uncertain. Typical findings include normal glucose, elevated protein in about 25%, mild pleocytosis (<50 monocytes), and an increase in immunoglobulin G (oligoclonal bands or free kappa chains). An MRI is far more sensitive and specific than a CT scan in diagnosing MS, and is the imaging study of choice. In patients with a known diagnosis, perform laboratory testing in a search for infections or other causes of weakness, if indicated.
- ■ *ED management.* This should focus on stabilizing any acute life-threatening conditions if fulminant disease is present as well as treating infections and fever aggressively. Consultation with a neurologist and ophthalmologist (if ocular symptoms are present) are indicated. Patients with routine exacerbations and stable vital signs can be admitted to a

Table 60–2   Multiple Sclerosis Manifestations

Ocular involvement	• inflammatory demyelination of the optic nerve (optic neuritis) • abnormal pupillary response • diplopia
Internuclear Ophthalmoplegia	• lesion of the median longitudinal fasciculus (MLF)
Transverse Myelitis	• acute *partial* loss of motor, sensory, autonomic, reflex, and sphincter function below level of the lesion
Acute Encephalitis	• acute onset of global CNS dysfunction
Spinal Cord involvement	• upper motor neuron (UMN) symptoms (paralysis, spasticity, hyperreflexia) • bladder, bowel, sexual dysfunction
Cerebellar involvement	• disequilibrium • truncal ataxia • intention tremor
Neuropsychological impairment	• poor attention span and memory • depression

regular floor. Intensive care admission is indicated for fulminant MS or disseminated encephalitis.

- *Helpful hints and pitfalls.* Consider this diagnosis in young, otherwise healthy patients who have isolated neurologic problems such as optic neuritis, transverse myelitis, internuclear ophthalmoplegia, or paresthesias.

Myasthenia Gravis (MG)

- *Background.* This is a rare (incidence approx 10-15/100,000) auto-immune disease characterized by formation of auto-antibodies to the acetylcholine (ACh) nicotinic postsynaptic receptors at the myoneural junction.
- *Pathophysiology.* Auto-antibodies bind to the Ach receptors, and inhibit cholinergic nerve conduction to striated (skeletal) muscle. Patients usually become symptomatic once the number of unaffected receptors is reduced to 25% to 30%. Smooth and cardiac muscles have different antigenic properties, and are not affected.
- *History.* Most patients with MG will be aware of their diagnosis and on medications for its treatment. Many factors affect symptom severity, and multiple common medications (beta-blockers, calcium channel blockers, macrolides, flouroquinolones, and so forth) provoke acute MG exacerbations. In the patient without a diagnosis of MG, question the patient about diplopia, blurry vision, ptosis, difficulty swallowing, and dysarthria, as MG often most prominently affects the bulbar muscles. Patients also may complain of proximal muscle weakness, or, more ominously, difficulty breathing or coughing.

■ *Physical examination.* Patients with MG may come to the ED with a wide variety of complaints, and the clinical syndromes due to excessive (cholinergic crisis) or inadequate medication (myasthenia crisis) are nearly indistinguishable. In mild exacerbations, ptosis or diplopia may be the only symptoms. Weakness will be intensified with repetitive testing. In severe exacerbations, patients may have a pronounced facial droop, marked proximal muscular weakness, and respiratory difficulty.

■ *Diagnostic testing.* Laboratory testing for presence of the auto-antibody to Ach receptor will not be available in the ED, and in those patients who do not yet have a confirmed diagnosis of MG, the diagnosis must be suspected on the basis of the clinical syndrome. The Tensilon (edrophonium) test can be used to confirm the diagnosis, and to delineate cholinergic from myasthenic crisis. It is performed by first fatiguing the patient with a task that is readily clinically apparent. Next, 1 mg of Tensilon IV is given as a test dose followed by 9 mg. A positive test involves rapid recovery of symptoms over the next 2 minutes. In patients with known MG, failure of symptomatic improvement represents a cholinergic crisis. This test should always be administered with cardiac monitoring due to the risk of severe bradycardia and hypotension. In patients in severe crisis, a chest radiograph should be done to evaluate for aspiration pneumonia, and forced vital capacity (FVC) should be measured. Normally these values range from 60 to 70 ml/kg. As the FVC approaches 15 ml/kg, intubation is often necessary. An easy bedside assessment used to follow ventilatory status is to have the patient count from 1 to 25 with one breath. With sequential performance of this, a decline in respiratory function will be detected as the patient fails to count as high as on the prior attempt.

■ *ED Management.* Myasthenic crisis is a medical emergency characterized by respiratory failure from diaphragm weakness, or severe oropharyngeal weakness leading to aspiration. Management should focus on the treatment of airway and respiratory compromise. Patients may need suctioning of secretions, and supplemental oxygen should be given. Intubation decisions can be guided by pulmonary function testing as mentioned above. Obtain consultation with a neurologist. Admission to an intensive care unit is indicated for intubated patients, and for severe exacerbations with the potential for respiratory compromise. Cholinesterase inhibitors (CEIs) are safe first-line therapy in all patients. Inhibition of acetylcholinesterase (AChE) reduces the hydrolysis of ACh, thus increasing the amount of ACh at the nicotinic postsynaptic membrane. Pyridostigmine (Mestinon) is the most widely used CEI for long-term oral therapy. Corticosteroids are used in patients with moderate to severe, disabling symptoms that are refractory to CEI. Several other immunosupressive agents have also been used. Plasmapheresis removes acetylcholine receptor antibodies, and is indicated in patients requiring rapid improvement. High dose intravenous immunoglobulin (IVIG) is also associated with rapid improvement. It is easier to administer than plasmapheresis, but is more expensive.

■ *Helpful hints and pitfalls.* Changes in pulmonary function tests may be subtle. Patients requiring intubation may be resistant to succinylcholine, but hypersensitive to nondepolarizing neuromuscular blocking agents.

Noninvasive ventilation has been used with success. One technique available at some hospitals is intrapulmonary percussive ventilation, which assists with ventilation and drainage of secretions. Patients with myasthenic crisis tend to have more respiratory symptoms and neurologic symptoms that improve with edrophonium. Patients with cholinergic crisis have more gastrointestinal symptoms, pinpoint pupils, and excessive secretions. These patients worsen with edrophonium.

Myelopathy

- This refers to primary diseases of the spinal cord. Most pathologic processes causing a myelopathic syndrome are acute in nature, and result in interruption of ascending tracts from below the lesion, and descending tracts from above the lesion.
- There are multiple etiologies that produce the characteristic constellation of symptoms by mass effect (tumor, epidural abscess/hematoma), demyelination (multiple sclerosis), interruption of vascular supply (anterior spinal artery syndrome), or disruption of the spinal cord (trauma). Spinal trauma and cord syndromes are reviewed in Chapter 12. See Chapter 21 for other diseases involving the spinal cord.

Myopathy

- *Background.* *Myopathy* is a general term used to describe primary diseases of skeletal muscle without involvement of the nerves. Although there are exceptions, myopathies are characterized by proximal shoulder and hip girdle muscle weakness. Loss of distal muscle strength is less pronounced, and strength is often completely preserved. They are rare diseases, and often not fatal.
- *Pathophysiology.* There are many different etiologies, including congenital, inflammatory, immunologic, toxicologic/drug-induced, and endocrine, that all result in intrinsic muscular dysfunction.
- *History.* The diagnostic focus depends on the suspected etiology. In infants, inquire about poor feeding, weak cry, breathing difficulty, and decreased movement or hypotonia. Note that some patients with congenital myopathies may not become symptomatic until adolescence. In adults with a suspected acquired myopathy, explore the social habits, medication use, and potential toxic exposures. Patients with polymyositis and dermatomyositis may present with a known diagnosis (see Chapter 71).
- *Physical.* In general, myopathies result in proximal limb weakness (affecting all limbs equally) with preserved distal strength. They are easily distinguished from neuropathies by preservation of sensation with normal reflexes. Inflammatory myopathies may cause tenderness and weakness of affected areas. Patients with dermatomyositis have a characteristic heliotrope rash: erythema with or without edema of the periorbital skin. Cardiopulmonary abnormalities rarely occur in dermatomyositis and polymyositis, but are poor prognostic indicators.
- *Diagnostic testing.* The CPK is typically elevated. The diagnosis is usually confirmed with a muscle biopsy, though not performed in the ED. Electromyography and nerve conduction studies may also be done.

- **ED management.** In most cases, ED management should focus on supportive care because most myopathies are benign. Consultation with a neurologist should be sought. Inflammatory myopathies may be treated with steroids or intravenous immunoglobulins. With an increasing number of patients on lipid controlling drugs (e.g., Lipitor), there are an increasing number of patients presenting with muscle cramps and weakness.
- **Helpful hints and pitfalls.** Sometimes these patients will present with myopathy determined only by obtaining an elevated CPK as the patient is asymptomatic, and the test was ordered for an unrelated reason.

Teaching Points

Weakness is a common and often dreaded complaint by emergency physicians. It may represent a somatizing syndrome, such as chronic fatigue syndrome, and not a serious threat to the patient, but can be very hard to manage. Conversely, it is the presenting complaint of some very serious diseases.

Distinction between the two ends of the spectrum often lies with changes in vital signs, with aspects of the history, and with neurologic deficits discovered on physical examination. Some of the hardest cases to diagnose are metabolic in origin because the patient often does not recognize the length of time of the symptoms, and may only be aware of not feeling well. The elderly patient often complains of weakness rather than pain, and this may mask the presence of a very serious disease such as heart attack or impending stroke.

Suggested Readings

Bannwarth B. Drug-induced myopathies. Expert Opin Drug Saf 2002;1:65–70.

Noseworthy JH, Lucchinetti C, Rodriguez M, Weinshenker BG. Multiple sclerosis. N Engl J Med 2000;343:938–952.

Saguil A. Evaluation of the patient with muscle weakness. Am Fam Physician 2005;71:1327–1336.

Shearer P, Jagoda. Neuromuscular disorders. In: Marx JA, Hockberger RS, Walls RM (editors). Rosen's Emergency Medicine: Concepts and Clinical Practice (6th ed). Philadelphia: Mosby, 2006, pp 1702–1710.

SPECIALIZED EMERGENCY MEDICINE

CHAPTER 61

Dental Emergencies

Steve Lim ■ Trevor J. Mills

Overview

Most dental problems seen in the ED are relatively benign; however, some can progress to life-threatening situations.

Dental complaints can be thought of as traumatic or nontraumatic in nature. Before addressing traumatic dental complaints ensure that the patient has been adequately assessed for other possible traumatic injuries, specifically to the head, face, and neck (see Chapter 10).

Tooth fractures involving pulp exposure require immediate intervention. An avulsed tooth can be successfully re-implanted if replaced within 30 minutes. The odds of successful re-implantation are decreased by 1% for every minute a tooth is left out of its socket. Soft-tissue injuries in dentoalveolar trauma are repaired after the teeth have been stabilized. In children, do not replace avulsed primary teeth because they may ankylose or fuse to the alveolar bone causing deformity of the dentofacial bone, or prevent eruption of the permanent tooth.

Dental caries and periodontal disease constitute most nontraumatic dental complaints. Familiarity with dental analgesia, antibiotic use, and outpatient referral are the mainstay of ED interventions in most of these patients. Patients who are toxic from sepsis should be evaluated for deep-space infections from an odontogenic source.

Dental Anatomy

- *Primary (or deciduous) teeth.* Primary teeth differ from secondary teeth in many ways. Specifically, there are 20 primary teeth (8 incisors, 4 cuspids, and 8 molars). Incisors are the first primary teeth to erupt, and usually do so between 6 and 9 months. The last teeth usually grow in by 24 months.
- *Secondary teeth.* There are 32 secondary teeth (8 incisors, 4 cuspids, 8 premolars, and 12 molars). The first secondary tooth to erupt is the first molar, usually around 6 years of age. The third molar is the last to erupt emerging around the age of 21 years. All other teeth are usually present by the age of 14 years.
- The Universal/National system for numbering adult teeth is as follows: (#1) is the patient's upper right third molar, and follows around the upper arch to the upper left third molar (#16), descending to the lower left third

molar (#17), and follows around the lower arch to the lower right third molar (#32) (Figure 61–1). To avoid confusion, some prefer to identify the offending tooth by quadrant and name (i.e., right upper lateral incisor). Starting from the midline and moving posterior, each quadrant consists of a central incisor, a lateral incisor, a canine, two premolars, and three molars.

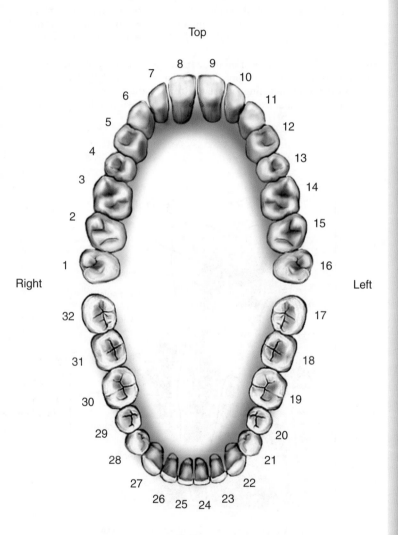

Top

Right

Left

Bottom

Figure 61–1. Adult dental numbering system. *(Adapted from American Dental Association. Current Dental Terminology Third Edition [CDT-3] © 1999.)*

- The pulp is in the center of the tooth, and serves as its neurovascular supply. It produces dentin, which hydrates and cushions the tooth during mastication.
- The coronal portion of the tooth is the visible part of the tooth, and is covered with enamel, the hardest substance in the body.
- The tooth's attachment apparatus consists of cementum, the periodontal ligament, and alveolar bone. Cementum covers the part of the root covered by the gingival tissues. It is not designed for exposure in the oral cavity. The periodontal ligament forms a cap around the root, and produces both cementum and alveolar bone to anchor the tooth in place (Figure 61–2).
- Specific terminology is used to describe the oral cavity: medial (midline), distal (toward the temporomandibular joint [TMJ]), buccal (points toward the cheek), lingual/palatal (toward the tongue), apical (toward the root), coronal (toward the crown and occlusal (the biting surface).

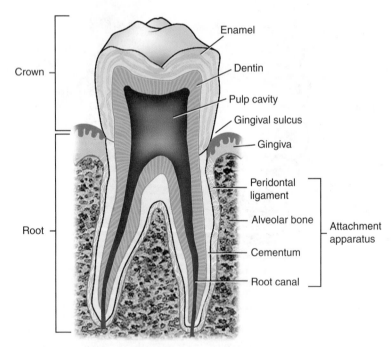

Figure 61–2. The dental anatomic unit and attachment apparatus. *(Reproduced from Amsterdam JT. Oral medicine. In: Marx JA, Hockberger RS, Walls RM [editors]. Rosen's Emergency Medicine: Concepts and Clinical Practice [6th ed]. Philadelphia: Mosby, 2006, p 1027.)*

Initial Diagnostic Approach
General

- ABCs (*a*irway, *b*reathing, and *c*irculation) should be assessed as discussed in Section II.
- ***Dental examination.*** If using a dental mirror, prevent it from fogging by touching the mirror to the patient's tongue. Consider the use of a tongue depressor or cotton swab in each hand, or use a bite block to examine the soft tissues in patients who may bite down on an examiner's fingers. Also consider using retractors, as opposed to fingers, to expose oral cavity landmarks before performing local dental blocks. Sudden movements by a patient can increase the risk of accidental needle sticks. Perform a systematic examination of the oral cavity starting with the soft tissues, progressing to the salivary ducts, the palate, and the teeth.
- Cellulitis or facial swelling of the buccal space may be impressive enough to appear to involve the submandibular spaces. Assess for submandibular/submental involvement by palpating under the tongue and the submandibular/submental spaces simultaneously.
- Percussing a tooth with a tongue blade or other instrument is a sensitive test to assess for a periapical inflammation.

Radiography

- ***Periapical/dental radiographs.*** These are the best imaging modality for radiographic evaluation of teeth, but they are often not available in the ED.
- ***Panoramic radiographs.*** These are useful alternatives to periapical/dental films, but are also not available in all EDs.
- ***Mandible series radiographs.*** Alveolar ridge fractures may be associated with concurrent mandible fractures. Because the mandible is essentially a ring structure, always look for a second fracture.
- ***Computed tomography (CT scan) of the face and neck.*** Use this imaging study, to define facial and mandibular fractures (without contrast) and to determine the extent of facial plane and deep-space infections (with contrast).

Emergency Department Management Overview
General

- Most patients with dental complains require analgesia and treatment for trauma or infection.

Medications

- ***Analgesia.*** Pain control is best achieved through oral analgesia, or the use of specific dental blocks. The most commonly used blocks are noted in Table 61–1. For temporary relief of pain before obtaining definitive dental care, the preferred agent is 0.5% bupvipacaine (longer acting) with 1:200,000 epinephrine. This provides 1 to 3 hours of dental pulp analgesia and 4 to 9 hours of soft-tissue analgesia. Duration of analgesia is less with supraperiosteal injections than with regional nerve blocks. A

Table 61–1 Common Dental Blocks*

Type of Block	Area Anesthetized	Procedure	Comments
Supraperiosteal injection (local infiltration)	Any maxillary tooth	See Figure 61–3. Aim at apex of the tooth to be anesthetized. The average adult tooth is 21- to 27-mm long; thus the apex is well above the gum line. Have the patient relax the face and close the jaw slightly. The mucous membrane is grasped with gauze and pulled out and downward in the maxilla. Orient the syringe parallel to the long axis of the tooth. With the bevel facing bone, insert the needle into the target area. Advance the needle until the bevel is at or a just beyond the apex of the tooth. Aspirate, if no blood, inject 2 ml of anesthetic over 30 to 60 s.	Easy to do and highly successful (95%). Not recommended for more than two adjacent teeth, infection, or if inflammation present. Does not work well on the mandible due to thickness of bone.
Posterior superior alveolar nerve block	Maxillary molar teeth first maxillary molar 70% of the time	See Figure 61–4. The puncture is made in the mucosal reflection just distal to the distal buccal root of the upper second molar. The needle is directed toward the maxillary tuberosity (i.e., upward, backward, and inward) and then along the curvature of the maxillary tuberosity to a depth of approximately 2 to 2.5 cm. On reaching this depth, the needle is aspirated and 2 to 3 ml of anesthetic solution is injected.	Significant risk of hematoma so frequent aspiration during injection is important.
Inferior alveolar nerve block	All mandibular teeth to midline; anterior two thirds of tongue and floor of oral cavity; distribution of mental nerve.	See Figure 61–5. The ramus is grasped between an intraorally placed thumb (positioned on the coronoid notch of the mandible) and extraorally positioned index finger. The pterygomandibular triangle may then be well visualized. The syringe should cross over the first and second premolars on the opposite side of the mandible. The operator should be able to feel the needle contacting the bony surface of the inner mandible. The injection is 1 cm *above* the level of the teeth. Directing the needle too far posteriorly will result in entry into the area of the parotid gland. Anesthesia of the seventh nerve may result. An alternative is to use a 25-gauge 1.5-inch needle, bent 30 degrees with the needle guard.	May need a longer (1.5 inch) needle. Probably the most widely used anesthetic technique in dentistry. Failure rate of 15%-20%, but extremely useful when effective.

Refer to Chapter 94 for other facial blocks.

1.5-inch, 25- to 27-gauge needle should be used. When an intra-oral block procedure is performed, the needle should not be inserted to its full length at the hub in case inadvertent breakage occurs. Use caution when performing local infiltration in an infected area. If possible, an intra-oral block should be used with the injection site located outside of the infected area. As with other forms of infiltration, the direction of a needle should not be changed while the needle is deep in the tissue. One should always aspirate before injection to avoid intravascular injection. To decrease pain associated with the procedure, apply topical anesthetics on mucous membranes, and dry the area to be injected before performing infiltrating with a needle (See Figures 61–3, 61–4, and 61–5 for illustrations of the most common dental blocks). Avoid injecting a cold anesthetic solution, and inject slowly to minimize pain. Topical anesthesia is applied with a cotton-tipped applicator generously coated with 20% benzocaine (Hurricaine) or 5% to 10% lidocaine. Non-steroidal anti-inflammatory drugs (NSAIDs) and oral opiate combinations can supplement local blocks provided the patient can swallow safely (see Chapter 90.1). Never block the mandible bilaterally as the patient will then cause major chewing destruction of lip tissues without being aware of it until the block wears off.

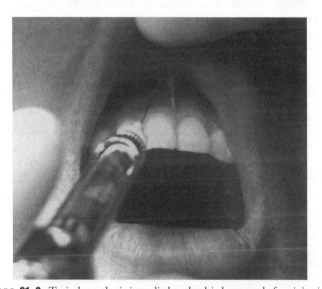

Figure 61–3. Topical anesthetic is applied to the dried mucosa before injection. Supraperiosteal injection technique above the incisors for anesthesia of the upper lip or individual teeth. The aim is to deposit the anesthetic right next to the periosteum at the level of the apex (area of the root tip) of the tooth. The palatal side of the tooth may also be injected. *(From Amsterdam JT, Kilgore KP. Regional anesthesia of the head and neck. In: Roberts JR, Hedges JR [editors]. Clinical Procedures in Emergency Medicine [4th ed]. Philadelphia: Elsevier, 2004, p 557.)*

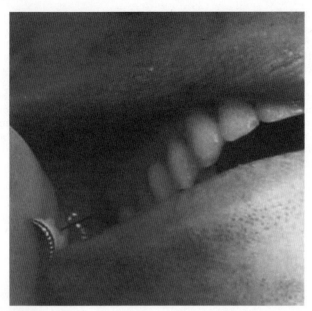

Figure 61–4. Posterior superior alveolar nerve block. *(From Amsterdam JT, Kilgore KP. Regional anesthesia of the head and neck. In: Roberts JR, Hedges JR [editors]. Clinical Procedures in Emergency Medicine [4th ed]. Philadelphia: Elsevier, 2004, p 557.)*

- *Antibiotics.* Beta-lactams (e.g., penicillin) are the antibiotics of choice for treatment of oral infections. Minor infections respond to oral formulations while more serious infections require high-dose IV formulations. In the beta-lactam–allergic patient, clindamycin oral or IV is an effective alternative.

Emergency Department Interventions

- *Incision and drainage.* Emergency physicians are able to drain abscesses of dental origin that do not extend into the deep spaces, and have well-defined boundaries that are easily accessible by intra-oral or external drainage. Incision and drainage may be a temporizing or definitive treatment for oral cavity abscesses, depending on their size.
- *Periodontal pack.* This is used to temporarily splint avulsed or subluxed teeth in position. Mix the resin and catalyst paste together then mould the mixture over the buccal and lingual surfaces of the involved tooth. Extend the splint to two or three adjacent teeth. Avoid placing splint material on occlusal surfaces if possible as this will place undue stress on the involved tooth during biting.
- *Suture splints.* This is an alternative to a periodontal pack. Several cross loops are made with 4-0 silk suture around the involved tooth, and then secured to the adjacent teeth.

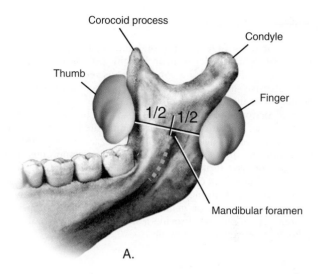

A.

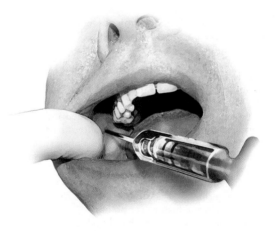

B.

Figure 61–5. When administering the inferior alveolar block, the target area **(A)** lies on the medial surface of the mandibular ramus at the mandibular foramen (inferior alveolar nerve and blood vessels course through), halfway between the thumb and forefinger. **B,** Injection site. The syringe should cross over the first and second premolars on the opposite side of the mandible. *(Reproduced from Hermann HJ. Dental and facial emergencies. In: Auerbach PS. Wilderness Medicine [4th ed]. New York: Mosby, 2001, p 570.)*

Disposition

■ *Consultation.* Consult with the oral and maxillofacial surgery (OMFS) or general dentistry department for any patient with significant oral cavity disease. Early OMFS consultation is required for oral infections with extensive facial cellulitis or deep-space involvement. In most communities, any isolated tooth trauma, alveolar ridge involvement, or localized periodontal infections are managed by general dentistry (and referred as an outpatient), whereas complicated periodontal infections and facial fractures, including the mandible, are seen by OMFS.

■ *Admission.* Admit patients who are immunocompromised, toxic, or septic or who have facial plane or deep-space involvement.

■ *Discharge.* Aside from complicated periodontal infections, most patients with dental complaints may be discharged home with next-day follow-up with an oral surgeon or general dentist after appropriate ED interventions are completed. Provide a limited supply of oral prescription analgesics to encourage follow-up.

Specific Problems: Dental Trauma
Dental Fractures

■ *Definitions.* See Box 61–1, "Classification of Dental Fractures".

■ *Epidemiology and risk factors.* Falls, followed by sporting injuries, altercations, and motor vehicle crashes are commonly implicated in dental trauma. The maxillary central incisors are involved in 70% of cases. Children are more likely to have pulp involvement because a larger proportion of the tooth is pulp. Adults have fully formed roots; thus fractures that extend into the root may compromise the tooth's attachment apparatus, and ultimately may make the tooth unsalvageable.

■ *Pathophysiology.* Exposure of pulp or dentin allows bacteria, saliva, and other substances to enter the tooth's interior. Pulp exposure is a true dental emergency. Dentin exposure is an emergent issue; however, approximately 2 mm of dentin may prove somewhat protective. These injuries cause an inflammatory reaction within the dentin and pulp that cause pain, and may ultimately lead to death of the tooth.

■ *History.* The most common history is of blunt trauma to the oral cavity. With dentin or pulp involvement the tooth becomes exquisitely sensitive.

■ *Physical examination.* The dentin appears pale yellow on examination. Pink tissue or blood that appears after wiping the fractured surface with

---

BOX 61–1   Ellis Classification of Dental Fractures

Ellis type 1
• Fractures involving the enamel only
Ellis type 2
• Fractures extending into the dentin (70% of cases)
Ellis type 3
• Fractures involving the pulp

sterile gauze indicates pulp involvement. Fractures involving the pulp require significant force, and are commonly associated with total crown or root involvement. The tooth may be displaced lingually or palately with an associated alveolar ridge fracture. Alveolar ridge fractures may require significant force to reposition.

- *Diagnostic testing.* Mandible and periapical films may be required to rule out an associated mandible fracture or alveolar ridge fractures (especially in type 3 Ellis fractures).
- *ED management.* The management of dental fractures depends on the patient's age and the extent of the fracture. Pulp exposure in the adult and pulp or dentin exposure in the pediatric patient require an immediate dressing of calcium hydroxide paste or sterile gauze soaked in sterile water covered by metal foil or an enamel-bonded plastic. Both adult and pediatric patients require immediate consultation or urgent next-day follow-up by a general dentist, endodontist, or pedodontist. If a displaced alveolar ridge fracture is to be reduced in the ED, materials to splint the fracture in place must be available. A Coe-Pak (GC America, Alsip, IL) or temporary paste made of a resin and catalyst is placed on both the buccal and palatal/lingual surface of the involved teeth and on several adjacent teeth on either side, after the alveolar ridge has been reduced. If no such materials are available, the fractured tooth should still be managed appropriately in the ED with urgent follow-up with a general dentist for the alveolar ridge fracture. Guidelines for tooth reimplantation are listed in Box 61–2.

Specific Problems: Odontogenic Infection
Acute Necrotizing Ulcerative Gingivitis (ANUG)

- *Epidemiology and risk factors.* Risk factors for ANUG include age younger than 25 years, smoking, poor oral hygiene, stress, loss of sleep, change in diet, malnutrition, and immunocompromised status.
- *Pathophysiology.* ANUG is a gingivitis caused by overgrowth of fusiform bacteria and spirochetes, along with other anaerobic oral bacteria.
- *History.* The patient will usually report a rapid progression of painful gingival irritation, sloughing, and bleeding.
- *Physical examination.* Oral examination will reveal gingival ulceration, bleeding, swelling and sloughing off of dead tissue. The gums may have irregular boarders or a "punched out" appearance. A grey pseudo-membrane overlying the gingival may be present. Most patients complain of (or present with) fetid halitosis.
- *Diagnostic testing.* ANUG without suspicion of concurrent deep-space spread requires no diagnostic testing in the ED.
- *ED management.* Urgent dental referral and administration of antibiotics, usually penicillin. Chlorhexidine 0.12% oral rinse may be used in addition to oral antibiotics. Pain control can be achieved with NSAIDS or oral opiate combinations.
- *Helpful hints and pitfalls.* Other names for this disease include trench mouth, Vincent's angina, acute membranous gingivitis, fusospirillary gingivitis, fusospirillosis, fusospirochetal gingivitis, and phagedenic gingivitis.

BOX 61–2 Guidelines for Tooth Reimplantation

- The tooth should be stored in appropriate media (milk and the commercially available Save-A-Tooth) if reimplantation is delayed for any reason.
- Handle the tooth by only by the crown and not the root.
- Perform a supraperiosteal dental infiltration before the manipulation or replacement of teeth to make the procedure more comfortable for the patient and easier for the clinician to perform.
- Check the oral cavity for trauma. If an alveolar ridge fracture is present or the socket is significantly damaged, the tooth should not be reimplanted.
- Suction the socket with a Frasier suction tip to remove the accumulated clot. Be careful not to damage the walls of the socket as this can further damage periodontal ligament fibers. Gentle irrigation should follow suctioning. If the clot is not removed, reimplantation and realignment will be difficult. Any debris on the tooth should be rinsed, not scrubbed, with saline. The tooth can then be implanted into the socket using firm, but gentle, pressure.
- Having the patient gently bite down on gauze may help to align the tooth. The tooth may require splinting after replacement. If significant mobility is present such that temporizing splints are not adequate, wiring or arch bars may need to be placed by the dental consultant.
- Tetanus should be updated as necessary. A liquid diet should be prescribed until seen in follow-up.

Deep-Space Infections of the Head and Neck

- ***Epidemiology and risk factors.*** Individuals with poor dental hygiene, human immunodeficiency virus (HIV), other immunosuppressive diseases, trauma, and IV drug abuse are at added risk for deep-space infections. Two thirds of all deep-space neck abscesses are polymicrobial. The most common isolated organisms in deep neck abscesses are *Streptococcus viridans*, *Staphylococcus aureus*, and *Staphylococcus epidermidis*. Mixed staphylococcus/streptococcus infections are common and may result in an overgrowth of anaerobic gas producing organisms.
- ***Pathophysiology.*** Odontogenic deep-space abscesses most often arise from periapical/alveolar infections. Extension through the subperiosteum and various muscle attachments within the maxilla and mandible allow entry into the deep spaces of the face and neck. Maxillary infections can spread to the canine, buccal, and infraorbital spaces. Anterior maxillary teeth abscesses tend to extend into the canine spaces with further extension into the infraorbital spaces. Contamination of this space can result in spread to facial venous system, resulting in cavernous sinus thrombosis (CST). Maxillary molar infections spread into the buccal space. Mandibular odontogenic infections can access the submental, submandibular and sublingual spaces of the neck. Bilateral involvement of submandibular spaces, the sublingual and submental space is called Ludwig's angina (see Chapter 64). Further extension

into the parapharyngeal space may result in epiglottis (see Chapter 76) involvement and airway compromise. Any involvement of the internal pterygoid muscles or masseter muscles may result in trismus.

- *History.* Patients report progressive facial or neck swelling typically preceded by odontogenic pain. In Ludwig's angina, patients may report dysphonia, odynophagia, drooling, trismus, fever, and other systemic signs of infection. CST presents initially after a periorbital and orbital cellulitis, progressing to cranial nerve abnormalities, vision, headache, and nuchal rigidity.
- *Physical examination.* Patients with deep-space infections may appear toxic with marked facial (or neck) swelling and cellulitis. Signs of respiratory distress—tachypnea, use of accessory muscles of respiration, and falling SaO_2—herald impending airway occlusion. Trismus may limit the ability to perform an adequate oral cavity examination. Classic findings in CST include chemosis, proptosis, ptosis, and cranial nerve findings. Patients may have meningeal irritation, clinical signs of sepsis, and altered level of consciousness. Less severe spread of odontogenic infections may only involve a single facial or deep space.
- *Diagnostic testing.* Obtain a CT scan of the face and neck to assess the extent of deep-space involvement if the patient is stable. A lateral soft-tissue neck radiograph can reveal the extent of airway narrowing and the presence of gas-producing organisms.
- *ED management.* Assess for airway patency. Start high-dose IV penicillin. Anaerobic gas producing infections may require extended-spectrum penicillins, clindamycin, or metronidazole. Consult OMFS or ENT emergently for toxic-appearing patients, extensive soft-tissue infection, or airway compromise. In any patient with trismus and in patients with Ludwig's angina, it may be impossible to obtain active airway management through the mouth; these patients may require a cricothyrotomy. It is therefore wise to be aggressive in achieving active airway management in the patient with Ludwig's angina before airway anatomic distortion occurs (see Chapter 5). Give IV dexamethasone in the first 48 hours. Steroids are beneficial in decreasing edema, increasing airway integrity, and enhancing antibiotic penetration. Intensive care unit admission is required for all cases of Ludwig's angina, CST, and those requiring close monitoring. Admit patients who are immuno-compromised, present with trismus, or an infection requiring surgical drainage with IV antibiotics. Very localized and superficial infections may be drained by emergency physicians. These patients are discharged with a prescription for oral antibiotics and instructions for close outpatient follow-up.
- *Helpful hints and pitfalls.* Odontogenic infections require aggressive treatment. Determine which infection is localized, confined, and easily accessible, or whether it is more complicated and extensive, requiring more aggressive therapy including specialist consultation, IV antibiotics, and admission.

Dental Caries, Pulpitis, and Periapical Abscess

- *Background.* *Dental caries* is a bacterial disease of the teeth with demineralization of the tooth enamel and dentine. Caries are initially asymptomatic until there is pulp involvement. Disease of the pulp can occur from trauma or dental procedures, or the cause may be unknown. The most frequent cause is invasion of microorganisms after carious destruction of the enamel. The tooth is usually exquisitely tender at this point. As the enamel is destroyed, caries development progresses more rapidly through the dentin and into the pulp chamber causing an inflammatory response, referred to as *pulpitis*. A severely inflamed pulp will eventually necrose, causing apical periodontitis, which is inflammation around the apex of the tooth. A *periapical abscess* is a localized, purulent form of apical periodontitis. It originates in the dental pulp.

- *History.* The patient has dental pain, usually without systemic complaints. Acute pulpitis is usually associated with severe tooth pain. The tooth becomes sensitive to hot, cold, and pressure, such as might occur with chewing.

- *Physical examination.* There is obvious decay of one or many teeth, and percussion tenderness of the abscessed tooth. Decay can be visualized as opaque white areas of enamel with grey undertones or as brownish, discolored cavitations. There may be localized redness, swelling, and tenderness. A periapical abscess will follow the path of least tissue resistance if not treated. This may be through the alveolar bone and gingiva, and into the mouth or into the deep structures of the neck. There may be fluctuant buccal or palatal swelling, with or without a draining fistula. Regional adenopathy is usually present.

- *Diagnostic testing.* Abscesses in the periapical region are usually visible on dental radiographs, and less commonly on a Panorex.

- *ED management.* Antibiotics are unnecessary in the absence of cellulitis or abscess formation. Antibiotic coverage should include typical oral flora. Penicillin and clindamycin are good choices. Analgesia should be provided as well. A supraperiosteal infiltration (tooth block) using a long-acting anesthetic can be performed for temporary relief. Dental abscesses can be drained by the emergency clinician if they are localized and easily accessible, the patient is not toxic, there is no airway compromise, and there are no signs of trismus. Regional blocks or dental blocks, or local infiltration may be performed. Needle placement should not track already infected tissues into healthy areas. A simple stab incision for periapical abscesses is an effective alternative to dental scaling and curettage. Direct the stab incision toward the alveolar bone and extend through the periosteum. Use a mosquito hemostat to bluntly dissect the area of induration. Irrigate the wound. In a moderate-to-large abscess, consider the use of a Penrose drain, piece of iodoform gauze, or portion of sterile glove fingertip held in place with a 4-0 silk suture.

- *Helpful hints and pitfalls.* Avoid creating too large an incision because this exposes too much alveolar bone.

Periodontal Disease

- *Background.* Periodontal disease refers to infection of the attachment apparatus of the teeth: the gingiva, the periodontal ligament, and the alveolar bone. Gingivitis is an inflammation of the gingiva caused by bacterial plaque. As the disease progresses, the gingiva becomes red and inflamed, and tends to bleed easily. With chronic periodontal disease, an abscess can form when organisms become trapped in the periodontal pocket. The purulent material usually escapes through the gingival sulcus; however, occasionally it invades the supporting tissues, the alveolar bone, and the periodontal ligament (periodontitis). Pericoronitis is a localized inflammation that occurs when gingiva overlying erupting teeth becomes traumatized and inflamed (e.g., third molar).

- **History.** Periodontal disease is not usually symptomatic, and, therefore, rarely is a primary reason to come to the ED. Patients with pericoronitis may develop erythema, edema, pus, and foul breath. The symptoms of a peridontal abscess are similar to a periapical abscess, although pain may not be as severe.
- **Physical examination.** There is erythema and swelling over the affected tissue. The tooth may be tender to percussion and have increased mobility.
- **Diagnostic testing.** No imaging studies are required.
- **ED management.** Periodontal abscesses that are not draining spontaneously through the sulcus can be drained in the ED. Saline rinses are encouraged to promote drainage. Antibiotics should be reserved for severe cases, or for abscesses that cannot be drained. If it is uncertain whether the abscess is from the pulp or the periodontium, antibiotics should be prescribed even if the abscess is drained. If pericoronal infection is localized, local or nerve block anesthesia is followed by removal of submucosal debris. Saline rinses and oral antibiotics are prescribed with dental follow-up in 24 to 48 hours. More extensive infections require specialist consultation as mentioned in preceding sections.

Teaching Points

There are many visits to the emergency department for dental emergencies, in part because there are few dentists available in the evening or at nighttime. In most instances, the patient will have an early infection from caries, often with swelling near the involved tooth, and with tenderness elicited by tapping the involved tooth. Most of these patients can be treated with analgesics and oral antibiotics, and referred for dental care the next day.

More serious oral infections are also seen, and present in a wide spectrum of oral involvement along with the various planes of the head and neck. These patients often require admission, intravenous antibiotics, and emergency oral surgery, otolaryngologic, plastic, or neurosurgical consultation for surgical drainage.

Patients with Ludwig's angina will often require active airway management. This should be achieved before there is anatomic compromise from edema and inflammation that will prevent a rapid sequence oral intubation.

Suggested Readings

Amsterdam JT, Kilgore KP. Regional anesthesia of the head and neck. In: Roberts JR, Hedges JR (editors). Clinical Procedures in Emergency Medicine (4th ed). Philadelphia: Elsevier, 2004, pp 552–566.

Amsterdam JT. Oral medicine. In: Marx JA, Hockberger RS, Walls RM (editors). Rosen's Emergency Medicine: Concepts and Clinical Practice (6th ed). Philadelphia: Mosby, 2006, pp 1026–1043.

Benko K. Emergency dental procedures. In: Roberts JR, Hedges JR (editors). Clinical Procedures in Emergency Medicine (4th ed). Philadelphia: Elsevier, 2004, pp 1317–1340.

Douglass AB, Douglass JM, Common dental emergencies. Am Fam Physician 2003;67:511–516.

Lewis C. Dental complaints in emergency departments: a national perspective. Ann Emerg Med 2003;42:93–99.

CHAPTER **62**

Dermatology

ANGELA J. KENNEDY ■ SHIREEN VICTORIA GUIDE ■ LYNN P. ROPPOLO

Overview

The focus of this section is to review the most common dermatologic complaints, to highlight those that require immediate treatment in the ED, and to offer an algorithmic approach to the diagnosis of dermatologic disease.

Describing the Lesions

Proper terminology is important in describing the lesions. Primary lesions are described as macular, papular, and so forth. Secondary lesions have developed over the natural course of a disease or are altered from the primary lesion's appearance by infection, scratching, or by the natural course of the disease. They are described with words like *scale, crust, erosion, ulcer*, etc. (Table 62–1). For our purposes, there are several main categories of dermatologic disease. These are described in the tables. Please be aware that the presentation can often overlap into multiple categories, as is the case with tinea, for example. These categories are simply a way of grouping disorders together by common presentation.

1. *Papulosquamous or psoriasiform lesions. Papulo* means elevated, and *squamous* means scaly. The borders of the plaques of psoriasis and superficial fungal infections are usually well defined. Common

Table 62–1 Basic Dermatologic Terminology

Term	Definition
Primary lesions	
Macule	*Flat* lesion; diameter <1 cm
Patch	*Flat* lesion; diameter >1 cm
Papule	*Elevated* lesion; diameter <1 cm
Plaque	*Elevated* lesion with a flat top/surface change; diameter >1.0 cm
Nodule	*Elevated* lesion with a round shape; diameter >1 cm
Vesicle	Small blister; diameter <1 cm
Bulla	Large blister; diameter >1 cm
Secondary lesions	
Cyst	Nodule filled with expressible material
Pustule	Vesicle filled with cloudy or purulent material
Scale	Layer of epidermal cells visible on skin surface
Crust	Dried superficial exudates of dead cells/blood adhered to skin below
Purpura	Extravasation of red blood cells into dermis resulting in nonblanchable lesions. Petechiae and ecchymoses are examples; classic is vasculitis
Erosion	Superficial denudation of epidermal layer of skin.
Ulcer	Defects extending to dermis and sometimes subcutaneous fat layer.
Wheal	Papule or plaque of dermal edema, often with central pallor and irregular borders
Other terms	
Erythema	Red appearance of the skin due to vasodilatation of superficial dermal blood vessels; the skin blanches when compressed
Induration	Dermal thickening and firmness often seen with inflammation or infection
Morbilliform	Beginning discreetly, then coalescing to form more diffuse lesion; resembling measles; both macular and papular (i.e., drug reaction)
Lichenification	Epidermal thickening characterized by visible and palpable skin thickening and accentuated skin markings
Annular	Round or ring-shaped lesions, often with a central clearing

papulosquamous diseases include psoriasis, pityriasis, lichen planus, seborrheic dermatitis, syphilis, and fungal infections. Several of these are discussed in Table 62–2 (Figure 62–1).

2. ***Eczematous diseases.*** When the term *eczema* is used alone, it usually means atopic dermatitis. *Dermatitis* and *eczema* are often interchangeable terms, and *eczematous* usually connotes some measure of scaling or crusting in addition to itching and erythema. Erythematous papules, dry skin, and small vesicles may be present. The scales are usually not as thick as in psoriasis. Patches of inflammation or plaques usually have indistinct borders. Acute inflammation is caused by contact with specific allergens such as Rhus (e.g., poison ivy, oak) or chemicals. In the id reaction, vesicular or papular reactions occur at a distant site during or after a fungal infection, stasis dermatitis, or other acute inflammatory processes. Table 62–3 discusses disorders that can present like atopic dermatitis, and includes contact dermatitis and candidiasis (Figure 62–2).

3. ***Annular lesions.*** These are round or ring-shaped lesions, often with a central clearing, and include erythema multiforme, erythema chronicum migrans, and fixed drug eruption (Table 62–4 and Figure 62–3).

4. ***Inflammatory papular or nodular lesions.*** See Table 62–5. Erythema nodosum is a classic example (Figure 62–4).

5. ***Vesiculobullous lesions.*** These are blistering diseases of the skin and mucous membranes, ranging from relatively benign (herpes simplex, Figure 62–5) to life-threatening (Stevens-Johnson and toxic epidermal necrolysis, Figure 62–6). These diseases require admission, intensive care, and early dermatology consultation (Table 62–6).

6. ***Pediatric lesions and viral exanthems.*** We include an overview of common dermatologic presentations in children, including varicella

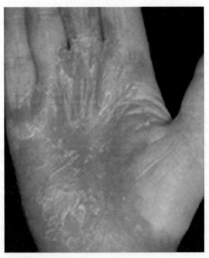

Figure 62–1. Psoriasis of the hand. *(From Habif TP. Clinical Dermatology [4th ed]. Philadelphia; 2004, Mosby, p 215.)*

Table 62–2 Papulosquamous or Psoriasiform Lesions

Problem	Risk Factors/Epidemiology	Clinical Presentation	Management
Pityriasis rosea	Spring and fall Young population Postulated viral (HHV-7) association Acute onset 7-10 d following oval "herald patch" appearance	Oval shaped plaques, plaques in "Christmas tree" pattern on trunk, sparing distal extremities and face, usually present for 1-8 wk.	Sunshine/UVB phototherapy Oral antihistamines Mid-potency topical steroids
Psoriasis	Family history Disease triggers: psychological stress, skin injury, infection	Red, scaly papules, plaques mainly on extensor surfaces, scalp, with relapsing/remitting course Removal of the scale causes pinpoint bleeding (Auspitz sign)	Emollient creams Topical steroids, PUVA radiation therapy or UVB light Generalized pustular psoriasis (GPP) presents with many sterile pustules especially on palms/soles; potentially dangerous with fever No oral steroid taper
Seborrheic dermatitis	Cold weather Alcoholism Hospitalization Bimodal distribution: infancy and fourth to seventh decades of life	Red/yellow greasy scaling at nasolabial folds, scalp, eyebrows, behind ears, central chest, back	Shampoo (selenium sulfide, zinc pyrithione, ketoconazole, salicylic acid) Steroid solution for scalp Low potency topical steroids for face Tacrolimus (steroid-sparing, as for patients with concurrent rosacea)

Continued

Table 62–2 Papulosquamous or Psoriasiform Lesions—*cont'd*

Problem	Risk Factors/Epidemiology	Clinical Presentation	Management
Tinea, or "ringworm" Four main types: • Capitis (head) • Corporis (body) • Cruris (groin/genital) • Pedis (feet)	Direct contact with infected person, pet, or surface Pedis: Hot, humid weather, occlusive footwear Infection with *Trichophyton*, *Epidermophyton*, or *Microsporum* species-fluoresces under Wood's lamp (i.e., kitten exposure)	Capitis: Scaling alopecia with short broken hairs, can look like "black dots"; can lead to kerion formation Corporis: Annular plaques with peripheral scale, central clearing Cruris: Red or hyperpigmented scaling confluent plaques with scrotal sparing and an advancing edge Pedis: Usually lateral web spaces, scaling/maceration of soles in "moccasin distribution" Diagnosis: KOH prep or fungal culture using one or two plucked hairs	Keep clean, dry Topical antifungals for 1-3 wk; use Lamisil (check liver function tests first), add miconazole if suspected concurrent Candida Capitis: Above plus Griseofulvin 10-20 mg/kg/d by mouth for 6-8 wks (children) or 250-500 mg by mouth twice daily for 1-2 mo (adults) Kerion: if very inflamed, can use prednisone 1 mg/kg/d for first 2 wk of antifungal therapy.
Lichen planus	Skin trauma (Koebner phenomenon)	Flat-topped sharply demarcated papules, often with white lines on the surface (Wickham's striae). The three "P's" that describe lichen planus are "purple, polygonal, papules."	Topical corticosteroids; can use mid to high potency, avoid face/axillae/groin Tacrolimus (steroid sparing)

ASO, antistreptolysin O; GPP, generalized pustular psoriasis; KOH, potassium hydroxide; PUVA, photochemotherapy; psoralen orally or topically followed by ultraviolet A radiation; UVB, ultraviolet B radiation.

Problem	Risk Factors/ Epidemiology	Clinical Presentation	Diagnosis	Management
Contact dermatitis Two types: • Allergic • Irritant	Allergic: Delayed hypersensitivity, lesions appear 48-72 h after exposure; occurs in genetically predisposed individuals Irritant: Occurs within hours of exposure; everyone is at risk	Red edematous plaques with vesicles Allergic: Distribution may correspond exactly to contactant; linear streaks with poison ivy Irritant: Borders indistinct	Clinical findings Allergen patch testing (referral)	Identification, removal of allergen/irritant Wet dressing/dome Burow's solution (aluminum acetate) to dry out vesicles Oral antihistamines Treat secondary infection Use mid to high potency topical steroid to localized lesions twice daily for a limited duration Oral prednisone taper for 3 wk
Atopic dermatitis "The itch that rashes"	Personal or family history of allergic rhinitis, hay fever, asthma (atopy) Extreme humidity, temperature, stress • Sensitive skin has increased reactivity • IgE overproduction	Usually presents in childhood	Clinical findings	Avoid scratching or rubbing Moisturizing creams or ointments Mild soaps, if any Oral antihistamines Treat secondary infection Mid- and low-potency corticosteroids to localized lesions OR Tacrolimus ointment (steroid sparing)
Superficial skin candidiasis	Diabetes mellitus Obesity Friction, heat, moisture in intertriginous areas	Bright marginated red areas with maceration, satellite lesions and pustules in intertriginous areas	KOH prep Fungal culture	Check for diabetes Keep area clean , cool, dry Topical antifungal twice daily to involved area until cleared
Tinea	See Table 62–2			

HSV, herpes simplex virus; PABA, para-amino benzoic acid' HCTZ, hydrochlorothiazide; KOH, potassium hydroxide preparation, used to identify fungus or yeast microscopically; TCN, tetracycline

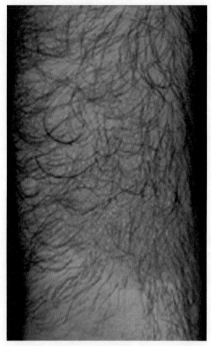

Figure 62–2. Acute eczematous inflammation. Numerous vesicles on an erythematous base. *(From Habif TP. Clinical Dermatology [4th ed]. Philadelphia; 2004, Mosby, p 42.)*

(Figure 62–7), scarlet fever, and measles (Figure 62–8, Table 62–7). Henoch-Schönlein's purpura is discussed in Chapter 77.

7. **Skin neoplasms.** This includes melanoma, squamous and basal cell carcinoma, and Kaposi sarcoma (Table 62–8).

8. **Skin changes associated with internal malignancy.** Dermatologic findings can often herald malignancy (see Table 62–9).

9. **Skin lesions associated with systemic disease.** Often a dermatologic finding will be consistent with undiagnosed or known disease. Table 62–10 lists skin findings associated with some common diseases.

10. **Causes of purpura.** Purpura denotes extravasation of red blood cells into the dermis resulting in nonblanchable erythema or purple discoloration. Purpura can be palpable (elevated) as in leukocytoclastic vasculitis (LCV) or Henoch Schonlein Purpura (HSP) or flat as seen in petechiae or ecchymoses. The etiologies are divided into thrombocytopenic and nonthrombocytopenic categories (Table 62–11).

11. **Disorders causing dermatologic manifestations on the palms and soles.** A variety of disorders cause palm and sole involvement, but these disorders can often be differentiated by lesion type. For instance, toxic shock syndrome, scarlet fever and Kawasaki disease often cause desquamation, whereas Rocky Mountain spotted fever is usually

Table 62–4 Annular Lesions

Problem	Risk Factors/Epidemiology	Clinical Presentation	Diagnosis	Management
Erythema chronicum migrans	*Borrelia burgdorferi* carried by Ixodes tick Bite precedes symptoms by 1-3 wk	Slow annular enlargement of the erythematous papule, with clear center; often with migratory arthritis "Lyme disease"	Clinical findings	Antibiotics (amoxicillin, doxycycline, cefuroxime) Supportive care
Erythema Multiforme (many forms = "multiforme") Stevens-Johnson syndrome (SJS) and toxic epidermal necrolysis (TEN) are reviewed in Table 62–6.	Adolescents, young adults Etiologies include (usually) infection, most notably herpes simplex virus; and mycoplasma medications (especially in severe cases) Involvement of two or more mucous membranes is termed SJS, between 10-30% BSA involvement is considered SJS/TEN overlap, and greater than 30% BSA involvement is considered TEN regardless of concomitant mucous membrane involvement.	Discrete, symmetric pink/red macules, usually on palms/soles, extensor surfaces Target lesions have three zones: dusky center, surrounding pale area, outer erythema May present with constitutional symptoms NOT SCALY	Clinical findings Confluent purpura should make you think of impending TEN	Remove precipitating cause Check liver function tests Usually benign clinical course Recurrent outbreaks of EM may warrant systemic antiviral therapy

BSA, body surface area.

Continued

Table 62–4 Annular Lesions—*cont'd*

Problem	Risk Factors/Epidemiology	Clinical Presentation	Diagnosis	Management
Fixed drug eruption	HIV infection Occurs within 1-3 wk of drug initiation most common causes: sulfa, ASA, ibuprofen, tetracycline, barbiturates	One to several round red patches occurring at same location each time drug is ingested Not scaly	Clinical findings	Stop the offending medication Symptomatic treatment
Granuloma annulare	Age <40 y Subcutaneous and perforating forms usually found in children	Flesh-colored or erythematous papules in a ringed pattern, upper extremities more often than lower	Clinical findings	Treatment generally not required, most cases spontaneously resolve Generalized form most protracted course, least likely to resolve, refractory to treatment
Sarcoidosis	Young adult, usually <40 y Blacks and females Lofgren's syndrome: Erythema nodosum, hilar adenopathy, migratory polyarthralgias, fever	Lupus pernio: chronic, violaceous indurated papules on face, plaques on limbs, back, or buttocks Erythema nodosum common	Clinical findings Skin biopsy shows noncaseating granulomas	Generally nonemergent unless major organ system compromise Steroids by mouth, injected, topical Antimalarials Immunosuppressive agents
Systemic lupus erythematosus (SLE)	See Chapter 71 for a detailed discussion.			
Tinea, or "ringworm"	See Table 62–2			

ASA, aspirin.

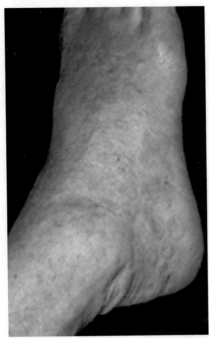

Figure 62–3. Erythema multiforme. *(From Habif TP. Clinical Dermatology [4th ed]. Philadelphia; 2004, Mosby, p 629.)*

petechial; scabies has web space involvement and typical linear burrows (Table 62–12).

12. ***Miscellaneous skin lesions.*** These include sebaceous cysts, hidradenitis suppurativa, and molluscum contagiosum (Table 62–13).

Allergic reactions are covered in Chapter 19, "Allergic Reactions."

Skin ulcers (venous stasis and diabetic foot ulcer) are discussed in Chapter 54, "Soft-Tissue Infections and Ulcerations."

Skin findings associated with biological weapons are briefly mentioned in Chapter 86, "Disaster."

Dermatologic problems associated with infestations such as scabies and lice are discussed in the Chapter 65, "Environmental Emergencies."

Tick born illness is covered in Chapter 67, "Infectious Disease."

Sexually transmitted diseases are discussed in Chapter 67 "Infectious Disease". HIV is discussed in Chapter 37.

Table 62–5 Inflammatory Papular or Nodular Lesions

Problem	Risk Factors/Epidemiology	Clinical Presentation	Diagnosis	Management
Erythema Nodosum	Females>Males Young adult population (18–34 y) May occur in association with multiple systemic diseases or drug exposure	Acute, painful, nodular, erythematous lesions are usually limited to extensor surface of lower legs Progress in color from red to bluish to yellow Often concomitant arthritis	Clinical findings Elevated ESR and ASO titers can support the diagnosis and point to strep infection as cause.	Self-limited Remove underlying cause Rule out sarcoid, infection Symptomatic relief using NSAIDS, cool wet compresses, elevation, and bed rest Intralesional steroid injection Restrict activity if arthritis is a factor.
Folliculitis, furuncles, boils	Other skin disorder with itching, introduction of bacteria Hair bearing regions of skin Infection usually with Group A strep or staph, can be pseudomonal ("hot tub"), fungal	Raised, painful, warm, erythematous lesion, often with underlying fluctuance Drainage from one or multiple sites	Clinical findings Can culture material from inside lesion Blood cultures if worried about systemic involvement	Drainage if necessary Warm compresses Bactroban to lesion Antibiotic choices include cephalexin, dicloxacillin or erythromycin (if PCN allergic). If there is extensive involvement, treat for MRSA.
Lice (pediculosis)	See Chapter 65.			
Scabies	See Chapter 65.			

ASO, *anti-streptolysin O*; ESR, *erythrocyte sedimentation rate*; NSAIDs, *nonsteroidal anti-inflammatory drugs*; OCPs, *oral contraceptive pills*.

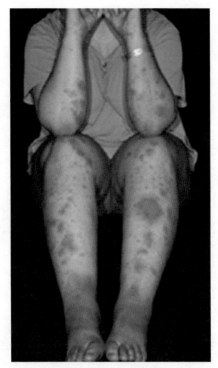

Figure 62–4. Erythema nodosum. *(From Habif TP. Clinical Dermatology [4th ed]. Philadelphia; 2004, Mosby, p 635.)*

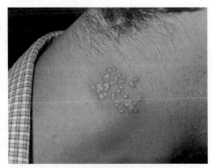

Figure 62–5. Herpes simplex of the skin: vesicular stage. The uniform size of the vesicles helps differentiate from herpes zoster, in which the vesicles vary in size. The local distribution of the vesicular lesions helps differentiate it from smallpox in which the distribution in diffusely spread throughout the body. *(From Habif TP. Clinical Dermatology [4th ed]. Philadelphia; 2004, Mosby, p 386.)*

Table 62–6 Vesiculobullous Lesions

Problem	Risk Factors/Epidemiology	Clinical Presentation	Diagnosis	Management
Herpes simplex	Immunosuppression Infection with HSV-1 or HSV-2	Painful ulcerated lesions on primarily mucosal surfaces (mouth, genitalia) present for up to a week Sometimes lymphadenopathy	Clinical presentation Tzanck smear Viral culture PCR studies	Avoid skin to skin contact Viral shedding still occurs during remission Antiviral therapy (daily use with recurrent disease) Eye involvement is an emergency because it can lead to blindness (see Chapter 69)
Pemphigus vulgaris	Sixth and seventh decades of life (any age can be affected) Autoimmune disorder	Painful blisters/erosions anywhere on skin surface, often preceded by mucous membrane involvement Often intertriginous involvement	Definitive diagnosis requires biopsy	Oral prednisone Immunosuppressants Consult if ocular, oropharyngeal, ophthalmologic involvement Manage severely affected patients as burn patietns Refer to dermatology because it can be associated with severe morbidity/mortality
Staphylococcal scalded skin syndrome (SSSS)	Most commonly age < 2yrs but can occur in adults with renal impairment Staphylococcal infection	Sudden onset fever, skin tenderness, blisters (especially at perioral, intertriginous areas), irritability; can lead to widespread desquamation	Clinical presentation, confirmed by staphylococcal culture and skin biopsy	EMERGENT IV dicloxacillin or nafcillin IV fluid/electrolyte support Topical emollients Low mortality rate, usually from pneumonia/sepsis Can completely heal in 5-7 d

Table 62–6 Vesiculobullous Lesions—cont'd

Problem	Risk Factors/Epidemiology	Clinical Presentation	Diagnosis	Management
Stevens-Johnson Syndrome (SJS)/bullous erythema multiforme	Skin, mucous membrane lesions of EM enlarge, with necrosis and crusting. Hypersensitivity reaction to infection, medication, other	Mucous membrane involvement; wheals, macules, papules, bullae "target lesion"~ 5% Mortality~ 5%	Clinical findings; skin biopsy not typically performed in the ED.	EMERGENT IV fluid/electrolyte support Burn care. Avoid silver sulfadiazine as this may precipitate TEN Consult dermatology, burn, or plastic surgery for severe cases; other specialists depending on system involvement Opthalmologic consult (risk for blindness)
Toxin Epidermal Necrolysis (TEN)	Speculated to be on a spectrum with SJS as a single disease entity. Initially seen with SJS–like mucous membrane disease and progresses to diffuse, generalized detachment of the epidermis through the dermoepidermal junction Nearly all cases are medication induced Pathophysiology largely unknown	Often involves at least 30% skin surface, usually with mucous membrane involvement Ocular and respiratory involvement may occur. Skin lesions may present as a generalized popular exanthem, purpuric macules, atypical targetlike lesions, bullae, or erosions. Lesions may rapidly form large blisters that may wrinkle and separate with slight pressure (Nikolsky sign)	Clinical findings; skin biopsy not typically performed in the ED. Grade 1: SJS mucosal erosions and epidermal detachment < 10% Grade 2: Overlap of SJS/TEN epidermal detachment between 10% and 30% Grade 3: TEN epidermal detachment > 30%	EMERGENT Treatment is the same of SJS but more agressive as these patients are more ill-appearing

Continued

Table 62–6   Vesiculobullous Lesions—*cont'd*

Problem	Risk Factors/Epidemiology	Clinical Presentation	Diagnosis	Management
Herpes zoster virus (varicella zoster virus)	Initial infection produces chicken pox, usually during childhood; reactivation of dormant viral infection then produces shingles Can produce Ramsay Hunt syndrome (involvement of the 7th cranial nerve, geniculate ganglion), postherpetic neuralgia Decreased cellular immunity	Vesicular rash in single dermatome (along dorsal root ganglion innervation) usually on trunk, causing pain, paresthesia If >1 dermatome involved, may be disseminated and may lead to varicella pneumonia	Clinical findings	Tzanck smear DFA (direct fluorescent antibody)- 2 swabs in viral culture to micro Wet dressings with water or Burow's solution (aluminum acetate) Symptomatic treatment

DFA, direct fluorescent antibody; EM, erythema multiforme; HSV, herpes simplex virus; TEN, toxic epidermal necrolysis; NSAIDS, nonsteroidal anti-inflammatory drugs.

*Note: Although EM, SJS, and TEN are often listed separately, there is controversy regarding whether they are all a part of a spectrum of disease that involves skin and mucous membranes, and induced by exposure to infection or medications. However, SJS and TEN are more similar to each other than to EM, and as they tend to have a more serious clinical course.

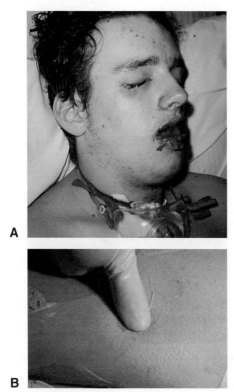

A

B

Figure 62–6. *A,* Stevens Johnson syndrome. Lesions are present on the conjunctiva and in the mouth. *B,* Toxic epidermal necrolysis. Large sheets of full-thickness epidermis are shed. With slight thumb pressure, the skin wrinkles, slides laterally, and separates from the dermis (Nikolsky's sign). *(From Habif TP. Clinical Dermatology [4th ed]. Philadelphia; 2004, Mosby, pp 631, 633.)*

Initial Diagnostic Approach

■ The patient with a skin complaint requires a history and a physical examination that emphasizes an assessment of the entire skin as well as mucous membranes, hair, scalp, and nails. Good lighting should be used, and the patient should be examined while disrobed for all but the most localized complaints. Important to the history taking is the progression of lesion morphology, family history, occupational exposure, and medication history.

■ In diagnosing dermatologic disease, a useful method is the grouping of disorders in terms of lesion morphology. For our purposes, there are several main categories of dermatologic disease. These are described under "Describing the Lesions" above.

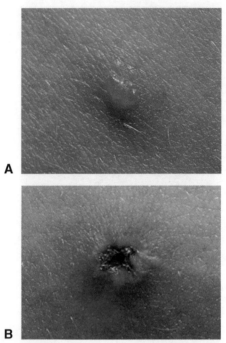

Figure 62–7. *A,* Varicella (chicken pox) lesion. "Dewdrop on a rose petal." Early lesions are thin-walled vesicles with clear fluid on a red base. The rash begins on the trunk (centripetal distribution) and spreads to the face and extremities (centrifugal spread). *B,* Varicella (chicken pox) lesion. The vesicle fluid becomes cloudy. A crust eventually forms in the center. The rash begins on the trunk (centripetal distribution) and spreads to the face and extremities (centrifugal spread). *(From Habif TP. Clinical Dermatology [4th ed]. Philadelphia; 2004, Mosby, p 389.)*

■ By the end of the physical examination it should be possible to narrow the diagnosis to one or two of the above categories. Some disease presentations can fit into a couple of categories, depending on the stage of the disease (for instance, atopic dermatitis can appear eczematous or vesicular). From here you can perform whatever diagnostic tests (scrapings, microscopic inspection, etc.) are necessary to help you arrive at a definitive diagnosis. In most cases, diagnosis is based on history and the clinical appearance of the rash. Consult dermatology and contact the burn unit immediately for suspicion of toxic epidermal necrolysis (TEN) and Stevens Johnson syndrome (SJS).

Emergency Department Management Overview

■ Topical corticosteroids are commonly used in the treatment of a multitude of dermatologic disorders. The basic mechanism is a decrease in local

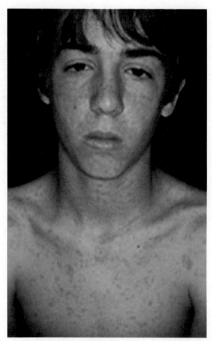

Figure 62–8. Measles. Lesions begins on the face and spreads to the trunk and extremities. Eruption has become confluent on the face. *(From Habif TP. Clinical Dermatology [4th ed]. Philadelphia; 2004, Mosby, p 461.)*

inflammation leading to symptomatic relief secondary to local immuno-suppression and down-regulation of pro-inflammatory cytokines. Therefore the most logical use is in those disorders where inflammation is the primary source of symptoms. Because topical steroids so often provide relief, they can be overused, and, if used in the wrong situation, can worsen the patient's initial problem (i.e., scabies, and fungal infections often flourish with the use of topical corticosteroids, and systemic steroid therapy can cause an even worse psoriasis flare once it is discontinued). The reason for caution in potency choices is twofold: Potent steroids on thin skin can cause further thinning and changes in appearance, and there can be increases in systemic absorption depending on the thinness and vascularity of the area to which the steroid is applied. There are seven categories, with potency inversely related to category number (i.e., category seven is least potent). In general, high-potency steroids are reserved for severe disease and for areas of more thickened skin (hands, elbows, knees, thighs), and kept away from more delicate areas (face, eyelids, intertriginous areas). Lower potency steroids are used for nonspecific dermatitis, and can be applied to areas with thinner skin. Note: If a patient has an allergic reaction to a certain prescribed steroid,

Table 62-7	Pediatric Lesions and Viral Exanthems			
Problem	**Risk Factors/Epidemiology**	**Clinical Presentation**	**Diagnosis**	**Management**
Henoch-Schönlein's purpura	See Chapter 77.			
Measles (rubeola)	Exposure to infected person Single-stranded RNA paramyxovirus Decrease in frequency with vaccine administration	Usually a child with recent fever, cough, coryza, conjunctivitis, 10 d after exposure to virus; Koplik spots in oral mucosa, rash appears/resolves from head down, involves palms and soles	Clinical findings	Supportive care Treat secondary infection Immune globulin to the immunocompromised and pregnant within a week of exposure
Herpangina	Exposure to coxsackie virus, enterovirus, usually through fecal/oral route	Fever and vesicular lesions in posterior oropharynx	Clinical findings	Supportive care Antipyretics
Varicella (VZV)	Late winter/early spring Usually <age 10	Faint red macules starting on trunk/face outward, sparing palms/soles teardrop vesicles on an erythematous base	Clinical findings Tzanck smear shows multinucleated giant cells or giant cells with margination of chromatin	Supportive care for uncomplicated cases No aspirin (Reye's syndrome) Aggressive antiviral therapy for the immuno-compromised Send DFA to distinguish HSV from VZV
Roseola infantum	Children 6 mo to 3 y	Abrupt onset high fever lasting 3-5 d followed by discrete centralized rash that blanches	Clinical findings	Supportive care Acetaminophen for fever

Table 62-7 Pediatric Lesions and Viral Exanthems—cont'd

Problem	Risk Factors/Epidemiology	Clinical Presentation	Diagnosis	Management
Erythema infectiosum (fifth disease)	Spring Children 5-15 y Infection with human parvovirus B19	Abrupt appearance of fiery red rash on cheeks ("slapped cheek" appearance); reticulated lacy blanchable patches on arms/trunk; associated arthralgias	Clinical findings	Supportive care Pregnant adults who acquire parvovirus B19 carry risk of hydrops fetalis Adults with HIV are at risk for aplastic anemia
Rubella	Spring Inadequate immunization	Pink macules/papules on face, spreads centrifugally after 1- to 5-d prodrome (fever, malaise, HA, sore throat) Lymphadenopathy (suboccipital/posterior auricular nodes)	Clinical findings History of inadequate immunization	Supportive care
Scarlet fever (erythema marginatum; gyrate erythema)	Group A beta-hemolytic streptococci produces toxin	Red oropharynx White and red "strawberry tongue" Red, punctuate, blanching "sandpaper" rash Desquamation of hands/feet	Clinical findings Throat culture Check ASO titer (>160 is abnormal)	Penicillin to reduce risk of rheumatic fever, nephritis Macrolide for penicillin allergic Supportive care
Hand, foot, and mouth disease	Cocksackie virus A16 infection	Fever, anorexia, malaise, sore mouth followed by small vesicles in mouth which rupture and ulcerate, spread to palms/soles, dorsal feet/hands, buttocks	Clinical findings	Supportive care

ASO, anti-streptolysin O; DFA, direct fluorescent antibody; HSV, herpes simplex virus.

Table 62–8 Skin Neoplasms

Problem	Risk Factors/Epidemiology	Clinical Presentation	Diagnosis	Management
Melanoma	Sun exposure Family history Immunosuppression Multiple atypical nevi Thought to grow radially before vertically; best chance for cure in radial growth phase	Black or dark brown spot changing in color/size or new itching/bleeding A: Asymmetry B: Border irregularity C: Color irregularity D: Diameter ≥ 5 mm Dark E: Evolving lesion	Biopsy	*Referral to dermatologist Thorough examination for other lesions/signs of metastasis (chest radiograph, lymph node examination, lactate dehydrogenase) Excision
Basal cell carcinoma Two main types: • Superficial • Nodular	Sun exposure Radiation Heredity Immunodeficiency	Slowly growing pearly papules, often with depressed center/central ulceration and telangiectasias, in sun-exposed area (most commonly found on head and neck, ears) Usually middle aged/elderly patient	Biopsy	*Referral to dermatologist Close follow-up with frequent examinations Skin check every 6 mo
Kaposi's sarcoma	See Chapter 37.			
Squamous cell carcinoma	Immunosuppression Transplant recipients HIV patients Sun exposure	Slowly enlarging lesion on usually sun-exposed cutaneous or mucosal surfaces Often associated with pain/bleeding Present for months to years	Clinical suspicion with biopsy confirmation	*Referral to dermatologist Excision of invasive lesions Malignant potential, especially involving mucosal surfaces

AIDS, acquired immunodeficiency syndrome; HIV, human immunodeficiency virus.

Table 62–9   Skin Changes Associated with Internal Malignancy

Skin Lesion	Clinical Presentation	Associated Malignancy
Acanthosis nigricans	Velvety, hyperpigmented plaques most often found on axillae and neck, often with skin tags	Most commonly adenocarcinoma, usually of gastric origin
Acquired ichthyosis	Symmetrical scaling of the skin, which varies from barely visible roughness and dryness to strong horny plates More common in lower extremities and mostly on extensor surfaces	Hodgkin's lymphoma
Dermatomyositis (DM)	Heliotrope rash (periorbital), ragged cuticles, proximal muscle weakness, "tendon streaking"	Carcinomas of the breast, ovary, and female genital tracts, GI malignancies, thymoma, and multiple myeloma; refer for age-appropriate screening
Erythema multiforme	Symmetric pink/red painful/itchy macules (many forms; "multiforme") on palms/soles, extensor surfaces "Target/iris" lesions have three zones: dusky center, surrounding pale area, outer erythema May present with constitutional symptoms	Leukemia
Erythroderma	Usually rapid onset of generalized erythema and scaling over large portion of skin, often involving palms/soles	Cutaneous T-cell lymphoma, Hodgkin's disease and leukemia
Pruritis	Area of itching without a discernible rash	Hodgkin's disease, leukemia, adenocarcinoma or squamous cell carcinoma of various organs, carcinoid syndrome, multiple myeloma, and polycythemia vera; liver and renal disease, neuropsych
Purpura	Bleeding into the skin; ranges from petechiae to ecchymoses, and does not blanch with pressure	Leukemia, lymphoma, myeloma (see Table 62–11 for other causes)

GI, gastrointestinal.

Table 62–10 Skin Lesions Associated with Systemic Disease

Disease	Skin findings
AIDS/HIV	Kaposi sarcoma, HSV, VZV; molluscum contagiosum, fungal infection (Candida, Trichophyton), papillomavirus infection (warts), scabies, syphilis, severe seborrheic dermatitis or psoriasis
Diabetes	Cellulitis, furuncles, carbuncles, necrotizing fasciitis; candidiasis, onychomycosis
Hypothyroidism	Cool, rough, dry skin, pretibial myxedema (shins), vitiligo (loss of pigmentation)
Lyme disease	Erythema migrans (plaque with central clearing; the "target" lesion) followed in second stage by multiple annular lesions
Rocky mountain spotted fever	Maculopapular rash and petechiae spreading centripetally to trunk from hands, feet, wrists, ankles (Chapter 67)
Syphilis	Primary: Painless chancre on genitalia Secondary: Papular red-pink rash spreading from trunk/flexor surfaces to palms, soles "copper pennies"; always check for concomitant HIV infection
Toxic Shock	Diffuse, blanching rash fades, then full thickness desquamation of toes, fingers, soles, palms
Ulcerative colitis	Erythema nodosum, pyoderma gangrenosum, Behçet's disease
Vasculitis	Erythema nodosum, painful, palpable purpura

AIDS, acquired immunodeficiency syndrome; HIV, human immunodeficiency virus; HSV, herpes simplex virus; VZV, varicella zoster virus.

Table 62–11 Causes of Purpura

Thrombocytopenic:
- Aplastic anemia
- Drug-induced
- Idiopathic
- Malignant disease
- Sarcoidosis
- Splenomegaly
- Systemic lupus erythematosus
- Thrombocytopenic purpura
- Tuberculosis

Nonthrombocytopenic:
- Drugs
- Infection (meningococcemia, Rocky mountain spotted fever)
- Qualitative platelet defect
- Vasculitis

Table 62–12 Disorders Causing Dermatologic Manifestations on the Palms and Soles

Enteroviruses (coxsackie): Blisters
Erythema multiforme: Targetoid lesions
Kawasaki disease: Desquamation
Parvovirus B19: Reticulated/blanchable erythema
Rocky Mountain spotted fever: Petechiae
Scabies: Web-space involvement, lateral fingers, linear burrows, crusted papules
Scarlet fever: Desquamation
Secondary syphilis: Scaly papules; "copper pennies"
Small pox: Umbilicated papules
Toxic shock syndrome: Desquamation

try another before abandoning steroid therapy altogether. Patients are not allergic to steroids in general, only to a specific type (Table 62–14).

- If the patient should be spared steroid therapy, tacrolimus (Protopic) or pimecrolimus (elidel) can be used in many instances, especially in sensitive areas such as the face or groin.
- Other treatment options are disorder-specific and include emollient creams, shampoos, topical antifungals, ultraviolet light, and oral medications such as antihistamines, antibiotics, and occasionally oral corticosteroids.
- Topical medications are available in many forms. Generally, ointments which are the greasiest are the most effective and hydrating for very dry scaly lesions. Creams and lotions have a greater percentage of water with lotions being the least hydrating. For weepy ulcers or vesicular/bullous lesions, you may consider Dome Burrow soaks (aluminum and magnesium salts), which help dry out lesions and provide symptomatic relief.
- All patients should have follow-up with a primary care provider or dermatologist. It is useful to give an adequate amount of topical agents to tide the patient over until the follow-up appointment.
- If tumor is a concern (e.g., malignant melanoma), call the dermatologist to arrange a time for biopsy.
- Be careful not to overuse oral steroid therapy, especially if you are not sure of the diagnosis. For example, psoriasis often becomes much worse after withdrawal of initial steroid therapy.
- Even though most rashes are irritating and cause cosmetic concern, there are a small number of rare but very serious dermatologic problems. It is only prudent to consider these, and if uncertain about their presence, consult dermatology.

Special Considerations

- Children and the elderly can have variations from the normal presentation of diseases, and often have a less robust immune response to disease. Many diseases present predominantly during childhood, and because their appearances can be very similar, it is easy to mistake a serious rash for something else (e.g., thinking the patient has

Table 62–13   Miscellaneous Lesions

Problem	Risk Factors/Epidemiology	Clinical Presentation	Diagnosis	Management
Sebaceous cyst/ epidermal inclusion cyst	Sterile foreign body response Familial	Single lesion, usually above nipple line (scalp/face/back), present months to years, often with central punctum	Clinical findings	Definitive: surgical excision of entire lesion Incision and drainage if symptomatic Kenalog 3-10 mg/ml injection for inflammation Can use antistaphylococcal antibiotics
Hidradenitis suppurativa	Young adult population, obesity, acne Keratin blocks apocrine glands or hair follicles, then bacterial infection	Tender swellings usually axillae, anogenital region, breast Can drain foul-smelling material	Clinical findings	Oral and topical antibacterials (erythromycin, metronidazole, minocycline), bactroban to furuncles; peripubertal cases are good surgical candidates Check bacterial cultures; patients often have mixed resistant infections
Molluscum contagiosum	Common in children Molluscum poxvirus	Unbilicated papules, rarely involving palms/soles Genital involvement presumed to be sexually transmitted	Clinical findings	Cryotherapy Trichloroacetic acid Cantheridin Retinoids Curettage In autoimmune deficiency syndrome, lesions are persistent, refractory to treatment

Table 62-14   Topical Corticosteroids*

Steroid strength	Group	Generic name	Potency (%)	Disease treatment recommendation
High potency	1	Clobetasol propionate (Temovate)	0.05	Hands/feet Thick lesions Limit time of use
		Betamethasone dipropionate (Diprolene)	0.05	
	2	Halcinonide (Halog)	0.1	
		Flucinonide (Lidex)	0.05	
		Desoximetasone (Topicort)	0.25	
Mid potency	3	Betamethasone dipropionate (Alphatrex, Maxivate)	0.05	Severe dermatitis on face, arms, legs, trunk
		Triamcinolone acetonide (Aristocort, Kenalog, Trymex)	0.5	
	4	Mometasone furoate (Elocon)	0.1	
		Halcinonide (Halog)	0.025	
		Triamcinolone acetonide (Aristocort, Kenalog, Trymex)	0.1	
	5	Flurandrenolide (Cordran)	0.025	
		Triamcinolone acetonide (Aristocort, Kenalog, Trymex)	0.1	
Low potency	6	Triamcinolone acetonide (Aristocort, Kenalog, Trymex)	0.025	Lesions on face, intertriginous areas Areas with thinner skin
	7	Hydrocortisone (Hytone)	1, 2, 5	

Note: Never use steroids on tinea or scabies.

Henoch-Schönlein purpura when the rash is actually the petechiae of meningococcemia).

■ Exercise caution as well with the immunocompromised and pregnant; not only can disease present itself differently in these populations, but the fetus is a concern in the pregnant patient, and the immuno-compromised patient often easily succumbs to systemic involvement quickly. Medication will have to be more cautiously chosen in these populations.

■ Always consider the *great imitators* in your differential diagnosis list: Think of syphilis, leprosy, sarcoid, and so forth.

■ A terminology note: *Maculopapular* is a commonly used term, but often incorrectly used and nonspecific. It literally means having both flat and raised components. Morbilliform means "many forms," and the prototypical example is a drug rash, but this term is often misused as a description of a rash of unknown origin. Be as descriptive as possible, and unless you are describing a drug rash, it is best to stay away from this term.

Teaching Points

Rashes are an important aspect of emergency medicine. Most rashes are not serious problems in regard to causing life or limb threat, but are of concern to the patient because of cosmetics and the discomfort of pruritis.

The desquamating diseases are rare, but can produce the same intense loss of fluids as a bad burn. These need aggressive fluid resuscitation and intensive care management. If unsure that such a disease is presenting, do not hesitate to obtain a dermatology consultation along with arranging admission to a burn unit.

Suggested Readings

Cydulka, RK, Hancock M. Dermatologic presentations. In: Marx JA, Hockberger RS, Walls RM (editors). Rosen's Emergency Medicine: Concepts and Clinical Practice (6th ed). Philadelphia, Mosby, 2006, pp 1838–1867.

Ferrera PC, Dupree ML, Verdile VP. Dermatologic problems encountered in the emergency department. Am J Emerg Med 1996;14:588–601.

Fleischer AB, Feldman SR, MsConnell CF, et al. Emergency Dermatology: A Rapid Treatment Guide (1st ed). New York: McGraw-Hill, 2002.

Flowers FP, Krusinski P. Dermatology in Ambulatory and Emergency Medicine, (1st ed). Chicago: Year Book Medical Publishers, 1984.

Habif TP. A Color Guide to Diagnosis and Therapy (4th ed). Philadelphia: Mosby, 2004.

Joseph, MG. Dermatology for Clinicians: A Practical Guide to Common Skin Conditions. New York: Parthenon Publishing Group, 1996.

McKenna JK, Leiferman KM. Dermatologic drug reactions. Immunol Allergy Clin North Am 2004;50:399–423.

CHAPTER 63

Endocrine Emergencies

LISA D. MILLS

Overview

Endocrine emergencies are commonly encountered in the ED. The most common endocrine-related disorders are hypo- and hyperglycemia. A finger-stick glucose should always be checked in patients with altered mental status because symptoms of hypo- or hyperglycemia can mimic any neurologic emergency. Because they are both common presentations to the ED, hypo- and hyperglycemia are discussed in Chapter 38. Pheochromocytoma is discussed in Chapter 39.

This chapter will focus on the following: hypopituitarism, adrenal insufficiency, hypothyroidism, and hyperthyroidism. These endocrinopathies are usually gradual in onset, manifest with nonspecific inconsistent signs and symptoms, and are often unrecognized by both patient and physician. All of these can be precipitated by stress, and if untreated, can have life-threatening consequences.

The pituitary regulates endocrine function with stimulating hormones that affect the adrenal glands, thyroid gland, ovaries and testicles, and mammary glands. The system is regulated by a complex feedback loop. The pituitary gland consists of an anterior lobe (adenohypophysis), a rudimentary intermediate lobe, and a posterior lobe (neurohypophysis). The adenohypophysis contains five major distinct cell types: (1) corticotropes (maintenance of adrenal function, promotion of steroidogenesis); (2) lactotropes (prolactin: milk production, reproduction); (3) somatotropes (growth hormone: effect on growth as well as fat, carbohydrate, and protein metabolism); (4) gonadotropes (luteinizing hormone and follicle-stimulating hormone: induce gonadal steroid production and gametogenesis); and (5) thyrotropes (thyrotropin: synthesis and secretion of thyroid hormones). The posterior pituitary produces oxytocin (uterine contractions, milk production, and excretion) and vasopressin (water homeostasis), whereas the intermediate lobe of the pituitary produces melanocyte-stimulating hormone.

The adrenal gland has a cortex and a medulla. The medulla is responsible for production of epinephrine and norepinephrine in response to stress. The adrenal cortex is divided into three zones: the zona glomerulosa, the zona fasciculata, and the zona reticularis. The zona glomerulosa produces minerolocorticoids to regulate sodium and fluid homeostasis. The zona fasciculata produces glucocorticoids that regulate glucose homeostasis and to a lesser degree, acute stress response. The zona reticularis produces sex hormones. Cortisol is the major corticosteroid hormone made in the adrenal cortex, and is required for normal function of all cells in the body. It is required for metabolism of carbohydrates, proteins, and fats; immune function; synthesis and action of catecholamines; wound healing; vascular tone and permeability; and many other vital functions.

The formation of thyroid hormones (TH) requires iodine. Thyroid hormones function at the cellular level, and regulate many of the metabolic processes of the body. These thyroid hormones, thyroxine (T_4) and triiodothrinine (T_3), are released from the thyroid gland by the secretion of thyroid-stimulating hormone (TSH) from the anterior pituitary gland. TSH in turn is controlled by the secretion of thyroid-releasing hormone (TRH) from the hypothalamus and by the negative feedback loop of thyroid hormones on the pituitary. Both T_3 and T_4 are released from the thyroid gland, and circulate in the bloodstream by attachment to a binding protein named thyroid binding globulin (TBG). When bound, T_3 and T_4 are not biologically active. They must be unbound in the periphery to exert their influence. T_4 converts to T_3 in the periphery through the removal of an iodine molecule, and is responsible for most of the T_3 in the body. T_3 is more physiologically active than T_4, but has a shorter half-life.

Specific Problems
Hypopituitarism

■ *Epidemiology and risk factors.* Acute hypopituitarism is most commonly seen in patients with chronic hypopituitarism who have an acute physiologic or emotional stressor. *Pituitary apoplexy* (Sheehan's syndrome) is a life-threatening clinical syndrome that results from the sudden infarction via hemorrhage into the pituitary gland. Most patients arrive in the ED without a history of known tumor, but this is often the initial presentation of a pituitary adenoma. Precipitating factors include head trauma, radiation therapy, anticoagulation, bromocriptine therapy, diabetes mellitus, and the peripartum state.

■ *Pathophysiology.* Patients with hypopituitarism have hypogonadism, adrenal insufficiency, and hypothyroidism. When acute destruction of 90% of the pituitary occurs, panhypopituitarism occurs.

■ *History.* The symptoms range from a simple headache to sudden alterations in mental status. The headache may be sudden and severe. A meningitis-like picture may result with fever, nausea, vomiting, and meningismus. Patients usually do not have a history of hypopituitarism. An acute stressor may be identified in the history. Women will have amenorrhea and failure to lactate. Rarely, polyuria and polydipsia may be present if associated with diabetes insipidus (DI).

■ *Physical examination.* Depending on the direction and degree of sellar extension, the patient may have a variety of abnormalities, such as visual field defects and cranial nerve palsies. Compression of the hypothalamus may cause abnormal thermoregulation (fever), disturbed respiration, and hypertension. Adrenal insufficiency may cause hypotension.

- ***Diagnostic testing.*** Acutely, there is no way to distinguish panhypopituitarism from acute adrenal crisis. Furthermore, more common central nervous system (CNS) disorders (i.e., bacterial meningitis, subarachnoid hemorrhage) may mimic its presentation. If hypopituitarism is suspected, serum TSH, cortisol, and ACTH levels are ordered, but results will not be available in the ED. Hyponatremia may be present due to inappropriate antidiuretic hormone secretion or secondary to hypoadrenalism or hypothyroidism. A computed tomography (CT scan) can rapidly detect the presence of acute pituitary bleeding. Magnetic resonance imaging (MRI) has better sensitivity for pituitary pathology, and provides more anatomic detail.

- ***ED management.*** This consists of supportive management with stress-dose steroids (see "Adrenal Insufficiency") and neurosurgical consultation. Steroids may also help reduce intracranial swelling. The patient may require cardiopulmonary stabilization. Fluid and electrolytes should be monitored for the development of DI.

- ***Helpful hints and pitfalls.*** Consider panhypopituitarism in patients who are obtunded or hypotensive.

Acute Adrenal Insufficiency

- ***Epidemiology and risk factors.*** Primary adrenal insufficiency occurs when the adrenals glands independently fail. This is referred to as Addison's disease. Secondary adrenal insufficiency is a result of hypopituitarism. The adrenal glands fail secondary to a lack of stimulation from the pituitary gland. The most common cause of acute adrenal insufficiency is hypothalamic-pituitary-adrenal (HPA) axis suppression from long-term exogenous glucocorticoid therapy. Acute precipitating stressors include infection, surgery, and psychologic stresses. Acute adrenal insufficiency occurring in a previously normal HPA axis is unusual, and is produced by either pituitary or adrenal hemorrhage or infarction. The Waterhouse-Friderichson syndrome is a rare cause of primary adrenal insufficiency caused by hemorrhage into the adrenal cortex. This usually occurs during meningococcal or pseudomonal sepsis.

- ***Pathophysiology.*** In adrenal insufficiency, the lack of aldosterone from the zona glomerulosa, lack of cortisol from the zona fasciculata, and lack of epinephrine and norepinephrine from the medulla cause the clinical syndrome. Aldosterone insufficiency causes sodium wasting. Sodium lost in the urine pulls water into the urine. The result is a hyponatremia and profound dehydration. Potassium is retained in the hypoaldosterone state, leading to hyperkalemia. Loss of epinephrine and norepinephrine cause a decreased sympathetic tone, manifest by hypotension and orthostatic syncope. The lack of cortisol is responsible for loss of glucose homeostasis and resultant hypoglycemia. Insufficient cortisol levels also decrease response to epinephrine and norepinephrine, which also contributes to hypotension.

- ***History.*** Patients complain of vague symptoms including progressive lethargy, weakness, nausea, vomiting, anorexia, weight loss, diarrhea, orthostatic dizziness, and mental depression. Nonspecific abdominal complaints are often present, but the patient may have an acute abdomen. Patients with primary adrenal insufficiency may have hyperpigmentation and vitiligo. Patients with secondary adrenal insufficiency may have pallor, amenorrhea, decreased libido, scanty axillary and pubic hair, headache, or visual complaints. A history of recent steroid discontinuation, or a hospitalization for sepsis may be obtained. An acute exacerbating event, such as trauma, infection, or an emotional stressor, may be obtained in the history. Medication history should be reviewed for new medications, discontinued medications, and dosage adjustments.

- *Physical examination.* Patients with acute adrenal insufficiency look ill. They are often confused and obtunded. Vital signs show a bradycardia. Patients are dehydrated, and may have hypotension that is unresponsive to fluids and pressors.

- *Diagnostic testing.* Although cortisol levels should be tested in the mornings (when cortisol levels are the highest), a random cortisol test can be sent if acute adrenal insufficiency is suspected, and should be interpreted in light of the current stressful event, which could raise the cortisol level. A cortisol level less than 18 μg/dl, in a stressful clinical situation, implies decreased cortisol production. If steroids are given, 10 mg of dexamethasone is preferred as this does not alter the cortisol assay and the ability to carry out the cosyntropin stimulation test at a later time. If dexamethasone is available, hydrocortisone, methylprednisolone, and prednisone should be avoided within the first 24 hours because these agents can all be detected by cortisol assays. If dexamethasone is not available, an alternative steroid should be administered. The cosyntropin stimulation test uses a synthetic corticotropin analog. A low dose of cosyntropin (1 μg via intravenous [IV] line) is the preferred dose to decrease the frequency of false-negative results. Cortisol levels are measured immediately before and 60 minutes after administration. Adrenal function is considered normal if the basal or postinjection cortisol level is at least 20 μg/dl. Hyperkalemia is usually in the 4.5–5.0 mEq/L range, and is seldom greater than 7.0 mEq/L. Hyponatremia is seldom less than 120 mEq/L. Hypercalcemia is relatively common. Other metabolic abnormalities include azotemia and elevated hematocrit levels, both related to hypovolemia. A mild metabolic acidosis may be present.

- *ED management.* Treatment is aimed at glucocorticoid replacement, correction of electrolyte and metabolic abnormalities as well as hypovolemia, and treatment of the event precipitating event. Fluid resuscitation should begin immediately with normal saline. Patients should receive empiric antibiotics because sepsis mimics and causes acute adrenal insufficiency. Cortisol (glucocorticoid therapy) should be replaced with hydrocortisone (100 mg IV every 6 to 8 hours) or dexamethasone (4 mg IV every 6 to 8 hours) administered by the IV route. Dexamethasone is as effective as hydrocortisone, and has the benefit of not interfering with later tests of adrenal function. Dexamethasone has no mineralocorticoid effect. If the patient is known to have adrenal failure, hydrocortisone should be used. If IV access cannot be obtained, cortisone acetate, 100 mg intramuscularly (IM) every

6 to 8 hours may be used. The intramuscular dosing route is not as reliable as the IV route. If salt and water replacement is adequate, mineralocorticoid replacement is usually not needed. Mineralocorticoid supplementation is done with fludrocortisone acetate (Florinef), which replaces aldosterone. Hydrocortisone 100 mg has the salt-retaining effect of 0.1 mg of Florinef. If dexamethasone is used, Florinef should be added to prevent salt loss. Patients should be admitted to a monitored bed or the intensive care unit (ICU), depending on how ill they appear.

- *Helpful hints and pitfalls.* Consider acute adrenal insufficiency in patients with hypotension, hyponatremia, and hyperkalemia.

Hypothyroidism and Myxedema Coma

- *Epidemiology and risk factors.* The incidence of hypothyroidism is much higher in women. The most common causes are noncompliance with thyroid therapy, thyroid-removal surgery, radiation therapy for hyperthyroidism, and untreated autoimmune disease (Hashimoto's thyroiditis). Multiple medications cause hypothyroidism. Iodine deficiency is a rare cause of hypothyroidism in developed countries. Myxedema coma is the manifestation of extreme hypothyroidism. However most patients with severe hypothyroidism do not have myxedema, and are not in a comatose state. Most cases occur in patients who are over 60 years of age. Common precipitants include surgery, sepsis, burns, trauma, severe infections, and medications.
- *Pathophysiology.* In patients with hypothyroidism, physiologic or emotional stress may lead to a decompensated state. Every organ system in the body may be affected due to a lowered metabolic state.
- *History.* Patients may complain of fatigue, headache, cold intolerance, decreased appetite, dry skin, hoarse voice, constipation, decreased libido, menstrual irregularities, myalgias, paresthesias, memory deficits, and depression. Patients with severe hypothyroidism may be found minimally responsive with no available history.
- *Physical examination.* Patients manifest a profound slowing of all systems. Early in the course of disease, high diastolic pressures are found. Deep tendon reflexes show a prolonged relaxation phase. A paralytic ileus may be present. Psychosis or seizures are sometimes present. Myxedema is characterized by generalized nonpitting skin and soft-tissue swelling, often associated with periorbital edema; ptosis; macroglossia; cool, dry skin; or coarse, sparse hair. The voice may be hoarse. Frank coma is uncommon in myxedema coma. However, the diagnosis is unlikely in the absence of altered mental status. These patients may also present with hypothermia, bradycardia, and hypotension.
- *Diagnostic testing.* The diagnosis is confirmed with low (or undetectable) levels of T_4 (total and free) and T_3. TSH is usually elevated but may be normal or even low in the setting of hypothalamic-pituitary disease or advanced critical illness. Patients with an elevated TSH but normal T_4 and T_3 levels have subclinical hypothyroidism. Other laboratory findings include normocytic anemia, hyponatremia, hypoglycemia, azotemia, and elevated creatine kinase levels. Hypoxia, hypercapnea, and respiratory acidosis are common findings on arterial blood gas analysis.

- **ED management.** The usual therapy for clinical hypothyroidism is oral T_4 replacement with approximately 1.6 µg/kg/d. Lower doses should be used in the elderly and those with preexisting coronary artery disease. This should be done in coordination with an endocrinologist or the patient's primary physician. Myxedema coma must be thought of because the clinical presentation looks like sepsis or adrenal insufficiency. Thyroid studies often are not available in the ED, and the patient will need empiric treatment with intravenous thyroxine. Attention to the airway and cardiovascular stabilization are critical initial interventions. Mechanical ventilation may be necessary due to diminished respiratory drive. Intravascular volume depletion is common, but fluid resuscitation must be done with caution in patients with underlying congestive heart failure (CHF) or hyponatremia. A blood sample for TSH and free T_4 should be sent before administering thyroid hormone. Thyroid hormone in elderly patients with underlying heart disease should be used with caution as this can precipitate acute myocardial injury. Intravenous levothyroxine (T_4) is the treatment of most efficacy for myxedema coma. Give levothyroxine 5 to 8 µg/kg (300 to 500 µg) IV infused over 15 min, then 100 µg IV q24h. Although IV T_3 has quicker onset, there are more adverse cardiac effects. Glucocorticoids are recommended to prevent adrenal crisis as the administration of T_4 or T_3 can cause relative adrenal insufficiency. Stress-dose hydrocortisone, 100 mg IV every 8 hours, can be given but a random serum cortisol level should be sent before initiation. Hypothermia should be treated with passive rewarming using blankets and increased ambient temperatures. Hyponatremia can be treated with fluid restriction and thyroid hormone replacement. Hypertonic saline is used for severe hyponatremia (serum sodium <120 mEq/L) or associated seizures. As infection is a common cause of hypothyroidism, empiric antibiotics are indicated. If there is reason to suspect panhypopituitarism, appropriate treatment should be initiated (see "Hypopituitarism"). Patients with myxedema coma require admission to the intensive care unit. Stable patients with mild hypothyroidism can be discharged with close follow-up arranged as an outpatient.
- **Helpful hints and pitfalls.** Hypothyroidism is a great imitator of many common complaints encountered in the ED.

Hyperthyroidism and Thyroid Storm

- **Epidemiology and risk factors.** The incidence in women is 10 times higher than that of men. The most common causes are Grave's disease, toxic multinodular goiter, and adenoma. Other causes are factitious (exogenous intentional intake), lithium (high iodine concentration favors formation of T_3 and T_4), amiodarone treatment (also high in iodine content), and autoimmune disease (Hashimoto's thyroiditis). Thyroid storm is a hyperthyroid emergency usually seen in patients with untreated or previously undiagnosed hyperthyroidism. Thyroid storm is usually induced by physiologic or emotional stress, such as illness, infection, pregnancy, acute myocardial infarction, surgery, and cerebral vascular events. Noncompliance with antithyroid therapy is a risk factor for thyroid storm. Apathetic hyperthyroidism occurs in older patients in whom end-organ responsiveness is attenuated compared with younger patients.

- ■ *Pathophysiology.* Excessive release of thyroid hormones from the thyroid creates hyperadrenergic state. The pathophysiologic mechanisms underlying both thyrotoxicosis and the shift from uncomplicated hyperthyroidism to thyroid storm are not entirely clear. Thyroid storm probably reflects the addition of adrenergic hyperactivity, induced by a nonspecific stress, into the setting of untreated or undertreated hyperthyroidism.

- ■ *History.* Symptoms include heat intolerance, agitation, weight loss, tremor, nervousness, sweating, bulging eyes (exopthalmos). Fatigue and weakness may be present. Patients often have gastro-intestinal complaints including hyperphagia, abdominal pain, vomiting, or diarrhea. Patients in thyroid storm may complain of tachycardia, palpitations, or chest pain. They will feel hot and anxious.

- ■ *Physical examination.* Tachycardia is often present. Patients with Graves' disease may have ophthalmopathy and goiter. Eye findings include upper-lid retraction, staring, lid lag, exophthalmos, and extraocular muscle palsies. The severity of ophthalmopathy does not necessarily parallel the magnitude of thyroid dysfunction, but reflects the responsible autoimmune process. Fever is often present in thyroid storm. Behavioral abnormalities include agitation, anxiety, and restlessness. A significant number of patients have confusion or delirium. Elevations in systolic blood pressure and the pulse pressure may be noted, leading to a dicrotic or water-hammer pulse. High-output CHF is possible, and indicates severe illness. Hepatic dysfunction with jaundice may be present. The skin is typically flushed with warm, moist skin; hair is fine and straight. Hyperpigmentation, vitiligo, or alopecia may occur, especially when an autoimmune mechanism is responsible for the disease. Pretibial myxedema may be present in 5% of cases. Elderly patients with apathetic hyperthyroidism classically present with depressed mental function and cardiac complications.

- ■ *Diagnostic testing.* TSH and free T_4 levels are the most commonly obtained thyroid function tests. Thyroid storm is often a clinical diagnosis, since treatment should not be delayed to obtain laboratory test results. Serum free T_4 levels can be measured directly or indirectly by calculation of the free-thyroxine index. TSH is suppressed except where hyperthyroidism is pituitary-dependent. An elevated T_4 is seen in 95% of patients. An increased serum free T_3 and normal T_4 occurs in fewer than 5% of patients (T_3 toxicosis). Total T_4 includes the T_4 bound to circulating plasma proteins, primarily thyroxine-binding globulin (TBG), and a portion that circulates freely. It can be difficult to interpret due to alterations caused by thyroid binding proteins, and thus, is not routinely used. An EKG should be ordered as atrial fibrillation, atrial flutter, or premature atrial contractions may occur with or without underlying heart disease. Blood cultures should be obtained in the febrile thyrotoxic patient.

- ■ *ED management.* Treatment is summarized in Table 63–1 and is divided into five general components: supportive therapy, blocking TH synthesis

Table 63–1	**Overview of Management of Thyroid Storm**
Supportive therapy	Tachypnea: Oxygen therapy Hyperkinesis: Benzodiazepines, barbiturates Hyperthermia: Intravenous (IV) fluids, cooling blanket, antipyretics (no aspirin) Dehydration: IV fluids with dextrose and electrolyte replacement; use with caution if congestive heart failure is present (use diuretics sparingly)
Block thyroid hormone synthesis and release	Thioureas: Block new hormone synthesis • Propylthiouracil (PTU): Load 600-1000 mg, then 1200 mg/d, given as 200-300 mg by mouth (PO) q4-6h • Methimazole (tapazole): 20 mg PO q4h (not available in parental form but can be given rectally) Inorganic iodine: Block release of preformed hormone (give at least 1 h after thiourea) Saturated solution of potassium iodide: 4-8 drops PO q6-8h Lugol's solution: 4-8 drops PO q6-8h Ipodate (contrast dye): 0.5-1.0 g PO q12h Iohexol (contrast dye): 0.6 g IV q12h For iodine allergy: Lithium carbonate: 300 mg PO q6h, adjust to maintain serum lithium level of 1 mEq/L.
Block peripheral conversion of T_4 to T_3	PTU (see previous section) Propranolol (see next section) Corticosteroid: hydrocortisone 50-100 mg IV q6-8h or dexamethasone 2 mg IV q6h
Block peripheral effects of thyroid hormone	Beta blockade: • Propranolol: 0.5-1.0 mg IV q15 min, or 40-80 mg PO, q4-8h • Esmolol: 250-500 mg/kg IV load, then 50-100 mg/kg/min IV Beta blockade contraindicated (bronchospasm or severe congestive heart failure): • Guanethidine 30-40 mg PO q 6 hrs *OR* Reserpine 2.5-5 mg via intramuscular injection q4h (both contraindicated if hypotension present)
Treat underlying cause	Search for source of infections. Empiric antibiotic use is not recommended.

and release, blocking peripheral TH conversion, blocking peripheral effects of TH, and identifying and treating the precipitating event. Supportive therapy includes respiratory support, sedation, and management of hyperthermia. Benzodiazepines are the more commonly used sedative in the ED. However, phenobarbital has the additional benefit of enhancing clearance of TH by inducing hepatic microsomal enzymes.

Patients usually are dehydrated, and require fluid resuscitation. The tachycardia and hyperadrenergic state decreases heart filling time and can result in high-output CHF, even in the setting of dehydration. In the setting of high-output CHF, continue fluid resuscitation, as indicated. Administer beta-blocking agents to slow and relax the heart. The increased filling time will improve the high-output CHF. Tylenol is the antipyretic of choice. Aspirin exacerbates thyroid storm. Antithyroid therapy is instituted in two phases. The first phase results in blockade of new TH synthesis with the thioureas, propylthiouracyl (PTU) or methimazole. PTU is safe in pregnancy. The second phase is to block release of thyroid hormone with iodine. Iodine is administered 2 hours after PTU or methimazole. Administering iodine before PTU or methimazole will worsen the thyroid storm. Glucocorticoids block conversion of T_4 to T_3, and provide stress doses of glucocorticoids. Dexamethasone is the most effective glucocorticoid. Blocking the peripheral affects of TH is accomplished with beta-blockers. Options include propranolol (oral or IV) or esmolol IV. A beta-blocker and antithyroid medication are the sole agents used for stable patients with mild symptoms of hyperthyroidism. Patients may be safely discharged from the ED, if their tachycardia can be controlled and close follow-up can be arranged. In life-threatening cases or when medical therapy is not effective, plasmapheresis, plasma exchange, charcoal plasma perfusion, and peritoneal dialysis have all been successfully used to remove TH. The mortality in the storm state of hyperthyroidism can be as high as 40%. Severe cases require admission to the intensive care unit.

- *Helpful hints and pitfalls.* Thyroid storm is a clinical diagnosis. Thyroid function tests will be normal. Administer PTU or methimazole 2 hours before giving iodine. Evaluate for inciting causes.

Other

- Carcinoid tumors arise from neuroendocrine cells, and produce amines and peptides such as serotonin, bradykinin, and histamine. The release of these substances produces a symptom complex that is characterized by paroxysmal vasomotor disturbances, diarrhea, and bronchospasm.
- Pheochromocytoma is discussed in Chapter 39.

Special Considerations
Elderly

- Geriatric patients more commonly develop myxedema coma.
- Geriatric patients present obtunded from infection, acute myocardial infarction, cerebral vascular accidents, and other stressors. All of these stressors can induce the initial presentation or cause decompensation of endocrine disorders.

Women and Pregnancy

- Look for Sheehan's syndrome in postpartum women with hypotension. Pregnancy can induce glucose intolerance.

Teaching Points

Metabolic emergencies are often hard to identify. There is no commonality of symptoms, and the patient and the physician are often confused by the presentation. Think metabolic disease if the patient looks ill, but the history is trivial.

All metabolic emergencies are accompanied by loss of fluid. Therefore, it is always prudent to establish intravenous access, and commence resuscitation with normal saline or lactated Ringers solutions. Always check a finger-stick glucose level because hypo- or hyperglycemia can cause an altered mental status, *and* mimic any neurologic emergency.

Most endocrinopathies have subtle presentations, and many times patients will have to be treated empirically without being able to prove the diagnosis in the emergency department. This is particularly true for adrenal crisis: look for hyponatremia along with hyperkalemia. In thyroid emergencies, look for cardiac manifestations in the elderly, usually presenting with atrial fibrillation and congestive heart failure in hyperthyroidism, or bradycardia and congestive heart failure in hypothyroidism.

All metabolic emergencies can be precipitated by sepsis, cardiac emergencies, or surgical emergencies, and these often require simultaneous investigation and management.

Suggested Readings

Goldberg PA, Inzucchi SE. Critical issues in endocrinology. Clin Chest Med 2003;24:583–606.

McKeown NJ, Tews MC, Gossain VV, Shah SM. Hyperthyroidism. Emerg Med Clin N Am 2005; 23:669–685.

Sherman. Clinical & socioeconomic predisposition to thyrotoxicosis. Am J Med 1996; 101:192–198.

Tews MC, Shah SM, Gossain VV. Hypothyroidism: mimicker of common complaints. Emerg Med Clin N Am 2005;23:649–667.

Torrey SP. Recognition and management of adrenal emergencies. Emerg Med Clin N Am 2005; 23:687–702.

CHAPTER 64

Ear, Nose, and Throat
Emergencies

LISA G. LOWE ■ THEODORE C. CHAN ■ DANIEL L. BAMBER

Overview

Many ENT patients can be completely cared for by the emergency physician, and discharged with appropriate follow-up. Some will have concerning presentations requiring immediate attention such as airway compromise, inability to tolerate oral secretions, significant dehydration, a septic or toxic appearance, unstable vital signs, and hemorrhage. Patients at the extremes of age, immunocompromised patients, and those who are pregnant lack compensatory reserves and have special considerations.

Many related subtopics requiring acute or outpatient management by an ENT specialist are covered elsewhere, including Chapter 10 (maxillofacial trauma), Chapter 33 (nasal and ear foreign bodies), Chapter 35 (sinusitis), Chapter 55 (sore throat), and Chapter 59 (vertigo).

The most common ENT problems in the ED will be discussed in the following sections.

Specific Problems: Ear
Auricular Hematoma

■ A hematoma forms separating the perichondrium from the cartilage of the ear, most commonly around the auricle. The cartilage is devoid of its blood and nutrient supply (perichondrium). Without drainage, the hematoma can lead to long-term complications including cartilage necrosis, abscess formation and permanent auricular deformity (*cauliflower ear deformity*). It is commonly associated with blunt trauma to the ear.

■ Drainage of auricular hematomas is necessary to prevent permanent deformity from loss of the cartilage. This may be done in the operating room in cases of severe trauma requiring operative debridement and repair of the ear. If performed in the ED, anesthetize the pinna using local infiltration of 1% lidocaine (without epinephrine), or perform complete auricular block by injecting anesthetic around posterior base of ear and tragus. Make a scalpel incision into most dependent portion and fully drain hematoma. Hematoma reaccumulation is common. Daily rechecks should be arranged. A well-placed compression dressing reduces the risk of reaccumulation. Use of a rubber drain may help prevent the reaccumulation. Needle aspiration without incision doesn't work as effectively as open drainage. Prophylactic antibiotics are not necessary.

Mastoiditis

- **Epidemiology and risk factors.** This is mostly a disease of the very young, peaking in those aged 6 to 13 months. The greatest risk is associated with immunocompromised hosts, including diabetics, and those patients with cholesteatoma (accumulation of keratin-producing squamous epithelium in the middle ear) or recurrent OM.
- **Pathophysiology.** The organisms that cause mastoiditis are those most commonly associated with bacterial OM. The most common bacterial isolates include *Streptococcus pneumoniae*, *Streptococcus pyogenes*, and *Staphylococcus aureus*. Middle ear inflammation spreads to the mastoid air cells, resulting in inflammation, infection, and destruction of the mastoid bone. Complications include subperiosteal abscess, meningoencephalitis, facial paralysis, labyrinthitis, or intracranial involvement.
- **History.** Classic acute mastoiditis is linked to a recent or concurrent episode of acute OM. There will be otalgia, posterior auricular pain, and fever. In latent mastoiditis, there may be accounts of chronic OM or recurrent otalgia. Both types can present with only nonspecific symptoms, especially in young infants, and include vomiting, lethargy, diarrhea, irritability, and poor feeding.
- **Physical examination.** These may include findings of acute OM, tenderness to palpation, erythema, and edema over the mastoid area. There may also be posterior auricular fluctuance, or protrusion of the auricle. Patients with latent mastoiditis often lack evidence of mastoid inflammation with normal appearing tympanic membranes, but may have recurrent or persistent fevers. The neurologic examination is usually nonfocal, unless suppurative intracranial complications exist.
- **Diagnostic testing.** The diagnosis of mastoiditis is clinical; however imaging studies may be helpful adjuncts. Plain radiographs, although unreliable, may reveal clouding of the mastoid air cells. Computed tomography (CT scan) may demonstrate a fluid-filled middle ear and mastoid as well as demineralization of the mastoid trabeculae. It can also detect the presence of any intracranial complications. Any suspicion of intracranial extension warrants an immediate CT scan. Magnetic resonance imaging (MRI) is indicated in patients suspected of having intracranial involvement that is not confirmed by a CT scan. Lumbar puncture to look for meningitis is required if meningeal irritation is present.
- **ED management.** Admit for IV antibiotics. Recommended therapy includes a third-generation cephalosporin or the combination of a penicillinase-resistant penicillin and an aminoglycoside. If a patient is allergic to penicillin (history of anaphylaxis), clindamycin can be used instead of penicillins. An ENT consultation is indicated. The most common surgical treatment is myringotomy or tympanostomy tube insertion. Mastoidectomy is performed when medical management fails, particularly for mastoid osteitis, a subperiosteal abscess, intra-cranial involvement, or lack of improvement after 24 to 48 hours of treatment.

■ *Helpful hints and pitfalls.* Mastoiditis must be treated aggressively since delayed management may result in serious complications.

Otitis Media: Acute

■ *Epidemiology and risk factors.* Acute OM is characterized by acute inflammation of the inner ear. This is due to infection by viral or bacterial pathogens, and is often associated with an effusion. This has also been called acute suppurative otitis media. Otitis media with effusion (OME) has an effusion without signs or symptoms of an acute infection. Myringitis is inflammation of the TM. Risk factors for acute OM include younger age and related anatomy because children have a more horizontal and narrower ear canal. Ethnicity, family history, exposure to tobacco smoke, and lower socioeconomic status have been linked to an increased incidence in OM. Also bottle-feeding, pacifier use, and daycare attendance have been shown to increase risk of disease.

■ *Pathophysiology.* The main pathogens are *Streptococcus pneumoniae* (25%-50%), nontypable *Haemophilus influenzae* (12%-25%), and *Morexella catarrhalis* (5%-15%). The exact incidence of viral etiology is unknown, but is common. Complications include labyrynthitis, cranial nerve VII palsy, deafness, ossicular damage, brain abscess, epidural abscess, meningitis, mastoiditis, and lateral sinus thrombosis.

■ *History.* The signs and symptoms are often nonspecific, and may include ear pain, discharge, fever, irritability, anorexia, and vomiting. There are often symptoms associated with an upper respiratory tract infection (URI). Young children may pull on their ears, or have a decreased appetite. In infants, a fever often heralds the onset of acute OM, but this sign may be absent in older children. Conversely, OME may be completely asymptomatic.

■ *Physical examination.* The classic signs of acute OM are redness and bulging of the TM. In OME, the TM will often be retracted, the malleolus is prominent, and landmarks are obscured, especially in the presence of significant fluid. Additional signs of effusion include lack of TM mobility (one of the most sensitive indicators), air-fluid levels, bubbles behind the TM, decreased mobility, color change, or TM opacification. A comparison examination of the other ear may be helpful in confirming suspected infection. In neonates, the TM appears thickened and opaque normally in the first few weeks of life, and the TM is in a highly oblique position. With tympanostomy tubes, in the absence of infection, the TM may have decreased mobility, altered landmarks, opacity, or dullness.

■ *Diagnostic testing.* OM is typically a clinical diagnosis made from an otoscopic examination and insufflation as discussed above.

■ *Management.* The treatment of OM with antibiotics varies in different countries and institutions within countries. Many believe that most cases of otitis media do not require antibiotics, but that by not using them, there is a higher incidence of mastoiditis. Most physicians in the United States will use antibiotics when there is fever, dullness of the TM, lymphadenitis, or appearance of toxicity. When there is only some reddening of the TM or simple OME, the patient can be observed for worsening signs or symptoms before starting antibiotics. Recommended therapies are listed in Table 64–1.

Table 64–1 Recommended Therapy for Otitis Media	
First-line antibiotic	High-dose amoxicillin (80-90 mg/kg/d divided into twice-daily dosing)
History of nonanaphylactic penicillin allergy	Cefdinir Cefpodoxime Cefuroxime
History of anaphylactic penicillin allergy	Azithromycin Clarithromycin
Severe illness, immuno-suppression, diabetes, or treatment failure	Amoxicillin-clavulanate Ceftriaxone
Watchful waiting (no antibiotics)	Observation is an option for (and should be limited to) otherwise healthy children age 6 months or older with nonsevere illness at presentation and an uncertain diagnosis. Excluded from the guidelines are patients with recurrence within 30 d or underlying conditions that alter the natural course of acute otitis media
Other	Analgesics and antipyretics

Otitis Externa

- *Epidemiology and risk factors.* Otitis externa (OE) is inflammation of the external auditory canal. Swimmers, patients with narrow canals or abnormal anatomy including post-surgical or perforated TMs are at an increased risk. Patients with allergies, trauma, foreign bodies, or abnormal cerumen production are more likely to have superinfection of already edematous TMs. Diabetics, elderly patients, and those with immunodeficiencies or dermatological diseases such as eczema and psoriasis are at a particular risk of developing complications from OE such as necrotizing otitis externa.
- *Pathophysiology.* Disruption of the squamous epithelium of the auditory canal or alteration in pH increases susceptibility to bacterial invasion leading to inflammation and symptoms. Excess moisture (e.g., water sports, bathing, and excessive cleaning) cause epithelial damage. Bacterial pathogens include *Pseudomonas* species, *S. aureus*, gram-negative rods, and group A streptococcus. Necrotizing otitis externa is a necrotizing bacterial infection of the external auditory canal caused by *P. aeruginosa* that is characterized by a progression of the infection from the external auditory canal through periauricular tissue toward the base of the skull.
- *History.* Typical symptoms include pruritis, otalgia, feeling of fullness, fluid leak, and hearing loss that develops over days. Patients with necrotizing otitis externa complain of severe otalgia that worsens at night, and otorrhea.
- *Physical examination.* Tenderness to palpation of the tragus or pinna traction is often a clue to the diagnosis. On otoscopic evaluation there

may be erythema and edema of the canal, purulent or other discharge from canal, and sloughing of the epithelium in the external auditory canal with a characteristically normal TM. Clinical findings of necrotizing otitis externa include granulation tissue in the external auditory canal, especially at the bone–cartilage junction. Facial and other cranial nerve palsies indicate a poor prognosis

- *Diagnostic testing.* OE is a clinical diagnosis. There are no commonly performed laboratory or radiologic studies for OE. If the clinical presentation suggests necrotizing otitis externa, WBC count, ESR, cultures of blood and canal discharge, and a CT scan or MRI study are used to evaluate for osteomyelitis.
- *ED management.* Inflammatory debris should be gently removed from the external auditory canal by curettage with a cotton-tipped wire applicator. Occasionally suction with a Fraser tip may be necessary. Ear washes with sterile saline, 2% acetic acid irrigation, or hydrogen peroxide can be performed in the ED. Treatment is with topical antibiotic drops with corticosteroid (typically a combination of polymyxin, neomycin, and hydrocortisone), to be applied in the ED and at home. For concurrent OM, oral antibiotics are indicated. Treat immunocompromised patients with oral ciprofloxacin, and follow closely for symptoms of necrotizing OE. Management of necrotizing otitis externa includes ENT consultation, IV antibiotics, and hospitalization. If TM perforation is suspected, suspensions of these medications should be used in place of solutions. If the canal is edematous, it is often helpful to insert a wick after cleaning. Patients should be instructed to keep ears dry and clean, and to use acetaminophen or ibuprofen for analgesia.
- *Helpful hints and pitfalls.* Swelling can impair antibiotic drop penetration. A wick can be placed for 24 hours to facilitate entry. Earplugs can be used for swimming and water sports as a preventive measure. Patients may have a sensitivity reaction to neomycin. Ofloxacin 0.3% otic solution should not be used in infants younger than 1 year. Topical glycerin is useful for drying the canal and the relief of discomfort.

Specific Problems: Mandible
Mandible Fracture and Mandibular Dislocation

- See Chapter 10.

Temporomandibular Joint Dysfunction

- Temporomandibular joint (TMJ) is a neuromuscular disturbance thought to result from occlusal disturbances and disharmonies of the TMJ anatomy. Trauma, psychological stress, jaw clenching, and bruxism (grinding of the teeth) exacerbate the disorder.
- Patients may present complaining of unilateral facial pain that is nonspecific, and somewhat regionalized to the TMJ area. The pain is achy and dull, and often worsens over the course of the day. Symptoms frequently increase with chewing, and the patient often notes an ear clicking or popping sensation. Patients may complain of earache, headache, or neck pain. There may be a history of jaw or facial trauma or

psychiatric disease. Muscle spasm of the masseter and internal pterygoid muscle is common. Jaw opening is often limited, and there is frequently tenderness to palpation of the TMJ via the external auditory meatus. In advancing disease, crepitus or popping may be felt over the TMJ, and there may even be lateral deviation of the mandible. Radiologic studies are most often normal, or show chronic degenerative disease of the TMJ.

- Nonsteroidal anti-inflammatory drugs (NSAIDs) and benzodiazepines are often helpful for symptomatic relief. Patients should follow-up with an otolaryngologist.

Specific Problems: Nose
Epistaxis

- *Epidemiology and risk factors.* Anterior epistaxis accounts for 90% of all nosebleeds, and usually involves Kiesselbach's plexus on the anterior-inferior nasal septum. Epistaxis is usually unilateral, and can be controlled with anterior packing. Posterior epistaxis accounts for 10% of nosebleeds, and usually arises from a posterior branch of the sphenopalatine artery. It is not controlled even with a well-placed anterior pack, and often requires a posterior packing. Posterior bleeding is rare in children.
- *Pathophysiology.* The multiple etiologies for epistaxis can be classified as local, idiopathic, or systemic. Examples of systemic factors include hypertension (controversial), vascular disease, or a coagulopathy. There is little evidence that hypertension causes epistaxis, but it probably worsens the bleeding if present. Local factors are the most common, and include upper respiratory infection and trauma, either accidental or iatrogenic (i.e., nose picking).
- *Diagnostic testing.* Hematologic testing is rarely useful, and is not required for most patients. If the bleeding is significant, a CBC, coagulation studies, and type and screen should be ordered.
- *ED management.* Resuscitative measures such as ABC assessments should be performed as needed. A large-bore IV line and fluid boluses should be administered, if the patient is symptomatic from blood loss, or if the blood loss is significant. Hypertension does not require treatment until the bleeding is controlled, and the pain or anxiety of the situation is resolved. However, in patients with significant blood pressure elevations or if presenting with other signs of a hypertensive emergency, the blood pressure should be treated. Parenteral sedation or analgesia should be given as needed, but with close monitoring. Indications for packing are persistent epistaxis from a diffuse anterior source, high risk of rebleeding, and posterior epistaxis. If possible, the bleeding site should be located and cauterized. Blindly placed packing is less likely to control bleeding. Topical thrombin is an alternative to cautery for diffuse bleeding. Contraindications to anterior packing include suspected cribriform plate fracture or evidence of cerebrospinal fluid (CSF) rhinorrhea. The procedure for anterior nasal packing is described in Table 64–2. There are now a number of commercial anterior nasal packs available that consist of a self-expanding sponge that absorbs and expands upon insertion (see Figures 64–1). The sponges are inserted along the nasal cavity floor,

Table 64–2	**Procedure for Anterior Nasal Packing**
Equipment	• Personal protective equipment: face mask with shield, gown, and gloves for the physician; gown or drape for patient • Other equipment: chair with headrest, suction device, bayonet forceps, nasal speculum, head lamp, tongue depressors, scissors, emesis basin, silver nitrate sticks or electrocautery, pediatric Foley catheters • Packing: Vaseline gauze 1/4-, 1/2, or 0.5-inch Nu-Gauze packing, nasal tampons, dual balloon pack • Medications: topical antibiotic, topical anesthetic (4% cocaine, 4% lidocaine, or 1% tetracaine; lidocaine used for laceration repair does not work), topical vasoconstrictor such as 0.05% oxymetazoline (Afrin)
Preparation and initial hemostasis	• Position the patient sitting upright in the sniffing position with the neck flexed and head extended. • Have the patient hold emesis basin to collect blood or emesis of swallowed blood. • Ask the patient to blow the nose to remove residual clots. • Ask the patient to hold external pressure by either pinch grasp or compression device to the alae just inferior to the nasal cartilage for 5-10 min. • Insert the nasal speculum horizontally, and open in superoinferior access to view the nasal cavity. Evacuate any blood. • If no bleeding is found, pack the nose only if epistaxis is recurrent. • If the bleeding is minimal, attempt to localize it; inject the mucosa at the base of the bleeder with 2% lidocaine with 1:100,000 epinephrine via a tuberculin syringe to promote hemostasis and anesthesia before cautery. If an anterior source is found, cautery is indicated as long as it is not done over large areas or on both sides of the nasal septum. Silver nitrate may be used to cauterize by holding the stick gently against the bleeding site or identified blood vessel for 4-5 s. Remember, this will not work in an actively bleeding area. Electrocautery penetrates more quickly. No packing is necessary if hemostasis is achieved. Vaseline or antibiotic ointment should be applied to prevent dessication. • If the bleeding is profuse, soak a cotton pledget with a local vasoconstrictor and topical anesthetic agent, place in the nose, and ask the patient to clamp the nostrils to promote contact for 5-10 min. • If bleeding continues and no anterior source is found, assume a posterior source, and pack the nose with an anterior and posterior nasal pack.
Anterior nasal packing	• Place antibiotic ointment around the nares or around device prior to insertion to facilitate passage, prevent desiccation, crusting, and infection. Use the bayonet forceps to facilitate insertion. • Traditional gauze packing: Applied in an accordion fashion such that each layer extends the entire length of the nasal cavity. Each layer should lie anterior and superior to the previous layer in order to prevent the gauze from falling posteriorly into the nasopharynx. Up to 6 feet of gauze may be needed.

Continued

Table 64–2	**Procedure for Anterior Nasal Packing—*cont'd***
	• Preformed nasal tampon: Trim the edges as needed with scissors or a scalpel. Advance the packing along the floor of the nose. Once inside the nasal cavity, expand the packing with 5-10 ml of saline. • Nasal balloon catheters: Insert such that the posterior aspect of the balloon rests in the nasopharynx. Inflate the balloon with saline (air may deflate slowly) as directed.
Aftercare for anterior nasal packing	• Systemic antistaphylococcal antibiotics are recommended for patients with unilateral packing, and are mandatory for bilateral packing to prevent bacterial superinfection and complications. • Patients should apply petroleum jelly to nares regularly and use humidified air in an effort to prevent drying. • Follow-up with removal of the packing is done at 48-72 h. Nasal tampons should be hydrated with saline before removal.

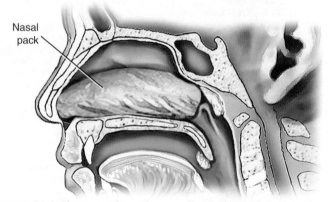

Figure 64–1. Placement of a nasal sponge for anterior nasal packing. *(From Gray, Henry. Anatomy of the Human Body. Philadelphia: Lea & Febiger, 1918.)*

parallel to the palate. Bilateral anterior packing should be used in cases of severe bleeding, or if there is an unstable nasal septum. If bleeding recurs, the patient should be instructed to pinch the nostrils closed for 20 minutes, and to return to the ED if unsuccessful. Anterior packing does not provide hemostasis for a posterior bleed. This is achieved with direct compression of the sphenopalatine artery with posterior packing. Posterior packing is always combined with anterior packing. Two common procedures currently used for posterior packing are listed in Table 64–3 and shown in Figures 64–2 and 64–3. Patients should not take aspirin or nonsteroidal medications until at least 4 days after the epistaxis. Antibiotics (amoxicillin, trimethoprim-sulfamethoxazole) are prescribed with any packing left in the nose because of the risk of sinusitis and

Table 64–3	Common Procedures for Posterior Nasal Packing
Foley catheter method	• The balloon is tested with sterile saline several times, both to ensure that the balloon and valve are functioning properly, and to stretch the balloon, which facilitates inflation after it has been placed; the amount of resistance with inflation should be noted. If significantly more resistance is encountered after the catheter is in place, this may indicate that the balloon is in the posterior nasal cavity rather than the proximal nasopharynx. • The Foley catheter is lubricated and advanced along the floor of the nasal cavity until the tip and the balloon are entirely in the nasopharynx (about 8-10 cm from the nares). The patient may be asked to open his or her mouth, and, once the tip is visible, the catheter should be pulled back 2-3 cm. • After the catheter is in the appropriate location, the balloon is filled with enough sterile saline (usually 5-10 ml) to allow it to be pulled snugly against the posterior nasal choana with anterior traction on the catheter. After anterior traction has been applied, another 3-5ml of saline is instilled to prevent the balloon from migrating anteriorly. • After the posterior pack has been positioned, the anterior pack is placed. After the anterior pack is in place, the Foley catheter is secured; this is accomplished by applying gentle traction on the catheter and placing an umbilical clamp or a c-clamp on the catheter at the level of the nasal ala. Several cotton eye pads are placed between the pad and the ala to prevent pressure injury (and subsequent necrosis) to the nasal ala (Figure 64–2)
Preformed anterior and posterior packing	Most of these preformed packs are composed of separate anterior and posterior balloons, which are inflated with saline through separate ports. Several variations exist, but configuration is shown in Figure 64–3.

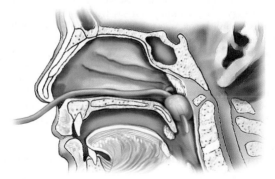

Figure 64-2. Positioning of a balloon (Foley catheter) for posterior nasal packing. *(From Schaefer SD. Rhinology and Sinus Disease: A Problem-Oriented Approach. St Louis, MO: Mosby, 1998, p 47.)*

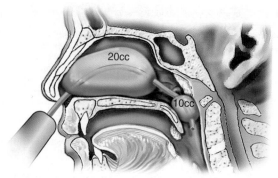

Figure 64–3. Placement of a nasal balloon for anterior and posterior nasal packing. *(From Marks SC. Nasal and Sinus Surgery, Philadelphia: Saunders, 2000, p 462.)*

toxic shock syndrome. Decongestants may be prescribed to decrease secretions. Patients with posterior packing and those with bilateral anterior packing require admission.

■ *Helpful hints and pitfalls.* Complications of nasal packing range from nasal injury and local infection to airway obstruction, respiratory arrest, sinusitis, and toxic shock syndrome.

Specific Problems: Oropharyngeal Infections
Ludwig's Angina

■ *Epidemiology and risk factors.* This is a life-threatening infection of the floor of the mouth that most commonly stems from an odontogenic infection such as involving the second or third molars. Infections in children are less commonly from a dental source. Other risk factors include IV drug injection into neck structures, oral lacerations or tongue piercings, sialadenitis, peritonsillar abscess (PTA), or mandibular fractures.

■ *Pathophysiology.* This condition arises from a rapidly spreading, often gangrenous cellulitis or necrotizing fasciitis of the sublingual, submandibular, or submaxillary spaces. Pathogens are polymicrobial, consisting mainly of *Streptococcus viridans*, *Staphylococcus aureus*, *Staphylococcus epidermidis*, and anaerobes of which *Bacteroides* species is the most notable. There are four cardinal aspects: bilateral involvement of more than one deep-tissue space; the infection spreads by fascial planes and not lymphatics; gangrene occurs with a serosanguinous, putrid infiltrate; and there is connective tissue, fasciae, and muscle involvement sparing glandular structures.

■ *History.* The patient complains of submandibular pain, fevers, drooling, and may have had a recent dental abscess, AOM, or other head and neck infection.

■ *Physical examination.* The patient is febrile, often tachycardic and tachypneic with the tongue elevated and often protruding. There may be associated trismus, anxiety, stridor, and drooling, and the patient will try to sit forward in the "sniffing" position. The submandibular area may have a woody induration that is exquisitely painful.

- *Diagnostic testing.* A CBC with differential and blood cultures are recommended. Imaging studies that may aid in diagnosis are soft-tissue films of the neck and a CT scan or MRI to detect severe cellulitis, thoracic extension, and abscess/fluid collections. An ultrasound study can locate a fluid collection. Chest radiograph studies and the Panorex are additional studies to consider in looking for intrathoracic spread and dental infections, respectively.
- *ED management.* Rapid airway obstruction can occur, and therefore active airway management should be established before anatomical distortion occurs. There are many ways to manage the airway, but with any sign of anatomic distortion, it is most prudent to utilize a surgical approach. If the patient is stable, this can be achieved in the operating room, where a semi-emergency tracheostomy can be performed. If the patient is in airway distress, a cricothyrotomy must be performed in the ED. If the patient is seen early before there is anatomic distortion, intubation can be performed with a fiberoptic scope and topical or local tracheal anesthesia, or via a rapid sequence oral intubation with anticipation of a difficult airway (Chapter 5). Initiate broad-spectrum antibiotics including clindamycin or penicillin G plus metronidazole, cefoxitin, ticarcillin/clavulanate, piperacillin/tazobactam, or ampicillin/sulbactam. Urgent ENT consultation should be obtained in the ED. Admit all patients to an intensive care unit (ICU).
- *Helpful hints and pitfalls.* Intubation before anatomical distortion develops is the most prudent management.

Peritonsillar Abscess (PTA)

- *Epidemiology and risk factors.* PTA is the most common head and neck abscess, and usually affects adolescents and young adults. One-third are pediatric patients.
- *Pathophysiology.* PTA is an infection of the peritonsillar space located between the capsule of the palatine tonsil and the pharyngeal muscles. It may arise de novo or from exudative tonsillitis. Pathogens are usually mixed, including both aerobes and anaerobes. *S. pyogenes* makes up 30% of all cases, followed by aerobes such as *S. milleri*, *H. influenza*, and *S. aureus* combined with anaerobes such as *S. viridans*, *S. sanguis*, and *Fusobacterium* species.
- *History.* Symptoms usually start 3 to 5 days before arrival in the ED, and may include sore throat, headache, dysphagia, fevers, malaise, neck pain, and otalgia. The pain is usually progressive and lateralizes to one side.
- *Physical examination.* The patient may be drooling, have trismus, appear toxic, speak with a muffled "hot potato voice," or even have airway compromise. Visualization of the oral cavity may reveal a uvula displaced away from the lesion, and the affected tonsil is usually anteromedially displaced. There are cases of bilateral peritonsillar abscesses, and in these, the uvula will remain in the midline.
- *Diagnostic testing.* There is no need to send the aspirate for culture. The diagnosis of PTA can be made without radiologic imaging. If the

aforementioned findings are lacking, it can difficult to differentiate from peritonsillar cellulitis. If a patient with suspected PTA appears toxic or has an unclear diagnosis after examination, a CT scan or ultrasound studies are indicated.

- **ED management.** Indications for drainage of PTAs in the ED are a fluctuant peritonsillar abscess or pus collection. Contraindications include trismus and a toxic-appearing patient requiring admission or drainage in the operating room. The carotid artery is only 2.5 cm posterior and lateral to the tonsil. Patient cooperation is important because there is minimal room for error. The abscess can often be aspirated in a cooperative patient avoiding a formal and more difficult incision and drainage. Many patients are successfully treated with aspiration only, and outpatient antibiotics. The recurrence rate following needle aspiration is 10%, and its cure rate is about 94%. Fewer than 10% of cases require repeated aspiration. The technique for aspiration or incision and drainage is described in Table 64–4 and Figure 64–4. Usually 2 to 6 ml of pus is obtained. If more than 10 ml is obtained, this may be an indication for repeated aspiration, incision and drainage, or hospital admission. IV antibiotics can be started before the procedure, and the patient can be given supplemental oxygen and sedation. Following needle aspiration or incision and drainage, patients should be observed for bleeding and the ability to take oral fluids. Most patients can be discharged with 24-hour follow-up. Penicillin, clindamycin, or cephalosporins are first-line antimicrobial agents. Alternative choices include penicillin plus rifampin or a penicillinase-resistant antibiotic such as amoxicillin-clavulanic acid for severe cases. Erythromycin and other macrolides are used in those patients with penicillin allergies. Any patient with marked dehydration or appearing toxic should have an urgent ENT consultation and be admitted.

- **Helpful hints and pitfalls.** In very young, uncooperative or complicated patients, surgical drainage in the OR may be necessary. Complications include bleeding, damage to the internal carotid artery or a dry tap. A negative aspirate does not rule out a PTA. Needle aspiration is effective for most PTAs presenting to the ED. It is much easier to perform, and has fewer complications than incision and drainage.

Retropharyngeal Abscess (RPA)

- **Epidemiology and risk factors.** This is the second most common deep neck infection, and generally afflicts children 6 months to 4 years old, with a decreasing incidence in older children due to regression of the posterior pharyngeal nodes. However, RPA has been seen in any age group.

- **Pathophysiology.** An infection lying between the middle cervical and alar fascia anterior to the prevertebral space characterizes this disease. Bacterial pathogens are mainly gram-positive organisms and anaerobes, but occasionally RPA will be caused by mycobacteria or gram-negative bacteria, and may arise as a complication of a recent URI, OM, airway trauma, foreign body (FB), instrumentation, or from cervical osteomyelitis.

Table 64–4   Procedure for Draining a Peritonsillar Abscess

Positioning and equipment	• Have the patient seated with the head in a slightly extended and well supported position. • Maximize visibility by having an assistant retract the cheek. • A head lamp provides optimal lighting. • Anesthetic 1% lidocaine with 1:100,000 epinephrine • Needles and syringes: 27-, 18- or 20-gauge long needle; 2-, 5-, and 10-ml syringes • No. 11 or 15 blade scalpel • Kelly clamp and No. 9 or 10 Frazier suction tip or tonsil suction tip • Suction and airway equipment are an important part of the drainage procedure as the patient may have a large volume of pus, and active airway management may be necessary.
Analgesia and sedation	• Parenteral narcotic analgesia and mild sedation may be helpful. • Anesthetize the area with topical Cetacaine spray or 4% to 10% lidocaine. • Identify the fluctuant area of the abscess, and locally infiltrate with 1-2 ml of 1% lidocaine with 1:100,000 epinephrine via a 27-gauge long needle to allow visualization. Infiltrate intramucosally until a blanching area is seen on the mucosal surface.
Needle aspiration	• Prepare an 18- to 20-gauge long needle and syringe with the cap on the needle but with 1cm of the tip cut off. The plastic cap acts as a stop gauge for the needle's entrance into the PTA, and prevents damage to deeper structures. • Insert the needle into the most fluctuant (or prominent) area, which is most commonly the superior pole of the tonsil. The tonsil itself is not aspirated, as the abscess develops in the surrounding peritonsillar space. The needle is advanced in the sagittal plane, and not directly laterally where it may injure the carotid artery. If aspiration is negative, repeat aspiration in the middle pole of the tonsil; 1cm caudal to first aspiration. If negative again, a third and final attempt should be made at the inferior pole. If pus is not obtained at 1-cm depth, deeper penetration is discouraged.
Incision and drainage	• Prepare a No. 11 or 15 scalpel blade by taping over all but the distal 0.5 cm of the blade to prevent deeper penetration. • Incise the area of maximal fluctuance, or where preceding aspiration located pus. • Suction the purulent material with a No. 9 or 10 Frazier suction tip or tonsil suction tip. • Insert a closed Kelly clamp into the incision, and gently open to break up loculations.
Postprocedure	• The patient should be allowed to rinse the mouth with normal saline or water after the procedure. • Observe the patient for 1 h for any bleeding, and to assess the ability to tolerate oral fluids.

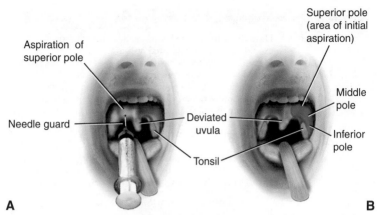

Superior pole
(area of initial
aspiration)

Aspiration of
superior pole

Needle guard

Deviated
uvula

Tonsil

Middle
pole

Inferior
pole

A   **B**

Figure 64–4. *A,* Needle aspiration of a peritonsillar abscess. Anesthetize the posterior pharynx with topical lidocaine spray. Blanch the mucosa with lidocaine/epinephrine with a 27-gauge (ga) needle on a long syringe (to allow visualization of the site) in the area to be aspirated. Advance an 18- or 20-ga needle with needle guard into the area of greatest fluctuance, usually the superior pole. Aspirate as you advance the needle. Advance the needle in the sagittal plane. Do not direct the needle laterally toward the carotid artery or jugular vein. *B,* The superior pole is aspirated first, but the middle and inferior poles should be aspirated if pus is not obtained initially. Note that the tonsil itself is not aspirated. The peritonsillar space contains the abscess. *(From Roberts JR and Hedges J. Clinical Procedures in Emergency Medicine (4th ed). New York: Elsevier, 2004, p 1285.)*

- *History.* Patients may complain of fever, dysphagia, recent URI, or OM. In the infant, parents often report vague symptoms of irritability and poor feeding, or apparent pain upon moving the neck.
- *Physical examination.* The patient may appear toxic or drooling with an inspiratory stridor. The examiner may see erythema and bulging of the posterior pharynx, trismus, or meningismus. Often dysphagia and decreased oral intake occur before respiratory distress. Up to 70% of patients will have torticollis or refusal to move the neck. Patients have cervical lymphadenopathy. A rapidly fatal airway obstruction can occur from rupture of an abscess. Aspiration pneumonia, empyema, bacterial spread to the mediastinum, and jugular vein or carotid artery erosion are possible complications.
- *Diagnostic testing.* Laboratory workup includes a CBC with differential, blood cultures, and a throat culture if the patient is stable. Imaging studies are crucial in making the diagnosis. The infection can be visualized on a plain lateral soft-tissue neck radiograph taken in inspiration with partial neck extension. Widening of more than 7 mm (less than half of the width of the vertebra at the retropharyngeal space just anterior to C-2) makes the diagnosis. Widening of the retrotracheal space anterior to C-6 also fits criteria, and is considered diagnostic if it is more than

14 mm in children younger than 6 years and more than 22 mm in adults. Chest radiograph is used to rule out mediastinal widening or aspiration. A CT scan of the neck with contrast can delineate the extent of deep-space involvement, and differentiate RPA from cellulitis as well as detect abnormalities of adjacent vertebra and vasculature.

■ ***ED management.*** As with any throat pathology, active airway management should be established if there is any question of anatomic distortion or breathing difficulty. Palpation of the neck should be gentle and limited, and the patient should be allowed to sit in a comfortable position of choice, and be kept calm. Broad-spectrum antibiotics should be started, and may include one or more of the following: a second- or third-generation cephalosporin, clindamycin, and ampicillin/sulbactam. The presence of a fluid collection should be ascertained, and a surgical consultation obtained for incision and drainage or aspiration. Patients should have nothing by mouth, and be given supplemental IV hydration.

■ ***Helpful hints and pitfalls.*** The child with airway compromise may need an airway secured prior to IV placement. Allow the child to sit in a parent's lap who gives supplemental oxygen. Intubation can then be accomplished in the operating room. If it cannot await a surgeon and anesthesiologist, use ketamine as a conscious sedating agent, and be prepared for a surgical airway. Avoid palpation of the posterior pharynx. All patients require hospital admission. Half of pediatric cases occur in children under 12 months of age.

Specific Problems: Neck Masses

■ The differential diagnosis of a single neck mass is extensive, but can be simplified by division into four categories that include: inflammatory, congenital, neoplastic, or vascular. The probable etiology varies with age. Most neck masses in people under 40 are due to inflammatory or congenital disorders, whereas most neck masses in people over 40 are due to neoplastic or vascular disorders. Any mass can become infected, expand, and interfere with the airway.

■ Inflammatory etiologies for neck masses include lymphadenitis, reactive lymphadenopathy, and deep space infections.

■ Branchial cleft cysts and thyroglossal duct cysts are the most common congenital neck masses. Congenital neck masses are typically chronic, painless, round and smooth unless infected (see above). Thyroglossal duct cysts are located midline and inferior to the hyoid, while branchial cleft cysts are found laterally between the auricle and the clavicle anterior to the sternocleidomastoid. Either may have an external sinus tract opening to the skin with mucopurulent drainage.

■ The "80% rule" states that 80% of adults with nonthyroid neck masses are neoplastic, and 80% of these are malignant; 80% of neck masses in children are benign. The differential diagnosis for neoplastic neck masses include (a) malignant: thyroid, parathyroid, or metastatic squamous cell carcinoma, lymphoma, sarcoma, and salivary gland neoplasia; (b) benign: lipoma, fibroma, neural tumor, hemangioma, atrioventricular malformation, and lymphangioma. The incidence increases with age, alcohol or tobacco use, history of syphilis, history of herpes simplex virus, sunlight exposure, HIV, exposure to industrial chemicals, neck irradiation, multiple endocrine neoplastic syndromes, thyroiditis, and goiter.

■ It is very rare for the carotid arteries to develop aneurysmal swelling. Clues are restless pain that is many times not relieved by customary doses of analgesics. Vascular masses can also result from penetrating or blunt trauma, and the episode of trauma can be months to years prior, confusing the diagnosis. Depending on the length of time of symptoms, and how impaired is the vessel flow, there may be focal neurologic findings compatible with a hemiplegic stroke. If there is simultaneous involvement of the vertebral arteries, there may be an inability to walk, to balance, or to perform cerebellar functions such as rapid hand alternation and position recognition.

Teaching Points

There are many ear, nose, and throat emergencies that vary from minor to life threatening. Many of them involve infections, and although most are easy to manage, some may rapidly progress to become life-threatening.

The key to virtually all the emergencies is early protection of the airway. If there is any question of possible or early airway distortion, active airway management should immediately be established. Early in the course of many ear, nose, and throat problems, it may be possible to achieve a safe and effective rapid sequence intubation, but when airway distortion occurs, this will be impossible. Surgical airway management will be necessary but will also be very difficult. It is therefore best to manage the airway actively before any disturbance of the anatomy can occur.

Suggested Readings

Ganiats, TG, Leiberthal, AS. Diagnosis and management of acute otitis media. Pediatrics 2004;113:1451–1465.

Hickner JM, Bartlett JG, Besser RE, et al. Principles of appropriate antibiotic use for treatment of acute respiratory tract infections in adults. Ann Emer Med 2001;37:690–697.

Kazzi AA, et al. Peritonsillar abscess, Emedicine; August 7, 2004.

Kahn J, et al. Retropharyngeal Abscess, Emedicine; July 27, 2004.

Kozyrskyj AL, Hildes-Ripstein GE, Longstaffe SE, et al. Treatment of acute otitis media with a shortened course of antibiotics: a meta-analysis. JAMA 1998;279:1736.

Massick D, Tobin. Epistaxis. In: Cummings CW, Flint PW, Haughey BH, et al (editors). Otolaryngology: Head and Neck Surgery (4th ed). Philadelphia: Mosby, 2005, pp 942–960.

Riviello RJ. Otolaryngologic procedures. In: Roberts JR, Hedges JR (editors). Clinical Procedures in Emergency Medicine (4th ed). Philadelphia: Elsevier, 2005, pp 1280–1316.

Schwetschenau E, Kelley DJ. The adult neck mass. Am Fam Physician 2002;66:831–838.

CHAPTER 65

Environmental Emergencies

65.1 Altitude Illness

Karen Van Hoesen ■ Kelly Pettit

Acute Mountain Sickness

- *Background.* The incidence and severity of acute mountain sickness (AMS) depends on rate of ascent, altitude attained, level of exertion, and physiologic susceptibility. Susceptible individuals have a relative hypoventilation at altitude with fluid retention, impaired gas exchange, and vasogenic edema leading to increased intracranial pressure (ICP) in moderate to severe AMS (and high-altitude cerebral edema [HACE]).
- *Clinical presentation.* The hallmark symptom is headache (throbbing, bitemporal) with fatigue, anorexia, and dizziness. Other symptoms include nausea, vomiting, dyspnea on exertion, and irritability. Specific physical findings are lacking in mild AMS. Tachycardia, bradycardia, and postural hypotension have been reported. Retention of fluid may be present. Ataxia or change in consciousness indicates progression to HACE.
- *Diagnostic testing.* Oxygen saturation should be checked, otherwise there is no specific testing.
- *ED management.* Mild AMS can be treated with acetazolamide, which speeds acclimatization. Symptomatic therapy includes aspirin, acetaminophen, or ibuprofen for headache, and prochlorperazine or promethazine for nausea and vomiting. Low-flow oxygen is effective. Dexamethasone should be given for moderate to severe cases of AMS.
- *Helpful hints and pitfalls.* AMS is often misdiagnosed as a viral flu illness, exhaustion, hangover, or dehydration. Any symptom of AMS should be considered due to altitude. If symptoms worsen despite 24 hours of acclimatization and treatment, descent to lower altitude is mandatory. Any neurologic changes or pulmonary edema requires immediate descent.

High-Altitude Cerebral Edema (HACE)

- *Background.* HACE is an extreme form of AMS representing a progression of AMS to cerebral edema and encephalopathy. High altitude pulmonary edema (HAPE) commonly occurs with HACE. This is similar to AMS with vasogenic edema of the brain. As HACE becomes more severe, intracellular (cytotoxic) edema develops.

- *Clinical presentation.* HACE may include all the symptoms of AMS with ataxia, severe lassitude, and altered consciousness (confusion, drowsiness, and coma). Seizures, hemiparesis, hemiplegia, and cranial nerve palsies are reported.
- *Diagnostic testing.* Computed tomography (CT scan) or magnetic resonance imaging (MRI) can show evidence of white matter edema.
- *ED management.* Initial treatment includes supplemental oxygen and dexamethasone. Comatose patients require intubation and mild hyperventilation. Furosemide may reduce brain edema, but careful attention must be given to maintain intravascular volume and perfusion pressure. Hyperbaric chambers can be used to simulate descent.
- *Helpful hints and pitfalls.* If possible, descent should be started at the first sign of ataxia or change in the level of consciousness.

High-Altitude Pulmonary Edema (HAPE)

- *Background.* HAPE is the most common cause of death related to high altitude, and usually occurs within the first 2 to 4 days of ascent to altitudes above 2500 m (8202 feet), but symptoms may be apparent within a few hours. Physical exertion, rate of ascent, altitude attained, individual susceptibility, and degree of cold are all important factors. Although the exact mechanism is unknown, elevated pulmonary artery pressure (PAP) is the hallmark of HAPE. Some areas of the lung are overperfused, leading to capillary stress failure and leak.
- *Clinical presentation.* Initial symptoms include fatigue, weakness, and dyspnea on exertion. Signs of AMS are often present. Worsening symptoms include dyspnea at rest and audible chest congestion. Pink frothy sputum and hemoptysis are late findings. Elevated temperature, tachycardia, tachypnea are usually present. Unilateral or bilateral rales can be auscultated. Altered levels of consciousness suggest concurrent HACE. Cyanosis may be noted.
- *Diagnostic testing.* Arterial blood gases (ABGs) shows a respiratory alkalosis and marked hypoxemia. The infiltrates are fluffy (alveolar) and patchy in distribution. Pleural effusion is rare. Chest radiograph finding of cardiomegaly, bat-wing distribution of infiltrates, and Kerley B lines, which are typical of cardiogenic pulmonary edema, are absent in HAPE. There is a predilection for the right middle lung field for infiltrates. Signs of acute pulmonary hypertension can be seen on EKG, and include right axis deviation, right bundle branch block, right ventricular hypertrophy and P wave abnormalities. Echocardiography studies demonstrate high estimated pulmonary artery pressures, pulmonary vascular resistance, and normal left ventricular function.
- *ED management.* Oxygen at 4 to 6 L/min and descent are the main treatment for HAPE. Hyperbaric oxygen can be used to simulate descent. Nifedipine can be used to reduce pulmonary vascular resistance. Furosemide, 80 mg twice daily, combined with morphine may result in clinical improvement due to diuresis.
- *Helpful hints and pitfalls.* ABG results may be misleading in patients taking acetazolamide because this drug causes metabolic acidosis.

Special Considerations for Altitude Illness

- **Pulmonary disease.** Severe chronic obstructive pulmonary disease (COPD) is a contraindication to traveling to high altitudes. Persons with asthma should be at maximum function prior to high-altitude ascent. Pulmonary hypertension is a relative contraindication to high-altitude exposures.
- **Sickle cell disease.** High altitude can precipitate vaso-occlusive crisis.

Teaching Points

High altitude illness is common and occurs in young, otherwise healthy people as an acute problem developed in reaction to sudden ascent. Most patients do not develop problems until an altitude greater than 8000 feet is reached, but older patients with concomitant pulmonary and cardiac disease can become symptomatic at lower altitudes.

Serious illness can be prevented by the use of acetazolamide orally; slower ascent; maintenance of hydration; minimal activity at altitude, and preservation of renal function. The earliest signs seen are headache, irritability, nausea, and vomiting. If unresponsive to initial therapy, descent must be arranged. Non-cardiogenic pulmonary edema and cerebral edema usually develop concomitantly, and require descent.

Suggested Readings

Gallagher SA, Hackett PH. High-altitude illness. Emerg Med Clin North Am. May 2004:22:329–355.

Yaron M, Honigman B. High-altitude medicine. In: Marx JA, Hockberger RS, Walls RM, eds. Rosen's Emergency Medicine, Concepts and Clinical Practice. 6th ed. Philadelphia: Mosby, 2006:2296–2311.

65.2 Barotrauma

Karen Van Hoesen   ■   Kelly Pettit

Overview. As a diver descends in the water, pressure on the diver increases with depth. The greatest pressure change is in the first 33 feet of sea water, hence the majority of injuries due to barotrauma occur in shallow depths. The diver's body is generally unaware of this pressure, except in the air-containing spaces of the body. The gases in these spaces obey Boyle's law, which states that the pressure of a given quantity of gas varies inversely with its volume. Thus air in the face mask, middle ear, paranasal sinuses, lungs, and gastrointestinal tract is reduced in volume during descent under water, and expands during ascent. Trauma due to the expansion or contraction of these gas spaces within the body is called barotrauma.

Face-Mask Barotrauma

- **Background.** As a diver descends, the volume of air inside the face mask will decrease. If the diver forgets to exhale through the nose, a negative pressure in the mask can rupture capillaries, causing damage to periorbital tissues. Orbital hemorrhage is rare.
- **Clinical presentation.** Skin ecchymosis, subconjunctival hemorrhage, lid edema, and rarely hyphema may be seen. Visual acuity is almost never affected. Orbital hemorrhage is rare, but can be associated with diplopia, proptosis, and visual loss.
- **Diagnostic testing.** MRI to look for orbital hemorrhage.
- **ED management.** Provide supportive care with cold compresses and analgesics if needed. Ophthalmology consultation should be obtained for suspected orbital hemorrhage due to potential for permanent vision loss from elevated intraocular pressure.

Sinus Barotrauma

- **Background.** If the sinus ostia are blocked by mucosal congestion or polyps, the volume of air in the sinus will decrease during descent, causing mucosal edema and bleeding into the sinus cavity. The diver experiences pain in the sinuses during descent. On ascent, the remaining gas in the sinus expands, and may force mucus and blood into the nose and mask. The frontal sinus is most commonly affected followed by the maxillary sinus. There may be pain in the upper teeth.
- **Clinical presentation.** Tenderness to percussion over the affected sinuses. If the maxillary sinus is involved, there may be numbness over the cheek due to compression of the posterior superior branch of the fifth cranial nerve, which runs along the base of the maxillary sinus.
- **ED management.** Treat with systemic (e.g., pseudoephedrine) and topical vasoconstrictors (e.g., phenylephrine or oxymetazoline), analgesics, abstinence from diving until resolved, and antihistamines if needed. On rare occasions, drainage of the affected sinus by an otolaryngologist is required for persistent pain.

Middle Ear Barotrauma

- **Background.** Middle ear barotrauma occurs when the diver does not equalize the pressure in the middle ear during descent. A relative vacuum in the middle ear develops leading to mucosal swelling, bleeding, and retraction of the tympanic membrane (TM) with possible rupture of the TM.
- **Clinical presentation.** Symptoms of middle ear barotrauma (squeeze) include ear pain during descent, a sensation of fullness, reduced hearing in the affected ear, mild tinnitus, or vertigo. With TM rupture, the pain is relieved but the stimulation of seawater entering the middle ear cavity causes severe vertigo with nausea, vomiting, and disorientation underwater.
- **ED management.** Decongestants and analgesics may be helpful, although most cases will clear spontaneously in 3 to 7 days without complication.

Antihistamines may be used if the eustachian tube dysfunction has an allergic component. Divers should abstain from diving until the condition has resolved. For rupture of the TM, fluoroquinolone drops should be used. Most TM ruptures will heal spontaneously within 1 month. If the TM has not healed, referral to an otolaryngologist is indicated for surgical repair.

Inner Ear Barotrauma

- ■ *Background.* This results from labyrinthine window rupture, usually due to a sudden increase in middle ear pressure by a forceful Valsalva. This pressure disequilibrium may cause several types of injury to the cochleovestibular apparatus.
- ■ *Clinical presentation.* The diver experiences roaring tinnitus, vertigo, and hearing loss. In addition, a feeling of fullness or "blockage" of the affected ear, nausea, vomiting, nystagmus, pallor, diaphoresis, disorientation, or ataxia may be present in varying degree. Otoscopic findings on physical examination may be normal or may reveal signs of middle ear barotrauma.
- ■ *ED management.* Bed rest (with the head elevated to 30 degrees), avoidance of any strenuous activity or any straining that can lead to increased intracranial pressure, and symptomatic measures as needed. Deterioration of hearing, worsening of vestibular symptoms, or persistence of significant vestibular symptoms after 48 hours requires otolaryngologic evaluation, and possible surgical exploration.

Pulmonary Barotrauma

- ■ *Background.* This is usually associated with a rapid ascent to the surface. Air within the alveoli expands causing rupture. Air can dissect along the bronchi to the mediastinum causing *pneumomediastinum* (most common). Rarely, air escapes between the pleura resulting in a *pneumothorax* or tension pneumothorax. *Arterial gas embolism (AGE)* occurs when expanding air enters the pulmonary capillaries, travels to the left atrium and ventricle, then out the aorta and is distributed systemically. Air bubbles may enter the coronary arteries, travel up the carotid and vertebral arteries to the brain, and embolize systemically.
- ■ *Clinical presentation.* Patients may be asymptomatic or complain of substernal chest pain. If the air dissects from the mediastinum up to the neck, the diver may experience hoarseness and neck fullness. Subcutaneous emphysema may be present, and palpated as crepitance under the skin of the neck and anterior chest. In severe cases, the diver may complain of marked chest pain, dyspnea, and dysphagia. A Hamman's sign (a crunching, rasping sound, synchronous with each heartbeat) may be heard. There are varied clinical symptoms depending on the amount and distribution of air. Neurologic manifestations of AGE are typical of an acute stroke, although hemiplegia and other purely unilateral brain syndromes are infrequent.
- ■ *Diagnostic testing.* Radiographs may show extra-alveolar air in the neck, mediastinum, or both. The presence of air on the radiograph may be very

subtle, and should be looked for along the pulmonary artery and aorta and along the edge of the heart.

- **ED management.** Treatment of pneumomediastinum is conservative, consisting of rest, avoidance of further pressure exposure (including flying in commercial aircraft), and observation. Supplemental oxygen administration may be useful in severe cases. Recompression is indicated only in cases associated with AGE. If a pneumothorax occurs with AGE, a chest tube must be placed before recompression treatment, because a simple pneumothorax can expand into a tension pneumothorax during ascent in the hyperbaric chamber. AGE produces hemoconcentration so 1 to 2 L of normal saline fluid should be given via intravenous (IV) line. Recent data suggest lidocaine may be cerebroprotective in AGE, and can be used as an adjunct (100 mg IV push). A diving and hyperbaric specialist must be consulted for any suspected case of AGE. Diving medicine consultation is available 24 hours per day through the Divers Alert Network (DAN) at (919) 684-8111.

Teaching Points

The majority of injuries due to barotrauma occur in shallow depths as this is where the greatest pressure difference is located. The most common manifestation of barotrauma is middle ear barotrauma that is usually a benign condition, but may cause severe vertigo and disorientation under water. The most devastating consequence of barotrauma is an arterial gas embolism. Any diver that presents with acute neurologic signs and symptoms or loss of consciousness during ascent or in the first 10 minutes after surfacing must be considered to have an arterial gas embolism. These patients must be referred for recompression treatment. A 24 hour a day diving medicine consultation can be obtained by calling the Divers Alert Network (DAN) at 919-684-8111.

Suggested Readings

Kizer K, Van Hoesen KB. Diving Medicine. In: Auerbach PS editor. Wilderness Medicine. 5th ed. Philadelphia: Mosby, in press.

Kuo DC, Jerrard DA. Environmental insults: smoke inhalation, submersion, diving, and high altitude. Emerg Med Clin North Am 2003;21:475–497.

Neuman TS: Arterial gas embolism and pulmonary barotrauma. In Brubakk AO, Neuman TS (eds): Physiology and Medicine of Diving, Philadelphia: WB Saunders, 2003, p 557.

65.3 Burns and Electrical Injuries

Jeffrey Druck ■ Stephen V. Sherick

Burns

■ *Background.* A burn is defined as a denaturation and destruction of skin proteins and other components by thermal or chemical means. Burns are characterized by the size of the area that is exposed, and the length of time that the area is exposed. Tissue destruction from severe burn injury results in increased capillary permeability with extravasation of fluid to the surrounding tissues. Inordinate amounts of fluid are also lost by evaporation from the damaged surface that is no longer able to retain water. This increase in capillary permeability, coupled with evaporative water loss, causes hypovolemic shock.

■ *Clinical presentation.* Rapidly assess ABCs. Rapid extravasation of fluid may be seen in burned patients. Patency of the airway may be compromised with this swelling. Hypotension may be present from fluid shifts and hypovolemic shock. The patient also may be in respiratory distress if an inhalation injury or facial burn is present. Concerning clinical findings include stridor, wheezing, tachypnea, hypoxia, soot in the nares and oropharynx, and airway edema. If possible look for direct laryngoscopic evidence of injury (e.g., fiberoptic bronchoscopy to evaluate for swelling and soot in more distal parts of the airway). The entire skin should be inspected for burn injury. Burns are defined by the combination of the depth of the affected tissue, the breadth of the destruction, and the location of this injury. Burns involving the head and neck, or circumferential burns should raise concerns for airway and circulatory compromise, respectively. There are four degrees of burn injury, based on cellular landmarks in the affected integument (Table 65.3–1). The *rule of nines* is a common method for estimating the extent of body surface area (BSA) involved in a burn injury (see Figure 65.3–1). The area of a patient's palm represents approximately 1% of the BSA, and can be helpful in calculating scattered areas of involvement. In estimating the extent of burn injury, the extent of involvement of each anatomic area (e.g., an arm or leg) must be calculated separately, and the total derived from the simple addition of the burned anatomic sites. The difference between the BSA of the adult and infant reflects the size of the infant's head, which is proportionally larger than that of the adult, and the legs, which are proportionately smaller than those of the adult. The modified Lund-Browder chart is a modified scale for the young to account for the much greater size of the head (Table 65.3–2).

■ *Diagnostic testing.* Severe burns require a complete laboratory workup including a CBC, electrolytes, renal function, arterial blood gases with carboxyhemoglobin, coagulation studies, type and screen, creatine phosphokinase (CPK), and urine myoglobin (in electrial injuries). The initial chest radiograph rarely shows significant findings of smoke inhalation.

Table 65.3–1 Burn Classification

	Description	Comment
First-degree (superficial) burn	Affects only the epidermis layer, and is most commonly seen in sunburns. They are tender, dry, erythematous, and they will blanch to pressure.	Usually heal in less than 1 wk
Second-degree burn (partial thickness)	Divided into superficial or deep partial thickness depending on whether or not deep structures are severely injured. Superficial partial-thickness burn (SPTB) is sensitive to air and temperature, with blistering, weeping, blanching. Deep partial-thickness burn (DPTB) is sensitive to pressure only, blisters but does not blanch.	SPTB heals in one to three weeks usually without a scar. DPTB heals in over 3 wk with a scar.
Third-degree or full-thickness	Epidermis and dermis, usually painless with a white-to-gray appearance that will not blanch.	Healing is slow, and skin grafting is often required. Scarring is extensive.
Fourth-degree burn	Involves nerve, muscle and bone tissue and is a severe injury in all cases.	May require amputation of an extremity.

Table 65.3–2 Modified Lund-Browder Scale by Age

Part of Body	<1 Year Old	1-4 Years Old	5-9 Years Old	10-14 Years Old	15 Years and Older
Head	19	17	13	11	9
Neck	2	2	2	2	2
Trunk (face)	13	13	13	13	13
Buttock	2.5	2.5	2.5	2.5	2.5
Genitalia	1	1	1	1	1
Upper arm	4	4	4	4	4
Lower arm	3	3	3	3	3
Hand	2.5	2.5	2.5	2.5	2.5
Thigh	5.5	6.5	8	8.5	9
Lower leg	5	5	5.5	6	6.5
Foot	3.5	3.5	3.5	3.5	3.5

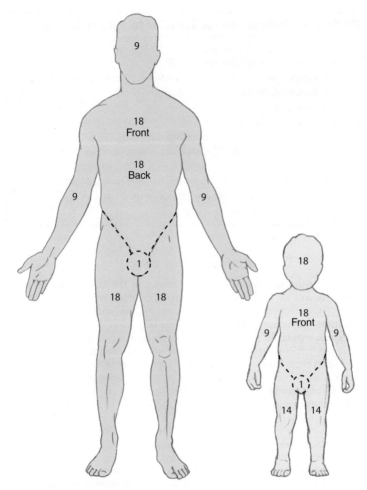

Figure 65.3–1. The "rule of nines" for estimating percentage of area burned. Note that adults and children are different. This formula frequently overestimates the extent of a burn in clinical practice. *(Source: Bethel C, Krisanda TJ. Burn care procedures. In: Roberts JR, Hedges JR (editors). Clinical Procedures in Emergency Medicine (4th ed). Philadelphia: Elsevier, page 7511.)*

- **ED management.** Airway management should always be the first priority. A difficult airway should be anticipated (Chapter 5). The American Burn Association has established criteria for referring patients to a burn center (Box 65.3–1). The airway should be secured, and any necessary escharotomies should be performed prior to transfer. Patients with significant traumatic injuries should be transferred to a burn center with this capability. Disposition should be a decision made in

BOX 65.3–1 Indications for Transfer to a Burn Center

- Second-degree burns great than 10% TBSA
- Third-degree burns greater than 5% TBSA
- Second-degree or third-degree burns involving critical areas (e.g., hands, feet, face, perineum, genitalia, major joints)
- Burns with associated inhalation injury
- Electrical or lightning burns
- Severe burns complicated by coexisting trauma
- Preexisting disease that could complicate management of the burn injury
- Chemical burns with threat of cosmetic or functional compromise
- Circumferential burns on the extremities or the chest
- Children with severe burns

TBSA, total body surface area.

concert with burn specialists if the status of the burn is in question. Management of burn injuries at the early phase of treatment should emphasize symptomatic pain treatment and anti-inflammatory administration. Intravenous narcotic analgesia (e.g., morphine sulfate) should be given especially during care of the burn wounds. Protection of the site and patient should include application of antibiotic ointment to any open burn sites, with variance in type of antibiotic for each type of burn as dictated by each institution's protocol; however, if the patient is being transferred to a burn center, the application of topical agent can be left to the burn center, and the burned areas should be covered with a dry sheet. For closed minor burn wounds, an aloe vera and topical analgesic lotion formula is appropriate. For second degree burns, intact blisters should be left alone, but those located in areas that have a high likelihood of rupture should be sharply debrided. Burn care for most of these wounds involves washing affected areas, debridement, topical antibiotics and a dressing. Topical agents used on the face include Neosporin and Bacitracin. Most facial burns do not require a dressing. Topical antibiotics, such as Silvadene, or bacteriocidal solutions such as 0.5% silver nitrate are used to cover the deep burn wounds. Second-degree burns should be covered with a layer of Adaptic, then Kerlix or Kling dressings. Patients who are discharged should be instructed to change the dressing daily. If Silvadene is used, it needs to be changed every 12 hours. Most importantly, discharged patients should be educated about concerning signs of infection, and close follow-up should be arranged. Check the tetanus status of all patients, and administer tetanus immunization (Td) as appropriate. Some patients may also require tetanus immune globulin (Hypertet). Adult burns greater than 20% of BSA require fluid resuscitation. Adult burns less than 15-20% total BSA without inhalation injury are usually not enough to initiate the systemic inflammatory response, and these patients can be rehydrated successfully, primarily via the oral route with modest IV fluid supplementation. IV fluid resuscitation is usually required in pediatric patients with smaller burns (in the range of 10-20%). The Parkland formula is used as a guideline for total volume during the first 24 hours of fluid resuscitation (with Ringer lactate [RL] solution): approximately 4 mL/kg body weight per percentage burn TBSA; half the volume is given in the first 8 hours postburn, with the remaining volume delivered over 16 hours.

Electrical and Lightning Injuries

- *Background.* Electricity is defined as the flow of electrons through a conductor. When the human becomes a conductor, injuries tend to happen. The nature and severity of electrical burn injury are directly proportional to the current strength, resistance, and duration of current flow. Current strength is expressed in amperes, and is a measure of the amount of energy flowing through an object. Current is determined by the voltage and resistance. Resistance is determined by the current's pathway through the body. Nerves, blood, mucous membranes, and muscle have the least resistance, whereas bone, fat and tendons have the most. High voltage is defined as 600 V or higher. In the United States, homes are wired for 110 V at the outlets, and 220 V for large appliances. There are two types of circuits, direct current (DC) or alternating current (AC). High-voltage DC causes a single muscle spasm, often throwing the individual from the source. AC is three times more dangerous than DC, and causes continuous muscle contraction or tetany. Common complications to watch for include cardiovascular issues like dysrhythmia or vascular injury, neuronal injury, cutaneous burns, rhabdomyolysis, and multiorgan injury. An electrical injury should be treated like a crush injury, rather than a thermal burn, because of the large amount of tissue damage that is often present under normal-appearing skin. Injury from lightning injuries occur by direct strike, contact with an object that is part of the pathway of the lightning current, side splash as the lightning jumps from the primary strike object to a nearby person on the way to the ground, the electrical potential that develops between the person's feet as the current spreads radially through the ground, or blunt trauma.
- *Clinical presentation.* See Table 65.3–3 for injury patterns in electrical and lighting injuries.
- *Diagnostic testing.* Obtain an EKG. Laboratory assessment should be focused on the patient's complaints and specific injuries as with any trauma or burn patient. A complete blood count, metabolic panel, ABG, and myoglobin levels or serum creatine kinase levels may be appropriate, based on symptoms or history.
- *ED management.* The patient should initially be placed on a cardiac monitor, have IV access placed, and have an EKG performed. Depending on the individual case, this may need to be repeated serially. Muscular injuries can cause a compartment syndrome (Chapter 17) or rhabdomyolysis (Chapter 49). A fasciotomy may be needed to de-compress the compartment pressures and prevent necrosis. Cutaneous burns should be treated with antibiotic dressings such as sulfadiazine

Tables 65.3–3   Patterns of Electrical and Lightening Injuries

	Electrical	Lightning
Head and neck	Cataracts Head is common point of contact	Blunt trauma Ruptured tympanic membrane Cataracts and other eye injuries
Cardiovascular	Cardiac arrest from asystole or ventricular fibrillation Electrocardiogram (other): sinus tachycardia, transient ST elevation, reversible QT prolongation, premature ventricular contractions, atrial fibrillation, bundle branch block.	Cardiac arrest from electrical shock or induced vascular spasm. Multiple dysrhythmias, nonspecific ST-T wave changes, and QT prolongation. Elevation of cardiac enzymes
Skin	Burns most severe at contact point (e.g., hands and skull) and ground (e.g., heel), flash burns, and "kissing" burn on flexor creases.	Deep burns are less common. Superficial burns such as linear, punctate, feathering (fern pattern from electron shower), or thermal.
Extremity	Muscle necrosis with rhabdomyolysis Compartment syndrome Numerous fractures and dislocations.	May have cold, blue, mottled, and pulseless extremity from severe vasospasm lasting up to a few hours. Numerous fractures and dislocations.
Nervous system	Loss of consciousness, confusion Head injury Seizures Spinal cord injury Weakness and paresthesias	Keraunoparalysis (temporary paralysis) Paresthesias

silver (Silvadene) and debridement as necessary. Tetanus toxoid and tetanus immunoglobulin should be given depending on immunization history. Indications for continuous cardiac monitoring include cardiac arrest, loss of consciousness, an abnormal EKG, history or significant risk factors for cardiac disease, hypoxia or chest pain. Patients who are totally asymptomatic, have a normal physical examination, a normal EKG, and no urinary pigment can be reassured, and then discharged without performing any ancillary tests. Pregnant patients should have obstetric consultation due to the risk of stillbirth with electrical injuries. Most patients with significant electrical burns should be stabilized, and transferred to a regional burn center for burn care and extensive occupational and physical rehabilitation.

Special Considerations

- Treatment for tar burns requires special attention. Debridement is often required, and is a balance between removing the foreign body (tar) and exposing the injured skin for evaluation and treatment. Applying ointments, such as polymicrobial antibiotic ointment, petroleum jelly, or mineral oil, can facilitate tar removal.
- Electric and chemical burns often have delayed appearance of the severity of their damage. These patients need continued observation to respond to delayed vascular injuries and worsening of the burns. Chemical burns often look more superficial than they will prove to be. They require extensive amounts of irrigation, and depending on the mechanism of injury, may require debridement. Fluoride burns often require injection of calcium chloride to control the intense pain that they cause (mentioned briefly in Chapter 72).
- Circumferential third-degree burns often form a stiff, nonelastic eschar that may impede circulation, and when on the chest, respiration. Escharotomy may have to be performed to relieve pressure and restore circulation. This is rarely necessary in the emergency department, but should be achieved before transfer to a burn center if this is necessary. The procedure is performed along the lateral aspect of the extremity. Use of an electrocautery simplifies the procedure, and can reduce the amount of bleeding. The incision should go completely through the eschar. The subcutaneous fat will appear to bubble up into the escharotomy wound.

Teaching Points

Burns, whether by flame, chemical, or electricity, cause intense psychologic as well as physiologic damage. It is helpful to immediately provide adequate analgesia and appropriate sedation. Deep burns produce marked sequestration of body fluids, and require aggressive resuscitation, which should start in the ED. Remember the Parkland formula for IV fluid resuscitation and use 4 ml/kg × % BSA (for second and third degree burns); half of this should be given in the first 8 hours with the remaining volume given over the next 16 hours. Electric and chemical burns often have delayed appearance of the severity of their damage, and these patients need continued observation to respond to delayed vascular injuries and worsening of the burns.

Suggested Readings

Gatewood MO, Zane RD. Lightning injuries. Emerg Med Clin North Am 2004;22:369–403.
Koumbourlis AC, Electrical injuries, Critical Care Medicine 2002;S424–S430.
Monafo WW. Initial management of burns. New Engl J Med 1996;335:1581–1586.

65.4   Near-Drowning and Submersion

Karen Van Hoesen ■ Kelly Pettit

■ *Background.* Near-drowning is one of the leading causes of accidental death in the world and is associated with high morbidity and mortality despite improved efforts of prevention and treatment. See Table 65.4–1 for terminology. Toddlers are at greatest risk for drowning. Infants younger than 1 year of age have the highest drowning rate, followed by teenaged boys. Child abuse and homicide must be considered in cases of pediatric submersion, particularly in any bathtub drowning. Alcohol use is a major risk factor in adult submersion accidents. Drowning is the most common cause of death in SCUBA divers and near-drowning is a complication of pulmonary barotrauma. Other risk factors that predispose to drowning and near-drowning include seizures, syncope, suicide, boating accidents (in particular, not wearing a personal flotation device), hypothermia, and home swimming pools. Cervical spine injuries and head trauma must be suspected in all unwitnessed events, particularly those in shallow water. Regardless of whether seawater or freshwater is aspirated, the final common pathophysiologic consequence of submersion is hypoxemia. The most important parameter in improving morbidity and mortality from drowning and near-drowning is prevention.
■ *Clinical presentation.* The diagnosis is usually made by report of the patient, bystanders, and emergency medical service (EMS) personnel. In victims found unconscious in the water, one needs to consider the possible cause of the near-drowning. The near-drowning victim may vary from being fully alert and without complaints to being comatose. Coughing, cyanosis, tachypnea and tachycardia are commonly seen. The chest examination may reveal rhonchi, rales, or wheezes. A detailed neurologic examination is important, particularly in SCUBA divers who have lost consciousness in the water, and victims with potential cervical spine injury. Evaluate all such patients for potential head and neck trauma. See Table 65.4–2 for complications.

Table 65.4–1 Terminology of Submersion Incidents	
Term	**Definition**
Drowning	Death from suffocation by submersion in a liquid
Secondary or delayed drowning	Death 24 h after submersion from complications (acute respiratory distress syndrome, infection)
Near-drowning	Loss of consciousness due to submersion with survival. May be associated with or without aspiration.
Aspiration syndromes	Effects of aspiration from submersion without loss of consciousness

Table 65.4–2   **Complications of Near-Drowning**

Early (within 4 h)	Late (after 4 h)
Hypoxia	Acute respiratory distress syndrome
Respiratory acidosis	Aspiration pneumonia
Metabolic and lactic acidosis	Lung abscess
Bronchospasm	Renal failure
Vomiting with aspiration	Sepsis
Fluid and electrolyte disturbances (rare)	Anoxic–ischemic encephalopathy
Seizures	Rhabdomyolysis
	Myoglobinuria

- *Diagnostic testing.* An ABG should be obtained in all submersion victims. The ABG often shows hypoxemia and a combined metabolic and respiratory acidosis. Serum bicarbonate may be decreased due to lactic acidosis from tissue hypoxia. Electrolytes and hemoglobin levels are usually normal. Urine drug screen and blood alcohol level (BAL) should be obtained. Cardiac enzymes may be useful in elderly patients, those with known coronary artery disease, or significant submersion time. An EKG may reveal sinus tachycardia or bradycardia, ventricular ectopy, fibrillation, myocardial ischemia, and asystole. In cases of concomitant hypothermia, a J or Osborn wave may be seen (see Chapter 65.5). Obtain a chest radiograph in all patients with suspected submersion. Chest radiograph findings will be normal in approximately 20% of near-drowning victims. Findings include perihilar opacities, pulmonary edema, or fine alveolar infiltrates. Diffuse interstitial infiltrates, segmental atelectasis, or air bronchograms are seen in severe cases. Cervical spine films should be obtained in anyone with suspected neck injury, e.g., the patient was diving into the water, or those who cannot give a reliable history. A noncontrast computed tomography (CT) of the head should be obtained on any unconscious victim pulled from the water to look for head trauma. Victims of near-drowning with prolonged hypoxemia often have evidence of cerebral edema on CT.
- *ED management.* First-line treatment is adequate ventilation and correction of hypoxia. Victims who are awake and breathing spontaneously should receive supplemental oxygen. Victims in respiratory distress may benefit from continuous positive airway pressure (CPAP). Cardiac irritability usually responds to correction of hypoxia and acidosis. A loop diuretic (furosemide, 0.5-1 mg/kg) can be used for diuresis in cases of pulmonary edema. Sodium bicarbonate should be administered if the pH is below 7.25 and not improving with aggressive respiratory management. If severe hypothermia exists, the patient will need to be rewarmed before successful defibrillation is possible. In intubated patients, PEEP improves ventilation by increasing lung volume, shifting interstitial pulmonary water into capillaries, increasing diameter of large and small airways, and reducing intrapulmonary shunting. CPAP counteracts the effects of pulmonary edema and atelectasis, and can increase PaO_2. The use of CPAP can delay or eliminate the need for intubation, and should be considered if the PaO_2 is below 55 mm Hg and

the patient is unlikely to aspirate. Admit all patients with abnormal vital signs, radiographic findings or abnormal findings on ABG measurements. Asymptomatic adults with no radiologic abnormalities or evidence of hypoxia may be discharged with appropriate follow-up after a period of 4 to 6 hours of observation in the ED.

Teaching Points

Near drowning is common in infants, children, and young adults who consume alcohol with their water recreations. The best treatment is prevention. Some patients will look well initially, but then subsequently deteriorate. Clues are any abnormality of the initial vital signs, any pathology seen on a chest x-ray study, or any alteration in the level of consciousness. These patients should be admitted to a critical care unit, given supplemental oxygen, and may require endotracheal intubation. There is no benefit to using steroids or antibiotics.

Suggested Readings

Model JH. Drowning. N Engl J Med 1993;328:253–256.
Olshaker JS. Emerg Med Clin North Am 2004;22:357–367.

65.5 Heat and Cold Exposure

Christopher L. Dunnahoo ■ Lawrence B. Stack

Heat Exhaustion

- *Background.* Heat exhaustion is the most common heat-related illness. The physiology and predisposing factors are the same as for heat stroke (see "Heat Stroke"). There is water and salt depletion. Water depletion is caused by inadequate fluid replacement when working in a hot environment and can progress to heat stroke. On average, individuals only consume approximately two thirds of what they lose to perspiration, leading to a relative dehydration. Salt depletion is caused by a large volume of sweat replaced by hypotonic solution. It tends to take longer to develop and results in hyponatremia, hypochloremia, and low urinary chloride and sodium. Body temperature remains near normal.
- *Clinical presentation.* Signs and symptoms include lightheadedness, weakness, fatigue, nausea, vomiting, headache, myalgias, syncope, orthostasis, sinus tachycardia, tachypnea, diaphoresis, hyperthermia (variable core temperature), and normal mental status.
- *Diagnostic testing.* Hepatic transaminase elevations of several thousand units may be seen in heat exhaustion or healthy runners after a marathon,

whereas in heat stroke such levels are usually in the tens of thousands after 24 hours.

- ***ED Management.*** For mild cases, rest in a cool environment and an oral electrolyte solution may suffice. Patients with significant volume depletion or electrolyte abnormalities generally require IV fluids. Free water deficits should be replaced slowly over 48 hours or slowly enough so as not to decrease serum osmolality more than 2 mOsm/h. Too-rapid correction of hyponatremia is associated with seizures and cerebral edema. Young, healthy patients with mild heat exhaustion and mild laboratory abnormalities can be discharged home. Discharge instructions should include drinking plenty of fluids and avoiding heat exposure for the next 24 to 48 hours. Older patients, those with severe heat exhaustion, or significant laboratory abnormalities should be admitted.

Heat Stroke

- ***Background.*** Heat stroke consists of a triad of core temperature greater than 40.5° C (104.9° F), central nervous system dysfunction, and anhidrosis. The body has several mechanisms to transfer heat to the environment (Table 65.5–1). Predisposing factors for heat stroke include increased internal heat production (e.g., physical activity, febrile illness and certain drugs such as amphetamines, cocaine, aspirin), external heat gain (e.g., increased temperature and humidity), and decreased ability to disperse heat (dehydration, extremes of age, cardiovascular disease, obesity, skin disease, inappropriate clothing, and certain drugs such as anticholinergics, diuretics, phenothiazines, cardiovascular drugs, sympathomimetics). Classic or epidemic heat stroke occurs during prolonged increased ambient temperature and humidity. Typically it involves poor, elderly patients living in poorly ventilated homes without central air conditioning who have chronic diseases, alcoholism or schizophrenia. Exertional heat stroke typically occurs in young, healthy patients whose heat management mechanisms are unable to keep up with endogenous heat production.

Table 65.5–1 Mechanisms of Heat Loss	
Conduction	The transfer of heat by direct physical contact with a cooler object. It results in only 2% of total body heat loss.
Convection	The transfer of heat to air and water vapor molecules that encompass the body. When the ambient temperature is greater than the body temperature, heat is actually gained.
Radiation	The transfer of heat by electromagnetic waves. It results in 65% of heat loss in cool environments and is the major source of heat gain when the ambient temperature is greater than the body temperature.
Evaporation	The transfer of heat through conversion of a liquid to a gas. As the ambient temperature increases, evaporation becomes the major mechanism of heat loss. High humidity prevents evaporation.

- **Clinical presentation.** The clinical presentation includes central nervous system dysfunction (irritability, bizarre behavior, combativeness, hallucinations, seizures, coma, etc.), tachycardia, hypotension, right-sided heart failure, and tachypnea. Sweating may or may not be present. Multiorgan system failure can occur, resulting in encephalopathy, acute renal failure, acute respiratory distress syndrome, disseminated intravascular coagulation (DIC), rhabdomyolysis, and hepatocellular injury. Lack of sweat does not reliably differentiate between heat stroke and heat exhaustion.

- **Diagnostic testing.** This should include CBC (hemoconcentration), a metabolic panel (hyponatremia, hypochloremia, variable potassium and magnesium, acute renal failure), liver function tests (should be increased; if normal, the diagnosis of heat stroke should be questioned), CPK (rhabdomyolysis), urinalysis (myoglobinuria), coagulation panel (coagulopathy, DIC), lactate (lactic acidosis), arterial blood gas (respiratory alkalosis). Thyroid function tests, blood cultures, and head CT should be ordered as clinically indicated.

- **ED management.** Address the ABCs and IV fluid (be alert for right-sided heart failure). Treat rhabdomyolysis (see Chapter 49) if present and evaluate for DIC. Evaporative cooling is very effective and can be performed with spray bottles filled with tepid water and fans. Immersion in ice-water baths is another method but, it is difficult to monitor patients while immersed. Ice packs to the groin and axilla can be used. Benzodiazepines and phenothiazines should be used for shivering. Cooling measures should be stopped at 39° C to avoid overshoot. All patients should be admitted to a monitored or ICU bed. The management of other types of heat-related illness are summarized in Table 65.5–2.

Frostbite

- **Background.** Risk factors for frostbite include dehydration, hypoxia, wet or constrictive clothing, alcohol use, decreasing ambient temperature, increasing wind chill, hypovolemia, anemia, and diabetes. Frostbite occurs when tissue temperature drops below O° C. Two types of tissue injury exist: ice crystal formation with microvascular thrombosis and stasis.

- **Clinical presentation.** Similar to burns, frostbite can be divided into four degrees. *First-degree* consists of partial-thickness skin freezing. Erythema, mild edema with no blister formation, and occasional desquamation may also be present. Patients may complain of stinging or burning paresthesias. *Second-degree* consists of full–skin thickness freezing, and increasing edema and erythema with clear blister formation that desquamates to form black, hard eschar. Patients describe numbness, aching, and throbbing of the involved tissue. *Third-degree* consists of damage to the subdermal plexus. Hemorrhagic blisters form and the skin has a blue–gray discoloration. The extremity feels like a "block of wood." Patients also complain of burning, throbbing, and shooting pains. *Fourth-degree* consists of damage of the subcutaneous tissues including muscle, bone, and tendon. The tissue has little to no edema, and appears mottled

Table 65.5–2	Other Types of Heat-Related Illness	
	Description	**Management**
Heat syncope	Type of postural hypotension occurring in nonacclimatized patients and is secondary to volume depletion, peripheral vasodilatation, and decreased vasomotor tone.	Remove the patient from the heat source. Rehydrate with IV or PO fluids and allow the patient to rest. Other causes of syncope should be ruled out. Rarely needs hospitalization.
Heat tetany	Hyperventilation occurring in a hot environment and resulting in respiratory alkalosis. This causes carpopedal spasm and paresthesias of distal extremities and perioral area.	Remove the patient from the heat source and decrease the respiratory rate.
Heat cramps	Painful, involuntary, spasmodic skeletal muscle contractions which are thought to be a deficiency in sodium, potassium and fluid. Occurs in the first few days of working in a hot environment with a large amount of sweat replaced by copious amounts of hypotonic fluid. Usually involves calves, thighs, and shoulders.	Consists of rest, oral fluids (IV rarely needed), and salt replacement.
Prickly heat (heat rash, miliaria rubra, lichen tropicus)	A pruritic, erythematous, maculopapular rash over clothed areas of the body that is caused from blocked sweat pores with subsequent inflammation.	Includes antihistamines and a chlorhexidine wash. Antibiotics can be used if a *Staphylococcal* superinfection is present. Prevention includes wearing clean, light, loose fitting clothing and avoiding sweat production.
Heat edema	Dependent edema of the hands and feet secondary to vasodilatation and orthostatic pooling. It tends to occur during the first few days of heat exposure in elderly, non-acclimatized patients.	Includes elevation and compression stockings. Heat edema resolves spontaneously but may take up to 6 weeks for full resolution.

IV, intravenous; PO, by mouth.

with nonblanching cyanosis progressing to deep mummified black eschar. Patients tend to complain of a deeper aching, joint-type pain.

■ *ED management.* Rapidly rewarm the injured tissue using 40 to 42° C circulating water for 10 to 60 minutes or until the injured part is pliable and distal erythema is present. Avoid reexposure to cold with subsequent refreezing of the rewarmed extremity. Warm compresses should be used for facial frostbite. Local wound care consists of elevation and wrapping in sterile gauze. Affected digits should be separated. Clear blisters may be unroofed followed by application of topical treatment with aloe vera every 6 hours; avoid unroofing hemorrhagic blisters. Hemorrhagic blisters indicate deeper damage to the subdermal venous plexus and unroofing these blisters can further damage the vascular network. Topical aloe vera may be applied to affected areas every 6 hours. Additionally, ibuprofen should be given every 6 to 8 hours. Prophylactic antibiotics are unnecessary. The rewarming process is quite painful and adequate analgesia with narcotics is warranted. Tetanus immunization should be updated. Surgical intervention should be delayed for 3 to 4 weeks until demarcation occurs. Except for minor cases, most patients should be admitted for observation in order to better define the extent of injury.

Hypothermia

■ *Background.* Hypothermia occurs when the body's core temperature drops below 35° C (95° F). Hypothermia can result from environmental exposure and includes immersion and nonimmersion. Exposure to a profoundly cold environment is not needed for hypothermia to occur. Immersion hypothermia can occur in water at 60 °F to 70 °F. However, many different metabolic emergencies may lower body temperature including: hypothyroidism, hypopituitarism, adrenal insufficiency and hypoglycemia. Additionally, central nervous system dysfunction (head trauma, stroke, or tumor) can lower body temperature. Several medications (alcohol, insulin, sedatives, and phenothiazines) can result in hypothermia. Sepsis, diabetic ketoacidosis, burns, and dermatologic diseases can also lower body temperature.

■ *Clinical presentation.* Patients present with altered mental status, initial tachycardia progressing to bradycardia, dysrhythmias, hypotension, initial tachypnea progressing to hypoventilation, bronchorrhea, apnea, abdominal rigidity mimicking an acute abdomen, ataxia, hyporeflexia, impaired judgment, rigidity, shivering, erythema, and cyanosis. The clinical presentation often reflects the degree of hypothermia. In mild (32 °C-35° C) hypothermia, tachypnea, tachycardia, dysarthria and shivering may be present. In moderate (28 °C-32 °C) hypothermia, there may be loss of shivering and decreasing level of consciousness. In severe (<28 °C) hypothermia, decreased reflexes, coma, and ventricular fibrillation may occur.

■ *Diagnostic testing.* EKG changes include T-wave inversions; increased PR, QRS and QT intervals; and J or Osborne waves (Figure 65.5–1). Dysrhythmias also occur, with the most common types being sinus bradycardia, atrial fibrillation or flutter with slow ventricular response,

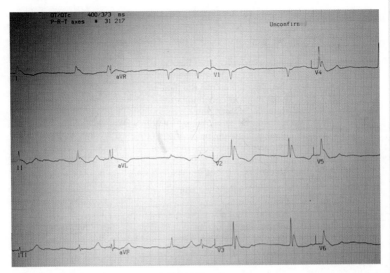

Figure 65.5–1. Osborne waves in hypothermia.

nodal rhythms, atrioventricular block, premature ventricular contractions, ventricular fibrillation, and asystole. Additionally, the EKG findings that suggest hyperkalemia are not reliable in the setting of hypothermia. With respect to arterial blood gases (ABG), the pH rises and the PaO2 and PaCo2 fall as body temperature drops. The ABGs should be interpreted uncorrected for temperature because the ABGs are warmed to body temperature before being processed. Patient results are compared to normal values. The hematocrit should increase 2% for every 1° C fall. Various electrolyte abnormalities can occur. Hypokalemia is the most common electrolyte abnormality. Hyperglycemia suggests acute hypothermia. Hypoglycemia suggests subacute or chronic hypothermia. Enzyme action is depressed by low body temperature resulting in a coagulopathy.

- ***ED management.*** Use low-reading rectal thermometers to obtain accurate temperature readings. Patients should be handled carefully due to risk of ventricular fibrillation. Warm oxygen and IV fluids should be used. Thiamine and glucose should be given to alcoholic patients. Treat signs of coagulopathy with rewarming rather than fresh frozen plasma. Most dysrhythmias convert spontaneously during rewarming. Bretylium 10 mg/kg is the drug of choice for ventricular fibrillation. Amiodarone is a second choice. Due to low fibrillatory threshold, avoid transvenous pacing for bradycardia. Transcutaneous pacing should be used instead. Rewarming techniques are summarized in Table 65.5–3. Sudden cardiopulmonary collapse may result from the afterdrop, a paradoxical decrease in core temperature from rapid peripheral, and loss of more heat.

Table 65.5–3	**Rewarming Techniques**	
	Description	**Comment**
Passive external	Requires patients to be able to produce enough heat to warm themselves. Remove the patient from the cold environment. Remove any wet clothing and insulate the patient with blankets. Provide insulating material to prevent further heat loss. Must be able to generate heat for rewarming to occur.	Rewarming rate of 0.5° C to 2 °C/h
Active external	Includes forced-air warming (Bair Hugger), arteriovenous anastomosis rewarming (immersion of hands, forearms, feet, and calves in water warmed to 44 °C-45 °C, which opens atrioventricular anastomosis and returns warm venous blood to the core), radiant heat and heated objects (blankets and water bottles). Complications include rewarming shock (peripheral vasodilatation and pooling of blood) and rewarming acidosis (lactic acid washout).	Bair Hugger rewarming rates up to 2.5 °C/h without afterdrop.
Active core	Includes heated intravenous (IV) fluid (D5NS at 40 °C-42 °C), inhalational rewarming, bladder or gastrointestinal tract lavage, thoracic lavage, peritoneal lavage and extracorporeal (cardiopulmonary bypass, continuous arteriovenous or venovenous rewarming, and hemodialysis).	Rewarming rates: airway 1°C to 2.5 °C/h; warm IV fluids 2.9 °C/h; peritoneal dialysis and lavage up to 6 °C/h; mediastinal mediastinal lavage 3 °C/h; hemodialysis 6 °C/h; arteriovenous 2.5 °C/h, venovenous up to 5.4 °C/h; cardiopulmonary bypass 9.5 °C/h.

Table 65.5–4   Other Cold-Related Illness

	Definition	Characteristics	Treatment
Frostnip	Superficial cold injury with lack of extracellular crystal formation and no progressive tissue loss.	The skin appears pale. The involved area may be painful. Symptoms resolve with rewarming and no tissue loss is present.	See frostbite treatment.
Chilblains (pernio)	Caused by chronic intermittent exposures to a dry, nonfreezing environment.	Involves the hands, ears, lower legs, and feet. Skin findings include localized edema, vesicles, bullae and ulcerations. Patients may also complain of pruritus and burning paresthesias. After rewarming, blue nodules often develop.	See frostbite treatment. Topical and oral steroids have been used as well as nifedipine.
Trench foot	Caused by chronic exposure to a damp, nonfreezing environment.	Initially, the skin appears pale, mottled, anesthetic, pulseless and immobile; paresthesias may be present. Initially no change occurs with rewarming. A hyperemic phase then develops with burning paresthesias. Proximal sensation returns. Over the next 2-3 d hyperemia worsens and bullae develop. Later, cold sensitivity and hyperhidrosis develop.	Care is mostly supportive. Keep the patient warm and dry and elevate feet. Preventive measures include good shoe fit, changing socks several times a day, keeping feet dry, and never sleeping in wet socks or boots.

Otherwise healthy patients with mild hypothermia (32 °C-35 °C) due to exposure can be discharged home to a warm environment. More severely hypothermic patients and patients with co-morbid illness should be admitted to a monitored bed. Other types of cold-related illness are summarized in Table 65.5–4.

Teaching Points

Like many other phases of human physiology, temperature must be maintained within a narrow range. Deviations above and below are often signs of serious disease, and therefore temperature is one of the vital signs and should be measured in all patients.

The skin is very sensitive to low temperatures, and will develop changes that simulate burns of the skin. Before freezing and crystallization of water in the skin occurs, there will be blanching, anesthesia, and a striking physical appearance of whiteness. The skin can be rewarmed rapidly with no subsequent problems.

As ice crystals form, there is great danger of permanent damage to the skin. Rapid rewarming is still the best therapy, but only if the patient is capable of being protected against another episode of cooling. The skin will go through a phase of blistering, erythema, and eschar formation that will look very ominous, but there should be great patience exercised in the amputation of cold-induced gangrene, since many of these patients will recover. They may have persistent problems with cold exposure.

Hypothermia also produces significant metabolic and physiologic changes. Mild to moderate hypothermia can be managed with self rewarming and external heat sources, but severe hypothermia will require active rewarming. This includes warmed IV fluids, warmed humidified air, and if it is readily available, extracorporeal circulation.

Hyperthermic episodes are equally significant in regards to the extremes of age, and morbidity and mortality. Rapid cooling is best achieved by moistening, fans, ice bags, and shivering suppression. The patient will often have severe dehydration as well and require IV replacement. The presence or absence of sweating is less helpful than mental status changes. Any degree of confusion should be treated as heat stroke.

Suggested Readings

Danzl DF. Accidental Hypothermia. In: Marx JA, Hockberger RS, Walls RM, eds. Rosen's Emergency Medicine, Concepts and Clinical Practice. 6th ed. Philadelphia: Mosby, 2006:2236–2254.

Lugo-Amador NM. Heat-related illness. Emerg Med Clin North Am 2004;22:315–327.

Ulrich AS. Hypothermia and localized cold injuries. Emerg Med Clin North Am 2004; 22:281–298.

Vicario S. Heat illness. In: Marx JA, Hockberger RS, Walls RM, eds. Rosen's Emergency Medicine, Concepts and Clinical Practice. 6th ed. Philadelphia: Mosby, 2006:2254–2267.

65.6 Common Bites and Envenomations

Stephan E. Russ ■ Lawrence B. Stack

Venomous Reptile Bites
Overview

■ Venomous reptiles of North America include numerous snakes and two closely-related venomous lizards. The venomous snakes of North America fall into two families: Viperidae (crotalids such as rattlesnakes, copperheads, and water moccasins) and Elapidae (coral snakes), with at least one species of venomous snake found in all lower 48 states except Maine.

■ Fang marks may appear as a scratch or single wound, rather than the classic pair of puncture wounds. The extent of tissue swelling and ecchymosis should be documented in a quantifiable manner to allow comparison over time. Special attention should be paid to the patient's vital signs, including assessing for orthostatic hypotension. A thorough examination is necessary, with particular emphasis on the cardiovascular, respiratory, neurological, and any hemorrhagic skin or mucous membrane findings. Repeat assessments of both local tissue reaction and systemic cardiovascular stability should be performed frequently.

■ The most crucial step in prehospital care of the envenomated patient is rapid transport to an appropriate medical facility. Many of the field treatments advocated by various sources, such as locally applied electric shocks, cryotherapy, and incising the bite, have been proven to increase morbidity. Venom extraction devices that seal over a wound and use mechanical suction have been shown to extract an insignificant amount of venom while possibly worsening local tissue damage. Acceptable prehospital care includes splinting and elevating the bitten extremity. Applying a constriction band proximal to the bite that occludes lymphatic flow while sparing arterial and venous flow has been shown to be helpful in reducing systemic absorption in animal models, but can easily become a dangerous tourniquet if not applied and monitored carefully.

■ Antivenom therapy must be initiated as soon as possible for envenomations that have resulted in systemic symptoms or moderate-to-severe local symptoms. Hypotension should be treated with aggressive fluid resuscitation using first crystalloids and then colloid preparations if necessary. Fresh frozen plasma or platelets should be reserved for significant bleeding. The wound should be cleaned, copiously irrigated with normal saline, and placed in a padded splint and elevated above the level of the heart. Prophylactic antibiotics are not necessary. Tetanus immunization should be given as for any wound.

Crotalids

■ *Background.* Most venomous snakebites in the United States are due to species of the crotaline family, also known as pit vipers for the heat-sensing organs present between the pupils and nostrils. Crotalids include rattlesnakes, copperheads, cottonmouths, and cantrils. Rattlesnakes are widely distributed in North America with the exception of Alaska, Maine, and the northern parts of Canada, whereas copperheads and cottonmouths are found in the Southeast, Mid South and Mid Atlantic United States and parts of Mexico. Cantils are a venomous species similar to copperheads that are located throughout Mexico.

■ *Clinical presentation.* Crotalid venom is a complex mixture of enzymes that cause tissue necrosis, endothelial and red blood cell (RBC) damage, and a consumptive coagulopathy. As a general rule, crotalid venom has very few neurotoxic effects and systemic symptoms are usually secondary to the hypovolemic shock from increased vascular permeability and coagulopathy. Notable exceptions are a few subspecies of Mohave Rattlesnakes that have neurotoxic venom that can cause a clinical syndrome similar to corral snake envenomation.

■ *ED management.* Approximately one in four crotalid bites will not result in envenomation, even when at least one fang punctured the skin. Patients with no local or systemic symptoms and no laboratory abnormalities after 8 hours may generally be discharged if they have reliable follow-up the next day with repeated laboratory studies. Patients with bites that may possibly be from a neurotoxic subspecies should be observed for a minimum of 24 hours. Antivenom therapy is the cornerstone of treatment. Indications for antivenom therapy include systemic symptoms, compartment syndrome, or evidence of ongoing envenomation such as progressive swelling. Two formulations are currently available for North American crotalid bites. Antivenom (Crotalidae) Polyvalent is refined from the serum of horses that have been immunized with four different species of crotalids and gives various degrees of protection from a large range of North and South American crotalid species. Because antivenom is produced from equine serum, it has the potential for severe adverse reactions such as anaphylaxis and serum sickness. The manufacturer recommends that patients should be skin tested first, but consult your local toxicologist. All patients receiving the antivenom should be adequately fluid resuscitated and pretreated with diphenhydramine and a histamine-2 (H_2) blocker. Pretreatment with corticosteroids is not recommended because this may worsen tissue damage at the site of the envenomation. Dosing of the antivenom is determined by the severity of the patient's symptoms and needs to be adjusted on the basis of clinical response to treatment. CroFab is a refined preparation of ovine immunoglobulin Fab fragments with a similar spectrum of activity as Polyvalent Antivenom but with fewer adverse reactions. The initial dose is four to six vials. It is effective if given within 6 hours of the snake bite. Patients treated with CroFab should still be monitored for anaphylactic reactions and carefully observed for resurgence in symptoms because redosing is frequently necessary.

Elapids

■ *Background.* Coral snakes are found in the extreme southern portions of the United States and throughout Mexico. Several other species of snakes imitate the coloring pattern of coral snakes, but rather than having wide red and black bands interposed by narrow yellow bands, the imitators have wide red and yellow bands interposed by narrow black bands. These coloring differences have lead to the adage "red touching yellow kill a fellow, red touching black venom lack." Coral snakes are reclusive and relatively uncommon. Furthermore, coral snakes have small fangs that penetrate skin poorly with less than half of all bites actually resulting in envenomation. Coral snakes are often reported as "chewing" on their prey over several seconds to a minute to inject a sufficient amount of venom.

- *Clinical presentation.* The coral snake carries a neurotoxin that blocks acetylcholine from binding on the postsynaptic portion of the neuro-muscular junction, resulting in muscle weakness. Systemic symptoms predominate with little local tissue damage. Generally envenomations first produce nonspecific symptoms such as nausea, abdominal pain, paresthesias, and altered mental status that progress to muscle weakness, resulting in dysphagia, diplopia, ptosis, and ultimately respiratory insufficiency.

- *ED management.* Systemic symptoms may not occur until almost 18 hours after a bite and can be difficult to manage if treated late. Therefore, although more than half of all bites are "dry," careful consideration should be made regarding antivenom administration even in the absence of symptoms. At a minimum, all patients should be closely observed for 24 hours. Patients who have begun to exhibit respiratory compromise should be intubated early for airway control. Equine antivenom is available from Wyeth with activity against the two medically relevant species of coral snakes in the United States. The patient should be observed closely for anaphylactic reactions and serum sickness (see section on crotalid antivenin for further discussion). The duration of respiratory depression is typically 24 to 72 hours.

Helodermatid lizards

- Bites from lizards such as the Gila Monster and the Mexican beaded lizard are rare and usually not life-threatening in a healthy individual. Both species produce a venom that is similar in composure and effect to crotalid venom. Tissue damage from the bite alone can be substantial, since the lizards will frequently hold on to their victims tenaciously. Systemic manifestations and treatment of lizard envenomation are similar to that of Crotalid bites.

Marine Bites and Envenomations

- As most marine envenomations in North American waters result in only local injury, an extensive laboratory workup in an otherwise healthy individual with no systemic effects is not necessary. However, these wounds are at high risk for infection and should be copiously irrigated and debrided. A careful search should be undertaken for foreign bodies; most organic debris is radiolucent.

- In general, primary wound closure with sutures should not be carried out to minimize the risk of infection. General wound care can otherwise be given with tetanus immunization as for all wounds. Prophylactic antibiotics are used except in minor abrasions and superficial wounds in the healthy adult. *Staphylococcus* and *Streptococcus* species still cause a large portion of aquatic associated wound infections. Freshwater wound infections may be caused by a wide variety of gram-negative organisms including *Pseudomonas, Aeromonas, Serratia, Enterobacter* and *Acinetobacter*. Infections caused by *Aeromonas* species bear special mention as they cause an aggressive cellulitis that can develop into a severe necrotizing gas-forming infection. Saltwater infections are also associated with gram-negative organisms such as Vibrio genus. Common marine bites and envenomations are summarized in Table 65.6–1.

Insect and Arthropod Bites and Stings

- Most insect and arthropod bites and stings result in only a mild local reaction that can be best treated by washing the wound with soap and water, elevation, cold compresses and diphenhydramine or topical corticosteroids for pruritis. Bites can occasionally serve as a nidus for infection such as cellulitis, but the risk is too small to warrant prophylactic antibiotics.
- Anaphylactic reactions are an infrequent but potentially life-threatening effect of insect bites, particularly hymenoptera. Treatment of anaphylaxis includes fluid resuscitation, steroids, diphenhydramine, cimetidine, and epinephrine if symptoms are severe enough (see Chapter 19).

Brown Recluse Spider (Loxoceles reclusa)

- ***Background.*** Commonly known as the *brown recluse* or *fiddleback spider*, Loxoceles reclusa are found in the areas surrounding the Mississippi River valley. They are small venomous brown spiders with a leg span roughly the size of a quarter, a characteristic violin–shape, and a dark brown marking on the dorsum of their cephalothorax. Known for being shy and preferring dark undisturbed locations, brown recluse spiders usually bite humans only in defense.
- ***Clinical presentation.*** The bite is sometimes described as a pinprick, but may be initially painless. Most bites do not evolve beyond a tiny papular lesion, but in some cases the wound will progress within 24 hours to a wide erythematous ring around a dark sunken necrotic core with a middle zone of vasoconstriction. Over the next several weeks, the necrotic center will slough to form an ulcer that is typically 1 to 3 cm in diameter but may be larger. It is estimated that 10% of patients with brown recluse envenomation develop systemic loxoscelism, manifested by malaise, and in severe cases, fever and hemolysis. The natural history of ulcerated brown recluse bites is slow gradual healing via secondary intention over 4 to 6 weeks.
- ***ED management.*** Debridement of the central core is generally not necessary. The erythema around the bite does not represent cellulitis and antibiotics are not indicated. If an infection is thought to be present the diagnosis of a spider bite must be seriously reconsidered. The use of dapsone is not recommended because of the high incidence of side effects such as methemoglobinemia.

Table 65.6–1 Marine Bites and Envenomations

	Mechanism	Clinical Presentation	Treatment	Comments
Jellyfish	Nematocysts on tentacles release toxin which causes inflammation and autonomic dysfunction. Worst cases in South Pacific.	Localized skin irritation with a linear raised erythematous rash, intense stinging, paresthesias that radiate proximally.	Rinse area with normal saline, soak in 5% acetic acid solution (white vinegar) for 30 min, and remove remaining nematocysts with adhesive tape or shave with razor (apply shaving cream). Cold packs and oral analgesia for pain.	Avoid vigorous rubbing or contact with fresh water (causes discharge of nematocysts). Systemic symptoms more likely in very young and old.
Sponges	Cause dermatitis due to implantation of small inorganic spicules or an allergic dermatologic reaction.	Pruritis, burning sensation, edema, local joint swelling, bullae, fever, malaise, muscle cramps.	Remove spicules with adhesive tape or rubber cement and soak in dilute acetic acid for 30 min. Hydrocortisone cream and antihistamines for itching. Systemic steroids if severe.	Rarely, a more severe allergic reaction such as anaphylaxis or erythema multiforme may require more aggressive immuno-modulatory treatment.
Echinoderms (starfish and sea urchins)	Spiny appendages may be filled with venom.	Puncture wound is erythematous and edematous. Systemic symptoms if severe: nausea, paresthesias, neuromuscular dysfunction, and hypotension.	Hot water immersion to tolerance for at least 30 min or until pain mostly resolves as some of the toxins are heat-labile. Evaluate for foreign body.	As always, orthopedics should be called if there is joint involvement.

Continued

Table 65.6-1 Marine Bites and Envenomations—*cont'd*

	Mechanism	Clinical Presentation	Treatment	Comments
Stingrays	Patients usually step on an unsuspecting stingray and the spine on their tail is embedded in the patient's foot. Glands on either side of the spine can cause an envenomation.	Trauma is caused by the spine with local hemorrhage and necrosis, may have systemic symptoms such as autonomic dysfunction, syncope, and arrhythmias.	Place wound in non-scalding hot water for one hour to help denature the toxins and debride the area. Delayed primary closure is utilized due to the very high rate of infection. Monitor for systemic symptoms for 6 h after the injury.	
Coral	Mechanical abrasions or lacerations. Some species have nematocysts which cause mild envenomation.	Localized skin irritation. Intense stinging if nematocysts envenomate.	Aggressive irrigation, scrubbing to remove foreign particles, rinse with hydrogen peroxide and water to remove small coral particles. Topical and PO antibiotics recommended.	Poor wound healing (up to 8 weeks) is common. Follow-up is essential as many wounds get infected or require debridement.

Black Widow Spider (Latrodectus Mactans)

- *Background.* The female spider is the one that bites humans. They are small black spiders with a red, hourglass-shaped mark on their ventral abdomen and a leg span the size of a dime. Black widows are found outdoors typically in outbuildings, woodpiles, and thick vegetation.
- *Clinical presentation.* Bites are painful and most cause only a small papule with no systemic symptoms. The 25% of bites that will result in systemic symptoms typically cause severe chest or abdominal pain, sustained muscle spasms, facial swelling, and autonomic dysfunction causing hypertension. Symptoms last from 12 hours to 3 days and rarely result in serious sequelae in otherwise healthy adults.
- *ED management.* Treatment of systemic symptoms consists of IV narcotics and benzodiazepines with IV nitrates or calcium channel blockers to control severe hypertension. Calcium gluconate was used in the past in an effort to ease muscle spasms but more recent studies have cast doubt on its efficacy. Equine-based antivenom is available and should be considered in cases of seizures, respiratory distress, priapism, pregnancy, or severe, uncontrolled hypertension.

Hymenoptera

- *Background.* Wasps, bees, and fire ants are the more common stinging insects that belong to the order hymenoptera. Hymenoptera are of great medical significance as they are the cause of the vast majority of deaths in the developed world due to envenomation.
- *Clinical presentation.* Most stings cause only local release of histamine resulting in a wheal and flare reaction. However, a spectrum of systemic reactions from mild urticaria to life-threatening anaphylactic reactions can occur (Chapter 19). Large numbers of stings may also cause severe systemic reactions. Life-threatening anaphylaxis usually occurs within the first 30 minutes after a sting and death is due to airway compromise or hypotension.
- *ED management.* Treatment for local reactions includes removal of any retained stingers, cold compresses, and oral diphenhydramine. Treatment for systemic reactions includes IV diphenhydramine, cimetidine, corticosteroids, and aggressive fluid resuscitation. Patients with hypotension or respiratory symptoms should be treated with epinephrine at increasing doses until symptoms are tolerable (see Chapter 19). Patients who have sustained a large number of stings must be monitored for renal failure, cardiac ischemia, and coagulopathy.

Scorpions

- *Background.* Most scorpion stings cause only mild local tissue reaction; however, a few species can cause a more severe envenomation. In the United States and Mexico, only the stings of the Centruroides species are medically noteworthy and actually cause more deaths than snakebites primarily due to a small but significant mortality in Mexican children. These nocturnal small brown scorpions are found in the desert southwest and hide in ground debris and rock crevices.

■ *Clinical presentation.* Stings result in immediate pain at the affected site, but little inflammation. Mild envenomations produce only local pain whereas more severe envenomations lead to autonomic dysfunction including hypertension, bronchospasm, and hypersalivation and skeletal muscle hyperactivity such as ptosis, saccades, dysphagia, tremors, and chorea.

■ *ED management.* Pain and paresthesias at the site of the bite are best treated with local anesthetic infiltrated directly or via a nerve block, and if no systemic symptoms have occurred within 6 hours the patient may be safely discharged. Patients with systemic symptoms should be managed in consultation with a toxicologist. An antivenom is available but can cause anaphylaxis.

●●● Cat, dog, and human bites are briefly discussed in Chapter 94, "Wound
●●● Care."

Teaching Points

Envenomations are rare injuries often caused by pet snakes. If the patient has no symptoms, the probability is that this was a dry bite, and no treatment other than local wound care is necessary. With symptoms, it is prudent to call the local toxicology service for advice on when and how to give an antivenin, and where to obtain it.

Spider envenomations are often painful, and may cause tissue destruction. Without secondary overgrowth, these do not require antibiotics. Marine wounds tend to be very contaminated and have a different flora than land wounds. For any dirty wound, it is safer to not close the wound primarily.

Suggested Readings

Gold BS, Barish RA, Dart RC. North American snake envenomation: diagnosis, treatment, and management. Emerg Med Clin North Am 2004;22:423–43.
Singletary EM, Rochman AS, Bodmer JCA, Holstege CP. Envenomations. Med Clin North *Am* 2005;89;1195–1224.

65.7 Infestations

Clay B. Smith ■ Lawrence B. Stack

Overview

■ Infestations are defined as a "parasitic attack or subsistence on the skin and its appendages, as by insects, mites, or ticks; sometimes used to denote parasitic invasion of the organs or tissues, as by helminths." As the definition indicates, the cardinal features of most infestations are dermatologic. See Chapters 62 for a discussion of more dermatological problems.

Swimmer's Itch (Cercarial Dermatitis)

- *Epidemiology and risk factors.* Cercarial dermatitis, or swimmer's itch, occurs more often in fresh or brackish water and tends to affect only exposed skin. Exposure to water inhabited by both the definitive avian or mammalian host and the intermediate host, the snail, is necessary for human infestation.
- *Pathophysiology.* Non-human *Schistosoma* spp. and other avian fluke cercariae are the causative organisms. The eggs are shed into the water via bird or mammalian feces, develop into miracidia, infect snails, are released from snails as cercariae, and penetrate exposed human skin in an attempt to find their definitive mammalian or avian host. Skin penetration produces an intense inflammatory response and re-exposure elicits an even more profound hypersensitivity response.
- *Clinical presentation.* The usual history is one of bathing or wading in shallow, warm waters cohabited by snails and various aquatic birds or mammals, with the onset of itching within minutes to hours after emerging from the water and subsequent development of a papular, intensely pruritic rash. Erythematous papules, vesicles, or urticarial lesions will be present only on exposed skin, sparing skin covered by swimwear.
- *ED management.* Vigorous towel drying after swimming in suspect areas may prevent some cercariae from penetrating. After the rash is present, soap and water cleansing and application of topical antipruritics will be soothing. In severe cases, a short course of oral prednisone may be indicated.

Chiggers

- *Epidemiology and risk factors.* One of the most common infestations, chigger bites occur during warmer weather when mites are active. Bites are much more likely to occur in brushy outdoor areas.
- *Pathophysiology.* The adult mite lays eggs in the soil. These larvae crawl onto an unsuspecting host, preferring areas with tight fitting clothing. The bite is usually painless, but after a few hours, pruritis occurs at the site, and often a wheal. The larval mites may remain on the skin for up to 3 days but are easily brushed off the skin, and usually have fallen off by the time the rash is noted. In a previously sensitized individual, the rash may not remain a simple papule, but may progress to papular urticaria or vesiculation. The rash may persist for up to three weeks. New lesions may form up to two days post exposure.
- *Clinical presentation.* Typically patients present with complaints of intense pruritis, rash in areas of tight-fitting clothing, and a history of outdoor exposure in the warmer months. The rash may vary from small 1 to 2 mm papules to larger wheals at each bite site. Papular urticaria

may occur as a result of type IV hypersensitivity causing persistent papules. Lesions may vesiculate and cause localized lymphadenopathy. The rash is usually concentrated in areas where clothing fits snugly, such as the ankles, waistline, groin, or wrist under a watchband.

■ *ED management.* Preventing bites with DEET-containing insect repellent is the best treatment. Keeping the skin cool and dry helps with the pruritis. Antihistamines, particularly those which are sedating, may be helpful as well. Low-potency topical steroids may be needed in cases with severe pruritis. Despite its popularity as a home remedy, there is no evidence that clear nail polish applied to lesions is effective in treating chigger bites.

Cutaneous Larva Migrans

■ *Epidemiology and risk factors.* This is often referred to as a "creeping eruption," and many other colloquialisms. Cutaneous larva migrans can occur in anyone exposed to soil contaminated with dog or cat feces. Most cases occur in warmer climates.

■ *Pathophysiology. Ancyclostoma braziliense*, the dog and cat hookworm, is the most common cause in the United States. Humans are incidental hosts in true cutaneous larva migrans. The hookworm larvae lack the enzymes to penetrate the collagen layer present in human skin and consequently migrate through the subcutaneous tissues between the stratum corneum and stratum germinativum layers, leaving in their wake a serpiginous, palpable tunnel that elicits a robust inflammatory response from the host. The larvae tend to be 1-2 cm ahead of clinically detectable lesions at all times, and can live and migrate in the skin for days to weeks, leaving behind erythematous, pruritic, serpiginous, often vesicular tracts in the skin. This "creeping eruption" may manifest almost immediately or be delayed for months.

■ *Clinical presentation.* The above exposure history will be present in addition to great alarm from the patient at the expanding, intensely pruritic lesions the larvae leave behind. Excoriation may lead to secondary impetigo, crusting, and pain. The rash is very characteristic, and presents as an erythematous ribbon-like rash in the subcutaneous tissues, with the advancing edge having the most intense erythema and often vesiculation. The trailing end of the rash begins to fade in intensity and may crust or scale.

■ *Diagnostic testing.* Rarely does cutaneous larva migrans cause an eosinophilia, as its penetration is quite superficial. Attempts to retrieve the larvae from the skin by excision are ill advised, as the exact location of the larva ahead of the lesion is unknown and less invasive treatments are highly effective.

■ *ED management.* Ninety-eight percent of cases respond to topical 15% thiabendazole cream twice a day, with cessation of migration within 24 hours, and resolution of pruritis and healing of the skin lesions in one to two weeks. For refractory cases, oral thiabendazole may be necessary. Topical glucocorticoids may be helpful for severely pruritic lesions as well as oral antihistamines.

Fleas and Bedbugs

- *Epidemiology and risk factors.* Fleas most often arise from infested pets that live in the house. Bedbugs are most often found in areas with warmer climates. Bedbugs hide in floors, walls, furniture, and in any other crack or crevice, and come out only at night to feed. Bedbugs can not fly or jump, and can run only when temperatures are warm enough.
- *Pathophysiology.* Both produce papular pruritic lesions, and both are common causes of papular urticaria. As they bite, the saliva elicits a robust immune response from the host, leading to the characteristic rash.
- *Clinical presentation.* At times, a papular rash is the presenting complaint, and the clinician is faced with a rash of unclear etiology. A history of pets in the home is usually present in those with fleas. Residing or visiting areas with a warmer climate may be part of the history in those affected by bedbugs, but they can be transported in luggage to new locations. Bedbugs may bite numerous times in one feeding, producing a linear array of bites. The bites may produce pinpoint areas of bleeding that may be noticed as stains on the sheets. Fleshy pruritic papules or, at times, vesicles may be noted.
- *ED management.* Topical steroids and antipruritic agents, oral antihistamines, and good hygiene are usually sufficient to relieve itching. Definitive treatment involves removing the fleas or bedbugs from the home and from pets, and an experienced exterminator or veterinary assistance is essential.

Lice (Pediculosis Capitis, Pediculosis Pubis, and Pediculosis Corporis)

- *Epidemiology and risk factors.* Pediculosis capitis (*Pediculus humanus capitis*) is the most common parasitic infection of children in the United States, with 6-12 million new cases occurring every year. Close contact with affected individuals may result in disease transmission. Epidemics can occur in schools. Pubic lice (*Phthirus pubis*), or "crabs," are most often transmitted sexually. Body lice (*Pediculus humanus corporis*) are encountered during conditions of severe deprivation, such as homelessness, war, natural disaster or in refugee camps where poor hygiene and overcrowding are prevalent.
- *Pathophysiology.* Lice feed by sucking blood from the host. Bites lead to pruritic papular lesions, excoriation, and often impetiginization. The body louse is a common vector for systemic disease, such as trench fever, epidemic typhus (Chapter 67), and relapsing fever.
- *Clinical presentation.* The presenting history is pruritis and a papular rash in the affected area. Head lice are often few in number and difficult to detect, as they hide close to the scalp; but the nits are readily seen attached to hair shafts. Nits that contain live larvae fluoresce with a Wood's lamp. Pubic lice are extremely small and difficult to detect without a magnifying glass. Some patients are very adept at finding the lice and may be able to show them to the examiner. A rash in the pubic area or other hairy areas of the body can alert the clinician to inspect more closely for lice and nits. Maculae ceruleae are small, bluish macules at bite sites due to punctate bruising from the bites. These may be seen

in both pubic and body lice. Body lice are less common but may be suspected in individuals with a characteristic, widespread papular rash who have poor hygiene. The lice will likely not be seen, as they hide in the clothing but nits may be found on clothing, particularly in the seams of clothing.

- *ED management.* Those with lice should be appropriately isolated from other patients. Placing a surgical cap on those with heavy infestations of head lice may help minimize transmission. Often head lice are detected in patients needing hospital admission or medical clearance for psychiatric admission. These patients can be treated in the ED with 1% permethrin cream applied to the scalp for 10 minutes, then rinsed; the treatment is repeated in 1 to 2 weeks to ensure that any nits that may have survived initial treatment and hatched can not reinfect the patient. Of course, the same therapy can be prescribed for outpatient treatment as well, and many topical pyrethrins are available over-the-counter. The entire household should be treated simultaneously. The home should be thoroughly cleaned and all clothing and bedding washed in hot water and dried. Items not able to be laundered can be stored in a sealed plastic bag for a month. Combs, brushes, and other toiletry items should be soaked in alcohol for one hour and washed in hot water. Treatment is highly effective, and one may be assured that treated patients are no longer contagious. Pubic lice are treated similarly to head lice, except that medication is applied to all hair bearing areas. Pubic lice affecting eyelashes should have an occlusive coating of petrolatum applied to the lashes twice a day for ten days. Sexual contacts and others in close contact must be treated as well. Homeless patients will greatly benefit from laundering and drying of their clothes and bedding before discharge to prevent immediate recurrence. Allowing them to shower and apply a topical pyrethrin preparation and rinse is a merciful practice, and may prevent the spread of serious systemic disease. Decontamination of the ED simply consists of thorough cleaning of the room and laundering of all blankets and pillowcases in hot water.

Myiasis

- *Epidemiology and risk factors.* This is a condition of having fly larvae feeding on or in the body and is commonly referred to as "maggots". Open wounds or extremely poor hygiene may result in larvae being deposited on the body or in a wound.
- *Pathophysiology.* Flies are attracted to dead and decaying organic matter, land there to feed, and lay their eggs there to develop. Fly larvae, or maggots, then develop and grow, feeding on the organic matter upon which they were deposited. At times they are deposited on the skin or clothing of individuals with poor hygiene. They may even be deposited in the nasopharynx, paranasal sinuses, anal or vaginal area, or just about anywhere else in or on the body.
- *Clinical presentation.* Homeless people with filthy, soiled clothing are subject to infestation with maggots, as is anyone with an open wound. A maggot infestation is readily apparent on the skin or in the wound. They appear as small, whitish, motile, wormlike objects. Lesions caused

by botfly larvae look strikingly similar to a common furuncle, but on closer inspection one may notice the central breathing pore, bubbling from the wound, or movement of the larva itself inside the lesion.

- *ED management.* Maggots can be brushed off the skin or gently irrigated from a wound. While they may be unsavory in appearance, maggots are highly effective at debridement of necrotic debris from a wound, and often the appearance of a wound that has been infested with maggots is quite clean, free of necrotic debris, with good granulation tissue. The botfly is not gotten rid of so easily. It comes equipped with rows of spines around its body that prevent it from slipping backwards out of the wound. The breathing pore may be occluded for 24 hours with occlusive petrolatum, suffocating the larva. It may then emerge or be manually expressed, but often a small cruciate skin incision and extraction of the larva is necessary. If signs of cellulitis are present, then antibiotics are needed.

Scabies

- *Epidemiology and risk factors.* Scabies is also known as the "seven year itch," as it causes intense pruritis that may go undiagnosed for long periods of time. Scabies tends to occur more commonly in conditions of overcrowding and in institutionalized patients. Close contacts of individuals with scabies are also at a much higher risk of infestation.
- *Pathophysiology.* Scabies is caused by the arachnid *Sarcoptes scabiei*, var. *hominis*. It is an obligate human parasite and can only live for three days without contact with a human host. They are freely mobile on human skin at body temperature, are unable to fly or jump from host to host, and can only be transmitted by direct contact with a host or, less commonly, by contact with recently contaminated fomites. Female mites cause human disease by burrowing into the skin and laying eggs behind in the newly formed tunnel. Scybala, or feces, is also deposited in the burrows. Presence of these antigens elicits a type IV hypersensitivity response, causing severe pruritis. Often bite sites become excoriated and may become superinfected by bacteria.
- *Clinical presentation.* Pruritis, especially at night, is usually the chief complaint. Patients may also complain of a rash. Pruritis may precede the rash by several weeks in some cases. Often, family members are affected as well. The burrow made by the female mite is the most characteristic lesion. Burrows tend to be 2-3 mm in length, may have a small papule at the end, are slightly raised, and distributed on the finger and toe webs, hands, knees, arm flexure surfaces, groin (including the scrotum and penis), perianal area and buttocks, waistline, and axillae, sparing the head and neck. Nodular scabies occurs less than 10% of the time and consists of fleshy colored nodules at burrow sites. Norwegian, or crusted scabies, are hyperkeratotic and, as the name suggests, crusted; lesions were mistaken for leprosy. Lesions may be vesicular, papular, or pustular. Most burrows will be excoriated and are often eczematous or impetiginous in appearance. Superimposed bacterial infection is common. Infants tend to have more mites, more widespread lesions, and lesions involving the head, neck, face, palms and soles. Pustular lesions are more common in

infants as well. Infants may present with fussiness, poor sleep, or with rubbing together of the hands and feet.

- **Diagnostic testing.** An intact burrow is covered with mineral oil and scraped with a scalpel blade or back of a scalpel blade. The scrapings are then viewed with or without a cover slip under low power microscopy. Findings of a mite, ova, or scybala are diagnostic for infestation.
- **ED management.** Topical permethrin 5% cream is applied from head to toe, completely covering all skin and nail surfaces, overnight for 8 to 14 hours, and then washed off. The treatment should be repeated in one week. Infants less that 2 months and pregnant or lactating women should be treated with precipitated sulfur 5% to 10% in petrolatum daily for 3 consecutive days. Treatment with the sulfur compound is foul-smelling and can stain clothing. Oral ivermectin 200mcg/kg has been used to treat Norwegian scabies or refractory cases, especially in immunocompromised patients, and has been shown to have equal efficacy to topical permethrin when the ivermectin dose is repeated in 2 weeks. All family members and close contacts within the past month should be treated, whether or not they are symptomatic. All clothing and bedding should be washed in hot water and dried on the hot cycle or dry cleaned. Larger items that are not amenable to washing, such as pillows, should be sealed in an airtight bag or kept from human contact for over 72 hours.

Teaching Points

Infestations of human skin are common in lower socioeconomic groups, institutionalized patients, children, and immunocompromised patients. A generalized pruritic rash usually follows the infestation. Look carefully, it may require a magnifying glass, in all body hair, especially the scalp and the pubic hair.

Treatment may require topical or oral steroids, antihistamines to control the pruritis, or antimicrobial agents. Treatment of all contacts is helpful in preventing recurrence.

Suggested Readings

Huynh TH, Norman RA. Scabies and pediculosis. Dermatol Clin 2004;22:7–11.
Brimhall CL, Esterly NB. Uninvited guests: skin infestations of childhood. Cont Peds 1990;7:18–57.
Steen CJ, Carbonaro PA, Schwartz RA. Arthropods in dermatology. J Am Acad Dermatol 2004;50:819–842.
Fitzpatrick TB, Johnson RA, Wolff K, Suurmond D. Color Atlas & Synopsis of Clinical Dermatology: Common and Serious Diseases. 4th ed. New York: McGraw-Hill, 2001.

CHAPTER 66

Hematologic-Oncologic Emergencies

LISA D. MILLS ■ GRANVILLE A. MORSE, III

Overview

The hematologic-oncologic patient often has many complex processes occurring simultaneously.

Aggressively control pain in patients with cancer presenting to the ED. Obtain a thorough history including chemotherapy and radiation history, staging, and current treatment. Most of these patients are immunocompromised. Evaluate for the presence of neutropenia, and implement reverse isolation precautions in these patients. The presence of a fever is a true emergency, and almost always a sufficient reason to admit the patient. Nonspecific complaints such as shortness of breath, abdominal pain, weakness, and headache have extensive differential diagnoses in these patients due to a predisposition to mass lesions, cytopenias, infection, electrolyte disorders, hyperviscosity syndrome, and thromboembolic disorders.

Hematologic disorders that may present to the ED include anemia, thrombocytopenia, neutropenia, and abnormal hemostasis. Neutropenia is defined as a neutrophilic granulocyte count of less than 1500/mm^3 and is calculated as follows:

$$\text{Absolute neutrophil count} = \text{white blood cell (WBC) count} \times$$
$$(\% \text{ bands} + \% \text{ mature neutrophils}) \times 0.01$$

Anemia is a common problem seen in the ED. It is more of a symptom than a disease itself, and is mentioned in various chapters of this book (see Chapter 34 "Gastrointestinal Bleed", Chapter 43 "Lightheaded and Dizzy", and Chapter 60 "Weakness"), but will be briefly discussed here. Sickle cell anemia is discussed in Chapter 53. Although a rare event, the porphyrias are briefly mentioned here due to the wide spectrum of manifestations of the disease that may be mistaken for other, more commonly, seen diagnoses (e.g., surgical abdomen).

Specific Problems: Oncologic Emergencies
Airway Obstruction

■ Patients with cancers involving the neck, oropharynx, thyroid, bronchial tree, or the mediastinum are at risk for this emergency.

- Obstruction of the trachea from mechanical compression of the airway by tumors causes airway compromise. If the circumstances mandate an emergent airway in the ED, have multiple airway options available (see Chapter 5).

Cardiac Tamponade

- *Epidemiology and risk factors.* These are most commonly due to the spread of lymphoma, leukemia, melanoma, breast, and lung cancer to the pericardium.
- *Pathophysiology.* The mechanism of effusion is unknown. The consequence of the effusion depends on the rate of accumulation. If fluid accumulates slowly, the pericardium stretches to accommodate the fluid, causing little impact on cardiac function. If the fluid accumulates rapidly, the pericardium cannot stretch to accommodate the fluid. The volume usually cannot exceed 250 ml. In this case, the result is increased pressure in the pericardial sac. When this pressure exceeds pressures in the heart, chambers of the heart collapse. The right atrium has the lowest pressures and collapses first. Right atrial collapse impairs cardiac filling. The result is decreased cardiac output and hypotension. The initial response is a tachycardia; however, just before arrest, the heart will slow. At this point it will be necessary to perform a thoracotomy to effect drainage of the pericardial sac; a pericardiocentesis won't be effective at this stage.
- *History.* The patient's complaints can be related to the pain of local malignant infiltration, or to decreased cardiac output. The patient may present with cough, chest pain, dyspnea, edema, nausea, paroxysmal nocturnal dyspnea, orthopnea, and hoarseness. If the fluid accumulation has been gradual, patients provide a history of progressive shortness of breath or dyspnea on exertion.
- *Physical examination.* Beck's triad is the classic physical examination finding in tamponade. The triad includes jugular venous distention, muffled heart tones, and hypotension. Patients may not have all three of these present. In addition the patient may be tachypneic. If the process has been gradual, the patient may have lower extremity edema.
- *Diagnostic testing.* Although the EKG may show a diagnostic finding of electrical alternans, it is more prudent to establish the diagnosis with a cardiac ultrasound study. Bedside ultrasound will also assist in needle placement for a therapeutic pericardiocentesis. If accumulation of fluid has been gradual, the chest radiograph shows a "water bottle" heart. If accumulation of the fluid has been rapid, the cardiomediastinal silhouette will be normal. The radiograph will also help identify other causes of shortness of breath including infection, airway compression, or pulmonary metastatic disease. An echocardiogram will show pericardial effusion with right atria collapse.
- *ED management.* An IV fluid bolus may temporarily improve blood pressure while preparing for pericardiocentesis (see Chapter 91). Cardiac tamponade requires emergent pericardiocentesis. Ultrasound guidance should be used when available. The patient's oncologist should be notified. Cardiothoracic surgery should be consulted for a pericardial

drain or pericardial window for definitive therapy. These patients require admission to the intensive care unit.

■ *Helpful hints and pitfalls.* A patient presenting in pulseless electrical activity (PEA) with distended neck veins should have an emergent pericardiocentesis.

Hypercalcemia

■ Hypercalcemia occurs in 10% to 20% of patients with cancer, and is considered the most common metabolic emergency of malignancy. It is most often associated with metastatic spread from breast, lung, and renal carcinoma, but is also associated with hematologic cancers.

■ See Chapter 88 for ED management.

Hyperviscosity Syndrome (HVS)

■ *Epidemiology and risk factors.* This occurs in patients with Waldenström's macroglobulinemia (85%-90% of cases), multiple myeloma (5%-10% of cases), and high cell count leukemias.

■ *Pathophysiology.* Increased serum viscosity occurs from hyperproteinemia and rigid cells. This causes hematologic sludging and cell clumping at small vessels. The result is microvasculature hypoperfusion.

■ *History.* A symptomatic triad of bleeding, visual disturbances, and neurologic manifestations is a classic presentation of HVS. Hypoperfusion of the brain leads to neurologic deficits that can be waxing and waning but has a sudden onset. Patients may complain of fatigue, shortness of breath, or headache.

■ *Physical examination.* Mucosal bleeding, epistaxis, and "sausage-like" retinal veins are pathognomonic for the hyperviscosity syndrome. Retinal exudates, hemorrhage, and papilledema are late findings. Patients may have focal neurologic findings that mimic an acute cerebrovascular accident.

■ *Diagnostic testing.* A CBC with peripheral smear may show leukocytosis and rouleaux (stacking of erythrocytes) formation. Renal function should be evaluated for damage from hypoperfusion. Electrolytes should be evaluated as a cause of the patient's symptoms. In multiple myeloma, significant hypercalcemia may also occur, and with high M protein fractions, a factitious hyponatremia may be present. Serum and urine protein electrophoresis should be done with all suspected dysproteinemias. A large spike on the serum electrophoresis supports the diagnosis. The laboratory may be unable to perform chemical tests on the blood because of the serum stasis and increased viscosity that clogs analyzers.

■ *ED management.* The goal of therapy is to decrease the serum viscosity. Isotonic intravenous fluid is the mainstay of treatment in the ED. The patient's oncologist should be consulted to arrange exchange transfusion. Emergent phlebotomy is a temporizing measure when exchange transfusion is not emergently available. Admit these patients to the hospital.

■ *Helpful hints and pitfalls.* Consider a hyperviscosity syndrome in patients with malignancy and bleeding, visual changes, or neurologic deficit. If blood cannot be processed in the laboratory machines, suspect hyperviscosity.

Neutropenia

- *Epidemiology and risk factors.* Neutropenia is an absolute neutrophil count (ANC) less than 1500 neutrophils per microliter (see calculation in the "Overview"). The absolute neutrophil count can be classified as mild (1,000 to 1,500 cells/mm^3), moderate (500 to 1,000 cells/mm^3), and severe (<500 cells/mm^3) risk levels for infection. Patients are at risk for neutropenia if they are undergoing chemotherapy or radiation, or they have a cancer that can infiltrate the marrow. The mortality rate has been reported as high as 50%.

- *Pathophysiology.* Chemotherapeutic drugs will destroy blood cell lines, especially the granulocytic line (e.g., neutrophils). Neutrophils function to phagocytose and destroy microbes. Loss of neutrophil response leaves patients with an impaired inflammatory response to infection and an impaired immune system. Patients with neutropenia may not have classic presentation of illness. Infection is most commonly from gram-positive organisms, especially *Staphylococcus aureus*. If a patient develops fever following a course of broad-spectrum antibiotics, fungal infections should be considered.

- *History.* Symptoms may be vague and difficult for the patient to localize due to the impaired inflammatory response. As a result, patients may only have generalized complaints such as weakness or lethargy. A detailed review of systems should be performed in an attempt to localize the infection.

- *Physical examination.* Due to an impaired inflammatory response, neutropenic patients may not develop a fever in the presence of significant infection. Be aware of other signs of the inflammatory response such as hypothermia, tachycardia, tachypnea, and hypotension. Patients with neutropenia should undergo a thorough examination with all clothing removed. Common sites for hidden infection are the ocular fundus, oropharynx, dentition, esophagus, covered portions of the skin, perianal, perineum, and periungual areas. Do not perform a rectal examination on patients with neutropenia, as this can produce a bacteremia that the patient cannot respond to because of the immunosuppression.

- *Diagnostic testing.* CBC with differential will show ANC below 1500/mm^3. Two sets of blood cultures and a urinalysis with cultures should also be obtained. Obtain cultures from any indwelling lines. Send stool studies if the patient is having diarrhea. A chest radiograph is a standard part of the evaluation of a neutropenic patient who is sick or has a fever.

- *ED management.* Apply neutropenic precautions to patients, including masks, stringent hand washing, and dietary precautions. Do not delay antibiotic therapy. Once allergies are established, the choice of antimicrobial therapy should be broad spectrum antibiotics to include coverage for *P. aeruginosa*. Empiric antibiotic therapy should also be directed toward the patient's risk factors for infection, and should be chosen in recognition of local resistance patterns. Antibiotic monotherapy can be given with either a carbapenem (e.g., imipenem-cilastatin, meropenem) or an extended-spectrum antipseudomonal cephalosporin, such as ceftazidime or cefepime. Piperacillin/tazobactam may also be effective as monotherapy. Duotherapy is useful with a combination of an aminoglycoside and antipseudomonal penicillin or cephalosporin. Vancomycin should be used for high-risk patients: catheter-related infection, blood culture positive for gram-positive bacteria, known colonization with methicillin-resistant *S. aureus,* and hypotension or shock without identified pathogen. Empiric antifungal treatment is not indicated. If the patient has a history of fungal infection or recently discontinued broad-spectrum antibiotics, antifungal therapy may be warranted. Patients with neutropenia and suspected infection should be admitted to the hospital.

Spinal Cord Compression

- This occurs in almost 5% of all cancer patients. The most common causes are metastatic breast, lung, and prostate cancers. Multiple myeloma, lymphoma, melanoma, sarcoma, or renal cancers cause spinal cord compression by local extension. The most common site is the thoracic spine followed by the lumbar spine. The presentation may be similar to other conditions causing spinal cord compression (see Chapters 12 and 21).
- MRI is the optimal imaging study. If an emergent MRI is not available or contraindicated because of implanted metallic foreign bodies (e.g., certain heart valves), a CT scan with contrast is an alternative imaging study. Plain films of the spine may show osteolytic lesions.
- This is a true emergency, as delays in decompression may lead to irreversible nerve damage. Consult with the neurosurgical and radiation oncology services as soon as cord compression is suspected. The definitive therapy is radiation or surgical decompression. IV steroids decrease edema, and decrease compression on the spinal cord in the interim. If urinary retention is present, place a urinary catheter. These patients require admission, often to an ICU.

Superior Vena Cava Syndrome

- *Epidemiology and risk factors.* This entity is most commonly caused by invasive tumors of the lungs, such as small cell carcinoma, but may also be caused by lymphomas, leukemias, or metastases from breast or prostate cancer. The incidence is approximately 2% to 4% of all patients with cancer, with lung cancer the leading cause (65%) of all superior vena cava (SVC) syndromes.
- *Pathophysiology.* A mass compresses, or a tumor infiltrates the SVC. This prevents return of blood from the arms, head, and neck to the heart. Accumulation of blood leads to edema of the head and neck, and to an increased venous pressure in the head. This can lead to edema of the airway with eventual airway compromise. Although life-threatening SVC syndrome effects such as airway obstruction or laryngeal or cerebral edema are rare, they do occur and must be addressed early.

- **History.** The onset of SVC syndrome is insidious, with the gradual development of facial and neck swelling. Patients report dyspnea, cough, and orthopnea.
- **Physical examination.** Face and neck swelling are common findings. Upper extremity swelling may be present. Venous plethora of the neck and shoulder may be noted. Jugular venous distention is present, and may be the first sign of the syndrome, as well as the first sign the patient notices. Occasionally patients have signs of respiratory distress such as tachypnea, stridor, or use of accessory muscles of respiration. This indicates impending airway failure. As described above, invasion of the trachea or bronchi often coexists with an SVCS.
- **Diagnostic testing.** A chest radiograph may reveal a mass in the mediastinum. A CT scan with IV contrast of the neck and chest will define the mass, and delineate involved structures.
- **ED management.** Provide supplemental oxygen, limit fluids, and elevate the head of the bed. Steroids may decrease edema in the mass, decreasing compression of the SVC. In patients with impending airway failure, immediate measures should be taken to obtain a definitive airway. Radiation therapy is the treatment of choice in most cases of SVC syndrome. Patients with any airway compromise should be admitted to the ICU. Patients without signs or symptoms of airway involvement can be admitted to the hospital, but do not require ICU care.
- **Helpful hints and pitfalls.** Be prepared for a difficult airway.

Syndrome of Inappropriate Antidiuretic Hormone Secretion

- The syndrome of inappropriate antidiuretic hormone secretion (SIADH) occurs in only 1% to 2% of cancer patients. Patients with small cell cancers comprise almost 60% of the cases. There is an ectopic secretion of antidiuretic hormone from oat cell, pancreatic, prostate, adrenal, and esophageal cancers. This causes retention of free water in the kidney. Metastatic disease to the brain is also associated with SIADH. Vincristine and cyclophosphamide are implicated in SIADH. Symptoms are due to cellular edema, particularly in the brain.
- The presentation depends on the severity of hyponatremia (see Chapter 88). The patients appear euvolemic. Mental status changes vary from mild confusion to coma.
- Fluid restriction (500 ml to 1 L per 24 hours) is the mainstay of treatment. Reserve 3% normal saline for patients with seizures. Do not correct the sodium faster than 0.5 to 1.0 mEq/L/h to avoid central pontine myelinolysis. Demeclocycline has been shown to help in refractory patients, but usually fluid restriction and treatment of the underlying cause, will bring resolution. These patients require admission to a telemetry unit. Patients with severe hyponatremia deserve ICU admission. Patients with mild, incidental, asymptomatic hyponatremia can be discharged home with fluid restriction instructions and follow-up with the oncologist.

Tumor Lysis Syndrome

- **Epidemiology and risk factors.** Tumor lysis syndrome occurs in rapidly multiplying tumors, large tumor burdens, and with depressed renal function. It most often affects patients with lymphomas and leukemias. Radiation and chemotherapy, especially induction regimens, cause tumor lysis syndrome.

- *Pathophysiology.* There are metabolic abnormalities consisting of hyperkalemia, hyperuricemia, hyperphosphatemia, and hypocalcemia. These occur secondary to the rapid breakdown of the cells with destruction and release of RNA, DNA, and uric acid.

- *History.* Patients usually present within a week of induction chemotherapy. Their complaints will vary dependant on which metabolic derangement is most prominent. They may have altered mental status, seizures, muscle spasms, fatigue, weakness, or a combination of any of these.

- *Physical examination.* The patients are often dehydrated, and may have an altered mental status. Cardiac dysrhythmias can occur.

- *Diagnostic testing.* A CBC will help to reveal other causes of these general complaints, including hyperviscosity syndrome, infection, and anemia. Electrolytes and serum uric acid levels should be drawn. Usually hyperkalemia, hyperuricemia, hyperphosphatemia, and hypocalcemia are present. The blood urea nitrogen (BUN) and creatinine may also be elevated. An EKG may reveal severe electrolyte disorders and dysrhythmias.

- *ED management.* Monitor the patient on a cardiac monitor. Aggressive intravenous fluid rehydration is important. Treat electrolyte disorders as appropriate (see Chapter 88). Severe cases will require emergent dialysis. These patients are admitted to the ICU. Early involvement of an oncologist is advisable.

- *Helpful hints and pitfalls.* These patients can decompensate quickly. Suspect tumor lysis syndrome in patients who have recently received chemotherapy or radiation treatment.

Specific Problems: Hematologic Emergencies
Anemia

- *Epidemiology and risk factors.* Anemia is the most common hematologic problem presenting to the ED. The causes can be classified as blood loss, decreased production (hypoproliferative), or increased destruction (hemolytic). Iron deficiency is the most common cause of anemia in the ED. It is the most common anemia in women of child-bearing age. Occult blood loss should be suspected in older individuals. Except in the setting of acute blood loss, the new onset of anemia in an adult is more commonly associated with a hypoproliferative process rather than a hemolytic one. Nutritional deficiencies are the most common cause of hypoproliferative anemia worldwide, and affect both adult and pediatric patients. It is estimated that 4% of women in the United States have iron deficiency anemia. Anemia of acute or chronic inflammation (rheumatoid arthritis, chronic infections), hypoendocrinism (hypothyroidism, hypopituitarism, hypoadrenalism), and anemia of renal disease are other common causes of hypoproliferative anemia. Malignancies that infiltrate the bone marrow or red blood cell aplasia are less common examples of a hypoproliferative anemia. Hemolytic anemias may be congenital or acquired. The congenital causes often present early in childhood (e.g., β-thalassemia, sickle cell anemia) or are provoked by stressors later in life (e.g., glucose-6-phosphate dehydrogenase deficiency). Aplastic anemia is rare condition that can affect all cell lines, and is related to drug or chemical exposure in 50% of cases. Other causes include viral hepatitis, radiation, pregnancy, or an autoimmune problem.

■ *Pathophysiology.* In response to acute or chronic blood loss, there is decreased oxygen delivery to the kidney resulting in increased erythro-poietin, which then stimulates red blood cell (RBC) production in the bone marrow. Provided that there is an adequate supply of folate, vitamin B_{12}, iron, and other nutrients, the marrow responds by increasing the production and release of erythrocytes into the circulation. Erythro-poietin stimulates the proliferation and differentiation of stem cells in the bone marrow resulting in the release of reticulocytes into the circulation. Within 1 day, reticulocytes transition into mature red blood cells that circulate for 100 to 120 days, at which time they are removed from the circulation by macrophages in the spleen and other reticuloendothelial tissues. Hypoproliferative anemias are the result of decreased RBC production from acquired nutritional deficiencies or systemic disease. Both impair erythropoiesis in the bone marrow. Anemia of renal disease, for example, is due to a deficiency of erythropoietin. Common causes of iron deficiency anemia are uterine and gastrointestinal sources. Hemolytic anemia is due to an accelerated breakdown of RBCs. Hemolytic anemias may be caused by processes intrinsic or extrinsic to the cell membrane (Table 66–1).

■ *History.* Symptoms of significant acute blood loss include thirst, altered mental status, and decreased urine output. Patients may complain of fatigue, weakness, headache, lightheadnesses, shortness of breath, or chest pain. Identify any potential sources of bleeding such as rectal bleeding, hematuria, or vaginal bleeding in females of reproductive age. Medical history that might suggest the source of anemia or might complicate the anemia (i.e., cardiac disease) should be elicited. Any previous blood transfusion should be ascertained. Ask about drug use as certain medications may be associated with bone marrow depression or the development of autoimmune hemolytic anemia. Occupational and environmental exposures should be determined, as lead or other poten-tially marrow toxic agents can cause anemia. Social history, such as risk factors for HIV, and dietary history should be assessed. Family history of anemia should be assessed to determine risk for inherited forms of anemia such as hereditary spherocytosis and sickle cell anemia.

■ *Physical examination.* Patients with acute blood loss may present with tachycardia, decreased blood pressure, postural hypotension, and increased respiratory rate. Pallor may be present. Patients with slowly developing anemia are hemodynamically stable. Angular cheilitis (cracking at the edges of the lips) and koilonychia (spooning of the nails) may accompany iron deficiency anemia. Splenomegaly may be present in young patients with congenital hemolytic anemia, such as thalassemia, sickle cell disease, or hereditary spherocytosis. In older patients splenomegaly with an acquired disorder, such as autoimmune hemolytic anemia, lymphoproliferative disease, or agnogenic myeloid metaplasia may be present. A systolic cardiac murmur may be present in patients

Table 66–1	**Classification of Hemolytic Anemias**	
	Problem	**Example**
Intrinsic	Enzyme defect	Pyruvate kinase deficiency G6PD deficiency
	Membrane abnormality	Spherocytosis Paroxysmal nocturnal hemoglobinuria
	Hemoglobin abnormality	Sickle cell anemia Thalassemia
Extrinsic	Immunologic	ABO incompatibility Autoimmune
	Mechanical	Microangiopathic hemolytic anemia (thrombocytic thrombocytopenia, disseminated intravascular coagulation, and malignant hypertension) Prosthetic valve disease
	Environmental	Drugs (sulfa drugs, oral hypoglycemic agents, quinidine, high doses of penicillin and cephalosporins, d-, methyldopa) Toxins (brown recluse spider or snake bite) Infection (Malaria and *Clostridium* sepsis) Hyperthermia
	Abnormal sequestration	Hypersplenism

with anemia itself, but may be increased in patients with a perivalvular leak or prosthetic dysfunction. Neurologic manifestations such as loss of vibration or position sense may be a clue to vitamin B_{12} deficiency. The skin should be evaluated for petechiae, ecchymoses, pallor, jaundice, or diaphoresis. A rectal examination should be performed to evaluate for overt or occult bleeding.

■ *Diagnostic testing.* The most important laboratory test used in diagnosing anemia is the CBC. Age and sex-related differences in hemoglobin and hematocrit levels are listed in Table 66–2. An attempt

Table 66–2	**Hemogram Normal Values**		
Age	Hemoglobin (g/dl)	Hematocrit (ml/dl)	Red blood cell count ($\times 10^6$)
3 mo	10.4–12.2	30–36	3.4–4.0
3–7 y	11.7–13.5	34–40	4.4–5.0
Adult man	14.0–18.0	40–52	4.4–5.9
Adult woman	12.0–16.0	35–47	3.8–5.2

should be made to determine the patient's baseline levels. In the setting of acute blood loss, it may hours before the hematocrit accurately reflects the degree of blood loss. The mean corpuscular volume (MCV) is the most commonly used RBC index, and reflects average cell size. It is calculated by dividing the hematocrit by the RBC count. The normal range is 81 to 100 μm^3. Microcytic anemia with an MCV of less than 70 fL is most commonly due to iron deficiency anemia or thalassemia. Values between about 70 fL and the lower limit of normal may be associated with the anemia of chronic disease, hyperthyroidism, or other causes. Macrocytic anemias, with an MCV of greater than 120 fL, are associated with folate or vitamin B_{12} deficiency. Otherwise, MCV values above the upper limit of normal suggest the possibility of increased ethanol intake, liver disease, or bone marrow failure states such as aplastic anemia or myelodysplastic syndromes. The most commonly encountered normocytic hypoproliferative anemia in adults is that of chronic disease, which includes anemia due to renal disease and inflammatory causes. If the diagnosis is still uncertain, the reticulocyte count and peripheral blood smear are very helpful. The reticulocyte count is a marker of RBC production. When reported as a percentage (instead of an absolute number), it needs to be adjusted for the total number of RBCs present. This correction can be achieved by multiplying the reticulocyte count by the patient's hematocrit divided by an age- and gender-appropriate normal hematocrit. A corrected reticulocyte count of less than 2% or absolute reticulocyte count of less than 100,000/μL are associated with hypoproliferative anemias, whereas values above these are associated with either an appropriate response to blood loss or with hemolytic (hyperproliferative) anemias. Aplastic anemia may extend to all cell lines and manifests as a normocytic anemia and a low reticulocyte count. Severe aplastic anemia is present when two of the following are present: the ANC is less than 500/mm^3, platelets are less than 20,000/mm^3, or the reticulocyte count is less than 40,000/mm^3. The peripheral smear may be a clue to the cause of the anemia. Commonly encountered findings that can be seen in red blood cells on the peripheral blood smear are listed in Table 66–3. The typical cell seen in intravascular hemolysis is the schistocyte. A spherocyte is the classic cell identified in extravascular hemolysis. Additional diagnostic testing for hemolysis includes haptoglobin levels (decreased when saturated with hemoglobin), fractionated bilirubin (both conjugated and unconjugated bilirubin are increased), lactate dehydrogenase (increased with RBC breakdown), plasma-free and urine hemoglobin (increased), and direct (tests antibody or complement on RBC membrane) and indirect Coomb's test (measures antibody titers in serum). A bone marrow biopsy is sometimes required, but need not be performed in the ED. Hematologic disorders such as myelodysplasia, leukemia, lymphoma, or myeloma may be identified.

- **ED management.** Several factors will influence the management of patients with anemia such as the underlying etiology, rate of onset, ongoing bleeding, symptomatology (e.g., chest pain, shortness of breath, orthostasis), the hemodynamic reserve, and the degree of anemia of the patient. Anemia from an acute gastrointestinal bleeding is discussed in Chapter 34. Sickle cell anemia is covered in Chapter 53. Trauma is

Table 66–3 Features of the Peripheral Blood Smear

Red Blood Cell Morphology	Definition	Interpretation
Polychromasia	Large, bluish red blood cells lacking normal central pallor on peripheral blood smear; bluish stain is the result of residual ribonucleic acid.	Rapid production and release of red blood cells from marrow; elevated reticulocyte count; most commonly seen in hemolytic anemia.
Basophilic stippling	Many small bluish dots in portion of erythrocytes; comes from staining of clustered polyribosomes in young circulating red blood cells.	Seen in a variety of erythropoietic disorders, including acquired and congenital hemolytic anemias, and occasionally in lead poisoning (lead inhibits pyrimidine 5'-nucleotidase, which normally digests the residual RNA).
Pappenheimer bodies	Several grayish, irregularly shaped inclusions in a portion of erythrocytes visible on peripheral smear; composed of aggregates of ribosomes, ferritin, and mitochondria.	Erythropoietic malfunction in congenital anemias such as hemoglobinopathies, particularly with splenic hypofunction or acquired anemias such as megaloblastic anemia.
Heinz bodies	Several grayish, round inclusions visible after supravital staining with methyl crystal violet of the peripheral blood smear, represent aggregates of denatured hemoglobin.	Indicative of oxidative injury to the erythrocyte, such as occurs in G6PD deficiency, or less commonly of unstable hemoglobins.
Howell-Jolly bodies	Usually one or at most a few purplish inclusions in the erythrocyte visible on the routine peripheral blood smear; represent residual fragments of nuclei containing chromatin.	Associated with states of splenic hypofunction or after splenectomy.

Continued

Table 66–3   Features of the Peripheral Blood Smear—*cont'd*

Red Blood Cell Morphology	Definition	Interpretation
Schistocytes	Red blood cells that are fragmented into a variety of shapes and sizes, including helmet-shaped cells; indicative of shearing of the erythrocyte within the circulation.	Associated with microangiopathic hemolytic anemias, including disseminated intravascular coagulation, thrombocytic thrombocytopenia, hemolytic uremic syndrome, as well as other mechanical causes of hemolysis, such as prosthetic valves.
Spherocytes	Red blood cells that have lost their central pallor and appear spherical; indicative of loss of cytoskeletal integrity due to internal or external causes.	Associated with hereditary spherocytosis, autoimmune hemolytic anemia; may also be observed in addition to schistocytes in the presence of microangiopathic hemolytic anemia.
Teardrop cells	Pear-shaped erythrocytes visible on peripheral blood smear; indicative of mechanical stress on the red blood cell during release from the bone marrow or passage through the spleen.	Seen in a variety of conditions, including congenital anemias such as thalassemia and acquired disorders such as megaloblastic anemia; may also suggest a more ominous process such as myelophthisis (marrow replacement).
Burr cells (echinocytes)	Red blood cells that have smooth undulations present on the surface circumferentially; pathogenesis unknown.	Indicative of uremia when present on a properly made peripheral blood smear.
Spur cells (acanthocytes)	Red blood cells that have spiny points present on the surface circumferentially; reflective of abnormal lipid composition of red blood cell membrane.	Most commonly indicative of liver disease when present in significant numbers; also seen in betalipoproteinemia and in red blood cells lacking the Kell blood group antigen.

covered in Section III of this text. TTP is discussed in a subsequent section of this chapter. The treatment for other causes of anemia is listed in Table 66–4. For aplastic anemia, the possible offending agent is discontinued. Blood transfusion is given only in life-threatening situations. Definitive treatments include stem cell transplantation or immunosuppression. Stable patients should be admitted if they develop any cardiac (chest pain, shortness of breath) or neurologic symptoms, have an unexplained hemoglobin level less than 8 to 10 g/dL, or a hematocrit less than 25% to 30% especially if the patient is elderly or has underlying cardiovascular or cerebrovascular disease. Patients with poor social circumstances may also require admission.

- *Helpful hints and pitfalls.* Children and young adults may tolerate a significant blood loss with unaltered vital signs until a precipitant hypotensive episode occurs. The elderly, on the other hand, often have a decreased ability to compensate and underlying co-morbidities that are affected by the anemia.

Disseminated Intravascular Coagulation

- *Epidemiology and risk factors.* Disseminated intravascular coagulation (DIC) most commonly occurs in patients with sepsis. Other risk factors for DIC are labor and delivery, acute leukemia, multisystem trauma, liver disease, and massive transfusion.
- *Pathophysiology.* The coagulation cascade and the fibrinolytic system are simultaneously activated without regulatory factors. There is massive consumption of platelets and clotting factors. Thrombosis and bleeding disorders result.
- *History.* Severely ill patients who develop diffuse bleeding or new focal neurologic deficits should be suspected of having DIC.
- *Physical examination.* Hallmarks of DIC are petechiae, ecchymoses, purpura, or distal ischemia and gangrene (i.e., scrotum and fingertips). Additionally, there may be mental status changes, respiratory distress, focal neurologic deficits, gastrointestinal bleeding, or oliguria.
- *Diagnostic testing.* A peripheral smear will show evidence of cellular damage, schistocytes and red cell fragments, thrombocytopenia, and anemia. The prothrombin time (PT), partial thromboplastin time (PTT), and thrombin times will be elevated. Fibrinogen levels will be low, reflecting consumption. There may be an increase in fibrin split products. Renal function should be assessed for damage due to microvascular ischemia. Hepatic function tests may show elevation of liver enzymes. A chest radiograph is indicated to evaluate for acute respiratory distress syndrome.
- *ED management.* The primary problem that led to DIC must be addressed. If bleeding predominates, transfuse platelets, fresh frozen plasma, and cryoprecipitate (see Chapter 84). If clotting predominates, heparin may be beneficial. These patients require admission to an ICU.
- *Helpful hints and pitfalls.* Look for DIC in acutely decompensated, critically ill patients. The fibrinogen may be falsely elevated as this is an acute phase reactant. Do not exclude DIC based on a normal fibrinogen level.

Table 66–4 Anemia Encountered in the Emergency Department Based on RBC Indices

	Background	Diagnosis	Treatment
		Microcytic Anemia	
Iron deficiency anemia	Most common anemia in women of childbearing age. An occult bleed should be sought in older patients.	Low serum iron, low serum ferritin, and increased iron binding capacity. A low MCV may not be present.	Ferrous sulfate is the most cost effective treatment. It may cause constipation and black stools. Reticulocytosis takes 3-4 d in children and up to a week in adults.
Thalassemia	Autosomal defect resulting in decreased synthesis of globin chains. Homozygous β-chain thalassemia (major) occurs in Mediterranean populations, and is the most severe type. Heterozygous β-chain thalassemia (minor) is a much milder form of the disease. Patients with α-thalassemia may be completely asymptomatic.	Severe anemia with homozygous β-chain type. There is a microcytic hypochromic anemia with target cells on peripheral smear. Hemoglobin electrophoresis and genetic testing.	Blood transfusions to correct anemia, suppress erythropoiesis, and decreased GI absorption of iron.
Lead poisoning	The toxic affects of lead primarily affect the hematopoietic (anemia), neurologic (causes segmental demyelination and axonal degeneration), renal (nephropathy), and GI systems (abdominal pain, constipation, nausea, vomiting)	Normochromic (normocytic) or hypochromic (microcytic) anemia. Lead levels greater than 10 μg/dl are toxic for children. Anemia occurs at a level of 70 μg/dl in adults. In children with chronic exposure, plain radiographs of the wrist and knees may show a characteristic "lead band" or "lead line" of increased metaphyseal activity in the distal ulna and fibula.	If GI symptoms or CNS problems are present, hospitalization with parenteral chelation therapy is indicated. More aggressive therapy is used in children.

	Background	Diagnosis	Treatment
Microcytic or Macrocytic Anemia			
Sideroblastic anemia	A congenital or acquired disorder causing altered production of the heme component of the hemoglobin. The hereditary form is rare, and seen in the elderly. Acquired causes include toxin exposure and systemic disease such as hemolytic anemia, infection, malignancy, and rheumatoid arthritis.	There is a paradoxical finding of hyperferremia, and nearly total transferrin saturation in a patient with a hypochromic anemia; microcytic is more common in hereditary form, and macrocytic is more common in acquired forms. Rare RBCs containing siderotic granules, or Pappenheimer bodies, also may circulate in the peripheral blood. Ring sideroblasts (iron deposits within mitochondria) are found on bone marrow aspirate.	Pyridoxine is may be used mostly for the heredity form of the disease. Iron removal may be of benefit. Transfusions are used for relief of symptomatic anemia in the acquired form. Prolonged support with RBC transfusions may lead to secondary hemochromatosis, and require chelation therapy with deferoxamine.
Macrocytic Anemia			
Megaloblastic anemia	Defective DNA synthesis most commonly caused by a lack of the coenzyme forms of vitamin B_{12} and folic acid. Vitamin B_{12} deficiency can also cause neurologic involvement such as paresthesias, loss of proprioception and vibratory sense, weakness and spasticity of the lower extremities, and variable mental status changes.	Macrocytic anemia with an MCV greater than 100 μm^3. On peripheral smear, large oval RBCs (macro-ovalocytes) and hypersegmented polymorphoneutrophils are usually present. Vitamin B_{12} and folic acid levels. Note: liver disease, alcoholism, hemolysis, and hypothyroidism are macrocytic anemias that do not have megaloblastic changes.	Folate 1 mg by mouth per day. Malabsorption is the most common cause of B_{12} deficiency and is usually required to correct the anemia.
Normocytic Anemia			
Chronic disease	Malignancy, chronic inflammation, uremia, and infection are common causes.	Low serum iron, low TIBC, normal or elevated ferritin. A normochromic, normocytic anemia is common, but a microcytic anemia may also be present.	Therapy is usually not required because the hematocrit is seldom less than 25% to 30%.

CNS, central nervous system; GI, gastrointestinal; MCV, mean corpuscular volume; RBC, red blood cell; TIBC, total iron binding capacity.

Hemophilia A & B

- *Epidemiology and risk factors.* Hemophilia A and B are genetically inherited, X-linked recessive bleeding disorders. Bleeding can be mild, moderate or severe. Mild hemarthroses and muscle hematomas comprise 90% of all bleeding episodes.
- *Pathophysiology.* Factor VIII deficiency defines hemophilia A. Factor IX deficiency defines hemophilia B. Severity of the disease depends on the deficiency of each factor. Severe disease results when there is less than 1% of factor activity, and mild disease occurs when there is approximately 6% to 60% of factor activity. Minor bleeds include hematuria, early hemarthrosis, muscle hematomas, and excessive bleeding in lacerations. Moderate bleeds include late hemarthroses, and persistent bleeding after dental trauma. Major bleeds include intracranial bleeding, gastro-intestinal bleeding, and excessive bleeding accompanying major trauma.
- *History.* Patients have spontaneous bleeding or excessive bleeding following trauma. Spontaneous bleeding includes painless hematuria, gastrointestinal bleeding, hemarthroses, and muscle hematomas. Patients may have persistent bleeding after lacerations or minor musculoskeletal trauma. Patients with minor trauma to the head may present for prophylactic factor, or may present with signs or symptoms of intracranial hemorrhage.
- *Physical examination.* The physical examination findings depend on the site of bleeding. Retroperitoneal bleeding may show a Gray-Turner's sign (discoloration of the flank) or a Cullen's sign (discoloration around umbilicus), hypotension, tachycardia, and back or abdominal pain. Gastrointestinal bleeding will show hematemesis, coffee-ground vomitus, melena, or bright-red blood per rectum. Musculoskeletal bleeding may not have any significant physical findings, but patients frequently complain of joint pain with a hemarthrosis. Signs of intracranial bleeding range from a normal examination to coma.
- *Diagnostic testing.* Obtain a CBC to evaluate for anemia. A PT and international normalized ratio (INR) will be normal. The PTT and bleeding time will be prolonged. In severe bleeding, a type and cross match for packed red blood cells should be sent. A CT scan is always necessary, even with minor head trauma, in any patient with hemophilia or on anticoagulation therapy.
- *ED management.* Patients with hemophilia A require factor VIII. Patients with hemophilia B require factor IX. Treatment may be tailored to the type of bleed. For mild bleeding, administer 18 U/kg IV of the factor. For moderate bleeding, administer 26 U/kg IV of the factor. For major bleeding, administer 50 U/kg IV of the factor. For minor surgery, such as incision and drainage of a superficial abscess, prophylactically treat as a moderate bleed with 26 U/kg. If emergent major surgery is required, prophylactically treat as a major bleed with 50 U/kg. Patients with any head trauma should be treated with factor prophylactically before a head CT scan is obtained. Patients with minor bleeding can be discharged home if hemostasis is achieved and factor levels are replaced. Patients with moderate bleeding, such as a hemarthrosis or muscle bleeding, may also be discharged if symptoms do not progress after

treatment, and after factor replacement. If symptoms progress or patients exhibit any signs of a compartment syndrome, such as severe pain, admit the patient. Patients with major bleeding should be admitted to the hospital. If concentrated factor is not readily available, cryoprecipitate or fresh frozen plasma can be used. The limiting factor is the volume needed to achieve the same end. Cryoprecipitate also has large amounts of factor VIII, but larger volumes are required to achieve the same end. Fresh frozen plasma contains large amounts of all factors. The patient's hematologist can often determine the amount of factor to administer.

- *Helpful hints and pitfalls.* Administer factor, 50 U/kg, prophylactically for head trauma. This should be done prior to or while obtaining a CT scan of the head. Some patients may have antibodies to factor. Patients are usually able to tell the physician the name of their factor. Watch patients with muscle hematomas for the development of a compartment syndrome.

Porphyria

- There are several forms of porphyria, each due to a separate defect in the biosynthesis of heme. Only a few of the more common ones will be mentioned here. Porphyria cutania tarda is the most common. The vast majority of cases are inherited as an autosomal dominant or recessive trait. An exacerbation may be precipitated by certain stressors such as sunlight, alcohol, starvation, infections, and certain drugs, including estrogen.
- Most of the symptoms are a due to the accumulation and toxicity of porphyria precursors.
- Patients with porphyria cutania tarda (PCT) and erythropoietic protporphyria (EPP) primarily present with skin findings after sun exposure. Acute intermittent porphyria (AIP) is primarily associated with neurovisceral symptoms, with abdominal pain being the most common complaint. The diagnosis should be considered in patients with a long history of undiagnosed abdominal pain, somatic and autonomic neural complaints, and psychiatric concerns. Acute intermittent porphyria may easily be mistaken for an acute surgical abdomen.
- The primary role of ED management is recognition of the disease, and to help the patient avoid stressors that may induce an exacerbation (i.e., sunlight for PCT and EPP), and for symptomatic relief. For AIP, reversal of the enzymatic activity responsible for the disease manifestations is induced by increased carbohydrate intake.

Thrombocytopenic Purpura

Idiopathic Thrombocytopenic Purpura (ITP)
- *Epidemiology and risk factors.* ITP (also called immune thrombo-cytopenic purpura) can be acute or chronic. Both forms are caused by antibody-induced destruction of platelets. Both acute and chronic ITP are associated with bleeding. Acute ITP is more common in children from 2 to 6 years of age, and usually follows a viral infection. Acute ITP usually has a spontaneous, complete resolution. Chronic ITP is more common in middle-aged women. It is associated with malignancy in

geriatric patients, and autoimmune disorders in women. Chronic ITP has a waxing and waning course. Relapse is common.

- **Pathophysiology.** The inciting event for ITP is poorly understood. Increased antiplatelet antibodies mediate increased platelet destruction. The result is spontaneous bleeding, most commonly manifested as easy bruising, petechiae, and mucosal bleeding.
- **History.** Acute ITP occurs in a child usually with a recent mild viral syndrome. The parent notices easy bruising, mucosal bleeding, or petechiae. A patient with chronic ITP is usually a middle-aged woman who reports easy bruising, petechiae, gastrointestinal bleeding, mucosal bleeding, or abnormal vaginal bleeding.
- **Physical examination.** The patients are often well-appearing, with petechiae, purpura, mucosal bleeding, or gastrointestinal bleeding.
- **Diagnostic testing.** CBC with differential reveals thrombocytopenia, PT/PTT will be normal. Bleeding time is prolonged. Type and screen blood for platelet transfusion if severe bleeding is present.
- **ED management.** Platelet transfusion is generally withheld unless platelets are 10,000 to 20,000, the patient has severe bleeding, or emergent surgery is needed. The first choice for treatment is corticosteroids. IV immune globulin can also be used. Immunomodulating medications have been used in difficult cases. Splenectomy is avoided if possible. Decision to begin therapy should be made in consultation with a hematologist. Patients with severe bleeding or platelets less than 10,000 should be admitted to the ICU.
- **Helpful hints and pitfalls.** Distinguish ITP from TTP by the well appearance of the patient with ITP. Transfuse platelets after IV immune globulin for better response.

Thrombotic Thrombocytopenic Purpura (TTP)

- **Epidemiology and risk factors.** Sixty percent of cases occur in women. The disease tends to present following pregnancy, infection with *Escherichia coli*, and chemotherapy. If untreated, the mortality rate is as high as 98%, but drops to 10% to 20% with early recognition and treatment.
- **Pathophysiology.** TTP is an immune-mediated platelet aggregation that causes widespread microvasculature thrombosis, microangiopathic hemolysis, and platelet consumption. Patients have bleeding related to thrombocytopenia and ischemia due to thrombosis.
- **History.** patients may complain of fever, abdominal pain, or headache. Patients may be brought by family members who report an altered mental status. A history of prodromal flulike illness is usually present.
- **Physical examination.** These patients appear ill. The classic pentad of fever, acute renal failure, altered mental status, thrombocytopenic purpura, and microangiopathic hemolytic anemia is present in only 40% of patients with TTP. A patient may have jaundice from hemolysis. Mucosal bleeding and palpable purpura are common. The stool is often heme-positive. The neurologic examination may be normal or may reveal focal deficits, altered mental status, or coma.
- **Diagnostic testing.** CBC with differential shows thrombocytopenia and anemia. Urinalysis often shows hematuria. Renal function may be impaired, thus electrolytes should be evaluated. Liver function tests will

show elevated indirect bilirubin due to hemolysis. Patients may have elevated liver enzymes from thrombosis. A head CT scan is indicated for altered mental status.

- **ED management.** Plasmapheresis is the treatment of choice. Fresh frozen plasma can improve the coagulopathy. Do not transfuse platelets as they will be rapidly consumed, and may worsen the thrombosis. High dose corticosteroids should be initiated. Aspirin decreases platelet clumping. These patients should be admitted to the ICU.
- **Helpful hints and pitfalls.** Distinguish TTP from ITP by the ill-appearance of the TTP patient. Do not transfuse platelets.

von Willebrand's Disease

- **Epidemiology and risk factors.** von Willebrand's disease (vWD) is the most common genetic bleeding disorder, affecting approximately 1% of the general population. It is inherited in an autosomal dominant fashion. There is variable penetrance.
- **Pathophysiology.** There is a genetic deficiency of vWF that transports factor VII, and assists with platelet adherence to the endothelium. The result of this deficiency is easy bruising, increased bleeding from the mucous membranes, epistaxis, gastrointestinal bleeding, menorrhagia, and (rarely) hemarthroses.
- **History.** Patients usually report spontaneous epistaxis, menorrhagia, or bleeding after dental extractions. There should be a family history of vWD.
- **Physical examination.** The patients appear well. Patients may have areas of focal bleeding including mucosal, gastrointestinal, or vaginal bleeding. There will not be petechiae or purpura because these patients have normal platelet count and function.
- **Diagnostic testing.** The PT and INR will be normal. The PTT will be elevated. Bleeding time will be increased. A CBC with differential shows normal platelets and hemoglobin.
- **ED management.** Treatment depends on the severity of bleeding. Minor bleeding can be controlled with DDAVP at 0.3µg/kg IV over 30 minutes. For mild bleeding, DDAVP can be administered in a nasal dose of 300 mcg for adults and 150 mcg for children. Tranexamic acid and epsilon aminocaproic acid, which are antifibrinolytics, have both been used successfully to stop bleeding in these patients post dental procedures. More significant bleeding can be controlled with factor VIII, which contains large amounts of von Willebrand factor. Cryoprecipitate also has large amounts of von Willebrand factor, but larger volumes are required to achieve the same end point. Fresh frozen plasma contains large amounts of all factors.
- **Helpful hints and pitfalls.** Patients can have significant bleeding.

Special Considerations
Pediatric

- In regard to anemia, the normal ranges for red blood cell parameters are significantly different in infants and children, and do not reach adult levels until adolescence (see Table 66–2).

■ On identification of anemia, the likelihood of certain diagnostic entities is different in infants, children, and adults. In infants and children, anemia often represents a nutritional deficiency or a primary hematologic process, whereas in adults anemia more commonly is an indicator of systemic disease or malignancy.

Teaching Points

Oncologic emergencies are common, and often represent critical illness. Many of these patients are immunocompromised before any treatment, and especially so after radiation, bone marrow transplantation, or chemotherapy. The patient's ability to demonstrate disease may be limited by the immunocompromise. Therefore any fever in an immunocompromised patient must be aggressively investigated, and is a cause for admission in virtually all such patients.

Immediately after initiation of chemotherapy, patients may develop a lysis syndrome. This will not only alter many electrolytes, but may produce the symptoms of acute gouty arthopathy, confusion, and coma.

Patients with many different tumors may develop spinal cord syndromes. The rectal examination may show the earliest neurologic deficit with impairment of rectal sphincter tone. While the usual treatment is radiation therapy, a neurosurgical spinal decompression may be necessary to preserve function.

Hematologic emergencies are rare, but also represent critical illness. Among these, the more common cause for an ED visit is in the patient with hemophilia. These patients may have their own factor replacement with them, but still need to have it administered, and they may need imaging studies as well as analgesia. Any head trauma in such patients requires evaluation with computed tomography of the head.

Suggested Readings

Cines DB, Blanchette VS. Immune thrombocytopenic purpura. N Eng J Med 2002;346:995–1008.

Dombeck TA, Satonik RC. The porphyrias. Emerg Med Clin North Am 2005;23:885–899.

Hamilton GC, Janz TG. Anemia, polycythemia, and white blood cell disorders. In: Marx JA, Hockberger RS, Walls RM (editors). Rosen's Emergency Medicine: Concepts and Clinical Practice (6th ed). Philadelphia: Mosby, 2006, pp 1867–1891.

Hughes WT, Armstrong D, Bodey GP, et al. 1997 Guidelines for the use of antimicrobial agents in neutropenic patients with unexplained fever. Clin Infect Dis 1997;25:551–573.

Krimsky, WS, Behrens, RJ, Kerkvliet, GJ. Oncologic emergencies for the internist. Cleve Clin J Med 2002;69:209–222.

Pier MM. Treatment of von Willebrand's disease. N Eng J Med 2004;12;351:683–694.

Sadowitx PD, Amanullah S, Souid A. Hematologic emergencies in the pediatric emergency room. Emerg Med Clin North Am 2002;20:177–198.

CHAPTER 67

Infectious Disease

LARISSA S. MAY ■ TENAGNE HAILE–MARIAM

Overview

This chapter is a brief overview of infectious disease problems not discussed elsewhere. This is by no means a complete list of all potential infectious problems presenting to the ED. The approach to a patient with a fever is discussed in Chapter 31. Pediatric fever is discussed in Chapter 79. Human immunodeficiency virus (HIV) is covered in Chapter 37. See Chapter 54 for soft-tissue infections and ulcerations and Chapter 62 for other skin infections. See Chapter 24 for upper respiratory infections. Pharyngitis, diphtheria, epiglottitis, and laryngitis are covered in Chapter 55. Ludwig's angina and peritonsillar abscess are covered in Chapter 64. Chapter 61 briefly discusses dental infections. Dental related infections are discussed in Chapter 61. Chapter 69 briefly mentions ophthalmologic infections. Reference to other infections covered elsewhere in this book are listed by system below.

Viruses, bacteria, and fungi are microorganisms capable of causing disease. The Gram's stain and early culture results of infected fluid may provide clues to the offending organism. The morphological characteristics of bacteria are listed in Table 67–1.

Common antimicrobial therapy used in the ED is briefly summarized in Chapter 90.2.

Central Nervous System Infections
Botulism

■ **Background.** It is a syndrome of neuromuscular weakness and autonomic instability caused by toxins produced by *Clostridium botulinum*. See Table 67–2 for risk factors. Complications include airway compromise resulting in asphyxia. Autonomic dysfunction can result in hypotension. Fatality is low if appropriately diagnosed and treated.
■ **Clinical presentation.** See Table 67–2.
■ **Diagnostic testing.** This is initially a clinical diagnosis. Confirmatory laboratory tests include bacterial cultures and toxin assays of stool, blood, wound, and implicated foods. Electromyelography and nerve conduction studies may support the diagnosis.
■ **ED management.** Airway management and supportive therapy are the main components of treatment. Antitoxin is associated with a high

Table 67–1   **Morphologic Characteristics of Bacteria**

Morphology	Gram Positive	Gram Negative
Coccus (sphere)	Staphylococcus (clusters) Streptococcus (chain)	Neisseria
Bacillus (rod)	*Bacillus Clostridium Corynebacterium Listeria*	Enterics *(E. coli, Salmonella, Shigella, Klebsiella, Proteus, Yersinia), Pseudomonas, Bacteriodes Eikenella, Hemophilus, Legionella, Bordetella*
Spiral		*Treponema, Borrelia, Leptospira*
Fungi-like	*Actinomyces* Nocardia	
Pleomorphic		*Chlamydia, Rickettsiae*
No cell wall	*Mycoplasma* (neither gram positive or gram negative)	

Table 67–2   **Types of Botulism**

Type	Risk Factors	History	Physical Findings
Food-borne	Ingestion of home-canned or home-fermented foods containing toxin	May have gastrointestinal prodrome. Weakness, dysphagia, dysarthria. 1- to 3-d incubation period	Cranial neuropathies and descending symmetric weakness without sensory loss
Infant	Honey ingestion. Toxin is produced by spores in germinating in infant gut.	Weakness, drooling, constipation. Can develop over weeks	Upper airway obstruction, "floppy baby"
Wound	Chronic ulcers; heroin injection	Like food-borne but longer incubation period, and lacks gastrointestinal prodrome	Cranial neuropathies and descending symmetric weakness without sensory loss

incidence of hypersensitivity so skin testing precedes administration. Equine-derived trivalent botulinum antitoxin administration is given for food-borne and wound botulism. Human-derived pentavalent botulinum immune globulin is for infant botulism. Gastrointestinal decontamination and charcoal administration may be advised for food-borne botulism.

Only the U.S. Centers for Disease Control and Prevention (CDC) officials can authorize the release of the botulinum antitoxin to state health departments and physicians in the United States. These services are available 24 hours a day, and can be reached through local health departments as soon as the diagnosis of botulism is entertained. To contact the CDC directly, call (404) 639-2888 or (770) 488–7100.

Intracerebral Abscess

■ See Chapter 35.

Meningitis

■ *Background.* Acute bacterial meningitis is caused by infection of the subarachnoid space resulting in neurotoxicity and inflammation. Pathologic changes include cerebral vasculitis, edema, ischemia, and necrosis. The responsible organisms vary with the patient's age (Table 67–3). Since the advent of *Haemophilus influenzae* vaccine, the median age of patients with acute bacterial meningitis has changed from 15 months to 25 years. Complications of bacterial meningitis include seizures, coma, syndrome of inappropriate secretion of antidiuretic hormone, septic shock, cerebral edema, disseminated intravascular coagulation, respiratory arrest, and death. Possible long-term sequelae of bacterial meningitis include hearing loss, blindness, ataxia, and intellectual deficits. Viral meningitis also causes an inflammatory reaction

Table 67–3 Predominant Pathogens and Empiric Therapy for Bacterial Meningitis

Age Group or Risk Factors	Predominant Bacterial Pathogens	Empiric Antibiotic Choices
Neonates (0-4wk)	Group B strep., *E. coli*, *S. pneumoniae*, *L. monocytogenes*	Ampicillin plus aminoglycoside or cefotaxime
Infants (1-3 mo)	*H. influenzae, N. meningitidis, S. pneumoniae*, Group B strep, and *L. monocytogenes*	Vancomycin plus ceftriaxone or cefotaxime
Young children (3 mo-7 y)	*H. influenzae, S. pneumoniae*, and *N. meningitidis*	Vancomycin plus ceftriaxone or cefotaxime
Older children and adults (7-50 y)	*S. pneumoniae* and *N. meningitidis*	Vancomycin plus ceftriaxone or cefotaxime
Older adults (>50 y)	*S. pneumoniae, N. meningitidis*, and *L. monocytogenes*	Ceftriaxone plus ampicillin
Nosocomial (e.g., neurosurgery)	*S. aureus, S. epidermidis*, and Gram-negative bacilli	Vancomycin plus ampicillin plus ceftazidime or cefepime

that is usually self-limited. Herpes simplex virus (HSV), HIV, and mumps can all cause meningitis.

- *Clinical presentation.* Classic features are fever and headache, but patients can have seizures or changes in mental status. The patient may also have photophobia, lethargy, malaise, and vomiting. Beware of subtle presentations in patients at extremes of age or in the immuno-compromised patient. For example infants can have irritability and refusal to feed on presentation. Physical examination findings include fever, meningismus, Kernig's sign (reluctance to allow full extension of the knee when the hip is flexed to 90 degrees) or Brudzinski's sign (spontaneous flexion of the hips during passive flexion of the neck). Look for the petechial rash of meningococcal meningitis. The patient may also have an obvious source of infection such as pneumonia, mastoiditis, or a urinary tract infection.

- *Diagnostic testing.* Obtain cerebrospinal fluid (CSF), and evaluate for cell count, protein, glucose, Gram's stain and culture (see Chapter 91 for lumbar puncture procedure and Appendix 1 for CSF analysis). If incompletely treated meningitis is suspected in a patient who has started antibiotic therapy, antigen testing may be helpful. Although antigen tests may identify the bacterial pathogen, they do not provide information about the antibiotic susceptibility of the organism. Initial CSF samples, although frequently suggestive of the diagnosis, may not differentiate viral from bacterial meningitis. The CSF in patients with viral meningitis typically exhibits pleocytosis with 10 to 500 leukocytes (usually mononuclear cells), and a slightly elevated protein level (<100 mg/dl). Other causes for a mononuclear or aseptic meningitis include tuber-culosis, brucellosis, syphilis, Lyme disease, fungi, leptospirosis, infectious hepatitis as well as noninfectious agents such as chemical meningitis, collagen vascular disease and malignancy. Inadequately treated bacterial meningitis may also result in an aseptic meningitis. Classic CSF findings in bacterial meningitis include a predominance of polymorphonuclear (PMNs) cells, elevated protein, and low glucose. Blood cultures are positive in 60% of patients with bacterial meningitis. If the patient is immunocompromised, test for cryptococcus.

- *ED management.* Antibiotic therapy should not be delayed for a lumbar puncture to be performed (Tables 67–3 and 67–4). Chemoprophylaxis should be given for close contacts of patients with meningococcal meningitis (Table 67–5). Dexamethasone (0.15 mg/kg every 6 hours for 2 to 4 days in children >6 weeks old) may decrease the incidence of hearing loss and neurological damage in children, and has a beneficial role in some adults. Steroids should not be used in neonatal cases. Steroids should be initiated 10–20 minutes before or concomitant with the first antibiotic dose. Ceftriaxone is not recommended for neonates because it may displace bilirubin from albumin-binding sites.

- *Helpful hints and pitfalls.* Patients with viral meningitis may have the same signs and symptoms as patients with bacterial meningitis, but are usually less ill, and have a much better prognosis. Although patients with encephalitis may present in a similar fashion with meningeal irritation, all of them have an alteration in consciousness.

Table 67–4 Empiric Antibiotics Dosing for Suspected Bacterial Meningitis

Antibiotic	IV Adult Dose	IV Pediatric Dose
Ampicillin	2 gm q 4 hours	50-100 mg/kg q 6 hours
Cefepime or ceftazidime	2 gm q 8 hours	
Cefotaxime	2 gm q 6 hours	50 mg/kg q 6 hours
Ceftriaxone	2 gm q 12 hours	100 mg/kg q 24 hours (must be older than 3 months)
Chloramphenicol	1.0 gm q 6 hours	25 mg/kg q 6 hours
Gentamicin	2 mg/kg q 8 hours loading dose, then 1.7 mg/kg	2.5 mg/kg q 8 hours
Vancomycin	2-3 gm per day 500-750 mg q 6 hours	15 mg/kg q 12 hours

Table 67–5 Chemoprophylaxis for Close Contacts of Meningococcal Meningitis

Rifampin	Adults, 600 mg PO q12h for 2 d; children >1 mo, 10 mg/kg PO q12h for 2 d; children <1 mo, 5 mg/kg PO q12h for 2 d
Ciprofloxacin	Adults, 500 mg PO (single dose)
Ceftriaxone	Adults, 250 mg IM (single dose); children <15 y, 125 mg IM (single dose)

IM, intramuscular; PO, by mouth.

Rabies

- *Background.* This is a fatal viral zoonotic encephalitis that is a global health problem. There are a handful of cases annually in the United States, which are mostly associated with exposure to infected wild animals (bats, raccoons, and skunks). It is very rare in small rodents. There is progressive neurologic and systemic collapse resulting in death.
- *Clinical presentation.* The incubation varies from a few days to several years, although most fall in the 20- to 60-day range. A viral prodrome may be accompanied by pain or paresthesias at or near the bite site and is followed by progressive neuropsychiatric changes and tingling at the bite site develop into progressive neuropsychiatric changes from agitation and hallucinations to coma and death. Back pain and spasms are frequent. The furious form is the most common and includes agitation, pharyngeal spasms and hydrophobia (inability to swallow). The paralytic form accounts for less than a fifth of cases.
- *Diagnostic testing.* Rabies infection can be confirmed by isolating the virus, by identifying the antigen, or, detecting antibody in unvaccinated patients, by detecting antibody. Viral isolation from saliva, respiratory secretions, CSF, or brain biopsy is the ideal method of diagnosis.

- **ED management.** There is no effective treatment for rabies. Therapy is primarily supportive. Patients should be admitted to the intensive care unit.
- **Helpful hints and pitfalls.** Post exposure prophylaxis (see Chapter 94) is the most important ED intervention for this disease as it can be assumed to be uniformly fatal.

Tetanus

- **Definition.** This is a neurotoxic disease that results from infection with *Clostridium tetani*. Spores are very hardy and ubiquitous. Since adequate immunization is effective, the non-immunized patients (e.g., elderly, neonates, marginalized) are at risk.
- **Clinical presentation.** The initial insult might be a minor injury or super-infection of a chronic wound. Tetanus is often not thought of, and the patient's symptoms passed off as painful muscle spasms. Generalized tetanus is the most common and severe form of the disease. Trismus is often the presenting symptom. The characteristic sardonic smile (risus sardonicus) appears as other facial muscles are involved. Irritability, weakness, myalgia, muscle cramps, dysphagia, hydrophobia, and drooling may be present. The patient remains lucid. Patients may have spasms ranging from local muscle groups to opisthotonos. Spasm of laryngeal and respiratory muscles can lead to ventilatory failure and death. Sympathetic hyperactivity and cardiovascular instability can be seen. Cephalic tetanus presents with trismus plus cranial nerve palsies. Localized tetanus is a form of the disease characterized by persistent muscle spasms in proximity to the site of infection. Neonatal tetanus is found in underdeveloped countries where immunization is inadequate and contaminated material is used to cut umbilical cords. Symptoms develop in the first week of life and include irritability, poor sucking, and poor swallowing that can progress to opisthotonus and death.
- **Diagnostic testing.** All laboratory tests may be normal including CSF. This is a clinical diagnosis. Wound cultures are positive in only one-third of cases.
- **ED management.** Aggressive supportive care with careful attention to the airway, administration of antitoxin, elimination of toxin production, and active immunization are initial treatment priorities. Human tetanus immunoglobulin (3000-6000 U given IM is recommended for children and adults; 500 U IM for infants) and tetanus toxoid (0.5 ml IM for patients older than 7 years) should be administered to all patients with suspected tetanus. The tetanus toxoid vaccine should be given at a separate site. Local debridement and antibiotic therapy with metronidazole should also be initiated. Sympathetic overactivity can be treated with combined α- and β-adrenergic agents such as labetalol.
- **Helpful hints and pitfalls.** Localized tetanus can be mistaken for a muscle spasm. Tetanus can complicate a chronic wound. Clinical tetanus does not result in immunity, recovering patients should be immunized. Strychnine poisoning is similar to tetanus in that the patient develops opisthotonos while remaining awake. However, there are alternating

periods of relaxation, and trismus occurs later with cases of strychnine poisoning.

Viral Encephalitis

- **Background.** This is an infection of the brain parenchyma resulting in variable degrees of neurological and systemic illness. This disease often presents as a meningoencephalitis. Arthropod-borne causes of encephalitis show seasonal variability, and account for the majority of cases. Other causes of encephalitis include rabies, mumps (both rare in the United States), and HSV. Complications include seizures, coma, death, and long-term neuropsychiatric problems.

- **Clinical presentation.** All patients have an alteration in mental status. Fever, headache and mental status changes are classic findings, but meningismus, seizures, focal neurologic changes, and hallucinations may be present.

- **Diagnostic testing.** Patients with altered mental status, an immuno-compromised state, focal neurolgic findings, or papilledema should have a head CT scan before the LP is performed. CSF should be obtained for evaluation and sent for glucose, protein, Gram's stain, and culture (Chapter 91 and Appendix 1). A CSF pleocytosis usually occurs in encephalitis, but is not necessary for the diagnosis. White blood cell counts typically number in the 10s to 100s, although higher counts occur. The CSF glucose levels are usually normal although some viral etiologies (Eastern equine encephalitis) produce findings consistent with acute bacterial meningitis. Some viruses (HSV) produce a hemorrhagic necrosis, and the CSF reveals moderately high protein levels and evidence of red blood cells (RBCs). For some viruses (HSV, enterovirus, varicella zoster virus [VZV], JC virus), polymerase chain reaction (PCR) detection of viral nucleic acids from the CSF has replaced culture and brain biopsy as the standard for diagnosing encephalitis. Electro-encephalogram (EEG) changes precede CT or magnetic resonance imaging (MRI) evidence of encephalitis.

- **ED management.** The treatment is supportive. Antiviral therapy with acyclovir should be instituted if HSV encephalitis is likely.

- **Helpful hints and pitfalls.** The West Nile virus is becoming an important cause of epidemic encephalitis in the USA. HSV can cause necrosis in the temporal lobes. It often presents with olfactory hallu-cinations (i.e., the patient reports bad smells that are not experienced by other persons present in the same environment).

Respiratory
Pneumonia

- **Background.** This is an acute infection of the lung parenchyma with or without pleural effusion. It is the sixth leading cause of death in the United States. Community-acquired pneumonia can occur in any patient; however, patients who are immunosuppressed are at greater risk. A microbiologic etiology cannot be determined in up to 50% of cases.

The most common causes of CAP in patients requiring hospitalization includes *S. pneumoniae* and *H. influenzae*. Atypical organisms (Legionella, *Mycoplasma*, and *Chlamydia spp.*) and viruses account for an additional one-third of cases. Severe cases of CAP are due to *S. pneumoniae* (most), *Legionella sp.*, *S. aureus* and aerobic gram-negative bacilli. Nosocomial pneumonia is a hospital-acquired pneumonia that can be severe, and leads to increased morbidity, mortality, and length of hospital stay. Complications include empyema, bronchopleural fistula, abscess formation, and necrotizing pneumonia.

■ *Clinical presentation.* Patients most commonly complain of cough, shortness of breath, and fever. Viral and atypical pneumonias tend to be more indolent; whereas, bacterial pneumonia begins more suddenly, and may be more severe. Fever is usually present in 75% of patients. Tachypnea and tachycardia are present in half. Early in the course of the illness, the chest examination may be normal, or may reveal fine rales. Evidence of lung consolidation is highly suggestive of bacterial infection, but is absent in two thirds of patients. Physical findings of consolidation include dullness on percussion, bronchial breath sounds, and E to A changes. Egophany is noted when an "E" sound changes to an "A" sound during auscultation of a consolidated lung. Patients with viral or atypical pneumonia most often have normal physical examination findings despite impressive radiographic abnormalities.

■ *Diagnostic testing.* Chest radiographs are most useful when combined with the history and physical examination, but are frequently not helpful in determining the etiology of the pneumonia. Chest radiographs may show lobar consolidation, patchy interstitial infiltrates, cavitation, or pleural effusions. Microscopic examination and culture of expectorated sputum remain the gold standard for microbiologic diagnosis. Mucopurulent sputum is more common with bacterial infections, whereas scant or watery sputum is suggestive of viral or atypical infection. A chest CT scan is most helpful in evaluating recurrent pneumonia, or to delineate tumors or lung abscesses.

■ *ED management.* Outpatient treatment is safe in those less than age 50 with no significant co-morbid conditions such as malignancy, congestive heart failure, cerebrovascular disease, renal disease, liver disease, or HIV, and if the patient has adequate social circumstances. Admit patients who have the following findings on physical examination: altered mental status, pulse of 120 or greater beats per minute, respiratory rate of 30 or greater breaths per minute, systolic blood pressure below 90 mm Hg, temperature below 35°C or above 40°C, or hypoxia. It is also prudent to admit patients with multilobar pneumonia, patients with any significant comorbidity (e.g. diabetes), patients who are unable to eat or drink, or who have pain that cannot be relieved in the ED. Moderate and high risk patients can be classified by various scoring systems, and should be admitted to the hospital. Antibiotic treatment is generally recommended for 10 to 14 days (Table 67–6).

■ *Helpful hints and pitfalls.* Empiric therapy should be guided by suspected organisms based on clinical features, radiographic findings, and local antibiotic susceptibility patterns. Older children and younger adults are more likely to have viral or atypical pneumonia. Elderly patients,

Table 67–6	Pneumonia and Empiric Therapy	
Risk group	Initial Antibiotic Recommendations	Possible Organisms
Community acquired, non-immuno-compromised	Third-generation cephalosporin more likely than second-generation to be active against DRSP*. Add macrolide for atypical pathogens. Respiratory fluoroquinolones are for more complicated cases; covers both typical and atypical.	S. pneumoniae Atypicals: Mycoplasma pneumoniae, C. pneumoniae species Enteric gram-negative organisms Respiratory viruses
Suspected aspiration	Cefoxitin or cefotetan (best anaerobic activity of cephalosporins); β-lactam/β-lactamase inhibitor; clindamycin +/- amino-glycoside; or metronidazole + third-generation cephalosporin	Polymicrobial Anaerobic mouth bacteria (e.g., fusobacteria and Bacteroides species); Staphyloccocus aureus and gram-negative bacilli are common causes if hospital acquired
Severe pneumonia (intensive care unit patients)	Third-generation cephalosporin or fluoroquinolone; consider adding aminoglycoside for septic shock.	S. pneumoniae Legionella spp H. influenzae M. pneumoniae Enteric gram-negative organisms Pseudomonas aeruginosa M. pneumoniae Respiratory viruses Also consider C. pneumoniae, M. tuberculosis, and endemic fungi
Severe pneumonia with neutropenia, bronchiectasis or recent hospitalization	Antipseudomonal beta-lactam plus fluoroquinolone; add aminoglycoside for septic shock	P. aeruginosa, enteric gram-negative bacilli, S. aureus
HIV/AIDS (Chapter 37)	Trimethoprin/sulfamethoxazole for suspected PCP. Alternatives for sulfa allergy include: Pentamidine + third-generation cephalosporin, or clindamycin + primaquine	P. carinii is the most common; M. tuberculosis and common bacterial pathogens such as S. pneumoniae and H. influenzae.

DRSP, drug-resistant S. pneumoniae; PCP, pneumocystis carinii pneumoniae. See Chapter 90.2 for antibiotic dosing.

immunosuppressed patients and those with comorbid conditions are likely to be more ill and infected with more virulent or resistant organisms. For elderly and nursing home patients, obtain blood cultures and aggressively commence antibiotics.

Pulmonary Abscess

- *Background.* This is a suppurative cavity-forming infection of the lung parenchyma that can progress to necrotizing pneumonia. Anaerobic bacteria are the main infecting organisms, as lung abscess most often results from aspiration in patients with an altered level of consciousness, such as in alcohol intoxication.

- *Clinical presentation.* The patient may complain of several weeks or longer of malaise, low-grade fevers, and cough productive of purulent sputum, which is foul-smelling in about half of patients. Review of systems often reveals weight loss and anemia. The physical findings are similar to those in pneumonia, with or without a pleural effusion.

- *Diagnostic testing.* The diagnosis is most often made from the chest radiograph, showing a cavity with an air-fluid level or pneumonitis with small cavities in a dependent lung segment. A CT scan may show an obstructing endobronchial lesion. Because of the presence of large numbers of anaerobes as indigenous flora in the mouth, expectorated sputum is less useful for microbiologic diagnosis. Empyema fluid, if available, provides an excellent specimen. Blood cultures are infrequently positive.

- *ED management.* A prolonged course of antimicrobial therapy is often necessary. Empiric therapy should begin in the ED. The anaerobes involved in lung abscess are increasingly resistant to penicillin. Combinations of beta-lactam drugs and beta-lactamase inhibitors such as ticarcillin plus clavulanic acid and ampicillin plus sulbactam are active against essentially all anaerobes, have good activity against *S. aureus* and many gram-negative bacilli, and are a good first-line empiric therapy. Clindamycin is also active against most anaerobes. These patients should be admitted to the hospital. If tuberculosis cannot be ruled out, patients should be placed in respiratory isolation.

- *Helpful hints and pitfalls.* Lung abscess is on a continuum with necrotizing pneumonia, and often the distinction between the two cannot be made in the ED.

Tuberculosis (TB)

- *Background.* Many mycobacteria cause human disease, but *Mycobacterium tuberculosis* is most significant, and can infect any organ. M. avium complex (MAC) is the second most frequently encountered. It causes pulmonary disease in patients with parenchymal lung disease and disseminated infections such as AIDS. Disseminated tuberculosis can present with TB meningitis, osteomyelitis (Pott's disease), or genitourinary TB.

- *Clinical presentation.* Acute progression and dissemination is most likely to develop in the very young (<5 years) and in the immunocompromised.

Reactivation disease can happen in any organ, but is most commonly seen in the lung, most typically as progressive cavitary pneumonitis of an upper lobe. Systemic symptoms of weight loss and sweats often accompany progressive pneumonia. It is important to note that this presentation of "classic" reactivation tuberculosis may be altered especially at the extremes of age and with an immunocompromised state. Cough and mild hemoptysis may be present.

■ *Diagnostic testing.* Ninety percent of those with a response of more than 10 mm to the tuberculin test (PPD) are infected with *M. tuberculosis*. The gold standard for diagnosing active TB is by microscopic visualization of mycobacteria and culture results. Chest radiograph abnormalities are not limited to the classic upper lobe cavitary infiltrate. The chest radiograph may be normal if the patient is immunocompromised especially in those patients positive for HIV. Approximately 1% of immunocompetent adults may have a normal appearing chest radiograph. The white blood cell count is often normal in pulmonary TB.

■ *ED management.* The most important aspect of ED management is containment of infection. Place the patient with possibly active TB in respiratory isolation. Admit the patient for diagnosis and therapy of tuberculosis. First-line agents used in the treatment of TB include isoniazid (INH), rifampin, and pyrazinamide. Antibiotics for community acquired pneumonia should be initiated until the diagnosis of TB is confirmed.

■ *Helpful hints and pitfalls.* Acute miliary TB can be quickly fatal if undiagnosed. Healthcare workers are at high risk for acquiring TB. There is a growing incidence of multidrug-resistant TB. The chest radiograph may resemble bacterial pneumonia. Clinically, bacterial pneumonias usually present with more profound symptoms of systemic toxicity and have symptoms of shorter duration.

Cardiovascular
Infective Endocarditis (IE)

■ *Background.* This is an infection of endocardium (almost always involving one or more heart valves), and resulting in hematogenous spread of the infecting organism. Transient bacteremia is common after certain medical and non-medical procedures such as dental extraction and tooth brushing. Endocarditis is produced by a combination of an adherent organism and a breakdown of host defense mechanisms (e.g., damaged valve) to produce disease. The most common organisms are *Streptococcus viridans* and *S. aureus*, but the disease can be caused by other bacteria and fungi. High-risk groups include IV drug abusers and patients with congenital heart disease. Complications include myocarditis, valve rupture, and septic embolization. Emboli most commonly lodge in the skin, lungs (right-sided IE), the kidneys, the spleen, blood vessels, or the central nervous system.

■ *Clinical presentation.* Fever is reported by most patients. There may be a heart murmur, splenomegaly, or skin manifestations. A list of classic physical findings is noted in Table 67–7.

■ *Diagnostic testing.* Blood cultures are positive in 95% of cases; the ESR is elevated; and transthoracic or transesophageal echocardiography will

Table 67-7	Classic Findings of Endocarditis
Physical finding	**Description**
Janeway lesions	Septic emboli; small erythematous macules; painless
Osler's nodes	Small, red tender nodules on the finger or toe pads
Roth spots	Septic retinal emboli; necrotic areas with white centers.
Petechiae	Small hemorrhage; look for subconjuctival hemorrhage
Splinter hemorrhages	Small linear subungual hemorrhages

most likely reveal vegetation. The white blood cell count may or may not be elevated. Microscopic hematuria and proteinuria may be present. The EKG should be evaluated for conduction blocks concerning for an aortic ring abscess or other myocardial injury. The chest radiograph is often abnormal in right-sided endocarditis demonstrating consolidation, atelectasis, pleural effusion, or septic emboli. Other cases may reveal evidence of congestive heart failure.

- ***ED management.*** Obtain a minimum of three sets of blood cultures before institution of antibiotic therapy. Administer empiric antibiotics that are aimed at most likely organisms. Empirical coverage for patients with suspected native valve endocarditis include nafcillin-penicillin-gentamicin. Vancomycin-gentamicin is preferred for patients at risk for methicillin-resistant *S. aureus* (MRSA), such as IV drug abusers, and dialysis patients. Patients with prosthetic valves should be empirically treated with vancomycin, gentamicin, and rifampin for adequate coverage of *S. aureus* (including MRSA), coagulase-negative staphylococci, and gram-negative organisms. Admit to a monitored bed as patients can develop CHF and conduction abnormalities.
- ***Helpful hints and pitfalls.*** IE may be mistaken for a viral syndrome on multiple ED visits before the correct diagnosis is entertained.

Myocarditis

- ***Background.*** This is an infection of the myocardium, but is often accompanied by pericarditis (see Chapter 22). Most cases in the United States are assumed to be due to viruses (especially coxsackie virus). Other causes include bacteria, parasites, and fungi. Host inflammatory response is an important, poorly understood determinant of severity. The disease affects all age groups including infants. The rule of thirds states that one third recovers fully, one third has mild to moderate residual heart failure, and one third develops chronic severe congestive heart failure (CHF).

- *Clinical presentation.* There is typically an antecedent viral syndrome complicated by dysrhythmias or CHF. Edema, jugular venous distention, tachycardia, and a cardiac gallop may be noted on physical examination. Left ventricular aneurysm may occur.
- *Diagnostic testing.* The patient may have elevated cardiac enzymes. Echocardiogram is useful, but an endocardial biopsy may be necessary for definitive diagnosis. This procedure is not necessary in the ED.
- *ED management.* Patients should be admitted. Cardiovascular monitoring and support are prudent. Possible in patient therapies include antiviral and immunosuppressive agents.
- *Helpful hints and pitfalls.* Patients often present with myopericarditis, and can have pericardial effusions that can lead to tamponade. Patients with a fulminant clinical course may require cardiac transplantation.

Rheumatic Fever

- *Background.* This is a systemic inflammatory disease whose major manifestations include carditis, polyarthritis, erythema marginatum, chorea, and subcutaneous nodules. Prior group A streptococci upper respiratory infection is a risk factor. Complications include valvular dysfunction and CHF.
- *Clinical presentation.* An antecedent sore throat is often present. The patient may complain of fever and joint pain. Other manifestations are listed in Table 67–8.
- *Diagnostic testing.* ASO titers will rise, but the diagnosis is most often based on clinical findings. The diagnosis is based on the Jone's criteria. The presence of two major, or one major and two minor, criteria in the presence of supporting evidence of prior Group A Streptococcal infection is required to make the diagnosis. The major manifestations of the Jone's criteria are listed in Table 67–8. Minor manifestations for diagnosis include nonspecific laboratory findings such as an elevated ESR and nonspecific clinical findings such as fever and arthralgia. An echocardiogram may be helpful.

Table 67–8   J♥NES Criteria for Rheumatic Fever (Major Manifestations Only)

Clinical Manifestation	Characteristics
Joints	Migratory polyarthritis. Usually large joints
Carditis	Appears in the first 3 ws of illness. Pancarditis. Only serious complication of ARF. Major cause of heart disease in the developing world
Nodules	Painless subcutaneous nodules on extensor surfaces over bony prominences; associated with carditis
Erythema marginatum	Evanescent enlarging serpiginous eruption. Can come and go over weeks
Syndenham's chorea	Involuntary choreiform movements

- **ED management.** Supportive care is used to decrease inflammation, decrease fever and toxicity, and control cardiac failure. The mainstays of treat-ment are salicylates, corticosteroids, and medications to treat CHF. Rheumatic patients are at extremely high risk of developing recurrent acute rheumatic fever after immunologically significant streptococcal upper respiratory infections. Benzathine penicillin G (1,200,000 units IM every 4 weeks) is the drug of choice. Oral penicillin V or erythromycin (if penicillin allergic) are also acceptable prophylactic agents.

Gastrointestinal

- See Chapter 18 for intra-abdominal infections, Chapter 27 for infectious diarrhea, Chapter 41 for hepatitis, and Chapter 48 for rectal abscess.
- Peritonitis and hepatic abscess are summarized in Table 67–9.

Genitourinary

- See Chapter 50 for testicular and scrotal infections and Chapter 58 for urinary tract infections. Sexual transmitted diseases are summarized in Table 67–10.

Bone

See Chapter 42 for septic joint.

Osteomyelitis

- **Background.** This refers to infection in any part of the bone. It results from hematogenous seeding, seeding from a contiguous source of infection, or direct inoculation of bone from surgery or trauma. S. *aureus* is the leading cause in all age groups. Polymicrobial osteoarthritis is more common in diabetics, after trauma, or from chronic infection. *E. corrodens* and *P. multocida* are the organisms associated with human or animal bites. Patients with sickle cell disease are at risk for *Salmonella* species. In chronic osteomyelitis (complicating a chronic ulcer, diabetes, or vascular insufficiency), the infection is often polymicrobial. *Pseudomonas* bacteria are responsible in the setting of puncture wounds to the foot, prosthetic devices, and IV drug abusers. Tuberculosis may cause vertebral osteomyelitis (Pott's disease). Fungal infections are rare. A rare form of osteomyelitis that may occur in HIV patients is bacillary angiomatosis, a gram-negative rickettsia-like organism that frequently leads to osteolytic bone lesions.
- **Clinical presentation.** There is pain over the infected bone. Fever (more common in children), localized warmth, swelling, and erythema may be present. Headache, fatigue, malaise, and anorexia may be noted by the patient. In advanced cases, sinus tracts that drain through the skin may be present.
- **Diagnostic testing.** The WBC is often elevated. The ESR is elevated in over 90% of cases. The C-reactive protein (CRP) increases early (within

Table 67–9   Intra-Abdominal Infections

	Peritonitis	Hepatic Abscess
Definition	Infection of the peritoneal cavity and membranes. Can be spontaneous or from rupture of viscous intrabdominal abscess or intestinal perforation	Can be due to pyogenic bacteria or parasites (e.g., amoeba, echinococcus)
Risk factors	Ascites, cirrhosis, peritoneal dialysis, bowel obstruction	Cholangitis, liver trauma, travel
Clinical presentation	Fever, abdominal pain, and tenderness	Fever, right upper quadrant tenderness
Diagnostic testing	Paracentesis for suspected SBP : Fluid should be evaluated for cell count, gram stain and culture. Gram stain often negative. Obtain radiologic studies to evaluate for bowel obstruction or free intraperitoneal air. Ancillary testing is useful but not diagnostic	Ultrasound and computed tomography are useful for diagnosis, and for guided aspiration to determine etiology
Emergency department management	Supportive care, intravenous: third-generation antibiotics: e.g., cephalosporins, broad-spectrum penicillins. Infection associated with peritoneal dialysis can be treated with locally instilled antibiotics after "washout" with dialysate, and often does not require that the peritoneal dialysis catheter be removed. Consult surgery if concerned for surgical disease (e.g., bowel perforation).	Drainage is often required for cure, so need early surgical consultation. If amebic abscess is suspected, treat with metronidazole. If suspect pyogenic abscess, treat with antibiotics that cover *Enterobacteraciae* and *B. fragilis*.

SBP: spontaneous bacterial peritonitis.

24 hours of infection), and peaks within 48 hours. Both the ESR and CRP decrease in response to therapy. Less than one third of patients have abnormalities on plain radiographs in the first 7 to 10 days after the onset of symptoms because 30% to 50% of bone mineral must be lost before lucent areas can be detected. Early findings include lucent lytic areas of cortical bone destruction and periosteal reaction (elevation of the periosteum). Soft tissue edema may be present within 3 to 5 days from the onset of infection. Bone scanning is more useful in the early diagnosis, and can detect osteomyelitis within 48 to 72 hours after the

Table 67–10 Sexually Transmitted Diseases

Disease	Organism	Clinical presentation	Diagnostic Testing	Management
Chancroid	*Haemophilus ducreyi*, a gram-negative rod.	1-2 cm *painful* erythematous papule that erodes into a pustule and ulcerates. Painful, suppurative lymphadenopathy may form an inguinal abscess or bubo.	A clinical diagnosis that is difficult to culture, and no serologic tests are available.	Single-dose ceftriaxone 250 mg IM or azithromycin 1 g PO; ciprofloxacin 500 mg PO twice daily for 3 d.
Chlamydia	*Chlamydia trachomatis*, an obligate, intracellular parasite. The most common of all STDs.	70% asymptomatic or mild symptoms. May present as urethritis, cervicitis, pelvic inflammatory disease (PID), chronic pelvic pain.	Immunological tests on endocervical swab, and urethral swab	Azithromycin 1 g PO for one dose, or doxycycline 100 mg PO twice daily for 7 d; also levofloxacin 500 mg PO for 7 d (do not use if pregnant and children).
Genital warts (condylomata acuminata)	Human papilloma virus (HPV), mostly types 6 and 11, which are not associated with malignancy.	Cauliflower-like lesions may coalesce to form pedunculated growth called condyloma acuminata; may be pruritic.	Polymerase chain reaction (PCR) testing of a genital swab; subtle lesions will appear as shiny white areas with application of 5% acetic acid.	Referral for cryotherapy or TCA (trichloroacetic acid) treatment. A topical antiviral cream such as imiquimod or podofilox may also be prescribed.

Table 67-10 Sexually Transmitted Diseases—*cont'd*

Disease	Organism	Clinical presentation	Diagnostic Testing	Management
Gonorrhea	*N. gonorrhoeae*, a gram-negative diplococci	May cause infection of the pharynx, anal canal, or conjunctivae, but genital infection is the most common (see Chlamydia). Epididymitis and prostatitis may occur. Disseminated gonococcal infection: arthritis-dermatitis syndrome, meningitis, and endocarditis.	Culture on Thayer Martin media; DNA testing is more accurate and reliable in females. For men, a Gram's stain showing the organism is sufficient to make the diagnosis.	Ceftriaxone 125 mg IM, ciprofloxacin 500 mg PO, levofloxacin 250 mg PO, or Cefixime 400 mg PO. Spectinomycin, 2 g IM, is indicated in patients who cannot take cephalosporins or quinolones. Treatment for *C. trachomatis* because of coinfection in up to 60% of cases.
Granuloma inguinale (Donovanosis)	*Calymmatobacterium granulomatis*, intracellular gram-negative bacterium. Rare in the United States; endemic to Africa, India, and New Guinea.	Painless, progressively enlarging ulcers. The ulcers are "beefy red" in color and are highly vascular and bleed easily. Painless lymphadenopathy may or may not accompany the ulcers.	A clinical diagnosis. A biopsy of the ulcers may identify Donovan bodies (monocytes engulfing clusters of organisms that look like microscopic safety pins).	Doxycycline 100 mg PO BID for 3 wk, or trimethoprim-sulfamethoxazole DS PO twice daily for 3 wk. Alternative regimens include ciprofloxacin or azithromycin.

Continued

Table 67–10 Sexually Transmitted Diseases—*cont'd*

Disease	Organism	Clinical presentation	Diagnostic Testing	Management
Herpes simplex	70%-80% of infections are caused by HSV-2, while the remaining are caused by HSV-1 (causative agent of oral herpes).	Painful, pruritic, tingling red papules that coalesce to form clear fluid-filled vesicles that progress to crusted ulcerations; unilateral inguinal lymphadenopathy; dysuria and urinary retention; fever and headache. Complications: aseptic meningitis, encephalitis, and autonomic nervous system dysfunction (especially in immuno-compromised).	Primarily a clinical diagnosis; viral antigen detection via PCR or direct fluorescent antibody testing. Viral culture is the best proof of the infection. The Tzank smear, looking for multinucleated giant cells, is less common.	For primary infection, a 7-10-d course of acyclovir (400 mg TID), famciclovir (250 mg TID), or valacyclovir (1 g BID) is indicated. A 5- to 7-d course is indicated for recurrent infections. Patients with severe systemic symptoms, particularly if immunosuppressed, should be admitted for intravenous acyclovir at (5-10 mg/kg QID).
Lympho-granuloma venerium (LGV)	*Chlamydia trachomatis* immunotypes L1, L2, and L3. Rare entity in the United States.	Primary stage: asymptomatic in most but may develop small, painless chancres. Second stage: painful unilateral inguinal lympha-denopathy that may become fluctuant and suppurative. "Groove sign"; palpable lymphadenopathy on opposite sides of the inguinal ligament.	The mainstay of laboratory testing for LGV is culture and serology.	Painful, fluctuant buboes may be drained with needle aspiration. Treatment consists of doxycycline 100 mg PO BID for 3 wk.

Disease	Organism	Clinical presentation	Diagnostic Testing	Management
Syphilis	Spirochete *Treponema pallidum*. It enters via mucus membranes and small breaks in the skin.	Primary (1-3 wk): Painless chancre with indurated borders. Secondary (3-6 wk after primary): Papular mucocutaneous rash, beginning on the trunk, and spreading distally to involve the palms and soles; condyloma lata (flat wartlike lesions); fever, malaise, sore throat, and lymphadenopathy. Tertiary (20 y later): Granulomatous lesions or gummas, cystic medial necrosis, and aortitis of the aorta, and thoracic aortic aneurysm; central nervous system involvement (meningitis symptoms, dementia, tabes dorsalis*)	Spirochetes may be visualized in the scrapings via dark-field microscopy. Serologic testing includeg nontreponemal assays (RPR, VDRL) and more specific treponemal tests (FTA). Usually negative in primary syphilis. Treponemal tests may remain positive for life. The nontreponemal tests may be falsely negative or positive but are quantitative and are useful in assessing response to treatment. The VDRL test is the test of choice in cerebrospinal fluid for neurosyphilis, but is not positive in all cases of neurosyphilis.	Treatment for both primary and secondary syphilis consists of benzathine penicillin, 2.4 million units IM for one dose. Penicillin-allergic patients may be treated with doxycycline, 100 mg PO BID for 15 d, erythromycin 500 mg PO q6h for 15 days, or ceftriaxone 1g IM daily for 10 days. Tertiary or latent syphilis is treated with benzathine penicillin, G 2.4 million units IM for 3 weeks plus aqueous crystalline penicillin G 3-4 million units IV q4h for 10 days. There are no proven effective alternatives for neurosyphilis. Patients allergic to penicillin should be desensitized.

BID, twice daily; IM, intramuscular; IV, intravenous; PO, by mouth; TID, three times daily; QID, four times daily.

*Tabes dorsalis: affecting the dorsal columns of the spinal cord and peripheral nerves, characterized by paroxysmal pain, particularly in the abdomen and legs; sensory ataxia; normal strength; autonomic dysfunction, and Argyll-Robertson pupils (pupil reacts poorly to light but well to accommodation).

onset of infection. A CT scan has the same limitations in detecting early cases, but can help to localize bony lesions found on bone scan. An MRI scan is comparable to skeletal scintigraphy in terms of early detection of osteomyelitis. A bacteriologic diagnosis in acute osteomyelitis may be found in up to 80% to 90% of cases. Cultures of infected bone by needle aspiration or surgical resection is the most effective method. Other potential sites of infection should be cultured (e.g., blood, urine, CSF).

- **ED management.** If the clinical presentation strongly suggests osteomyelitis, a lengthy diagnostic workup should not delay treatment. Patients should be admitted, and empiric IV antibiotic treatment started preferably after cultures are obtained. A penicillinase-resistant penicillin (oxacillin, nafcillin, methicillin, amoxicillin-clavulanate) and third-generation cephalosporin (e.g., ceftriaxone, cefotaxime, cefamandole, ceftizoxime, cetizoxime, moxalactam) are the initial coverage for the most common pathogens that include *S. aureus*. Vancomycin should be used if concerned for MRSA. Antipseudomonal coverage should be given for those at risk such as gentamycin, ceftazidime, cefepime, piperacillin-tazobactam, or ticarcillin-clavulanate. Clindamycin is a good alternative for patients with a penicillin allergy. Surgical debridement should be performed on all devitalized bone and tissue.

Tick-Borne Illness
Lyme Disease

- **Background.** Lyme disease is the most common vector-borne disease in the United States. It is caused by the spirochete *Borrelia burgdorferi*. The tick is almost always of the genus *Ixodes*. Lyme disease is a multisystem disorder that begins with a rash and flulike illness, and can cause early disseminated disease (neurologic and cardiac problems), or late disseminated disease (chronic arthritis and neurologic changes). Endemic areas in the United States include the coastal Northeast, the Midwest, and the West. One third of patients do not recall a tick bite. Complications include meningoencephalitis, cranial neuropathies, chorea, radiculopathy, cardiac conduction abnormalities, and chronic arthritis.

- **Clinical presentation.** Erythema chronicum migrans (ECM) is the characteristic rash, and manifests as an erythematous macule or papule with central clearing. Constitutional symptoms include fatigue, malaise, and fever. Symptoms of meningeal irritation (headache, photophobia and neck stiffness), and hepatitis (anorexia, right upper quadrant pain) may occur. In acute disseminated infection, patients may have cranial nerve palsies (cranial nerve VII), fluctuating meningoencephalitis, and lightheadedness, palpitations, or syncope from high-degree atrioventricular block. Later in the course, relapsing and remitting arthritis and arthralgias may be present.

- **Diagnostic testing.** This is primarily an epidemiologic and clinical diagnosis. Serologic testing is inconclusive, and the confirmation of the disease will be based on the ELISA test.

- **ED management.** Doxycycline is the drug of choice for men, nonpregnant or lactating women, and children over 8 years of age. Amoxicillin is an alternative for those in whom tetracyclines are contraindicated. For patients with neurologic symptoms or severe cardiac disease, parenteral antibiotic therapy with ceftriaxone or penicillin G is indicated.

Rocky Mountain Spotted Fever (RMSF)

- *Background.* This is a tick-borne illness spread by the *Dermacentor variabilis* or *Dermacentor andersoni* tick. The *Ixodes* tick is endemic to much of North America; 30-40% of patients cannot recall a tick bite. Complications include pneumonitis, renal failure, gangrene with loss of digits, and circulatory collapse.
- *Clinical presentation.* Patients may be asymptomatic. The classic triad is fever, rash, and headache; myalgias, malaise, and neurologic symptoms may be present. A maculopapular rash develops, which then becomes petechial, and involves the palms and soles. In severe cases gangrene may occur.
- *Diagnostic testing.* Patients may have thrombocytopenia and elevation of liver enzymes. In severe disease, renal insufficiency occurs. The diagnosis is clinical in the early stages, but serology is usually positive after 10 days. A skin biopsy can aid in diagnosis.
- *ED management.* Because of the high mortality associated with a delay in diagnosis, empiric treatment should begin in the ED for all patients suspected of having RMSF. Mild disease can be treated as an outpatient. Patients with neurologic symptoms, renal failure, vomiting or hemodynamic instability should be admitted. Doxycycline is the first line antimicrobial therapy, even in children. Therapy should be continued for 7 to 10 days or until 2 days after defervescence.

Tick Removal and Other Tick Borne Illness

- Any tick should be removed by grasping it with blunt forceps or tweezers and steady upward traction. Avoid touching the tick with bare hands or crushing the tick. Ticks should be flushed down the toilet.
- Other tick borne illnesses are described in Table 67–11.

Diseases of the Returning Traveler

- Determine any possible exposures to infections such as which areas were visited (and when), the type of travel (e.g., back packing, camping), eating patterns, insect bites, fresh water exposures, and contacts with animals or other humans. Ask about timing of symptoms because the incubation periods of infections, such as dengue fever or traveler's diarrhea, are days, hepatitis A can be several weeks, and tuberculosis or intestinal worms can be many months. Inquire about prophylaxis medications and immunizations. Malaria is less common (although still possible) among those who take antimalarials, and hepatitis A is extremely rare in those who have been immunized properly.
- No "routine" laboratory tests need to be performed on all returning travelers; these should depend on the particular clinical presentation.

Table 67–11 Other Tick-Related Illnesses

	Transmission	Clinical Presentation	Diagnosis	Treatment
Babesiosis	Deer tick; may also be transmitted by infected blood.	Fever, chills, anorexia, fatigue, emotional lability, photophobia, myalgias, arthralgias, dark urine, hyperesthesia. A rash is not characteristic of the disease. Splenomegaly may be present. Complications: hemolytic anemia, renal insufficiency, acute respiratory distress syndrome, and DIC.	Giemsa-stained or Wright-stained blood smears; serology	Clindamycin for severe disease and splenectomized.
Tularemia	Hares and rodents	Ulceroglandular is most common type (fever, headache, ulcerated skin lesions, painful regional lymphadenopathy). Oculoglandular (painful conjunctivitis). Typhoidal and pulmonary (pleuropneumonitis). Complications: pericarditis, meningitis, endocarditis, peritonitis, appendicitis, perisplenitis, osteomyelitis, Guillain-Barré. Death from respiratory failure and sepsis.	Blood or wound cultures, sputum, or conjunctival smears; bacterial agglutination or ELISA	Streptomycin or gentamycin. Standard isolation precautions necessary for pneumonic tularemia

	Transmission	Clinical Presentation	Diagnosis	Treatment
Erlichiosis	Salivary glands and midguts of tick vectors	Fever, headache, or myalgias. A rash may be present. Complications: ARDS, DIC, meningitis, pancarditis, renal failure, cognitive and neurologic deficits.	Peripheral blood smears (clusters inside leukocytes). PCR in the acute phase. IgG antibodies with IFA is confirmatory. Leukopenia, thrombocytopenia, and elevated liver enzymes in up to 50%	Doxycycline or tetracycline
Tick born relapsing fever	Infected saliva of arthropod vectors	Abrupt high fever, chills, headache, arthralgias, a macular or petechial skin rash (trunk > extremities), myalgias, nausea, and vomiting. A pruritic eschar at the bite site is rare. Delirium and peripheral neuropathy. Febrile episode lasts 3 d, asymptomatic period for 7 d, then relapse. Hepatomegaly, splenomegaly, and jaundice may occur. Death is rare and is limited to infants and elderly persons.	Spirochetes are visible on a routine blood smear stained with Wright's or Giemsa stain during an acute febrile episode.	Tetracycline or erythromycin. A Jarisch-Herxheimer–type reaction may occur in 30% after treatment (fever, severe rigors, hypotension).
Tick paralysis	Neurotoxin released when an adult female tick attaches	4 to 7 d after tick attaches, cerebellar dysfunction or an ascending paralysis ensues. Bulbar involvement and respiratory failure. Fever and sensory deficits are rare.	Clinical diagnosis	Complete recovery within 48 h of tick removal.

ARDS, acute respiratory disease syndrome; DIC, disseminated intravascular coagulation; ELISA, enzyme-linked immunosorbent assay; IFA, immunofluorescent assay; PCR, polymerase chain reaction

Eosinophilia may be present with human intestinal helminthes, such as *Ascaris*, hookworm, whipworm, and *Strongyloides*, or may be due to hypersensitivity reactions to drugs, such as antimalarials.

■ The most common infection among travelers is diarrhea, particularly from developing countries such as Latin America, Asia, Africa, and parts of the Middle East. Bacteria are the most common etiology, followed by viruses and parasites (see Chapter 27).

■ Common causes of fever in returned travelers include malaria, dengue, typhoid (Table 67–12), and hepatitis (see Chapter 41). Other possible travel-related causes of fever are extraintestinal amebiasis (most commonly hepatic abscess, Table 67–9), acute schistosomiasis, and leptospirosis (Table 67–12). Influenza (see Chapter 24), pneumonia (discussed above), urinary tract infection (see Chapter 27), and sexually transmitted diseases (Table 67–10) are also commonly encountered.

■ The viral hemorrhagic fevers (e.g., Ebola virus, Lassa fever, Hantavirus) are characterized by fever, mucosal and gastrointestinal bleeding, edema, and hypotension. These are caused by RNA viruses that result in severe and potentially fatal disease. They present as a severe multi-system syndrome with vascular compromise and hemorrhage. Treatment is primarily supportive as there is no cure.

■ The pattern of fever may provide diagnostic clues. *P. vivax* malaria causes tertian fever (fever spike every other day) and *P. malariae* causes a quartan pattern (fever spike every 3 days). A biphasic fever (brief afebrile period occurs between periods of fever) is seen in several flavivirus infections, such as dengue and yellow fever. A relative bradycardia (i.e., less than the expected 15 beats per minute increase for every 1°C elevation in temperature) may be seen in typhoid fever, yellow fever, and Legionnaire's disease.

■ Maculopapular rashes that are associated with fever may occur in dengue fever, viral hemorrhagic fevers, or early meningococcemia. Petechiae, ecchymoses, or hemorrhagic lesions are red flags to the clinician that the underlying illness may be life-threatening; meningococcemia, dengue, leptospirosis, and RMSF are possible causes.

■ Febrile patients who are jaundiced should raise concern for serious illness, such as *P. falciparum* malaria, typhoid fever, or leptospirosis. Patients who have one of the primary hepatitides (A-E) have fever typically in the prodromal, nonicteric phase that resolves with the onset of jaundice but may persist for a few days longer.

■ New onset of seizures may be the first manifestation of the parasitic CNS infection neurocysticercosis (*T. solium*), which is relatively common in those areas of the United States with immigrants from Latin America, and is caused by eating undercooked pork with encysted parasites. Latent syphilis and HIV (primary CNS disease, toxoplasmosis, and lymphoma) are other infectious disease causes of seizures.

Sepsis Syndrome

■ *Background.* Bacteremia is the presence of bacteria in the blood, as confirmed by culture. It may be transient or associated with sepsis and organ failure. Sepsis syndrome is defined as infection plus evidence of a

Table 67–12 Causes of Fever in the Returned Traveler

	Malaria	Typhoid (Enteric) Fever	Dengue	Leptospirosis	Schistosomiasis
Etiology	Protozoan parasite *Plasmodium*.	*Salmonella typhi*	Dengue virus (flavivirus)	Spiral bacteria (genus *Leptospira*)	Trematodes (flatworms); genus *Schistosoma*.
Incubation period	*P. falciprum:* <2 weeks *P. vivax, P. ovale:* may be months or years	Up to 3 wk	3–10 d	15 d	5–7 wk
Risk factors	Travel to any area where malaria is endemic; 90% of malaria cases originate in Africa. Transmitted by mosquito bite	Fecal-oral transmission. Travel to endemic areas such as Mexico, India, the Philippines, Pakistan, El Salvador, and Haiti.	Travel to endemic areas, particularly Mexico, the Caribbean, and Central and South America. Transmitted by mosquito bite.	Contact through abraded skin, mucous membranes, or conjunctiva following contact with urine-contaminated soil or water.	Fresh water in endemic areas: Africa, Eastern Mediterranean, South America, southeast Asia, and the western Pacific.
Clinical presentation	Fevers, diaphoresis, malaise, headaches, myalgias, vague abdominal pain; nausea, vomiting, and diarrhea in 25%; jaundice and hepato-splenomegaly.	Diarrhea early, constipation later. Fever, abdominal pain, pulse-temperature dissociation with relative bradycardia. Rose spots (bacterial emboli to the skin; sparse blanching maculopapular rash).	"Breakbone fever". Fever, headache and myalgias. Eye pain.	High fever, headaches, myalgias, conjunctivitis, maculopapular rash, hepato-splenomegaly; jaundice, azotemia, hypotension in 10% (Weil's syndrome)	Fever, chills, abdominal pain, diarrhea, nausea, vomiting, cough, headache, urticaria, hepato-splenomegaly, and lymphadenopathy.

Continued

Table 67–12 Causes of Fever in the Returned Traveler—*cont'd*

	Malaria	Typhoid (Enteric) Fever	Dengue	Leptospirosis	Schistosomiasis
Diagnostic testing	Malaria smears; pancytopenia and abnormal liver enzymes may be present	Blood cultures	Antibody titers	Serologic tests. Blood, urine, and cerebrospinal fluid can be obtained for culture.	Serology or by identifying characteristic eggs in stool, urine, or mucosal biopsies
Emergency department management	Quinine or quinidine gluconate. Parenteral therapy for complicated cases. Alternative therapy: artemisinin derivatives. Do not give steroids for cerebral edema	Fluoroquinolones	Supportive and symptomatic care	Doxycycline, ampicillin, amoxicillin, or erythromycin.	Praziquantel
Complications	Untreated *P. falciparum* infection can cause hypoglycemia, renal failure, pulmonary edema, neurologic deterioration, and death	Pancreatitis, meningitis, orchitis, osteomyelitis. Chronic carrier state with risk for GI malignances.	Dengue hemorrhagic fever can be present with DIC, shock state	Aseptic meningitis, uveitis, or chorioretinitis	Bleeding esophageal or gastric varices, liver failure, pulmonary hypertension, glomerulonephritis, central nervous system involvement.

systemic response manifested by two or more of the following: temperature below 36° C or above 38°C; heart rate above 90 beats per minute; respiratory rate above 20 breaths per minute or arterial CO_2 tension <32 mm Hg; and WBC below 4000 or above 12,000 or with more than 10% bands. Severe sepsis is sepsis syndrome with associated organ dysfunction and one or more of the following: hypotension, confusion, oliguria, hypoxia (not explained by primary respiratory disease), lactic acidosis, disseminated intravascular coagulation (DIC), or hepatic dysfunction (not explained by primary liver disease). Septic shock is defined as sepsis syndrome plus hypotension despite adequate fluid resuscitation.

■ *Clinical presentation.* A thorough history and physical examination should be performed because there are a variety of presentations depending on the source of infection. Tachycardia, tachypnea, hyperthermia or hypothermia, and hypotension may be present. A septic patient will often have flushed skin with warm, well-perfused extremities secondary to the early vasodilatation and hyperdynamic state.

■ *Diagnostic testing.* Obtain two sets of blood cultures (including line cultures). Culture other sites as clinically indicated. An elevated serum lactate concentration identifies tissue hypoperfusion in patients at risk who are not hypotensive. A CBC, electrolytes, liver function tests, coagulation studies, and urinalysis should be sent.

■ *ED management.* This includes early source identification and control (e.g., drainage of abscess, removal of infected foreign body). Empiric IV antibiotic therapy (see Chapter 90.2) should be started within the first hour of recognition of severe sepsis, after appropriate cultures have been obtained. A fluid challenge is useful for patients with suspected hypovolemia. When an appropriate fluid challenge fails to restore adequate blood pressure and organ perfusion, therapy with vasopressor agents should be started. Either norepinephrine or dopamine (through a central catheter as soon as available) is the first-choice vasopressor agent to correct hypotension in septic shock (see Chapter 90.3). Early goal-directed therapy for sepsis-induced hypoperfusion includes all of the following as the treatment protocol: central venous pressure of 8 to 12 mm Hg, mean arterial pressure of 65 mm Hg, urine output of 0.5 mL/kg^{-1}/h^{-1}, and central venous (superior vena cava) ($ScvO_2$) or mixed venous oxygen (SvO_2) saturation of 70%. During the first 6 hours of resuscitation of severe sepsis or septic shock, if $ScvO_2$ of 70% or SvO_2 of 65% is not achieved with fluid resuscitation to a central venous pressure of 8 to 12 mm Hg, transfuse packed red blood cells to achieve a hematocrit of 30% or administer a dobutamine infusion (up to a maximum of 20 μg/ kg^{-1}/min^{-1}) to achieve this goal. Recombinant human activated protein C (rhAPC) is used in patients with high risk of mortality and no contraindications (e.g., risk of life-threatening bleeding). IV corticosteroids (hydrocortisone 200-300 mg/d, for 7 days in three or four divided doses or by continuous infusion) are recommended in patients with septic shock who, despite adequate fluid replacement, require vasopressor therapy to maintain adequate blood pressure (i.e., adrenal insufficiency).

Infections in the Immunocompromised Host

- *Background.* See Chapter 37 (HIV) and 66 (Neutropenic Fever). These infections are considered to be present when there has been a fever above 38.5° C (or above 38° C three times in a 24-hour period) and an absolute neutrophil count (ANC) below 500/mm^3. Infections are common in patients with cancer after chemotherapy.
- *Clinical presentation.* The patient may have fever, malaise, mental status changes. A careful examination should include the skin, mouth, and any indwelling catheter sites.
- *Diagnostic testing.* Obtain a CBC with differential to calculate the ANC (WBC × [% bands + % mature neutrophils] × 0.01). At least two sets of blood cultures should be obtained, one set from indwelling catheter if present. Obtain a chest radiograph if any respiratory complaints are present, a urinalysis, and culture all possible sites of infection.
- *ED management.* Do not delay the administration of antibiotics. Empiric regimens may include cefepime, imipenem-cilastatin or meropenem as monotherapy. Use vancomycin if MRSA is suspected, or the patient has an indwelling venous catheter. Use vancomycin in the initial regimen only in highly selected cases. Add vancomycin, amphotericin, or both if the patient is febrile after 5 days of empirical antibiotic therapy, and especially if there is evidence of progressive disease.
- *Helpful hints and pitfalls.* These patients often lack signs of localizing infection, or they can be subtle because of lack of inflammatory response.

Infection Control Guidelines

- Guidelines for infection control have been established to protect patients and healthcare workers from infectious diseases. All health care workers should practice standard precautions on all patients. The most common types of isolation precautions are described below.
- **Standard precautions:** Should be used when the health care provider expects exposure to blood and body fluids. Personal protective equipment (PPE) is to be used, including a gown, gloves, and mask with eye protection if splash anticipated.
- **Contact isolation:** PPE is required for all healthcare worker interactions, and patients are to be in private rooms, with the use of dedicated patient equipment and patient transport occurring only if necessary. Conventional diseases requiring contact precautions includes MRSA, vancomycin resistant enterococcus (VRE), *Clostridium difficile*, respiratory syncytial virus (RSV), parainfluenza, enteroviruses, enteric infections in the incontinent host, and skin infections (e.g., staphylococcal scalded skin syndrome, herpes simplex virus, impetigo, lice, and scabies).
- **Droplet isolation:** Droplet transmission involves contact with large-particle droplets containing microorganisms generated from a person who has a clinical disease, or who is a carrier of the microorganism. Transmission via large droplet particles requires close contact between source and recipient persons, because droplets do not remain suspended in the air, and generally travel only short distances. Because droplets

do not remain suspended in the air, special air handling and ventilation are not required to prevent droplet transmission. Health care providers are to use PPE including surgical masks at all times while providing patient care. This type of patient should be in a private room. Conventional diseases requiring droplet precautions include invasive *Haemophilus influenzae* and meningococcal disease, drug-resistant pneumococcal disease, diphtheria, pertussis, mycoplasma, Group A beta-hemolytic streptococcal (GABS), influenza, mumps, rubella, and parvovirus. Pneumonic plague is an example of a biothreat disease requiring this type of isolation.

■ **Airborne isolation:** This is for small infectious particles. PPE including N95 mask or PAPR (Powered Air-Purifying Respirator) should be worn at all times and the patient should remain in a private negative pressure isolation room with 6-12 air changes per hour. Conventional disease that require airborne precautions include measles, varicella, and pulmonary tuberculosis. Any suspicious for a bioterrorism threat from smallpox should also have airborne precautions.

■ **Reverse isolation:** This is a unique form of isolation designed to protect the patient from infection. This form of isolation is used most commonly in patients at risk for serious infection such as burn, transplant, and chemotherapy patients.

Teaching Points

When the patient is immunocompromised, has severe comorbidities, or is at the extremes of age, bacterial infections become more common, more dangerous, and less likely to present with easily recognizable signs and symptoms. It is therefore necessary to aggressively treat with broad spectrum antibiotics, admit the patient to the hospital, and try to intervene in the illness before serious manifestations become evident. Cultures and sensitivities will not provide useful information in the ED, but may guide inpatient management more rationally. Septic workups can be performed efficiently, but in sick patients, diagnostic information gathering should yield to the initiation of life-saving therapy such as starting the antibiotics and fluids in the patient who is ill, and then obtain needed diagnostic studies.

CHAPTER 68

Obstetrics and Gynecology

DIRK ALAN PERRITT ■ ELYSIA MOSCHOS

68.1 Approach to the Female Patient with a Genitourinary Complaint

Overview

In general, nongenitourinary complaints of male and female patients are treated without differentiation to gender. However, there are a myriad of physiologic and anatomic differences that differentiate the two genders, and must be understood to safely and accurately treat genitourinary (GU) complaints of the female patient. The most common GU problems presenting to the ED will be discussed in this chapter: pelvic pain (68.2), vaginal bleeding in the nonpregnant patient (68.3), genital infections (68.4), and pregnancy and pregnancy-related conditions (68.5).

Pelvic pain is a common complaint of female patients in the ED. The ED evaluation of any woman with abdominal pain must consider genitourinary-related sources. Concerning causes include salpingitis, ectopic pregnancy, ruptured corpus luteum cyst, adnexal torsion, tubo-ovarian abscess, and appendicitis.

Vaginal bleeding is the most common gynecologic complaint. There are multiple causes in the pregnant and nonpregnant patient. Vaginal bleeding may be the first manifestation of an ectopic pregnancy or concerning for a malignancy in the postmenopausal patient.

Genital infections are a common reason for visits to the ED, and a proper pelvic examination and testing must be performed on all women where there is suspicion for such diagnosis. Sexually transmitted diseases (STDs) are discussed in Chapter 67.

Pregnancy must always be considered in all women of reproductive age. Any failure to identify pregnancy may result in harm to both the fetus and the patient.

Initial Diagnostic Approach
General

■ Assesss the ABC's as discussed in Section II. All female patients of reproductive age presenting to the ED need to be evaluated for pregnancy, regardless of last menstrual period or birth control method. No contraception, including tubal ligation, is 100% effective. If pregnant, the physical examination should include an evaluation of both maternal and fetal well-being. In patients presenting with acute pelvic pain, early consideration should be given to potentially life-threatening or fertility compromising causes: ectopic pregnancy, ovarian torsion, salpingitis or tubo-ovarian abscess, as well as common non-gynecologic diseases such as appendicitis.

■ *Obstetric and gynecologic history.* An OB/GYN history should be routinely obtained on all female patients, regardless of age. This includes menstrual history, pregnancy history, vaginal and pelvic infections, gynecologic procedures, urologic history, sexual history, and contraceptive status. Ask about the presence of pelvic or vaginal pain, bleeding, or discharge.

■ *Symptoms.* Inquire about the characteristics of the pain if present. Diffuse pain extending bilaterally may be due to pelvic inflammatory disease, peritonitis, or intra-abdominal hemorrhage. Sudden onset of pain should be concerning for torsion, perforation, or rupture (ectopic pregnancy or cyst). Chronic or recurrent pain is commonly due to endometriosis, ovarian cyst, or mass. The presence of fever is more concerning as a source of sepsis. Nausea and vomiting may be present with early pregnancy, appendicitis, ovarian torsion, or ureteral colic. Pain in the mid cycle may be due to Mittelschmerz (ovulation pain). Ask about urination and bowel habits. Pelvic pain may occur with a urinary tract infection or constipation. Inquire about any vaginal discharge, vaginal pain, or vaginal bleeding.

■ *Physical examination.* Determine the presence of tenderness and evidence of diffuse peritonitis (pelvic inflammatory disease [PID], ruptured appendix, or hemorrhage). A rectal examination should be performed looking for blood or hard stool in the rectal vault.

■ *Pelvic examination.* Indications for pelvic examination include: menstrual abnormalities or abnormal bleeding, unexplained abdominal or pelvic pain, vaginal discharge, symptoms of infection, or pregnancy. Patients who are more than 20 weeks pregnant should have an obstetric consult if complaining of pelvic pain. A pelvic ultrasound should be performed to exclude the diagnosis of placental previa if the patient complains of vaginal bleeding. Both external and internal genitalia (speculum examination and bimanual) should be examined. However, refrain from performing a pelvic examination if placenta previa is suspected. An open os in a pregnant patient is indicative of an incomplete or inevitable abortion. Cervical motion tenderness may be caused by PID, ruptured ovarian cyst, ovarian torsion, or endometriosis. A pelvic mass is concerning for an ovarian cyst, ovarian torsion, tubo-ovarian abscess, ovarian tumor, or ectopic pregnancy. Pus from the cervical os is consistent with PID. The proper bacteriologic swabs (gonorrhea and chlamydia) should be sent for any patient where pelvic infection is of concern. It is also useful to employ microscopic examination of vaginal secretions in saline and 10% potassium hydroxide (KOH) solution for candida vaginitits (hyphae or pseudohyphae), trichomonas (flagellated trichomonads), or bacterial vaginosis (fishy odor and "clue" cells).

Laboratory

- Laboratory studies will depend on the chief complaint and the pregnancy status of the patient.
- A urinary pregnancy test should always be done on any woman of reproductive age regardless of the date of last menstruation. A urine dipstick should be done on all pregnant patients as screening for pre-eclampsia and urinary tract infections; however mild glycosuria and proteinuria are normal.
- For pregnant women in the first trimester with pain, vaginal bleeding, or in whom an ectopic pregnancy is otherwise suspected, order a quantitative beta-human chorionic gonadotropin (β-hCG) level, type and screen, Rh factor, complete blood count (CBC) (baseline hemoglobin), and urinalysis (evaluate for urinary tract infection [UTI]).
- For patients presenting in the second or third trimester, studies may include a CBC, liver function tests (LFTs), electrolytes, renal function tests, type and screen, and urinalysis particularly if concerned for pre-eclamsia.
- When there is clinical concern for fetomaternal hemorrhage (e.g., maternal trauma) a Kleihauer-Betke test should be performed to determine the extent of any feto-maternal transfusion so that the appropriate amount of RhoGAM may be given to prevent isoimmunization.
- Nonpregnant female patients with pelvic pain should have a CBC and urinalysis.
- Nonpregnant patients with vaginal bleeding should have a CBC, urine pregnancy test, type and screen or type and cross match if necessary, and coagulation studies.
- Patients with significant bleeding or hemodynamic instability should have blood sent for type and cross match. An initial hemoglobin and hematocrit level may not be indicative of acute blood loss so repeated hemoglobin testing should be done to ascertain a trend. A CBC, coagulation studies, d-dimer, and fibrinogen studies should be ordered to determine if a coagulopathy exists.
- A catheterized urinary specimen is preferred in patients with vaginal bleeding as the presence of vaginal blood may skew results.

Radiography

- ***Ultrasound.*** Pelvic ultrasound in the ED is a fast and inexpensive method of evaluating the female reproductive organs. A formal sonographic examination is used to evaluate for intrauterine pregnancy, uterine size and endometrial characteristics, and the adnexae for the presence of ovarian torsion, cysts, hydrosalpinx, neoplasms, or tubo-ovarian abscess. Identification of an intrauterine pregnancy excludes an ectopic pregnancy as the presence of a heterotopic pregnancy is rare. An intrauterine pregnancy should be evident on transvaginal ultrasound when the serum β-hCG is above 1500 mIU/ml or on transabdominal ultrasound when the β-hCG is above 6500 mIU/ml.
- ***Radiography.*** While it is wise to limit the radiation exposure of the fetus from imaging studies, this should not be done at the expense of failing

to obtain lifesaving information about the mother. Refer to Chapter 92 for radiation exposure in the pregnant patient.

Emergency Department Management Overview
General

- Patients who arrive with unstable vitals or show signs of shock should receive aggressive volume resuscitation with two large bore IVs, isotonic fluids, and blood products as needed. Emergent consultation with an obstetrics/ gynecology specialist should be arranged.
- All pregnant patients should have fetal heart tones assessed. Fetal heart tones can be heard by Doppler starting at 12 weeks, and by fetoscope at 18 weeks. The normal fetal heart rate is 120 to 160 beats per minute (bpm). All patients who have a viable pregnancy at 20 weeks or greater should be placed on fetal monitoring. The obstetrician/gynecologist on call should be notified when the patient presents with pain or vaginal bleeding.

Medications

- The pharmacologic effects of fetal drug exposure should always be considered in the pregnant patient before treatment. Teratogenesis has its most profound effects during the time of fetal organogenesis, which occurs between 3 and 9 weeks of gestation. The U.S. Food and Drug Administration (FDA) categories of drug safety in pregnancy are listed in Table 68.1–1. A list of common medications and use in pregnancy is listed in Table 68.1–2. Most drugs are safe during lactation, as subtherapeutic amounts appear in breast milk (approximately 1% to 2% of the maternal dose).
- *Analgesia.* Medicate for pain as described in Chapter 90.1. NSAIDs should not be used on the pregnant patient, but are commonly used to treat pelvic pain in the nonpregnant patient.
- *Antibiotics.* They are given for a variety of causes described in this chapter. Treatment for sexually transmitted disease is summarized in Chapter 67.
- *Estrogen.* Give 25-mg doses IV for severe uterine bleeding in the nonpregnant patient.
- *RhoGAM.* For an Rh-negative woman with antepartum bleeding, RhoGAM should be administered. A Kleihauer-Betke test should also be performed to determine the extent of any feto-maternal transfusion so that the appropriate amount of RhoGAM may be given to prevent isoimmunization. The approximate dose is 300 µg.
- *Betamethasone.* This corticosteroid is commonly given to promote fetal lung maturity prior to 34 weeks in any patient where preterm delivery is imminent (12 mg IM every 12 hours for two doses).

Emergency Department Interventions

- *Transfusion.* Any patient with an emergent cause of bleeding should immediately be typed and cross matched. If the patient is unstable, type O–negative blood may be started pending donor matched blood.

Table 68.1–1	**FDA Classification of Drug Safety During Pregnancy**
Category A	Controlled studies in women fail to demonstrate a risk to the fetus in the first trimester (and there is no evidence of risk in later trimesters), and the possibility of fetal harm appears remote.
Category B	Either animal reproduction studies have not demonstrated a fetal risk but there are no controlled studies in pregnant women, or animal reproduction studies have shown an adverse effect (other than a decrease in fertility) that was not confirmed in controlled studies in women in the first trimester (and there is no evidence of risk in later trimesters).
Category C	Either studies in animals have revealed adverse effects on the fetus (teratogenic or embryocidal or other) and there are no controlled studies in women, or studies in women and animals are not available. Drugs should be given only if the potential benefit justifies the potential risk to the fetus.
Category D	There is positive evidence of human fetal risk, but the benefits from use in pregnant women may be acceptable despite the risk (e.g., if the drug is needed in a life-threatening situation or for a serious disease in which safer drugs cannot be used or are ineffective).
Category X	Studies in animals or human beings have demonstrated fetal abnormalities or there is evidence of fetal risk based on human experience, and the risk of the use of the drug in pregnant women clearly outweighs any possible benefit. The drug is contraindicated in women who are or may become pregnant.

FDA, US Food and Drug Administration.
(From Briggs GG, Freeman RK, Yaffe SJ (editors). Drugs in Pregnancy and Lactation: a Reference Guide to Fetal And neonatal risk. 5th ed. Baltimore: Williams & Wilkins, 1998, pp 12, 577–578, 627–628.)

Transfusions are usually avoided in stable patients unless the hematocrit drops below 20%.

- **Urinary catheter.** Urine output should be closely monitored as a gauge of renal function and perfusion status in all emergent causes of vaginal bleeding.

Disposition

- **Consultation.** Obstetric and gynecologic consultation should be obtained whenever the diagnosis requires intervention (e.g., ectopic pregnancy, incomplete abortion, tubo-ovarian abscess, uncontrolled vaginal bleeding) and for any patient presenting to the ED in the second or third trimester with pregnancy related concerns. General surgery should be consulted for appendicitis.
- **Admission.** All patients requiring IV therapy or surgical intervention should be admitted. Any pregnant female with a viable pregnancy greater

Table 68.1–2   Common Medications Used During Pregnancy

	Safe for Pregnancy	Not Recommended	Comment
Analgesics	Acetaminophen Opiates (therapeutic use)	Aspirin NSAIDS*	NSAIDs may reduce the amount of amniotic fluid, and can prematurely close the ductus arteriosus.
Antibiotics	Penicillin and derivatives Cephalosporins Macrolides Nystatin Clotrimazole Isoniazid (INH) Ethambutol Rifampin	Sulfonamides (first and third trimesters) Tetracycline Fluoroquinolones Metronidazole (first trimester) Aminoglycosides.	The estolate salt of erythromycin has been associated with the development of hepatotoxicity. Sulfonamides are not recommended in the third trimester because of the risk of kernicterus in the newborn and their effects on folate metabolism. Fluoroquinolones are contraindicated in pregnancy due to the risk of arthropathy. Tetracycline is a teratogen, and can stain bones and decidual teeth. Aminoglycosides can cause fetal ototoxicity.
Anticoagulants	Heparin Low-molecular-weight (LMW) heparin	Warfarin	Warfarin can increase congenital anomalies, prematurity, and still birth.
Anticonvulsants	Magnesium sulfate (for eclampsia) Felbamate Gabapentin Clonazepam Lamotrigine	Phenytoin Carbamazepine Valproic acid Phenobarbital	All commonly used anticonvulsant agents have been associated with congenital anomalies. Patients maintained on an agent before pregnancy may continue therapy during pregnancy due to the negative effects of seizure on the fetus. Oral administration of vitamin K beginning a month before delivery is recommended to decrease the incidence of hemorrhagic disease of the newborn. All safe agents listed (except for magnesium sulfate) are category C.

Table 68.1–2 Common Medications Used During Pregnancy—*cont'd*

	Safe for Pregnancy	Not Recommended	Comment
Antiemetics	Promethazine Prochlorperazine Odansetron Pyridoxine		Most standard antiemetics are in FDA category C (promethazine, prochlorperazine), and are used successfully to treat hyperemesis gravidarum. Odansetron is category B, but more costly. Pyridoxine (category A) can be used as a single agent.
Acid suppressants	Ranitidine Omeprazole		
Cardiovascular drugs	Adenosine Digoxin Encainide/Flecainide Lidocaine Procainamide	Amiodarone	Lidocaine and procainamide levels should be monitored.
Antihypertensives	Beta blockers Calcium channel blockers Hydralazine Clonidine Methyldopa Nitroprusside	Angiotensin-converting enzyme inhibitors Thiazide diuretics	First trimester use of thiazides has been associated with congenital anomalies. Volume depletion with diuretics is an adverse effect that may have negative consequences on the fetus.
Antihistamines and decongestants	Diphenhydramine Topical nasal sprays	Brompheniramine	Drowsiness can be a problem. Long-term effects of decongestants are unknown.
Respiratory medications	Albuterol Terbutaline Prednisone		Prednisone during the first trimester has been associated with the increased incidence of oral clefts. Guaifenesin is commonly used, but may increase the risk of neural tube defects if used in the first trimester.

NSAID=non-steroidal anti-inflammatory drugs

than 20 weeks should be admitted to an obstetrics service for continued fetal monitoring and management.

■ ***Discharge.*** All patients should be given appropriate and clearly understandable discharge instructions, including directions for follow-up. All pregnant patients should receive timely access to prenatal care. Recommendations for prenatal care include initial obstetric evaluation between 6 and 8 weeks. Recommendations for proper nutritional supplementation (Folate 400 µg by mouth daily) and medications to avoid in pregnancy should also be given.

68.2 Acute Pelvic Pain

■ See Chapter 68.1 for initial diagnostic approach and overview of ED management.

■ Acute pelvic pain is the second most common gynecologic complaint after vaginal bleeding. The history and physical examination can narrow the differential diagnosis and direct diagnostic investigations (see Chapter 68.1).

■ Pelvic pain is due to a variety of different causes, many of which do not require definitive diagnosis or treatment on an emergent basis. No pathologic condition is identified in up to 20% of women. The goal is to identify those causes that are most likely to cause significant morbidity.

■ Box 68.2–1 lists the differential diagnosis of acute pelvic pain. Table 68.2–1 summarizes concerning causes of acute pelvic pain that must be identified in the ED. Recommended antimicrobial therapy for PID is listed in Table 68.2–2.

BOX 68.2–1   Differential Diagnosis of Acute Pelvic Pain

- Appendicitis
- Constipation
- Diverticulitis
- Ectopic pregnancy
- Endometriosis
- Gastroenteritis
- Inflammatory bowel disease
- Irritable bowel syndrome
- Mesenteric adenitis
- Ovarian cyst
- Ovarian torsion
- Pelvic inflammatory disease
- Renal colic
- Tubo-ovarian abscess
- Urinary tract infection

Table 68.2–1   Concerning Causes of Acute Pelvic Pain in the ED*

	Background	History	Physical Examination	Diagnostic Studies in the ED	ED Management
Ectopic pregnancy	Implantation of embryo outside of the endometrial cavity. 95% occur in the fallopian tubes. Risk factors: history of an ectopic or pelvic infection, IUD.	Sudden, sharp unilateral pelvic pain, but pain may be vague or bilateral. Vaginal bleeding is common; syncope and orthostatic changes may occur.	Adnexal mass and tenderness (+) CMT Hypotension, or peritonitis suggest rupture.	Pelvic ultrasound to look for IUP. Quantitative β-hCG (should double every 48 hours) Progesterone >25 ng/ml suggests a viable intrauterine pregnancy	Emergent gynecology consultation. Surgical removal or methotrexate (if unruptured and less than 4 cm in diameter).
Ovarian torsion	Pain is mostly due to ischemia. Risk factors: ovarian mass, pregnancy.	Acute, severe, intermittent and unilateral pain; may be related to abrupt change in position. Nausea and vomiting.	Adnexal mass and tenderness Possible peritonitis (+) CMT	Ultrasound with doppler flow studies	Emergent gynecology consultation.
Pelvic inflammatory disease (PID) and tubo-ovarian abscess (TOA)	PID includes endometritis, parametritis, salpingitis, oophoritis, pelvic peritonitis, tubo-ovarian abscess, periappendicitis, perihepatitis (Fitz-Hugh-Curtis syndrome), and perisplenitis.	Without TOA, pain usually bilateral. Fever, new or malodorous vaginal discharge, dyspareunia, dysuria, and abnormal uterine bleeding. Gonococcal PID is more fulminant than Chlamydia PID; occurs within one week of	Abnormal cervical or vaginal mucopurulent discharge. (+) CMT If peritonitis present usually bilateral adnexal mass with TOA.	Cervical cultures and smear Minimum criteria for diagnosis include uterine/ adnexal tenderness or CMT. Pelvic ultrasound or CT scan for TOA Laparoscopy is more accurate.	All require broad-spectrum antibiotics for 10-14 days (see Table 68–3). Hospitalize patients who are unable to comply with outpatient regiment, complicating

Table 68.2–1 Concerning Causes of Acute Pelvic Pain in the ED*—cont'd

	Background	History	Physical Examination	Diagnostic Studies in the ED	ED Management
	Risk factors: prior PID, unprotected sex, IUD, substance abuse. Complications: risk of ectopic pregnancy, chronic pelvic pain, infertility, sepsis. Mostly due to gonorrhea and chlamydia.	1 week of the onset of menses. Chlamydial PID is characterized by a subacute course with mild symptoms.			factors (pregnancy, HIV, TOA), or severe illness. Most TOAs resolve with medical therapy but surgery required in 25%.
Ruptured corpus luteum cyst	Less common than follicular cysts but clinically more important. Most occur between days 20 and 26 of cycle or may have a delay in menses.	Abrupt severe lateral pain. Patients may have cramping or lower abdominal pain 1-2 weeks before overt rupture. May have lightheadedness if bleeding is severe; rectal pain from fluid in cul-de-sac.	Hypotension and tachycardia if blood loss is significant.	Pelvic ultrasound	Emergent gynecology consultation.

*CMT, Cervical motion tenderness; RLQ, right lower quadrant; CT scan, computed tomography; IUD, intrauterine device; β-hCG, β-human chorionic gonadotropin; TOA, tubo-ovarian abscess; PID, pelvic inflammatory disease; *Appendicitis is discussed in Chapter 18, "Abdominal Pain."*

Table 68.2–2	Recommended Treatment of PID	
Oral treatment		
Regimen A		Ofloxacin 400 mg PO q12h for 14 d
	Plus	Metronidazole 500 mg PO q12h for 14 days
Regimen B	Either	Ceftriaxone 250 mg IM, or
		Cefoxitin 2 g IM plus probenecid 1 g PO in a single dose concurrently, or
		Other parenteral third-generation cephalosporin (e.g., ceftizoxime or cefotaxime)
	Plus	Doxycycline 100 mg PO q12h for 14 d
	Plus	Metronidazole 500 mg PO q12h for 7 d
Parenteral treatment		
Regimen A	Either	Cefotetan 2 g IV q12h, or
		Cefoxitin 2 g iv q6h
	Plus	Doxycycline 100 mg IV or PO q12h
This regimen should be continued for 48 hours after substantial clinical improvement. Doxycycline 100 mg PO q12h should then be administered for 14 d		
Regimen B		Clindamycin 900 mg iv q8h
	Plus	Gentamycin loading dose IV or IM (2 mg/kg body weight) followed by a maintenance dose of 1.5 mg/kg
	Followed by either	Doxycycline 100 mg PO q12h, or
		Clindamycin 450 mg PO q6h
This regimen should be continued for 48 hours after substantial clinical improvement. Doxycycline 100 mg PO q12h or clindamycin 450 mg PO q6h should then be administered for 14 d.		

Data from Centers for Disease Control and Prevention.

68.3 Vaginal Bleeding in the Nonpregnant Patient

Review of Normal Menstruation

- Normal menstrual cycles vary from 21 to 35 days (average of 28 days) and last from 2 to 6 days. The average volume of blood loss during menstruation is 20 to 60 ml per cycle.
- The first part of the menstrual cycle is the follicular or proliferative phase in which the ovarian follicles develop, and the endometrium thickens (in response to estrogen). After ovulation the ovarian corpus luteum produces progesterone to stabilize the endometrium.

- The second part of the menstrual cycle is the luteal phase and lasts 14 days. The endometrial secretory glands further develop and mature. If implantation of a fertilized egg does not occur, the corpus luteum decreases production of progesterone and involutes. The endometrium then begins to slough, causing menstruation to occur.
- Menopause occurs around 50 years of age. The ovaries begin to fail causing anovulatory cycles and irregular bleeding. Ovarian production of estrogen declines, follicular development ceases, and the endometrium lining thins.

Terminology

- Menorrhagia is excessive blood loss during menstruation exceeding 80 ml or more than 7 consecutive days of menstruation.
- Metrorrhagia is abnormal bleeding at irregular intervals or between cycles.
- Menometrorrhagia is prolonged or heavy bleeding at irregular intervals.

Causes of Vaginal Bleeding in the Nonpregnant Patient

- Vaginal bleeding is the most common gynecologic complaint. The history and physical examination can narrow the differential diagnosis and direct empiric therapy. See 68.1 for initial diagnostic approach and overview of ED management.
- The underlying disease process often goes undiagnosed during the initial ED evaluation. Conditions such as trauma, sexual abuse, infection, coagulopathy, or foreign body must be diagnosed and addressed in the ED. See Table 68.3–1 for causes of vaginal bleeding by different age groups in the nonpregnant patient. Vaginal bleeding in the pregnant patient is discussed in Chapter 68.5.
- Vaginal bleeding in the prepubertal female is always abnormal and should be investigated.
- Dysfunctional uterine bleeding (DUB) is the most common cause of menorrhagia. Anovulatory bleeding is the most common type. When anovulation occurs, no corpus luteum is formed, and no progesterone is produced exposing the endometrium to unopposed estrogen. The endometrium eventually outgrows its blood supply and begins to degenerate resulting in irregular and unpredictable bleeding. The causes of anovulation are often related to the hypothalamic-pituitary-ovarian axis. It is a diagnosis of exclusion after pregnancy, reproductive tract pathology, systemic illness, and coagulopathy have been ruled out. It is most common at the extremes of reproductive years. The patient may describe periods of amenorrhea interspersed with unpredictable heavy vaginal bleeding and intermenstrual spotting. This diagnosis cannot be proven in the ED setting.
- Postmenopausal bleeding is bleeding occurring after menopause, which is defined as cessation of menses for 12 months. Endometrial cancer is not the most common cause of vaginal bleeding in the postmenopausal female, but it is the most important. These patients should be referred for an endometrial biopsy.

Table 68.3–1	Causes of Vaginal Bleeding in the Non-Pregnant Patient
Causes of Vaginal Bleeding in the Non-Pregnant Patient	
Premenarchal	Exogenous hormones Inflammation/infection of vagina or vulva Foreign bodies Sexual abuse Trauma Tumor Urologic pathology Precocious puberty (sexual development before age 8)
Pre-Menopause	Vulvar/vaginal lesions Cervicitis/endometritis Endocervical/endometrial polyps Uterine fibroids and adenomyosis Dysfunctional uterine bleeding/anovulation Hormonal contraception/IUDs Pelvic cancer (i.e. cervix) Sexual intercourse/trauma/foreign body Coagulopathy Systemic diseases (i.e. thyroid disease)
Peri-Menopause	Same as Pre-Menopause, plus Endometrial cancer
Post-Menopause	Vaginal atrophy Cervicitis/endometritis Endometrial polyps Endometrial hyperplasia Pelvic cancers (i.e. vagina, vulvar, endometrial, ovarian) Exogenous hormones

Diagnostic Testing

- Studies that may influence ED therapy and disposition are indicated. These include a CBC, urine pregnancy test, type and screen or type and cross match if necessary, and coagulation studies.
- Thyroid studies and prolactin levels may be requested by the consulting physician.
- A pelvic ultrasound is indicated in the ED setting to evaluate for a foreign body in a prepubertal female or for the evaluation of pelvic pain or pelvic mass.

Emergency Department Management

- Any hemodynamically unstable patient requires emergent resuscitation before further workup.

- Estrogens are the treatment of choice for heavy uterine bleeding. For hospitalized patients, intravenous doses of conjugated equine estrogens can be given in 25-mg doses every 4 to 6 hours for 24 hours until bleeding has subsided. Then a progestin is added, and the patient switches to oral estrogens. For outpatients, estrogen can also be given by mouth at a dose of 8 mg/day in four divided doses (estradiol 2 mg PO q 4-6 hours). When bleeding stops, 10 mg of medroxyprogesterone acetate is also given each day for 7 to 10 days. A short-lived withdrawal bleeding episode can then be expected. For patients with minimal continuous bleeding and a history suggestive of chronic anovulation, oral medroxyprogesterone alone or as combination oral contraceptives can be used.
- Nonsteroidal anti-inflammatory drugs may increase endometrial hemostasis, and provide symptomatic relief for dysmenorrhea. These are often used to supplement therapy for most causes of vaginal bleeding in the nonpregnant patient. Several other agents are used by gynecologists for the treatment of menorrhagia but have little utility in the ED setting.
- There are many surgical techniques available to treat vaginal bleeding unresponsive to medical management. Dilation and curettage is the quickest surgical modality. In cases of severe, recurrent menorrhagia, a hysterectomy can be performed.
- Consultation with a gynecology specialist may be useful to assist with acute therapy. Perimenopausal and menopausal women should have an evaluation for possible uterine malignancy. Admit patients requiring blood products, surgical intervention, or intravenous pharmacotherapy. Patients who are orthostatic or whose hemoglobin is less than 7.0 should be transfused. Elderly patients or those with underlying medical conditions should have earlier administration of blood products.

68.4 Vaginitis and Genital Infections

- See 68.1 for initial diagnostic approach and overview of ED management.
- Genital infections are a common reason for presentation to the ED. Sexually transmitted diseases (STDs) are summarized in Chapter 67.
- Pelvic inflammatory disease and tubo-ovarian abscess are discussed in Table 68.2–1.
- Vaginitis commonly presents with abnormal vaginal discharge (increased volume, color change, or malodorous), vulvar itching or burning, and dyspareunia. The most common causes are due to infections or atrophic changes and are summarized in Table 68.4–1. Other causes include vulvar dermatologic conditions, trauma, neoplasms. Genital herpes can cause acute vulvar symptoms.

Table 68.4–1 Common Causes of Vaginitis

	Etiology	Clinical Presentation	Diagnosis	Management
Candida vaginitis	*Candida albicans*, a yeast (fungi) causes most. *Candida glabrata* and *Candida tropicalis* are more resistant to standard treatment Risk factors: birth control pills, spermicides, HIV, systemic steroids, antibiotics, tight clothing, diabetes.	Thick, white discharge, vulvar pruritis; vulvar swelling, dysuria. Most occur before menses or associated with intercourse.	Clinical presentation and microscopic examination of vaginal discharge in saline and 10% KOH: hyphae or pseudohyphae with budding yeast. Vaginal pH: < 4.5 Vaginal culture rarely indicated.	Antifungal intravaginal agents or oral agent. Fluconazole 150 mg (pregnancy category C) PO, 1 course is as efficacious as 7 days of intravaginal clotrimazole in uncomplicated cases. Low potency steroid discomfort from vulvitis.
Trichomonas vaginalis vaginitis	Due to motile protozoan *T. vaginalis*. Can be recovered from 70%–80% of male partners and is thus considered an STD.	Up to 50% may not report symptoms unless asked directly. Discharge is malodorous, copious, green, and frothy; vulvar irritation and pruritis. Punctation or "strawberry" cervix may be noted.	Vaginal pH >4.5. Saline wet mount: numerous leukocytes and motile, flagellated trichomonads.	There are multiple sites of infection (urethra, Skene glands, Bartholin's glands in addition to vaginal epithelium) requiring systemic therapy with metronidazole 2 g PO as a single dose or 500 mg PO BID for 7 d. Treat during pregnancy only if symptomatic as disease may cause low birth weight and pre-term labor.

Table 68.4–1   Common Causes of Vaginitis—*cont'd*

	Etiology	Clinical Presentation	Diagnosis	Management
Bacterial vaginosis	Normal levels of lactobacillus (needed to maintain normal pH < 4.5 and prevent proliferation of other organisms) are reduced and replaced by *Gardnerella vaginalis*, *Mycoplasma*, *Mobiluncus*, *Bacteriodes* species, and peptostreptococcus.	50% are asymptomatic. Most common presentation is malodorous gray discharge.	Vaginal pH >4.5. Wet mount preparation with saline reveals minimal or no leukocytes, many bacteria, and "clue cells," which are squamous cells in which coccobacillary bacteria have obscured the borders and cytoplasm. Positive "whiff" test: fishy odor when 10% KOH is added.	Metronidazole 500 mg BID for 7 days. Other options include 0.75% metronidazole intravaginally for 5 days or 2% clindamycin intravaginally for 7 days.
Atrophic vaginitis	Most common in postmenopausal women. Results from estrogen withdrawal because the vaginal epithelium depends on estrogen.	Atrophy and inflammation of vulvar structures; pruritis, burning, tenderness, dyspareunia. There is normal vaginal discharge.	Vaginal pH >4.5. Absence of infectious source of symptoms.	Topical estrogen vaginal cream every night for up to 2 wk. Hormone replacement therapy to be initiated by the patient's primary care physician.

68.5 Pregnancy and Pregnancy-Related Issues

- Pregnancy is associated with numerous adaptations of maternal physiology and anatomy. These changes are essential to understanding potential complications in pregnancy as well as interpreting laboratory tests (Table 68.5–1).
- Pregnant women can have the same surgical conditions as nonpregnant women, and should be treated appropriately for any emergent condition, regardless of pregnancy status. While purely elective and semi-urgent cases should be postponed until after delivery, any emergent condition, such as cholecystitis or appendicitis, should be treated in the same manner as a nonpregnant patient.

Table 68.5–1   Normal Physiologic Changes in Pregnancy

Organs System	Change	Potential Complications
Heme	Plasma volume ↑ with relative hemoglobin/hematocrit ↓ White blood cells ↑	Dilutional anemia
Cardiovascular	Arterial relaxation Venous dilatation Stroke volume↑, heart rate↑, cardiac output↑	↓ Blood pressure until 20 wk then rises Venous stasis → hypercoagulable state
Pulmonary	Minute ventilation ↑ Tidal volume ↑ Residual volume ↓	Physiologic hyperventilation, drop in $PaCO_2$ Respiratory alkalosis
Gastrointestinal	↓Gastric sphincter tone ↑Abdominal pressure ↓Gastric motility	Nausea, vomiting and gastric reflux Hemorrhoids Constipation
Renal	Dilatation of ureters/renal pelvis Glomerular filtration rate ↑, blood urea nitrogen/creatinine ↓ Mild glycosuria and proteinuria are normal	Increases risk of urinary tract infection and pyelonephritis
Endocrine	Insulin resistance	Gestational diabetes
Other	Erythrocyte sedimentation rate ↑ Alkaline phosphatase ↑	Poor indicators in pregnancy

Pregnancy Complications

- The complications that arise during pregnancy can be threatening to both the fetus and the mother.
- A summary of pregnancy complications are listed in Table 68.5–2. Pregnancy complications associated with vaginal bleeding are discussed in Table 68.5–3. Most patients presenting to the ED with vaginal bleeding are in their first trimester.
- Patients in their second or third trimester with possible pregnancy-related concerns are often brought directly to the obstetrical unit, thus bypassing the ED. However, given that these patients may present to the ED, concerning problems in this patient population are briefly discussed.

Vaginal Bleeding In The Pregnant Patient

- See Table 68.5–3 for the differential diagnosis of vaginal bleeding in pregnancy.
- If the patient is hemodynamically unstable, place on a cardiac monitor, insert two large bore IVs, infuse 1-2 liters of normal saline, and administer blood products as needed.

First-Trimester Bleeding: Spontaneous Abortion

- *Background.* Spontaneous abortion, commonly referred to as a miscarriage, is defined as the unexpected loss of a pregnancy before 20 weeks of gestation. Spontaneous abortions occur in 15% to 25% of clinically

Table 68.5–2	Complications of Pregnancy	
Trimester	**Fetal**	**Maternal**
First: 1-14 wk	Pregnancy failure • Spontaneous abortion • Fetal demise • Gestational trophoblastic disease	Ectopic pregnancy Anemia Hyperemesis gravidarum Urinary tract infection/ pyelonephritis
Second 15-27 wk	Disorders of fetal growth • Intrauterine growth restriction • Abnormal amniotic fluid volume Maternal/placental causes as well	Gestational diabetes Rh Incompatibility Urinary tract infection/ pyelonephritis
Third 28-40 wk	Vasa previa	Preterm labor/preterm rupture of membranes Preeclampsia/eclampsia Placenta previa Placental abruption Uterine rupture Deep venous thrombosis

Table 68.5–3 Causes of Vaginal Bleeding in the Pregnant Patient

Trimester	Nonemergent	Emergent
First (1-14 wk)	Implantation bleeding Cervicitis Cervical polyps/decidual reaction of cervix Cervical dysplasia/cancer Sexual intercourse/ vaginal trauma	Spontaneous abortion Ectopic pregnancy Gestational trophoblastic disease Placental abnormalities (previa, subchorionic hematoma)
Second (15-27 wk)	Cervicitis Cervical polyps/decidual reaction of cervix Cervical dysplasia/cancer Sexual intercourse/vaginal trauma	Spontaneous abortion Ectopic pregnancy Gestational trophoblastic disease Preterm labor Abdominal or pelvic trauma
Third (28-40 wk)	Bloody show Cervicitis Cervical polyps Cervical dysplasia/cancer Sexual intercourse/vaginal trauma	*Placental causes* • Placenta previa • Placental abruption *Maternal causes* • Uterine rupture • Coagulopathy • Abdominal or pelvic trauma *Fetal causes* • Vasa previa

recognized pregnancies. The most common cause of spontaneous abortion is chromosomal abnormalities, and the incidence is higher in women of advanced maternal age (>35 years). Other risk factors include maternal systemic disease, uterine abnormalities, and infection.

■ *Classification and management.* Spontaneous abortions are classified based on (a) whether any or all of the products of conception (POCs) have passed and (b) the dilatation of the cervix (Table 68.5–4).

First-Trimester Bleeding: Ectopic Pregnancy

■ *Epidemiology and risk factors.* The incidence of ectopic pregnancy has been increasing over the last 20 years, and now occurs in 1% of all pregnancies. It is the third leading cause of pregnancy-related deaths in the United States, and is the most common cause of maternal mortality in the first trimester. Any condition that results in scarring or adhesions of the fallopian tract, thereby negatively affecting the tubal transport mechanism, increases the risk of an ectopic pregnancy. Such conditions include previous STDs and PID, previous tubal surgeries or tubal ligation, and a history of ruptured appendicitis. The rise of ectopic pregnancy has also been attributed to the increasing use of assisted reproductive techniques and contraceptive methods that prevent intrauterine implantation, such as the intrauterine device.

Table 68.5–4 Classification of Spontaneous Abortion

	Septic	Threatened	Inevitable	Incomplete	Complete	Missed
Symptoms	Vaginal bleeding, endometritis, sepsis	Vaginal bleeding, possibly mild abdominal cramping	Gross rupture of membranes, may experience vaginal bleeding and mild abdominal cramping	Vaginal bleeding and abdominal cramping	Vaginal bleeding and abdominal cramping	May be asymptomatic, No fetal heart motion on sonogram
Products of conception (POCs)	Some retained POCs	No passage of POCs	No passage of POCs	Passage of some POCs	Passage of all POCs	Demise of fetus with retention of POCs
Cervix dilated	Maybe	No	Yes	Yes	No	No
Treatment	Emergent D&C for evacuation of retained POCs, broad-spectrum IV antibiotics; supportive care for shock and DIC	Observation Bed/pelvic rest RhoGAM if Rh negative	Observation IV Fluids RhoGAM if Rh negative	IV Fluids RhoGAM if Rh-negative D&C	Observation RhoGAM if Rh negative	Observation RhoGAM if Rh negative
Disposition	Admit to ICU, OB consult	Discharge Pelvic rest OB follow-up	Admit OB consult Nonemergent D&C	Admit OB consult Emergent D&C	Discharge OB follow-up	Discharge OB follow-up for D&C for retained POCs

D&C, dilation and curettage; ICU, intensive care unit; IV, intravenous; OB, obstetric.

- *Pathophysiology.* An ectopic pregnancy is any pregnancy that implants outside of the endometrial cavity. In nearly 95% of cases, the implantation occurs within the fallopian tube. The other sites for implantation include the uterus, cervix, and the abdomen. A heterotopic pregnancy is one in which there is both an intrauterine pregnancy (IUP) and an ectopic pregnancy. Heterotopic pregnancy is rare in the general population (1 in 30,000 pregnancies), but has an incidence of 8% in patients who use assisted reproductive technologies.

- *History.* Classically the symptom triad consists of amenorrhea, vaginal bleeding and abdominal pain. Patients most often complain of unilateral lower quadrant abdominal pain (90%). Only 75% of women with an ectopic pregnancy will report amenorrhea or a history of an abnormal last menstrual period and vaginal spotting. Heavy vaginal bleeding is not typical of an ectopic pregnancy. Elucidating key risk factors such as PID or previous pelvic surgery increase concerns for the diagnosis.

- *Physical examination.* Most patients will have lower quadrant abdominal tenderness, with one side more tender than the other. Other findings on physical examination may include cervical motion tenderness, an adnexal mass on bimanual pelvic examination (20%), and the observation of bleeding from the cervical os. Although most patients are afebrile, 10% may have a temperature above 38° C. If the ectopic pregnancy has ruptured, the patient may present with symptoms of hypovolemia (tachycardia and orthostatic blood pressure), and peritoneal signs on physical examination (rebound, guarding and shoulder pain).

- *Diagnostic testing.* The diagnosis of ectopic pregnancy is based on a high clinical probability from history and physical examination. Once pregnancy is detected by a urine β-hCG, a quantitative serum β-hCG must be drawn. This initial value will assist with interpretation of the sonographic evaluation, and may serve as a baseline for serial levels for patients without conclusive findings on ultrasound. The β-hCG should double every 48 hours in a normal pregnancy. A serum progesterone level may also be drawn. A value below 5 ng/ml is highly suggestive of a nonviable pregnancy but does not indicate location. A progesterone level of greater than 25 ng/ml is highly suggestive of an intrauterine pregnancy. RhoGAM should be administered if the patient is Rh-negative. Ultrasound is used to document an IUP. A transvaginal sonogram cannot detect an IUP until the β-hCG reaches a level above 1500 mIU/ml (β-hCG >6500 mIU/ml for transabdominal sonogram). Ultrasound findings highly suggestive for an ectopic pregnancy include absence of a gestational sac in the uterus, presence of blood in the cul de sac, an echogenic complex adnexal mass separate from the ovary, or documentation of fetal heart motion outside of the endometrial cavity.

- *ED management.* If the patient is unstable or presents with a ruptured ectopic pregnancy, the foremost goal is to stabilize the patient by starting IV fluids, ordering blood products, and obtaining an obstetric consultation for immediate exploratory laparotomy and ectopic resection. A patient who has an unruptured ectopic pregnancy and a β-hCG above 15,000 mIU/ml, should be scheduled for immediate laparoscopy, and observed for signs of rupture, which include increasing abdominal pain or shock. If a patient has an unruptured ectopic pregnancy and is stable, medical treatment with methotrexate can be utilized if the ectopic mass size is less than 3.5 cm and the β-hCG below 15,000 mIU/ml. Contraindications to methotrexate include the presence of fetal heart motion and maternal liver or kidney disease. If the patient is not a candidate for medical treatment, surgical management with laparoscopic resection of the ectopic pregnancy should be performed.

First-Trimester Bleeding: Gestational Trophoblastic Disease

- *Epidemiology and risk factors.* The incidence of molar pregnancy is about 1 in 1,000 pregnancies among whites in the United States. There is a higher incidence in Asian females in the United States (1 in 800 pregnancies), and an even higher incidence in Asian females in the Far East (1 in 200 pregnancies). Gestational trophoblastic disease occurs more commonly at the extremes of reproductive age (women <20 years and >40 years old).
- *Pathophysiology.* Gestational trophoblastic disease (GTD) is the result of the pathologic proliferation of placental (trophoblastic) tissue. The term GTD describes a spectrum of neoplasms that are grouped into one of four classifications: (a) benign hydatidiform molar pregnancy (80%); (b) invasive molar pregnancy (10%-15%); (c) choriocarcinoma (2%-5%); and (d) placental site trophoblastic tumor (rare). A malignant GTD includes invasive mole, choriocarcinoma and placental site trophoblastic tumor.
- *History.* The most common presenting symptom of molar pregnancy is irregular or heavy vaginal bleeding during the first half of pregnancy, along with severe vaginal pain. Other symptoms include the passage of molar vesicles, severe hyperemesis, symptoms of severe thyroid disease, and symptoms of preeclampsia before 24 weeks of gestation.
- *Physical examination.* Findings suspicious for hydatidiform molar pregnancy include vesicles seen in the vagina, a uterus larger than dates, and absence of fetal heart tones.
- *Diagnostic testing.* A quantitative β-hCG much higher than expected for pregnancy dating is the key to diagnosis. This initial β-hCG will also serve as a baseline to follow declining levels once dilatation and curettage (D&C) is performed. Confirmation is made by the classic finding of a "snowstorm" pattern on ultrasound, which represents swelling of the chorionic villi. A plain film of the chest should be obtained to screen for metastasis to the lung (most common site).
- *ED management.* Once the diagnosis of gestational trophoblastic disease is made, refer to an obstetrician/gynecologist for admission and further treatment, including D&C. After uterine evacuation is performed, serial β-hCG levels should be followed as an outpatient to identify recurrence or progression to malignant disease.

Third-Trimester Bleeding

- Third-trimester bleeding can result in profuse hemorrhage and therefore is potentially fatal to both the fetus and mother. As such, the patient with third-trimester bleeding should be considered an obstetric true emergency, and should be approached in the same manner as any critically ill patient. Never perform a pelvic examination on any patient in the third trimester until a sonogram has ruled out placenta previa or vasa previa because otherwise a cervical examination may result in uncontrolled hemorrhage.

- Third-trimester bleeding is usually separated into the broad categories of painful and painless bleeding (Table 68.5–5).

Other Pregnancy-Related Problems
Hyperemesis Gravidarum

- Nausea and vomiting are common in pregnancy especially during 6 to 20 weeks of gestation. A small percentage of pregnant women have a more profound course, with the most severe form being hyperemesis gravidarum, which causes persistent vomiting, dehydration, ketosis, electrolyte disturbances, and weight loss (more than 5% of body weight).
- Diagnostic studies are ordered to rule out nonpregnancy causes, evaluate for electrolyte abnormalities and ketonuria. Bilirubin and alkaline phosphatase can be mildly elevated but should return to normal levels after delivery.
- Most standard antiemetics are in FDA category C (promethazine, prochlorperazine), and are used successfully to treat hyperemesis gravidarum. Ondansetron and metoclopramide are category B. Pyridoxine or Vitamin B_6 (category A) can be used as a single agent. Doxylamine (Unisom) 10 mg three times a day is also effective in combination with vitamin B_6. Severe vomiting may require hospitalization, orally or intravenously administered corticosteroid therapy, and total parenteral nutrition.

Urinary Tract Infections

- Asymptomatic bacteriuria (ASB) is defined as significant bacterial colonization of the lower urinary tract without symptoms. Without treatment, ASB progresses to pyelonephritis in 20% to 40% of pregnant women. In contrast, progression to pyelonephritis in nonpregnant women is only 1% to 2%. With appropriate treatment in pregnancy, progression to pyelonephritis can be decreased to 3%. The causative organisms are similar in pregnant and nonpregnant women and include enterobacteriae, a group of gram-negative rods, which includes colonizing organisms, including *Escherichia coli*, the pathogen in most urinary tract infections (UTIs).
- Greater than 10 leukocytes per high-power field in the sediment from a clean-catch midstream urine specimen is considered positive. A urine culture should be sent on all pregnant patients with a UTI. The diagnosis of ASB is based on a clean-catch voided urine culture revealing greater than 100,000 colonies/ml of a single organism.
- Antibiotic choices for ASB and cystitis include cephalexin (500 mg PO four times daily), nitrofurantoin macrocrystals (100 mg PO four times daily), or amoxicillin/ampicillin (500 mg PO four times daily) for at least 3 days duration. Patients with pyelonephritis require IV hydration,

	Painless Bleeding		Painful Bleeding	
	Placenta Previa	Vasa Previa	Placental Abruption	Uterine Rupture
Epidemiology	1 in 200 pregnancies 20% of all antepartum hemorrhages	1 in 5000 pregnancies	1 in 200 deliveries	Rare
Mechanism	Placental implantation over the cervical os	Fetal vessels overlying the cervical os placenta	Premature separation of normally implanted placenta	Full thickness uterine wall tear, usually at site of prior uterine scar
Risk factors	Previous previa Prior cesarean delivery Advanced maternal age Multiparity Smoking	Velamentous (membranous) cord insertion	Hypertension Cocaine Trauma Previous abruption Preterm rupture of membranes	Uterine scar (cesarean delivery, myomectomy), marked uterine overdistention (multiple gestation, poly hydramnios), high parity, trauma
Diagnosis	Ultrasound is nearly 100% accurate	Nonreassuring fetal heart tones Ultrasound and color Doppler Detection of fetal red blood cells in vaginal blood	Clinical diagnosis Uterine tenderness Only 2% will be detected by ultrasound	Fetal heart rate decelerations Abrupt onset of abdominal pain Loss of fetal station
Treatment	Fetal monitoring Close observation and expectant management if stable Cesarean delivery if unstable or at term	Emergent cesarean delivery (50% perinatal mortality; increases to 75% if membranes also rupture)	Maternal-fetal monitoring and expectant management in mild cases Immediate delivery if unstable Check coagulation studies (primary cause of obstetrical disseminated intravascular coagulation)	Emergent cesarean delivery Repair of uterus

antipyretics, IV antibiotics, close monitoring of urine output, and hospital admission. During the first trimester, admission is not necessary if the patient receives an initial IV dose of antibiotics in the ED, can take oral fluids and medications, and is pain free. During the second and third trimester, the patient should be admitted. Initial antimicrobial treatment for pyelonephritis is empiric and includes cefazolin (1-2 g IV every 6 to 8 hours) or ampicillin (2 g IV every 6 hours) plus gentamicin (2 mg/kg load, then 1.5 mg/kg in three divided doses with monitoring of drug levels).

■ Complications that may result from untreated bacteriuria in pregnancy include premature labor, perinatal mortality, low birth weight, maternal anemia, cognitive delay in infants, and pyelonephritis. Pyelonephritis may result in septic shock, renal failure, or renal scarring.

Hypertensive Emergencies

■ The three types of hypertensive disease in pregnancy include gestational hypertension (pregnancy-induced hypertension), preeclampsia, and eclampsia. Gestational hypertension is defined as blood pressure of greater than 140/90 mm Hg, without the presence of proteinuria or edema. It occurs after 20 weeks of gestation or postpartum in a woman known to be previously normotensive. Preeclampsia is defined as hypertension with a blood pressure of 140/90 mm Hg or greater associated with the presence of proteinuria or pathologic edema. The proteinuria must be greater than or equal to 300 mg/24 hours or 1+ on a dipstick. As preeclampsia worsens, systemic involvement leads to increased blood pressure, worsening proteinuria, and a rise in serum creatinine to above 1.2 mg/dl. The hemolysis/elevated liver function tests/low platelets (HELLP) syndrome may develop in untreated pre-eclampsia. Eclampsia is the occurrence of seizures in pregnant women with preeclampsia that cannot be attributed to any other cause. The vasospastic complications of gestational hypertension affect the cardiovascular, renal, hepatic, and central nervous systems.

■ Patients with significant blood pressure elevation may present with epigastric or liver tenderness, visual disturbances, or headache. The edema of preeclampsia is usually generalized, involving the face and hands, and persists throughout the day.

■ Delivery is the definitive management of eclampsia and severe pre-eclampsia. Initial therapy includes controlling seizures with magnesium sulfate, and lowering blood pressure (after seizure control) if diastolic blood pressure is greater than 105 mm Hg. The urine output should be monitored. IV fluids are limited to ≤ 125 ml/hr, unless significant volume loss occurs. Diuretics and hyperosmotic agents should be avoided, because they cause further volume loss and compromise uterine/placental blood flow. Treat a persistent systolic pressure equal to or greater than 160 mm Hg or diastolic pressure greater than 105 mm Hg with hydralazine (5-10 mg IV every 15-20 minutes) or labetalol (20 mg, 40 mg, then 80 mg IV every 10 minutes; maximum dose of 220 mg). A satisfactory response is defined as a decrease in diastolic blood pressure to 90 to 100 mm Hg. If blood pressure is decreased more than this, placental perfusion may become compromised.

Labor and Delivery

- Labor is defined as the coordination of uterine contractions (usually 5 minutes apart and lasting 30-60 seconds) that cause cervical change in either dilatation or effacement. In 10% of all pregnancies, the placental membranes rupture at least 1 hour before the initiation of labor. False labor is any uterine contractions not associated with cervical change. The most commonly described contractions of false labor are Braxton Hicks' contractions. Unlike the contractions of true labor, Braxton Hicks' contractions are usually 10 to 20 minutes apart, fail to increase in intensity or frequency, do not lead to cervical dilatation, and cease with sedation. Braxton Hicks' contractions may persist for days and are treated with bed rest and hydration. The active phase of labor begins when the cervix is dilated 10 cm.

- Delivery of the pregnant patient is rare in the average ED, and accounts for fewer than 1% of all deliveries. In most institutions that have an obstetric service, patients greater than 20 weeks gestation optimally have an initial evaluation on the labor deck rather than in the ED.

- Vaginal delivery in the ED should only occur if there is no time to transport the patient to the delivery suite. Unfortunately, some hospitals have no obstetric service, and it may be necessary to transfer the mother in labor. In addition to routine vitals and examination, a rapid evaluation of the pregnant female should include an assessment of fetal lie and presentation. Lie is the relationship between the long axis of the fetus and long axis of the mother. Presentation refers to the fetal anatomy that overlies the pelvic inlet. The most common lie and presentation are longitudinal and cephalic, respectively. A cervical examination should be performed to assess for cervical dilatation, effacement, and station using a sterile glove especially if rupture of the membranes has occurred.

- If delivery is imminent, supplies and the procedure for vaginal delivery are discussed in Chapter 91. Neonatal resuscitation equipment should also be available. Complications of labor and delivery are listed in Table 68.5–6. These complications are categorized below based on their relation to delivery: before delivery (antepartum), during delivery (intrapartum), and after delivery (postpartum).

Table 68.5–6 Complications of the Perilabor and Delivery Period

Relation to Delivery	Condition	Definition	Diagnosis	Treatment
Antepartum	Premature rupture of membrane (PROM)	Rupture of the amnion and chorion before labor	Pooling of amniotic fluid in vagina with ferning pattern and positive nitrazine test of fluid	*Fettus >37 wk*: Induce labor *Fettus <37 wk*: Delivery risk assessment
	Preterm labor	True labor between 20 and 37 wk	Uterine contractions with cervical dilatation	Hydration/sedation Glucocorticoids (for fetal lung maturity) Tocolysis (magnesium sulfate, terbutaline)
Intrapartum	Chorioamnionitis	Infection of the amniotic fluid, due to extended duration of PROM	Fever, ↑WBC, uterine tenderness, ↑FHR, purulent vaginal discharge.	Broad spectrum IV antibiotics with group B streptococcus and *Escherichia coli* coverage (IV ampicillin or penicillin plus gentamycin). Hasten delivery
	Breech presentation	Fetal presentation of buttocks or legs first	Ultrasound	External version Cesarean delivery
	Shoulder dystocia	Impaction of the anterior shoulder behind the pubis	Anterior shoulder fails to deliver	McRoberts maneuver: The maternal hips are completely flexed, allowing the knees to rest on the abdomen Suprapubic pressure Delivery of the posterior shoulder first
Postpartum	Postpartum hemorrhage	Excessive blood loss following delivery	>500 ml blood loss for vaginal delivery (>1000 ml for cesarean delivery) in first 24 h	Laceration repair Manual removal of all POCs Oxytocin, carboprost, methylergonovine for uterine atony Hysterectomy for refractory cases
	Endometritis	Infection of the endometrium	Fever, tender uterus and foul-smelling lochia	Broad-spectrum IV antibiotics Hospital admission

Teaching Points

A pregnancy test should be performed on all females of reproductive age prior to treatment.

Fetal heart tones should be considered the fifth vital sign of all pregnant patients.

The possible teratogenic effects of any medication should be considered prior to administration to the pregnant patient.

Pregnant women can have the same surgical conditions as non-pregnant women, and should be treated appropriately for any emergent condition regardless of their pregnancy.

Any woman presenting with pelvic pain requires an evaluation to rule out potentially life-threatening or fertility compromising conditions.

UTIs during pregnancy should be treated regardless of symptomatology as asymptomatic bacteriuria may lead to pyelonephritis in up to 25% of untreated patients, which can result in sepsis and preterm labor/birth.

Any patient greater than 20 wk of gestation presenting with hypertension and proteinuria has preeclampsia until proven otherwise.

The first priority in the evaluation of vaginal bleeding is to determine whether the patient is hemodynamically stable, and if the patient is pregnant as this will dictate the priority of the patient as well as the differential diagnoses.

In patients with first trimester vaginal bleeding obtain a quantitative β-hCG, and a sonogram to document an intrauterine pregnancy.

RhoGAM should be administered to all pregnant women where maternal blood type is Rh-negative or unknown, and maternal/fetal blood exposure is possible to prevent isoimmunization.

Ultrasound should be performed in all patients with third trimester bleeding prior to pelvic examination to rule out placenta or vasa previa.

Suggested Readings

Abbrescia K, Sheridan B. Complications of second and third trimester pregnancies. Emerg Med Clin North Am 2003;21:695–710.

Coppolo PT, Coppola M. Vaginal bleeding in the first 20 weeks of pregnancy. Emerg Med Clin North Am 2003;21:667–677.

Daniels RV, McCuskey C. Abnormal vaginal bleeding in the nonpregnant patient. Emerg Med Clin North Am 2003;21:751–772.

Dart R. Acute pelvic pain. In: Marx JA, Hockberger RS, Walls RM (editors). Rosen's Emergency Medicine: Concepts and Clinical Practice (6th ed). Philadelphia: Mosby, 2006, pp 248–253.

Della-Giustina D, Denny M. Ectopic pregnancy. Emerg Med Clin North Am 2003;21:565–584.

Lawrence LL. Unusual presentations in obstetrics and gynecology. Emerg Med Clin North Am 2003;21:649–665.

Niebyl JR. Drugs in pregnancy and lactation. In: Gabbe SG, Niebyl, Simpson JL (editors). Obstetrics, Normal and Problem Pregnancies (4th ed). New York: Churchill Livingston, 2002, pp 221–245.

CHAPTER 69

Ophthalmology

SHARI SCHABOWSKI

Overview

Eye complaints represent common causes for visits to the ED. Yet many clinicians are apprehensive when approaching ophthalmologic emergencies. Most eye problems can be treated by emergency medicine physicians without ophthalmologic consultation in the ED.

A complete eye examination is essential to identify expected and unexpected complications. A functional examination of visual acuity is the first step in the evaluation of all eye complaints followed by a step by step inspection of the structures and their individual functions. Further evaluation using a slit lamp, fluorescein stain, pH testing, and tonometry provide additional diagnostic information.

Beware of ophthalmologic emergencies requiring immediate attention. Patients with chemical exposure to the eye or central retinal artery occlusion require prompt treatment before the diagnosis is confirmed. Other true ophthalmologic emergencies include globe rupture, retrobulbar hematoma, and acute angle-close glaucoma.

Eye Anatomy

- **Sensorimotor.** The sixth cranial nerve controls the lateral rectus (abducts eye or moves it laterally). The fourth cranial nerve controls the superior oblique (depresses eye AND moves eye laterally). The third cranial nerve controls all other extra-ocular movements, pupilary constriction, and upper lid elevation. The fifth cranial nerve is responsible for sensation of the eye through the supra-orbital and infraorbital nerves.
- **Conjunctiva.** This layer is a clear vascular tissue that supplies the eyelids and sclera with oxygen and nutrients.
- **Sclera.** This is the white, opaque, elastic collagen tissue that encompasses the globe from the cornea to the optic nerve, giving the eye its shape and form.
- **Cornea.** This is the clear avascular structure in front of the eye that must remain clear for good vision.
- **Iris and pupil.** This is the pigmented, round, contractile membrane of the eye that is suspended between the cornea and the lens, and is perforated by the pupil. The iris helps regulate the amount of light that enters the eye. The pupil is the dark aperture in the iris that determines how much light is let into the eye.

- *Lens.* The transparent structure inside the eye that focuses light rays onto the retina.
- *Aqueous chamber.* This is the space in the eye that is between the lens and the cornea. It is filled with a watery fluid known as the aqueous humor, and is divided anatomically by the iris into the anterior and posterior chamber.
- *Aqueous humor.* This is a substance produced by the ciliary body. It passes first into the posterior chamber, and then flows forward through the pupil into the anterior chamber of the eye.
- *Ciliary body.* The ciliary muscle changes the shape of the lens. The ciliary process produces the aqueous humor.
- *Uveal tract.* This consists of vascularized structures including the iris, the ciliary body, and the choroid (the dark-brown vascular coat of the eye between the sclera and the retina).
- *Vitrous humor.* This is located between the lens and the optic nerve and is surrounded by the retina. It is filled with gelatinous vitreous humor that aids in the structural integrity of the globe and retina.
- *Retina.* This is the neurosensory interface that lines the vitreous chamber. It senses light, and creates impulses that travel through the optic nerve to the brain. The outer third is supplied by a vascular layer called the choroids. The inner two thirds are supplied by the central retinal artery, the terminal branch of the ophthalmic artery. The macula is located roughly in the center of the retina, temporal to the optic nerve. It is a small and highly sensitive part of the retina, and is responsible for detailed central vision. The fovea is the depression in the center of the macula that is responsible for sharp central vision.

Initial Diagnostic Approach
General

- Any patient with eye trauma (ruptured globe), chemical contamination (alkaline burn), or sudden vision loss (central retinal artery occlusion) should have an expedited evaluation in an attempt to prevent permanent vision loss.
- *History.* Obtain the contributing history, baseline visual acuity and correction, ophthalmologic history, medical history, allergies, and medications. For patients with vision loss, important historical points include time of onset, quality and severity of visual loss, mono- or binocularity, duration of loss, and associated ocular and systemic diseases.
- *Physical examination.* This should include all of the important components listed below.

Eye Examination

- *Visual acuity.* This is the vital sign of the eye, and should be documented in every patient with an ophthalmologic complaint. In patients complaining of vision loss, emergent visual acuity assessment should first be performed beginning with the assessment of counting fingers, then hand motion, and finally, light perception. Each eye should be tested separately. Use corrective eyewear whenever possible, but never insert contact lens into an injured or infected eye. A hand-held chart in a less brightly lit room (Figure 69–1) may be more effective than the Snellen chart in a bright hallway for patients with eye pain, light sensitivity, or near-sightedness. A hand held chart is preferred for patients who are unable to stand. If eye pain is the predominant symptom, consider re-testing visual acuity after topical anesthetics have been administered. A pinhole device is helpful to reduce refractory errors in patients who have not brought their corrective glasses with them. Decreased visual acuity that does not improve with the pinhole device suggests that corneal refractive error is not the cause. Visual acuity is reported as two numbers separated by a slash. The first number, usually "20", is the standard distance from the chart to the individual being tested. The second number represents the distance that the average eye can see letters on a certain line of the eye chart. If an individual can read part of a line, that line is listed as the second number followed by a minus sign and the number of characters missed on that line. Formal visual acuity testing should never delay important therapeutic interventions such as eye irrigation. All patients with decreased visual acuity from their baseline require routine referral for further ophthalmologic follow-up; however, those patients with moderately or severely decreased visual acuity not explained by refractive error require prompt ophthalmologic consultation especially if the change is acute.

■ **Inspection.** Inspect the eyelashes, lids, lacrimal structures, and conjunctiva. The eyelid should be inverted to examine the undersurface of the lid. The patient maintains a downward gaze while the upper lid is flipped over a cotton tipped applicator. This facilitates complete evaluation of bulbar and palpebral conjunctiva, lid margins and lacrimal system. Look at the position of the globe. Enophthalmos (sunken eye) is seen with an orbital rupture or blowout fracture (Chapter 10). Proptosis (protruding eye) is seen with an orbital cellulitis or retrobulbar hematoma. A pinguecula is wedge-shaped thickening of the conjunctiva. If it extends onto the cornea, it is called a pterygium which can cause loss of vision if it crosses the cornea.

■ **Pupils.** Examine the pupils and ascertain the size, asymmetry, shape, direct and consensual response to light, and accommodation. A "teardrop" shaped pupil is seen with globe injury. See Table 69–1 for pupil abnormalities. In the patient with equal pupils, check for the presence of a relative afferent pupillary defect (APD) or Marcus-Gunn pupil. Take a light source and shine it back and forth between the two eyes. In a patient with an APD, when the light shines in the normal pupil, it constricts. The consensual reflex causes the pupil of the abnormal eye to constrict also. When the light swings over to the abnormal eye, the pupil of the abnormal eye appears to dilate. It is actually unable to perceive the light in front of it, and is just returning to its normal midrange size. An APD is caused by pathology of the optic nerve distal to the optic chiasm. This is opposed to the Argyle-Robertson pupil in which the pupil does not contract to light, but does contract with accommodation, and is seen in neurosyphilis.

■ **Ocular motility.** Evaluation of cardinal eye movements occurs as the patient follows object in the pattern of an H. Causes of impaired ocular

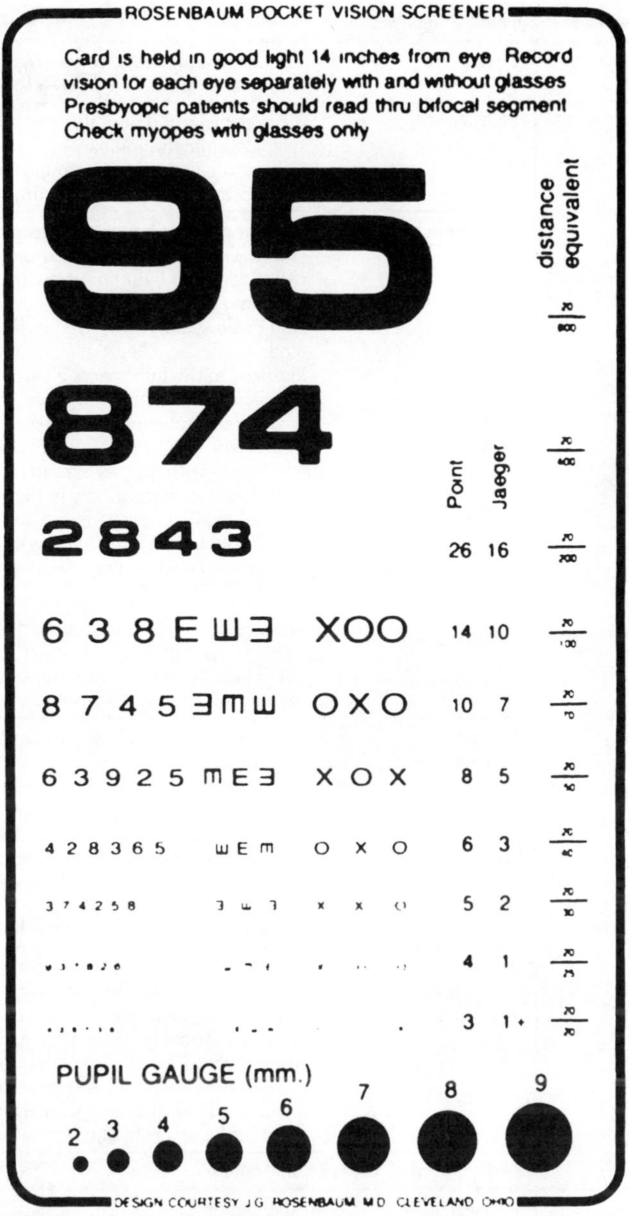

Figure 69-1. If the patient cannot stand or a formal eye chart is not available, ask the patient to read this "distance equivalent" chart by holding this figure 14 inches away from the patient. *(From Roberts: Clinical Procedures in Emergency Medicine (4th ed). Philadelphia: Elsevier, 2004.)*

Table 69–1	Pupil Abnormalities	
Anisocoria	Physiologic	20% of people may have anisocoria >0.4 mm. Anisocoria is rarely >1 mm.
	Pharmacologic mydriasis	Local administration of both sympathomimetic and para-sympatholytic agents. This pupil will not constrict with pilocarpine drops.
	Adies tonic pupil	Blurred near vision but normal distant vision. There is a dilated pupil that reacts poorly to light but better to accommodation. Seen in young women along with symmetrically reduced deep tendon reflexes. The damage is localized to the third nerve ciliary ganglion, and is usually due to a virus or other inflammatory processes. Pilocarpine (0.1%) causes an intense pupillary constriction as a result of cholinergic supersensitivity in the affected pupil. These patients need to be referred to an ophthalmologist for cholinergic agent therapy.
	Third nerve palsy	Dilated pupil, ptosis, and diplopia with extraocular muscle dysfunction. The involved eye will be turned down and out. The patient should be evaluated for a possible intracranial aneurysm.
	Horner's syndrome	Ptosis, miosis, and facial anhydrosis resulting from an interruption of sympathetic innervation. There is a dilatation lag in darkness. The anisocoria will be greater at 3 to 5 s of darkness. Some causes include central nervous system strokes and tumors, thyroid adenomas, and a Pancoast tumor (tumor in the apex of the lung).
	Afferent pupillary defect or Marcus-Gunn pupil	When the light shines in the normal pupil, it constricts. The consensual reflex causes the pupil of the abnormal eye to constrict also. When the light swings over to the abnormal eye, the pupil of the abnormal eye appears to dilate. Pathology of the optic nerve distal to the optic chiasm.
	Iritis	Miotic and red eye.
Irregular shape	Postsurgical	Most common cause is prior ocular surgery from cataracts.
	Globe rupture	A teardrop-shaped pupil is suggestive of ocular rupture, and the apex of the teardrop points to the laceration.

Table 69–1	Pupil Abnormalities—*cont'd*	
Irregular shape	Iris dislocation	D-shaped pupil
	Iritis	Synechiae or scarring from a prior iritis can cause an irregularly shaped pupil
	Argyll-Robertson	Pupil is a small, irregular pupil that does not react to light but does react to accommodation. Localization is to the mid brain and the cause is neurosyphilis.

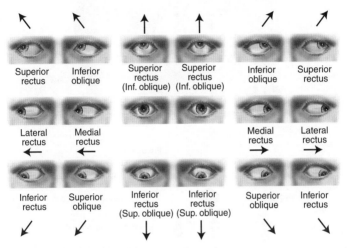

Figure 69–2. The principle actions of the extra-ocular muscles. (*From Palay DS, Krachmer JH. Ophthalmology for the Primary Care Physician. St. Louis, MO: Mosby Year Book, 1997.*)

motility include entrapment of a muscle (inferior oblique in a blowout fracture will prevent an upward gaze), direct muscle injury, orbital cellulitis, or cranial nerve palsy of cranial nerves II, IV, or VI. Defer extra-ocular muscle (EOM) testing if an open globe injury is suspected. Evaluate for diplopia. If diplopia disappears when either eye is covered, an EOM is dysfunctional. If it persists (monocular diplopia), a corneal or lens irregularity, or a malingering patient is the likely cause. See Figure 69–2 for the principle actions of the extraocular muscles.

■ *Visual fields.* Confrontational visual field testing is performed by having the physician and patient face each other, with the patient covering one eye, and the physician covering the eye directly opposite to the patient's covered eye. The patient should look at the physician's nose while the physician places and moves his or her fingers in all four quadrants, starting far away and moving progressively toward the nose. This is especially helpful for picking up hemianopic field defects (Figure 69–3).

R   L

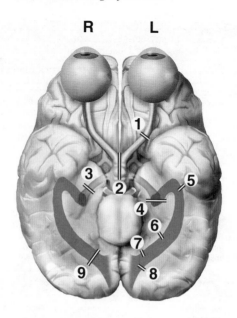

Field defect

Location	Left eye	Right eye	Comment
1 Left optic nerve			No light perception left eye
2 Chiasm			Bitemporal hemianopsia
3 Right optic tract			Incongruous left homonymous hemianopia
4 Left lateral geniculate nucleus			Right homonymous sectoranopia (lateral choroidal artery) or Incongruous right homonymous hemianopia
5 Left temporal lobe			Right homonymous upper quadrant defect ("pie in the sky")
6 Left parietal lobe			Right homonymous defect, denser inferiorly
7 Left occipital lobe (upper bank)			Right homonymous lower quadrantanopia (macular sparing)
8 Left occipital lobe (lower bank)			Right homonymous upper quadrantanopia (macular sparing)
9 Right occipital lobe			Left homonymous hemianopia (macular sparing)

Figure 69–3. Visual field defects. *(From Stein J [editor]. Internal Medicine [5th ed]. St Louis, MO: Mosby, 1998.)*

- *Funduscopy.* This is best performed through dilated pupils (use 1% tropicamide or 2.5% phenylephrine). Pupil dilatation should not be performed if serial neurologic examinations are required in elderly patients who have had cataract surgery (can cause iris-plane artificial lenses to become displaced), or if there is any possibility of acute angle-closure glaucoma. Phenylephrine is preferentially used in cases where future pupillary examinations will be necessary. Document any dilating drops administered. Direct ophthalmoscopy gives a good view of the optic nerve, macula, and vessels. The examiner's right eye should be used to examine the patient's right eye and visa versa. The patient should focus the non-tested eye on a distant point, approximately 15 degrees laterally (to the eye being examined) to facilitate visualization of the optic disc, which is located inferomedially. First find the red reflex. When black forms are seen against the red reflex background, or there is a decreased red reflex, the likely pathologies are corneal edema, vitreous hemorrhage, cataract, or retinal detachment. Focus anteriorly on the lids, cornea, conjunctiva, and iris. Then focus posteriorly through the vitreous humor to find the optic disc. The fovea is typically found about 2 disc diameters temporal to the disc. Indirect ophthalmoscopy is needed for the peripheral retinal examination. Examples of pathology seen on the funduscopic examination are listed in Table 69–2.
- *Slit lamp.* This device is useful to evaluate the lens and everything anterior to it. It evaluates abnormalities of the cornea, anterior chamber (i.e., hyphema, iritis), and iris. A direct ophthalmoscope with the +10 lens in place also works well. The viewing arm of the slit lamp contains the eye pieces and magnification elements. The illumination arm (IA)

Table 69–2	Abnormalities on Funduscopic Examination
Papilledema	Swelling of the optic disc and blurring of the disc margins, hyperemia, and loss of physiologic cupping. Flame-shaped hemorrhages and yellow exudates appear near the disc margins as the edema progresses.
Central retinal artery occlusion	Pale fundus with a cherry red spot at the macula. There arterioles are narrowed.
Retinal vein occlusion	Venous dilatation and diffuse, large hemorrhages throughout the retina.
Retinal detachment	The retina appears like a billowing sail at the area of the attachment. May be difficult to see at the periphery.
Vitreous hemorrhage	Reddish haze in mild cases to a black reflex in severe cases. Details of the fundus are usually difficult to visualize.
Diabetic retinopathy	Microaneurysms, small-vessel obstruction, cotton-wool spots or soft exudates (microinfarcts), hard exudates, and macular ischemia.

contains the lamp bulb, adjustments for the height and width of the beam. See Figures 69–4 and 69–5 for slit lamp controls and examination of the normal eye. The slit lamp examination procedure is summarized in Box 69–1.

■ *Intraocular pressure (IOP).* This pressure should not be measured if there is any possibility of globe perforation. Emergency IOP testing is not necessary if the patient has normal visual acuity, no signs and symptoms of glaucoma, normal chamber depth by illumination, and normal pressure by digital examination. Nevertheless, a normal IOP is reassuring that the patient does not have glaucoma. A normal IOP is about 12 mm Hg, and increases by 1 mm Hg per decade after age 40. The IOP in acute closed-angle glaucoma is >50 mm Hg. A Goldmann-type applanation tonometer (an adjunct to the slit lamp) is best but the portable Tonopen also works well. An alternative is the Schiotz tonometer. Topical anesthetic is required with any of these techniques. The patient must be in the recumbent position with the Schiotz, but can be in any position with the portable Tonopen (see Figure 69–6). Be careful not to apply any pressure on the globe during IOP measurements as this will alter the reading.

Emergency Department Management Overview

■ *Emergent interventions.* Patients with a ruptured globe, chemical contamination (alkaline burn), or central retinal artery occlusion require immediate attention in order to attempt to prevent permanent vision loss. See Table 69–3 for a summary of treatment of emergent problems.

BOX 69–1   Slit Lamp Examination

Start with unaffected eye.

Place the illumination arm (IA) on the lateral canthus side of the patient, about a 45-degree angle. (i.e., to examine the right eye, the IA should be on the patient's right side).

Low magnification, wide tall beam, medium intensity of light: Evaluate the lid, lid margins, the eyelashes, tarsal conjunctiva with lower and upper lid eversion.

Low magnification, narrow tall beam, medium intensity of light: Evaluate the cornea (clarity, infiltrates, foreign bodies, abrasions) and depth of anterior chamber (the iris should be flat and billowing out toward you).

High magnification, smallest beam, high intensity of light: Evaluate the anterior chamber for cells (specks of dust passing through a ray of sunlight) and flare (beam of light passing through fog). Always do this BEFORE staining with fluorescein.

Stain with fluorescein and view under cobalt blue light: Evaluate for corneal abrasions. An occult leak of aqueous humor from the laceration may be identified by the Seidel test. Application of fluorescein causing a stream of aqueous humor to fluoresce bright green is indicative of a positive result.

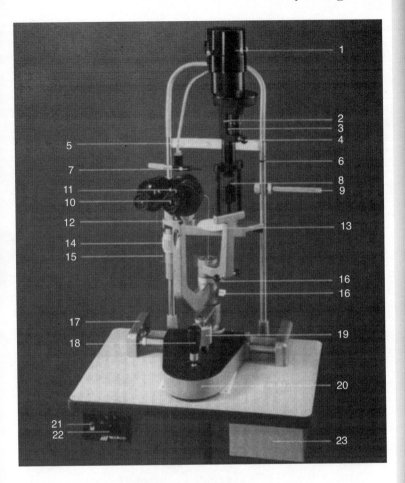

Marco I primary care slit lamp

Nomenclature

1. Cover for lamp bulb
2. Slit width controls (red-free filter)
3. Slit height control (cobalt blue filter)
4. Control of the rotation of slit
5. Headrest
6. Eye level marker
7. Fixation lighthead
8. Mirror
9. Examiner's handrest
10. Eyepieces
11. Knurled rings for refractive error adjustment
12. High-low magnification lever
13. Patient's chinrest
14. Headrest elevation control
15. Breath shield
16. Fixing screws for arm
17. Rail covers
18. Joystick
19. Elevation control
20. Slit lamp base
21. On-off switch
22. Intensity control
23. Accessory storage drawer

Figure 69–4. Slit lamp controls. *(From Operating Instructions for Slit Lamp Microscopes, Marco Equipment, Jacksonville, FL.)*

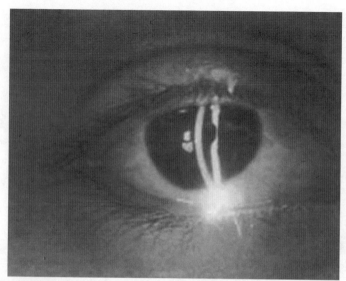

Figure 69–5. Slit lamp examination of the normal eye. Slit lamp photograph of a normal right eye under low power. The curved slit of light on the left is reflected off the cornea while the slit on the right is reflected off the iris. The depth of the anterior chamber can easily be appreciated under this low-magnification setup. *(Courtesy D. Price. From Roberts: Clinical Procedures in Emergency Medicine, 4th ed., Copyright © 2004 Elsevier, p 1273, Figure 64–45.)*

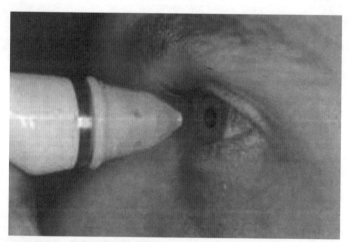

Figure 69–6. After topical anesthesia, the Tonopen is touched lightly and briefly to the cornea with a tapping motion, then withdrawn. Disposable tip covers are used to minimize any cross contamination. *(From Roberts J: Clinical Procedures in Emergency Medicine (4th ed). Philadelphia: Elsevier, 2004, p 1269.)*

Table 69–3	Initial Management of Ophthalmologic Emergencies
Condition	**Immediate Therapy**
Ruptured globe	Stabilize (do not remove) any foreign body Metal shield to eye; do not apply pressure to the globe Elevate head of bed 30 degrees or higher Tetanus prophylaxis and IV antibiotics No fluids or food by mouth Analgesia, antiemetic, and sedation as needed
Retrobulbar hematoma	Treat increased IOP Perform lateral canthotomy for vision loss (Table 69–5)
Retinal artery occlusion	Globe massage Paper bag breathing Carbogen inhalation (95% oxygen, 5% carbon dioxide)
Chemical burn	Topical anesthetic drops Immediate copious irrigation (prior to visual acuity testing)
Acute angle-closure glaucoma	IV or PO acetazolamide Topical pilocarpine and timolol

IOP, intraocular pressure; IV, intravenous; PO, by mouth.

- *Medications.* Topical anesthetics, systemic pain medication, and mydriatic agents are given when appropriate. Steroids should be given in consultation with ophthalmology, and should not be used if there is any chance of herpetic conjunctivitis.
- *Disposition.* Most patients can be discharged with outpatient follow-up with an ophthalmologist. Patients requiring an emergency ophthalmologic procedure or IV antibiotics require admission.

Specific Problems

- Common eye complaints presenting to the ED can be classified into three basic groups: infections (Table 69–4), trauma (Table 69–5), and visual impairments (Table 69–6).

Special Considerations
Pediatrics

- Ophthalmia neonatorum (neonatal conjunctivitis) is a peripartum infection acquired during vaginal delivery through an infected birth canal. The most common etiologies are: Gonorrhea, *Chlamydia trachomatis*, herpes simplex virus, group B *Streptococcus* and *Staphylococci*. While most of these can be life-threatening infections in the neonate, they can be prevented by instillation of silver nitrate or antibiotic drops. Patients present with purulent conjunctival inflammation within the first 7 days of life. It is often bilateral but may be asymmetric. Treatment is determined

Table 69–4   Eye Infections

	Etiology	Clinical presentation	Management
Conjunctivitis	Inflammation of the conjunctiva. Bacteria: *Streptococcus pneumoniae, Haemophilus influenzae, Staphylococcus* organisms, *Moraxella catarrhalis,* and *Neisseria gonorrhoeae.* Viruses: adenovirus Allergic	Discharge: Watery discharge (viral); mucopurulent or thick mucus and pus-containing (bacterial); watery with white, stringy mucus (allergic). Preauricular lymphadenopathy if viral. Gonococcal conjunctivitis has large amounts of mucopurulent discharge, progressing to lid swelling and pain. May lead to corneal ulceration and blindness. It is called keratoconjunctivitis if cornea involved.	Difficult and not cost effective to differentiate. Bacterial: Warm compresses, topical antibiotics (topical trimethoprim and polymyxin; fluoroquinolone for contact lens wearers) until 24–48 h after symptoms completely resolve (average 3–7 d). Remove and do not reapply contact lens until treatment is complete. Allergic/viral: Artificial tears, cool compresses, topical vasoconstrictor/antihistamine. For gonococcal conjunctivitis: hospital admission for IV antibiotics, saline irrigation, and topical ophthalmic antibiotics are warranted in moderate and severe cases. Also treat possible concomitant *Chlamydia trachomatis.*
Blepharitis	Inflammation along lid margins	Thickened, matted, red eyelid margins with pronounced blood vessels. Patients complain of burning, itching, tearing, foreign body sensation, and morning crusting of the eyelids.	Wash with dilute baby shampoo, and apply topical antibiotic ointment along lid margins. Discontinue use of causative cosmetic or ophthalmologic product

Table 69–4 Eye Infections—cont'd

	Etiology	Clinical presentation	Management
Hordeolum (i.e., stye)	Local infection or inflammation of the eyelid margin involving hair follicles of the eyelashes (i.e., external) or meibomian glands (i.e., internal). Due to *Staphylococcus aureus* in most cases.	Painful, erythematous, and localized. It may produce edema of the entire lid. Purulent material exudes from the eyelash line in external hordeola, while internal hordeola suppurate on the conjunctival surface of eyelid. Untreated, the disease may spontaneously resolve, or it may progress to chronic granulation with formation of a painless mass known as a chalazion.	Spontaneous rupture may occur, and most resolve with warm compresses applied for 15 min four to six times each day. Topical antibiotics (erythromycin) may be used. Incision and drainage are indicated for chalazia unresponsive to conservative therapy.
Dacryocystitis	Streptococcal species are currently the most common organisms.	Inflammatory mass adjacent to the medial canthus. Most commonly seen in infants and the elderly. Pressure on the mass results in purulent drainage from the puncta.	Topical nasal decongestants. Broad spectrum antibiotics and warm compresses.
Herpes simplex keratitis	Caused by HSV-1. Most common cause of infectious keratitis.	Unilateral photophobia, blurred vision, and a foreign body sensation. The most typical findings are characteristic dendritic figures with bulbar terminal endings. Recurrent infections can result in corneal scarring and blindness.	Refer promptly to ophthalmology. Treatment includes trifluridine eye drops, one drop every hour nine times a day for up to 21 d. The therapy is associated with a 95% cure rate. Vidarabine ointment can also be used. Topical acyclovir has been shown be as effective as vidarabine or trifluridine.

Continued

Table 69–4 Eye Infections—*cont'd*

	Etiology	Clinical presentation	Management
Herpes zoster kerato-conjunctivitis	Due to activation of the virus along ophthalmic division of the trigeminal nerve.	Red eye, photophobia, tearing, or decreased vision. Rash follows dermatomal patterns, involves the forehead and upper eyelid, and produces significant pain. Nasociliary nerve involvement: zoster lesions on the tip of the nose (Hutchinson sign), is associated with a 76% risk of ocular involvement. Branching dendritic figures can be seen in the epithelial layers that are similar to the lesions in HSV, but have tapered ends.	Ophthalmic zoster requires emergent ophthalmologic consultation. Treatment is complex, and depends upon the type, location, and degree of ocular involvement. Oral and topical antiviral and steroid agents as well as antibiotics are used.
Periorbital (preseptal) cellulitis	Infection lying anterior to the orbital septum. Streptococcal species are currently the most common organisms.	Swelling of the eyelid, discoloration of the orbital skin, redness, and warmth. Conjunctival injection, occasional discharge, fever, and leukocytosis are seen. Vision, extraocular movements, pupillary findings, and optometric examinations are normal.	Cool compresses for comfort. Typically responds to oral antibiotics. IV antibiotics for severe infections/treatment failures. Antipyretics and pain medication as needed.
Orbital cellulitis	Inflammatory process in the structures posterior to the orbital septum. Due to extension from an adjacent structure: Sinusitis is the most common cause. Streptococcal infections are the most common etiology.	Similar to preseptal cellulitis but more severe; proptosis, decreased ocular mobility, ocular pain, and tenderness on eye movement. A CT scan of the orbit is the most useful aid to determine retro-orbital involvement.	Treatment for orbital cellulitis includes hospitalization, IV antibiotics, and occasionally incision and drainage. Broad-spectrum antibiotic coverage of *H. influenzae*, *S. aureus*, *Streptococcus pyogenes*, and anaerobes is indicated.

Table 69-5 Traumatic Eye Injuries

	General Overview	Mechanism	Diagnostic Clues	Treatment	Comment
Corneal abrasions	Disruption of the corneal epithelium. Red, painful eye with foreign body sensation, excessive tearing, blepharospasm and photophobia.	Results from mild trauma to the eye: foreign body, dust, contact lens.	Topical anesthetics cause immediate relief and facilitate examination. Fluorescein staining and inspection with cobalt blue light delineates the lesion.	Cycloplegia for comfort, oral pain medication and topical antibiotics. Patching may be considered in severe abrasions.	Long term use of topical anesthetics retards healing and may lead to more severe damage. If eye patching is used the eye should be reexamined within 12-24 h.
Foreign body (FB)	Red, irritated eye with foreign body sensation. Excessive tearing, pain and blepharospasm are likely to be present if cornea is involved.	A history of exposure to high speed metal on metal or similar projectile injury should suggest the possibility of globe rupture or an intra-orbital foreign body.	Inflammation in the anterior chamber suggests ulceration of the cornea or penetration of the globe. Irregular pupil or bloody chemosis suggest globe rupture. Seidel test positive with corneal penetration.	Superficial FB can be removed with irrigation. Topical anesthesia and damp, cotton-tipped applicator may facilitate removal. Embedded metallic foreign bodies can be removed with a tuberculin syringe approached from the lateral aspect in a tangential plane. Ophthalmologist should be consulted if removal is difficult.	Multiple linear corneal abrasions suggest a retained foreign body under the upper eyelid "ice rink" sign. Metallic foreign bodies may lead to rust deposition in the cornea. Metallic foreign body should be removed to prevent progression. Rust ring can be removed at follow-up.

Continued

Table 69–5 Traumatic Eye Injuries—*cont'd*

	General Overview	Mechanism	Diagnostic Clues	Treatment	Comment
Chemical burns	Exposure to caustic materials can cause permanent visual loss. Present with severe pain, redness, blurred vision and blepharospasm.	*Alkali chemicals* cause liquefaction necrosis and therefore damage continues until agent is removed. *Acids* cause surface burns. Organic materials are less likely to cause severe burns.	Splash burns on the skin around the eye. Conjunctival, scleral and stromal edema, and erythema may be present.	Irrigation with copious amounts of normal saline with special attention to irrigating the cul de sacs where substance may be concentrated. Use a Morgan lens (an irrigating contact lens) Check pH and continue to irrigate until pH normalizes and remains normal on sequential readings.	Emergent ophthalmologic consultation. Do not attempt to neutralize with acid or alkaline.
Hyphema	Red blood cells are found within the anterior chamber caused by a sheering injury to the iris or ciliary body. May be associated with pain and blurred vision. Somnolence has been reported in children.	Typically caused by blunt ocular trauma. Commonly co-exists with other eye injuries. Globe rupture should be excluded.	Small hyphemas may be missed because of other distracting eye injuries. If patient remains in upright position, hyphema may form a meniscus at the lower aspect of the chamber. This is not seen when supine.	Check intraocular pressures via tonometry device. Controlling IOP changes to prevent secondary bleeding. Anti-emetics and rest. Eye shield should be placed. Analgesia, avoid aspirin.	Emergent ophthalmologic consultation. May re-bleed resulting in a threat to vision. Large or complete (eight ball) hyphemas may be associated with permanent visual loss due to corneal staining or secondary glaucoma. Patients with sickle cell disease are at

Table 69–5 Traumatic Eye Injuries—*cont'd*

	General Overview	Mechanism	Diagnostic Clues	Treatment	Comment
Globe rupture	Painful red eye. Decreased vision with blepharospasm.	Result of blunt or penetrating trauma.	Enophthalmos, bloody chemosis, irregular teardrop-shaped pupil that "points to the rupture."	Do not touch the eye. Metal shield for protection. Seidel test positive with corneal rupture. Consider a CT scan to evaluate for intra-orbital foreign body.	Emergent ophthalmologic consultation. Pressure on the globe or eye manipulation may result in herniation of intraocular contents.
Eyelid lacerations	The upper eyelid is relatively easy to suture. Lacerations to the lower eyelid are more complicated.	Result of blunt or penetrating trauma.	The significance of this diagnosis is determined by the location of the injury and the structures involved such as the tarsal plate and lacrimal system.	Injuries to the tarsal plate or lacrimal system should be evaluated and repaired by an ophthalmologist, most often in the operating room.	Lacerations that traverse the lid margin require exact realignment to avoid entropion or ectropion.

Continued

Table 69–5 Traumatic Eye Injuries—*cont'd*

	General Overview	Mechanism	Diagnostic Clues	Treatment	Comment
Retrobulbar hemorrhage	Retrobulbar hematoma results in acute rise in IOP that is transmitted to the globe and optic nerve.	Result of blunt trauma with injury to the orbital vessels.	Proptosis, limitation of ocular movement, visual loss, increased IOP. A CT scan will reveal a hematoma.	Immediate ophthalmologic consultation. Treat increased IOP with carbonic anhydrase inhibitors, topical beta blocker, and IV mannitol. Lateral canthotomy; apply local anesthesia and a clamp to the area to decrease bleeding. Using sharp scissors, cut laterally, dissecting carefully to the orbital rim/lateral fornix. Use blunt dissection to free the inferior lid margin and disinsert the inferior crus of the lateral canthal tendon.	A lateral canthotomy should be performed in the ED for severe symptoms (loss of sight) especially if ophthalmology is unavailable.

CT, computed tomography; ENT, ear, nose, and throat; IOP, intra-ocular pressure.

	Mechanism	Clinical Presentation	ED Management
		Painless Loss of Vision	
Retinal artery occlusion	Occlusion of retinal artery or branch of the retinal artery most often resulting from carotid or cardiac valvular emboli.	Abrupt and near complete unilateral visual loss. Vision often limited to hand movement or less. Relative afferent papillary defect. Distinct macular "cherry red spot."	Immediate orbital massage. Hypoventilate for vasodilatation. Emergent ophthalmologic consultation
Retinal vein occlusion	Most often idiopathic; hypertension, diabetes, hyperviscosity syndromes, and glaucoma are risk factors. Leads to edema, hemorrhage, and vascular leakage.	Prolonged visual obscurations. Loss of vision can range from minimal (nonischemic) to recognition of hand motion only (ischemic). Dilated and tortuous veins, retinal hemorrhages, and disc edema ("blood and thunder" appearance).	Treatment is complex, and includes lowering of intraocular pressure, topical steroids, cyclocryotherapy, and photocoagulation.
Retinal detachment	Rhegmatogenous (tear or hole in neuronal layer with vitreous leakage), exudative (fluid or blood leakage from retinal vessels), and tractional (traction of fibrous bands in the vitreous).	Visual loss may be preceded by flashes of light, floaters. May report visual loss or curtain covering part of visual field. Yellow–orange light reflex in affected eye.	Emergent ophthalmologic consultation
Vitreous hemorrhage	Underlying vascular process results in hemorrhages into the vitreous humor. Typically seen in systemic diseases such as diabetes.	May report spider webs in visual axis or recent onset floaters. If severe, decreased red reflex. Hemorrhages may be seen on direct ophthalmoscopy.	Urgent ophthalmologic referral
Ischemic optic neuropathy	Vasculitic occlusion of the arteries to the optic disk. Often associated with giant cell arteritis. May be seen in hypertension and older diabetics.	Visual loss may be extreme. Jaw claudication or scalp tenderness may be present. Afferent papillary defect common. Optic nerve swelling on funduscopic exam.	Corticosteroids. Temporal artery biopsy. Referral to ophthalmology and primary care. See Chapter 35 for temporal arteritis.

Continued

Table 69-6 Visual Disturbances—*cont'd*

	Mechanism	Clinical Presentation	ED Management
		Painful Loss of Vision	
Acute angle-closure glaucoma	The pupillary margin of the iris is pushed against the surface of the lens. Aqueous fluid can no longer flow forward through the pupil, resulting in an increase in the pressure behind the iris.	Onset associated with abrupt change from a constricted to a mid-dilated pupil. Unilateral severely painful injected eye with a midrange minimally reactive pupil; vision may be decreased due to corneal edema. Profound systemic complaints may include severe headache, nausea and vomiting. Intraocular pressure >20 mm Hg (usually 50 to 70).	Reduce obstruction to outflow: topical miotic agent (pilocarpine 1%) Reduce production of aqueous: topical beta-blocker (timolol 0.5%), carbonic anhydrase inhibitor (Diamox 500 mg IV) and osmotic agent (glycerol or mannitol -1 g/kg). Emergent ophthalmologic consultation.
Anterior uveitis (iritis)	Inflammation of the iris that can be precipitated by trauma or linked to some inflammatory disease process (sarcoidosis, tuberculosis). It may also follow an attack of acute angle-closure glaucoma. The inflamed iris releases cells and debris into the aqueous.	Eye pain, photophobia, ocular redness, injection around the limbus. The pupil is somewhat constricted. Vision is unaffected early on, but may decrease later on. On slit lamp examination, there are cells and flare in the anterior chamber. Keratitic precipitates may form from congregation of floating material onto the back surface of the cornea. The iris may form adhesions to the cornea or lens (synechia).	Topical or oral (if severe) steroids after consultation with ophthalmology. Mydriasis to reduce pain by keeping the iris still. Treat the underlying cause.
Optic neuritis	Most commonly associated with multiple sclerosis (see Chapter 60). Other causes include syphilis. This is inflammatory demyelination, whether or not MS is diagnosed clinically.	Visual loss over a few days. Evaluate for visual field defects. Dull pain with eye movements. Afferent papillary defect. Most have normal fundoscopic examination.	Ophthalmologic referral and MRI

ED, emergency department; IV, intravenous; MS, multiple sclerosis; MRI, magnetic resonance imaging.

by the infectious etiology. Gonorrhea requires systemic therapy and frequent lavage. Conjunctivitis presenting in the first day of life is usually iatrogenic.

Teaching Points

Vision should be tested on all patients presenting with eye complaints. An acute deterioration of vision suggests a significant ophthalmologic problem that needs immediate intervention.

Chemical exposures should begin lavage immediately without delay for registration, triage procedures, or medical evaluation.

Patients with a retinal artery occlusion should be aggressively treated. Look for eye injuries in patients with any trauma to the face.

A penetrating or ruptured globe injury is an ophthalmologic emergency that may be subtle in its presentation. If there is any history suggestive of a foreign body penetration (e.g., hammering upon metal), then an imaging study must be obtained. This can be done with plain radiographs, a CT scan, or with an ultrasound examination. The patient may have few symptoms at the onset of the injury. No pressure should be placed on the globe of an injured eye until completely evaluated for evidence of globe rupture. Routinely, any pressure applied when opening an eye should be directed over the bony structure of the orbit or lid retractors should be used.

Patients who complain of new flashes or multiple floaters require an investigation for a possible retinal detachment.

In the case of infectious processes, a contact lens should not be used until advised to do so after follow-up with an ophthalmologist. Premature use of contact lens may result in corneal ulcers and possible visual loss or perforation.

Suggested Readings

Barish RA, Naradzay JF. Ophthalmologic therapeutics. Emerg Med Clin North Am 1995;13:649–667.

Bertolini J, Pelucio M. The red eye. Emerg Med Clin North Am 1995;13:79.

Datner EM, Jolly BT. Pediatric ophthalmology. Emerg Med Clin North Am 1995;13:669–679.

Handler JA, Ghezzi KT. General ophthalmologic examination. Emerg Med Clin North Am 1995;13:521–528.

Knoop K, Trott A. Ophthalmologic procedures in the emergency department, III: Slit lamp use and foreign bodies. Acad Emerg Med 1995;2:224–230.

Kuckelkorn R, Kottek A, Schrage N, Reim M. Poor prognosis of severe chemical and thermal eye burns: the need for adequate emergency care and primary prevention. Int Arch Occup Environ Health 1995;67:281–284.

LaVene D, Halpern J, Jagoda A. Loss of vision. Emerg Med Clin North Am 1995;13:539–560.

Linden JA, Renner GS. Trauma to the globe. Emerg Med Clin North Am 1995;13:561–605.

Rothenhaus TC, Polis MA. Ocular manifestations of systemic disease. Emerg Med Clin North Am 1995;13:607–630.

Santen SA, Scott JL. Ophthalmologic procedures. Emerg Med Clin North Am 1995;13:681–701.

CHAPTER 70

Psychiatric Emergencies

HOLLYNN LARRABEE ■ ANDRA L. BLOMKALNS

Overview

Psychiatric emergencies are common, and frequently their care commences in the ED. Emergency physicians are often asked to medically clear patients thought to have primary mental disorders before their psychiatric care begins.

It is critical to differentiate organic from functional symptoms to ensure appropriate care for these individuals. *Organic disease* refers to nonpsychiatric pathology, while *functional disease* denotes symptoms derived from a psychiatric source.

Agitation is a common problem. Treatment of agitation involves both chemical and physical restraints. These patients require close monitoring. It should not always be assumed that they have a psychiatric etiology for the agitation.

Suicide continues to be the eighth leading cause of death in the United States. Unfortunately depression is often masked, and at times, not noted or understood by the patient. The risk for suicide requires discernment and experience to recognize its hidden and subtle presentations.

Every state provides for some form of emergency detention in which immediate psychiatric intervention is required, usually due to potential danger to self or others. Emergency detention is designed to provide for an assessment of a dangerous situation. It is generally limited to a brief period, usually 3 to 5 days; the period ranges from only 24 hours in a few states to 20 days in New Jersey.

Patients cannot be admitted to a mental health facility on the basis of substance-induced psychiatric symptoms. These patients usually detoxify in the ED after a period of close observation.

Psychiatric services should be consulted for outpatient follow-up for patients who can safely be discharged from the ED. Psychiatric consultation in the ED is required for patients who may be a threat to self or others.

Medical Clearance of the Psychiatric Patient
General

■ Emergency physicians are often asked to medically clear patients thought to have primary mental disorders before their psychiatric care begins.

Table 70–1 Common Causes of Secondary Psychiatric Disease

Cardiopulmonary	**Endocrine/metabolic**
Dysrhythmias	Adrenal disease
Chronic obstructive pulmonary disease	Hepatic disease
Heart failure	Hypoglycemia
Hypoxia	Thyroid disease
Myocardial infarction	Vitamin deficiency
Pulmonary embolization	
Neurologic	**Infectious**
Central nervous system tumors	Encephalitis
Hypertensive encephalopathy	Human immunodeficiency virus
Hydrocephalus	Meningitis
Intracranial hemorrhage	Pneumonia
Multiple sclerosis	Sepsis
Seizures	Syphilis
Stroke	Urinary tract infection
Renal/electrolyte	**Drug/toxin**
Dehydration	Alcohol
Hypercalcemia	Amphetamines
Hypernatremia	Anticholinergic
Hyponatremia	Carbon monoxide
Uremia	Drugs of abuse
	Jimson weed
	Polypharmacy
	Sedatives

- Nearly 10% of "psychiatric symptoms" in patients with a known psychiatric history are due to an underlying medical condition. See Table 70–1 for common causes of secondary psychiatric disease. Failure to identify underlying medical disorders may prevent appropriate treatment and result in complications of the disease.
- No laboratory investigations are required unless specifically indicated in patients who have an established psychiatric diagnosis, and who present with typical symptoms. In patients with underlying psychiatric disorders such as schizophrenia, agitation often results from noncompliance with maintenance therapy or disease progression.
- A thorough history (including review of systems), vital signs, physical examination, and cognitive examination (tests for orientation at a minimum) are the most important components of a medical screening examination. Focus the examination on organ systems that include common co-morbid conditions (neurologic, cardiovascular, pulmonary, gastrointestinal). A more thorough evaluation should be performed for specific groups of patients who may be at higher risk. These include the elderly, patients with a new onset of psychiatric symptoms, those with preexisting medical conditions or concurrent complaints, and those with substance use disorders.

Features Suggestive of a Medical Cause for Psychiatric Symptoms

- Late age of onset of the initial presentation
- Sudden onset of psychiatric symptoms
- Atypical presentation of psychiatric illness
- Nonauditory hallucinations
- Substance abuse or overdose
- Polypharmacy
- Treatment resistance
- Abnormal vital signs especially fever
- Neurologic or cognitive abnormalities on examination
- Signs of delirium, including waxing and waning mental status
- Trauma
- Headache
- Co-morbidities such as human immunodeficiency virus (HIV) or diabetes
- No personal or family history of psychiatric conditions

Diagnostic Studies

- ***Laboratory tests.*** These should be obtained as indicated by history, physical examination, and known medical conditions. Studies may include a complete blood count (CBC) with differential, electrolytes, blood urea nitrogen (BUN) level, creatinine level, glucose level, liver function tests, ammonia, urine toxicologic screen, blood alcohol level, medications levels, thyroid function tests, urinalysis, and a urine pregnancy test in females of reproductive age. A lumbar puncture may be indicated to rule out encephalitis or meningitis. Overdose and intoxication are leading causes of both medical and psychiatric emergency visits. Toxidromes must be rapidly recognized and treated. Refer to Chapter 72 for an in-depth discussion of treatment of the poisoned or intoxicated patient.
- ***Radiology.*** Computed tomography (CT scan) of the head should be performed if structural or traumatic pathology is suspected. Chest radiographs should be performed to help rule out active tuberculosis (TB) in patients with risk factors or symptoms suspicious for TB (e.g., cough). Identifying active TB is particularly important due to close person-to-person contact in psychiatric wards.

Approach to the Violent or Agitated Patient and Use of Restraints

- Assure a safe environment as agitated patients can be a risk to themselves and to staff caring for them. Use of physical and chemical restraints is often indicated for protection of the patient and staff.

Physical Restraint

- Restraints are used to prevent patients from hurting themselves, to protect families and staff from agitated or violent patients, and to allow for appropriate patient assessment and treatment.

■ Restraining patients crosses the boundaries of patient autonomy, and may lead to claims of battery. Restraining a patient may potentially result in physical or psychological damage, and requires justification. Restraints should never be used for convenience or discipline. Emergency care providers must consider the risks and benefits of restraining the patient and consider all viable options. Indications for patient restraint include protecting the patient from self-harm (intentional and unintentional); protecting patients' families and staff from harm; facilitating appropriate examination, testing, and treatment of uncooperative patients; and to prevent a patient from leaving during evaluation of suicidal or homicidal ideation.

■ The use of restraints is governed by federal and state law and hospital accreditation protocols. Restraint orders must be written by a physician, and need to include a time limitation, not to exceed 24 hours. Monitoring and reassessment of the need for restraints should be documented each time the restraints are renewed.

■ Soft wrist restraints are appropriate to prevent self-extubation in confused or sedated patients. A Posey restraint is used to prevent confused patients from falling out of bed. Limb restraints (soft, leather) are used to restrain potentially violent individuals. Limb restraints may be used on the upper or lower extremities.

■ Staff should be trained in restraint use to minimize risk to both patient and staff. Ideally, each team member immobilizes one extremity. Complications, including minor bruises and abrasions, are common. There is a risk of choking and aspiration, especially when using four-point restraints. Injuries to staff can occur as a result of patient spitting, biting, scratching, or kicking.

■ There is no form of physical restraint that is free from complications, and patients have died, or sustained fractures while restrained even in a very limited fashion. Any patient who requires physical restraint should be evaluated for the need for chemical restraint and closely monitored.

Chemical Restraints

■ Any medication used to prevent patients from harming themselves or others is considered a chemical restraint.

■ Advantages of chemical restraint include reduced need for physical restraints, and increased ability to perform examination and diagnostic tests.

■ Disadvantages include oversedation, resulting in respiratory depression, paradoxical increased agitation, and limited neurologic examination due to altered level of consciousness.

■ The ideal agent would be long-lasting, easily reversible, and cause no hemodynamic or respiratory alterations. Unfortunately, such a drug does not exist. Table 70–2 lists commonly used agents. Patients must be carefully monitored for respiratory depression. Dosing is variable and titration of sedating agents must be done gradually, with care to prevent over sedation.

Table 70–2   Medications for the Acutely Agitated Patient

Generic Name	Brand Name	Dose	Comments
Haloperidol	Haldol	5-10 mg IM or IV	Conventional antipsychotic. Prolongs QT interval, but has been widely and safely used especially for the control of violent patients. Extrapyramidal symptoms (dystonia, akathesia) are common, and occur in 10% of patients. These can be prevented with prophylactic benadryl (25–50 mg PO). In rare cases neuroleptic malignant syndrome occurs after the use of Haldol.
Ziprasidone	Geodon	10-20 mg IM	Atypical antipsychotic. Little to no extrapyramidal effects. May prolong QT.
Olanzapine	Zyprexa	5-10 mg IM	Atypical antipsychotic. Little to no extrapyramidal effects. May prolong QT.
Lorazepam	Ativan	0.5-2 mg IM/IV	Benzodiazepine. Adverse effects include respiratory depression and paradoxical excitatory reactions.

IM, intramuscular; IV, intravenous.

Evaluation of the Suicidal Patient
Risk Factors for Suicide

- Men commit successful suicide more frequently, but women have more attempts. Suicide rates peak in adolescent and elderly populations. People older than 65 years have the highest rate of suicide. Isolated individuals are at greater risk than those involved in their community. Married people have lower risk than single, divorced, or widowed individuals.
- Other risk factors include a family history of suicide, or a recent suicide by friends (especially in adolescence); a history of physical, sexual, or emotional abuse; and mental illness. Suicide rates are highest in the mentally ill population when they are "highly functioning," often after starting new medications. Individuals who talk about suicide are more

BOX 70–1   Risk Assessment for Suicide

- Persons with a definite plan to kill themselves
- Patients who appear to be "wrapping things up"—making a will, saying goodbye to loved ones, writing a suicide note or giving away personal belongings
- Anyone with a strong family history of suicide
- Access to a gun, especially a handgun
- Substance abuse, especially alcohol
- Recent unexpected loss of loved one, job, home
- Patients who appear isolated or withdrawn
- History of depression or schizophrenia
- Feelings of hopelessness
- Patient with progressive painful or terminal illness
- Patients recently discharged from psychiatric units.

likely to kill themselves. Having a definite plan for suicide increases the likelihood of a suicide.

Assessing the Risk for Suicide

- Determine whether the patient has suicidal ideation or plan for a specific method: purchasing a weapon, making out a will, or writing a suicide note should be considered very significant in risk assessment (Box 70–1).
- Don't be afraid to ask the patient why death is desirable. You will not introduce the idea of suicide to a patient who does not already harbor it, and the answer may provide an important clue to the psychiatric seriousness of the patient's suicidal tendencies. Other factors such as finances or family stress may be involved. Because suicide is an aggressive act, homicidal thoughts should be queried as well. Inquire about symptoms of depression, recent loss (especially of a spouse in an elderly patient), stresses, or substance abuse. Ask about prior attempts. Query emergency medical services personnel, family members, and friends for additional information.
- If there is no indication of physical illness, no laboratory tests may be needed. If an overdose is suspected a full toxicologic workup must be undertaken (Chapter 72).

Emergency Department Management of the Suicidal Patient

- The patient must never be left alone; involve family, friends, social workers, or hospital security if necessary. Make sure the environment is safe. Remove any object that the person may use for self-harm.
- Determine a risk management plan. Patients with no imminent risk of suicide may be referred for outpatient management. Hospitalization (emergency detention) is necessary if any serious psychiatric suicidal threat exists. Psychiatric consultation should be done for evaluation of patients who may be a threat to self or others. Patients who are suicidal

and require hospital admission for another medical condition will require a 24-hour attendant and inpatient psychiatric consultation.

Mental Competence and Involuntary Hospitalization
General

■ *Involuntary hospitalization* and *civil commitment* are synonymous terms defined by state laws.
■ Duty to hospitalize a patient involuntarily is founded on two traditional government powers/responsibilities: police power (responsibility to protect each citizen from harm from others) and parens patriae (the government assumes responsibility for the care of those unable to care for themselves). Failure to commit a patient who falls under these laws will be considered a breach of duty, however there must be documented reasons for undertaking this commitment.

Ethical Principles

■ Two basic principles govern the decision to curtail a patient's freedom: the presence of severe mental illness that impairs the individual's ability to make capacitated decisions (that is those that an ordinarily prudent person would make), and the likelihood of harm to self or others. While the patient in most situations is deemed to have the right to refuse care, even if it is life-saving, it is only in the act of suicide that our ethics have deemed it wise to interfere with that patient's autonomy. The reason is that with the treatment of severe depression, many patients will reverse the desire to end life. This differs from the patient with a terminal disease who no longer wishes to continue living, although in the USA, there is as yet no legal permission to conduct euthanasia, or permit suicide in these patients. Similarly, under careful consideration, these patients may be medicated against their will.

Informed Consent, Capacity, and Competence

■ The informed consent process requires that patients be given information about a proposed medical treatment in a way that is understandable so the patient can make meaningful choices about medical alternatives. Without both understanding and decision-making capacity, the informed consent process by definition cannot take place.
■ *Capacity* is a medical term, and refers to the patient's ability to make decisions. A patient may have the capacity to make some decisions but not others, and capacity may fluctuate over time. *Competence*, by contrast, is a legal term, and refers to a person's ability to perform certain functions. Competence is determined by a judge. From a legal perspective, patients are either competent or not competent. Judges determine whether the patient is still competent to make decisions, or whether the patient needs to have a surrogate person to consent.
■ When a patient lacks capacity, several options exist. These include an informal surrogate decision maker (close family member), an attorney-in-fact (a person granted durable power of attorney), or a conservator/guardian. Even when a surrogate decision maker is used, we suggest that

the patient sign the consent form if this can be arranged. A record should explain why the patient appears to understand and accept the recommended treatment, even in the presence of significant psychiatric disease. If family members are involved, certain circumstances may require a more formal arrangement. There may be disagreements between family members, between family and patient, or between family and physician. A physician is never obligated to use as a decision maker an individual who does not appear to be capacitated, or who does not appear to be acting in the best interest of the patient. For example, the spouse of the patient may be incapacitated by medical disease or neurologic deteriorations. Moreover, unless the spouse or other relative is a court appointed legal guardian who has the right to make decisions for the patient, no relative has the right to refuse life-saving care even if the patient is unable to consent (e.g., because of coma). In the circumstances of such disagreements, consensus between the parties may be assisted by obtaining an ethics consult.

■ In an emergency, a physician may be faced with a patient unable to make decisions when none of the options discussed in this chapter are available. When there is a risk of death or irreversible harm such as loss of limb, physicians have a right and a duty to act. Every effort must be made to respect individual autonomy. An emergency does not permit physicians to override known patient preferences: for example a Jehovah's Witness who is known to oppose transfusion under any circumstance may not be transfused against the patient's consent because the physician deems the transfusion to be life-saving.

Teaching Points

Always ensure a safe environment when dealing with psychiatric illness. Agitated patients can be a risk to themselves, and to staff caring for them. Physical and chemical restraints are often indicated for protection of the patient and staff.

Suicide attempts must be evaluated in regard to medical as well as psychiatric seriousness as the two may not coincide. If the patient expresses homicidal ideations, it is only prudent to hold the patient, and to warn the person being threatened.

Patients who present with apparent psychiatric issues require medical screening as nearly 10% have an underlying medical condition. Patients who have a previous psychiatric history and established psychiatric diagnosis require a basic history and physical examination for medical screening. No laboratory investigations are required unless clinically indicated.

Any patient who is a danger to self or others requires emergency detention and psychiatric intervention.

Determining if patients are capable of making health care decisions involves demonstrating that the individual can receive and understand information relevant to the decision, can understand the possible consequences of the choice and alternatives, can express a decision, and can discuss values and desires in relation to the medical advice provided. A psychiatric evaluation may be helpful especially when the assessment of a patient's capacity is not clear.

Suggested Readings

Annas GJ. The last resort-the use of physical restraints in medical emergencies. N Engl J Med 1999;341:1408–1412.

Currier GW, Allen MH. Emergency psychiatry: physical and chemical restraint in the psychiatric emergency service. Psychiat Serv 2000;51:717–719.

Desan PH, Powsner S. Assessment and management of patients with psychiatric disorders. Crit Care Med 2004;32(4 Suppl):S166–173.

Hillard R, Zitek B. Emergency Psychiatry. New York: McGraw-Hill, 2004.

Soreff S. Suicide. eMedicine.com Last updated March 14, 2005, accessed October 21, 2005. Available at http://www.emedicine.com/med/topic3004.htm.

Wigder HN, Matthews MS. Restraints eMedicine.com. Last updated September 14, 2005, accessed October 21, 2005. Available at http://www.emedicine.com/emerg/topic776.htm.

Williams ER, Shepherd SM. Medical clearance of psychiatric patients. Emerg Med Clin North Am 2000; 18:185–198.

CHAPTER **71**

Rheumatology

AUTUMN GRAHAM ■ ANDRA L. BLOMKALNS

Overview

Rheumatology covers a wide range of conditions from self-limiting but troublesome musculoskeletal problems (i.e., osteoarthritis), to progressive multisystem disorders (i.e., systemic lupus erythematosus [SLE]) with life-threatening complications.

Many of these patients may come to the ED with a non-rheumatologic problem, but may have a complicated course due to their immunosuppressed state from chronic steroid use.

Specific Problems

■ Many rheumatologic problems are covered elsewhere in this book. See Chapter 21 for causes of back pain other than the seronegative spondyloarthropathies. See Chapter 42 for osteoarthritis, crystal-induced synovitis (gout and pseudogout), septic joint, bursitis, and tendinitis. See Chapter 63 for adrenal insufficiency (secondary to acute steroid withdrawal) and Chapter 67 for Lyme disease and rheumatic fever.

Dermatomyositis and Polymyositis

- *Definition.* Both dermatomyositis and polymyositis represent inflammatory myopathies. Dermatomyositis is present when cutaneous manifestations accompany inflammatory myositis.
- *Epidemiology and risk factors.* The disease occurs in 1/100,000 people. Women are affected two times more often than men. It peaks in the teenage years, but rises again in the fifth decade. There is a possible association with prior coxsackievirus and toxoplasmosis infections. It may be associated with malignant tumors in 10% to 15% of cases.
- *Pathophysiology.* Dermatomyositis is thought to be an autoimmune disorder with immune complex deposition in vessels, associated with an increased risk of malignancy. Polymyositis is caused by T-cell–mediated damage to the muscle fibers.
- *Clinical presentation.* The disease is characterized by symmetric proximal muscle weakness of the hips, shoulders, pharynx, and neck. Other complaints include myalgias, systemic symptoms of fever, weight loss, and Raynaud's phenomenon (claudication of the fingers and toes with cold exposure). Two characteristic lesions of dermatomyositis are a heliotrope rash and Gottron papules. A heliotrope rash (faint, lilac-colored eruption) may be found over the eyelids with dermatomyositis. Gottron nodules are raised, red, or violaceous, sometimes scaly lesions overlying the metacarpophalangeal, proximal interphalangeal joints, elbows, and knees. There may be an erythematous macular rash on the face, neck, and upper chest. The usual clinical course is slow and progressive.
- *Diagnostic testing.* An elevated creatine phosphokinase, lactate dehydrogenase (LDH), myoglobin, and transaminases (AST/ALT) are common. The elevation and height of the elevated ESR does not correlate with severity. An antinuclear antigen (ANA) titer and extractable nuclear antigen titer will often be positive. Referral for electromyography may be needed. A muscle biopsy is diagnostic.
- *ED management.* Start corticosteroids 60 to 100 mg/d. Azathioprine is second-line therapy. If patient is able to function reasonably, and good follow-up can be arranged, it is safe for the patient to be discharged home. Admit the patient if unable to ambulate, there is concern for malignancy, or if the patient appears toxic or unstable.
- *Helpful hints and pitfalls.* Proximal symmetric muscle weakness is the dominant clinical feature, but the examination may be normal.

Fibromyalgia

- *Epidemiology and risk factors.* The disease affects women 10 times more often than men. The prevalence increases with age. The average age of presentation is between 30 and 55 years. This is one of the somatizing diseases that frequently present to an ED.
- *Pathophysiology.* The cause is largely unknown; however, the most widely accepted hypothesis is an abnormal pain perception leading to muscle inactivity and atrophy.
- *Clinical presentation.* It can be subclassified into five subgroups depending on predominant symptoms: (1) pain and fatigue; (2) anxiety,

stress and depression; (3) multiple sites of pain and tenderness; (4) numbness and swollen feeling; and (5) associated features such as headaches and irritable bowel syndrome. The reasons for presenting to the ED are often vague and difficult to determine.

- **Diagnostic testing.** Most patients seen in the ED will have already been given the diagnosis outside of an ED. The presence of 11 tender points of the 18 sites determined by the American College of Rheumatology are needed for diagnosis. These sites are nine symmetric points that include the medial fat pad of the knee and the proximal trapezius that have frequently been found in patients diagnosed with fibromyalgia.
- **ED management.** The major problem with patients who present to the ED, is to have repeated expensive and always negative workups. The patients do not want to hear that there is nothing wrong with them, and unfortunately develop the ability to present with complaints that mimic other diseases that require extensive workups and multiple ED visits. What seems to work the best is to tell the patient that the emergency physician is unlikely to be able to solve problems that have been ongoing for years. The patient has problems that will likely continue. Then ask the patient what will make them comfortable at that time; in most instances, that is all that is needed. The ED stay can be shortened, and the patient can be safely referred to a primary care provider.
- **Helpful hints and pitfalls.** Fibromyalgia is not a diagnosis of exclusion, and is not excluded by the diagnosis of concomitant illness. No laboratory finding is diagnostic, although routine blood work including thyroid evaluation can be helpful to rule out other nonsomatizing diseases.

Polymyalgia Rheumatica

- **Epidemiology.** Polymyalgia rheumatica (PMR) is a systemic inflammatory disease that is most common in women and patients older than 50 years.
- **Pathophysiology.** The exact etiology is unclear, but the disease is the result of a systemic inflammatory response.
- **Clinical presentation.** The onset is acute, but may progress over a month before a diagnosis is made. Constitutional symptoms are common. The patients classically present with proximal extremity pain and morning stiffness. There is bilateral synovitis of the large proximal joints (shoulders > hips). Bursitis may be present. There is full range of motion and normal strength of the affected areas. Some patients can present with distal extremity manifestations.
- **Diagnostic testing.** The diagnosis is made clinically, but the ESR will be above 40 mm/h. Patients with limited disease may have a mildly elevated or normal ESR. In these cases, the diagnosis is based on a rapid positive response to low dose corticosteroids.
- **ED management.** Corticosteroids are the mainstay of therapy. The usual starting dose of prednisone is 10 to 20 mg/d. This is continued for 1 month and is carefully tapered by 1 to 2.5 mg/mo to a dosage of 10 mg/d, based on clinical response. The patient should be referred to a primary physician or rheumatology for outpatient management.

■ *Helpful hints and pitfalls.* The disease is commonly associated with giant cell arteritis or temporal arteritis, which is discussed in Chapter 35 and is briefly mentioned in this chapter under "Vasculitis".

Rheumatoid Arthritis (RA)

■ *Epidemiology and risk factors.* Women are 2-3 times more likely to be affected with RA than men. The incidence is 30/100,000 people. The age of onset is between 30 and 50 years.

■ *Pathophysiology.* This is a chronic autoimmune disorder of the synovial fluid characterized by destruction of the joint.

■ *Clinical presentation.* Arthritis most often involves the wrists, interphalangeal joints and knees. The joint pain is symmetrical. Morning stiffness lasting greater than 1 hour over months is the most common complaint, and the duration of this complaint often separates it from other arthralgias. Systemic symptoms include malaise, anorexia, fever, myalgia, weight loss and Raynaud's phenomenon (see Dermatomyositis). Other findings include ulnar deviation of the carpometacarpal joint, valgus deformity of the knees, Baker's cysts, and instability of the atlantoaxial joint with laxity of the transverse ligament and cervical spine. Complications of RA are listed in Box 71–1.

■ *Diagnostic testing.* The diagnosis is based on the clinical course over months to years. At least four of seven clinical factors must be present to make the diagnosis: morning stiffness; arthritis of more than three joints; swelling of the proximal interphalangeal (IP), metacarpophalangeal (MCP) or wrist joint; symmetric arthritis; rheumatoid nodules; positive rheumatoid factor; and erosions on radiographs of the hands or wrists. Laboratory data such as rheumatoid factor is positive in 50% to 75% of cases. The ESR, complement levels, and other autoantibody titers may be helpful.

■ *ED management.* Joint rest and NSAIDs are the first-line therapy. A first-time diagnosis of RA will rarely be made in the ED. Management should be made along with the ongoing primary care provider to undertake the initiation of oral steroids and disease-modifying drugs such as

---

BOX 71–1 Complications of Rheumatoid Arthritis

Airway compromise secondary to cricoarytenoid joint involvement
Interstitial pulmonary fibrosis
Cervical spine instability
Pericarditis
Vasculitis: Most commonly small dermal vessels
Nerve entrapment (i.e., carpal tunnel syndrome)
Sjögren syndrome: dry eyes and mouth, arthralgias
Felty syndrome: Rheumatoid arthritis, neutropenia, and splenomegaly; patients prone to infection
Tendon rupture

antimalarial agents, sulfasalazine, gold salts, d-penicillamine, azathiprine, cyclophosphamide, chlorambucil, methotrexate, and arthroplasty. External heat may be helpful.

- **Helpful hints and pitfalls.** Arthrocentesis should be performed when a septic joint is a diagnostic possibility. RA is a risk factor for septic joint.

Scleroderma

- **Epidemiology and risk factors.** This is a rare disease. There is a female predominance with a 10:1 ratio. It usually presents in the late 30s and 40s.
- **Pathophysiology.** This is an autoimmune disease. There are a complicated series of processes that lead to immune system initiation, vascular damage, and increased deposition of collagen.
- **Clinical presentation.** Early symptoms are nonspecific and include fatigue, arthralgias (polyarthritis), myalgias, and Raynaud's phenomena (see Dermatomyositis). Scleroderma is clinically divided into systemic sclerosis (SSc) and localized scleroderma. Systemic sclerosis has two major subsets: limited (formerly known as calcinosis; Raynaud's phenomenon, esophageal dysfunction, sclerodactyly, and telangiectasia [CREST] syndrome), and diffuse (widespread skin thickening with cardiopulmonary and renal involvement). Myocardial fibrosis can lead to congestive heart failure. Pulmonary manifestations include fibrosis (dyspnea, nonproductive cough, and fine inspiratory crackles) and pulmonary hypertension. Renal involvements may manifest as malignant hypertension or rapid progressive renal failure. Localized scleroderma primarily affects the skin (circular or linear lesions, skin tightening, pigment changes, atrophy, hair loss). Patients with scleroderma may also have finger or hand swelling; associated carpal tunnel syndrome may be present.
- **Diagnostic testing.** The diagnosis is not typically made in the ED. Anemia and ESR are variable. Thrombocytopenia may be present. Nearly all patients with SSc have elevated serum antinuclear antibodies that are very specific for SSc. For example, anticentromere antibodies are positive in 10% of patients with systemic illness, and in up to 95% of the patients with limited scleroderma. Chest radiographs may show ground glass, honeycomb or basilar scarring.
- **ED management.** Management in the ED consists of identification of complications of the disease that require prompt therapy such as hypoxia or acute renal failure. The overall management of this disease is complex.

Seronegative Spondyloarthropathies

- These are characterized by sacroiliac involvement, peripheral inflammatory arthritis, pathologic changes at the enthesis (tendinous/ligamentous insertion points), negative rheumatoid factor, and association with HLA-B27.
- They are believed to have an underlying genetic etiology triggered by an environmental stimulus.
- See Table 71–1.

Table 71–1 Seronegative Spondyloarthropathies

	Epidemiology	Clinical Presentation	Diagnosis	Treatment	Complications and Prognosis
Reiter's syndrome	• Males 15-35 y • Reactive arthritis • Often described as triad of conjunctivitis/iritis, urethritis and arthritis	• Subacute • Follows urethritis or diarrheal episode by 2-6 wk • Large weight-bearing joints • Lower extremity • Polyarticular • Asymmetric • Involves mucosa oral or conjunctiva	• Synovial fluid evaluation is inflammatory with PMN predominance • CBC/ESR high • 80% HLA-B27 positive • RF negative • Asymmetric sacroiliitis	• NSAIDs (i.e., indomethacin) • Tetracycline for suspicion of chlamydial infection • Physical therapy	• Lasts 4-6 mo • Recurrent episodes • Chronic arthritis • Ankylosing spondylitis • Aortic insufficiency • Prognosis variable but good
Ankylosing spondylitis	• Presents in adolescence • Male predominance	• Subacute/chronic • Vague lower back pain with loss of ROM • Symmetric • Pain improves with exercise • Uveitis • Plantar fasciitis • Achilles tendinitis	• HLA-B27 positive • RF negative • Radiograph of the spine may reveal vertebral bodies that are square shape (bamboo spine) • Pain for >3 mo required	• Strengthening exercises • NSAIDS • Pain control	• Progressive • Variable prognosis • Complicated by decreased mobility and chronic pain

Continued

Table 71–1 Seronegative Spondyloarthropathies—*cont'd*

	Epidemiology	Clinical Presentation	Diagnosis	Treatment	Complications and Prognosis
Psoriatic arthritis	• Occurs in 20% patients with psoriasis	• Multiple forms • Asymmetric oligoarthropathy with sausage digits • Symmetric polyarthropathy • Asymmetric spondylitis • DIP involvement • Arthritis mutilans	• Inflammatory • Clinical diagnosis	• Treat inflammatory process • NSAIDs • May require steroids • Treat psoriasis	• Usually self-limited • Prognosis good
Colitis arthritis	• 20% of IBD patients affected • Corresponds with IBD exacerbation	• Acute • Migratory • Polyarticular • Asymmetric or symmetric • Large joints of lower extremity	• Clinical • No particular laboratory or radiologic studies required • Rule out septic joint	• Treat IBD exacerbation • NSAID therapy • Pain control	• Prognosis good • Generally no long-term complications if treat underlying cause

CBC, complete blood count; DIP, distal interphalangeal; ESR, erythrocyte sedimentation rate; IBD, inflammatory bowel disease; NSAID, nonsteroidal anti-inflammatory drug; PMN, polymorphonuclear; RF, rheumatoid factor; ROM, range of motion.

Systemic Lupus Erythematosus

- *Epidemiology and risk factors.* The prevalence of SLE is 1/2000 people, predominantly affecting women. Black women are more commonly affected.
- *Pathophysiology.* The etiology is unknown. It is believed to be an autoimmune disorder that triggers an inflammatory cascade involving complement complexes, chemotactic factors, and antibody-dependent cytotoxic leukocytes.
- *Clinical presentation.* The most common initial complaints are fatigue and arthralgias. The rash associated with SLE is described as an edematous, maculopapular butterfly rash over the cheeks and bridge of the nose that is worsened by the sun. Discoid lupus consists of an erythematous raised plaque with scales usually on the face, head, or neck. This can be associated with alopecia. Mucous membrane lesions can be seen with small, shallow ulcerations. Vasculitic lesions such as ulcerations, purpura, and digital infarcts may occur. Other problems include Raynaud's phenomenon (see Dermatomyositis), leukopenia, intestinal obstruction, pericarditis, myocarditis, endocarditis, diffuse interstitial pneumonia, psychosis, depression, glomerulonephritis, aseptic meningitis, pleurisy, pulmonary embolism, pulmonary fibrosis, pneumonitis, stroke, neuropathy, and lupus cerebritis.
- *Diagnostic testing.* Antinuclear antibodies (ANAs) are positive in 95% of patients. Antibodies to dsDNA and anti-Smith's antigen are most specific for SLE. Complement levels are depressed. Patients with disease flares may show an increase in the ANA or dsDNA titers. Decreases in complement levels for C3 and C4 also correlate with disease flares in certain patients. The ESR is a very poor index of disease activity. A normochromic, normocytic anemia is common in SLE. Leukopenia is common with disease flares as well. Thrombocytopenia occurs in up to 25% of patients. The remainder of tests should be aimed at ruling out the serious complications of SLE and its treatment. Evaluation of new-onset monoarthritis should include arthrocentesis to rule out a septic joint. Because antiphospholipid antibodies are associated with SLE, patients are at high risk for clotting disorders, and they often require a search for deep venous thrombosis or pulmonary embolism.
- *ED management.* NSAIDs and lifestyle modification (i.e., smoking cessation, diet, and exercise) are first-line therapy. NSAIDs should be avoided in patients with severe gastrointestinal complications, thrombocytopenia, or renal impairment. Acetaminophen can be used for mild to moderate pain. Lupus cerebritis and acute worsening of lupus nephritis should be treated with methylprednisolone 1 g via IV. Less threatening flare-ups may be treated with as much as 100 mg or as little as 10 mg prednisone by mouth daily (or other agents in equivalent dosage), tapering gradually according to clinical symptoms, with an increase of 10% to 20% during the taper if clinical disease flares again. Alternative treatments such as antimalarial medications, azathioprine, or cyclophosphamide should be added or changed with the rheumatologist who will follow the patient. Sulfonamides, possibly penicillins, and estrogen-containing drugs should be avoided because they can exacerbate disease.

Tight control of hypertension is advised, as synergistic damage with SLE occurs. Admit patients for severe exacerbation, serious complications, any suggestion of sepsis, and signs of acute renal failure. Rheumatology consultation should be involved in the management of these patients. Stable patients may be followed up as outpatients by a primary care provider or rheumatologist.

■ ***Helpful hints and pitfalls.*** An ANA test can be ordered to rule out the diagnosis when the results of other tests are negative. Discontinue medications if you suspect a drug-induced SLE. Commonly associated medications are isoniazid, procainamide, minocycline, diltiazem, hydralazine, penicillamine, interferon alpha, methyldopa, and chlorpromazine. Lupus cerebritis should be considered in any patient with SLE who exhibits a change in behavior or mental status. Patients with SLE may have a false-positive VDRL or RPR test.

Vasculitis

■ Vasculitis syndromes are a spectrum of diseases whose common denominator is inflammation of the vessel wall. They are primarily due to an inflammatory response resulting from deposition of immune complexes in the vessel walls, activation of the complement system, vessel wall damage, and necrosis.

■ Since vasculitis can involve any vessel in the body, it can result in a wide variety of signs, symptoms, and laboratory abnormalities.

■ If an underlying disease is the cause of the vasculitis, such as SLE or RA, the blood vessel disorder is a secondary vasculitis. All others are considered primary. Some vasculitides can be both primary and secondary. Polyarteritis nodosa can be idiopathic (primary) or may be secondary to a multitude of viruses (hepatitis B and C, HIV, herpes zoster, cytomegalovirus) or a malignancy.

■ Suspect vasculitis in any patient who presents with an unexplained systemic illness, or has symptoms of organ-specific ischemia.

■ Consultation with a rheumatologist is helpful.

■ It is important to differentiate thrombosis and vasculitis, because the treatments are different.

■ The clinical manifestations of common primary vasculitides are listed in Table 71–2.

Table 71–2 Overview of Common Primary Vasculitides

	Primary Vessel Involved	Epidemiology	Clinical Presentation	Comments
Giant cell arteritis or temporal arteritis	Large	Age >50 y Prevalence is 200/100,000 people Risk factor: Tobacco use	Headache, jaw claudication, abrupt visual loss (early finding), arm claudication, polymyalgia rheumatica, unexplained fever or anemia	Late complications include aortic aneurysm or dissection Characterized by very high ESR >85
Takayasu's arteritis	Large	Female predominance Age of onset 10–40 y Asian descent 1–3 cases/million	Arthralgia/myalgias, fever, weight loss, claudication in extremities usually upper extremities, decreased pulsation in one/both brachial arteries, bruit over subclavian artery	Chronic disease with waxing and waning severity Glucocorticoids are the mainstay of therapy Standard angioplasty/bypass grafts for limb-threatening disease
Behçet's disease	Medium to small	Middle/Far Eastern descent Rare disease	Key finding: Oral aphthae. Also urogenital ulcers on scrotum and vulva, erythema nodosum, thrombophlebitis, palpable purpura, nodules, pyoderma gangrenosum, posterior or anterior uveitis, hypopyon, arthritis of medium to large joints	Cyclosporine and azathioprine may be protective for eye disease that often progresses to blindness Penicillin may be helpful for arthritis
Kawasaki's disease	See Chapter 79			

Continued

Table 71–2 Overview of Common Primary Vasculitides—*cont'd*

	Primary Vessel Involved	Epidemiology	Clinical Presentation	Comments
Polyarteritis nodosa	Medium to small	Male predominance Incidence 3–4/100,000 Age at onset: 40–60 y	Asymmetric polyneuropathy with motor and sensory deficits, livedo reticularis, skin ulcers, palpable petechiae, usually involving lower extremities, colicky abdominal pain, hypertension, renal insufficiency, weight loss, myalgias	Prognosis poor in untreated patients. Early treatment can increase 5-y survival Treatment includes corticosteroids and cyclophosphamide
Wegener's granulomatosis	Medium to small	Slight male predominance Most common major vasculitides Affects all ages	Respiratory and renal involvement (glomerulonephritis) Persistent rhinorrhea, purulent/bloody nasal discharge, oral/nasal ulcers, polyarthralgias, myalgias, sinus pain, cough, dyspnea, hemoptysis, pleuritic chest pain, hematuria, renal insufficiency Respiratory symptoms almost universal	High mortality (90%) if untreated Chest radiograph may show alveolar opacities, parenchymal lung nodules (classic finding) or pleural opacities Associated with antineutrophil cytoplasmic antibodies
Buerger disease	Small	See Chapter 25		
Churg-Strauss vasculitis	Small	Prevalence unknown No gender predominance Age of diagnosis 50 years old	Prodromal phase: 20-30 year olds; atrophic disease, allergic rhinitis, asthma Eosinophilic phase: Blood eosinophilia Vasculitic phase: Systemic	Clinical diagnosis with lung biopsy confirmation Steroids are the mainstay of therapy Asthma usually severe

Table 71-2 Overview of Common Primary Vasculitides—*cont'd*

	Primary Vessel Involved	Epidemiology	Clinical Presentation	Comments
Goodpasture's disease	Small	Children: median age 16 y Adults peaks in 20s-30s, and then again in 50s-60s White, and male predominance	Gross hematuria, hemoptysis, cough, edema, diaphoresis, tachypnea, exertional dyspnea, fatigue, fevers, cyanosis, inspiratory crackles, anemia, hypertension, pallor Usually no generalized vasculitis	Clinical diagnosis supportive laboratory studies: UA, CBC, renal panel, ESR, anti-glomerular basement membrane titer, pANCA titer Treat with steroids, fluid restriction and sodium restriction
Henoch-Schönlein's purpura	Small	See Chapter 77		
Erythema nodosum	Small	Annual incidence is 1-5/100,000 people Female predominance Age of onset between 15 and 40 y Recent streptococcal infection often present	Painful, red–violet subcutaneous nodules usually in pretibial location on bilateral legs. Can evolve into bruiselike lesions that resolve in 2-8 wk	Clinical diagnosis with ESR, biopsy, tuberculosis test, chest radiograph; ASO titer recommended May occur with sarcoidosis, streptococcal pharyngitis, tuberculosis, leprosy, histoplasmosis, inflammatory bowel disease, and medications such as birth control. Treat underlying cause and symptomatic relief

ASO, anti-streptolysin O; CRP, C-reactive protein; ESR, erythrocyte sedimentation rate; pANCA, perinuclear antineutrophilic cytoplasmic antibody.

Teaching Points

Rheumatoid diseases often present with involvement of one or many joints. It is rare that the diagnosis of the specific type will be made in the ED. A common error is to underestimate the seriousness of the flare-up, or the involvement of concomitant diseases that are triggering the flare-up (e.g., the presence of a septic joint in a patient with rheumatoid arthritis that is not searched for because it is thought to only be another episode of rheumatoid arthritis). These patients all have a form of immunosuppression, and therefore may have minimal signs and symptoms of sepsis. Despite the chronicity of their diseases, it is necessary to use the same criteria for admission as in any immunosuppressed patient.

Suggested Readings

Amor B. Eiter's syndrome: diagnosis and clinical features. Rheum Dis Clin North Am 1998; 24:677–695.

Boumpas DT, Austin HA 3rd, Fessler BJ, et al. Systemic lupus erythematosus: emerging concepts, I: Renal, neuropsychiatric, cardiovascular, pulmonary and hematologic disease. Ann Intern Med 1995;122:940–950.

Boumpas DT, Austin HA 3rd, Fessler BJ, et al. Systemic lupus erythematosus: emerging concepts, I: Dermatologic and joint disease, the antiphospholipid antibody syndrome, pregnancy and hormonal therapy, morbidity and mortality, and pathogenesis. Ann Intern Med 1995; 123:42–53.

Jain R, Lipsky PE. Treatment of rheumatoid arthritis. Med Clin North Am 1997;81:7–84.

Mitchell H, Bolster MB, LeRoy EC. Scleroderma and related conditions. Med Clin North Am 1997;81:129–149.

Nash P, Mease PJ, Braun J, van der Heijde D. Seronegative spondyloarthropathies: to lump or split? Ann Rheum Dis 2005;64(Suppl 2):ii9–13.

Strand V. New therapies for systemic lupus erythematosus. Rheum Dis Clin North Am 2000; 26:389–406.

Targoff IN. Dermatomyositis and polymyositis. Curr Prob Dermatol 1991;3:131–180.

Van der Linden S, Van der Heijde D. Ankylosing spondylitis: clinical features. Rheum Dis Clin North Am 1998;24:663–676.

Yunus MB. A comprehensive medical evaluation of patients with fibromyalgia syndrome. Rheum Dis Clin North Am 2002;28:201–217.

CHAPTER 72

Toxicology

72.1 General Approach to the Poisoned Patient

Ellen J. O'Connell ■ Larissa I. Velez

Overview

Toxic exposures must be considered in the differential diagnosis of multiple complaints, ranging from altered mental status to trauma. Comorbidities not only complicate the outcomes, but confuse the presentation.

Treat all patients as having a potentially life-threatening exposure, until proven otherwise. Some poisons do not display any signs or symptoms until late in the exposure.

Regional poison centers are an invaluable resource in the management of the poisoned patient. The national phone number that connects the caller to the closest poison control center (PCC) is (800) 222-1222. This number will enable you to obtain information on any toxic exposure and to reach a toxicologist if needed.

Initial Diagnostic Approach
General

■ The A/B/C/D/E (*a*irway, *b*reathing, *c*irculation, *d*isability, and *e*xposure) is useful in the approach to a poisoned patient (Table 72.1–1).
■ Clinical clues may assist with the identification of the toxic substance. A *toxidrome* is a term for the constellation of specific signs and symptoms that occur with exposure to a given substance. These findings may be dose or time-since-exposure dependent. The toxidromes are primarily based on vital signs; ocular signs such as nystagmus, pupillary size, and reactivity; skin color and moisture; absence or presence of bowel sounds and pulmonary secretions; and mental status changes (Table 72.1–2).
■ The history may come from patients, family, friends, paramedics, or scene witnesses. Unfortunately, the patient often cannot or will not give an accurate history, and one may not be available from other sources. Important points in the history of present illness include time of exposure, route of exposure, amount of exposure (e.g., pill counts), and patient access to any medications or other toxic substances.

Table 72.1–1   General Approach to the Toxicology Patient

Airway protection and **A**ntidote administration	Decreased mental status and respiratory depression with loss of the protective airway reflexes are common after overdoses. Antidote administration must be considered early in some cases, and may precede airway protection (e.g., naloxone for opioid intoxication).
Breathing	Ventilatory failure, hypoxia, and bronchospasm are known effects of many toxins.
Circulation	Many drugs affect the autonomic nervous system, manifesting as blood pressure and heart rate changes.
Disability and **D**econtamination	Initial evaluation of disability includes either the AVPU (alert, voice, pain, unresponsive) or the Glasgow Coma scale (Appendix 2). Evaluate the need for external or gastrointestinal (GI) decontamination.
Exposure and **E**nhanced elimination	Always undress the patient, looking for clues in the physical examination and ensuring that no injuries go undetected. Assess the need for enhanced elimination such as multi-dose activated charcoal (MDAC), hemodialysis, or urinary alkalinization.

■ A complete physical examination should be performed focusing on vital signs, respiratory status, skin findings, pupil size and reactivity, and the presence or absence of bowel sounds. In addition, evaluate reflexes and muscle tone; note any particular odors; and whether there is urinary retention.

Laboratory

■ Electrolytes, glucose, blood urea nitrogen (BUN), creatinine, serum osmolality, liver function tests (LFTs), complete blood count (CBC), clotting tests (prothrombin time [PT], partial thromboplastin time [PTT], international normalized ratio [INR]), total creatine phosphokinase (CPK) and urinalysis are commonly ordered in evaluation of the poisoned patient. These should be ordered selectively depending on the clinical circumstances. A urine pregnancy test should be performed on all women of childbearing age.

■ Serum acetaminophen and salicylate concentration should be measured on all drug exposures, as both are found in many over-the-counter preparations and prescription combinations.

■ Drugs and toxins with readily available serum concentrations include ethanol, methanol, ethylene glycol, lithium, digoxin, phenytoin, valproic acid, carbamazepine, phenobarbital, theophylline, lead, and iron.

Table 72.1–2 Toxindromes

Toxidrome	Clinical Findings	Common Agents	Management	Antidotes
Anti-cholinergic	Remember the mnemonic "red as a beet, dry as a bone, blind as a bat, mad as a hatter, and hot as a hare," referring to the symptoms of flushing, dry skin and mucous membranes, mydriasis with loss of accommodation, altered mental status (AMS), and fever, respectively. Tachycardia, hypertension, and urine retention may also be present	"anti" drugs: Antiemetics Antipsychotics Antihistamines	Supportive Avoid neuroleptics Benzodiazepines for agitation	Physostigmine 1-2 mg IV slow Avoid physostigmine if QRS or PR interval is wide (possible TCA poisoning)
Cholinergic*	Remember the mnemonic "DUMBELS" for muscarinic effects: defecation, urination, miosis, bradycardia and bronchorrhea, emesis, lacrimation, and salivation. Remember the mnemonic MTWtHFS (similar to days of the week) for nicotinic effects: muscle cramps, tachycardia, weakness, hypertension, fasciculations and paralysis, and sugar (hyperglycemia)	Organophosphate Carbamate insecticides Nerve agents Black widow spider venom	Supportive External decontamination if indicated	Atropine: 2-4 mg IV slow; use enough to dry bronchial secretions. Pralidoxime (2-PAM) 1 g IV over 15-30 min. May need an infusion at 500 mg/h.

Continued

Table 72.1-2 Toxindromes—cont'd

Toxidrome	Clinical Findings	Common Agents	Management	Antidotes
Sympatho-mimetic	Tachycardia, hypertension, ↑ temperature, tachypnea, diaphoresis, agitation, mydriasis	Epinephrine, cocaine, amphetamines, ephedrine	Supportive Benzodiazepines for agitation	None
Opiate	Pinpoint pupils, respiratory depression, CNS depression	Heroin, morphine, fentanyl, meperidine	Supportive	Naloxone 1-2 mg IV for respiratory depression In opiate-dependent patients, use lower doses (0.2-0.4 mg IV) to avoid precipitating withdrawal.
Sedative-hypnotic	Sedation Respiratory depression	Benzodiazepines Ethanol Barbiturates GHB	Supportive	Flumazenil is the antidote for the benzodiazepines, but should be used with extreme caution. Do not use in patients with seizure disorders, at risk for seizures, or in patients habituated to benzodiazepines. The dose is 0.1 mg/min to a maximum of 1 mg.
Opiate withdrawal	Yawing, piloerection, rhinorrhea, anxiety, diarrhea, abdominal cramping	Excessive opiate antagonist	Supportive	None
Sedative-hypnotic withdrawal	Agitation, diaphoresis, tachycardia, seizures, tremors	Abrupt stopping of benzodiazepines, barbiturates, ethanol, or GHB	Supportive	Benzodiazepines to control the agitation. Chlordiazepoxide can be used for very mild cases.

CNS, central nervous system; GHB, gamma hydroxybutyrate; IV, intravenous; TCA, tricyclic antidepressant.

- A urine drug screen for drugs of abuse is a common part of the workup of a poisoned patient, but the results rarely impact the immediate care of the patient. A positive test only identifies recent exposure to substances, and should not be used to definitively diagnose an acute intoxication, as it remains positive for days to weeks after the exposure.

EKG

- The electrocardiogram (EKG) is a useful tool in evaluating the poisoned patient. It is suggestive but rarely diagnostic of any single substance (e.g., paroxysmal atrial tachycardia [PAT] with block or bidirectional, ventricular tachycardia are commonly seen with digitalis toxicity). The EKG may be helpful in revealing the magnitude of an exposure such as the demonstration of QRS widening with a tricyclic antidepressant overdose.

Imaging Studies

- A chest radiograph is useful to evaluate for foreign body ingestions, the presence of noncardiogenic pulmonary edema, or aspiration pneumonitis. Abdominal radiographs can identify radio-opaque substances, such as iron tablets and other metallic objects. It can also sometimes identify drug packets in the intestines and bezoars.
- Computed tomography (CT scan) of the brain is often indicated in the patient with altered mental status to look for etiologies other than toxins. It can also be used to evaluate for complications of the drug (e.g., hemorrhagic stroke after the use of cocaine) or associated trauma.

Emergency Department Management Overview
General

- The ABCDEs should be addressed as discussed in previous sections.
- Decontamination techniques and enhanced elimination techniques are summarized in Table 72.1–3 and 72.1–4. A summary of management of some toxidromes is listed in Table 72.1–2. An antidote is a remedy, agent, or treatment used to counteract the effects of a poison or toxin (Table 72.1–5).
- Immediate interventions may include oxygen for documented or suspected hypoxemia, dextrose for hypoglycemia (if finger-stick glucose test is low), naloxone for opioid-induced altered mental status with respiratory depression, and thiamine in the alcoholic or vitamin deficient patient.
- The PCC (800-222-1222) is available 24 hours a day to help in the management of any poisoned patient.

Disposition

- Any patient who remains symptomatic from an ingestion or withdrawal state, requires ongoing medical treatment, or requires serial or frequent evaluations needs to be admitted.

Table 72.1–3 Decontamination Techniques

Name	Method and Dose	Indications	Contraindications	Complications
Skin and mucous membrane	Wear protective garment and gloves Remove clothes Brush particles Copious water or saline irrigation	All skin and mucous membrane exposures	None	None, in general Hypothermia if done outdoors in cold climate
Oral gastric lavage (OGL)	Place patient in left lateral decubitus, with the head down about 15-20 degrees (Trendelenburg) Insert tube (adults: 36 to 40 Fr; children 24 to 28 Fr) through mouth, confirm placement, irrigate with normal saline, and withdraw fluid	Recent (<1 h), life threatening ingestions only	Hydrocarbon ingestions Corrosive ingestions Unprotected airway Agitated or combative Pediatric (relative)	Aspiration, perforation, hypoxemia, trauma tracheal placement, hypothermia, fluid or electrolyte disturbance, lower esophageal spasm (may be relieved by glucagon)
Activated charcoal (AC)	Approximately 1 g/kg, or 10:1 charcoal to drug ratio	Substances that don't bind to charcoal* Recent ingestions within 4-6 hours Awake enough to drink it	Unprotected airway Caustic ingestion Risk for aspiration Ileus or perforation	Aspiration Emesis
Whole bowel irrigation (WBI)	Needs placement of NGT Use polyethylene glycol as the irrigant Children 9 mo to 6 y: 500 ml/h Children 6-12 y: 1 L/h >12 y and adults: 1.5-2 L/h	Sustained-release or enteric coated Body packers Substances not adsorbed by activated charcoal*	Unprotected airway Ileus or obstruction GI perforation GI hemorrhage	Nausea, vomiting, abdominal bloating, abdominal cramping

GI, gastrointestinal; NGT, nasogastric tube; PO, by mouth.

Table 72.1-4 Enhanced Elimination

	Method/Dose	Indications	Contraindications	Complications
Hemodialysis (HD)	Semipermeable membrane, which divides fluid and the patient's blood	Isopropyl alcohol, salicylates, theophylline, uremia, methanol, phenobarbital, lithium, ethylene glycol, ethanol	Hemodynamic instability	Bleeding
Hemoperfusion	Similar to HD, but uses cartridge with an adsorbent	Theophylline, salicylate, valproic acid	Same as for HD	Same as for HD Adsorbent emboli
Multidose activated charcoal (MDAC)	1 g/kg initial dose 0.5 g/kg every 4-6 h of plain activated charcoal	Phenobarbital, dapsone, quinine and quinidine, salicylate, theophylline, carbamazepine	Same as for single dose charcoal	Same as for single dose activated charcoal
Urinary and serum alkalinization	Initial dose of 1-2 mEq/kg Three ampules of Na HCO$_3$ in 1 L D5W, at 1.5 ml/kg/h (up to 250 ml/h in adult) Supplemental K+ Keep urine pH at 7-8 and serum pH at 7.5-7.55	Salicylates Phenobarbital Tricyclic antidepressants	Inability to tolerate sodium or volume loads Renal failure	↓ K+ and Ca++, tetany Coronary vasoconstriction Decreased oxygen disassociation

Table 72.1–5 Antidotes

Antidote	Toxin	Dose	Adverse Effects
Atropine	Organophosphate Carbamate Muscarinic mushroom Bradycardia from calcium channel blocker or beta blocker	0.5–2 mg IV High doses may be required for organophosphates and carbamates	Anticholinergic toxicity
Calcium salts (chloride and gluconate)	Calcium channel blocker or beta-blocker Hydrofluoric acid	10 ml of 10% CaCl (1 g/10 mL or 13.6 mEq/g) IV via central line only 10 ml of 10% calcium gluconate IV (1 g/10 mL or 4.65 mEq/g) 20 mg/kg or up to 1 g in children Can repeat q 5 min; infusion of 1–2 g/h	Hypercalcemia Extravasation of the chloride salt results in tissue necrosis
Crotalinae antivenom (CroFab)	Crotaline snake envenomations	Four to six vials initially, then two vials every 6 h for 18 h	Allergies (rare) Recurrence of venom effects (if follow-up doses are not used)
Deferoxamine	Iron poisoning	15 mg/kg/h, not to exceed 6 g in 24 h	Hypotension (rate related) Abdominal discomfort, nausea, vomiting, local irritation
Dextrose	Hypoglycemia due oral hypoglycemics or insulin	0.5–1 g/kg of D50W in adults, D25W in children, and D10W in neonates	Rare Vein sclerosis

Table 72.1–5 Antidotes—*cont'd*

Antidote	Toxin	Dose	Adverse Effects
Digoxin antibody (DigiBind)	Digoxin Digoxin-like cardiac glycoside (e.g., Foxglove)	Empiric dosing: 10–20 vials for an acute ingestion Three to six vials (adult) and one to two vials (pediatric) for chronic poisoning Note: also based on amount ingested (see text) or serum digoxin level	Rare
Flumazenil	Benzodiazepine	0.1 mg/min to a maximum of 1 mg	Benzodiazepine withdrawal and seizures; avoid if chronic benzodiazepine use or abuse, seizure disorder, ingestion of substances that decrease seizure threshold
Fomepizole	Ethylene glycol Methanol	15 mg/kg IV loading (maximum 1 g) 10 mg/kg IV q12h for 48 h 15 mg/kg IV q12h for the remainder of treatment	None
Glucagon	Hypoglycemia Calcium channel blocker Beta blocker	0.5–1 mg IV for hypoglycemia 50 to 100 μg/kg IV bolus (max 10 mg) and continuous infusion of 2 to 5 mg/h (children: 0.05 to 0.1 mg/kg bolus, then 0.05 to 0.1 mg/kg/h) for calcium channel and beta blocker poisoning. Follow with an infusion at the response dose per hour	Nausea and vomiting (premedicate with ondansetron)

Continued

Table 72.1–5 Antidotes—*cont'd*

Antidote	Toxin	Dose	Adverse Effects
Methylene blue	Methemoglobinemia	1-2 mg/kg IV Maximum dose of 7 mg/kg	Hemolysis in G6PD-deficient individuals and at high doses False decrease in pulse oximetry readings
N-Acetylcysteine (NAC, Acetadote)	Acetaminophen	Oral: 140 mg/kg loading dose, then 70 mg/kg q 4 hours for 17 doses IV Acetadote : (for acute toxic ingestions when enteral therapy cannot be tolerated) 150 mg/kg LD, then 50 mg/kg in 500 ml D5W infused over 4 hours, and 100 mg/kg in 1 L D5W over 16 hours	Anaphylactoid reactions (rate-related) Nausea and vomiting with oral dosing
Naloxone	Opioids, clonidine	0.4-2 mg IV, IM, SQ	Opioid withdrawal. Use lower dose in patients chronically on opiates.
Octreotide	Hypoglycemia due to sulfonylureas	50-100 μg SQ every 6-12 hours IV infusions have been used	Rare
Physostigmine	Anticholinergic delirium	1-2 mg IV over 5 minutes. Do not use if widened QRS	Can cause cholinergic excess
Pralidoxime	Organophosphate Carbamate	1 gram IV over 15-30 minutes. May require an infusion at 500 mg/h. Should be used with atropine	Hypertension Rapid IV administration can result in cardiac or respiratory arrest

- If the patient has had a minor, unintentional exposure and is asymptomatic after an observation period (usually 6-8 hours), and has appropriate follow-up, the patient may be discharged home.
- All patients with an intentional ingestion should have a psychiatric evaluation.
- The parents of children who have accidentally ingested a toxic substance should be educated about poison safety at home.

72.2 Common and Concerning Toxicities

Neil Harris ■ Jeremy J. Brywczynski

Specific Problems
Acetaminophen (Tylenol; also called APAP, derived from acetyl-para-aminophenol)

- ***Mechanism of toxicity.*** Peak serum levels occur within four hours in acute overdose. The toxic dose of single acute ingestion is 150 mg/kg or approximately 7 g in adults. The toxic dose may be lower in susceptible populations, such as persons with alcohol abuse. Under normal body conditions, 5% of metabolism by cytochrome P450 enzymes generates the toxic byproduct, *N*-acetyl-para-benzoquinoneimine or NAPQI, which is bound by glutathione and detoxified by oxidation. In overdose, glutathione stores are depleted and NAPQI concentrations increase, resulting in cellular injury and eventual hepatic necrosis. NAPQI is also produced to a lesser extent in the kidney. Therefore, toxic amounts can lead to acute renal failure.
- ***Clinical presentation.*** **Initial stage (0-24 hours)** is predominantly asymptomatic, but may have nausea and vomiting. In the **latent stage (12 hours-2 days)**, the patient may have right upper quadrant pain and a rise in transaminase and bilirubin levels. In the **hepatic stage (1-4 days)**, vomiting, jaundice, and altered mental status may occur. Laboratory values may reveal a coagulopathy, hypoglycemia, and renal failure. The **recovery stage (4 days-2 weeks)** occurs in patients who recover without need for liver transplant; hepatic dysfunction generally resolves within 2 weeks.
- ***Diagnostic testing.*** A 4-hour postingestion level should be obtained and the Rumack-Matthew nomogram (Figure 72.2–1) can help determine the need for antidotal treatment (>140 mg/L). If the time of ingestion is unknown, a serum level should be drawn immediately, and then again in 4 hours. However, this type of practice is controversial. The nomogram is only valid in a single acute ingestion with a known time of ingestion. Liver function tests should be obtained to detect any early liver toxicity.
- ***ED management.*** A single dose of activated charcoal reduces the serum acetaminophen level if given within 1 hour of an acute ingestion. There may be benefit after 1 hour if the ingestion involves an agent that delays gastric emptying or slows GI motility. *N*-acetylcysteine (NAC) is the

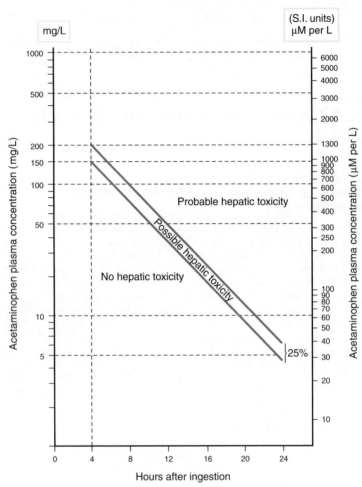

Figure 72.2–1. Rumack-Matthew nomogram for acetominophen poisoning. *(Modified from Rumack BH, Matthew H. Acetominophen poisoning and toxicity. Pediatrics 55:871–876, 1975.)*

antidote to prevent hepatotoxicity and is described in Table 72.1–5. It repletes glutathione stores. It may also enhance sulfate conjugation of any unmetabolized APAP. In patients who present **<8 hours after ingestion**, NAC can rapidly detoxify toxic metabolites or prevent their formation. Administer NAC if the presentation is close to 8 hours postingestion, or if the acetaminophen level will not be available within

8 hours postingestion, and if the history is unclear but toxic acetaminophen ingestion is suspected. A presentation **after 8 hours** should not preclude NAC administration if the history or presentation suggests potential toxicity. NAC has been shown to decrease mortality in late-presenting patients with fulminant hepatic failure, even in the absence of measurable serum acetaminophen levels. Patients with a non-acute overdose or chronic overdose are those individuals who ingest more than the manufacturer-recommended dose (usually >4 g and typically >10 g per day). In this situation, patients with detectable APAP or abnormal AST and ALT should be treated with a course of NAC. For extended release APAP, check 4-, 6-, and 8-hour acetaminophen concentration levels. Begin NAC therapy if any level crosses above the nomogram treatment line. If the 6-hour level is greater than the 4-hour level, begin NAC therapy.

- *Helpful hints and pitfalls.* The "Rule of 150" states that the toxic dose of a single ingestion is 150 mg/kg, the 4-hour serum level requiring treatment is 150 mg/L, and the oral loading dose of NAC is 150 mg/kg (intravenous [IV], 150 mg/kg). The NAC loading dose is sometimes reported as 140 mg/kg but 150 mg/kg is easier to remember and more NAC will not harm the patient.

Beta-Blockers

- *Mechanism of toxicity.* Beta-blocker overdose causes blockade of β_1 and β_2 receptors, thereby decreasing intracellular cyclic adenosine monophosphate (CAMP). β_1 blockade results in decreasing myocardial contractility, sinus rate, cardiac electrical conduction, and renin release. β_2 blockade also results in bronchoconstriction.
- *Clinical presentation.* Patients may present with hypotension, bradycardia, conduction abnormalities, and pulmonary edema. Neurologic effects include lethargy, coma and seizures, especially with lipid-soluble agents such as propranolol. Other less common presentations include hypoglycemia and bronchospasm.
- *Diagnostic testing.* An EKG may reveal a sinus bradycardia, atrioventricular (AV) nodal blockade, prolonged QTc, or conduction delays. A bedside glucose level may reveal hypoglycemia.
- *ED management.* Gastric lavage may be beneficial if the patient presents to the ED within 1-2 hours of ingestion. Some recommend that gastric lavage be undertaken after pretreatment with atropine to avoid the potential for increased vagal tone. Activated charcoal (AC) is generally recommended. Multidose charcoal or whole bowel irrigation (WBI) can be considered in extended release preparations. Atropine (0.5 mg for adults, 0.02 mg/kg for children, minimum 0.15 mg) and crystalloids should be given for bradycardia, hypotension, or AV block. Glucagon, which does not depend on β-receptors for its action to increase intracellular cAMP concentrations, has both inotropic and chronotropic effects. The dose is described in Table 72.1–5. If hypotension or bradycardia persists, other cardioactive drugs are indicated such as isoproterenol, dobutamine, dopamine, epinephrine, or norepinephrine. Phosphodiesterase inhibitors such as amrinone (5 μg/kg/min) have been

used. Refractory bradycardia may respond to an external or transvenous pacemaker. Propranolol overdoses with prolonged QRS (>100 milliseconds), acidosis, or persistent hypotension despite these therapies should be given a trial of sodium bicarbonate. High dose insulin therapy 0.5-1 units/kg/hr with dextrose have been suggested in cases of refractory shock. All patients with symptomatic β-blocker overdose should be admitted to a monitored setting, as should any patient with an ingestion of a sustained release product. Asymptomatic patients should be monitored for 6 hours in the ED. If the patient remains stable, but the ingestion included an immediate release product, the patient can be deemed to be cleared medically.

■ *Helpful hints and pitfalls.* Although calcium administration has been advised, it should be given cautiously and less aggressively than for calcium channel blocker overdose.

Calcium Channel Blockers (CCBs)

■ *Mechanism of action.* These drugs inhibit calcium influx across voltage-dependent channels resulting in sinoatrial (SA) and atrioventricular (AV) nodal depression, decreased contractility and smooth muscle relaxation.

■ *Clinical presentation.* The presentation is similar to that of β-blocker overdose with hypotension, bradycardia, conduction delays, lethargy, coma, and seizures.

■ *Diagnostic testing.* Sinus bradycardia, AV nodal blockade, or other conduction abnormalities may be present. Electrolytes and renal function should be assessed, and may reveal a metabolic acidosis with hyperglycemia (CCBs inhibit insulin release).

■ *ED management.* Treatment is similar to that of β-blocker overdose with AC, WBI, atropine, crystalloid infusion, glucagon, use of catecholamines, and admission criteria. Calcium salts are utilized to treat CCB overdose. Calcium chloride may be preferable to calcium gluconate because the calcium concentration is approximately three times greater (see Table 72.1–5). Ionized plasma calcium concentrations should be maintained between 2.0 and 3.0 mEq/L.

■ *Helpful hints and pitfalls.* Higher doses of calcium are given for CCB overdose compared with β-blocker overdose. Calcium should not be used if concomitant cardiac glycoside (e.g., digoxin) toxicity is possible. Gastric lavage has not been shown to change outcome after overdose of these agents and can induce an unwanted vagal response.

Carbon Monoxide

■ *Mechanism of toxicity.* Carbon monoxide (CO) binds hemoglobin with an affinity 200 times greater than that of oxygen. Fetal hemoglobin binds CO with even greater affinity. CO also binds myoglobin and inactivates cytochrome oxidase. The end result is tissue ischemia as oxygen delivery and utilization by cells is impaired.

■ *Clinical presentation.* Mild exposures can cause headache and dizziness, whereas more significant exposures can result in altered mental status, focal neurologic symptoms, ataxia, seizures, visual changes, and coma.

Cardiovascular symptoms include chest pain, dyspnea, syncope, and dysrhythmias. Gastrointestinal complaints include nausea and vomiting. The carbon monoxide is supposed to cause a cherry-red skin, however, this is not observed before the patient is dead. Patients may present in groups as exposures may occur in common buildings, cars, etc.

- **Diagnostic testing.** Check a carboxyhemoglobin (COHb) level from an arterial or venous blood gas. Pulse oximetry will be normal since it cannot discriminate carboxyhemoglobin from oxyhemoglobin. Obtaining a COHb level via co-oximeter confirms the diagnosis. If the clinical picture suggests CO poisoning, patients should be treated with 100% oxygen by nonrebreather mask until a level can be obtained. Normal levels are less than 5% in a nonsmoker, but can be elevated as high as 10% in an urban smoker. While COHb levels can aid in making the diagnosis, they do not always correlate with prognosis or severity of exposure. All patients should have a CBC to evaluate for an existing anemia. Any female patient of child-bearing age should have a pregnancy test.

- **ED management.** Administration of oxygen at the highest possible concentration is the goal of therapy. Hyperbaric oxygen (HBO) therapy should be used when possible for severe CO exposures. Indications include syncope, altered mental status, neurologic deficits, seizures, chest pain, or an abnormal EKG, and pregnancy with CO-Hgb levels >15–20%. Special consideration should be given to patients with cardiovascular compromise (ischemia, infarction, dysrhythmia), metabolic acidosis, extremes of age, an elevated CO-Hgb level (>25–40%), abnormal neuropsychometric testing results, or persistent symptoms despite normobaric oxygen. Consult with a toxicologist or a hyperbaric medicine expert. Admission should be arranged for symptomatic patients, those with elevated COHb levels, pregnancy, and those with significant exposures.

- **Helpful hints and pitfalls.** Remember the "Rule of 1/3": the half-life of CO with hyperbaric O_2 therapy (~30 min) is one third of the time of a patient on a 100% nonrebreather face mask (~90 minutes), which is one third compared to a patient on room air (~270 minutes). CO exposure should be suspected in patients with headache and nausea during the winter months, especially if family members, co-workers, or pets are symptomatic.

Cyanide

- **Mechanism of toxicity.** Cyanide inhibits cytochrome oxidase, the enzyme involved in the final step of oxidative phosphorylation. Blockade of this enzyme disrupts the ability of the cell to use oxygen, resulting in tissue anoxia, increased anaerobic metabolism, and the rapid development of lactic acidosis. Exposures are seen in some cases of smoke inhalation, with industrial chemical exposure, and in suicide attempts.

- **Clinical presentation.** Patients can rapidly become unstable with altered mental status, severe lactic acidosis, dyspnea, hypoxia, bradycardia, CNS disturbance, and hypotension. The patient may present with anxiety, agitation, seizures, and coma. Cardiac effects include sinus tachycardia, followed by bradycardia that can progress to asystole. There is typically no cyanosis in patients who are still breathing, and the retinal arteries and veins are equally red upon funduscopic examination. Both of these findings are due to the tissue's inadequate oxygen use. There may be an odor of bitter almonds; however, many people are unable to detect this odor.

■ *Diagnostic testing.* This is a clinical diagnosis. The pulse oximetry reading is usually normal. Severe lactic acidosis is an important clue.

■ *ED management.* Treatment is with the cyanide antidote kit. First, methemoglobinemia is induced (methemoglobin binds CN avidly) with nitrites, using inhaled amyl nitrite and intravenous sodium nitrite. There is no need to administer amyl nitrite if IV access has been established enabling rapid administration of sodium nitrite. Second, intravenous sodium thiosulfate is given to convert CN to less toxic thiocyanate.

■ *Helpful hints and pitfalls.* Sodium thiosulfate can be given without the nitrites in smoke inhalation (if carbon monoxide exposure is likely or in hypotensive patients). Patients are not cyanotic unless pulmonary edema is present or apnea has occurred.

●●● See Table 72.2–1 for a brief listing of other common or concerning agents
●●● that may cause toxicity.

Digitalis

■ *Mechanism of toxicity.* Digitalis inactivates the sodium-potassium ATPase-dependent pump. This allows efflux of potassium out of the cell and influx of sodium and calcium into the cell. This results in enhanced excitability and contractility of the myocardium. Digitalis also increases cardiac vagal tone resulting in decreased conduction velocity.

■ *Clinical presentation.* Bradycardia, AV block, ventricular dysrhythmias and hypotension may occur. Anorexia, nausea, vomiting, abdominal pain, altered mental status, weakness, and visual disturbances (e.g., abnormal color perceptions) may be present.

■ *Diagnostic testing.* The most common EKG finding in digitalis over-dose is ventricular ectopy. Other findings include down-sloping ST depression, bradycardias, junctional rhythms and varying degrees of AV block. Specific findings include atrial tachycardia with AV block, slow atrial fibrillation, and bidirectional ventricular tachycardia. In an **acute ingestion** levels peak at 2 hours after ingestion, but toxicity correlates best with levels drawn 6 hours after ingestion. Levels drawn early ($\leq$ 2 hours) can confirm the exposure, but cannot predict toxicity. Levels drawn at 6 hours postingestion that exceed 2 ng/ml are considered toxic, and levels above 10 ng/ml, can cause severe toxicity. In **chronic ingestions**, levels should be obtained but they correlate poorly with toxicity. Clinical judgment must be the basis of therapy. In acute ingestions, hyperkalemia can be present, and is an indicator of poor prognosis. However, in chronic toxicity, hypokalemia has a worse prognosis since it causes increased glycoside binding to the Na-K pump.

■ *ED management.* Activated charcoal is indicated in acute ingestions within the first 2 hours. The antidote for digitalis toxicity is antibody

	Examples	Clinical Presentation	Management
Antihistamine	Diphenhydramine (Benadryl)	Sedation, anticholinergic effects	Treatment consists mainly of supportive care and observation.
Antihypertensives	ACE inhibitors	Hypotension	Supportive measures with IV hydration and pressor agents; angiotensin II infusions or naloxone in severe cases.
	Clonidine	Hypotension, bradycardia, altered mental status. Hypertension can be seen.	Treatment includes high-dose naloxone.
Anticonvulsants	Carbamazepine (Tegretol)	Anticholinergic effects, seizures, altered mental status, QRS widening.	Serum levels should be obtained. Supportive care; multi-dose activated charcoal if airway secured. Charcoal hemoperfusion if life-threatening
	Gabapentin (Neurontin)	CNS depression	Supportive care.
	Valproic acid (Depakote)	CNS depression, GI and pulmonary symptoms; elevation of ammonia levels (chronic use)	Treatment is mostly supportive, although high-dose naloxone has been utilized. Hemodialysis for levels > 850 mg/L.
Benzodiazepines	Lorazepam (Ativan) Diazepam (Valium)	CNS depression.	Supportive. Flumazenil is rarely indicated as it may precipitate benzodiazepine withdrawal, and can cause seizures.
Hydrocarbons	Toluene Propane Gasoline	Aspiration pneumonitis; dysrhythmias, CNS depression, agitation	Respiratory support, decontamination (external). Avoid exogenous catecholamines due to myocardial sensitivity.
Antidiabetic agents	Sulfonylureas: Glipizide Glyburide Nonsulfonylureas: Metformin Acarbose Rosiglitazone	Recurrent hypoglycemia can be subtle and not observed until the patient seizes or has a loss of consciousness.	Treat hypoglycemia (Chapter 38). Ingestions of sulfonylureas should be admitted if (a) hypoglycemia develops; (b) it is a deliberate overdose; and (c) the patient is a child. Lactic acidosis secondary to metformin use should be admitted. IV octreotide is effective for suppressing endogenous insulin secretion.

Continued

Table 72.2–1 Other Common or Concerning Agents—*cont'd*

	Examples	Clinical Presentation	Management
Miscellaneous	Hydrofluoric acid	Exposures are generally via skin contact. Dermal exposures may not cause pain until 24 h after the exposure.	Treatment includes copious irrigation and topical application of a calcium gluconate gel to the burn area. Severe cases may require intradermal, maybe intra-arterial calcium.
	Isoniazid (INH)	Causes seizures and an anion gap metabolic acidosis in overdose.	Treatment is intravenous pyridoxine. If the amount of INH ingested is known: 1 g pyridoxine for 1 g of INH IV/PO, initial dose not to exceed 5 g/30 min IV. Administer remaining dose in increments of 1 g/30 min until total dosage completed. If unknown amount of INH ingested: 70 mg/kg IV, not to exceed 5 g/30 min; once seizures are controlled, administer remaining dose over 4-6 h. May repeat initial IV dose q5-20 min until seizures are controlled.
	Isopropyl alcohol	Similar to ethanol but metabolized slower; GI and CNS complaints; fruity breath odor, GI and mucosal irritation but GI bleeding is uncommon. Ketosis without metabolic acidosis.	Care is primarily supportive. Use dialysis for serum levels greater than 400 mg/dl.
	Strychnine	Patients are awake during these contractions. Patients may require intubation and paralytics.	Sedate with benzodiazepines.
	Theophylline	Can cause seizures, hypokalemia and dysrhythmias.	Theophylline levels should be obtained, and treatment is directed at the presenting symptoms.

ACE, angiotensin-converting enzyme; CNS, central nervous system; GI, gastrointestinal; INH, isoniazid.

fragments known as Digibind. Indications for Digibind include dys-rhythmias, hyperkalemia (K >5.0 mEq/L) in acute ingestion, hemo-dynamic instability, or a steady-state digitalis level above 10 ng/ml. Empiric dosing is described in Table 72.1–5. All symptomatic patients, patients with elevated serum levels, and those who received Digibind should be admitted to a monitored bed. Those with dysrhythmias, hemodynamic compromise, or life-threatening electrolyte abnormalities should be admitted to an intensive care unit. Asymptomatic patients with nontoxic serum levels at 6 hours and normal potassium levels can be discharged home. The formula to calculate the dose of antibody fragments based on weight and steady state serum level is as follows:

$$\text{No. vials of Fab fragment} = \frac{\text{Serum digitalis level (ng/dl)} \times \text{body weight (kg)}}{100}$$

■ *Helpful hints and pitfalls.* Cardiac glycoside–containing plants include oleander, foxglove, and lily of the valley. Serum digitalis levels are misleading after the administration of digibind, unless free digoxin levels are available. A common cause of chronic toxicity is worsening renal function. A much rarer current cause is the use of a long acting digitalis product.

Iron

■ *Mechanism of toxicity.* Iron affects multiple organ systems by disrupting oxidative phosphorylation and catalyzing the formation of free radicals. Ingestions of greater than 20 mg/kg of elemental iron are considered toxic, and those above 60 mg/kg are severely toxic.
■ *Clinical presentation.* **Stage I (0.5-6 hours):** GI tract symptoms predominate including abdominal pain, vomiting, diarrhea, hematemesis, and hematochezia. **Stage II (4-12 hours):** Symptoms improve, often misleading the physician about the level of danger in the overdose. An anion gap metabolic acidosis may be present. **Stage III (6-72 hours):** Most deaths occur in this stage, characterized by shock and worsening metabolic acidosis. Altered mental status and seizures occur. Elevated transaminase levels and azotemia are common findings. **Stage IV (12-96 hours):** This is the hepatotoxic stage that develops in severely poisoned patients and is evidenced by liver failure, jaundice, coagulopathy, and altered mental status. **Stage V (2-4 weeks):** If the patient survives the acute stages, bowel obstructions are common within the next month. The presenting symptoms are generally vomiting with abdominal pain.
■ *Diagnostic testing.* Abdominal radiographs may reveal iron tablets in the GI tract. Patients may have negative radiographs with significant iron ingestions if they ingested a solution, a chewable tablet (many pediatric forms) or if the iron tablets have already dissolved. Serum iron levels should be obtained at 2 to 4 hours after ingestion. Toxicity may occur with levels above 100 μg/dl. Significant iron toxicity occurs with levels greater than 500 μg/dl. Levels drawn more than 4 hours after ingestion are unreliable as the iron migrates intracellularly. Total iron binding capacity levels do not correlate with toxicity and should not routinely be ordered. A type and screen, coagulation panel, and CBC

should be ordered as GI bleeding is common. Liver function studies, chemistry panel, renal function, and arterial blood gases should be evaluated.

- **ED management.** If iron tablets are seen on abdominal radiographs, whole bowel irrigation can be utilized. Other forms of GI decontamination are not indicated. Although deferoxamine is the antidote for iron poisoning, the most important acute intervention for iron toxicity is intravenous fluid resuscitation with crystalloids. Indications for deferoxamine include patients with symptoms beyond mild nausea and vomiting (including all patients with GI bleeding, hypotension, altered mental status, or metabolic acidosis). All of these patients should be treated, regardless of their serum levels. Patients with serum levels greater than 500 µg/dl should also be treated. The dose is described in Table 72.1–5. All symptomatic patients, those with a metabolic acidosis, evidence of iron tablets on radiograph, or those with elevated serum iron levels should be admitted. Patients with severe symptoms, GI bleeding, shock, altered mental status, or levels above 1000 µg/dl should be admitted to an intensive care unit.
- **Helpful hints and pitfalls.** Virtually all patients develop GI symptoms.

Lithium

- **Mechanism of action.** Lithium is a cation that partially substitutes for extracellular sodium and intracellular potassium. Lithium can affect essentially any organ system.
- **Clinical presentation.** Patients may present with nausea, vomiting, diarrhea, tremors, fasciculations, movement disorders, decreased mental status, seizures, visual disturbances, slurred speech, and ataxia. In moderate to severe toxicity, hyperreflexia, seizures, coma, and signs of cardiovascular collapse may be present. Hypotension can be seen as well as QTc prolongation and dysrhythmias. Patients with chronic toxicity can develop diabetes insipidus, hypothyroidism, or hyperthyroidism.
- **Diagnostic testing.** Serum lithium levels should be obtained. However, levels correlate poorly with toxicity in chronic ingestion. The therapeutic level is 0.6 to 1.2 mEq/L and a level above 2.0 mEq/L is considered toxic, but toxicity can occur with lower levels. Serum electrolytes and renal function should also be obtained. Thyroid function tests should be considered in the appropriate clinical setting. An abdominal x-ray study may be helpful as lithium is heavy metal.
- **ED management.** Charcoal does not bind lithium. Whole bowel irrigation may be useful in patients ingesting sustained release lithium. Patients with altered mental status or seizures, milder symptoms in the setting of renal insufficiency, and symptomatic patients with serum levels greater than 4.0 mEq/L in acute overdose are candidates for dialysis. Symptomatic patients, those with sustained release ingestions and patients with serum levels greater than 2.0 mEq/L in chronic ingestions should be dialyzed as well.
- **Helpful hints and pitfalls.** Chronic ingestions are more severe than acute ingestions because lithium is already in the brain.

Salicylates (Aspirin)

- *Mechanism of toxicity.* Acute salicylate ingestions of 150 to 200 mg/kg produce mild symptoms, whereas 300 to 400 mg/kg can produce serious toxicity. An ingestion of 100 mg/kg/day for only 2 days can produce symptoms of chronic toxicity. Toxicity causes central medullary respiratory stimulation, constriction of the auditory vasculature, and uncoupling of intracellular oxidative phosphorylation. Late consequences occur such as cerebral and pulmonary edema as well as alterations in platelet function and bleeding time. Death is the result of severe acidosis and dysfunction of bodily enzymatic functions.

- *Clinical presentation.* Vital sign abnormalities include hyperpnea, tachycardia, and hyperthermia. Hypotension and dysrhythmias may also be present. Noncardiogenic pulmonary edema may occur. The patient may be diaphoretic and appear dehydrated. The most common gastrointestinal (GI) tract complaints include nausea, vomiting, and abdominal pain. Gastrointestinal hemorrhage, intestinal perforation, pancreatitis, and liver failure may also occur. Central nervous system (CNS) symptoms include tinnitus, altered mental status, seizures (from cerebral edema or low glucose), and coma.

- *Diagnostic testing.* Toxicity correlates poorly with serum levels, particularly in chronic ingestion. Toxicity in acute ingestion occurs with serum levels exceeding 25 mg/dl. The Done nomogram is seldom used anymore as it is not useful in the vast majority of cases of acute or chronic salicylism. It may be misleading when there is an incorrect time of ingestion, ingestion of more than a single dose, use of enteric-coated preparations, or long-term use of salicylates. A respiratory alkalosis and anion gap metabolic acidosis are common findings in overdose. Glucose and calcium levels should be obtained and are frequently low. Potassium levels should be monitored as hypokalemia often ensues during therapy, and will preclude proper management. EKG abnormalities (e.g., U waves, flattened T waves, QT prolongation), may reflect hypokalemia. Prothrombin and bleeding times may be prolonged.

- *ED management.* In patients requiring intubation, care must be taken to maintain the preintubation minute ventilation (tidal volume and respiratory rate) to avoid a precipitous rise in P_{CO_2} resulting in a worsening acidemia. Activated charcoal should be given in repeated doses every 4 to 6 hours. Urinary alkalinization, which may be difficult to achieve in hypokalemic states, may increase renal excretion of salicylate and reduces acidemia as described in Table 72.1–4. Indications for hemodialysis include renal failure, worsening acidemia, hypotension, seizures, altered mental status, pulmonary edema, cerebral edema, or congestive heart failure. Serum levels >100 mg/dl will typically necessitate hemodialysis, but the intervention may be required with lower levels if signs of end-organ toxicity are exhibited. Any patient with an aspirin overdose requiring bicarbonate or hemodialysis should be admitted to an intensive care unit. Asymptomatic patients with rising serum levels, patients with serum levels greater than 25 mg/dl, or any symptomatic patient regardless of serum level should be admitted for monitoring.

■ *Helpful hints and pitfalls.* Common management pitfalls include relying on serum levels to determine toxicity or the false sense of security of one isolated negative level, underventilating intubated patients, and not considering chronic salicylate overdose in elderly patients with altered mental status. An aspirin overdose should be considered in any patient presenting with a mixed anion gap acidosis and respiratory alkalosis. Depending on the laboratory, salicylate levels may be reported as either mg/dl or mg/L. This 10 fold difference must be considered when interpreting all salicylate levels.

Toxic Alcohols: Ethylene Glycol (EG)

■ *Mechanism of action.* Ethylene glycol can cause inebriation similar to other alcohols; however, its main toxicity is due to its metabolites. Ethylene glycol is first metabolized to glycoaldehyde, and this is catalyzed by alcohol dehydrogenase. Glycoaldehyde can then be metabolized to glycolate. Aldehyde dehydrogenase catalyzes this reaction. Finally, glycolate can be metabolized to oxalate. The formation of glycolate causes an anion gap metabolic acidosis and renal toxicity, while oxalate can crystallize in the urine, causing further renal insult. Ingestion of as little as one mouthful of a 99% EG antifreeze solution by either a child or adult may lead to toxic signs and symptoms. The lethal dose in adults is 1-1.5 mL/kg.

■ *Clinical presentation.* Although there is often overlap, the clinical presentation can be divided into three different stages. **Stage I (0.5-12 hours):** Neurologic symptoms predominate in this stage, with central nervous system (CNS) depression, altered mental status, and seizures. Co-ingested ethanol may delay the onset of ethylene glycol toxicity. **Stage II (12-48 hrs),** metabolites produce severe acidosis with compensatory hyperventilation. The acidosis is primarily the result of an increase in glycolic acid, although glyoxylic, oxalic, and lactic acids also contribute in small part. Calcium oxalate crystals are deposited in the brain, lungs, kidneys, and heart. ARDS and CHF can occur with hypoxia and multisystem organ failure. Death commonly occurs during this stage. **Stage III (24-72 hrs),** the direct toxic effects of ethylene glycol metabolites in the kidneys can cause acute renal failure.

■ *Diagnostic testing.* An anion gap metabolic acidosis is concerning for a toxic ingestion regardless of serum levels. A serum ethylene glycol levels should be obtained. A level greater than 20 mg/dl is considered toxic. Since these results are usually not readily available in the ED, ethylene glycol exposure level is often estimated through measurement of the serum osmolality and calculation of the osmolar gap (see Chapter 83). The osmolar gap should be less than 10 mOsm/L. A large increase in the osmolar gap suggests the presence of small osmotically active molecules such as propylene glycol, methanol, isopropyl alcohol, or ethylene glycol. Of these, only methanol and ethylene glycol cause a significant and persistent acidosis, owing to their conversion to toxic acid metabolites. A normal osmolar gap does not rule out the presence of a toxic alcohol. The urine should be examined for calcium oxalate crystals. Urine that fluoresces under ultraviolet light (a wood's lamp may be used) indicates probable ethylene glycol ingestion. However, this is often unreliable as only 15% of cases will fluoresce.

- *ED management.* Treatment is aimed at the inhibition of alcohol dehydrogenase, and can be achieved by use of either ethanol or fomepizole. Fomepizole is preferred because there is no CNS depression, it can be given as a single dose every 12 hours and serum levels do not have to be followed. Indications for antidote treatment include the clinical picture of ethylene glycol ingestion accompanied by any one of the following: serum level greater than 20 mg/dl, an osmolar gap greater than 10 mOsm/L, an anion gap metabolic acidosis or calcium oxalate crystals in the urine. The dose of ethanol is 0.8 g/kg load then 130 mg/kg/h IV with a goal blood alcohol level of 100 mg/dl or greater. The dose of fomepizole is described in Table 72.1–5. Cofactors can aid in the metabolism of ethylene glycol via nontoxic pathways and have few side effects. These include pyridoxine (50 mg IV), thiamine (100 mg IV), and magnesium sulfate (2 g IV). Indications for hemodialysis include the presence of a significant metabolic acidosis or renal insufficiency. Some authors suggest dialysis for anyone with an ethylene glycol level greater than 50 mg/dl. Patients require admission to an ICU.
- *Helpful hints and pitfalls.* Initially, patients have an increased osmolar gap and a normal anion gap. Later, the osmolar gap decreases, and the anion gap increases. Oxalate crystals do not cause urine to fluoresce, but antifreeze additives can. Find out if your laboratory tests routinely for ethylene glycol and methanol when you request a blood alcohol test. It may require a special determination. Ethanol infusions are difficult to titrate and maintain at a therapeutic serum concentration.

Toxic Alcohols: Methanol

- *Mechanism of toxicity.* Methanol is first metabolized to formaldehyde, catalyzed by alcohol dehydrogenase. Formaldehyde is metabolized to formate. The formation of formate causes the majority of toxicity, mainly by inhibiting the cytochrome oxidase complex. Formate concentration in the vitreous humor and optic nerve causes ocular toxicity. The estimated lethal dose is 1 g/kg or 1 ml/kg in adults.
- *Clinical presentation.* Symptoms may not develop for up to 30 hours after ingestion, depending on factors such as amount of co-ingested ethanol. Manifestations include headache, vertigo, altered mental status, seizures, coma, cerebral edema, infarcts or hemorrhages of the basal ganglia, blurred vision ("looking into a snow field"), hyperemia of the optic discs, nausea, vomiting, abdominal pain, pancreatitis, significant acidosis, and shock.
- *Diagnostic testing.* A serum methanol level greater than 20 mg/dl is considered toxic. An anion gap metabolic acidosis indicates a toxic ingestion regardless of serum methanol levels. Check for the presence of an osmolar gap as mentioned previously under "ethylene glycol."
- *ED management.* Treatment is focused upon the inhibition of alcohol dehydrogenase, and can be achieved by use of either ethanol or fomepizole as discussed under ethylene glycol. Indications for fomepizole therapy include a history of methanol ingestion with an anion gap

acidosis >20, a suspected methanol ingestion with an osmolar gap >10, a blood methanol level >20 mg/dl, a symptomatic patient with history of methanol ingestion or a methanol level that is not readily available and suspect concurrent ethanol ingestion, which may be masking symptoms. Ethanol therapy may be used in the absence of fomepizole therapy. Monitor blood glucose, especially in children. Adjunct therapy with folate and folinic acid (Leucorvorin) can be initialized. This will metabolize any formed formic acid to carbon dioxide and water. Initial dosing is Leucorvorin 50mg IV followed by Folate 50 mg IM or IV q 4 h. Folinic acid is the active form of folate. Indications for hemodialysis include the presence of a significant metabolic acidosis, ocular symptoms or hemodynamic instability. Dialyze anyone with a methanol level greater than 50 mg/dl. Patients with methanol ingestions require admission to an ICU.

- **Helpful hints and pitfalls.** Methanol ingestion should be considered in any patient with inebriation and visual complaints. Therapy should not be delayed awaiting methanol levels.

Tricyclic Antidepressants

- **Mechanism of action.** The toxic effects of tricyclics are results of their 4 main pharmacologic properties: Inhibition of norepinephrine and serotonin reuptake at nerve terminals (seizures), anticholinergic activity, alpha-adrenergic blockade (hypotension), and sodium channel blockade (QRS widening). Anticholinergic symptoms may be present (Table 72.1–2).
- **Clinical presentation.** The onset of symptoms typically occurs within 2 hours of ingestion, which corresponds to the peak TCA serum level, which may range from 2-12 hours. Neurologic symptoms include altered mental status, coma and seizures. Anticholinergic effects are commonly seen, but are not predictors of life-threatening toxicity. Patients who present with wide complex rhythms have a high mortality.
- **Diagnostic testing.** The EKG is the most accurate predictor of toxicity in acute TCA overdose. Common findings include sinus tachycardia, a widened QRS (>100 ms), and an R wave in aVR greater than 3 mm.
- **ED management.** The patient should be closely monitored for rapid deterioration of mental functioning, airway compromise, or hemodynamic instability. The airway should be secured if gastric lavage or charcoal administration is to be performed in a patient with a decreasing level of consciousness. The use of gastric lavage in TCA overdose should be limited to serious toxicity presenting soon after the ingestion has occurred. Activated charcoal is recommended in acute overdose within the first two hours. Indications for sodium bicarbonate include a QRS duration longer than 100 milliseconds, dysrhythmias, and hypotension unresponsive to crystalloids. The initial dose is 2 mEq/kg IV and is further described in Table 72.1–4. Ventricular dysrhythmia refractory to sodium bicarbonate may require treatment with lidocaine, magnesium sulfate, or both. Class I-A (e.g., quinidine, procainamide, disopyramide) and class I-C (e.g., flecainide, propafenone) drugs are contraindicated because they may worsen sodium channel inhibition. Class III drugs (e.g., amiodarone, bretylium, sotalol) are contraindicated because they

can further prolong the QT interval, leading to ventricular dysrhythmia. Class II beta-blockers (e.g., propranolol, esmolol, metoprolol) and class IV calcium channel blockers (e.g., verapamil, diltiazem, nifedipine, nicardipine) are contraindicated because they may potentiate or worsen hypotension. Seizures should be treated with benzodiazepines immediately to avoid worsening acidosis. Barbiturates and propofol are second and third line interventions for TCA induced seizures. Phenytoin is not recommended. For hypotension refractory to intravenous saline, vasopressors with an alpha-agonist effect, such as Neo-Synephrine or norepinephrine may be used. Patients requiring treatment should be admitted to an intensive care unit. Asymptomatic patients with a normal EKG and no tachycardia should be observed on a cardiac monitor for 6 hours before being deemed medically safe.

■ *Helpful hints and pitfalls.* Flumazenil should not be used in any patient with suspected TCA overdose, as it may cause seizures and death. Physostigmine is a short-acting cholinesterase inhibitor used for the reversal of anticholinergic symptoms. It should not be used in treating TCA toxicity because of the reported cases of physostigmine-induced bradycardia and asystole.

Special Conditions

■ *Methemoglobinemia* is caused by exposures to nitrates, dapsone, pyridium, benzocaine (oragel), and sulfa drugs. Methemoglobin (MetHb) has an oxidized ferric (Fe^{3+}) form of iron instead of the ferrous (Fe^{2+}). Increasing levels of MetHb causes a functional anemia in which the MetHb does not allow oxygen to bind to hemoglobin. Patients can have cyanosis, headache, altered mental status, and shock. Pulse oximetry is typically in the middle to high 80s (86%-89%) and does not respond to supplemental oxygen. MetHb levels can be measured by co-oximetry. Treatment with methylene blue is recommended for symptomatic patients with elevated levels.

■ *Neuroleptic malignant syndrome (NMS)* can be seen in patients beginning, or on increasing dose of neuroleptics or other dopamine-blocking agents. The clinical presentation includes fever, hypertension, tachycardia, diaphoresis and extrapyramidal features, including rigidity. An elevation in serum creatine kinase is often seen. Treatment includes withdrawal of the neuroleptic (or dopamine-blocking agent), and aggressive supportive management that includes intravenous fluids and benzodiazepines. Dantrolene and bromocriptine have also been used. Neuromuscular blockade may be necessary if rigidity affects respiratory function. Patients should be admitted to an intensive care unit for close monitoring.

■ *The serotonin syndrome* can be seen with selective serotonin reuptake inhibitors (SSRIs) overdose (or therapeutic use) and in particular with the combination of other serotonergic agents (dextromethorphan, tricyclic antidepressants, lithium, MAO inhibitors, meperidine). Clinical presentations include tremor, rigidity, hyperthermia, tachycardia, diaphoresis and altered mental status. If a neuroleptic drug has recently been started or the dose increased, then neuroleptic malignant syndrome

(NMS) should be the diagnosis rather than serotonin syndrome but this is difficult to exclude. Management of a serotonin syndrome is predominantly supportive along with administration of benzodiazepines. The serotonergic agent should be withdrawn. In select cases, cyproheptadine and chlorpromazine may be utilized.

72.3 Drugs of Abuse

Rais Vohra ■ Matthew Cook ■ Binh T. Ly

Body Packing and Body Stuffing

- ■ **Background.** The intentional, planned transportation of illicit substances within the GI tract is known as *body packing*. In contrast, the hasty ingestion of poorly packaged drugs or paraphernalia to conceal these items from law enforcement personnel is called *body stuffing*. Due to limited time available for packaging the drugs for ingestion, only small amounts of drugs are typically ingested in this scenario.
- ■ **Clinical presentation.** Because the onset of symptoms is usually within a few hours following ingestion, and the quantity of drug ingested is small with body stuffers, these situations rarely cause severe life-threatening complications. In contrast, the onset of toxic symptoms in a body packer may be delayed, and herald an imminent catastrophe. The presence of symptoms in the body-packing situation is concerning because a packet containing potentially lethal amounts of drug may be leaking into the GI tract allowing for systemic absorption. Occasionally, body packers may have symptoms of bowel obstruction.
- ■ **Diagnostic testing.** Routine urine drug screens may be helpful in identifying the class of drug responsible for the clinical presentation in symptomatic patients (see Table 72.3–1). Plain abdominal radiographs may reveal ingested packets, but so often miss packets that there is no meaningful information gathered from a negative x-ray study. Serial radiographs may be helpful in following the progression of packets through the GI tract, and may provide an endpoint for decontamination. A contrast CT scan or an MRI find more packets but can also miss some.
- ■ **ED management.** Asymptomatic and stable symptomatic patients should be given activated charcoal followed by whole bowel irrigation (WBI). Symptomatic patients may require aggressive resuscitation and supportive care. The effects of cocaine are generally short-lived. Body stuffers require monitoring for several hours until they are no longer tachycardic and hypertensive (because of the drug), and until they are calm and cooperative. Patients who have normal vital signs and normothermia may be discharged home after observation for up to 6 hours. However, symptoms suggestive of drug intoxication may require admission for further monitoring and decontamination. Body packers may require hours to days of hospitalization until all the packets have been passed. Surgical intervention is needed if patients present with serious signs or

Table 72.3–1 Important Reminders for Urine Drug Screen Interpretation*

Drugs	Agents That May Give False Positives	Agents That May Not Be Detected by Screen	Detection Window
Amphetamines, methamphetamine	Decongestants (ephedrine, pseudoephedrine), Vick's inhaler (L-methamphetamine), Ecstasy (MDA, MDMA), phentermine, selegiline, sertraline, trazadone, bupropion, chlorpromazine, labetolol, ranitidine	Ecstasy (MDMA, MDA)	1-4 d
Cocaine metabolite (benzoylecgonine)	Reliable screen, coca leaf teas possible	Reliable screen	2-7 d
Barbiturates	Reliable screen	Reliable screen	2-4 d, phenobarbital detectable up to 4 wk
Marijuana (THC)	Passive marijuana smoke exposure, dronabinol, naproxen, ibuprofen, fenoprofen, promethazine	Reliable screen	1-30 d depending on use/exposure
Opiates	Poppy seeds (actually a true positive), ofloxacin, rifampin, dextromethorphan	Semisynthetic opiates (hydrocodone, oxycodone, hydromorphone), fentanyl, methadone, propoxyphene, meperidine, diphenoxylate, loperamide, tramadol	1-4 d
Phencyclidine (PCP)	Dextromethorphan, diphenhydramine, possibly ketamine	Reliable screen	1-7 d
Benzodiazepines	Oxaprozin	Lorazepam, alprazolam, triazolam, midazolam, estazolam, quazepam, flurazepam	1-30 d

*Findings are variable depending on dose, screening method, and manufacturer.

symptoms or intestinal obstruction. Benzodiazepines should be given agitation especially in the setting of cocaine use.

- *Helpful hints and pitfalls.* Patients should be closely monitored for progression of symptoms.

Dissociatives

- *Background.* These agents include phencyclidine (1,1-phenylcyclo-hexylpiperidine or PCP) and ketamine, which is structurally and pharmacologically similar to PCP but only possesses about 10% of PCP's potency. Dissociative agents are compounds that inhibit the normal communication of sensory inputs to the higher cortical centers. Antagonism of N-Methyl-D-aspartate (NMDA) receptors is thought to be the underlying mechanism for "dissociation" of the somatosensory cortex from higher centers in the brain. Low doses antagonize the NMDA glutamate receptor, but escalating doses cause reuptake blockade of dopamine and norepinephrine, and stimulation of sigma opioid receptors, muscarinic and nicotinic acetylcholine receptors, and GABA receptors.

- *Clinical presentation.* Symptoms range from sedation to profound agitation and violent delirium, particularly with PCP. Sympathetic signs such as diaphoresis, tachycardia, and hypertension are common. Vital organ function and protective reflexes are usually preserved. Motor abnormalities include cerebellar signs such as nystagmus (rotatory nystagmus is classic), ataxia, incoordination, or dysarthria. In contrast to PCP, symptoms of ketamine intoxication are comparatively brief, lasting 4 to 8 hours with ingestion. As effects of ketamine wane, a phenomenon called the "emergence reaction" characterized by bizarre behavior, agitation, vivid dreams, hallucinations, or frank psychosis may occur.

- *Diagnostic testing.* PCP is detectable by most immunoassay urine toxicology screens unless the amount used is too low. False-positives in the PCP assay include dextromethorphan and diphenhydramine. Ketamine does not cross react with all urine bioassays for phencyclidine, but its presence can be confirmed with gas chromatography-mass spectrometry. Because rhabdomyolysis is a pontential complication, skeletal muscle creatine phosphokinase levels should be checked.

- *ED management.* Treatment is supportive, and measures to prevent injury to the patient and medical staff should be undertaken. Severely agitated patients are at risk for sudden death, and liberal administration of benzodiazepines should be used. Treat rhabdomyolysis (Chapter 49) if present.

- *Helpful hints and pitfalls.* A minority of patients have cholinergic signs or sedation with higher doses.

Hallucinogens

- *Background.* These agents include *lysergic acid diethylamide* (LSD) and *hallucinogenic mushrooms* such as *Psilocybe cubensis, Gymnophilus, Panaeolus, Amanita muscaria* and *Amanita pantherina*. A few other examples of hallucinogens include ololuiqui (morning glory), jimsonweed, nutmeg,

Mexican mint (*Salvia divinorum*), khat (*Catha edulis*), N,N-dimethyltryptamine (DMT), and mescaline (*Lophophora williamsii* or peyote).

- *Clinical presentation.* The hallmark of hallucinogenic intoxication is alteration in mood, perception, and cognition. Micropsia and macropsia (the illusion of objects growing large or small), and visual afterimages (tracers) are typical of a LSD "trip." Patients report alterations in perception, shape and color distortion, and synesthesias. Sympathomimetic signs, seizures, anxiety, nausea, vomiting, and tremors may be noted. Rare complications may include hyperthermia, rhabdomyolysis, and subsequent myoglobinuric renal failure.
- *Diagnostic testing.* Hallucinogenic compounds are not detected by routine urine assays. The sinus tachycardia that is usually present provides no diagnostic clues.
- *ED management.* Initial therapy is geared toward minimizing stimuli to prevent further agitation. Most cases respond well to a quiet, calm environment. Benzodiazepines should be used in patients who are agitated or violent.
- *Helpful hints and pitfalls.* Patients should be monitored closely for safety and oversedation from chemical restraint.

Marijuana

- *Background.* The psychoactive substance contained in marijuana is Δ-9-tetrahydrocannabinol or THC. THC and other cannabinoids have activity at specific cannabinoid receptors in the cerebral cortex, but the exact mechanisms responsible for clinical manifestations are not completely understood.
- *Clinical presentation.* The drug can cause tachycardia, mild hypertension, dyspnea, conjunctival injection, altered sensorium, euphoria, labile affect, lethargy, ataxia, weakness, inattentiveness, loss of motor dexterity, increased appetite, and dry mouth. Individuals with underlying psychiatric dysfunction may be at increased risk of psychosis or paranoia with acute intoxication. Duration of effects is typically 1 to 4 hours with smoking.
- *Diagnostic testing.* Cannabinoids are detected by most urine immunoassays.
- *ED management.* Supportive care and reassurance from familiar persons are the mainstays of treatment for intoxications.
- *Helpful hints and pitfalls.* Chest radiography may be helpful in detection of pneumothorax or pneumomediastinum in patients complaining of chest pain after heavy smoking as marijuana users will often perform forceful Valsalva maneuvers to maximize absorption through the lungs.

Opioids

- *Background.* Opioids stimulate specific receptors in the CNS and GI tract.
- *Clinical presentation.* Lethargy, decreased bowel sounds, and pinpoint pupils may be noted initally. Larger overdoses may cause respiratory

depression, hypotension, bradycardia, coma, and muscle flaccidity, which along with aspiration may result in death. Poisoning with imidazoline derivatives such as clonidine, oxymetazoline (Afrin), naphazoline (Naphcon), and tetrahydrozoline (Visine) may present similarly to opioid intoxications. Noncardiogenic pulmonary edema (NCPE) may also occur as a result of opioid intoxication. **Methadone** is long-acting with duration of effect lasting 12 to 24 hours. **Fentanyl** is rapid-acting with potent analgesic action (50-100 times stronger than morphine) and short duration of effect (0.5-2 hours). **Propoxyphene** has fast sodium channel blocking (type 1A) activity that can cause QRS prolongation and predispose users to dysrhythmias and seizures. **Meperidine** is metabolized to normeperidine, which is eliminated renally. In individuals with renal insufficiency or after high dose therapy, normeperidine can accumulate to cause delirium, myoclonus, and seizures. Meperidine is also a potent serotonin reuptake inhibitor and may precipitate a serotonin syndrome when used with other serotonergic agents. Meperidine abusers may have equivocal pupillary findings in contrast to the miosis typical to most opioid intoxications. **Diphenoxylate** and **loperamide** are meperidine analogues used as antidiarrheals owing to their poor oral absorption and gut-slowing effects. Also, diphenoxylate is typically formulated in combination with atropine. Thus overdosed patients may exhibit an antimuscarinic toxidrome. **Tramadol** is a unique drug with both opioid and nonopioid effects. Seizures are a known effect of this drug even in therapeutic dosing. Like meperidine, tramadol is also a serotonin reuptake inhibitor. **Dextromethorphan** (DXM) is a complex drug commonly abused by teenagers as it is available without prescription in many cough and cold preparations.

- *Diagnostic testing.* Most urine immunoassays reliably detect morphine, heroin, and codeine. Semisynthetic and synthetic opioids are variably detected. Because DXM is a hydrobromide salt, there may be falsely elevated chloride concentrations due to cross interference of the bromide ion in analysis for chloride concentrations. The QRS duration may be prolonged with propoxyphene poisoning. A chest radiograph is useful in evaluation of patients suspected of having pulmonary aspiration or NCPE.

- *ED management.* Naloxone is the primary opioid antagonist and can reverse opioid-induced respiratory depression. The dosing is described in Table 72.1–5. The effect lasts only 1 to 2 hours and thus it may need to be redosed or given as a continuous IV infusion with longer acting opioids. When appropriate, an IV infusion of naloxone should be started at two-thirds of the effective bolus dose per hour. Nalmephene and naltrexone are long-acting opioid receptor antagonists with little role in the ED. Oxygen is the first-line treatment for NCPE. Positive end-expiratory pressure should be applied to patients with NCPE requiring mechanical ventilation. Diuretics and nitrates are not helpful in NCPE. Propoxyphene overdoses with QRS prolongation longer than 0.100 seconds should be treated with IV sodium bicarbonate boluses.

- *Helpful hints and pitfalls.* Be careful with the use of naloxone in the opioid dependent patient. Use lower dosages.

Sedative-Hypnotics

- *Background.* Benzodiazepines are sedative-hypnotics with anxiolytic, muscle relaxant, and anticonvulsant effects. Barbiturates have been used for induction of anesthesia and as anticonvulsants. The barbiturates can be subdivided as ultra–short-acting (thiopental, methohexital), short-acting (pentobarbital, secobarbital), intermediate-acting (butalbital), and long-acting (phenobarbital) agents. Most commonly abused preparations contain butalbital and phenobarbital. Gamma-hydroxybutyrate (GHB, Georgia homeboy, liquid ecstasy, easy lay, grievous bodily harm) became popular among bodybuilders due to its purported ability to enhance secretion of growth hormone. GHB is currently FDA approved for treatment of cataplexy in association with narcolepsy. The drug is abused by many for its soporific, hallucinogenic, and euphoric effects. It has also been implicated in drug-facilitated sexual assaults. All of these agents are agonists at the GABA receptor, the major CNS inhibitory neurotransmitter.

- *Clinical presentation.* Effects of sedative-hypnotics include anxiolysis, sedation, muscle relaxation, and seizure termination. In large overdoses or in combination with other sedatives, slurred speech, nystagmus, lethargy, ataxia, coma, hypotension, bradycardia, hypothermia, respiratory depression, and respiratory arrest can occur. Skin bullae, sometimes referred to as "barb blisters," may be present, and are thought to be pressure-induced due to prolonged immobilization. These bullae are not specific to barbiturate poisoning but can result from coma of any etiology. With GHB, there is a high incidence of profound obtundation and bradycardia. Myoclonic jerks and seizure-like activity may also be observed. Loss of protective airway reflexes may occur, increasing the likelihood of airway obstruction and aspiration. The effects of all sedative-hypnotics are enhanced by concurrent alcohol use, and death can occur with this combination.

- *Diagnostic testing.* Most urine immunoassay drug screens detect oxazepam and the benzodiazepines that are metabolized to oxazepam (diazepam, temazepam, and chlordiazepoxide). Because many benzodiazepines are not metabolized through this pathway, these agents may not be routinely detected with typical urine immunoassays. Urine immunoassay screens can more reliably detect exposures to barbiturates. Serum phenobarbital levels are also available from most hospital laboratories. GHB and its analogs are not detected on urine immunoassay drug screens, and serum levels are not readily available from most hospital laboratories.

- *ED management.* Management is supportive. Flumazenil is a specific benzodiazepine receptor antagonist, but is not used in the overdose setting secondary to the possibility of precipitating withdrawal. Activated charcoal should not be used because of the risk of aspiration when a sedative has been ingested. Hypotension can be treated with IV crystalloid boluses or pressors. Multiple-dose activated charcoal, urinary alkalinization, and hemodialysis have been shown to enhance elimination of phenobarbital. However, decreasing serum levels do not appear to have appreciable benefit clinically. Treatment is largely supportive although patients may remain obtunded for several days with severe phenobarbital intoxication.

Sympathomimetics

- **Background.** These agents include cocaine and amphetamines. A multitude of "designer" amphetamine and methamphetamine derivatives exist and include 3,4-methylenedioxymethamphetamine (MDMA, Ecstasy, Adam, XTC), 3,4-methylenedioxyamphetamine (MDA, love drug), and 3,4-methylenedioxyethamphetamine (MDEA, Eve), among others. Cocaine inhibits presynaptic reuptake of dopamine and serotonin in the CNS, leading to accumulation of these neurotransmitters at synaptic clefts. Peripherally, cocaine inhibits presynaptic reuptake and may stimulate release of catecholamines, especially norepinephrine, again leading to accumulation at synaptic clefts and sympathomimetic effects. Another mechanism of cocaine toxicity is mediated through the sodium channel blocking (Type 1A) effects of the drug. This blockade is responsible for the local anesthetic effect of cocaine but can also result in EKG abnormalities such as QRS prolongation. Sodium channel blockade and excessive sympathetic activity can predispose the affected individual to seizures and ventricular dysrhythmias. Amphetamines exert their primary effect in a manner similar to cocaine but do not cause sodium channel blockade.
- **Clinical presentation.** Includes mydriasis, diaphoresis, muscle rigidity, rhabdomyolysis, myoglobinuric renal failure, hyperthermia, tachycardia, hypertension, cardiac dysrhythmias, and cardiac ischemia. Intracranial hemorrhage can occur in the setting of severe uncontrolled hypertension. Chest pain may be a result of chest wall rhabdomyolysis, coronary artery spasm or thrombosis, aortic dissection, pneumothorax, or pneumo-mediastinum (caused by aggressive breath-holding during crack smoking). Central effects include euphoria, delirium, anxiety, paranoia, tremulousness, psychomotor agitation, and seizures.
- **Diagnostic testing.** Sympathomimetics are typically detected with most urine immunoassays, but positive amphetamines assays occur commonly due to over-the-counter decongestants (e.g., pseudoephedrine), prescription drugs (e.g., methylphenidate, selegiline) and herbal agents (e.g., ephedra).
- **ED management.** Treatment is supportive. Benzodiazepines are first-line management for most central and peripheral sympathomimetic effects and should be used liberally. Sodium bicarbonate is the treatment of choice for sodium channel blockade as evidenced by QRS prolongation of more than 0.120 seconds. Lidocaine may be helpful in treating ventricular dysrhythmias. Beta-blockers, including labetolol, should be avoided as unopposed alpha adrenergic effects can lead to severe hypertension. Nitroprusside or phentolamine IV may be used for hypertension refractory to treatment with benzodiazepines. Patients with persistently abnormal vital signs, altered mental status, rhabdomyolysis, intracranial hemorrhage, or those suspected to have ischemic complications of sympathomimetic use should be admitted to a monitored setting.

Teaching Points

There are a myriad of overdose and poisoning causes. Common to all of them is a requirement of a good history, as the diagnosis will never be considered without information to trigger the thought. Think of overdose with any sudden change in behavior, mental status, or onset of seizure activity. The clue to many poisonings is the presence of disease in more than one patient (e.g., carbon monoxide or methanol ingestion), and the sudden appearance of bizarre behavior. Be quick to consult the Poison Control Center and a toxicologist because details of management are difficult to retain for the whole spectrum of poisonings.

Attention to the principles of emergency resuscitation, and prudent directed therapies work best for most drugs. The use of gastrointestinal decontamination has diminished, and is reserved for special overdose situations. Charcoal is still widely used, but may be risky when given to a patient with increasing somnolence such as from benzodiazepine overdose. Routine use of certain antidotes should be avoided (e.g., flumazenil) since they may increase rather than reverse problems.

With children, even small ingestions can be very dangerous, and longer periods of observation or even hospital admission is often prudent. Safety counseling should be given to parents, and the need for a child protective services evaluation should be investigated.

Many drugs of abuse produce visits to the ED. Although there are a number of recognizable toxidromes, patients often abuse multiple drugs, and toxic effects may be additive, or canceling, and often are confusing. It is often helpful to obtain a toxicology consultation. In any patient with altered sensorium, a drug screen may be part of the evaluation, but just because it is positive, it does not necessarily account for the patient's presentation.

Suggested Readings

Eldridge DL, Dobson T, Brady W, Holstege CP. Utilizing Diagnostic Investigations in the Poisoned Patient. Clinics in Laboratory Medicine 2006. 26:13–30, vii.

Erwin M, Deliargyris E. Cocaine-associated chest pain. Am J Med Sci 2002;324:37–44.

Freese T, Miotto K, Reback C. The effects and consequences of selected club drugs. J Subst Abuse Treat 2002;23:151–156.

Goldfrank L, Flomenbaum N, Lewin N, Howland M, Hoffman R, Nelson L (editors). Goldfrank's Toxicologic Emergencies. 7th ed. New York: McGraw-Hill Medical Publishing Division, 2002.

Judge BS. Metabolic Acidosis: Differentiating the Causes in the Poisoned Patient. Med Clin North Am 2005;89:1107–1124.

Olson K, Anderson I, Benowitz N, Blanc P, Clark R, Kearney T, Osterloh J. (editors). Poisoning & Drug Overdose. 4th ed. New York: McGraw-Hill Medical Publishing Division, 2004.

Traub S, Hoffman R, Nelson L. Body packing—the internal concealment of illicit drugs. NEJM 2003;349:2519–2526.

PEDIATRICS

CHAPTER 73

General Approach to the Pediatric Patient

JAYSON PEREIRA ■ M. OLIVIA TITUS

Overview

Children have a unique physiology. There are anatomic, physiologic, pharmacologic, and emotional differences from adults that are critical to recognize for proper assessment and care.

All children are not the same. The spectrum of pediatric diseases varies with age. The differential diagnosis should reflect this spectrum. For example, toxic and infectious exposures vary with age, and different congenital abnormalities classically present at different ages.

Approach the patient as part of a family. Address the concerns of both the parents and the child, realizing that they may be quite different.

Regardless of the patient's age, the initial assessment always begins with the ABCs (*a*irway, *b*reathing, and *c*irculation). Recognize signs of abuse and always consider non-accidental trauma as part of the differential diagnosis in the pediatric patient (see Chapter 82).

Differential Diagnosis

Keep in mind the general categories of disease when evaluating a pediatric patient. The mnemonic "CHILDREN" may be helpful.
■ Congenital
■ Hematologic/vascular
■ Infectious/inflammatory
■ Lactation/pregnancy
■ Drugs/toxic exposures
■ Recent trauma/abuse
■ Endocrine/metabolic
■ Neoplastic

Initial Diagnostic Approach
History

■ Gathering historical information can be a challenge. Young children are not able to characterize symptoms, nor even generate a clear chief complaint. Collect information from as many sources as possible.

- Take the parents' concerns seriously. Parents know their children well, and often recognize subtle onsets of disease that will not be apparent to the physician seeing the child for the first time.
- Obtain information about the pregnancy and birth of the child, immunization status, hospitalizations, general developmental progress, and any possible toxic exposures. Current immunization requirements may be found at www.immunizationed.org and are listed in Table 73–1.
- A social history (including recreational drug use, menstrual history, and sexual relations) may be the most important component of a conversation with an adolescent, and should be obtained privately away from the parents.

Physical Examination

- Be familiar with "normal" vital signs for a child (Table 73–2). The lower limit of systolic blood pressure should be less than 60 mm Hg for neonates; 70 mm Hg from 1 month to 1 year; 70 mm Hg + (2 × age in year) from 1 to 10 years; and more than 90 mm Hg if older than age 10 year.
- Unless the child is acutely ill, several moments spent establishing a rapport can make the rest of the examination much easier. If possible, the physician should sit or kneel at the child's level, and assume a non-threatening manner. Avoid separating the young child from the parents. A young child will often be most cooperative for examination while seated in the mother's lap.
- The physician should observe first, without direct touching. Determine if the patient's physical characteristics and behavior are appropriate for the level of development (Table 73–3), keeping in mind that children tend to regress emotionally when sick.
- Perform the least invasive parts of the examination first (i.e., auscultation), and leave the potentially aggravating maneuvers (i.e., otoscopy) for the end.
- Watch the patient for signs of discomfort or anxiety, and modify the examination accordingly. Distraction can be an invaluable tool when examining a young child.
- Older children and adolescents should be given the choice of being examined with the parents out of the room. A chaperone should always be present when the genitalia are examined.

Laboratory

- Only order tests that are necessary for diagnosis or to guide treatment.
- Interpret all results within the context of age adjusted normal values.

Radiography

- Although radiation exposure should be minimized as much as possible, the information from appropriate imaging studies can be life saving.
- Consideration of the technical adequacy of the film and age-related differences are especially important in pediatrics. This is particularly important with regard to orthopedic imaging (Chapter 81).

Table 73-1 DEPARTMENT OF HEALTH AND HUMAN SERVICES • CENTERS FOR DISEASE CONTROL AND PREVENTION
RECOMMENDED CHILDHOOD AND ADOLESCENT IMMUNIZATION SCHEDULE UNITED STATES • 2006

Vaccine ▼　　Age ▶	Birth	1 month	2 months	4 months	6 months	12 months	15 months	18 months	24 months	4-6 years	11-12 years	13-14 years	15 years	16-18 years
Hepatitis B	HepB	HepB	HepB	HepB		HepB					HepB series			
Diphtheria, Tetanus, Pertussis			DTaP	DTaP	DTaP		DTaP	DTaP		DTaP	Tdap		Tdap	
Haemophilus influenzae type b			Hib	Hib	Hib	Hib	Hib							
Inactivated Poliovirus			IPV	IPV	IPV	IPV				IPV				
Measles, Mumps, Rubella						MMR				MMR	MMR			
Varicella						Varicella					Varicella			
Meningococcal							Vaccines within broken line are for selected populations		MPSV4		MCV4		MCV4	MCV4
Pneumococcal			PCV	PCV	PCV	PCV	PCV		PCV		PPV			
Influenza					Influenza (yearly)		Influenza (yearly)				Influenza (yearly)			
Hepatitis A									HepA Series					

Range of recommended ages　　　Catch-up immunization　　　11-12 year old assessment

This schedule indicates the recommended ages for routine administration of currently licensed childhood vaccines, as of December 1, 2005, for children through age 18 years. Any dose not administered at the recommended age should be administered at any subsequent visit when indicated and feasible. Indicates age groups that warrant special effort to administer those vaccines not previously administered. Additional vaccines may be licensed and recommended during the year. Licensed combination vaccines may be used whenever any components of the combination are indicated and other components of the vaccine are not contraindicated, and if approved by the Food and Drug Administration for that dose of the series. Providers should consult the respective ACIP statement for detailed recommendations. Clinically significant adverse events that follow immunization should be reported to the Vaccine Adverse Event Reporting System (VAERS). Guidance about how to obtain and complete a VAERS form is available at **www.vaers.hhs.gov** or by telephone, **800-822-7967.**

Table 73–2   Vital Signs at Various Ages

Age	Heart Rate (beats/min)*	Blood Pressure (mm Hg)†	Respiratory Rate (breaths/min)
Premature	120-170	55-75/35-45	40-70
0-3 mo	100-150	65-85/45-55	35-55
3-6 mo	90-120	70-90/50-65	30-45
6-12 mo	80-120	80-100/55-65	25-40
1-3 yr	70-110	90-105/55-70	20-30
3-6 yr	65-110	95-110/60-75	20-25
6-12 yr	60-95	100-120/60-75	14-22
>12 y	55-85	110-135/65-85	12-18

*In sleep, infant heart rates may drop significantly lower, but if perfusion is maintained, no intervention is required.

†A blood pressure cuff should cover approximately two thirds of the arm; too small a cuff yields spuriously high pressure readings, and too large a cuff yields spuriously low pressure readings.

(From Behrman RE, Kliegman RM, and Jenson, HB. Nelson Textbook of Pediatrics (17th ed). Philadelphia: Elsevier, 2004, p 280.)

- On chest x-ray study, the thymus will appear most prominently in infants and toddlers as a homogeneous, soft tissue density projecting from the superior mediastinum bilaterally.

EKG

- The standard electrocardiogram (EKG) equipment can be used for children; however, smaller-sized electrodes should be used with young children to avoid artifacts related to lead overlap.
- Tracing artifacts are common, and include respiratory variations at baseline, skeletal muscle electrical activity, and diaphragmatic electrical activity.
- The tracings should be interpreted within the context of age-adjusted values. In general, expect higher resting rates, more rightward axis, shorter PR intervals, and longer QTc values in infancy and early childhood.
- An EKG should be obtained in all children presenting with syncope, presyncope, chest pain, pallor, easy fatigability, or possible toxic exposure.

Emergency Department Management Overview
General

- All unstable or ill-appearing children should be placed on a cardiac monitor and pulse oximetry. Pediatric advanced life support (PALS) guidelines are located in Chapter 74.
- Achieving vascular access in a child can be a challenge. If time allows, the use of topical anesthetics can serve as a useful adjunct to minimize pain and anxiety. The liberal use of distraction can also be effective.

Table 73–3   Developmental Milestones in the First 2 Years of Life

Milestone	Average Age of Attainment (mo)
Gross Motor	
Head steady in sitting	2.0
Pull to sit, no head lag	3.0
Hands together in midline	3.0
Sits without support	6.0
Rolls back to stomach	6.5
Walks alone	12.0
Runs	16.0
Fine Motor	
Grasps rattle	3.5
Reaches for objects	4.0
Palmar grasp gone	4.0
Transfers object hand to hand	5.5
Thumb-finger grasp	8.0
Turns pages of book	12.0
Scribbles	13.0
Builds tower of two cubes	15.0
Communication and Language	
Smiles in response to face, voice	1.5
Monosyllabic babble	6.0
Inhibits to "no"	7.0
Follows one-step command with gesture	7.0
Follows one-step command without gesture	10.0
Speaks first real word	12.0
Speaks four to six words	15.0
Speaks 10-15 words	18.0
Speaks two-word sentences	19.0
Stares at own hand	4.0
Bangs two cubes	8.0
Uncovers toy (after seeing it hidden)	8.0
Egocentric pretend play (e.g., pretends to drink from cup)	12.0
Pretend play with doll (gives doll bottle)	17.0

From Behrman RE, Kliegman RM, and Jenson, HB. Nelson Textbook of Pediatrics (17th ed). Philadelphia: Elsevier, 2004, p 280.

Medications

- Medication errors have the potential for significant morbidity and mortality. The distinct physiology and pharmacokinetics of children affect toxic and therapeutic levels of drugs, and render certain drugs inappropriate.
- The patient's weight should be confirmed when giving medicine in weight-based dosages. All dose calculations should be double-checked. For critically ill children, the use of the Broselow Tape or a similar device is recommended to determine the appropriate drug dosing.

Disposition

■ Parental education and clear follow-up is a critical part of the disposition of pediatric patients. The primary physician should be notified when possible.

Special Considerations in the Evaluation of the Ill Child

■ When evaluating and treating the ill child, one should consider several important physiologic and anatomic distinctions:

■ *Respiratory effort.* Muscle retractions in the chest and neck, and flaring of the nostrils during inspiration are signs of an abnormally high level of effort required to move air into the lungs. Grunting is a moaning, crying-like noise during expiration, associated with generation of positive pressure to maintain alveolar patency.

■ *Low ventricular compliance.* Children increase cardiac output primarily via tachycardia. An elevated heart rate in a child must always be considered serious, and needs to be logically explained rather than dismissed as normal for age.

■ *Highly reactive vasculature.* Children are able to maintain a perfusing blood pressure despite significant intravascular depletion through vasoconstriction and tachycardia. A "stable" blood pressure may in fact represent an unstable, compensated state. If this physiologic state is allowed to persist it can result in significant intracellular hypoxemia and acidosis. When hypotension does manifest, it is often profound and resistant to resuscitative efforts.

■ *Large surface-to–body mass ratio.* Exposure should be limited as much as possible during resuscitation. Children are particularly susceptible to hypothermia.

■ *Immature immune system.* Sepsis is common in critically ill children. Early antibiotic treatment is an important step in resuscitative efforts.

■ *Low functional residual capacity.* Neonates and infants often have a limited ability for ventilatory adaptation, and require early intubation.

■ *Unique airway anatomy.* The smaller airways of a child are more susceptible to obstruction with a foreign body, mucous, inflammation, or edema. Children younger than 10 years old display a distinct airway anatomy that is important to consider when attempting intubation (see Chapter 74).

■ *Reduced hepatic glycogen stores.* Hypoglycemia is common in the critically ill child, and signs may often be nonspecific. Rapid serum glucose determination is a critical step in the initial assessment of the patient.

Teaching Points

Children require special attention to size, age, stage of development, and age-related disease. They may present in different ways, depending on their age and stage of development. It is necessary to rely on the parents for history, and to assist with the management of the child. Parental concerns are often different from the child's, especially in teenaged children. Drugs and therapies are usually weight-related, and cannot be assumed safe for children because they are safe in adults. Do not forget the possibility of nonaccidental trauma, and think of it even in the most unlikely situations.

Suggested Readings

Barkin RM. Pediatrics. A potpourri of clinical pearls. Emerg Med Clin North Am 1997; 15:381–388.

Fernandez CV, Gillis-Ring J. Strategies for the prevention of medical error in pediatrics. J Pediatr 2003;143:155–162.

Givens T. The ten commandments of pediatric emergency medicine. J Emerg Med 2004; 27:193–194.

Hedlund GL, Kirks DR. Emergency radiology of the pediatric chest. Curr Probl Diagn Radiol 1990;19:133–164.

Losek JD. Hypoglycemia and the ABC'S (sugar) of pediatric resuscitation. Ann Emerg Med 2000; 35:43–46.

Parker MM, Hazelzet JA, Carcillo JA. Pediatric considerations. Crit Care Med 2004; 32:S591–S594

Schroeder JK. Pediatric electrocardiography in the emergency department. J Emerg Med 1993; 11:543–553.

Wright JL, Patterson MD. Resuscitating the pediatric patient. Emerg Med Clin North Am 1996; 14:219–231.

CHAPTER **74**

Pediatric Resuscitation

TIMOTHY G. GIVENS ■ CHRISTINE KEYES

Overview

Pediatric cardiac arrest is most often the terminal event of progressive shock or respiratory failure, rather than a sudden collapse due to dysrhythmia, as is most common in adults.

The approach to the critically ill or injured child requires rapid cardiopulmonary assessment, establishment of treatment priorities, and timely intervention to reverse progression to cardiopulmonary failure.

Respiratory failure in children may be caused by airway, pulmonary, or neuromuscular disease that impairs oxygen exchange (oxygenation) or carbon dioxide (CO_2) elimination (ventilation). Pediatric patients have a higher oxygen demand per kilogram of body weight due to higher metabolic rates. Thus, hypoxia can develop more rapidly in a child compared to adults.

Differences in the pediatric circulatory system compared with the adult exist. In neonates, infants, and young children, cardiac output is primarily dependent on heart rate, rather than stroke volume. Children have tremendous compensatory vasoconstriction, and can maintain normal blood pressure despite the loss of 40% to 50% of their circulatory volume, making hypotension a late and ominous sign.

Initial Diagnostic Approach
General

- The ABCs (*a*irway, *b*reathing, and *c*irculation) should always be addressed first, and the presence or absence of vital signs noted. See Chapter 73 for vital signs at various ages.
- Infants and children at risk for respiratory arrest may demonstrate increased respiratory rate, increased respiratory effort, diminished breath sounds, decreased level of consciousness, poor skeletal muscle tone, or cyanosis. The presence of retractions, grunting, stridor, wheezing, or prolonged exhalation are concerning for significant respiratory compromise.
- Compensated shock is defined as the presence of a normal blood pressure with signs or symptoms of inadequate perfusion. Early signs of shock include tachycardia, thready or diminished peripheral pulses, mottling, capillary refill longer than 2 seconds, peripheral cyanosis, mental status changes, and decreased urine output (normal is 1 to 2 ml/kg/h in children). Hypotension may be defined by the following limits: systolic blood pressure (SBP) less than 60 mm Hg in term neonates (<28 days), SBP less than 70 mm Hg in infants, SPB less than 70 mm Hg + (2 × age in years), or a SBP less than 90 mm Hg in older children.

Diagnostic Studies

- Infants and small children, especially if they have been chronically ill, are predisposed to hypoglycemia because they have limited glycogen stores. A rapid bedside glucose should be checked on all pediatric resuscitations.
- Laboratory studies, a chest radiography, and an electrocardiogram (EKG) are needed if return of spontaneous circulation occurs. Laboratory studies may include an arterial blood gas, complete blood count, electrolytes and renal function tests, coagulation studies, and urinalysis. Blood and urine cultures may also be obtained.

Emergency Department Management Overview
General

- The most common cause of cardiac arrest in children is respiratory insufficiency, and the first priority is to provide adequate ventilation and oxygenation. After the airway is opened and two initial rescue breaths are given, signs of circulation are checked. This includes adequate breathing, coughing, or movement detected by lay rescuers or the presence of a pulse (brachial pulse in an infant; carotid pulse in a child). If a pulse is felt but the heart rate is less than 60 bpm, chest compressions should be initiated.

■ Basic life support (BLS) techniques are summarized in Table 74–1.

■ A length-based resuscitation tape (Broselow) should be used on all pediatric resuscitations for easy reference to precalculated drug dosages, fluid volumes, and resuscitation equipment.

■ Refer to Figures 74–1 through 74–5 for Pediatric Advanced Cardiac Life Support (PALS) Algorithms.

Airway and Breathing

■ See Box 74–1 for indications for endotracheal intubation in pediatric patients.

■ Bag-valve-mask (BVM) ventilation is an effective means of providing temporary but effective emergency ventilation. Choose a mask to provide an airtight seal. It should extend from the bridge of the nose to the cleft of the chin, and should cover the nose and mouth. Deliver enough tidal volume to make the chest rise and fall. Ventilation rates are listed at the bottom of Table 74–1.

■ Rapid-sequence intubation is the preferred technique for intubation. The sequence is similar to the adult population (see Chapter 5) with some minor differences (see Table 74–2). Atropine may be used to prevent bradycardia associated with direct laryngoscopy and the use of succinylcholine. The best position to maintain an open airway is the neutral sniffing position. The following formula is used as an estimation of endotracheal tube (ETT) size in children older than 1 year: (Age [years] + 16)/4. The width of the patient's little finger (5th digit) can also be used to estimate ETT size. Direct visualization of cords (orotracheal route) using a straight laryngoscope blade is the preferred technique especially in young children. Airway adjuncts such as pediatric laryngeal mask airways are available in most hospital settings, and are used as a rescue airway device in patients who are difficult to intubate. Other emergency airway techniques such as transtracheal jet ventilation and emergency cricothyrotomy are rarely required. Cricothyrotomy cannot be performed on a child less than 8 years of age because of the diminutive

---

BOX 74–1 Indications for Endotracheal Intubation in Pediatric Patients

Inadequate central nervous system control of ventilation
Functional or anatomic airway obstruction
Loss of protective airway reflexes (cough, gag)
Excessive work of breathing, concern for fatigue
Need for high peak inspiratory pressure to maintain alveolar gas exchange
Need for airway protection, controlled ventilation during sedation for
   diagnostic studies
Potential for any of the above during patient transport

Table 74–1 Basic Cardiac Life Support

	Older Child >8 Y*	Child (1-8 Y)*	Infant (<1 Y)	Newborn (< 4 weeks)
Pulse check	Carotid	Carotid	Brachial or femoral	Umbilical
Compression technique	Lower half of sternum; heel of one hand; other hand on top	Lower half of sternum; heel of one hand	Lower half of sternum; one finger's width below intermammary line; two thumb–encircling hands for two-rescuer or two-finger technique	Lower half of sternum; one finger's width below intermammary line; two thumb–encircling hands for two-rescuer or two-finger technique
Compression depth	Approximately one third to one half the anteroposterior diameter of the chest	Same as older child	Same as older child	Same as older child
Compression to ventilation ratio (this is the same for all age groups)	No advanced airway in place (compression: ventilation) 30:2 (1 rescuer) 15:2 (2 rescuer)			
	Advanced airway in place Compression rate of 100/min 8-10 breaths/min			
	Perfusing rhythm but not breathing 12 to 20 breaths/min (1 breath every 3-5 sec)			

*Children > 1 year, lay rescuers should use automatic external defibrillator (AED) after 5 cycles of CPR; in a witnessed collapse, use the AED as soon as it is available.

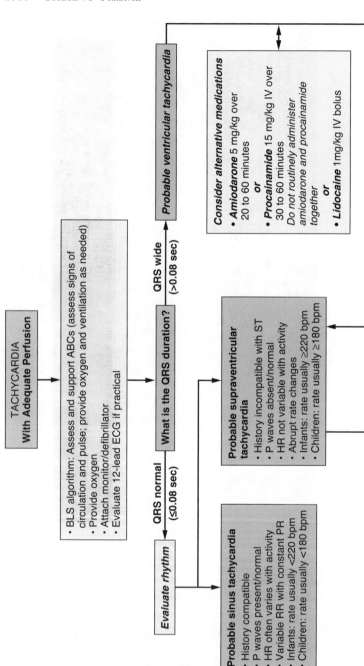

TACHYCARDIA
With Adequate Perfusion

- BLS algorithm: Assess and support ABCs (assess signs of circulation and pulse; provide oxygen and ventilation as needed)
- Provide oxygen
- Attach monitor/defibrillator
- Evaluate 12-lead ECG if practical

What is the QRS duration?

Evaluate rhythm

QRS normal (≤0.08 sec)

QRS wide (>0.08 sec)

Probable ventricular tachycardia

Consider alternative medications
- **Amiodarone** 5 mg/kg IV over 20 to 60 minutes
  or
- **Procainamide** 15 mg/kg IV over 30 to 60 minutes
  Do not routinely administer amiodarone and procainamide together
  or
- **Lidocaine** 1mg/kg IV bolus

Probable supraventricular tachycardia
- History incompatible with ST
- P waves absent/normal
- HR not variable with activity
- Abrupt rate changes
- Infants: rate usually ≥220 bpm
- Children: rate usually ≥180 bpm

Probable sinus tachycardia
- History compatible
- P waves present/normal
- HR often varies with activity
- Variable RR with constant PR
- Infants: rate usually <220 bpm
- Children: rate usually <180 bpm

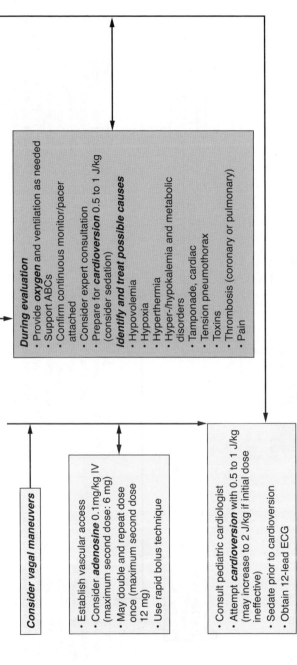

During evaluation
- Provide **oxygen** and ventilation as needed
- Support ABCs
- Confirm continuous monitor/pacer attached
- Consider expert consultation
- Prepare for **cardioversion** 0.5 to 1 J/kg (consider sedation)

Identify and treat possible causes
- Hypovolemia
- Hypoxia
- Hyperthermia
- Hyper-/hypokalemia and metabolic disorders
- Tamponade, cardiac
- Tension pneumothorax
- Toxins
- Thrombosis (coronary or pulmonary)
- Pain

Consider vagal maneuvers

- Establish vascular access
- Consider **adenosine** 0.1mg/kg IV (maximum second dose: 6 mg)
- May double and repeat dose once (maximum second dose 12 mg)
- Use rapid bolus technique

- Consult pediatric cardiologist
- Attempt **cardioversion** with 0.5 to 1 J/kg (may increase to 2 J/kg if initial dose ineffective)
- Sedate prior to cardioversion
- Obtain 12-lead ECG

Figure 74-1. Algorithm for pediatric tachycardia with adequate perfusion. *Reproduced with permission. PALS Provider Manual © 2002, American Heart Association..*

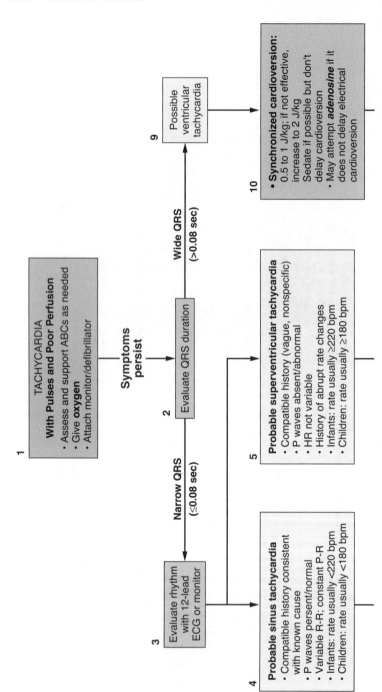

1
TACHYCARDIA
With Pulses and Poor Perfusion
• Assess and support ABCs as needed
• Give **oxygen**
• Attach monitor/defibrillator

Symptoms persist

2
Evaluate QRS duration

Narrow QRS
(≤0.08 sec)

Wide QRS
(>0.08 sec)

3
Evaluate rhythm with 12-lead ECG or monitor

9
Possible ventricular tachycardia

4
Probable sinus tachycardia
• Compatible history consistent with known cause
• P waves persent/normal
• Variable R-R; constant P-R
• Infants: rate usually <220 bpm
• Children: rate usually <180 bpm

5
Probable supraventricular tachycardia
• Compatible history (vague, nonspecific)
• P waves absent/abnormal
• HR not variable
• History of abrupt rate changes
• Infants: rate usually ≥220 bpm
• Children: rate usually ≥180 bpm

10
• **Synchronized cardioversion:**
0.5 to 1 J/kg; if not effective, increase to 2 J/kg
Sedate if possible but don't delay cardioversion
• May attempt **adenosine** if it does not delay electrical cardioversion

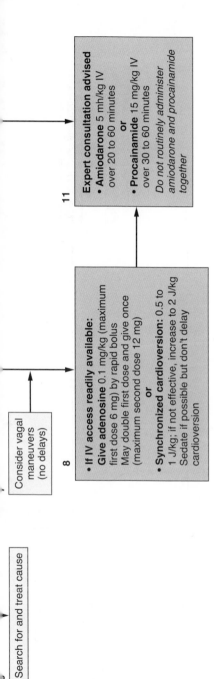

Figure 74-2. Algorithm for pediatric tachycardia with poor perfusion. *Reproduced with permission. 2005 American Heart Association Guidelines for Cardiopulmonary Resuscitation and Emergency Cardiovascular Care, Part 4: Adult Basic Life Support. Circulation. 2005;112 (suppl. IV):IV-58,68,70,90* © 2005, American Heart Association.

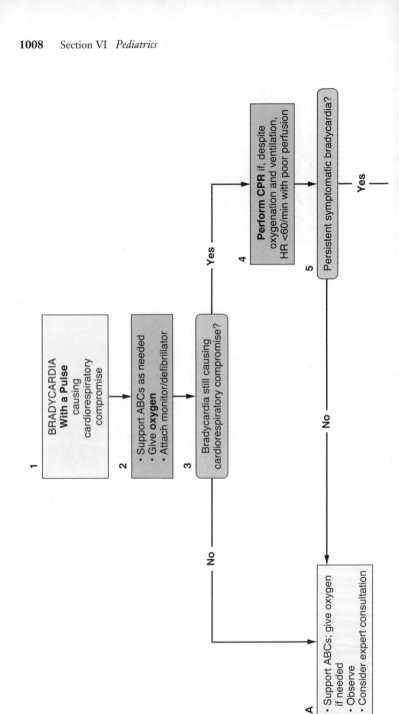

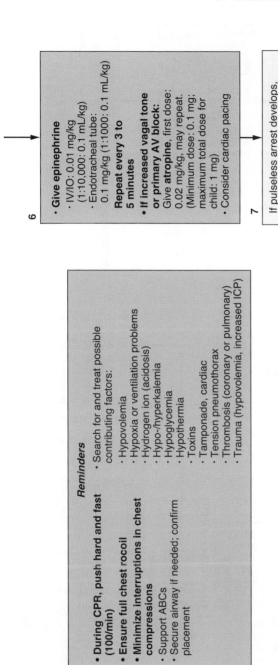

6

Give epinephrine
- IV/IO: 0.01 mg/kg
  (1:10,000: 0.1 mL/kg)
- Endotracheal tube:
  0.1 mg/kg (1:1000: 0.1 mL/kg)
Repeat every 3 to 5 minutes
- **If increased vagal tone or primary AV block:**
  Give **atropine**, first dose: 0.02 mg/kg, may repeat. (Minimum dose: 0.1 mg; maximum total dose for child: 1 mg)
- Consider cardiac pacing

7

If pulseless arrest develops, go to Pulseless Arrest Algorithm

Reminders

- **During CPR, push hard and fast** (100/min)
- **Ensure full chest recoil**
- **Minimize interruptions in chest compressions**
- Support ABCs
- Secure airway if needed; confirm placement

- Search for and treat possible contributing factors:
  - Hypovolemia
  - Hypoxia or ventilation problems
  - Hydrogen ion (acidosis)
  - Hypo-/hyperkalemia
  - Hypoglycemia
  - Hypothermia
  - Toxins
  - Tamponade, cardiac
  - Tension pneumothorax
  - Thrombosis (coronary or pulmonary)
  - Trauma (hypovolemia, increased ICP)

Figure 74–3. Pediatric bradycardia algorithm. *Reproduced with permission. 2005 American Heart Association Guidelines for Cardiopulmonary Resuscitation and Emergency Cardiovascular Care, Part 4: Adult Basic Life Support. Circulation. 2005;112 (suppl. IV):IV-58,68,70,90 © 2005, American Heart Association.*

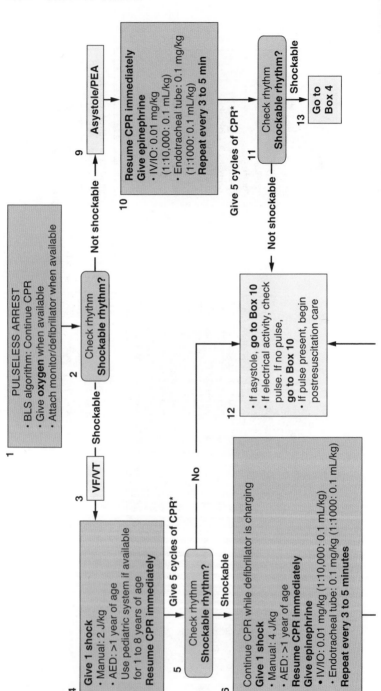

1
PULSELESS ARREST
• BLS algorithm: Continue CPR
• Give **oxygen** when available
• Attach monitor/defibrillator when available

2
Check rhythm
Shockable rhythm?

3
VF/VT — Shockable

9
Asystole/PEA — Not shockable

4
Give 1 shock
• Manual: 2 J/kg
• AED: >1 year of age
Use pediatric system if available
for 1 to 8 years of age
Resume CPR immediately

5
Check rhythm
Shockable rhythm?
Shockable

6
Continue CPR while defibrillator is charging
Give 1 shock
• Manual: 4 J/kg
• AED: >1 year of age
Resume CPR immediately
Give epinephrine
• IV/IO: 0.01 mg/kg (1:10,000: 0.1 mL/kg)
• Endotracheal tube: 0.1 mg/kg (1:1000: 0.1 mL/kg)
Repeat every 3 to 5 minutes

Give 5 cycles of CPR*

No

10
Resume CPR immediately
Give epinephrine
• IV/IO: 0.01 mg/kg (1:10,000: 0.1 mL/kg)
• Endotracheal tube: 0.1 mg/kg (1:1000: 0.1 mL/kg)
Repeat every 3 to 5 min

Give 5 cycles of CPR*

11
Check rhythm
Shockable rhythm?

13
Go to Box 4
Shockable

Not shockable

12
• If asystole, **go to Box 10**
• If electrical activity, check pulse. If no pulse,
go to Box 10
• If pulse present, begin postresuscitation care

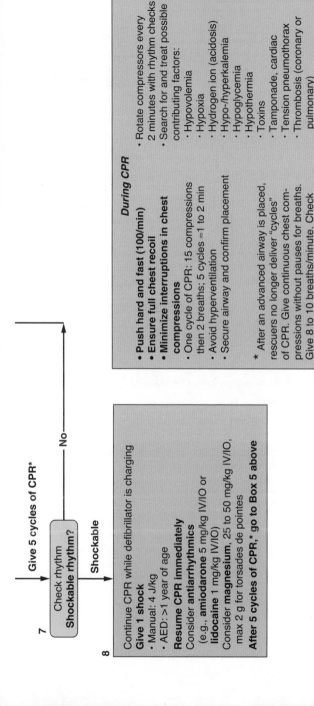

Figure 74–4. Pediatric pulseless arrest algorithm. *Reproduced with permission. 2005 American Heart Association Guidelines for Cardiopulmonary Resuscitation and Emergency Cardiovascular Care, Part 4: Adult Basic Life Support. Circulation. 2005;112 (suppl. IV):IV-58,68,70,90 © 2005, American Heart Association.*

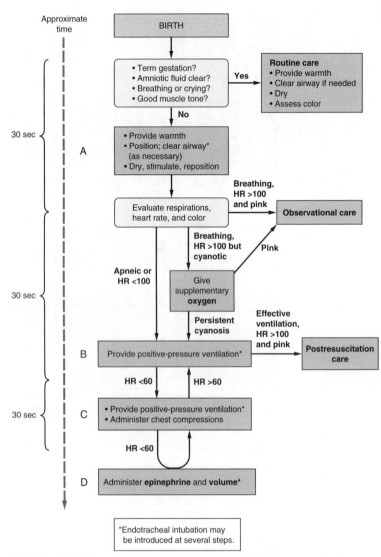

Figure 74–5. Neonatal flow algorithm. *Reproduced with permission. 2005 American Heart Association Guidelines for Cardiopulmonary Resuscitation and Emergency Cardiovascular Care, Part 4: Adult Basic Life Support. Circulation. 2005;112 (suppl. IV):IV-58,68,70,90 © 2005, American Heart Association.*

Table 74–2 Special Considerations for Pediatric Airway Management

Differences in Children	Special Considerations
Prominent occiput with a tendency to flex the head in the supine position—can occlude the airway.	Place a towel under the neck or shoulders to prevent head flexion but avoid hyperextension.
Large tongue is the most likely cause of airway	Chin-lift: Carefully place fingers under the mandible and avoid obstruction. compressing soft tissues under the chin, which can compress the airway Jaw thrust: Preferred if cervical spine injury suspected or if airway partially obstructed. Oral or nasal airway: Use correct size to avoid increasing airway obstruction.
The larynx is relatively cephalad and anterior in position.	Blind nasotracheal intubation is contraindicated until age 10 y. Cricoid pressure is a key component of tracheal intubation.
The narrowest portion of the child's airway is at the level of the cricoid cartilage (subglottic).	Use uncuffed endotracheal tubes (ETs) for younger than 8 y. The size is similar to the patients little finger or nares. A 2.5 or 3.0 uncuffed tube is used for preterm infants. A 3.0-3.5 uncuffed tube is used for term infants. A 3.5-4.0 cuffed tube is used for infants 6 mo to 1 y. For children older than 1 y: (Age [years] + 16)/4. Depth of ET insertion: position at the lips, 2 to 3 times the internal diameter of the ET tube in mm.
The epiglottis is long, narrow, and floppy in infants and young children.	A straight laryngoscopic blade is preferable to elevate the epiglottis in young children. Use a Miller size 0 for premature infants, size 1 for normal sized infants, and size 2 for older children.
The airway is smaller in diameter and shorter in length, with increased resistance to airflow and easier obstruction.	Surgical cricothyrotomy: contraindicated until age 8 y. Combitube: only if over 4 feet (1.2 m) tall. Other alternatives to endotracheal intubation: laryngeal mask airway (LMA) or needle cricothyrotomy.
The most clinically important difference between the adult and pediatric patient is the potential for desaturation, even with adequate preoxygenation. There is a much higher metabolic rate, higher oxygen consumption, and less physiologic reserve in pediatric patients.	High airway pressures may inflate the stomach in patients who are not intubated. Give 1 breath every 3-5 sec An adequate tidal volume is determined by the presence of normal chest rise, auscultation of good air-movement, and improvement of color. Air trapping: if the patient has bronchiolitis, asthma, or another airway disease characterized by air trapping, it is important to ventilate at a relatively slow rate to permit adequate time for exhalation.

These differences are most apparent in children younger than 8-10 y and are most notable in the infant.

anatomy. If a surgical airway is necessary, a tracheostomy will have to be performed.

Circulation
Vascular Access

■ Two large-bore, short-length vascular catheters are preferred for peripheral venous access in any pediatric resuscitation situation. Intraosseous (IO) access (proximal tibia, distal femur, anterior superior iliac spine) is an effective alternative for rapid drug delivery, and is commonly used to resuscitate pediatric patients. To minimize complications, IO needles should not be placed in fractured long bones or into the same extremity where a needle was previously placed, and then displaced to prevent infiltration of any drug or fluid into the tissues. Other options include central venous access using the femoral, external/internal jugular or subclavian vessels via the Seldinger (guide wire) technique or a peripheral venous cutdown. These latter techniques are less commonly used compared with the adult population.

■ Vascular access is often necessary to administer epinephrine in the pulseless patient. Central venous access is ideal, but not practical in the arrest situation. Effective chest compressions and flushing the intravenous (IV) catheter with 5 ml of saline will help deliver the drug to the central circulation.

Fluids

■ Fluids should be given for hypotensive patients in a bolus (20 ml/kg) of isotonic crystalloid (normal saline or ringer's lactate). Repeat boluses of 20 ml/kg (maximum of 50 ml/kg) as necessary if hypotension persists.
■ If myocardial dysfunction is present, use 5 to 10 ml/kg initially.
■ Avoid dextrose-containing solutions, as they may induce osmotic diuresis or aggravate hypokalemia. Glucose-containing solutions (5% Dextrose) are appropriate for maintenance fluids.
■ Transfuse blood (10-15 ml/kg packed red blood cells) if perfusion remains inadequate after two to three boluses of crystalloid in trauma victims.
■ For patients in full cardiac arrest, IV lines are used as the entry port for drug delivery, and should be maintained at a keep open rate. Give repeat fluid boluses of 20 ml/kg for hypotension occurring in the immediate postresuscitation period.

Vasoactive Medications

■ These are indicated for fluid-refractory shock (i.e., after two to three boluses of 20 ml/kg). They should be titrated to the patient's response (Table 74–3).
■ If no vascular access has been attained, lipid-soluble medications may be administered via the endotracheal tube (ET): *l*idocaine, *e*pinephrine, *a*tropine, *n*aloxone (LEAN). See Table 74–3 for drug dosages. The ET route requires about 10 times the amount of drug given IV to achieve equal plasma concentrations and peak drug action. For example, the dose

Table 74–3 Pharmacotherapy in Pediatric Resuscitation

Drug Availability	Dose/Route	Indications	Adverse Reactions	Comments
Adenosine	0.1 mg/kg rapid IV push (max first dose: 6 mg; max second dose: 12 mg)	Supraventricular tachycardia	Hypotension, chest pain, dyspnea, dysrhythmia, heart block	Decrease SA and AV node automaticity
Amiodarone	5 mg/kg IV/IO over 20–60 min; 15 mg/kg/d max For shock refractory VT/VF; 5-mg/kg rapid IV/IO bolus	Wide range of atrial and ventricular dysrhythmias and shock refractory VF/VT	Bradycardia, hypotension, prolonged QT and may increase risk for polymorphic VT	Do not use with other medications that can prolong QT (e.g., procainamide); can cause vasodilatation, heart block
Atropine	0.01–0.03 mg/kg/dose (min: 0.1 mg/dose; max: 2.0 mg) every 5 min as needed IV/IO; use 0.03 mg/kg for ET dose	Bradycardia, asystole, ↑ vagal tone Heart block (temporary)	Tachycardia, dysrhythmias, anticholinergic	Parasympatholytic; minimal dose of 0.1 mg/kg to avoid paradoxical bradycardia
Bicarbonate, sodium	1 mEq/kg/dose every 10 min as needed, IO	Metabolic acidosis Hyperkalemia	Metabolic alkalosis, hyperosmolality, hypernatremia	Incompatible with calcium, catecholamine infusion; monitor ABGs
Calcium chloride	20–30 mg (0.2–0.3 ml/kg/dose); (max: 500 mg/dose) every 10 min as needed IV slowly	Hyperkalemia Calcium channel blocker overdose	Rapid infusion causes bradycardia, hypotension Extravasation—necrosis	Inotropic; monitor; use caution with digitalized patient; probably no benefit in asystole or electromechanical dissociation
Dextrose (D50W–0.5 g/ml)	0.5–1.0 g (2–4 ml D25W or 1–2 ml D50W)/kg/dose IV	Hypoglycemia, with coma or seizure	Hyperglycemia	Check glucose; if possible use D25W

Continued

Table 74–3 Pharmacotherapy in Pediatric Resuscitation—cont'd

Drug Availability	Dose/Route	Indications	Adverse Reactions	Comments
Dobutamine (Dobutrex) (vial: 250 mg)	2–20 μg/kg/min IV	Cardiogenic shock	Tachycardia, dysrhythmia, hypotension, hypertension	Beta-adrenergic; positive inotropic. Use in cardiogenic shock but may cause hypotension
Dopamine (200 mg/5 ml)	Low: 2–5 μg/kg/min IV Mod: 5–20 μg/kg/min IV High: >20 μg/kg/min IV	Cardiogenic shock (moderate dose) Maintain renal perfusion Septic shock	Tachycardia, bradycardia, vasoconstriction (increase with higher doses)	Treat hypovolemia first
Epinephrine	Initial: 0.01 mg (0.1 ml; 1:10,000)/kg/dose (maximum: 10 ml/dose) IV Second or ET dose: 0.1 mg (0.1 ml; 1:1,000)/kg/dose every 3 to 5 min as needed	Asystole VF Anaphylaxis Significant bradycardia	Tachycardia, dysrhythmia, hypertension, decreased renal and splanchnic blood flow	Alpha- and beta-adrenergic; inotropic
Lidocaine	1 mg/kg/dose every 5 to 10 min IV/IO; ET dose 2 to 3 mg/kg	Alternative for recurrent VF/VF or wide complex VT	High doses may cause myocardial depression and seizures	
Naloxone (Narcan 0.4 mg/ml or 1 mg/ml)	For drug overdose: 0.1 mg/kg/dose (maximum 2.0 mg) IV; 0.2 mg/kg/dose ET	Narcotic overdose		Give empirically in suspected opiate overdose.
Procainamide	15 mg/kg over 15 minutes; 20 mg/kg/min drip	Hemodynamically stable SVT refractory to adenosine Resistant VT Atrial fibrillation or flutter	Prolonged QT, hypotension	Do not administer with amiodarone due to risk of hypotension and ventricular dysrhythmias

ABG, arterial blood gas; ET, endotracheal; IO, intra-osseous; IV, intravenous; VF, ventricular fibrillation; VT, ventricular tachycardia;

of epinephrine in the ET tube is 0.1 mg/kg, given as 0.1 ml/kg of the 1:1000 concentration. Drug administration through the ET tube should be followed by 2 to 5 ml of saline flush. It is important to follow drug administration with several deep positive-pressure breaths to help distribute the drug into the lower airways.

■ Epinephrine is the drug of choice in any pulseless patient, and should be administered to the pediatric patient once the airway and breathing are addressed. Epinephrine has α- and β-adrenergic actions, but the large doses used in cardiac arrest produce predominantly α-adrenergic effects resulting in increased blood flow to vital organs such as the heart and brain. Epinephrine is also helpful in reversing bradycardia. Children who do not have restoration of organized spontaneous cardiac activity with two rounds of epinephrine do not survive to leave the hospital.

■ Sodium bicarbonate can increase CO_2 production, which may worsen intracellular acidosis, even when the measured arterial pH improves. It should only be used to correct acidosis after the airway has been secured, the victim is hyperventilated, effective chest compressions are being delivered, and epinephrine administration and defibrillation are ineffective. It is also useful for patients with hyperkalemia and tricyclic antidepressant overdose as with the adult population.

■ Calcium is only indicated to (a) correct documented hypocalcemia, (b) antagonize the adverse cardiovascular actions of hyperkalemia and hypermagnesemia, and (c) reverse the hypotension produced by calcium channel blocker toxicity.

■ Magnesium is the drug of choice for torsades de pointes.

Special Situations
Apparent Life-Threatening Event

■ An apparent life-threatening event (ALTE) is an episode that meets at least one of the following criteria: significant apnea, which is defined as breathing cessation longer than 20 seconds or cessation of breathing (of any duration) associated with bradycardia, cyanosis, pallor, or hypotonia; marked change in muscle tone (usually limp or hypotonic, but may be hypertonic too); or gagging or choking.

■ Breath-holding spells are one common and benign cause of apnea in children between the ages of 1 week and 3 years old. They are frequently triggered by pain or rage, and look frightening to parents, with loss of consciousness, cyanosis, pallor, or hypotonia. The apnea is usually of shorter duration than an ALTE, but if there is any doubt, the emergency physician should assume the event is an ALTE and treat it as such.

■ Any patient with a history consistent with an ATLE should be admitted for further workup and evaluation.

Dysrhythmias

■ Primary dysrhythmias are unusual in children. Most rhythm disturbances encountered are secondary to hypoxia, acidosis, or metabolic derangements. Correction of ventilation and oxygenation through appropriate airway management is adequate therapy in most cases. Most pediatric patients in full arrest present with asystole and bradycardia. These patients usually have poor prognosis as they indicate extensive decompensation.

- **Tachycardia.** The most common causes are sinus tachycardia or supraventricular tachycardia (SVT). An "unstable tachycardia" is based on evidence of poor perfusion such as altered mental status, cyanosis, poor capillary refill or hypotension. A sinus tachycardia is usually a secondary phenomenon due to another condition such as that seen with dehydration. Supraventricular tachycardia is more likely in patients with underlying heart disease. Adenosine is the drug of choice in SVT. For cardioversion of tachydysrhythmias such as atrial fibrillation or supraventricular tachycardia, small energy doses of 0.25 to 1.0 J/kg can be used.
- **Bradycardia.** Hypoxia is the most common cause of bradydysrhythmias in pediatric patients. Prompt attention to oxygenation and ventilation is the focus of therapy. Epinephrine is the drug of choice for hypoxia induced bradycardia. Atropine may not be helpful in this setting.
- **Asystole.** Is the most common pediatric arrest rhythm. Epinephrine is the drug of choice.
- **Pulseless electrical activity.** There is electrical activity but no mechanical cardiac function. Epinephrine is the drug of choice in addition to treating possible underlying causes (H's and T's: Hypovolemia, Hypoxemia, Hypothermia, Hyper- or Hypokalemia, Tamponade, Tension pneumothorax, Toxins, Thromboembolism).
- **Ventricular fibrillation and pulseless ventricular tachycardia.** These are uncommon in the pediatric population. Defibrillation (2 J/kg) is the treatment of choice for both rhythms. The size of the paddles should allow adequate contact with the skin, but avoid contact of the paddles with each other.

Neonatal Resuscitation

- A targeted history aids preparation for delivery: number of fetuses, due date, maternal medications, membranes ruptured/color of fluid, bleeding, decreased fetal movement.
- Suction oro- and nasopharynx before delivery of the thorax.
- Warm the neonate, position the airway, suction the airway, dry the neonate to stimulate breathing, provide oxygen as necessary.
- Assist ventilation as necessary with bag-mask or endotracheal intubation.
- Chest compressions if heart rate remains less than 60 bpm with above maneuvers (see Figure 74–5).
- Give medications (epinephrine) via endotracheal tube/umbilical catheter if no response to cardiopulmonary resuscitation.

Teaching Points

Cardiac arrest in children is often an endpoint of diseases remote from the heart, most often respiratory. Therefore, arrests have a poor prognosis, and require aggressive management of the underlying problem as well as cardiac management.

Pharmacology is weight-guided in children, and interventional equipment must also be sized according to the child's weight and size. Intravenous access is often impossible in the arrested child, and quick utilization of the intra-osseous route may be the most efficient and optimal solution to this problem.

Suggested Readings

2005 American Heart Association Guidelines for Cardiopulmonary Resuscitation and Emergency Cardiovascular Care. In Circulation: Volume 112, Issue 24 Supplement; December 13, 2005.

Hazinski MF, Zaritsky AL, Nadkarni VM, et al. PALS Provider Manual. American Heart Association, 2002.

Gilligan BP, Luten RC. Pediatric resuscitation. In: Marx JA, Hockberger RS, Walls RM (editors). Rosen's Emergency Medicine: Concepts and Clinical Practice (6th ed). Philadelphia: Mosby, 2006, pp 97–118.

Morris MC, Nadkarni VM. Pediatric cardiopulmonary-cerebral resuscitation: an overview and future directions. Crit Care Clin 2003;19:337–364.

CHAPTER **75**

Pediatric Cardiology

STEPHANIE HORN RICHLING ■ **SEAN P. KELLY**

Overview

Cardiac disease in the pediatric patient is rare. The incidence of congenital cardiac disease is approximately 1%. Most lesions are silent until after the first week of life, when they may present to the ED. Pediatric patients with cardiac disease may present in many different ways. Those with mild disease may present with only an incidental murmur on physical examination. Those with severe disease may present in full cardiac arrest. Other possible presentations include poor feeding, failure to thrive, hypertension, hypotension, tachycardia, shock, syncope, lethargy, dysrhythmias, peripheral edema, dyspnea, and chest pain.

Neonatal circulation. At birth, when the infant takes its first few breaths, pulmonary arterioles dilate, resulting in a large increase in blood flow through the pulmonary circuitry. Pulmonary venous return and left ventricular output increase. Systemic blood pressure rises with the elimination of the placental circulation. The foramen ovale and ductus arteriosus close. Oxygen consumption and cardiac index are greater. Systolic reserve is limited. Fast heart rates compromise diastolic filling. Clinically, one sees a reduced cardiac reserve with limited ability to handle pressure or volume loads. This explains the greater incidence of congestive heart failure (CHF) in infancy.

The most common presentations of primary cardiac disease in the pediatric population can be divided into the following categories: benign heart murmurs, cyanotic heart disease, congestive heart failure, and chest pain.

This chapter will describe the general diagnostic and management approach to the pediatric patient with cardiac complaints, as well as focus on these four most important subsets of patient presentations.

Specific Problems: Heart Murmurs
Assessment of the Pediatric Patient with a Heart Murmur

- Useful parts of the history include birth history, feeding habits (volume, length, associated sweating or tachypnea), weight gain, cyanotic spells, breathing difficulties, and family history with regard to congenital abnormalities and heart defects. Concerning history includes failure to thrive, frequent respiratory infections, exercise intolerance, or family history of congenital heart disease.
- In any child with a murmur, obtain blood pressures in all four extremities. Also measure preductal (right arm) and postductal (either foot) oxygen saturations.
- Perform a complete cardiac examination. Palpate for a precordial bulge, heave, or thrill. Auscultate at the left lower sternal border for the first heart sound (mitral and tricuspid valves). Then auscultate at the left upper sternal border for the second heart sound (aortic and pulmonary valves). There should be a normal physiologic split that varies with respiration. A third heart sound may be auscultated at the apex or left lower sternal border. This may be normal in children. A fourth heart sound may be auscultated at the apex. This is always pathologic in children. Check peripheral pulses and capillary refill.
- A chest radiograph and EKG should be obtained.
- See Table 75–1 regarding the differential diagnosis of benign heart murmurs.

Emergency Department Management of Heart Murmurs

- Nonpathologic heart murmurs do not require emergent intervention, but some may require further outpatient follow-up.

Table 75–1 Benign Pediatric Heart Murmurs

Murmur	Etiology	Age	Type	Location	Increased Intensity
Peripheral pulmonic stenosis	Flow from PA to branches	<6 mo	1-2/6 SEM	LUSB to axilla, back	Supine, fever, anemia
Still's	Flow across normal AV	2-8 y	2-3/6 SEM	Apex	Supine, fever, anemia
Cervical venous hum	Flow from subclavian to SVC	3-6 y	1-2/6 continuous	Right infraclavicular	Sitting, fever, anemia
Pulmonary flow	Flow across normal PV	8-14 y	1-2/6 SEM	LUSB	Supine, fever, anemia

AV, atrioventricular; LUSB, left upper sternal border; PA, pulmonary artery; PV, pulmonic valve; SEM, systolic ejection murmur; SVC, superior vena cava.

- Cardiology should be consulted for an echocardiogram and definitive management.

Specific Problems: Cyanotic Heart Disease
Assessment of Cyanotic Heart Disease

- The underlying pathophysiologic derangement of cyanotic heart lesions is right-to-left shunting of blood.
- An important diagnostic clue in differentiating cyanotic heart disease from other forms of shock is that children with cyanotic heart disease often present with central cyanosis (their lips are blue, their extremities are warm, and their oxygen saturations are usually low). Children with sepsis, dehydration, or hypothermia usually present with peripheral cyanosis (their lips are pink, their extremities are pale, blue, cool, or mottled, and their oxygenation is often normal).
- To differentiate cyanotic heart disease from pulmonary pathology in patients with an abnormal oxygenation, a *hyperoxia test* can help. An arterial blood gas (ABG) should be obtained after placing the patient on 100% oxygen for 15 minutes. If the oxygenation remains low despite hyperoxygenation (<150 mm Hg), cyanotic heart disease should be suspected. If the oxygenation improves substantially (>150 mm Hg), pulmonary disease should be suspected.

Emergency Department Management of Cyanotic Heart Disease

- Supplemental oxygen should be avoided unless extreme hypoxia is present (oxygen saturations less than 75%). Oxygen is usually not helpful due to right-to-left shunting. Too much oxygen may actually be harmful by closing the ductus arteriosus and causing vasodilatation, therefore contributing to CHF.

- Correct metabolic acidosis and systemic hypoperfusion with fluid boluses and bicarbonate.
- Anemia should be treated with packed red blood cell transfusions. It is unclear what the optimal hemoglobin level is in a patient with cyanotic heart disease, but many providers maintain higher hemoglobin levels of 14 to 18 mg/dl in such patients.
- Prostaglandin E (PGE1) is used in newborn infants with suspected cyanotic heart disease. PGE1 works by opening or maintaining the patency of the ductus arteriosus. Functional closure of the ductus normally occurs at 10 to 15 hours of life. Fibrosis of the ductus usually occurs at 2 to 3 weeks of life. The dose of PGE1 is 0.05-2 µg/kg/min with an onset of 2-3 minutes. Side effects of PGE1 include apnea, fever, hypotension, and seizures.

Types of Cyanotic Heart Disease
Tetralogy of Fallot (TOF)

- The anatomy of TOF includes pulmonic stenosis and right ventricular hypertrophy, with an overriding aorta and a ventricular septal defect (VSD).
- These patients may present with cyanosis between 1 week and 4 months of life, depending on the degree of pulmonic stenosis.
- The physical examination reveals a single S_2 heart sound and a systolic ejection murmur heard best at the left upper sternal border.
- The EKG usually shows right axis deviation, right ventricular hypertrophy, and sinus tachycardia.
- The classic chest radiograph finding is a "boot-shaped heart." Approximately one third of patients will also have a right-sided aortic arch.
- "Tet spells" are hypercyanotic spells that occur with exertion or agitation. To manage a hypercyanotic spell, do the following: administer 100% supplemental oxygen. Place the patient in a knee-chest position (decreases venous return and increases left-sided resistance, lessening right-to-left shunting). Administer morphine 0.2 mg/kg IM or SQ (decreases venous return, and may directly relax the infundibulum). Avoid agitating the patient if possible, as this can worsen the condition. Administer a normal saline IV fluid bolus (right ventricular outflow is volume dependent and any hypovolemia adversely affects outflow). Administer propranolol 0.1 mg/kg IV (which may directly relax the infundibulum). Administer sodium bicarbonate to correct acidosis and transfuse packed red blood cells to correct anemia as needed.

Transposition of the Great Arteries (TGA)

- The anatomy of TGA involves two parallel circuits: systemic blood flows from the right ventricle to the aorta and body, then back to the right atrium. Pulmonary blood flows from the left ventricle to the pulmonary artery and lungs, then back to the left atrium.
- These patients present with cyanosis from birth to 1 week of life.
- The physical examination reveals a single S_2 heart sound and a systolic ejection murmur heard at the left lower sternal border.

- The EKG shows right axis deviation, right ventricular hypertrophy and an upright T in V_1.
- The classic chest radiograph finding is the "egg on a string."
- TGA must be accompanied by an atrial or ventricular septal defect or a patent ductus, to allow for mixing of blood in order for the patient to survive.

Tricuspid Atresia (TA)

- In TA, there is no blood flow from the right atrium to the right ventricle; the right ventricle is not fully formed. Blood from the right atrium must flow through an atrial septal defect to the left side of the heart.
- These patients present with cyanosis from 1 to 4 weeks of life.
- The physical examination reveals a single S_2 heart sound and a systolic ejection murmur heard best at the left lower sternal border (if there is a VSD).
- The EKG shows right atrial enlargement, left ventricular hypertrophy, and a leftward or superior QRS axis.
- The chest radiograph may be normal or reveal cardiomegaly.
- In addition to an atrial septal defect, TA may be accompanied by a ventricular septal defect or a patent ductus arteriosus.

Total Anomalous Pulmonary Venous Return (TAPVR)

- In TAPVR, pulmonary veins return to systemic veins instead of to the left atrium.
- These patients present with cyanosis from birth to 1 week of life.
- The physical examination reveals a fixed, split S_2. There may be a systolic ejection murmur at the left upper sternal border and a mid-diastolic murmur at the left lower sternal border.
- The EKG shows right axis deviation, right atrial enlargement and right ventricular hypertrophy.
- The classic chest radiograph finding of a "snowman in a snowstorm" is seen with supracardiac connections. Other findings include cardiomegaly, increased pulmonary markings (if nonobstructed), and pulmonary edema (if obstructed).
- TAPVR is accompanied by an atrial septal defect or a patent foramen ovale.
- TAPVR is the cyanotic lesion most commonly mistaken for lung disease.

Truncus Arteriosis

- In truncus arteriosus a single trunk from the heart supplies the systemic and pulmonary circulations. Truncus arteriosis is accompanied by a VSD.
- On physical examination, there may be an ejection click and a diastolic murmur.
- The EKG shows biventricular hypertrophy.
- Chest radiograph shows cardiomegaly. In 25% of patients, there is also a right-sided aortic arch.

Miscellaneous Cyanotic Heart Lesions

- Patients with hypoplastic left heart disease will usually present with shock. They have underdeveloped left ventricles, mitral and aortic valves.
- Ebstein anomaly consists of tricuspid regurgitation and an atrial septal defect. Patients present with cyanosis and CHF. A radiograph usually shows the classic "wall to wall heart." Ebstein anomaly is also associated with Wolff-Parkinson-White syndrome.

Specific Problems: Congestive Heart Failure
Assessment of Pediatric Congestive Heart Failure

- CHF in children is most often caused by the following conditions:
    - Congenital heart defects (CHDs)
    - Heart failure due to left-to-right shunting (Table 75–2)
    - Heart failure due to left-sided obstructive lesions (Table 75–3)
    - Cardiomyopathies: Metabolic, muscle disorders, infection, drugs
    - Postoperative complications following repair of CHD
    - Anemia
    - Dysrhythmias
    - Pulmonary pathology: pulmonary embolism, cystic fibrosis, chronic infection or aspiration, asthma
- The chest radiograph in CHF can provide important diagnostic information. Cardiomegaly on chest radiograph (defined as a cardiothoracic ratio greater than 0.55 in infants and greater than 0.5 in children older than 1 year), can reveal underlying cardiomyopathy or CHD. Increased vascular markings on chest radiograph are seen with pulmonary edema. Evidence of pneumonia, chronic aspiration, or asthma may also be noted.
- The EKG in CHF may be normal or show evidence of atrial or ventricular hypertrophy, as well as dysrhythmias or ischemia in severe cases.

Emergency Department Management of Pediatric Congestive Heart Failure

- Use IV fluids with caution. Up to 5 ml/kg over 30 minutes can be given only when the patient has a low preload. Significant anemia (hematocrit <20%) should be corrected by transfusion of packed red blood cells.
- Diuretics should be given in cases of fluid overload. Furosemide is the diuretic most commonly chosen.
- Adrenergic inotropes, such as dopamine or dobutamine, should be administered for any patient who has evidence of cardiogenic shock or hypotension. Digoxin is no longer in general use.
- Digoxin is contraindicated in idiopathic hypertrophic subaortic stenosis and TOF.
- Angiotensin-converting enzyme inhibitors have shown proven benefit in adults with ischemic cardiomyopathies; and they are probably also useful for pediatric patients. They are frequently used in the treatment of chronic CHF.
- PGE1 should be administered in any patient with a suspected congenital lesion and cyanosis.

Table 75–2   CHF Lesions Causing Left-to-Right Shunting

Lesion	Shunt	CHF Onset	Murmur	Important Info
ASD	Left atrium to right atrium	Usually asymptomatic into childhood	2-3/6 SEM at LUSB wide, fixed split S_2	Watch for atrial dysrhythmias, mitral valve prolapse
VSD	Left ventricle to right ventricle	2-12 wk (moderate to large defects)	2-5/6 SEM at LLSB	Eisenmenger complex with large VSD (right to left shunt, pulmonary hypertension)
Patent ductus arteriosus	Aorta to pulmonary artery	1 wk-childhood	1-4/6 continuous "machinery" murmur at LUSB bounding pulses	More common in preemies-indomethacin for closure (80% success rate)
AV canal	AV septal defect, common AV valve, VSD → increased pulmonary blood flow	2 wk-1 y	3-4/6 HSM at LLSB SEM at apex (mitral insufficiency)	Associated with Down syndrome (mongolism)

ASD, atrial septal defect; AV, atrioventricular; CHF, congestive heart failure; HSM, holosystolic murmur; LLSB, left lower sternal border; LUSB, left upper sternal border; SEM, systolic ejection murmur; SVC, superior vena cava.

Table 75–3   CHF Due to Outflow Tract Obstruction

Lesion	Pathophysiology	CHF Onset	Murmur	Important Information
Aortic stenosis	Thickened aortic valve → LV outflow tract obstruction	Usually asymptomatic unless critical stenosis (birth)	2-4/6 SEM at LLSB, apex systolic ejection click at apex	Chest radiograph usually normal Watch for exertional syncope
Pulmonary stenosis	Thickened pulmonary valve→ RV outflow tract obstruction	Usually asymptomatic unless severe (1 wk)	2-5/6 SEM at LUSB, neck and back click at LUSB	Chest radiograph with prominent pulmonary artery Watch for exertional syncope
Coarctation of the aorta	Constricted aorta→ LV outflow tract obstruction	1 wk-childhood	2-3/6 SEM at LUSB, back	Lower extremity blood pressure at least 10 mmHg less than right upper extremity pressure Rib notching seen on chest radiograph if older than 5 y Associated with Turner syndrome (ovarian agenesis)

CHF, congestive heart failure; LV: left ventricle; RV, right ventricle; SEM, systolic ejection murmur; LLSB, left lower sternal border; LUSB: left upper sternal border.

Specific Problems: Chest Pain
Assessment of Pediatric Chest Pain

- Most causes of chest pain in pediatric patients are benign. When considering all pediatric-range patients, the mean age of patients experiencing chest pain is between 11 and 13 years of age. Younger patients have a higher percentage of organic disease when compared with adolescents, who represent most of the patients with unknown or psychogenic etiologies of their chest pain. Less than 5% of chest pain in children is cardiac in origin.

- Chest pain associated with syncope, diaphoresis, pallor, or palpitations is concerning. Pain that is described as exertional, severe, tearing, or radiating to the back requires a thorough workup to look for cardiac ischemia or aortic dissection. Risk factors include Marfan syndrome, Kawasaki disease, congenital heart disease, or Ehlers-Danos syndrome.

- Most children without a known cardiac history and with normal vital signs and a normal physical examination have no significant morbidity or mortality.

- Helpful historical points include the quality, intensity, location, timing, duration, and alleviating or aggravating factors of the chest pain. Inquire about any associated symptoms such as fever, weight loss, fatigue, respiratory complaints, syncope, and gastrointestinal complaints.

- The physical examination should include vital signs, complete cardiac and pulmonary examinations, palpation of the chest wall, and maneuvers to try to reproduce the chest pain.

- When the history is negative for serious pathology and there is a normal physical examination, further testing is not necessary. A chest radiograph and EKG may be performed in some patients.

- *Idiopathic* is the most frequently encountered diagnosis for chest pain in pediatrics. The typical patient presents with a few weeks–to–1-month history of occasional episodes of chest pain. The pain is described as sharp, occurring with or without exercise, and usually is short in duration with no specific associated symptoms, except anxiety. The pain seldom interferes with activity. Recurrence is common, but long-term occurrences are not typical. The physical examination is normal, with the pain not being reproducible. Table 75–4 lists the differential diagnosis and management considerations of pediatric chest pain.

Emergency Department Management of Pediatric Chest Pain

- Reassurance to the patient and their parents is the mainstay of therapy in most cases due to the lack of serious pathology in the majority of pediatric patients with chest pain. A patient with a normal history and physical examination rarely has pathology, and routine tests or unnecessary referrals may be detrimental. Due to the recurrent nature of the chest pain, follow-up visits are important.

- Of course, chest pain related to organic causes needs appropriate treatment or referral. Chest pain that is associated with syncope, diaphoresis, pallor, nausea, palpitations, a sensation of a racing heart, or that occurs only with strenuous activity requires prompt referral to the pediatric cardiologist.

Table 75–4 Differential Diagnosis of Pediatric Chest Pain

	Examples	Comments
Cardiovascular	Coronary artery vasospasm	The pain described with these episodes is crushing, diffuse, and unrelenting. Associated features that can be seen with ischemic pain are diaphoresis, nausea, dyspnea, and syncope. Associated with cocaine use, but may occur in pediatric patients without predisposing risk factors.
	Anomalous coronary arteries	Patients usually present with chest pain during intense activity. Anomalous coronary blood supply can put patients at risk for myocardial infarction or sudden death.
	Kawasaki disease	Coronary artery aneurysms and stenosis can lead to cardiac ischemia.
	Hypertrophic cardiomyopathy	Chest pain is an unusual presenting symptom. Syncope is a more common presenting complaint. Physical examination usually reveals an aortic stenosis systolic ejection murmur that increases with standing or a Valsalva maneuver.
	Mitral valve prolapse (MVP)	It is not known how or even whether MVP causes pain. This should always be a diagnosis of exclusion.
	Aortic dissection	Marfan's syndrome (cystic medial necrosis of the aorta associated with long limbs) is an important risk factor leading to aortic dissection in the pediatric population. This is also seen with Ehlers-Danos syndrome (congenital connective tissue disorder), type IV, in which the vascular disease predominates over the other soft tissue defects.
	Tachydysrhythmias	Supraventricular tachycardia has been perceived as chest pain, especially in younger children. Palpitations, racing heart, syncope, or exercise intolerance are almost always present.
	Pericarditis	Associated findings include fever, friction rub on examination, and diffuse ST or T wave abnormalities, with PR depressions on the electrocardiogram.
	Myocarditis	Patients with myocarditis may present with an unexplained tachycardia and elevated cardiac enzymes.

Table 75–4 Differential Diagnosis of Pediatric Chest Pain—*cont'd*

	Examples	Comments
Pulmonary	Asthma	Asthma is one of the most common causes of chest pain in children. Pain is often pleuritic, and associated with wheezing or shortness of breath.
	Pneumonia	Another common cause of chest pain in children. Pain is often pleuritic, and associated with shortness of breath.
Gastrointestinal	Gastroesophageal reflux disease	Can lead to esophageal irritation, inflammation, and spasm, which cause burning or pressure-like chest pain.
Connective tissue	Marfan's syndrome	Aortic dilatation with the potential for aortic dissection and rupture exists.
Musculoskeletal	Chest wall muscle strain and costochondritis	Musculoskeletal pain is usually sharp in quality, and is worse with activity or inspiration. The onset of symptoms may be related to a respiratory illness or increased physical activity. On physical examination, the pain is reproducible.
	"Slipping rib" syndrome	The eighth through tenth ribs are joined by fibrous tissue. This fibrous tissue may pop or click as ribs slip over each other, causing the slipping rib syndrome.
		Pain is typically a dull ache and related to activity. To confirm the diagnosis, perform the "hooking maneuver": pain will be reproduced by lifting the involved ribs.
Other	Psychogenic	Chest pain is often associated with headache, abdominal pain, and panic attack. A stressful event nearly always precedes the pain.
	Idiopathic	This is the most frequent cause of chest pain in pediatrics. The pain is typically sharp and short in duration. There are usually no associated symptoms. The physical examination is normal. This is a diagnosis of exclusion.

MVP, mitral valve prolapse.

Teaching Points

Pediatric cardiac disease has a wide variety of presentations. The patient may be a normal baby with the only abnormal finding being that of a cardiac murmur. Conversely, the child may present during early infancy with heart failure, dysrhythmia, cyanosis, shock, and death.

In the youngest children, the history will more likely be that of inability to eat, failure to grow and develop normally, or the appearance of pneumonia. Depending upon the congenital anomaly, the child may or may not have cyanosis.

The "hyperoxia test" can help differentiate lung disease from cyanotic heart disease. Because pulmonary disease is much more common than cardiac, it is useful to give the child a test of high-flow oxygen. If the pO$_2$ does not improve with oxygen, the disease is more likely cardiac than pulmonary.

Newborns with cyanosis should have closure of the ductus arteriosus reversed or prevented with prostaglandin EI infusion.

Suggested Readings

Barkin RM (editor). Pediatric Emergency Medicine: Concepts and Clinical Practice (2nd ed). St Louis, MO: Mosby, 1997.

Cava JR, Sayger, PL. Chest pain in children and adolescents. Pediatr Clin N Am 2004; 51:1553–1568.

Devine SD, Anisman PC, Robinson BW. A basic guide to cyanotic congenital heart disease. Contemp Pediatr 1998;15(10):133–163.

Frommelt MA. Differential diagnosis and approach to a heart murmur in term infants. Pediatr Clin N Am 2004;51:1023–1032.

Kay JD, Colan SD, Graham TP. Congestive heart failure in pediatric patients. Am Heart J ournal 2001;142:923–927.

Woods WA, Schutte DA, McCulloch MA. Care of children who have had surgery for congenital heart disease. Am J Emerg Med 2003;21:318–327.

CHAPTER 76

Pediatric Respiratory Illnesses

Tarina Lee Kang ■ Leon D. Sanchez

Overview

Respiratory illnesses are very common in the pediatric population, accounting for the most visits to a pediatric ED. Most pediatric respiratory illnesses are not life-threatening. See Chapter 73 "General Approach to the Pediatric Patient."

A child's respiratory anatomy differs from adults in several ways. Children have a smaller oxygen reserve, so hypoxemia occurs more rapidly than in an adult. The resistance to air flow in a child's airway is inversely proportional to the fourth power of the airway radius. Therefore, small decreases in the radius can increase airway resistance substantially. Because a child's diaphragm is not fully developed, and the rib cage is more pliable, children are more susceptible to paradoxical respiration, which creates more work to breathe under duress. In addition, a child's lung tissue has less elastic recoil and thicker airway walls, which make children more prone to atelectasis and bronchoconstriction. Anatomical differences in airway anatomy are mentioned in Chapter 74.

When evaluating a pediatric patient with a respiratory illness, dyspnea, stridor, nasal flaring, abdominal breathing, and any other signs that the patient is working hard to breathe are indicative of more severe disease. Stridor is concerning for upper airway obstruction. Stridor from the nose and pharynx has a sonorous, gurgling, and coarse quality. The voice may be muffled or have a "hot potato" quality. An example of this is a retropharyngeal abscess (see Chapter 64). Stridor from the supraglottic and immediate subglottic trachea is inspiratory and high pitched. Viral croup is an example of this type of stridor. Biphasic stridor is heard on inspiration and expiration and may suggest a lesion at the glottis (vocal cords) or cricoid ring. Stridor from the lower trachea is usually expiratory. Bacterial tracheitis and a foreign body are examples. The presence of wheezing is concerning for lower airway disease, and can be found in patients with bronchiolitis, asthma, allergic reaction (see Chapter 19), aspiration, pneumonia, gastroesophageal reflux (see Chapter 77), cystic fibrosis, and cardiac failure (see Chapter 75).

This chapter will discuss some of the more common and concerning disease processes causing respiratory complaints in the pediatric population.

Specific Problems
Aspiration of Foreign Body (FB)

- *Epidemiology and risk factors.* Children between the ages of 1 and 3 years are at greatest risk for foreign body aspiration. Choking usually occurs during play or eating. The most common causes of foreign body aspiration in children are toys with small pieces, balloons, and foods such as grapes, peanuts, round candies, and hotdogs.
- *Pathophysiology.* The upper right main stem bronchus is shorter and larger in diameter than its left-sided counterpart, and departs from the trachea at a less acute angle than the left main stem bronchus. Therefore, foreign bodies are more commonly lodged in the right main stem bronchus.
- *History.* The history is a very important part of the diagnosis. Any history of a sudden onset of coughing, choking, or respiratory distress should be evaluated as a foreign body aspiration. No matter how well the child looks when first seen, a foreign body may still be present. Foreign body aspiration should also be considered in children who are suspected of having another respiratory illness, but who do not respond to therapy.
- *Physical examination.* Choking and coughing are the most common presentations. Inspiratory stridor, wheezing, and rhonchi may be heard on examination. Various findings indicating respiratory distress may also be seen.
- *Diagnostic testing.* Laboratory tests may be helpful in chronic cases. The white blood cell (WBC) count and sedimentation rate may be elevated. Chest radiographs (posteroanterior [PA] and lateral) should be obtained for foreign bodies. Atelectasis, focal pneumonia, air trapping, mediastinal shift, or compensatory emphysema on the contralateral side may be found, but unfortunately, the chest radiograph findings may be normal. A bronchoscopy should be done before concluding there is no foreign body aspirated. Coins and other flat foreign bodies can be visualized on PA and lateral chest radiograph. If in the trachea, the coin will appear in its largest anteroposterior diameter on the lateral film, and if in the esophagus, on the PA view. This is due to the tracheal rings that are incomplete, but render the diameter of the trachea larger in the anteroposterior axis and narrower in the lateral axis.
- *ED management.* As always, the airway is the first priority. Oxygen should be given for any patient with hypoxia or respiratory distress. Oxygen saturation levels should be monitored. An IV should be placed in any patient with an aspirated foreign body that needs to be removed.

A bronchoscopy to remove the foreign body will be done under general anesthesia. Steroids and antibiotics may reduce airway edema and infection. See Chapter 5 for management of complete airway obstruction.

- ■ *Helpful hints and pitfalls.* A FB should be sought in all young patients who have the sudden onset of coughing, wheezing, or asymmetric breath sounds on examination, or in those who do not respond to appropriate treatment for another presumed diagnosis.

Asthma Exacerbation

- ■ See Chapter 52 for additional information.
- ■ *History and physical examination. Mild exacerbation*: There is a history of wheezing or shortness of breath ongoing for hours, an increase in respiratory rate, a persistent tight hacking cough, expiratory wheezing; but good air exchange, with an oxygen saturation (O_2 sat) above 95%, peak expiratory flow rate (PEFR) or forced expiratory volume at 1 second (FEV_1) above 80% of personal best or predicted norm. *Moderate exacerbation*: Symptoms have been present for several days; there is an increased work of breathing, audible expiratory wheezes, with inspiratory and expiratory wheezes on auscultation; a $PEFR/FEV_1$ below 80% predicted value, and an O_2 sat low normal. *Severe exacerbation*: There will be marked respiratory distress, accessory muscle use, tachypnea, intercostal, tracheosternal retractions, breathlessness at rest, somnolence, hypoxia, or a $PEFR/FEV_1$ below 50% personal best/predicted. This can soon lead to respiratory failure, and the signs of impending respiratory arrest must be watched for and aggressively acted upon (e.g., bradycardia, profound hypoxia, and a quiet chest).
- ■ *Diagnostic testing.* Obtain a baseline SaO_2. Obtain a $PEFR/FEV_1$ in children 6 years and older. Use continuous pulse oximetry. Noninvasive end tidal CO_2 should be used, especially in severe attacks, or if there are any signs of fatigue. Clinical asthma scores (CASs) may be helpful in a decision to admit the patient. Blood gases should be obtained in persistently hypoxic children. A rising pCO_2 is an ominous finding, and indicates a need for active airway management. A chest radiograph is warranted to evaluate for a concurrent infectious process, pneumothorax, or aspirated foreign body, especially if the patient has a fever with cough, unequal breath sounds, or if this is the first presentation of wheezing.
- ■ *ED management.* Patient should be placed on oxygen, IV fluids, oxygen saturation monitoring, with expeditious medical intervention that includes β-agonists, ipratropium bromide, and steroids. Subcutaneous epinephrine or terbutaline are reserved for patients in extreme respiratory distress, or who are unresponsive to standard therapy. A ketamine bolus 2 to 4 mg/kg and subsequent drip may produce enough bronchodilatation to avoid intubation (see Chapter 90.6).
- ■ *Helpful hints and pitfalls.* Education and early, aggressive management is essential to successful treatment of asthma exacerbations in the ED. In young children, viral URIs are often correlated with asthma exacerbations. Oral antibiotics are not necessary.

Bacterial Tracheitis

- **Definition.** Bacterial tracheitis is a diffuse, inflammatory process involving the larynx, trachea, and bronchi, with adherent or semi-adherent mucopurulent membrane production that can obstruct the trachea.
- **Epidemiology and risk factors.** Bacterial tracheitis is most commonly seen in the fall and winter months. It is more common in the 7 to 16 year age group.
- **Pathogenesis.** Acute airway obstruction in bacterial tracheitis occurs when purulent membranous material produced by the inflammatory process occludes the trachea. It can be seen in all ages, but it may be more evident in younger children due to a narrower airway that is more quickly compromised by inflammation and swelling. It is most often secondary to a bacterial pathogen, such as *Staphylococcus aureus*.
- **History.** Onset can be acute, usually mimicking an upper respiratory infection, followed by a high fever, cough, and various degrees of inspiratory stridor, which can develop into respiratory distress in the later stages. Bacterial tracheitis can mimic symptoms of croup; however, it will not respond to the same treatment. Besides the difference in age, the child with bacterial tracheitis will appear more toxic, and is more likely to have a high fever and a high leukocytosis.
- **Physical examination.** The patient may exhibit a barklike cough, hoarseness, and various degrees of inspiratory or expiratory stridor.
- **Diagnostic testing.** Imaging studies are not essential in this diagnosis, and should only be obtained on patients with no airway compromise. Radiographs of the neck may show subglottic narrowing, clouding of the tracheal air column, or an irregular tracheal margin. Laryngotracheo-bronchoscopy is the definitive way to diagnose bacterial tracheitis because it allows direct visualization of the trachea and the pseudomembranous material. A culture and Gram's stain of tracheal sections should be obtained if possible.
- **ED management.** Be prepared to intubate, as over 50% of patients eventually require intubation. Once the airway is stabilized, IV fluids and antibiotics should be started. In rare cases, a cricothyrotomy or tracheostomy must be performed. Early consultation with the ear, nose, and throat (ENT) physician and a pediatric intensivist is warranted.
- **Helpful hints and pitfalls.** When evaluating a patient for croup, bacterial tracheitis should be part of the differential diagnosis.

Bronchiolitis

- **Definition.** Bronchiolitis is an inflammation of the bronchiolar epithelium by an acute infection. The inflammatory process causes desquamation of the epithelium with subsequent obstruction of the airway with cellular debris.
- **Epidemiology and risk factors.** Bronchiolitis is usually seen in children younger than 2 years, with a peak incidence in children 2 to 5 months old. Respiratory syncytial virus is the most common pathogen. Risk factors include age less than 6 months, living in crowded conditions,

not being breastfed, prematurity of birth (<37 weeks), and exposure to cigarette smoke.
- *History.* Usually there is a history of fever, rhinorrhea, and congestion before the onset of lower respiratory involvement of cough, wheezing, and tachypnea. The child may have decreased feeding or appetite, increased lethargy, or increased irritability. Important items in the history include the gestational age at birth, whether the mother breastfed the child, any perinatal complications or diseases, such as cystic fibrosis (CF), bronchopulmonary dysplasia, congenital heart malformations, or immunodeficiencies.
- *Physical examination.* This should include the overall appearance; whether the child is well appearing, playful, smiling, lethargic, irritable, or crying. The most important predictor of disease severity is the oxygen saturation. The respiratory rate, use of accessory muscles for breathing, and hydration status (moistness of membranes, capillary refill, and presence of tears) should be noted. Wheezes and crackles may be heard on the lung examination.
- *Diagnostic testing.* Chest radiographs are indicated for patients who present with an initial episode of wheezing or high fever. Hyperinflated lungs with flat diaphragms, increased radiolucency, a small heart size on anterior view, or peribronchial cuffing may be seen. Routine blood cultures and urine are unnecessary if the clinical presentation is consistent with bronchiolitis. Laboratory studies may be indicated for immunocompromised patients or patients with congenital heart disease.
- *ED management.* Supportive care is the mainstay of treatment. Patients should be allowed to remain in a position of comfort. Moist 100% oxygen should be given to any patients in respiratory distress. Secretions should be suctioned if copious amounts are present. Epinephrine should be given if the patient is in respiratory distress, or does not respond to beta agonists. Bronchodilators should be given in patients with a respiratory rate above 50 breaths per minute, increased work of breathing, or oxygen saturation less than 97%. Steroids have not been proven to be effective in bronchiolitis. Most patients with bronchiolitis do not require admission. Any patient who has not responded to treatment in the ED, exhibits increasingly severe airway compromise, or has a significant underlying medical illness should be admitted. Also admit the child for whom respiratory work is great enough that the child cannot suckle properly.
- *Helpful hints and pitfalls.* Children with mild illness can quickly progress to more severity. Cyanosis on physical examination occurs only with oxygen saturations < 85%.

Croup

- *Definition.* Croup, or laryngotracheobronchitis, is a clinical syndrome characterized by a barklike cough, hoarseness, inspiratory stridor, and various degrees of respiratory distress.
- *Epidemiology and risk factors.* The peak incidence of croup is 2 years old. It is most prevalent during the late fall and early winter months.

Patients who are at risk for croup are those who are younger than 3 years, have underlying respiratory problems such as asthma, recurrent respiratory infections, prior episodes of croup, a family member with croup, or attend a daycare center.

■ *Pathophysiology.* Croup is a viral infection transmitted via the nasopharynx, causing laryngeal and tracheal edema and erythema. Fibrinous exudate occludes the lumen of the trachea, and the vocal cords become edematous, causing inspiratory stridor and respiratory distress, hoarseness, and a barklike cough (sounds like a seal). The most common pathogen is the parainfluenza virus, although croup can also be caused by the adenovirus, respiratory syncytial virus (RSV), and influenza.

■ *History.* The patient often complains of cough, sore throat, low-grade fever, and coryza. This is often followed by hoarseness and a distinctive barking cough. Stridor may or may not be present.

■ *Physical examination.* The patient can present with a broad spectrum of signs, ranging from mild discomfort to respiratory distress. The lung examination may be normal, or demonstrate only mild expiratory wheezes. Evaluate the child with croup for any signs of imminent respiratory failure including nasal flaring, intercostal contractions, stridor, poor air movement, lethargy, agitation, tachycardia, tachypnea, or hypoxia.

■ *Diagnostic testing.* Croup is essentially a clinical diagnosis. A PA radiograph of the neck may show a steeple sign (gradual narrowing of the subglottic area secondary to tissue swelling).

■ *ED management.* The patient should be made as comfortable as possible. The parent should be allowed to stay in the room to decrease patient anxiety. Humidified oxygen should be delivered via face mask. If the patient exhibits any signs of respiratory distress, racemic or plain epinephrine (0.25-1 ml of a 2.25% solution in 3 ml of saline via a nebulizer) should be given to decrease mucosal swelling and respiratory compromise. Dexamethasone is routinely given to decrease mucosal inflammation and subsequent edema. If the patient is dehydrated, IV or oral hydration may be necessary. The patient should be observed in the ED for 3 to 4 hours after a treatment with steroids and epinephrine.

■ *Helpful hints and pitfalls.* If there is no response, or only partial response to treatment, the child should be admitted. It is at this time that bacterial tracheitis may be deemed a more appropriate diagnosis than croup, and antibiotics started.

Epiglottitis

■ *Definition.* Epiglottitis, also known as supraglottitis, is a bacterial infection of the epiglottis and aryepiglottic folds that causes inflammation and swelling. It is acute in onset and life-threatening if not treated properly.

■ *Epidemiology and risk factors.* Epiglottitis predominantly affects children between the ages of 3 and 7 years. However, the disease has been seen in older children and adults. Its incidence has dramatically decreased since the *Haemophilus influenzae* (Hib) vaccine was introduced in 1985. There is a male-to-female predominance of 2.5:1. The most common pathogen causing epiglottitis is *H. influenzae*. Other common causes are

S. aureus and *Staphylococcus pneumoniae*, as well as by viral infections. Epiglottis can also be caused by any mechanism that causes inflammation and swelling in this area, such as thermal injury or direct trauma. Crowded living conditions, poor medical care access, and lack of immunizations are risk factors.

- *Pathophysiology.* The supraglottis, false vocal cords, and aryepiglottic folds are invaded by a bacterial or viral pathogen causing swelling, inflammation, and respiratory distress.
- *History.* The classic presentation is the triad of drooling, dysphagia, and respiratory distress. Initially, the child may complain of a sore throat and fever. The patient may refuse to eat due to odynophagia, and with increasing inflammation and swelling, may not be able to swallow secretions, leading to drooling. Eventually, the patient's airway can occlude from inflammation and secretions, leading to respiratory distress and death.
- *Physical examination.* The patient may be febrile, toxic appearing, anxious, or irritable. In cases where there is significant respiratory compromise, the patient may exhibit stridor, or other signs of upper airway obstruction. The patient can be observed sitting upright, leaning forward in a sniffing position. Drooling may be noted on examination. The patient may also have a muffled sounding voice. Cough is rare.
- *Diagnostic testing.* Although they should not be performed if they delay or compromise patient care in any way, soft-tissue lateral neck radiographs may show an enlarged epiglottis and swollen aryepiglottic folds (known as a *thumbprint sign*).
- *ED management.* Be ready to intubate or perform a tracheostomy or cricothyrotomy emergently. An ENT and intensivist should be consulted early. The operating room may be needed for intubation. The patient should sit upright in a comfortable position with the parent present. A "stable" patient maintaining a patent airway and adequate oxygenation should not be agitated until preparations are made to secure the airway if needed. Direct visualization of epiglottis is not recommended unless the patient is stable and the diagnosis is in doubt. Airway equipment and experienced personnel should be immediately available to intubate should the patient decompensate. IV access should be obtained by the most experienced person available but the airway takes precedence. Empiric antibiotic treatment should be started immediately.
- *Helpful hints and pitfalls.* Direct visualization of the epiglottis in the ED is not recommended. It is better to involve an ENT specialist, and take the patient to the operating room for direct visualization of the airway and intubation.

Pertussis

Refer to Chapter 24.

Pneumonia

- *Epidemiology.* Children with cystic fibrosis (CF), aspiration syndromes, immunodeficiencies, or congenital or acquired pulmonary malformations are at higher risk for pneumonia. The newest heptavalent pneumococcal conjugate vaccine (approved to age 5) is directed against seven serotypes, the major strains that cause invasive disease.

■ *Pathophysiology.* There is an inflammatory reaction in the lungs in response to inhalation or aspiration of pathogens. It less commonly results from hematogenous spread. See Table 76–1 for most common organisms stratified by age group.

■ *History.* There may be a history of a preceding upper respiratory infection. The patient presents with mild, nonspecific symptoms such as emesis, cough, malaise, rhinorrhea, lethargy, chest pain, and abdominal pain to severe respiratory difficulty. Fever may be present. Milder symptoms are present with atypical pneumonias.

■ *Physical examination.* Fever, tachypnea, decreased breath sounds, crackles, or rales may be present. Wheezing may be noted with viral or atypical pneumonias. Neonates typically present with tachypnea (respiratory rate above 60 breaths per minute), grunting, retractions, poor feeding and irritability; hypothermia may be present.

■ *Diagnostic testing.* Bacterial pneumonias are more likely to have an alveolar or lobar infiltrate with air bronchograms. Viral pneumonias are characterized by diffuse interstitial infiltrates, hyperinflation, or atelectasis. Infiltrates due to aspiration may be seen in the right upper lobe in infants, and in the posterior lobes or bases of the lung in older children. Pleural effusions are more common with *S. pneumoniae* and *S. aureus* but may be seen with *M. pneumoniae.* Many tests performed on nasopharyngeal samples, such as enzyme-linked immunosorbent assays or direct fluorescent antibody assays, are very accurate in detecting viral etiologies of lower respiratory disease such as RSV and influenza. One exception is the cold agglutinin test, but while less accurate than the antibody assays, is more pragmatic in that it can be performed at the bedside for children older than 3 years with suspected mycoplasmic pneumonia. Blood cultures are rarely positive. Sputum cultures may be obtained in older children. Pulse oximetry should be useful to support the diagnosis of pneumonia, and to influence management decisions such as admission or outpatient treatment.

■ *ED management.* See Table 76–1 for antimicrobial therapy. Patients who do not respond to outpatient therapy, or those with a poor social situation, concerning clinical signs such as respiratory distress, dehydration or hypoxia, or significant co-morbidities should be admitted.

■ *Helpful hints and pitfalls.* The exact cause of pneumonia is almost always unknown in the ED. Treatment should be based on epidemiologic, seasonal, clinical, and radiologic findings.

Age	0-4 Wk	4-8 Wk	8-12 Wk	12 Wk-4 Y	5 Y-Adolescence
Etiology (in order of prevalence)	Group B strep gram-negative enteric bacteria *Listeria monocytogenes*	*C. trachomatis* Viruses (RSV, parainfluenza) *Staphylococcus pneumoniae* *Bordetella pertussis* Group B streptococcus Gram-negative enteric *L. monocytogenes*	*C. trachomatis* Viruses (RSV, parainfluenza) *S. pneumoniae* *B. pertussis*	Viruses (RSV, parainfluenza, influenza, adenovirus, rhinovirus) *S pneumoniae* *Haemophilus influenzae* (non-type b) *M. catarrhalis* Group A streptococci *M. pneumoniae* *M. tuberculosis*	*M. pneumoniae* *C. pneumoniae* *S. pneumoniae* Viruses (RSV, parainfluenza, influenza, adenovirus, rhinovirus) *M. tuberculosis*
Treatment: Outpatient (in order of initial choice)	Not applicable	For pertussis or chlamydial infection: erythromycin or other macrolides	For pertussis or chlamydia: erythromycin or other macrolides or sulfonamides — For *S. pneumoniae*: See next column	Amoxicillin or amoxicillin/ clavulanate or cefuroxime Macrolides	Macrolides or tetracyclines (>8 y) Fluoroquinolones (>16 y)
Treatment: inpatient	Neonatal pneumonia or sepsis: ceftriaxone or cefotaxime plus ampicillin	Neonatal pneumonia or sepsis: ceftriaxone or cefotaxime plus ampicillin	Penicillin or ampicillin or cefuroxime Cefotaxime or ceftriaxone Clindamycin Vancomycin until alternative susceptible agents identified	Penicillin or ampicillin or cefuroxime Cefotaxime or ceftriaxone Clindamycin Vancomycin until alternative susceptible agents identified	Cefuroxime plus macrolides Macrolides plus cefotaxime or ceftriaxone or clindamycin Vancomycin Fluoroquinolones (>16 y)

RSV, respiratory syncytial virus.

(From Liebenstein R, Suggs AH, Campbell J. Pediatric pneumonia. *Emerg Med Clin North Am* 2003;21:437–4.)

Teaching Points

There are many forms of respiratory disease in children, which may vary with age. The greatest responsibility in the management of any of the causes is to define the child in respiratory distress severe enough to warrant active airway management. This will be indicated by how hard the child is working to breathe, a falling O_2 saturation, intercostal or sternal retractions, cyanosis, as well as a rising pCO_2. Many patients with mild respiratory disease will not have to be admitted, and can be improved satisfactorily in the ED, but it is prudent to observe the child in the ED under treatment for several hours before concluding the disease is not getting worse.

The child has much less airway reserve than the adult, and it is respiratory disease that is the most common cause of pediatric cardiac arrest.

Suggested Readings

Allen JY, Macias CG. The efficacy of ketamine in pediatric emergency department patients who present with acute severe asthma. Ann Emerg Med 2005;46:43–50.

Bolte RG. Emergency department management of pediatric asthma. CPEM 2004;5;256–269.

Darr CD. Lower airway obstruction. In Marx JA, Hockberger RS, Walls RM (editors). Rosen's Emergency Medicine: Concepts and Clinical Practice (6th ed). Philadelphia: Mosby, 2006, pp 2532–2554.

Lichenstein R, Suggs AH, Campbell J. Pediatric pneumonia. Emerg Med Clin North Am 2003;21:437–451.

Manno M. Upper airway obstruction and infection. In: Marx JA, Hockberger RS, Walls RM (editors). Rosen's Emergency Medicine: Concepts and Clinical Practice (6th ed). Philadelphia: Mosby, 2006, pp 2519–2531.

CHAPTER **77**

Pediatric Gastroenterology

CRISTINA MARIA ESTRADA ■ STEPHEN JOHN CICO

Overview

Abdominal pain in children is a dynamic process requiring reassessment, including serial abdominal examinations, especially after any therapeutic intervention or change in the patient's condition.

Early surgical consultation is often necessary because many pediatric gastrointestinal (GI) tract problems are surgical in nature, and can rapidly become life-threatening.

Rectal examinations are not imperative in a child with abdominal pain. They have not been shown to be helpful in diagnosing appendicitis in the pediatric population. They are helpful, however, in the diagnosis of GI tract bleeding, intussusception, rectal abscess, or fecal impaction.

Bilious vomiting, especially in a young infant, may signify a bowel obstruction that warrants immediate surgical consultation.

This chapter will briefly discuss GI problems unique to the pediatric population.

Specific Problems
Acute Pancreatitis

- The etiologies in children include trauma (22%), structural (15%), drugs/toxins (13%), systemic illness (13%), and infection (11%). In almost 30% of cases, the precipitating factor is unknown. The mortality rate is 14%.
- Because of its frequently atypical presentation in children, pancreatitis should be considered in all children with blunt abdominal trauma, epigastric pain associated with nausea or vomiting, unexplained shock, ascites or pleural effusions of unknown origin. It is often associated with or caused by nonaccidental trauma (see Chapter 82). Patients with cystic fibrosis (diagnosed or undiagnosed) have a higher incidence of pancreatitis.
- Diagnostic testing and management is similar to the adult patient population (see Chapter 18).

Allergic Colitis

- *Epidemiology and risk factors.* It presents in the first year of life after the introduction of cow's milk into the diet, and may affect the upper or lower GI tract. The most common antigens implicated are proteins in cow's milk, soy, and infant feedings. Breast-fed infants are also susceptible as they are affected by immunogenic proteins in the maternal diet.
- *Pathophysiology.* This is an immune-mediated condition associated with the ingestion of foreign proteins that cause diffuse inflammation of the rectum and colon.
- *History.* A sudden onset of blood-streaked, mucoid, or diarrheal stools are common.
- *Physical examination.* Infants are afebrile and appear well, without dehydration or weight loss. Stools are usually hemoccult positive.
- *Diagnostic testing.* Verify bleeding with rectal examination and hemoccult testing of the stool. Peripheral eosinophilia or eosinophils in stool samples stained with Wright stain is suggestive of the diagnosis. Hypoalbuminemia is a sensitive marker. The hematocrit should be normal. Flexible proctosigmoidoscopy should be performed only for gross bleeding that persists 5 to 7 days after therapy.

■ *ED management.* Removal of cow's milk from the diet leads to re-solution of symptoms within 3 to 7 days. Infants should be changed to a formula containing casein hydrosylate as the protein source. In exclusively breast-fed infants, elimination of the offending protein from the mother's diet also leads to clinical improvement, and breast-feeding can usually be continued.

■ *Helpful hints and pitfalls.* A third of infants with allergy to cow's milk protein are also allergic to proteins in soy formula. They may be able to tolerate goat's milk.

Anal Fissures

■ Anal fissures are the most common proctologic disorder occurring during infancy and childhood, and are the most common cause of infantile rectal bleeding. Most occur in infants younger than 1 year. Multiple anal fissures are associated with group B hemolytic streptococcus.

■ The ED management is similar to adults (Chapter 48). Injection of the fissure with marcaine may resolve the pain and rectal spasm, and allow quicker healing.

■ All patients with peri-anal excoriation, multiple anal fissures, recurrent anal fissures, or fissures resistant to conservative management should have perianal cultures for group B hemolytic streptococcus.

Appendicitis

■ It is the most common nontraumatic surgical emergency in children. The peak age of incidence is between 9 and 12 years, but although it is uncommon in children younger than 5 years, it does occur, even in infants. Because the history is so hard to obtain in the younger children, it often presents with an already ruptured appendix.

■ The diagnosis can be difficult in the very young (i.e., those under 5 years old), patients who have been symptomatic for more than 2 or 3 days, and adolescent girls aged 13 to 18 years. A normal white blood cell (WBC) count does not rule out acute appendicitis. In the obese child, computed tomography (CT scan) is the preferred imaging study. Ultrasound may show a noncompressible appendix in thin children.

■ The management of appendicitis in children is similar to the adult population: surgical consultation and intravenous (IV) antibiotics (see Chapter 18).

Biliary Tract Disease

■ In children, gallstones are associated with hemolytic disease, cystic fibrosis, total parenteral nutrition, sepsis, and dehydration. Ceftriaxone has also been associated with sludging and biliary disease, particularly in neonates. Acute acalculous cholecystitis has been associated with Rocky Mountain Spotted Fever and a variety of bacterial infections from *Salmonella* and *Shigella* organisms. Hydrops of the gallbladder is associated with viral upper respiratory or gastrointestinal infections,

Kawasaki disease, streptococcal pharyngitis, mesenteric adenitis, nephrotic syndrome, and leptospirosis.
- Pigment stones occur in childhood, whereas cholesterol stones usually occur in adolescence. Pigment stones result from the excess breakdown of red blood cells, and are most commonly seen in hemolytic anemias such as sickle cell disease and spherocytosis. Gallstones occurring in infants are usually associated with abdominal surgery, sepsis, necrotizing enterocolitis, or administration of total parenteral nutrition. Adolescents form gallstones in association with oral contraceptives, pregnancy, obesity, or underlying hemolytic disease.
- Laboratory abnormalities and management are similar to the adult population (see Chapter 18).

Constipation

- *Epidemiology and risk factors.* Constipation in children usually does not reflect an underlying pathologic condition. It affects up to 37% of children, and is functional in origin for approximately 95% of cases. Excessive intake of cow's milk, inadequate fluid intake, malnutrition, medications, and underlying illnesses such as neuromuscular disease or a recent viral illness (gastroenteritis) may also lead to constipation. Other causes include hypothyroidism, lead poisoning, and infant botulism. Encopresis refers to the passage of feces in inappropriate places after a chronological age of 4 years. It may have a constipation component. Many of these children have abnormal anal sphincter physiology, but some may have behavioral or psychiatric problems.
- *Pathophysiology.* For many children, it may begin early in life following an acute problem with uncomfortable stool passage. These children learn to withhold their stools to avoid pain. Increased stool retention distends the rectum, and, over time, the sensory threshold for stool volume in the rectum increases. In addition, rectal and sphincter muscles weaken, which increases the risk for incomplete evacuation and soiling accidents in between stool attempts. Overflow incontinence of watery stool is also common. In some children, constipation is a reaction to early or too insistent toilet training.
- *History.* Patients often complain of uncomfortable stool passage, infrequent, larger-caliber outputs of stool that may clog the toilet, soiling accidents, and signs of stool withholding.
- *Physical examination.* A palpable abdominal mass is occasionally present; it is usually soft, mobile, and nontender or minimally tender without guarding or rebound. Rectal examination often reveals normal sphincter tone. Stool impaction may be noted.
- *Diagnostic testing.* A large amount of stool or gas in the colon on plain films corresponds with, but does not prove, the diagnosis.
- *ED management.* Disimpact of the rectum if necessary. Oral medications include mineral oil (1 to 4 ml/kg/dose bid, but should not be used in infants, or those at risk for aspiration); lactulose (1 to 2 ml/kg/dose bid); milk of magnesia (1 to 3 ml/kg/dose bid); docusate (5 to 10 mg/kg/day); or senna extract (5 to 10 ml daily). Hypertonic phosphate and tap water enema should not be used in infants or toddlers

due to electrolyte abnormalities. Maintenance therapy includes increased fluid and fiber intake.

- *Helpful hints and pitfalls.* If the patient's examination reveals a distended or tympanitic abdomen, a bowel obstruction should be suspected. Altered lower extremity reflexes, absent anal wink, pilonidal dimple, or hair tuft may be indicative of a spinal cord abnormality, and should be evaluated further. Some children may have a normal soft stool every 2-3 days without difficulty; this is not constipation.

Foreign Bodies

- *Epidemiology.* Most of the GI foreign bodies occur in the toddler age as they explore the world by putting everything into their mouths. Coins are the most common GI foreign body in children; food is the most common in adults.
- *Pathophysiology.* Esophageal foreign bodies may become lodged in any of three areas of normal physiologic narrowing: upper esophageal sphincter (cricopharyngeus muscle)/thoracic inlet (C6 to T1), the aortic arch/ tracheal bifurcation (T4 to T6), and the lower esophageal sphincter/ diaphragmatic hiatus (T10 to T11). In general, 80% to 90% of objects that have made it into the stomach will be passed without difficulty. Perforation is uncommon, even with very sharp objects such as straight pins. Distally, the ileocecal valve is the most common site for perforation, and occurs in fewer than 1% of patients.
- *History.* The actual ingestion of the foreign body may not be witnessed. The child may be asymptomatic, or have symptoms ranging from persistent gagging to drooling and dry heaves. Rapidly progressive symptoms of dysphagia, pain, respiratory distress, or fever raise the possibility of a perforation.
- *Physical examination.* An aspirated object will cause persistent coughing, wheezing, or increased work of breathing (see Chapter 76).
- *Diagnostic testing.* Plain films are the most common diagnostic study to identify a GI foreign body. Films should include two views of the chest (see Chapter 76, "Aspiration of Foreign Body"), neck, and abdomen. Repeated films are helpful to follow the passage of the foreign body such as button batteries. Contrast studies may be helpful to delineate the non–radio-opaque foreign bodies or evaluate for perforations.
- *ED management.* Button batteries in the esophagus should be removed in as rapid a manner as possible because erosions and mediastinitis will occur quickly. Button batteries in the stomach usually pass without difficulty, and do not require removal unless they fail to pass the pylorus in a reasonable period. Foreign bodies that remain in the esophagus need to be removed (e.g., endoscopically). Indications for surgical removal of gastric foreign bodies include objects greater than 2 cm in width, length greater than 5 cm, and those that are sharp.
- *Helpful hints and pitfalls.* Foreign bodies that have made it into the stomach usually pass without difficulty and require no further follow-up. Button batteries are the exception and require follow-up films to document passage beyond the pylorus.

Gastroenteritis

- *Epidemiology and risk factors.* In many parts of the world, acute gastroenteritis (AGE) is the leading cause of childhood mortality. In the United States, children experience two to three diarrheal episodes per year, and up to five illnesses per year if attending a day care center. Other risk factors include young age, immunocompromise, poor personal hygiene, and travel. Viruses are the organisms most commonly found in children in the United States. Rotavirus is the most common virus. Norwalk virus is responsible for up to 40% of diarrheal illness in older children.

- *Pathophysiology.* Inflammation of the intestinal tract interferes with intestinal absorption and secretion of fluids and electrolytes. Surface area is decreased by destruction of mucosal cells. Toxins promote fluid secretion into the gut lumen, blocking some absorptive functions. Increased osmolality of luminal fluid and increased transit time lead to production of watery stools.

- *History.* Patients often describe vomiting or diarrhea, abdominal pain, weight loss, or recent antibiotic use.

- *Physical examination.* This often may reveal fever, tachycardia, hypotension, and lethargy. Tachypnea may be present if the patient is acidotic. The abdomen is usually soft and nondistended with hyperactive bowel sounds and diffuse tenderness on palpation (although no localized or rebound tenderness). Skin turgor may be decreased, and mucous membranes may be dry. A relative bradycardia, splenomegaly and a macular rash, or rose spots, are detectable in up to a third of patients with *Salmonella* infection.

- *Diagnostic testing.* Electrolyte abnormalities including hypo- or hypernatremia, hypokalemia, low serum bicarbonate levels, hypoglycemia, and an elevated blood urea nitrogen (BUN) level may occur depending on the degree of dehydration. Patients who are moderately to severely dehydrated (Chapter 80) or very young (<6 mos old) should have electrolytes drawn. Stool cultures should be obtained for bacterial pathogens in febrile or toxic children under 1 year of age, or in those with more than 5 WBCs per high power field (HPF) in their stool, presence of a hemoglobinopathy, bloody stools, or immunosuppression.

- *ED management.* A fluid deficit can be calculated. Oral (PO) or IV hydration should be given (see Chapter 80). Urinary output should be monitored. Antiemetics should be given for persistent emesis. Antibiotics should be not be given for presumed viral AGE or until *E. coli* 0157:H7 has been excluded (see Chapter 78, Hemolytic Uremic Syndrome).

- *Helpful hints and pitfalls.* Antidiarrheal agents are only indicated for unusually severe or prolonged cases of gastroenteritis, after excluding a cause that would respond to specific therapy.

Gastroesophageal Reflux Disease

- *Epidemiology and risk factors.* Approximately 50% of infants 0 to 3 months of age have at least one episode of reflux per day. Gastroesophageal reflux disease (GERD) spontaneously resolves in 55% of infants by age 10 months. Risk factors include prematurity, birth asphyxia, perinatal stress, and congenital GI anomalies.

- *Pathophysiology.* Occurs as a result of an incompetent lower esophageal sphincter, resulting in regurgitation of stomach contents into the esophagus.
- *History.* Infants generally present with nonbilious, nonprojectile emesis or "spitting up." Weight gain is appropriate. It may be associated with stereotyped opisthotonic movements known as Sandifer's syndrome. In this syndrome, children exhibit extension and stiffening of the arms and legs, extension of the head, and often a shrill or guttural cry. It may also be associated with a brief period of apnea and pallor as formula is refluxed into the esophagus.
- *Physical examination.* This is usually normal.
- *Diagnostic testing.* An upper GI is performed in recalcitrant cases to ensure that there is no anatomic obstruction to gastric emptying, such as a duodenal web or annular pancreas. Direct visualization via endoscopy, or recording the esophageal pH with a pH probe may help quantify the severity of reflux, but these tests are not performed in the ED.
- *ED management.* Assess dehydration, and observe feeding. If there is no associated apnea, pallor, stiffening or bilious emesis, most infants respond to conservative measures such as smaller feedings, frequent burping, thickening of formula with rice cereal (1 tsp cereal per ounce of formula), and maintaining a semi-upright position for 45 minutes to 1 hour after feeding. Pharmacologic regimens (ranitidine and metoclopramide) are reserved for more severe cases.
- *Helpful hints and pitfalls.* Reflux associated with weight loss, apnea, or Sandifer's syndrome necessitates consultation for further evaluation.

Henoch-Schönlein Purpura (HSP)

- *Epidemiology and risk factors.* Peak incidence between 4 and 11 years of age, although adults may also be affected. Up to 70% of patients with HSP have GI complaints. Prolonged renal impairment occurs in 25% of patients.
- *Pathophysiology.* This is a small-vessel vasculitis that mainly affects arterioles and capillaries. There is immune complex deposition involving immunoglobulin A (IgA), with antigens to drugs, infectious agents, foods, insect bites, and immunizations.
- *History.* Presenting symptoms include rash; arthralgias of the lower extremities, most commonly the ankles; hematuria; and GI complaints such as abdominal pain, scrotal pain, nausea, vomiting, and diarrhea, associated with blood and mucus per rectum. Nervous system involvement is rare.
- *Physical examination.* This typically reveals abdominal tenderness, scrotal edema, swollen and tender joints, and petechiae or palpable purpura on the buttocks and lower extremities.
- *Diagnostic testing.* Most are diagnosed clinically on the basis of the appearance of a classic rash, abdominal pain, microscopic hematuria, and mild arthralgias. Screening studies should include a CBC with differential count and platelets, urinalysis, blood culture, and sedimentation

med specialties

FM - broad knowledge
- challenge
- be part of community

PROG - 1:1 support - faculty advisors
- weekly
- procedure log
- evaluations
- electives
- rotate thro hospitals
- pt allocated - cont' care

GOOD POINTS - hard work,g
- team work
- persistent
- prioritize
- limits

MISTAKE - IV w/ K+

?/ longitudinal electives
?/ med student teaching
?/

Godi apu

rate. Children with severe abdominal pain require a CT scan to rule out intussusception.

- **■ *ED management.*** Treatment of the inciting infection, or discontinuation of the drug and supportive care is the mainstay of therapy. Prednisone at 1 mg/kg/d (60 mg daily in adults) orally may help severe cases. Admit patients who are ill-appearing with severe abdominal pain or vomiting.
- **■ *Helpful hints and pitfalls.*** The syndrome is often relapsing and remitting over several weeks, and may be associated with arthralgias. Meningococcemia should be considered in the differential. The child is typically more ill-appearing, and the treatment requires aggressive therapy with IV antibiotics.

Hirschsprung's Disease

- **■ *Epidemiology and risk factors.*** This congenital disease occurs in approximately 1 in 5000 live births. It occurs more frequently in males. There is an increased association with chromosomal abnormalities, including trisomy 21.
- **■ *Pathophysiology.*** There is an absence of intramural parasympathetic ganglion cells from the rectum to the sigmoid or proximal colon, due to incomplete neural crest cell migration. In the aganglionic segment, normal colonic relaxation does not occur, and dysmotility and spasm result in constipation or acute obstruction.
- **■ *History.*** There is often a failure to pass meconium within the first 24 to 48 hours of life. Some infants present after the newborn period with severe chronic constipation. Patients may also present in full-blown sepsis from enterocolitis, causing toxic megacolon, characterized by fever, bilious vomiting, explosive diarrhea, abdominal distention, and shock.
- **■ *Physical examination.*** This presents most commonly in the newborn with abdominal distension, tenderness, and sometimes bilious vomiting. An empty rectal vault may also be found in older children.
- **■ *Diagnostic testing.*** Plain films may show signs of obstruction with dilated loops of bowel and air-fluid levels. A barium enema may show the cone-shaped transition zone and dilated segment of the proximal colon and smaller distal segment. This study may be normal in cases of total aganglionosis. Suction rectal biopsy demonstrates an absence of ganglion cells in the rectal submucosa. Anal manometry may reveal increased intraluminal pressures.
- **■ *ED management.*** The patient should have nothing by mouth, a rectal tube should be inserted, and IV fluids should be started. Broad-spectrum antibiotics should be given early if enterocolitis is suspected. Surgery should be consulted in any patient with suspected Hirschsprung's disease.
- **■ *Helpful hints and pitfalls.*** Complete intestinal obstruction in Hirschsprung's disease is more likely to present in early infancy, and only rarely in older age groups.

Intussusception

- **■ *Epidemiology and risk factors.*** This is the most common cause of intestinal obstruction between 3 months and 6 years of age. Male infants are most commonly affected. In children younger than 5 years, a pathologic lead point is found in fewer than 10% of cases, and include hypertrophied Peyer's patches secondary to a viral infection, a polyp, ileal duplication, Meckle's diverticulum, lymphoma, and HSP.

- **Pathophysiology.** There is telescoping of a proximal limb of the intestine (the intussusceptum) into the adjacent distal intestine (intussuscipiens). It involves the terminal ileum in 90% of cases. The pathologic process of intussusception involves the compression of the invaginated mesentery, resulting in lymphatic obstruction, venous congestion with subsequent bowel wall swelling, mucus overproduction, and ischemia.

- **History.** The history often reveals a previously well-appearing child who suffers a sudden onset of episodic crampy or colicky pain, accompanied by screaming, flexed limbs and straining. Episodes of pain generally occur 10 to 20 minutes apart, and often last for several minutes. The infant may seem asymptomatic between episodes. These painful episodes gradually become more frequent, and are often accompanied by fever, irritability, lethargy, bilious emesis, dehydration, and hemoccult-positive (early) or currant-jelly stools (late). Parents may not appreciate the significance that the early episodes of pain and leg flexion may present, and the child may present to the ED as a "limp," unresponsive baby.

- **Physical examination.** This may reveal a soft, nontender abdomen early in the course of the illness, or a palpable, vertically oriented, sausage-shaped mass in the right upper quadrant. Currant-jelly stools are bloody, mucous-like stools that are usually not present until 12 hours after the onset of pain. They may pass after the child has become asymptomatic.

- **Diagnostic testing.** There are no laboratory tests that confirm the diagnosis, and in a sick child, therapy should not be delayed to obtain these studies. Flat and upright plain films may show a normal gas pattern early in the course of the illness, or with more advanced disease, signs of intestinal obstruction, including distended bowel with air-fluid levels proximal to the obstruction and a paucity of gas distally. The head of the intussusception may be seen as a soft-tissue mass (if seen head-on, it is called the target sign and if seen at 90 degrees, it is called the crescent sign). Free air may be seen in cases complicated by perforation. Air or barium contrast enema is the gold standard for diagnostic and therapeutic study. Classic signs are a cervix-like mass as the barium reaches the intussusception or a coiled-spring appearance on the evacuation film. Ultrasound is a useful study when an enema is contraindicated (for example, if there is free peritoneal air).

- **ED management.** The patient should have nothing by mouth, a nasogastric tube should be placed, and IV hydration started. Surgery should be consulted immediately, and an air/contrast enema performed (if there are no signs or symptoms of bowel perforation). Antibiotics covering bowel flora should be given in cases of perforation.

- **Helpful hints and pitfalls.** The classic triad of colicky abdominal pain, vomiting, and currant-jelly stools is present in only 21% of cases. Currant-jelly stools occur in only 50% of cases, and their absence does not exclude the diagnosis of intussusception.

Malrotation and Midgut Volvulus

- **Definitions.** *Malrotation* is an abnormal rotation of the bowel mesentery. *Volvulus* is a complete twisting of a loop of bowel about its mesenteric base of attachment. It is the most common and dangerous complication of malrotation in infants.
- **Epidemiology and risk factors.** The incidence is 1 in 500 live births. In the newborn period, there is a male predominance that disappears after 1 year of age. Associated congenital GI anomalies are found in up to 50% of cases.
- **Pathophysiology.** Abnormal rotation or inadequate fixation of the midgut results in obstruction of the blood supply from the superior mesenteric artery to the bowel, resulting in necrosis of the involved segment.
- **History.** It may present in different ways including sudden onset of bilious or bloody vomiting and bloody stools with no prior history of GI problems; the abrupt onset of bilious vomiting in a child who previously seemed to have feeding problems and finally; failure to thrive because of intolerance to feedings.
- **Physical examination.** Examination may reveal a rigid, discolored, diffusely tender abdomen. A dilated loop of bowel is sometimes palpated, but abdominal distention may be minimal if the obstruction is high, and the bowel is decompressed by vomiting. Blood from the rectum is an ominous sign, and indicates bowel ischemia.
- **Diagnostic testing.** Upright, flat plate, and cross-table lateral abdominal radiographs examinations may demonstrate a small-bowel obstruction, including air-fluid levels, a paucity of bowel gas distally, dilated loops overlying the liver shadow, and a markedly dilated duodenum and stomach. However, sometimes the radiographs may appear gasless or relatively normal despite serious pathology. An upper GI may reveal narrowing at the site of the obstruction, spiraling of the small bowel about the superior mesenteric artery, and a malrotated small intestine occupying the right side of the abdomen. Ultrasound may show duodenal distention, intraluminal fluid, and bowel edema. An air-contrast study may reveal a double bubble sign signifying gastric and duodenal dilatation. A CT scan and an MRI may be useful in equivocal cases to demonstrate the abnormal orientation of the mesenteric vessels inside the twisted pedicle.
- **ED management.** The patient should be given nothing by mouth. A nasogastric tube should be placed. IV fluids and antibiotics that cover bowel flora should be administered. Surgery should be consulted for emergent laparotomy.
- **Helpful hints and pitfalls.** Evaluation by a pediatric surgeon in unstable patients should not be delayed for confirmatory contrast studies. The upper GI series is the gold standard diagnostic study in stable patients.

Meckel's Diverticulum

- **Epidemiology and risk factors.** This is the most common congenital malformation of the small intestine and follows the "Rule of 2s." It occurs in 2% of the population but only 2% of affected patients ever become symptomatic. Approximately one half of all patients with the condition become symptomatic by age 2 years, and most present by the second decade (age 20). The diverticulum is 2 cm wide, 2 cm long, and usually located within 2 feet of the ileocecal valve.

- *Pathophysiology.* The diverticula contain bowel wall with heterotopic tissue; the most common is gastric mucosa. Bleeding occurs when acid secretion from ectopic gastric mucosa causes ulceration and erosion. Complications may include intussusception, obstruction, perforation, and peritonitis.
- *History.* Painless rectal bleeding and abdominal cramping may be present. The bleeding is often described as brick red in color.
- *Physical examination.* Mild abdominal tenderness may be present. The stool is bright red or contains occult blood.
- *Diagnostic testing.* A technetium scan, also known as a Meckel's scan, is the diagnostic modality of choice, and is very accurate when ectopic gastric mucosa is present. Definitive diagnosis is confirmed by laparoscopy or laparotomy.
- *ED management.* Children with minor bleeding and normal screening laboratory studies may be followed closely as outpatients. Children with more active bleeding should be admitted, and followed by either pediatric surgery or pediatric gastroenterology.
- *Helpful hints and pitfalls.* Patients are classically boys under the age of 5 who present with an acute onset of massive, painless rectal bleeding. GI bleeding in children is uncommon.

Necrotizing Enterocolitis

- *Epidemiology.* Necrotizing enterocolitis (NEC) is typically a disease of premature infants, and is the most common cause of intestinal perforation occurring during the newborn period.
- *Pathophysiology.* The exact mechanism is unknown. There is inflammation or injury to the intestinal wall, which begins in the mucosa and then extends transmurally.
- *History.* Feeding intolerance and emesis. Emesis may be either nonbilious or bilious; hematemesis may occur.
- *Physical examination.* The abdomen may be distended from dilatation of individual loops. Infants may appear ill with shock and hematochezia.
- *Diagnostic testing.* Early on, abdominal plain films may reveal dilated loops of bowel, which are a common but nonspecific finding. Intramural air (pneumatosis intestinalis) is more specific for NEC. Portal venous gas is present.
- *ED management.* Keep the patient on nothing by mouth, give IV fluid hydration, and decompress the stomach with a naso- or oro-gastric tube. Broad-spectrum triple antibiotic (ampicillin, gentamycin, and either clindamycin or metronidazole) therapy should be administered, and emergent consultation should be obtained from a pediatric surgeon. Patients with evidence of perforation, peritonitis, or gangrenous bowel require immediate surgical intervention.

- *Helpful hints and pitfalls.* This is typically a diagnosis made in the neonatal intensive care unit, but some patients with NEC may present acutely ill to the ED. Malrotation usually has a paucity of small bowel air, whereas NEC usually has diffusely dilated loops of small bowel.

Pyloric Stenosis, Infantile Hypertrophic

- *Epidemiology and risk factors.* This is the most common disorder requiring abdominal surgery in infancy, occurring in 1 in 250 births. Whites are affected more often than any other race. Boys are afflicted more frequently than girls. Firstborn boys are particularly prone.
- *Pathophysiology.* Elongation and thickening of the circular layer of the antral-pyloric muscle results in progressive gastric outlet obstruction.
- *History.* Usually presents as progressive, nonbilious, forceful or projectile vomiting associated with weight loss at around 3 weeks of age. Emesis occurs just after or near the end of a feeding. Afterwards the infant will refeed hungrily. Constipation may be present. The baby may become dehydrated.
- *Physical examination.* The presentation varies from well-appearing to lethargic, with signs of dehydration and recent weight loss. A gastric peristaltic wave passing from left to right across the upper abdomen just before the baby vomits, or a palpable olive-shaped mass (representing the hypertrophic pyloric muscle in the epigastrium) may be present.
- *Diagnostic testing.* Vomiting and profound fluid loss may cause electrolyte abnormalities, and a hypokalemic, hypochloremic metabolic alkalosis will develop. If the olive can be palpated, further imaging studies are unnecessary. Ultrasound demonstrates an increased pyloric diameter, a thickened muscle wall, and an elongated pyloric canal. When the ultrasound study is negative, but there is still a strong clinical probability, an upper GI study should be obtained. It reveals delayed gastric emptying, indentation of the antrum by the olive, and elongation and narrowing of the pyloric channel (the string sign). Endoscopy may prove the diagnosis in younger infants, but is rarely necessary.
- *ED management.* The patient should have nothing by mouth. Surgery should be consulted for a pyloromyotomy, IV hydration should be initiated, and electrolyte abnormalities should be treated.
- *Helpful hints and pitfalls.* Many disorders produce vomiting, but GERD is the one that is most often confused with pyloric stenosis. In contrast to pyloric stenosis, GERD can occur earlier in life, is usually not severe, and does not tend to be as characteristically progressive.

Inflammatory Bowel Disease

- Inflammatory bowel disease is discussed in Chapter 27.

> ### Teaching Points
>
> Abdominal pain has a myriad of causes, many of which are age related. For example, congenital anomalies produce disease at an early age, whereas appendicitis is more often seen in children older than 5 years. It can occur in younger children, but because of the difficulties in obtaining histories from these youngsters, it often presents with the appendix already ruptured.
>
> Many adult gastrointestinal tract entities can occur in children, and are often overlooked because they are thought to be adult problems only. For example, pancreatitis is highly associated with nonaccidental trauma, and should be investigated in all children with pancreatitis.

Suggested Readings

Halter J. Common gastrointestinal problems and emergencies in neonates and children. Clin Fam Pract 2004;6:731.

Hostetler MA. Gastrointestinal disorders. In: Marx JA, Hockberger RS, Walls RM (editors). Rosen's Emergency Medicine: Concepts and Clinical Practice (6th ed). Philadelphia: Mosby, 2006, pp 2601–2623.

McCollough M, Sharieff G. Abdominal surgical emergencies in infants and young children. Emerg Med Clin North Am 2003;21:909–935.

CHAPTER **78**

Pediatric Jaundice

KHARY HARMON ▪ **STEVEN RILEY**

Overview

Jaundice is a yellowish discoloration of the tissues and body fluids, resulting from an excessive amount of bilirubin. Bilirubin is formed from the breakdown of hemoglobin. Unconjugated bilirubin binds to albumin in the blood, and is carried to the liver where it is conjugated by glucuronyl transferase and excreted into bile.

Jaundice develops from excessive production of bilirubin or diminished ability to metabolize or excrete bilirubin. Jaundice may be caused by increased amounts of either unconjugated (indirect) or conjugated (direct) bilirubin, and becomes clinically apparent when bilirubin levels reach 5 mg/dl. See Table 78–1 for examples of each. Some disease entities that cause pediatric jaundice may also present in the adult patient (see Chapter 41).

Every newborn with jaundice should have a total and direct bilirubin level checked, as well as a blood type and direct Coomb's test. A Coomb's test is a direct antiglobulin test (DAT) that can be used to detect immunoglobulin attached to the red cell surface. A positive test suggests an autoantibody or alloantibody may be responsible for the anemia. Other tests to obtain include a complete blood count (CBC), peripheral smear, reticulocyte count, and a glucose-6-phosphate dehydrogenase (G6PD) level (depending on ethnic origin). If a hemoglobinopathy is suspected, hemoglobin electrophoresis should be obtained. Newborn screen results should be checked, as well as urinary reducing substances (galactosemia), and thyroid function tests. In an ill infant, blood cultures, urine culture, and cerebrospinal fluid (CSF) studies should be obtained. If the direct bilirubin is elevated in infants older than 3 weeks, evaluate for causes of cholestasis. If the total serum bilirubin does not decrease or continues to rise in an infant who is receiving intensive phototherapy, this strongly suggests the presence of hemolysis. Indications for further evaluation of jaundiced infants are listed in Box 78–1.

The differential diagnosis of jaundice in a newborn is uniquely different from the remainder of the pediatric population. Neonatal jaundice is a frequent presenting complaint to the ED. Distinguish between physiologic and pathologic jaundice in this population. Direct hyperbilirubinemia in infants is always pathologic, and requires a detailed workup. High levels of bilirubin are neurotoxic, and may cause encephalopathy and the development of kernicterus. The preponderance of kernicterus cases occur in infants with high bilirubin (more than 20 mg/dl). Kernicterus, or bilirubin encephalopathy, is a potentially fatal condition caused by bilirubin toxicity to the basal ganglia and various brainstem nuclei.

Most cases of unconjugated hyperbilirubinemia in older children and adolescents are due to a hemolytic disorder.

This chapter will briefly discuss selected problems that may present with jaundice in the pediatric patient.

Special Problems
ABO-Rh Incompatibility

■ *Epidemiology and risk factors.* ABO incompatibility occurs in approximately 12% of pregnancies with evidence of fetal sensitization in 3% of live births. Rh isoimmunization tends to produce hemolysis after the first pregnancy with an Rh-positive fetus. Rh isoimmunization generally produces more severe hemolysis than ABO incompatibility. Hemolytic disease is present in only 3% of patients with ABO incompatibility.

■ *Pathophysiology.* Although theoretically a closed system, mixing of maternal and fetal blood occurs. The mother develops antibodies against

Table 78–1   Causes of Jaundice in an Infant and Children

	Etiology	Example
Unconjugated	Physiologic	Physiologic jaundice of the newborn; breast milk jaundice
	Hemolysis	ABO incompatibility Physiologic breakdown of birth trauma hematomas Sickle cell anemia Spherocytosis Pyruvate kinase deficiency Thalassemia Glucose-6-phosphate dehydrogenase deficiency Microangiopathic hemolytic anemia
	Infection	Urinary tract infection Sepsis TORCHS infections (toxoplasmosis, rubella, cytomegalovirus, herpes, syphilis)
	Obstructive	Duodenal atresia Hirschsprung's disease Meconium ileus Pyloric stenosis
	Metabolic	Galactosemia Gilbert's syndrome Crigler-Najjar syndrome Congenital hypothyroidism
Conjugated	Infection	Urinary tract infection Sepsis TORCHS infections Hepatitis
	Obstructive	Biliary atresia, bile duct strictures, gallstones
	Metabolic	Galactosemia, neonatal hypopituitarism, glycogen storage disease
	Other	Cirrhosis Drugs (acetaminophen)

an antigen on fetal red blood cells. This can occur in an Rh-negative mother and Rh-positive fetus, or a blood type O mother and a blood type A, B, or AB fetus. The antibodies formed cross the placenta, and bind to the specific antigen on the fetal red blood cells, thereby destroying them.

- *History.* Jaundice is often apparent before hospital discharge. The patient may be asymptomatic or have lethargy, irritability, and poor feeding. It may be difficult to differentiate historically from breast-feeding jaundice.
- *Physical examination.* It is impossible to accurately assess the true bilirubin level by visual estimation. The infant usually appears jaundiced.

BOX 78–1   Indications for Further Evaluation in Jaundiced Infants

- Jaundice appearing within 24 hours of birth.
- All conjugated hyperbilirubinemias.
- Rapidly rising total serum bilirubin unexplained by history or physical examination.
- Total serum bilirubin approaching exchange level or not responding to phototherapy.
- Jaundice persisting longer than age 3 weeks.
- Sick-appearing infant.

(From Hostetler MA. Gastrointestinal disorders. In: Marx JA, Hockberger RS, Walls RM [editors]. Rosen's Emergency Medicine: Concepts and Clinical Practice [6th ed]. Philadelphia: Mosby, 2006, pp 2601–2623.)

Table 78–2   Management of Hyperbilirubinemia in the Healthy Term Newborn

	TSB Level, mg/dl (pmol/L)			
Age, h	Consider Phototherapy*	Phototherapy	Exchange Transfusion if Intensive Photo-therapy Fails†	Exchange and Transfusion Intensive Phototherapy
≤24‡	—	—	—	—
25-48	≥12 (210)	≥15 (260)	≥20 (340)	≥25 (430)
49-72	≥15 (260)	≥18 (310)	≥25 (430)	≥30 (510)
>72	≥17 (290)	≥20 (340)	≥25 (430)	≥30 (510)

From Subcommittee on Hyperbilirubinemia. Management of hyperbilirubinemia in the newborn infant 35 or more weeks of gestation. Pediatrics 2004;114:297–316.

TSB, total serum bilirubin.

*Phototherapy at these TSB levels is a clinical option, meaning that the intervention is available and may be used on the basis of individual clinical judgment.

†Intensive phototherapy should produce a decline of TSB of 1 to 2 mg/dl within 4-6 hours, and the TSB level should continue to fall and remain below the threshold level for exchange transfusion. If this does not occur, it is considered a failure of phototherapy.

‡Term infants who are clinically jaundiced at 24 hours old or less.

If dehydrated, one will observe tachycardia and poor skin turgor. Acute bilirubin encephalopathy may cause hypertonia, retrocollis, opisthotonus, and a shrill cry.

- **Diagnostic testing.** Total and conjugated bilirubin, infant's blood type, and direct Coomb's test should be measured. It is helpful to know the mother's blood type. Other laboratory tests include a CBC, peripheral smear, and reticulocyte count.

- **ED management.** The goal of management is to prevent acute bilirubin encephalopathy and kernicterus (Table 78–2). Exchange transfusion is only required in fewer than 0.1 %. The patient should be admitted or transferred to a pediatric intensive care unit if an exchange transfusion is indicated. IV fluids should be started if the patient is dehydrated.

■ *Helpful hints and pitfalls.* If there is a positive Coomb's test, ABO or Rh incompatibility is a likely cause for the jaundice. Most other causes of hemolysis will be Coomb's negative.

Biliary Tract Disease

■ See Chapters 18 and 77.

Breast-Feeding Jaundice

■ *Epidemiology and risk factors.* This entity occurs in 5% to 10% of breast-fed infants.

■ *Pathophysiology.* Breastfeeding jaundice is caused by insufficient breast milk intake secondary to poor lactation, late milk production, or ineffective feeding. Poor feeding leads to decreased caloric intake, dehydration, and increased enterohepatic circulation of bilirubin.

■ *History.* Jaundice starts at 2 to 3 days of life, and peaks at approximately 1 to 2 weeks. Patients often have a decreased urinary output and number of stools.

■ *Physical examination.* All patients have jaundice; some may have tachycardia and poor skin turgor if dehydrated. The physical examination is otherwise normal for a newborn.

■ *Diagnostic testing.* Total and conjugated bilirubin, infant's blood type, and a direct Coomb's test should be obtained to rule out ABO/Rh incompatibility. It is helpful to know the mother's blood type.

■ *ED management.* Frequent breast feeding should be encouraged. If the infant appears dehydrated, the diet should be supplemented with formula, and breast feeding should be continued. The mother should be encouraged to follow-up with a lactation specialist. Phototherapy may be required (Table 78–2).

■ *Helpful hints and pitfalls.* Make certain ABO/Rh incompatibility or another pathological process is not the etiology of the jaundice.

Breast Milk Jaundice

■ *Epidemiology and risk factors.* Occurs in 1% to 2% of breast-fed infants.

■ *Pathophysiology.* Different causes have been hypothesized. Substances in breast milk may competitively inhibit glucuronyltransferase enzyme, thereby decreasing bilirubin conjugation.

■ *History.* Jaundice develops at 4 to 7 days of life, and lasts for 3 to 10 weeks. The infant should otherwise be healthy.

■ *Physical examination.* The examination usually reveals jaundice, with an otherwise normal examination.

■ *Diagnostic testing.* Total and conjugated bilirubin should be obtained.

■ *ED management.* The mother should be encouraged to continue breast feeding. She may need to alternate breast feeding with formula feedings until the bilirubin level begins to decline. This type of jaundice usually does not require phototherapy.

- *Helpful hints and pitfalls.* Inform the parents of the potential duration of jaundice, and emphasize the importance of follow-up with the infant's pediatrician.

Congenital Hypothyroidism

- *Epidemiology and risk factors.* The incidence of congenital hypo-thyroidism based on newborn screening is 1/4000. Most cases are sporadic. Maternal history of a thyroid disorder, and the mode of treatment should be ascertained.
- *Pathophysiology.* This disorder is most commonly caused by a deficiency in the formation or the migration of thyroid tissue or an inborn error in thyroid hormone metabolism.
- *History.* There may be few clinical manifestations in the first month of life. Signs and symptoms often include decreased activity, poor feeding, jaundice, and constipation.
- *Physical examination.* Physical findings may or may not be present at birth. Findings include enlarged tongue, coarse facies, hoarse cry, a large fontanelle, and an umbilical hernia. Prolonged jaundice is common.
- *Diagnostic testing.* Total or free T_4 and a thyroid-stimulating hormone (TSH) level help confirm the diagnosis. A low total or free T_4 and elevated TSH are diagnostic of hypothyroidism. Congenital hypo-thyroidism is part of the newborn screen in the United States.
- *ED management.* Consultation with a pediatric endocrinologist is important to assist in the proper treatment with thyroid hormone.
- *Helpful hints and pitfalls.* Prompt diagnosis is important. The affected patient's resulting IQ is lower with a delay in treatment.

Crigler-Najjar Syndrome

- See Chapter 41.

Galactosemia

- *Epidemiology and risk factors.* The incidence of galactosemia is 1/60,000. This is the most common error of carbohydrate metabolism. It is part of the newborn screen, but severely affected individuals often have symptoms before screening results are complete.
- *Pathophysiology.* Galactosemia is caused by a mutation in the galactose-1-phosphate uridyltransferase gene that inhibits the ability to convert galactose, formed from the breakdown of lactose, to glucose. Galactose accumulates in and damages tissues including the brain, eyes, kidneys, and liver.
- *History.* Patients often have vomiting, failure to thrive, hepatomegaly and jaundice, which occur days after exposure to lactose. Hypoglycemia and seizures can occur.
- *Physical examination.* Failure to thrive, dehydration, jaundice, hepatomegaly, and cataracts may be present.
- *Diagnostic testing.* Urinalysis should be sent to test for reducing sub-stances. Definitive testing requires enzyme deficiency screening assays.

- **ED management.** Treat dehydration (Chapter 80). Hypoglycemia should be treated with 2 to 4 ml/kg of 25% dextrose. Management involves complete exclusion of galactose from the patient's diet using lactose-free formula.
- **Helpful hints and pitfalls.** Galactosemia confers increased risk of gram-negative sepsis.

Gilbert's Syndrome

- See Chapter 41.

Glucose-6-Phosphate Dehydrogenase Deficiency

- **Epidemiology and risk factors.** This is an X-linked recessive disorder that affects males primarily. There is a greater prevalence in those of African and Mediterranean ancestry. Infections and medications such as antimalarials and sulfonamides can precipitate hemolysis. The severity of hemolysis depends on the degree of enzyme deficiency.
- **Pathophysiology.** G6PD helps maintain reduced glutathione within red blood cells. Reduced glutathione helps protect red blood cells against oxidative stress. If G6PD is absent or reduced within the red blood cells, oxidative stress causes hemoglobin to denature and red blood cells are lysed.
- **History.** Ethnicity is important in prompting G6PD deficiency as a part of the differential diagnosis. There is a wide spectrum of disease manifestation based on the degree of enzyme deficiency. It most commonly presents as an acute onset of jaundice and pallor. It can present at any age, including the newborn period. Individuals with mild enzyme deficiency may be largely asymptomatic.
- **Physical examination.** Tachycardia, pallor, and jaundice due to hemolytic anemia may be present. Splenomegaly may be present.
- **Diagnostic testing.** Obtain a CBC and peripheral smear and lactate dehydrogenase, haptoglobin, reticulocyte count, total, and conjugated bilirubin levels. The G6PD assay may be normal if obtained during the acute hemolytic event, as reticulocytes and younger red blood cells may have a higher level of enzyme present.
- **ED management.** Treat dehydration (Chapter 80). For symptomatic anemia, 10 ml/kg of packed red blood cells should be given. Neonates may require phototherapy and exchange transfusions. Obtain consultation with a neonatologist. Do not forget to attempt identification of the precipitating factor.
- **Helpful hints and pitfalls.** Ethnicity and family history assists in making the diagnosis.

Hemolytic Uremic Syndrome (HUS)

- **Epidemiology and risk factors.** This syndrome consists of a microangiopathic hemolytic anemia, thrombocytopenia, and acute renal failure. It is the most common cause of acute renal failure in children. The mean age of presentation is 3 years. The most common offending agent is an exotoxin produced by *E. Coli* 0157:H7. Other causes include *Shigella* organisms, *S. pneumoniae*, HIV, and drugs.

- **Pathophysiology.** In the case of *E. Coli* 0157:H7, the toxin enters the systemic circulation and damages endothelial cells, particularly in the kidney. Thrombi develop as a result of endothelial cell damage. Red blood cells passing through the injured vessels are damaged resulting in hemolysis. Thrombocytopenia also occurs as a result of vessel injury.
- **History.** A previously healthy child develops abdominal pain and diarrhea that subsequently becomes bloody. After several days, the child develops pallor, fatigue, oliguria or anuria. Neurologic symptoms occur in 20% to 30% of affected individuals.
- **Physical examination.** Vital signs may demonstrate fever and tachycardia. Hypertension is present in approximately 50% of patients with HUS. The patient may appear pale, dehydrated, and have abdominal tenderness. Jaundice is variably present. Petechiae may be present if there is significant thrombocytopenia.
- **Diagnostic studies.** A CBC will show normal or elevated white blood count, anemia, and thrombocytopenia. Schistocyte, helmet, and burr cells are often found on a peripheral smear. There is often an elevated total and unconjugated bilirubin, elevated lactate dehydrogenase, and low haptoglobin levels due to hemolysis. A negative Coomb's test suggests hemolysis that is not immune mediated. A basic metabolic profile shows metabolic acidosis, and an elevated potassium, BUN, and creatinine. Hematuria and proteinuria are usually present unless the patient is anuric.
- **ED management.** Treatment is primarily supportive. Aggressive hydration should be avoided due to concomitant renal failure. Treatment of hypertension should commence (e.g., calcium channel blockers or labetolol). Obtain consultation with a pediatric nephrologist. Packed red blood (5 mg/kg over 4 hours) cell transfusion may be necessary for symptomatic anemia (hemoglobin <6 g/dL). Dialysis is indicated for BUN above 100, volume overload, or severe hyperkalemia. Benzodiazepines and phenytoin should be used for seizures. Treatment of the colitis is supportive because antimotility agents may lead to toxic megacolon. Antibiotics may enhance the release of exotoxin from the bacteria and, therefore, should be avoided.

Sickle Cell Anemia

- See Chapter 53.

Teaching Points

Jaundice is a frequent occurrence in the newborn. Although usually detected before discharge from the delivery suite, it may present initially in the ED. One cannot predict an accurate level of bilirubin from observation alone, therefore it is necessary to obtain serum levels of both direct and indirect bilirubins.

Continued

> ### Teaching Points—cont'd
>
> If the jaundice is due to an underlying metabolic defect, it is often accompanied by hypoglycemia, therefore it is prudent to obtain a finger-stick or heel-stick glucose level early in the patient's course.
>
> Hemolysis is another common cause of hyperbilirubinemia, and may be the clue to underlying hemolytic disease such as sickle cell disease. Most of these children will require admission to an intensive care unit.

Suggested Readings

Claudius I, Fluharty C, Boles R. The emergency department approach to newborn and childhood metabolic crisis. Emerg Med Clin North Am 2005;23:843–883.

Hostetler MA. Gastrointestinal disorders. In: Marx JA, Hockberger RS, Walls RM (editors). Rosen's Emergency Medicine: Concepts and Clinical Practice (6th ed). Philadelphia: Mosby, 2006, pp 2601–2623.

Stanley I, Chung M, Kulig J. An Evidence-Based Review of Important Issues Concerning Neonatal Hyperbilirubinemia. Pediatrics 2004;114:e130–e153.

Subcommittee on Hyperbilirubinemia. Management of hyperbilirubinemia in the newborn infant 35 or more weeks of gestation. Pediatrics 2004;114;297–316.

CHAPTER 79

Pediatric Fever

ADAM Z. BARKIN ■ ANDREW J. CAPRARO

Overview

Febrile children can be challenging patients to evaluate and treat in the ED. Most febrile children have benign, self-limited illnesses that can be treated with supportive care such as hydration and antipyretics. Nevertheless, some diseases present with fever that will be life-threatening if not recognized and treated immediately (see Chapter 67 for meningitis and Chapter 76 for pneumonia).

Young children present unique challenges, because they are often unable to communicate with their parents or physician. The history and physical examination are often nonspecific, and usually require parental participation.

Evaluation of pediatric fever generally varies by age group: neonates aged 0-28 days, infants 29-90 days, infants and children 3 to 36 months, children 4 to 7 years, and children and adolescents 8 to 18 years of age. Fever in normal infants and toddlers is defined as rectal temperature of 38° C (100.4° F) or higher. During the first 3 months of life, any fever will have great clinical importance.

Most cases of fever are due to underlying infection. In young infants, serious bacterial infection may exist despite normal clinical findings. These children have a less developed immune system compared to older children. Critical diagnoses to be evaluated for in the ED include occult bacteremia, sepsis syndrome, and meningitis (Chapter 67). Kawasaki's disease is a concerning cause of fever in the pediatric population, and will be briefly mentioned here. Other concerning causes of fever in children include upper respiratory infection and pneumonia (see Chapter 76), appendicitis and gastroenteritis (see Chapter 77), heat-related illness (see Chapter 65), and otitis media (see Chapter 64).

Febrile seizures are an occasional consequence of high fever in the pediatric population, and will be briefly discussed in this chapter.

This chapter will discuss the general approach to the febrile pediatric patient. Selected problems unique to this population will be reviewed.

Initial Diagnostic Approach
General

- Any patient who appears toxic, is in respiratory distress, has an altered mental status, or other concerning clinical finding (a petechial rash of meningococcemia) should receive immediate attention. Continuous cardiac monitoring, pulse oximetry, and intravenous (IV) access should be obtained. However, take caution to not worsen a precarious situation. For example, if epiglottitis is suspected, IV access should be delayed until preparations are made for securing the airway (see Chapter 74).
- Certain aspects of the history are crucial when approaching a child who cannot provide a thorough history. These include the degree of fever, how the temperature was obtained (oral, rectal, tympanic, subjective), treatment for the fever, localizing symptoms (cough, congestion, pulling or rubbing ears), rashes, hydration status (fluid intake, stool and urine output), behavior change, activity level, sick contacts or travel, immunization status (see Chapter 73), medical history, and underlying medical illnesses. In the newborn period, key historical elements of the birth history are important, including prematurity, perinatal maternal fever, mother's group B strep and herpes status, the length of time the amniotic membranes were ruptured before delivery, and fluid intake.
- Whenever there is concern for a fever, a rectal temperature should be performed, especially in infants and toddlers. A tympanic temperature is unfortunately not reliable. It would appear to be easy to obtain, but in children in particular, it is often difficult to get an accurate otic temperature measurement.

Laboratory

- Depending on the age of the child and the presenting signs and symptoms, different laboratory tests may be indicated. These tests include a complete blood count (CBC), blood cultures, urinalysis and urine culture, cerebrospinal fluid (CSF) evaluation, and stool examination.
- High (>15,000/mm³) or low (<5000/mm³) white blood cell (WBC) counts may indicate serious disease. An increased proportion of polymorphonuclear (PMN) leukocytes and bands (immature forms) or a *left shift* occurs more commonly with bacterial illness but may be present early on in viral disease. There is typically a predominance of lymphocytes and monocytes (right shift) in viral illness. Toxic granulations and vacuolizations of PMN leukocytes correlate with bacterial illness.
- An erythrocyte sedimentation rate (ESR) is elevated in localized bacterial infections and inflammatory disease, but may occasionally be elevated in illness due to viral disease.
- Blood cultures for aerobic and anaerobic organisms should be obtained in any patient suspected of having bacteremia.
- Urine cultures should be obtained from all febrile boys younger than 6 months, and all acutely febrile girls under 2 years of age who are to be treated with antibiotics. The presence of a documented urinary tract infection (UTI) in these patients mandates a subsequent radiographic evaluation of the genitourinary tract to exclude anomalies and reflux. The urinalysis may be normal in the presence of infection especially in infants who may not be able to mount a pyuric response. Thus a culture should always be sent regardless of urinalysis results in these patients. A Gram's stain of the urine sediment is the most sensitive screening test (99%). In addition, urine collection should precede the other invasive steps of the fever workup in an infant as noxious stimuli will often cause the baby to void.
- A disseminated intravascular coagulation (DIC) panel should be performed if there are petechiae or other bleeding diasthesis because DIC is a common complication of meningococcemia. This includes fibrinogen, fibrin split products, d-dimer, prothrombin time, partial thromboplastin time, and platelets.
- Fecal leukocytes are concerning for bacterial infection. A stool culture should be sent if blood or white cells are noted in the stool sample of a febrile child to rule out *Shigella*, *Salmonella*, *Campylobacter*, toxigenic *Escherichia coli*, and *Yersinia* species.

Radiography

- ***Plain films.*** A chest radiograph is indicated if the patient has respiratory symptoms, and is often part of the evaluation of a child with fever of unknown etiology. In young children, pneumonia may be present in absence of any physical examination findings. Chest radiography should be considered a routine diagnostic test in children with a temperature of 39° C or greater, and WBC count of 20,000/mm³ or greater without an alternative major source of infection.

- *Ultrasound.* An ultrasound study may be indicated if there is suspicion for appendicitis or another intra-abdominal process. It may also be useful in the initial evaluation of a child with a documented urinary tract infection to rule out obstruction, hydronephrosis, or abscess.
- *Computed tomography (CT scan).* A CT scan may be indicated if there is concern for appendicitis or other intra-abdominal process. A head CT scan may be helpful in the patient with altered mental status and evidence of an intracranial infection, as well as febrile patients with a full anterior fontanelle.

Emergency Department Management Overview
General

- Very young infants and ill-appearing older children require aggressive management. Oxygen should be administered to all febrile children who are toxic appearing, those in respiratory distress, and children with a pulse oximetry of less than 95%.

Medications

- *Antipyretics.* All febrile children should be treated initially with anti-pyretics. Preferred choices are acetaminophen (15 mg/kg) or ibuprofen (10 mg/kg), which may be given sequentially or concurrently. Avoid aspirin in the febrile children due to the risk for Reye's syndrome (encephalopathy, fatty liver degeneration, and transaminase elevation).
- *Analgesia.* Analgesia should be administered as needed for pain. Acetaminophen and ibuprofen should be initially used in the rectal or oral form.
- *Antibiotics.* Antibiotics should be initiated empirically in any febrile child who is toxic, or who is on the verge of cardiopulmonary compromise. Antibiotics should also be used to treat identified infections or suspected occult bacteremia. Ideally, this is initiated after cultures are obtained.

Emergency Department Interventions

- *Urinary catheter.* Urinary catheterization may be indicated to obtain urine for testing. Clinicians may need to monitor urine output as an indi-cation of hydration status, which may be done by an indwelling catheter or a urine bag, depending on the circumstances. A urine specimen may also be useful in evaluating hydration status by assessing the specific gravity.

Disposition

- *Consultation.* Consultation with pediatric hospitalists/intensivists, surgeons, or infectious disease specialists may be required.
- *Admission.* Depending on the clinical presentation of the febrile child, admission may be required. In all infants less than 1 month of age, admission is mandated for any fever.

- **Discharge.** Febrile children who are nontoxic appearing may be safely discharged if follow-up with a pediatrician is assured in the next 24 hours or sooner as indicated.

Specific Problems
Febrile Seizure

- **Epidemiology and risk factors.** Febrile seizures are defined as seizures that occur in children with fever aged 6 months to 5 years, not associated with evidence of intracranial infection or other CNS disease. Febrile seizures occur in 2% to 5% of all children, and account for about 30% of all seizures in children. Simple febrile seizures are self-limited, lasting no longer than 15 minutes, are generalized, tonic–clonic, and do not recur within 24 hours. Complex (atypical) febrile seizures are described as lasting more than 15 minutes, are focal or recur within 24 hours. There is a genetic component to febrile seizures. A sibling of a child with a history of febrile seizures has 3.5 times increased risk of having a febrile seizure.
- **Pathophysiology.** The etiology of febrile seizures is unknown.
- **History.** Important historical information includes onset of the seizure (when, where, associated trauma or ingestions), type of seizure (tonic–clonic, myoclonic, generalized, focal), duration of seizure, recent illness, recent immunizations, sick contacts, medical history, previous neurologic and developmental status, medications, and any family history of seizures.
- **Physical examination.** The physical examination should be complete with emphasis on the neurologic examination. In infants, a neurologic examination includes examining the child's muscle tone, whether the eyes track, movement of extremities, deep tendon reflexes, and inter-action with parents and health care providers. Older children should have motor, sensation, reflexes, and cerebellar examinations. Gait is an important component of the neurologic examination in children old enough to walk. Parents serve as excellent resources in telling the provider when gait, interactivity or another component of the neurologic examination differs from baseline.
- **Diagnostic testing.** An LP should be performed in infants under 12 months of age with a first febrile seizure. Most children over 12 to 18 months of age who have brief, generalized convulsions, and who appear playful and nontoxic after the postictal period can be treated without an LP. If a child greater than 18 months of age has a tonic–clonic, general-ized single seizure in the setting of a fever and a normal neurologic examination, generally there is no diagnostic testing required beyond those appropriate to determine the source of the infection. Remember that a febrile seizure is generally caused by a febrile illness, and the same diagnostic strategies discussed above regarding febrile children apply to children with febrile seizures. A head CT scan should be performed in children with focal seizures, prolonged seizures, or if there is concern for intracranial injury secondary to trauma (especially nonaccidental).
- **ED management.** Initial management of a febrile seizure should be directed at protecting the child's airway. Often, the seizure has stopped

by the time the child arrives in the ED. Fever control should be aggressively initiated. The child is often postictal, and may be obstructing the airway with a large tongue or tonsils. A jaw–thrust or head tilt–chin lift maneuver should be performed to open an obstructed airway. If vomiting is imminent or occurring, place the child in the lateral decubitus position to prevent aspiration. If the patient is still seizing, airway and breathing need to be stabilized, followed by consideration of administration of anticonvulsant agents.

- *Helpful hints and pitfalls.* If the child is toxic appearing, and there is concern for serious bacterial infection or meningitis, do not delay the administration of antibiotics. A child with a febrile seizure has an approximately 1% increased risk of developing epilepsy versus the general population.

Kawasaki's Disease (Mucocutaneous Lymph Node Syndrome)

- *Epidemiology.* Eighty percent of patients are younger than 5 years old, but occasionally teenagers and adults are affected. Asians are at highest risk, but the disease can occur in any ethnic group. Approximately 20% of untreated patients develop coronary artery abnormalities such as aneurysms, coronary artery thrombosis, and myocardial infarction. Other cardiac complications include pericarditis and myocarditis.
- *Pathophysiology.* The cause remains unknown but appears to be infectious in origin. The disease causes a severe vasculitis of all blood vessels, but predominantly affects medium-sized arteries with a predilection for the coronary arteries.
- *History.* There is a history of prolonged high spiking fevers (to 40° C or greater).
- *Physical examination.* Characteristic findings include high fever, bilateral conjunctival irritation usually without exudates, erythema of the oral and pharyngeal mucosa with "strawberry tongue," dry and cracked lips, erythema and swelling of the hands and feet, a polymorphous rash (maculopapular, erythema multiforme), and a unilateral nonsuppurative cervical lymphadenopathy (>1.5 cm). There may be perineal and periungal desquamation. The child may be irritable from other less common features of the disease such as aseptic meningitis, diarrhea, mild hepatitis, hydrops of the gallbladder, urethritis and meatitis with sterile pyuria, otitis media, and arthritis. Tachycardia out of proportion to fever (14 beats/min increase for each degree centigrade increase in fever) is concerning for myocarditis. Pericarditis may manifest as muffled heart sounds and a friction rub.
- *Diagnostic testing.* The diagnosis of Kawasaki's disease is based on demonstration of characteristic clinical signs (Box 79–1). Atypical or incomplete cases in which a patient has fever with fewer than four other features of the illness, and then develops coronary artery disease, have been described worldwide. They are most frequent in infants, who unfortunately have the highest probability of developing coronary artery disease. No specific diagnostic test for Kawasaki's disease exists, but certain laboratory findings are characteristic. The WBC count is normal to elevated, with a predominance of neutrophils and immature forms.

BOX 79-1   Diagnostic Criteria of Kawasaki's Syndrome

Fever above 38.5° C for at least 5 days AND the presence of FOUR of the following:

- Changes in the extremities (edema, erythema, desquamation of hands and feet)
- Rash (polymorphous exanthema)
- Conjunctival injection, bilateral
- Changes in mucosa of the oropharynx, including injected pharynx, cracked lips, strawberry tongue
- Cervical lymphadenopathy >1.5 cm, usually unilateral

The illness should not be explained by another known disease process.

Elevated ESR, C-reactive protein, and other acute-phase reactants are almost universally present in the acute phase of illness, and may persist for 4-6 weeks. A normocytic anemia is common. The platelet count is generally normal in the first week of illness, and rapidly increases by the second to third weeks of illness, sometimes exceeding 1,000,000/mm^3. Sterile pyuria, mildly elevated transaminases, and CSF pleocytosis may be present. Echocardiography and angiography are used to evaluate for cardiac abnormalities. In the presence of this diagnosis, it is prudent to obtain consultation with a pediatric cardiologist.

- ***ED management.*** Treatment is with IV immunoglobulin 2 g/kg over 10 to 12 hours, and with aspirin 80 to 100 mg/kg per 24-hour period divided every 6 hours orally until day 14 of illness. All patients should be admitted to an ICU.
- ***Helpful hints and pitfalls.*** Treatment should be initiated as soon as the diagnosis is suspected.

Occult Bacteremia/Sepsis

- ***Epidemiology and risk factors.*** Children are at risk for serious bacterial infections in the neonatal period because their immune system is not fully developed. Infants born prematurely, and those with congenital heart defects or other congenital defects, are at particular risk for serious infection. Children undergo a series of immunizations to specific diseases during their first 5 years of life to provide protection; susceptibility exists until the series are completed. The number of serious bacterial infections among infants has declined with the introduction of new vaccinations. The *S. pneumococcus* (Prevnar) and Hib vaccines have substantially decreased the incidence of these bacterial infections. Depending on the age of the child, different bacteria are most prevalent. In infants 0 to 28 days old, group B streptococcus, *Listeria monocytogenes*, *E. coli*, *H. influenza*, *S. pneumococcus* and *Chlamydia* are most common. Children older than 28 days are susceptible to *S. pneumococcus*, *H. influenza*, and *N. meningitidis*.

- ■ *Pathophysiology.* Bacteremia is defined as the presence of bacteria within the circulating bloodstream. Bacteremia along with any other infection can trigger a systemic inflammatory response. This progresses to severe sepsis when there is evidence of end-organ dysfunction. Septic shock occurs when hypotension is not responsive to fluid resuscitation. The final pathway is multi-organ dysfunction syndrome (MODS) when more than one organ system fails. Secondary to the immature immune system in the neonate, localized infections can easily spread, and lead to serious bacterial infections and sepsis. As a result, the febrile neonate requires close monitoring and workups as discussed.
- ■ *History.* A thorough history is useful. Patients may have a decreased level of activity, altered behavior, poor fluid intake, decreased urine output, as well as rashes, vomiting, diarrhea, headache, abdominal pain, cough, and many other nonspecific symptoms. Birth history should be obtained on the febrile neonate.
- ■ *Physical examination.* Depending on the age of the child, the norms of heart rate, respiratory rate, and blood pressure vary (Chapter 73). Abnormalities in heart rate beyond those anticipated with an elevated temperature often indicate a systemic infection or fluid deficit. In infants 2 to 12 months of age, the pulse rate increases linearly with body temperature, with a mean increase of 14 beats per minute for each 1° C increase in body temperature.
- ■ *Diagnostic testing.* Depending on the age of the patient, the diagnostic evaluation of a febrile patient varies (Table 79–1). While a shaking chill is often clinical evidence of a bacteremia, the only conclusive evidence is a positive blood culture. Unfortunately, blood cultures are often negative depending on when and how they are drawn.
- ■ *ED management.* Management of patients with suspected occult bacteremia depends on the age of the patient and the degree of fever (Table 79–1).
- ■ *Helpful hints and pitfalls.* Defervescence on antipyretic therapy does not imply the absence of bacteremia. Urinalysis and urine culture should be performed via catheterization because "bagged urine" has a high number of false positives. A normal urinalysis result in children younger than 8 weeks of age does not exclude a urinary tract infection. Otitis media is not enough to explain a young child's fever with altered behavior—especially in children aged 90 days or less. Antibiotics should be given before diagnostic testing if the patient appears toxic or is hemodynamically unstable.

Special Considerations
The Immunocompromised Patient

- ■ The evaluation and treatment of immunocompromised children does not follow the same algorithms as otherwise healthy infants and children. Children on steroids, other immunosuppressants or who have congenital or acquired immunodeficiency may not have classic signs and symptoms of infection. Perform a full sepsis workup in these children, and initiate appropriate administration of antibiotics regardless of their age.

Table 79-1 Evaluation of Patients with Fever and No Obvious Source

All neonates aged 0-28 d with a fever >38.0° C	Need a full sepsis evaluation: CBC, blood culture, urinalysis and urine culture, lumbar puncture, chest radiograph, and stool testing (as indicated).
	Empiric IV antibiotics: ampicillin 100 mg/kg/d divided q6h plus gentamycin 5 mg/kg/d divided q8h or ampicillin, 100 mg/kg/d divided q6h, plus cefotaxime 100-150 mg/kg/d divided q8-12h.
	Admission required until cultures are proven negative.
	Neonatal herpes infection has a high morbidity and mortality, and is very difficult to diagnose. For the febrile neonate with a vesicular rash or significant unexplained red blood cells in the CSF, acyclovir should be given for presumed herpes at a dose of 60 mg/kg/d divided q8h.
Infants aged 29-90 d with a fever >38.0° C	These patients should also receive a full sepsis workup. If there are any clinical signs or diagnostic testing consistent with meningitis: Treat with ampicillin 100 mg/kg IV first dose, then 50 mg/kg q6h IV plus cefotaxime 50mg/kg IV q8h or ceftriaxone 100 mg/kg IV.
	If the child is a well-appearing, low-risk patient with good follow-up within 24 h, discharge home.
Infants and children aged >3-36 mo	Fever less than 39.0° C and who appear nontoxic: Treat with antipyretics and supportive care if no source of fever is discovered on history and physical examination.
	Fever is greater than 39.0° C: The child should have a CBC. If the WBC >15,000 or absolute neutrophil count >10,000, send a blood culture and treat the child with ceftriaxone 50 mg/kg IV or IM and arrange follow-up within 24 h. For these children with fever >39° C, a urinalysis should be performed by straight catheterization. Chest radiographs are recommended for children with respiratory symptoms including tachypnea or oxygen saturation <95%. Some studies have recommended chest radiograph in all children with WBC >20,000. All of these children need good supportive care with antipyretics and hydration and follow-up medical care within 24 h if being discharged. The patients in this age group with recognizable viral illnesses (bronchiolitis, croup, stomatitis, and varicella) do not require this workup because their risk for bacterial superinfection is quite low.

Table 79–1	**Evaluation of Patients with Fever and No Obvious Source—*cont'd***
	A WBC count is relatively insensitive for *Haemophilus influenzae* and *Neisseria meningitidis* infections, thus obtain blood cultures and administer ceftriaxone to patients who appear clinically ill, but who are not sick enough to warrant an immediate septic workup, even when the WBC count is normal. Because bacteremia becomes less common after 24 mo of age, a CBC and blood culture should not be routinely obtained unless the child has a fever of 40° C or higher, or appears ill.
	Empiric antibiotic therapy: cefotaxime 50 mg/kg q6h or ceftriaxone[‡] 50 mg/kg q12h IV or IM. If *Streptococcus pneumoniae* is a potential pathogen, vancomycin 10 to 15 mg/kg q6-8h should also be initiated pending sensitivities.

CBC, complete blood count; CSF, cerebrospinal fluid; IM, intramuscular; IV, intravenous; WBC, white blood cell.

*Ampicillin is needed in addition to a cephalosporin until at least 6 to 12 weeks of age to treat Listeria monocytogenes and enterococci.

[†]Criteria for low-risk patients: (a) WBC >5,000 but <15,000; (b) total band count >1500 cells/mm³ or band/neutrophil ratio <0.2; (c) urine WBC <10 per high-power field (hpf); (d) stool WBC count <5/hpf; (e) no evidence of soft-tissue infection or abscess.

[‡]Do not use ceftriaxone during the first 30 to 60 days of life if there is clinical jaundice; the antibiotic displaces bilirubin from its serum binding sites.

Hyperpyrexia

■ Hyperpyrexia is defined as fever greater than 41° C. In addition to serious infectious causes (meningitis, pneumonia, Kawasaki's disease), consider noninfectious causes such as malignant hyperthermia secondary to anesthetics (see Chapter 31) and heatstroke (see Chapter 65). Toxic ingestions can cause hyperpyrexia. Common examples include aspirin, anticholinergics, and beta-adrenergics (see Chapter 72).

Teaching Points

Fever is a common presentation in children presenting to the ED. Early control of the fever with antipyretics is prudent and justified because it increases the child's ability to maintain normal hydration, and eat and drink well.

Under the age of 1 month, do a complete sepsis workup, including a lumbar puncture, and admit to the intensive care unit.

Older children can have modified septic workups depending upon presentation, immunization status, and social context. Immunologically deficient children all require a full sepsis workup, early administration of antibiotics, and admission to the hospital.

Suggested Readings

American Academy of Pediatrics, Provisional Committee on Quality Improvement, Subcommittee on Febrile Seizures. The neurodiagnostic evaluation of the child with a first febrile seizure. Pediatrics 1996;97:769–775.

American College of Emergency Physicians Clinical Policies Committee; American College of Emergency Physicians Clinical Policies Subcommittee on Pediatric Fever. Clinical policy for children younger than three years presenting to the emergency department with fever. Ann Emerg Med 2003;42:530–545.

Avner JR, Baker MD. Management of fever in infants and children. Emerg Med Clin North Am 2002;20:49–67.

Bachur R, Perry H, Harper MB. Occult pneumonias: empiric chest radiographs in febrile children with leukocytosis. Ann Emerg Med 1999:33:166–173.

Baker MD, Bell LM, Avner JR. Outpatient management without antibiotics of fever in selected infants. N Engl J Med 1993;329:1437–1441.

Baraff LJ. Editorial: Clinical policy for children younger than three years presenting to the emergency department with fever. Ann Emerg Med 2003;42:546–549.

Baskin MN, O'Rourke EJ, Fleisher GR. Outpatient treatment of febrile infants 28-89 days of age with intramuscular administration of ceftriaxone. J Pediatr 1992;120:22–27.

Chávez-Bueno S, McCracken GH. Bacterial meningitis in children. Pediatr Clin North Am 2005;52:795–810, vii.

Melendez E, Harper MB. Utility of sepsis evaluation in infants 90 days of age or younger with fever and clinical bronchiolitis. Pediatr Infect Dis J 2003;22:1053–1056.

Warden CR, Zibulewsky J, Mace S, Gold C, Gausche-Hill M. Evaluation and management of febrile seizures in the out-of-hospital and emergency department settings. Ann Emerg Med 2003;41:215–222.

CHAPTER **80**

Pediatric Dehydration

CHRISTOPHER S. AMATO

Overview

Dehydration is one of the leading causes of morbidity and mortality in the pediatric population. In the United States, approximately 400 children aged 1 month to 4 years die annually as a result of volume depletion.

Despite its devastating effects, consensus on how to treat it remains a controversy. The key to its treatment begins in its diagnosis.

Volume depletion denotes contraction of the total intravascular plasma pool, whereas dehydration denotes loss of plasma-free water disproportionate to loss of sodium, the main intravascular solute. The distinction is important because volume depletion can exist with or without dehydration, and dehydration can exist with or without volume depletion. For the purpose of this chapter, dehydration will refer to volume depletion.

Most patients presenting to the ED with dehydration resulting from diarrhea and vomiting due to a variety of causes, most commonly due to viral or bacterial infections. This chapter will provide a general approach to the dehydrated pediatric patient.

Initial Diagnostic Approach
General

- Any child who is ill-appearing, has a depressed level of consciousness, or has altered vital signs should receive immediate attention. Be more conservatives and cautious with young children. Infants and young children have a higher surface-to-volume ratio, a higher metabolic rate, a smaller fluid reserve, and a higher total body water turnover within a 24-hour period. This makes them more vulnerable to the small changes in their body fluid homeostasis.

- The child's history and physical examination guide the clinician toward making an ultimate diagnosis, and assessing the degree of dehydration. The parents should be asked about any fluid losses such as vomiting, diarrhea, and urine output; type and amount of oral intake; medications and other possible ingestions; activity level and how it differs from baseline. On physical examination, the vital signs should be noted. Although pain and fever (pulse may increase 14 beats per degree Celsius of temperature elevation above reference range) may cause a tachycardia, it is also an early sign of significant volume depletion. The blood pressure will remain normal until severe volume depletion exists.

- Many assessment strategies are used to determine the degree of dehydration in pediatric patients. It is difficult to determine the level of dehydration from the clinical examination. No single finding is predictive. The gold standard of degree of dehydration is still the change in weight of the child from baseline to the dehydrated state. When this is not known, other clinical indicators can be used to guide the physician. Stool should be examined visually, tested for blood, and the presence or absence of urine should be noted. Capillary refill longer than 2 seconds, dry mucous membranes, absent tears, and ill appearance correlate with dehydration, with the presence of two or more indicating a degree of dehydration of at least 5%. See Table 80–1 for clinical parameters to assess dehydration status. The amount of fluid deficit can be calculated by the percentage of dehydration (e.g., 10%) by the weight of a child. For example, a 10-kg child who is 10% dehydrated has a total deficit of 1000 ml or 100 ml/kg.

- In stable older patients, orthostatic blood pressure and pulse should be obtained in the recumbent and standing (or sitting position). A decrease of 15 mm Hg in blood pressure or an increase of 20 beats per minute in pulse rate after 2 to 3 minutes in the upright position is significant. These changes can occur in the absence of hypovolemia.

Table 80–1 Clinical Parameters to Assess Dehydration Status

	Mild (3-5%)	Moderate (6-9%)	Severe (>10%)
Fluid Loss in ml/kg	0-50 ml/kg	60-90 ml/kg	>100 ml/kg
General	Alert	Restless, Irritable	Lethargic/ unconscious
Blood pressure	Normal	Normal	Normal, decreased
Quality of pulse	Normal	Normal, slightly decreased	Moderately decreased
Heart rate	Normal	Increased	Increased
Skin turgor	Normal	Decreased	Decreased
Fontanelle	Normal	Sunken	Sunken
Mucus membranes	Slightly dry	Dry	Dry
Eyes	Normal	Sunken	Deeply sunken
Extremities	Warm, normal cap refill	Delayed cap refill*	Cool, mottled
Urine output	Slightly decreased	< 1 ml/kg/hr	<< 1 ml/kg/hr
Thirst	Slightly increased	Moderately increased	Increased/ Decreased

Capillary refill > 2 seconds.

Laboratory

- Laboratory studies are rarely indicated for mildly dehydrated patients.
- The serum sodium is not predictive of degree of dehydration but can identify the presence of iso-, hypo-, or hypernatremic states for appropriate choice of therapy (Table 80–2).
- Serum urea (blood urea nitrogen [BUN]) and bicarbonate levels are the most helpful in determining the degree of dehydration. The BUN may be relatively low in malnourished patients because of low protein.
  - Mild to moderate dehydration: BUN up to 40 mg/dl and bicarbonate above15 mg/dl
  - Moderate to severe dehydration: BUN more than 100 mg/dl and bicarbonate less than 15 mg/dl
- A potassium deficit is present in all patients with volume depletion: This is not usually clinically significant. However, failure to correct for a potassium deficit during volume repletion may result in clinically significant hypokalemia.
- A mild metabolic acidosis is common, especially in infants. Causes include bicarbonate loss in stool and ketone production, decreased tissue perfusion with increased lactic acid production, and decreased hydrogen (H+) ion excretion from decreased renal perfusion. Arterial blood gas analysis is only needed in severe cases of dehydration. The acidosis is

usually corrected with volume restoration (as increased renal perfusion permits excretion of excess H+ ions in the urine). Administration of glucose-containing fluids further decreases ketone production.

- An initial glucose level (a finger-stick or capillary glucose) is important because children may develop hypoglycemia with dehydration. It may also reveal a hyperglycemia, and a cause for the dehydrated state.
- The specific gravity of the urine is typically elevated (≥ 1.020) in dehydrated patients. Urine electrolytes and osmolarity may be useful to further evaluate extrinsic fluid loss.
- A complete blood count is ordered to evaluate for an elevated white blood cell (WBC) count if there is concern for infection.

Emergency Department Management Overview
General

- Early intervention is important to prevent progression to shock and cardiovascular collapse. Immediate resuscitation should include 20 ml/kg of 0.9% saline (or other appropriate isotonic crystalloid solution) via intravenous (IV) line at a rapid rate to reverse signs of shock. Reevaluate at 15 minute intervals, and repeat administrations of 20 ml/kg if needed until clinical improvement occurs. Volume requirements greater than 50 ml/kg without signs of improvement suggest other conditions such as septic shock or hemorrhage.
- Interosseous routes should be used if venous access is not immediately available.
- For more stable patients, although oral rehydration therapy (ORT) may be used for mild-to-moderate dehydration, especially in less developed countries, the length of ED stay required for ORT and easy availability of IV access has made IV hydration the more common approach in the United States.

Oral Rehydration Therapy

- ORT can be as successful as IV hydration in an ED. Volume replenishment using ORT generally occurs over 8 hours. It is useful for mild-to-moderate dehydration in patients with acute diarrheal illness with or without vomiting. It is also used in non-Westernized countries for severe dehydration. The parents must be taught how to use ORT, amount to offer based on the clinical status and the amount of output, and to start other appropriate dietary intake during the maintenance phase.
- Early use at home may avoid a trip to the ED, and an appropriate diet should be continued. Infants should be fed or nursed more often.
- For mild dehydration, have parent administer 50 to 60 ml/kg of an oral replacement solution (ORS) over a 4-hour time period. For moderate dehydration, parent will administer 80 to 100 ml/kg over 4 hours; the parent (or caregiver) may administer with a spoon or syringe every 1 to 2 minutes. Administer 25% of the volume of ORS to be replaced each hour for the first 4 hours. If the rehydration is going well, consider discharge after 2 hours if the parent can continue the remainder at home.

- There are different types of ORS available. Oral rehydration solutions should contain 45-90 mmol/L of sodium and 74-140 mmol/L of glucose. Acceptable, commercially available ORS include: Naturalyte, Pedialyte, Infalyte, Rehydralyte, WHO Oral Rehydration Salts, and Pediatric Electrolytes. Cereal-based ORS is also available, and has been shown to decrease diarrhea by 20-30% compared to glucose-containing ORS. Rehydralyte is the most appropriate ORS that is easily available.
- Some vomiting is not a contraindication, and is also not an indication of failure of ORT. Emesis (volume-for-volume) and stool (5 ml/kg) are estimated and added to the replacement volume on an hourly basis. Anti-diarrheal and antiemetic agents are not routinely recommended; however, studies have demonstrated short-term benefits with ondansetron (Zofran) 0.2 mg/kg by mouth.
- If successfully rehydrated, discharge the patient home with reinstitution of an age-appropriate diet as tolerated.

Intravenous Hydration

- *IV access.* There are many choices for placement sites, although it is often difficult to place an IV in the dehydrated child. If IV access is needed, the typical sites in young pediatric patients include superficial veins in the dorsum of the hand, antecubital fossa (median cephalic or basilic veins), dorsum of the foot, and scalp veins. Intra-osseous access in the proximal tibia or distal femur may be used. Central venous access sites include femoral, internal jugular (may be difficult because of short neck in infants and young children), and subclavian veins. Umbilical vein catheterization may be difficult, and usually is not recommended for neonates who have been discharged from the hospital and are returning to the ED. A venous cutdown at the ankle saphenous vein is useful and is described in Chapter 91. Standard 19- to 22-gauge angiocaths are useful for this purpose.
- The fluid of choice for initial IV hydration is usually isotonic normal saline. A resuscitation bolus of fluid should be given in the presence of abnormal mental status, lethargy, poor muscle tone, a history of decreased urine output, decreased capillary refill, tachycardia at rest (not caused by fever, pain, or anxiety), bradycardia, or any other indication of shock. Caution should be used in a child with cardiac or renal disease where excess fluid can cause further clinical deterioration. For those cases a 10-ml/kg infusion should be performed with close re-evaluation. Often fluid infusions of 60 to 80 ml/kg are required for the severely de-hydrated child. Generally one half of the total fluid deficit is given during the first 8 hours of repletion. The remainder of the deficit is replaced in over the next 16 hours. Please see Table 80–2 for considerations in fluid replacement therapy.
- Once the child has begun to respond and vital sign abnormalities are corrected, initiate maintenance fluid therapy. If the patient weighs less than 10 kg, give 100 ml/kg/d. If the patient weighs between 10 and 20 kg, give 1000 ml/d plus 50 ml/kg/d for each kilogram between 10 and 20 kg. If the patient weighs more than 20 kg, give 1500 ml/d, plus 20 ml/kg/d

Table 80–2 Dehydration Status and Sodium Level

	Problem	Etiology	Therapy
Isonatremic volume depletion	Volume depletion without dehydration: There is contraction with solutes (mostly sodium) and solvents (mostly water) lost in proportionate quantities.	The result of vomiting or diarrhea with no replacement of fluids or solute.	The most common presentation in patients presenting with dehydration. Treat with saline or other isotonic solutions.
Hyponatremic volume depletion	Plasma volume contraction with free water excess.	Giving tap water to replete diarrheal losses. Free water is replenished, but sodium and other solutes are not.	For hyponatremia associated with dehydration and GI losses, rehydrate with isotonic saline over 24 hours. Serum sodium levels less than 120 mEq/L may result in seizures. If intravascular free water excess is not corrected during volume replenishment, the shift of free water to the intracellular fluid compartment may cause cerebral edema. In severe hyponatremia with decreased total body water in symptomatic patients, give 3% saline 4 ml/kg IV over 10 min and reassess.
Hypernatremic volume depletion	Volume depletion exists concurrently with true dehydration in which there is a disproportionate further free water loss. Dehydration, or excess free water loss, is present when plasma osmolarity increases. Osmolarity is the measure of solute concentration in a fixed solvent volume.	Diarrhea illness in which fluid is replenished with hypertonic liquid (e.g., soup or improperly diluted infant formula). Volume has been restored, but free water has not.	Do not administer hypotonic fluid at too fast a rate because water will equilibrate across the cerebral blood-brain barrier almost immediately (long before the sodium is corrected), creating increased intracranial pressure. D5W, D5W 0.2% NS, or D5W 0.45% NS are all acceptable if infused at a conservative rate, correcting deficits over 48 hours.

D5W, dextrose 5% in water; NS, normal saline.

for each kilogram over 20 kg. Adjust for fever (add 10% for each 1 °C over 37 °C), stool loss (5 ml/kg) or vomiting (volume for volume).

- Daily sodium and potassium requirements are each 2 to 3 mEq/kg/d. Full correction of severe sodium abnormalities usually should be staged over 24 hours or longer to decrease central nervous system complications resulting from rapid correction of the osmolar gradients.

- If the serum glucose is low (<50 mg/dl), glucose should be provided. For children in whom IV access cannot be obtained, oral or nasogastric glucose is an option, as is intramuscular glucagon (for nonketotic hypoglycemia). Once IV access is obtained, a small bolus 0.25 to 0.5 g/kg of dextrose should be given. For infants younger than 3 months of age, give 2-4 mL/kg of D10, but D25 is also safe if the IV is secure in a large vein at a dose of 2 mL/kg. The bolus should be followed by an infusion using a dextrose-containing solution such as D10 with 0.2NS drip at 1.5 times maintenance. It is prudent to use a dextrose-containing solution for maintenance fluid replacement.

- If a patient is acidotic with a bicarbonate level of 10 mEq/L or a pH below 7.1 on the basis of metabolic acidosis, one third of the sodium may be administered as sodium bicarbonate. In the presence of acidosis, serum potassium does not reflect total body deficit.

Nutrition

- *Gut rest* is not an appropriate approach to the child with diarrhea. Returning to full diet will reduce stool output and duration of diarrhea by up to 50%. An acquired lactase-deficiency, due to decrease in the enzyme found in the intestinal brush-border, has been shown in 88% of admitted patients with rotavirus diarrhea. Thus the use of milk-containing nutrition is best avoided.

- One can start with the classic BRAT diet (*B*ananas, *R*ice, *A*pplesauce, and *T*oast), but children should be started back on a regular diet as soon as tolerated. Avoid foods high in simple sugars (soda, undiluted apple juice, sugary cereals) and foods with high fat (fast food, butter).

Disposition

- **Consultation.** It is helpful to communicate the details of the visit to the primary care physician, and to help arrange an early follow-up visit.

- **Admission.** Admission is warranted when the patient is severely dehydrated, does not respond clinically to rehydration within the ED, continues to have significant output of emesis or diarrhea while in the ED, significant alteration in the patient's serum electrolytes, or significant coexisting illness (e.g., acute renal failure). If there are concerns about follow-up or concerns regarding the social situation of the patient, admission is also warranted.

- **Discharge.** Most patients will be discharged after hydration. Follow-up is prudent with the PCP as well as instructions to return to the ED if unable to tolerate oral hydration at home.

Teaching Points

Pediatric dehydration is common, serious, and sometimes lethal. It is easy to underestimate because there are few clinical reliable findings to guarantee the level of hydration.

Signs of moderate-to-severe dehydration include lack of tears, lack of urination (no wet diapers), poor skin turgor, slow capillary refill, and alertness of the child.

While oral rehydration is possible for mild-to-moderate dehydration, it is quicker and easier in most Westernized countries to use intravenous therapy. Start with a bolus of 20 ml/kg of normal saline.

All but severe dehydration can be safely treated in the ED, but it is also necessary to have good social circumstances, educable parents, and early and safe follow-up. If any of these are lacking, the child should be admitted.

Suggested Readings

Barkin RM, Ward DG. Infectious diarrheal disease and dehydration. In: Marx JA, Hockberger RS, Walls RM (editors). Rosen's Emergency Medicine: Concepts and Clinical Practice (6th ed). Philadelphia: Mosby, 2006, pp 2623–2635.

Duke T, Molyneux E, Intravenous fluids for seriously ill children: time to reconsider. Lancet 2003;362:1320–1324.

Egland AG. Pediatric dehydration. eMedicine. Accessed September 15, 2005, last updated July 27, 2005. http://www.emedicine.com/emerg/topic372.htm.

Mann C. Oral rehydration therapy. The American College of Emergency Physicians. Accessed September 15, 2005, last updated 2004. http://www.acep.org/webportal/MemberCenter/SectionsofMembership/PediatricEmergencyMedicine/DiarrheaandOralRehydrationTherapy/OralRehydrationTherapy.htm.

Yilmaz K, Karabocuoglu M, Citak A, Uzel N. Evaluation of laboratory tests in dehydrated children with acute gastroenteritis. J Pediatr Child Health 2002;38:226–228.

CHAPTER 81

Pediatric Orthopedics

BRIAN WILLIAM WALSH ■ CHRISTOPHER S. AMATO

Overview

Although many fractures in children are similar to those in adults, there are several important differences.

Pediatric bone is softer and more easily broken than adult bone.

The periosteal membrane in children is thicker and more "leathery," making pediatric bone less brittle. This feature frequently holds the ends of bone together, and makes reduction easier.

Remodeling, including correction in alignment or size, is more rapid.

The ligaments attaching to the bone are stronger than the bone itself. This leads to an overall increased number of fractures with a decreased incidence of dislocations, ligamentous injuries, and sprains. In general, a child younger than 12 to 14 years is more likely to fracture a bone than to sprain a ligament.

Because of the thick periosteal membrane and the rapid remodeling, many pediatric fractures can be treated with simple, even incomplete, closed reduction, and casting.

This chapter will discuss a practical approach to pediatric patients with orthopedic injuries. Problems unique to the pediatric population will be reviewed.

Initial Diagnostic Approach
General

■ Approach the child in a nonthreatening manner; leave the presumed area of discomfort for last to examine. There will be other areas of trauma that are missed when examinations are incomplete.
■ Due to growth plates, comparison views may be useful when a fracture is suspected, and the initial unilateral radiograph is difficult to interpret.
■ Children are not always capable of localizing pain. Therefore, getting radiographs of the joints above and below the suspected injury site is especially important. A parent or caretaker may be helpful in describing the initial trauma.
■ Always consider nonaccidental trauma in very young pediatric patients with orthopedic injuries.

Evaluating the Child with a Limp

- A limp is any alteration of the normal gait. Limping can be caused by problems with the lumbar spine, pelvis, hip, knee, ankle, or foot. In addition, neuromuscular diseases can also affect a child's gait.
- The most serious causes of a limp include septic arthritis, osteomyelitis, developmental dysplasia of the hip, slipped capital femoral epiphysis (SCFE,) or nonmusculoskeletal diseases such as appendicitis.
- The age of the child greatly affects the differential diagnosis of a limp (Table 81–1).

Laboratory

- In general, laboratory studies including a complete blood count (CBC), erythrocyte sedimentation rate (ESR), and C-reactive protein (CRP) can be useful in narrowing the differential diagnosis in patients with joint pain.
- Some studies suggest that a history of fever, nonweight-bearing, white blood count (WBC) count above 12,000/mm^3, and ESR more 40 mm/h can be used to differentiate between septic arthritis and transient synovitis.

Radiography

- *Plain films.* The presence of radiolucent epiphyses near the ends of long bones can cause difficulty when interpreting radiographs. Therefore, comparison views of the unaffected side may be helpful if initial radiographs are inconclusive. Injury can occur to the epiphysis and result in little, if any, radiographic findings. As the epiphysis is often weaker than the surrounding ligaments, caution should be exercised when diagnosing a sprain. Therefore, orthopedic referral for all suspicious injuries is important. As with adults, some fractures may not been seen on plain films until 7 to 10 days after the injury when absorption has occurred at the margins of the fracture. For patients with hip pain or possible *referred* knee pain, a frog-leg lateral view should be ordered in addition to the standard anteroposterior and lateral views. The frog-leg lateral shows the hip in a plane midway between the AP and lateral views, and is useful in diagnosis of disorders involving the hip such as slipped capital femoral epiphysis.
- *Computed tomography (CT scan).* Suspicious injuries with negative or equivocal plain films can be imaged with a CT scan to rule out a fracture. CT scan imaging is better able to define fractures by illustrating alignment, displacement, and fragmentation. CT scan imaging is especially useful to determine subtle fractures in traumatic cervical spine injuries.
- *Magnetic resonance imaging (MRI).* Although expensive and time consuming, and often not readily available for emergencies, MRI is the best technique for imaging soft-tissue structures like cartilage and ligaments. It is useful in evaluation of the spine and large joints like the shoulder and knee. As in adults, an MRI is typically not ordered from the ED for pediatric orthopedic injuries unless needed to diagnose potentially devastating injury such as a spinal cord syndrome (see Chapter 12).

Table 81–1	Differential Diagnosis of a Limp	
Age	**Location**	**Diagnosis: Common presentation**
Toddler	Bone	Fracture, including Toddler's fracture—oblique fracture of tibia
	Soft tissue	Osteomyelitis Foreign body Contusion/sprain
	Joint	Septic arthritis: fever, leukocytosis Juvenile rheumatoid arthritis: with or without swollen knee Transient synovitis of hip Developmental dysplasia of hip Congenital hip dislocation: side-to-side gait
	Other	Cerebral palsy: toe walking Muscular dystrophy Poor shoe fit
School aged	Bone	Tumor Fracture Osteomyelitis
	Soft tissue	Myositis Contusion/sprain
	Joint	Rheumatic disease: rheumatic fever, Henoch-Schönlein Septic arthritis Lyme arthritis Transient synovitis Baker's cyst in knee Avascular necrosis: Legg-Calve-Perthes Rickets
	Other	Appendicitis
Adolescent	Bone	Tumor Osteomyelitis
	Soft tissue	Tendinitis
	Joint	Septic arthritis: consider gonococcal Rheumatic disease: including inflammatory bowel Lyme arthritis Slipped capital femoral epiphysis Osgood-Schlatter Chondromalacia
	Other	Scoliosis Appendicitis

- *Radionucleotide bone scanning (scintigraphy).* Scintigraphy is used to detect bone lesions that may not be visible by other radiographic studies, such as stress fractures, osteomyelitis, and tumors. Scintigraphy detects reactive bone formation, and, therefore, cannot distinguish between fractures and other lesions. Furthermore, fractures are not visible for at least 24 to 48 hours.

Emergency Department Management Overview
General

- Most of these patients are stable. Pain management, although easily overlooked in nonverbal children, is the most important intervention in the management of these patients.

Medications

- *Analgesia.* Should be given as needed for comfort. Conscious sedation such as short-acting benzodiazepine (e.g., midazolam) and fentanyl or ketamine should be used for any significant orthopedic manipulation in the ED (see Chapter 90.1).
- *Antibiotics.* Should be given if there is concern for septic arthritis, osteomyelitis, or open fracture.

Emergency Department Interventions

- Splinting is described in Chapter 17. Even if the plain films are negative, patients with significant pain should be splinted in the event an occult fracture (such as the growth plate) is missed.

Disposition

- *Consultation.* With an orthopedic surgeon capable of taking care of pediatric injuries.
- *Admission.* Any patient with a suspected septic joint, any orthopedic injury requiring surgery, or for close observation (i.e., uncontrolled pain, frequent neurovascular monitoring).
- *Discharge.* Patients with minor injuries (e.g., closed, minimally displaced fractures) can be discharged with orthopedic follow-up.

Specific Problems
Osteomyelitis

- See Chapter 67.

Septic Joint

- Septic arthritis is more common in children than in adults. Two thirds occur in children less than 2 years old. The joints of the lower extremities (hips, knees) are most often affected.

- Infection of the joint space in children usually is a complication of bacteremia. It may also be a consequence of bacterial infection elsewhere in the body.
- See Chapter 42 for a more detailed discussion.

Transient (Toxic) Synovitis

- ***Epidemiology and risk factors.*** This is the most common cause of hip pain in childhood; it can also affect the knee. The peak incidence is between 3 and 6 years of age. It is bilateral in 5%.
- ***Pathophysiology.*** It is a self-limited inflammatory condition caused by a nonpyogenic inflammatory response of the synovium. The exact cause is unknown. At least half the children with transient synovitis have, or recently have had, an upper respiratory illness.
- ***History.*** The child may present with a limp. Hip and groin pain is the most common complaint, but referred pain to the medial thigh or knee is found in 10% to 30% of patients.
- ***Physical examination.*** The child is well appearing; a mild fever may be present. The leg is held in flexion with slight abduction and external rotation. Passive movement is usually pain free; however, there may be pain as well as a slightly decreased range of motion with extreme internal rotation or abduction.
- ***Diagnostic testing.*** This may reveal mild elevations in the white blood cell count and erythrocyte sedimentation rate (ESR), both consistent with a nonspecific inflammatory process. Plain films may reveal medial joint space widening, an accentuated pericapsular shadow, and Waldenstrom's sign, which is lateral displacement of the femoral epiphysis with surface flattening secondary to effusion. However, these findings can be found in Legg-Calvé-Perthe's disease. In unclear or atypical cases, ultrasonography, which is as accurate as a CT scan or an MRI for detecting effusions, can be used to look for an intracapsular effusion or guide hip joint aspiration.
- ***ED management.*** Management includes rest via avoiding weight-bearing, or, in cases of extreme pain, bed rest and anti-inflammatory medications. Orthopedic consultation should be obtained in questionable cases. The patient should have close outpatient follow-up within 24 hours. Most cases usually completely resolve within 4 weeks.
- ***Helpful hints and pitfalls.*** This is a diagnosis of exclusion. A septic joint must be ruled out.

Fractures and Other Problems

- ***Salter-Harris fractures.*** The epiphyseal plate (physis) is the growth cartilage of the long bones in children, and is located at or near the ends of bone. Injuries to the physis are concerning, because bone growth can be slowed or stopped after a physeal injury. The cartilaginous portion of the physis is not visualized on radiographs due to the radiolucency of cartilage. Thus, it is difficult to determine as to whether a fracture line is present. These injuries are relatively common during childhood as opposed to sprains or shaft fractures, and must always be considered in children with a "sprained ankle," because of the relative weakness of the

Table 81–2 Salter-Harris Fractures

Type	Description	Diagnostics	Management	Prognosis/Complications
I	Transverse fracture through the physis causing widening of the physis	Plain film Point tenderness at epiphyseal plate	Splint Orthopedic follow-up	Good: Usually no growth disturbance Often difficult to diagnosis on radiograph
II	Fracture through the metaphysis and physis Most common Salter-Harris fracture Metaphyseal spike is called *Thurston-Holland* sign	Plain film	Splint Orthopedic follow-up after discussion while in emergency department	Possible growth disturbance, but usually no disability
III	Fracture through the epiphysis and physis, involving the articular surface	Plain film	Splint Orthopedic follow-up after discussion while in emergency department Often requires surgery	Prone to chronic disability
IV	Fracture involving epiphysis, physis, and metaphysis	Plain films	Splint Orthopedic follow-up after discussion while in emergency department Often requires surgery	Prone to chronic disability and deformity
V	Crush injury of physis not involving epiphysis or metaphysis	Plain films	Splint Orthopedic follow-up after discussion while in emergency department Often requires surgery	Prone to chronic disability and deformity Difficult diagnosis: Look for these in the patient with axial-loading injuries

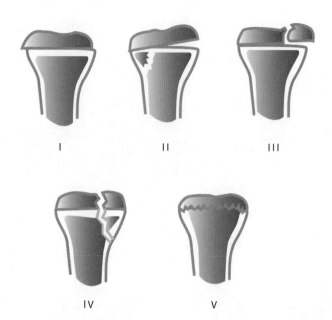

Figure 81–1. Salter-Harris classification of epiphyseal fractures in children. A type I fracture is straight across the epiphyseal plate, and may have some lateral displacement of the epiphysis. This occurs 5% of the time. A type II fracture involves a portion of the epiphyseal plate, and a corner fracture through the metaphysis. This occurs 75% of the time. A type III fracture involving part of the epiphysis occurs only about 10% of the time. A type IV fracture involving part of the epiphysis and part of the metaphysis occurs about 10% of the time. A type V fracture is direct impaction and has the most serious consequences for further growth. *(From Mettler F. Essentials of Radiology [2nd ed]. Philadelphia: Elsevier, 2005, p 308.)*

cartilaginous growth zone. Physis injuries should be described according to the Salter-Harris classification (Table 81–2, Figure 81–1). The fractures are diagnosed with plain films or CT scans or MRIs. Type I and V fractures are easily missed on plain films. All suspected Salter-Harris fractures should be treated with standard splinting techniques (see Chapter 17).

■ *Incomplete fractures.* Bones of children are soft and resilient, and therefore sustain a number of incomplete fractures (Table 81–3, Figure 81–2).
■ *Other extremity injuries.* Other commonly known pediatric orthopedic problems are briefly mentioned in Tables 81–4 and 81–5, Figures 81–3, 81–4, 81–5.

Table 81-3	Incomplete Fractures				
Type	**Description/Population**	**Mechanism/Presentation**	**Diagnostics**	**Management**	**Prognosis/Complications**
Torus	Also called *buckle* fractures Fractures over metaphyseal region causing bowing	Compressive forces in axis of affected bone, often involving distal radius	Plain film—no fracture seen— may see bowing Follow cortex curvature looking for area that departs from normal smooth line	Splint	Heal in 4-6 wk, usually with no complications
Greenstick	Fracture through tension side of bone, with "buckling" of other side	Compressive forces	Plain film—fracture seen does not go completely through bone	Splint Orthopedic follow-up after discussion while in emergency department	If more than 15 degrees of angulation, orthopedic referral for completion of fracture and reduction

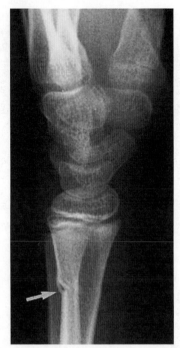

Figure 81–2. Torus fracture. A lateral view of the wrist shows "buckling" of the dorsal cortex. *(From Mettler F. Essentials of Radiology [2nd ed]. Philadelphia: Elsevier, 2005, p 367.)*

Nonaccidental Trauma

- Although no fracture pattern is absolutely pathognomonic of physical abuse, certain fracture patterns are seen more frequently than others. Fractures of almost any bone may occur; the extremities, skull, and rib cage are the most common sites of injury. Examples of fracture patterns seen in nonaccidental trauma (NAT) are listed in Box 81–1. Many of these fracture patterns are seen in both accidental and nonaccidental trauma. Diaphyseal fractures are the most common fractures in abused and nonabused children. Only 10% of abused children sustain fractures.
- A skeletal survey should be performed as part of the NAT workup in children younger than 5 years old.
- See Chapter 82 for a more detailed discussion of NAT.

Type	Description/Population	Mechanism/Presentation	Diagnostics	Management	Prognosis/Complications
Supracondylar fracture of humerus (Figure 81–3)	95% are the "extension" type fractures with posterior displacement of the capitellum. Ages 3–11 Most common elbow fracture in children Type I: nondisplaced. Type II: displaced fracture with intact posterior cortex Type III: displaced fracture with no cortical contact	Fall on an outstretched arm with the elbow in extension. Straight vertical forces tend to cause intercondylar fractures. If there is pain on flexion or extension of fingers, forearm tenderness, or pain that is disproportionate to the injury, compartment pressures should be measured immediately.	Plain films. May see posterior fat pad sign. Anterior humeral line will go through the anterior one third of the capitellum, or run completely anterior to it. May note carrying angle more than 12 degrees. Any manipulation should be avoided because movement may cause further neurovascular damage.	Posterior long-arm splint with elbow at 90 degrees. Careful neurovascular examination. Hospitalization required for type III. If more than 20 degrees of angulation or displacement, then emergent orthopedic consultation.	Limited extension and flexion of elbow if realignment not correct. Special attention to median nerve and brachial artery. 15% have associated nerve injury. Unrecognized ischemic injury can result in a Volkmann's ischemic contracture (from a "missed" compartment syndrome).
Lateral condyle fracture	Oblique, shearing fracture of the lateral joint.	Fall onto outstretched arm, driving the radial head into the capitulum.	Lack of complete ossification may make diagnosis difficult.	Highly unstable, usually Salter-Harris IV fractures. Often requires open reductions and fixation.	

Table 81–5 Pediatric Lower Extremity Problems

Type	Description/ Population	Mechanism/ Presentation	Diagnostics	Management	Prognosis/ Complications
Slipped capital femoral epiphysis (SCFE, Figure 81–4)	Femoral metaphysis is displaced downward and backward. Aged 10–16 y Most common hip disorder in adolescents Boys more often than girls Often affects obese children. 25% bilateral	Insidious onset in chronic SCFE (90% of cases), with months of painful limp. May present weeks to months after minor trauma with limp. Pain and decreased range of motion on internal rotation. A stable SCFE is one in which ambulation is possible (with or without crutches), and an unstable SCFE is one in which ambulation is not possible (with or without crutches).	With a stable slip, AP and frog-leg lateral pelvic radiographs should be obtained. When an unstable slip or a minimal slip is suspected, a cross table radiograph replaces the frog-leg lateral. Plain film shows "ice cream cone" sign. Look for Klein's line: a line drawn along the superior margin of the femoral neck. Normally, the line intersects or falls within the epiphysis, whereas in a hip with a SCFE, the line does not come in contact with the epiphysis.	The child should be made non–weight-bearing, either with crutches or a wheelchair, and an immediate orthopedic consultation should be obtained. All patients require admission. For a stable slip, definitive treatment may be delayed a few days. With an unstable slip, immediate fixation may be required.	Premature osteoarthritis – the greater the slip, the sooner degenerative changes begin. Avascular necrosis of femoral head with poor prognosis Chondrolysis: Degeneration of hip cartilage

Type	Description/ Population	Mechanism/ Presentation	Diagnostics	Management	Prognosis/ Complications
Legg-Calve-Perthes (Figure 81–5)	Avascular necrosis of femoral head Aged 4-10 y Boys more often than girls Often affects shorter children 15% bilateral	Insidious onset of limp. Often present as painless limp, although mild pain may occur with movement. Limited abduction and internal rotation. May see atrophy of thigh.	Initial plain film findings include a femoral head that appears smaller, widening of the medial joint space, a subchondral lucent zone (subchondral collapse), an irregular physeal plate, and a blurry and radiolucent metaphysis followed by increased radiolucency (fragmentation), increased radiodensity (new bone).	Orthopedic consultation. Treatment is not indicated in all cases. Primary therapy: "containment" of the femoral head within the acetabulum to assist with remolding of the femoral head via operative and nonoperative means.	Permanent deformity and decreased range of motion in a minority of cases. Worse prognosis with greater degree of deformity of the femoral head and acetabulum at maturity, disease onset in children 6-8 y or older, female sex, and prolonged duration of disease.
Osgood-Schlatter	Poor development of the tibial tuberosity caused by repetitive trauma. Girls aged 8-13 y Boys aged 10-15 y Boys more often than girls	Pain, swelling and tenderness of tibial tubercle.	Radiographs show fragmentation of lateral proximal tibia at attachment of patellar tendon 25% bilateral.	Rest, nonsteroidal anti-inflammatory drugs If severe, brace at 0 to 30 degrees.	Symptoms usually resolve when tubercle fuses to tibia (by age 18).

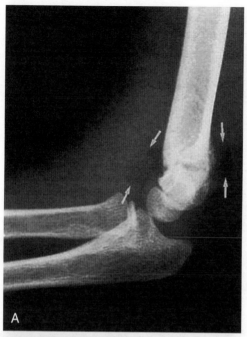

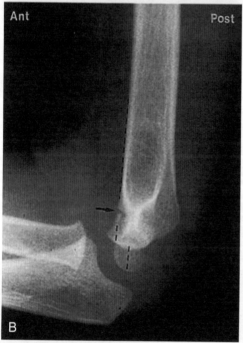

Figure 81–3.
Supracondylar fractures. This is the most common elbow fracture in children. *A,* A lateral view of the elbow shows marked anterior displacement of the anterior fat and visualization of the posterior fat pad (*arrows*), a sign that a fracture is almost certainly present. *B,* In a younger child, a fracture is seen because of the posterior displacement of the capitellum from the anterior humeral line. An incomplete cortical fracture also is seen (*arrow*). (*From Mettler F. Essentials of Radiology [2nd ed]. Philadelphia: Elsevier, 2005, p 365.*)

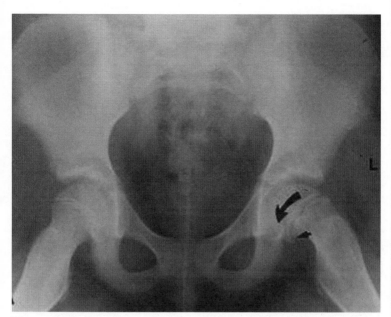

Figure 81-4. Slipped capital femoral epiphysis. An anteroposterior view of the pelvis in this overweight teenage boy shows slipping of the left femoral epiphysis relative to the femoral neck (arrows). *(From Mettler F. Essentials of Radiology [2nd ed]. Philadelphia: Elsevier, 2005, p 371.)*

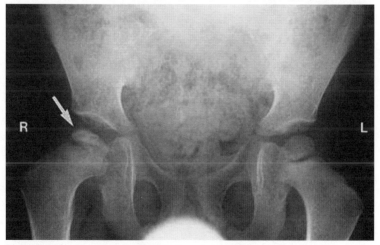

Figure 81-5. Legg-Perthes disease. An anteroposterior view of the pelvis demonstrates fragmentation and sclerosis of the right femoral epiphysis in this 6-year-old boy. *(From Mettler F. Essentials of Radiology [2nd ed]. Philadelphia: Elsevier, 2005, p 370.)*

BOX 81-1 Examples of Fractures in Nonaccidental Trauma

Multiple or bilateral fractures, especially of varying ages
Multiple or complex skull fractures
Sternum and rib fractures, especially posterior rib fractures
Scapular and clavicle fractures
Spiral fractures of femur or tibia in a nonambulatory infant
Spiral fracture of humerus; transverse long bone fractures are also common
Finger injuries in nonambulatory children
Metaphyseal or epiphyseal fractures (corner fractures, bucket-handle fractures, chip fractures), often caused by shaking
Avulsion fracture of clavicle and acromion process

Teaching Points

Children have special growth characteristics of their bones that make them susceptible to special kinds of fractures. They heal better than adults, and therefore are less often in need of open reduction and internal fixation.

Fractures, especially in the very young, should suggest nonaccidental trauma.

A limp is a very important sign of injury in a child, but it is often difficult to find the focus of injury because pain is not well localized by children. It is prudent to obtain radiologic studies of the joint above and below the suspected injury. Because of the differences in the timing of epiphyseal closure by age, it is often helpful to obtain comparison views of the uninjured side.

Suggested Readings

Kocher M, Zurakowski D, Kasser JR. Differentiation between septic arthritis and transient synovitis of the hip in children: an evidence based clinical prediction algorithm. J Bone Joint Surg 1999;81A:1662–1670.

Kocher MS, Mandiga R. Zurakowski D. Barnewolt C. Kasser JR. Validation of a clinical prediction rule for the differentiation between septic arthritis and transient synovitis of the hip in children. J Bone Joint Surg 2004;86A:1629–1635.

McQuillen KK. Musculoskeletal disorders. In: Marx, Hockberger, Walls, Rosen's Emergency Medicine: Concepts and Clinical Practice. 6th Ed. Philadelphia: Mosby; 2006:2689–2713.

Musgrave D, Mendelson S. Pediatric orthopedic trauma: principles in management. Crit Care Med 2002;30:431–443.

Sarwark J. What's new in pediatric orthopaedics. J Bone Joint Surg 2002;84A:887–893.

CHAPTER **82**

Pediatric Child Abuse (Nonaccidental Trauma)

LOIS K. LEE

Overview

Child abuse or nonaccidental trauma (NAT) can be categorized into four types: physical, sexual, neglect, or emotional/psychological. Specific definitions may vary by state.

The clinician should look for clues in the history or physical examination in all cases of pediatric trauma. With a NAT injury, the injury observed may be imcompatible with the history given; or the history may be inconsistent, either between caregivers, or when given to different evaluators. There may also be no explanation for the injury, or there may be a delay in seeking care for the injury. Another clue is the parent who is unreasonable about the care being given, and wants to take the child out of the ED when the evaluation is just beginning.

The injury, abuse, or neglect may be caused by the child's immediate caregivers, or others living in the same home as the child, such as family members, friends, or significant others. Physical abuse includes bodily injury that is not explained by the available medical history as being accidental. Sexual abuse may include statutory rape (sexual intercourse of a child younger than 14 years by a person 18 years or older), sexual assault, incest, rape, promotion of prostitution, or pornography, but this can vary by state law.

Physical neglect is the physical condition caused by prolonged or repeated lack of supervision, or failure to provide the essentials of life. Emotional or psychological abuse may cause a child to be chronically and significantly anxious, depressed, socially withdrawn, or psychotic, and may interfere with the child's ability to behave in a developmentally appropriate manner.

This chapter will briefly review a general approach to pediatric patients who may be victims of abuse.

Initial Diagnostic Approach
General

■ *History.* Information should be gathered from as many resources (e.g., caregivers, prehospital providers, social workers) as possible, especially in younger children. When interacting with the child, special consideration should be given to the age dependent appropriate developmental level.

Obtain the history via open-ended questions in a supportive and reassuring manner. Some children may express guilt for having "caused"
the abuse, or will worry about what will happen to the abuser. Make
efforts to gain the child's trust, and avoid making promises that cannot be
kept, such as saying the examination won't hurt. Information concerning
the perpetrator(s), time, date, and location of the abuse, and the specifics
of the abuse should be obtained. Additional information on the overall
family environment should be determined, and includes disciplinary
practices, substance abuse, domestic violence, recent stressors, and prior
child protection agency involvement. On occasion, the NAT is obscured
by the reality that while the child has had many visits to the ED due to
some trauma, the visits have always been to different EDs, so the
physician never has a chance to discover the multiplicity of the traumas.
- *Physical examination.* The physical examination should be comprehensive, covering not just areas that were allegedly injured, but all parts of
  the body, including the genitalia, regardless of the history obtained.
  Physical examination findings that may mimic physical abuse are listed in
  Table 82–1.

Laboratory

- Studies may include complete blood count (CBC) with differential,
  activated partial thromboplastin time, and prothrombin time. For high-
  risk child sexual abuse, the U.S. Centers for Disease Control and Prevention (CDC) recommends gonococcal and chlamydial cultures, and
  serology for syphilis, human immunodeficiency virus, and hepatitis B.
  Depending on the area of concern, lipase, liver function tests, urinalysis,
  or stool hemoccult may be indicated.

Radiography

- *Plain films.* For NAT, the skeletal survey is the standard radiographic
  imaging study for children less than 2 years; it includes 19 images (skull,
  long bones, hands, feet, thorax, pelvis, and spine). Additional views
  should be obtained for specific injuries with at least two views for each
  fracture. Once plain films of the acutely injured body part have been
  obtained, and there is no concern for another fracture needing acute
  attention, the rest of the skeletal survey may be completed after the child
  has been admitted to the hospital.
- *Computed tomography (CT scan).* A CT scan should be used for the
  evaluation of a possible intracranial hemorrhage or significant abdominal
  trauma. The CT scan may also be helpful in patients with significant
  spine or soft-tissue trauma. Magnetic resonance imaging (MRI) is more
  useful in determining injury from the NAT of a shaken baby, including
  shearing and diffuse axonal injuries.

Emergency Department Management Overview
General

- The ABCs (*a*irway, *b*reathing, and *c*irculation) should always be addressed
  as with any other trauma patients (see Chapter 8 and Chapter 74).

Table 82–1   Physical Examination Findings That May Mimic Physical Abuse

Bruises (Non NAT causes)	Burns	Fractures	Intracranial Hemorrhage
Mongolian spots	Photodermatitis	Birth injury	Coagulation disorders
Erythema multiforme	Drug eruption	Osteogenesis imperfecta	Arteriovenous malformation
Henoch-Schönlein purpura	Dystrophic epidermolysis bullosa	Nutritional/metabolic disorders (rickets)	Glutaric aciduria type 1
Coagulopathy/platelet function disorder	Staphylococcal toxin syndromes	Neoplasm	
	Folk medicine	Osteomyelitis	
Erythema nodosum	Contact dermatitis	Congenital syphilis	
Hypersensitivity vasculitis		Neuromuscular defects (cerebral palsy)	
Idiopathic thrombocytopenic purpura			
Ehlers-Danlos syndrome			
Leukemia			
Vitamin K deficiency			
Folk medicine (coining, cupping)			

Medications

- **Sedation.** May be required to perform the physical examination and for diagnostic studies.
- **Analgesia.** May be given by mouth or intravenous (IV) line as needed for the pain secondary to injury.
- **Antibiotics.** Should be administered if there is concern for a perforated viscus or other infection secondary to abuse.

Disposition

- **Consultation.** Early social work or child protective services consultation is necessary to obtain a thorough history by a trained professional, and for protection of the child. There is a legal mandate in all 50 states as well as ethical responsibility to report cases of suspected child abuse. Surgery consultation should be obtained for any visceral injury; neurosurgery consultation should be obtained for any intracranial hemorrhage, and orthopedics consultation should be obtained for most fractures. Ophthalmology should be consulted in all cases of physical NAT to obtain a thorough retinal examination (looking for hemorrhages), but this may be obtained once the child has been admitted to the hospital.
- **Admission.** Any child with a significant injury sustained from a mechanism suspi-cious for NAT should be considered for admission for further medical evaluation and treatment, and for ongoing social services, including protection of the child. Children without significant physical injury, but who are victims of NAT, may still need admission for protection, ongoing social services and placement.

Specific Problems
Child Neglect

- In nonorganic failure to thrive (FTT), the child may be described as eating a normal diet with no abnormal losses (i.e., emesis or diarrhea), and the parent(s) may not recognize the FTT. Medical neglect includes failure to seek timely medical care for an injury or illness or noncompliance with the prescribed therapies.
- Signs of malnutrition include increased or decreased pulse; decreased fatty tissue or prominent bony structures; pallor; protuberant abdomen; hepatomegaly; loose skin; heart murmur from anemia; and decreased activity. Evidence of poor hygiene includes diaper dermatitis; lice or scabies; or unkempt appearance.

Child Sexual Abuse

- The parent(s) and the child should be interviewed together and inde-pendently. History taking should be coordinated with the social worker to minimize the number of times the child has to provide details of the sexual abuse. Parents and caregivers may report behavioral changes in the child. The child may disclose the abuse.
- The supine frog-leg or prone knee–chest positions (child rests head in arms, abdomen sagging downward, knees bent 6-8 inches apart with

buttocks in the air) may maximize examination of the genital area of a prepubertal child. The diameter of the hymenal orifice alone cannot be considered evidence of sexual abuse. Concerning female findings include abrasions or bruising to the inner thighs and labia; scarring or tears of the labia minora or hymen; distortion, dilatation, or decreased hymenal tissue; injury to the posterior fourchette; or anal lacerations. Male findings of sexual abuse include penile shaft abrasions, petechiae, tears of the glans or frenulum, bruising, bite marks, and anal tears. There may be no physical evidence of abuse.

- Laboratory testing in cases of suspected sexual abuse must be guided by history and physical findings. Forensic evidence collection, prophylaxis for sexually transmitted diseases, and contraception are similar to the adult population (Chapter 40).

Cutaneous Manifestations

- The patterns of bruises or other lesions may not be consistent with the history or the developmental capabilities of the child, especially if the child is nonambulatory.
- Examination findings that are highly suspicious for NAT include bruises of the chest or abdomen in a nonambulatory child, patterns that look like loops (electrical cords/rope), human bite marks, hand prints, cigarette burns, circumferential wounds (especially around the wrists and ankles, which are indicative of restraint), and bruises around the neck. Suspicious burns include immersion burns with a symmetric "stocking or glove" distribution; presence of spared areas within the burned area (diaper area spared), or branding burns outlining the pattern of an object. If possible, photographs should be taken of the cutaneous findings for evidence.
- Laboratory tests to evaluate hematologic causes of bruising include CBC with differential, activated partial thromboplastin time, prothrombin time, bleeding time (children older than 1 year), and levels of von Willibrand factor antigen. In an infant or younger child with suspicious bruising, a skeletal survey to evaluate for fractures, and a head CT scan to evaluate for intracranial hemorrhage should be performed. If the child was shaken, an MRI is appropriate.
- Ask about family history of bleeding disorders or collagen vascular diseases. Certain cultural practices for healing, including cupping and coining, look like bruises, and should not be considered abuse. Mongolian spots and congenital lesions often occur on the back and buttocks, and can look like bruises. Inflicted burns tend to be deeper than those occurring from an accidental injury.

Head Trauma

- Intracranial lesions can present with seizures, irritability, poor feeding, emesis, lethargy, change in mental status, or apnea.
- Subdural and subarachnoid bleeding are common findings in intentional head trauma. Skull radiographs can reveal spreading of calvarial sutures when there is increased intracranial pressure. Physical evidence of a head injury without a history of trauma is a highly predictive historical feature for abuse. A history of another child with sudden infant death syndrome

in the family may be suspicious for abuse. The highest mortality in child abuse is from the shaken baby syndrome. Retinal hemorrhages do not occur from administering cardiopulmonary resuscitation.

■ Stabilize the airway, breathing, and circulation as needed. Neurosurgery should be consulted for any intracranial injury, and ophthalmology consulted for a complete eye examination to look for retinal hemorrhages or detachments.

Skeletal Injuries

■ The child may not be using the injured extremity, or may be limping. In cases of abuse, the injuries are often not consistent with the history or developmental level of child.

■ Radiologic studies should be taken of the injured area, followed by a complete skeletal survey if there is a question of NAT (see Chapter 81). Skull radiographs or a head CT scan should be performed to evaluate for skull fractures or intracranial injury, especially if a fracture is present. Calcium, phosphorous, and alkaline phosphatase levels may be sent to evaluate for rickets or other metabolic bone diseases.

Visceral Injuries

■ Symptoms may not manifest immediately after trauma. With intra-abdominal trauma there may be bruising, abdominal distention, tenderness, or no external findings at all. If there is significant bleeding, the patient may present in shock. Pulmonary injury may present with tachypnea, signs of respiratory distress, or decreased breath sounds.

■ Visceral organ injuries occur when the organ is compressed against the vertebrae from a direct blow (usually punching or kicking) to the abdominal area. The most common organs injured in order are the liver, spleen, duodenum/jejunum (rupture or hematoma), pancreas, vena cava, and kidney. Pancreatitis in a child is suspicious for NAT.

■ Refer to Chapter 14 for the evaluation and management of abdominal trauma.

Other Forms of Abuse

■ *Poisoning.* The child may present with a history of an accidental ingestion, or as a toxidrome with no history of ingestion. Commonly used poisons include ipecac, laxatives, salt poisoning, water intoxication, acetaminophen, aspirin, insulin, and oral hypoglycemic medications.

■ *Immersion.* Intentional immersion may be difficult to recognize due to a paucity of associated injuries. A history inconsistent with the child's developmental abilities strongly suggests NAT.

■ *Munchausen by Proxy.* This is defined as occurring when illness in a child is persistently faked or produced by a caregiver, and the child has repeated presentations for medical care. There is usually a history of multiple medical visits for poorly defined symptoms or illnesses, with no organic cause identified. There may be a history of illnesses or death of other children in the family.

Teaching Points

Nonaccidental trauma (NAT) is unfortunately more common than most physicians suspect. Inappropriate behavior on the part of the caregiver or parent when in the ED may signal the cause of the problem as NAT. Also, history of an injury that is inconsistent with the age and development of the child should suggest NAT. There is a legal obligation to report NAT in all 50 states.

Suggested Readings

Care M. Imaging in suspected child abuse: what to expect and what to order. Pediatr Ann 2002;31:651–659.

Heger AS, Emans SJ, Muram D (editors). Evaluation of the Sexually Abused Child (2nd ed). New York: Oxford University Press, 2000.

Ludwig S, Kornberg AE (editors). Child Abuse: A Medical Reference (2nd ed). New York: Churchill Livingstone, 1992.

Reece RM, Ludwig S (editors). Child Abuse: Medical Diagnosis and Management (2nd ed). Philadelphia: Lippincott Williams & Wilkins, 2001.

Sirotnak AP, Grigsby T, Krugman RD. Physical abuse of children. Pediatr Rev 2004;25:264–275.

SECTION VII

SPECIAL TOPICS

CHAPTER **83**

Acid-Base

COREY M. SLOVIS ■ NICOLE STREIFF MCCOIN

Overview

In this chapter, a five-step approach to the basic metabolic panel (BMP), and a three-step approach to the arterial blood gas (ABG), provide a succinct and simple method to diagnose acid-base disturbances. Subsequently, brief descriptions are provided of each particular acid-base disorder that may be found using these algorithms.

Five-Step Acid-Base Approach to the Basic Metabolic Panel

Step 1: Check the BMP values for abnormalities.
■ Know your normal laboratory value ranges (see Appendix 1).
Step 2: Calculate the anion gap (AG).
■ AG = sodium (Na) – (chloride [Cl] + bicarbonate [HCO_3]). In general, the normal range for AG = 5–12 ± 2 (thus an AG > 15 is elevated).
■ If an elevated AG is calculated, a wide-gap metabolic acidosis exists independent of the values of HCO_3 or pH.
■ Examples of AG calculation:
  (1) Na 140; potassium (K) 4.0; Cl 100; HCO_3 28
      AG = Na – (Cl + HCO_3) = 140 – (100 + 28) = 12 (This AG of 12 is within normal limits).
  (2) Na 140; K 5.0; Cl 100; HCO_3 10
      AG = Na – (Cl + HCO_3) = 140 – (100 + 10) = 30 (This AG of 30 represents an elevated anion gap, and, thus, a wide-gap metabolic acidosis exists independent of the pH.)
Step 3: If an acidosis is present, apply the Rule of 15 (Box 83–1).
■ The Rule of 15 states the following: HCO_3 + 15 should equal the partial pressure of CO_2 or PCO_2 (+/– 2). It is also approximately equal to the last two digits of the pH.

BOX 83–1   The Rule of 15

HCO_3 + 15 should = PCO_2 and the last two digits of the pH (7.XX)
(a) If PCO_2 = expected, simple compensation exists
(b) If PCO_2 < expected, a superimposed primary respiratory alkalosis exists
(c) If PCO_2 > expected, a superimposed primary respiratory acidosis exists

---

- The Rule of 15 yields a prediction of a patient's PCO_2 and pH by simply knowing the HCO_3 value.
- If the Rule of 15 is broken, a second primary process other than just a secondary respiratory compensation exists.
    (1) If the PCO_2 is appropriately depressed, simple compensation exists.
    (2) If the PCO_2 is lower than the expected value derived from the Rule of 15, a superimposed primary respiratory alkalosis exists.
    (3) If the PCO_2 is higher than the expected value derived from the Rule of 15, a superimposed primary respiratory acidosis exists.
- There is a corollary to the Rule of 15, which states that as the HCO_3 falls below 10 and approaches 5, the PCO_2 should equal 15. Alternatively, the Winter's formula can be used to calculate the expected PCO_2 when the HCO_3 falls below 10. The Winter's formula states that $HCO_3 \times 1.5 + 8$ = expected PCO_2 (±2). Examples of the application of the Rule of 15 are listed in Table 83–1.

Step 4: If an acidosis is present, check the delta gap.

- The delta gap relies on the 1:1 concept that for each rise of 1 in the AG, the HCO_3 should fall by 1 mmol/L. Observe the change in AG by using a normal reference value of 15 (the AG upper limit of normal). Observe the change in HCO_3 by using a normal reference value of 24 mmol/L.
- The delta gap searches for hidden metabolic processes (i.e., a second normal gap acidosis or a superimposed metabolic alkalosis). Examples are listed in Table 83–2.

Step 5: If unexplained wide-gap metabolic acidosis exists, check the osmolar gap.

- Osmolarity = $(2 \times Na)$ + (glucose/18) + (blood urea nitrogen [BUN]/2.8) + (ethanol [ETOH]/4).
- Osmolar gap = true osmolarity (value given in blood lab results) – calculated osmolarity (using the formula above). Normal osmolar gap is no greater than 10. If the osmolar gap is greater than 10, consider a toxic alcohol as a cause for the patient's wide-gap metabolic acidosis.
- Multiply osmolar gap × 3 = methanol in mg%.
- Multiply osmolar gap × 4 = ETOH in mg% (if not already used in the above calculated osmolarity equation.
- Multiply osmolar gap × 6 = isopropyl alcohol or ethylene glycol in mg%.
- Example: Na 140; K 6.0; Cl 100; HCO_3 8; BUN 30; creatinine 2.5; glucose 80; ETOH 240 mg%; MEASURED OSMOLARITY = 425 mOsm. Patient has consumed antifreeze and has evidence as above of renal failure. What is the osmolar gap? Can you calculate the patient's ethylene glycol level? Calculated osmolarity: $(2 \times Na)$ + (glucose/18) + (BUN/2.8) + (ETOH/4) = (2×140) + (80/18) + (30/2.8) + (240/4) = approximately 355. Osmolar gap = true osmolarity – calculated osmolarity = 425 – 355 = 70. Ethylene glycol (mg%) = osmolar gap × 6 = 70 × 6 = 420 mg%.

Three-Step Acid-Base Approach to the Arterial Blood Gas

Step 1: Determine if the patient has an acidosis or alkalosis.

- A pH of 7.35 or lower represents an acidosis. A pH of 7.45 or higher indicates alkalosis.

Table 83–1 Applying the Rule of 15

Example	Anion Gap	Rule of 15
Na 140; K 4.5; Cl 100; HCO₃ 20; Pco₂ 35; pH 7.35	AG = Na − (Cl + HCO₃) = 140 − (100 + 20) = 20 This AG of 20 represents an elevated anion gap, and, thus, a wide-gap metabolic acidosis exists independent of the pH.	HCO₃ + 15 = 20 + 15 = 35. Thus, the expected Pco₂ is 35 (±2), and the last two digits of the pH should approximate 35 (i.e., 7.35). Since the patient's given Pco₂ and pH values equal the expected values calculated using the Rule of 15, a pure wide-gap metabolic acidosis with an appropriate compensatory secondary respiratory alkalosis exists.
Na 140; K 4.0; Cl 110; HCO₃ 10; Pco₂ 20; pH 7.32	AG = Na − (Cl + HCO₃) = 140 (110 + 10) = 20. This AG of 20 represents an elevated anion gap, and, thus, a wide-gap metabolic acidosis exists independent of the pH.	HCO₃ + 15 = 10 + 15 = 25. Thus, the expected pCO₂ is 25 (±2), and the last two digits of the pH should approximate 25 (i.e., 7.25). However, the patient's given Pco₂ of 20, which is lower than the expected Pco₂ of 25. The patient is hyperventilating more than expected simply to compensate for the metabolic acidosis. Thus, there is a superimposed primary respiratory alkalosis.
Na 140; K 4.2; Cl 105; HCO₃ 10; Pco₂ 32; pH 7.14	AG = Na − (Cl + HCO₃) = 140 − (105 + 10) = 25. This AG of 25 represents an elevated anion gap, and, thus, a wide-gap metabolic acidosis exists independent of the pH.	HCO₃ + 15 = 10 + 15 = 25. Thus, the expected Pco₂ is 25 (±2), and the last two digits of the pH should approximate 25 (i.e., 7.25). However, the patient's given Pco₂ is 32, which is higher than the expected Pco₂ of 25. The patient is not compensating enough (not ventilating enough CO₂ from the body). Thus, there is a primary respiratory acidosis in addition to the primary wide-gap metabolic acidosis.
Na 140; K 4.2; Cl 110; HCO₃ 5; Pco₂ 20; pH 7.04	AG = Na − (Cl + HCO₃) = 140 − (110 + 5) = 25. This AG of 25 represents an elevated anion gap, and, thus, a wide-gap metabolic acidosis exists independent of the pH.	In this example, the HCO₃ has decreased below 10, and, therefore, the Pco₂ should equal 15 using the corollary to the Rule of 15. However, the patient's given Pco₂ of 15. The patient is not compensating enough (not ventilating enough CO₂ from the body). Thus, there is a primary respiratory acidosis in addition to the primary wide-gap metabolic acidosis.

Table 83–2   Calculating the Delta Gap

Example	Anion Gap	HCO₃	Comment
AG 22; HCO₃ 17	Change in AG = patient's AG –AG upper limit of normal = 22 – 15 = 7.	Change in HCO₃ = normal HCO₃ value – patient's HCO₃ = 24 – 17 = 7.	The AG has increased by 7, and the HCO₃ has decreased by 7. Thus, 7:7 = 1:1, and no hidden metabolic process exists.
AG 28; HCO₃ 20	Change in AG = patient's AG – AG upper limit of normal = 28 – 15 = 13.	Change in HCO₃ = normal HCO₃ value – patient's HCO₃ = 24 – 20 = 4.	The AG has increased by 13, and the HCO₃ has decreased by 4. Thus, the HCO₃ value is too high for this change in the AG. The only explanation for this relatively elevated HCO₃ is superimposed metabolic alkalosis in addition to the wide-gap metabolic acidosis.
AG 23; HCO₃ 12	Change in AG = patient's AG –AG upper limit of normal = 23 – 15 = 8.	Change in HCO₃ = normal HCO₃ value – patient's HCO₃ = 24 – 12 = 12.	The AG has increased by 8, but the HCO₃ has decreased by 12. Thus, the HCO₃ value is too low for this change in the AG. The only explanation for this relatively lower HCO₃ is a superimposed normal-gap acidosis in addition to the wide-gap metabolic acidosis.

AG, *anion gap.*

- Of note, a pH within normal limits may "hide" a combination of acidosis and alkalosis.

Step 2: Determine if the acidosis/alkalosis is a respiratory or metabolic process.

- In a respiratory process, the P_{CO_2} drives the pH in the opposite direction. In a metabolic process, the P_{CO_2} follows the pH in the same direction. Of note, normal P_{CO_2} is 40 and normal pH is 7.4.
- Examples:
  (1) pH 7.32; P_{CO_2} 50 mm Hg; P_{O_2} 83 mm Hg
      pH 7.32 = acidosis
      P_{CO_2} has increased to 50 mm Hg, and pH has decreased to 7.32.
      Respiratory acidosis.
  (2) pH 7.32; P_{CO_2} 30 mm Hg; P_{O_2} 80 mm Hg
      pH 7.32 = acidosis
      P_{CO_2} has decreased to 30 mm Hg, and pH has also decreased to 7.32.
      Metabolic acidosis.
  (3) pH 7.56; P_{CO_2} 20; P_{O_2} 83 mm Hg
      pH 7.56 = alkalosis
      P_{CO_2} has decreased to 20 mm Hg, and pH has increased to 7.56.
      Respiratory alkalosis.
  (4) pH 7.52; P_{CO_2} 60 mm Hg; P_{O_2} 80 mm Hg
      pH 7.52 = alkalosis
      P_{CO_2} has increased to 60 mm Hg, and pH has also increased to 7.52.
      Metabolic alkalosis.

Step 3: If a respiratory process exists, determine if it is a pure respiratory process, or if there is also a metabolic component.

- As stated above, in a respiratory process, the P_{CO_2} drives the pH in the opposite direction. In a pure respiratory process, a change of 10 mm Hg P_{CO_2} will result in a change of approximately 0.08 in the pH in the opposite direction.
- Examples:
  (1) In a pure respiratory process, if the P_{CO_2} decreases to 30 mm Hg (a decrease of 10 mm Hg), the pH should rise to approximately 7.48 (an increase of 0.08).
  (2) In a pure respiratory process, if the P_{CO_2} increases to 50 mm Hg (an increase of 10 mm Hg), the pH should decrease to approximately 7.32 (a decrease of 0.08).
  (3) In a pure respiratory process, if the P_{CO_2} decreases to 20 mm Hg (a decrease of 20 mm Hg), the pH should rise to approximately 7.56 (an increase of 0.08×2 = approximately 0.16).
- If the P_{CO_2} and pH do not follow the rule stating that a change in P_{CO_2} of 10 mm Hg should lead to a change in pH of approximately 0.08, a metabolic component may also exist. This is referred to as a mixed process. If the pH is higher than expected, metabolic alkalosis also exists. If the pH is lower than expected, metabolic acidosis also exists.
- Examples:
  (1) pH 7.47; P_{CO_2} 25 mm Hg; P_{O_2} 80 mm Hg
      pH 7.47 = alkalosis

PCO$_2$ has decreased to 25 mm Hg, and pH has increased to 7.47. Thus, a respiratory alkalosis exists.

Now, the PCO$_2$ has decreased 15 mm Hg. In a pure respiratory process, a PCO$_2$ drop of 15 mm Hg should lead to an increase in pH of approximately 1.5 × 0.08 = 0.12 (a pH increase of 7.40 + 0.12 = 7.52). However, the pH is 7.47, which is lower than it should be if only a pure respiratory process exists. Therefore, a second metabolic process must exist that is making the patient more acidotic. Thus, the patient has a primary respiratory alkalosis and a metabolic acidosis.

(2) pH 7.0; PCO$_2$ 60 mm Hg; PO$_2$ 55 mm Hg

pH 7.0 = acidosis

PCO$_2$ has increased to 60 mm Hg, and pH has decreased to 7.0. Thus, a respiratory acidosis exists.

Now, the PCO$_2$ has increased to 60 mm Hg. In a pure respiratory process, a PCO$_2$ increase of 20 mm Hg should lead to a decrease in pH of approximately 2 × 0.08 = 0.16 (a pH decrease of 7.40 − 0.16 = 7.24). However, the pH is 7.0, which is lower than it should be if only a pure respiratory process exists. Therefore, a second metabolic process must exist that is making the patient more acidotic. Thus, the patient has a primary respiratory acidosis, and a primary metabolic acidosis.

Specific Problems
Metabolic Acidosis

- **Wide-gap metabolic acidosis (WGMA).** Findings on BMP and ABG that signal the presence of a WGMA include an elevated AG (>15) independent of the value of the pH or HCO$_3$. The mnemonic "MUDPILES" is used to recall the causes of WGMA, which are listed in Box 83–2.
- **Normal-gap metabolic acidosis.** This is also known as hyperchloremic metabolic acidosis because the kidney retains Cl$^-$ ions in response to the loss of HCO$_3$. Findings on BMP and ABG that signal the presence of a normal-gap metabolic acidosis include an AG within normal limits (<15) (no unmeasured anions) in the setting of a metabolic acidosis indicating the presence of a normal-gap acidosis. Causes of a normal-gap metabolic acidosis are summarized using the mnemonic "HARD UP" (Box 83–2).

Metabolic Alkalosis

- If the metabolic alkalosis resolves with the administration of NaCl, a chloride-responsive metabolic alkalosis is present, and is due to the kidney retaining Na. In these patients, spot urine Cl$^-$ is less than 10. Those cases that do not respond to NaCl administration are termed chloride-unresponsive metabolic alkaloses. The majority of these chloride-unresponsive states are associated with endocrinologic abnormalities. Aldosterone stimulates the distal exchange site, resulting in increased H$^+$ and K$^+$ excretion in return for Na resorption (in the form of Na$^+$HCO$_3^-$).
- Causes of chloride-responsive and chloride-unresponsive metabolic alkaloses are summarized in Box 83–3.

BOX 83–2 Causes of Metabolic Acidosis

Wide-gap metabolic acidosis
Methanol
Uremia
Diabetic ketoacidosis / alcoholic ketoacidosis
Paraldehyde
Isoniazid / **I**ron
Lactic acidosis
Ethylene glycol
Salicylates

Normal-gap metabolic acidosis (hyperchloremic metabolic acidosis)
Hyperventilation
Acid infusion / **A**ddison's/**C**arbonic **A**nhydrase inhibitor
Renal tubular acidosis (RTA)
Diarrhea
Ureterosigmoidostomy (and ileal diversion)
Pancreatic drainage/fistula

BOX 83–3 Causes of Metabolic Alkalosis

Chloride-responsive metabolic alkalosis
  Nasogastric suction
  Vomiting
  Chloride-wasting diarrhea
  Villous adenoma
  Diuretics

Chloride-unresponsive metabolic alkalosis
  Cushing's disease
  Hyperaldosteronism (Barter's syndrome)
  Secondary hyperaldosteronism
  (congestive heart failure, chronic renal failure, liver failure)
  Steroids
  Bicarbonate ingestion
  Licorice overdose

- Compensation rules in metabolic alkalosis include the following: (1) In chronic metabolic alkalosis, the P_{CO_2} should rise 5 mm Hg for each rise of 10 meq HCO_3; (2) If the P_{CO_2} is greater than 55, respiratory failure is present. Remember, massive bicarbonate ingestions may cause severe metabolic alkalosis in patients with poor renal function, leading to sudden respiratory failure.

Respiratory Acidosis

- Findings on BMP and ABG that signal the presence of a respiratory acidosis include the following: an elevated P_{CO_2}, and the P_{CO_2} is not as low as expected in a patient with a metabolic acidosis.
- Causes of respiratory acidosis are summarized in Box 83–4.
- Compensation rules in respiratory acidosis are as follows: (1) The kidneys compensate for respiratory acidosis by retaining HCO_3 which begins at 12-16 hours, but maximal HCO_3 retention may take one week or longer; (2) Acutely, the HCO_3 should rise 1 meq for each rise of 10 mm Hg P_{CO_2} (remember, the pH falls by approximately 0.08 for each rise of 10 mm Hg P_{CO_2}); (3) Chronically, the HCO_3 should rise 3-4 meq for each rise of 10 mm Hg P_{CO_2}; (4) If HCO_3 is above 30, either a chronic respiratory acidosis is present, or there is a coexistent primary metabolic alkalosis.

Respiratory Alkalosis

- Findings on BMP and ABG that signal the presence of a respiratory alkalosis include a decreased P_{CO_2}; a P_{CO_2} that is not as high as expected in a patient with a metabolic alkalosis.
- Causes of respiratory alkalosis are summarized in Box 83–5.
- Compensation rules in respiratory alkalosis are as follows: (1) Respiratory alkalosis is the ONLY acid-base disturbance that may have full compensation; (2) Acutely, the HCO_3 should fall 2 meq for each fall of 10 mm Hg P_{CO_2} (remember, the pH rises by approximately 0.08 for each fall of 10 mm Hg P_{CO_2}); (3) Chronically, the HCO_3 should fall 5 meq for each fall of 10 mm Hg P_{CO_2}.

BOX 83–4   Causes of Respiratory Acidosis

Airway
    Obstruction
    Spasm
    Asthma
    Chronic obstructive pulmonary disease

Mass Effect
    Pneumothorax
    Massive pulmonary effusion
    Pulmonary edema
    Infection (pneumonia, aspiration, etc.)

Central Nervous System
    Drugs (sedative hypnotics, narcotics, etc.)
    Tumor
    Neuromuscular
    Myopathies (Muscular Dystrophy, potassium/phosphate deficiency)
    Neuropathies (Guillain-Barré)

BOX 83–5   Causes of Respiratory Alkalosis

Airway/Pulmonary: Any process causing hypoxia or a sensation of inadequate oxygenation or ventilation (pulmonary embolus, acute stages of asthma exacerbation, etc.)

CNS: Tumor

GI: Liver disease

Endocrine: Hyperthyroidism

Infectious: Fever, sepsis

Drugs: Aspirin, cocaine, beta-agonists, progesterone

Psychiatric: Anxiety

Miscellaneous: Pregnancy, pain, withdrawal

Teaching Points

Acid-base balance is maintained within a narrow range by the body's homeostatic mechanisms. The pH is maintained by a combination of sodium and potassium conservation mechanisms, as well as by respiratory compensations.

Although blood gas analysis is very helpful, it is possible to calculate bicarbonate, carbon dioxide, and pH measurements from a basic metabolic panel, and get an idea about the cause of the metabolic changes.

The presence of an anion gap can help narrow the differential diagnosis. If an osmolar gap is also present, look for toxic substances such as ethylene glycol.

Suggested Readings

Narins RG, Emmett M. Simple and mixed acid-base disorders: a practical approach. Medicine 1980;59:161–187.

Narins RG, et al. Diagnostic strategies in disorders of fluid, electrolyte, and acid-base homeostasis. Am J Med 1982;77:496–519.

Mennen M, Slovis CM. Severe metabolic alkalosis in the emergency department. Ann Emerg Med 1988;17:354–357.

Wrenn KD. The delta gap. Ann Emerg Med 1990;113:567–569.

Isenhour JL, Slovis CM. Arterial blood gas analysis: a simple 3-step approach. J Respir Dis 2001;22:289–296.

CHAPTER 84

Blood Transfusion Therapy

RIVA L. RAHL ■ KURT C. KLEINSCHMIDT

Overview

Blood and blood product transfusions are being used with increasing frequency in the ED.

The decision to transfuse should be based on the stability of the patient, the patient's co-morbidities, blood product availability, and the availability of alternative options of therapy for the underlying problem. Increasing the availability of oxygen to the circulating red blood cells (RBCs) enables greater oxygen delivery to the tissues.

There are many causes of anemia, acute blood loss, and coagulation disorders. Refer to Section III (Trauma), Chapter 34 (Gastrointestinal Bleed), and Chapter 66 (Hematology/Oncology).

This chapter will provide some general guidelines for transfusion therapy in the ED.

Initial Diagnostic Approach
General

■ Orthostatic vital signs (Chapter 2) may identify those with intravascular volume loss. Orthostatic vitals should not be obtained on a patient who is already hemodynamically unstable, or is unable to tolerate the procedure for other reasons.
■ Evaluate perfusion of end organs, such as the skin (cool, diaphoretic, mottled), brain (mental status), and kidneys (urine output).
■ The clinical examination should seek first to determine whether the patient has a local source for bleeding (i.e., bleeding from a gastric ulcer or trauma), or if it is more generalized bleeding suggesting a systemic coagulation defect.

Laboratory

■ The five laboratory tests that reflect basic parameters most important for blood volume and hemostasis are: hemoglobin and hematocrit, platelet count, prothrombin time (PT), activated partial thromboplastin time (PTT), and fibrinogen level. A type and cross match should be sent immediately to the blood bank to obtain the appropriate blood products for transfusion. A complete blood count (CBC), electrolytes, renal function, and coagulation tests should be sent in most situations.

- **Coagulation studies.** An elevated PT reflects an extrinsic pathway abnormality via factor VII deficiency. It is a sensitive gauge of hepatic function, and the efficacy of warfarin administration. An increased PTT reflects deficiencies of factors within the intrinsic coagulation system. They are the most common inherited abnormalities of the entire clotting system. Factor VIII, IX, and XI deficiencies account for 99% of inherited bleeding disorders. Both the PT and PTT are elevated in DIC; occasionally the PTT may be normal. Bleeding time is a measure of platelet function, and is indicated in a patient with mucocutaneous bleeding and normal PT, PTT, and platelet count. The bleeding time is prolonged in von Willebrand's disease and functional platelet disorders (e.g., uremia, aspirin).
- See Table 84–1 for laboratory clues to the diagnosis of anemia and bleeding.

Emergency Department Management Overview

General

- Patients who are hemodynamically unstable or require blood products should have two large–bore intravenous (IV) lines. A large-bore peripheral catheter (14- or 16-gauge) is preferred for rapid volume infusions unless an easily accessible venipuncture site is not available. A large-bore (8 French) introducer catheter is preferred over standard central venous catheters if large-volume infusion is required. Central venous access is preferred to peripheral access in the cardiac arrest or near-arrest situations because it provides a rapid and reliable route for the administration of drugs and blood products to the central circulation.
- Begin resuscitation with crystalloid infusion such as normal saline or lactated Ringers solution. Patients with ongoing blood loss, or those who fail to respond to initial crystalloid resuscitation, will need blood products.
- Attempt to treat the source of blood loss especially if actively bleeding (i.e., surgery, banding of varices). If there is visible or active bleeding, apply direct pressure to the source if possible.
- The threshold for transfusing packed RBCs depends on the clinical conditions. If the hematocrit is below 30%, and the patient is bleeding or hemodynamically unstable, packed RBCs should be transfused immediately. Stable patients can tolerate lower hematocrits, and aggressive transfusion may be detrimental. For example, healthy individuals may tolerate hemoglobin levels of 6 to 8 g/dl; whereas those with heart failure, pulmonary, renal, or vascular disease may benefit from levels closer to 10 g/dl. Patients with signs and symptoms of decreased oxygen delivery (e.g., shortness of breath, ischemic chest pain) should also be transfused earlier.
- The threshold for platelet transfusion is 10,000/μl if the patient is stable without signs of bleeding, is not on platelet inhibitors, has preserved renal function, and does not have DIC. If one of these risk factors is present, keeping the count more than 50,000/μl is reasonable.
- For a fibrinogen level below 100 to 125 mg/dl, transfusions of 10 units of cryoprecipitate should increase the plasma fibrinogen level by 100 mg/dl.

Table 84–1	**Laboratory Clues for Causes of Bleeding or Anemia**
Acute blood loss	Amount of blood loss may not be reflected in the hemoglobin or hematocrit Reticulocyte count is often not elevated for 3 to 4 d. Coagulopathy may contribute if present (e.g., preexisiting hepatic failure, anticoagulation therapy)
Hemolysis	Reticulocytosis (in the absence of bone marrow disease) Spherocytes or schistocytes on blood smear Unconjugated bilirubin ↑ Lactate dehydrogenase level ↑ Haptoglobin ↓ Hemoglobinuria
Disseminated intravascular coagulation	Platelets and fibrinogen ↓ Fibrin-related marker such as d-dimer ↑ Prothrombin time (PT) ↑ Partial thromboplastin time (PTT) ↑ (may be normal)
Idiopathic thrombocytopenic purpura (ITP)	Platelets ↓ (normal PT/PTT)
Thrombotic thrombocytopenic purpura (TTP)	Platelets ↓ (normal PT, PTT, fibrinogen) Hemolytic anemia (see "hemolysis" above; with schistocytes) Hematuria and proteinuria Renal function↓
von Willebrand's disease	PTT ↑ Bleeding time ↑ Factor VIII coagulant activity ↓ von Willebrand's factor (vWF) antigen or ristocetin cofactor ↓
Hemophilia	PTT ↑ Bleeding time usually normal (prolonged in von Willebrand's disease). Hemophilia A: reduced factor VIII:C level distinguishes hemophilia A from other causes of prolonged PTT; normal or increased vWF. Hemophilia B: reduced factor IX coagulant activity levels

↑, *increased;* ↓ *decreased; d, days; PT, prothrombin time; PTT, partial thromboplastin time.*

- In patients with an international normalized ratio (INR) above 1.6 to 2.0, or an abnormal aPTT, fresh frozen plasma (FFP) is given. Elevation of the aPTT above 1.8 times normal is associated with bleeding in trauma patients. Patients with marked abnormalities, such as an aPTT above twice normal, may require aggressive therapy of at least 15 to 30 ml/kg (4-8 units for an average adult) of plasma.
- For massive transfusions, some advocate the administration of 1 unit of FFP per each 5 units of packed RBCs in massively transfused patients.

However, it is not possible to predict the degree of coagulopathy. Therefore, monitoring the patient's coagulation status during massive transfusions is more accurate and beneficial.

■ All patients requiring transfusion therapy in the ED require hospital admission unless an observation unit is available. One exception at some institutions is the patient with a chronic illness who is being treated as an outpatient but requires intermittent transfusions.

Blood Products

■ Table 84–2 summarizes the commonly available blood products used in the ED.

Blood Typing

■ Patients who lack A or B red cell antigens have antibodies for the absent A (blood type B) or B (blood type A) antigen. Patients who lack both A and B antigens have antibodies against both A and B antigens (blood type O).

■ Because RBCs of type O blood are not hemolyzed by the recepient anti-A or anti-B antibodies, type O blood is considered the *universal donor*. It is used when blood is required immediately such as an unstable patient who has ongoing blood loss. Because O-negative blood exists in only 6% of the population, its use is often restricted to women of childbearing age who are at risk for Rh immunization against subsequent pregnancies. Universal donor group O-positive blood is recommended in all other patients.

■ ABO identification and compatibility are the most important step of the type and cross-match procedure because any incompatibility will cause the most severe transfusion reaction, acute hemolysis. Rh typing, antibody screening, and the testing of donor cells with recipient serum are also performed. Antibody screening is performed with recipient serum to discover agglutinating or nonagglutinating antibodies. Type-specific blood includes ABO and Rh typing. It is usually available within 10 to 15 minutes. ABO typing determines whether a blood type is A, B, AB, or O. Rh typing determines Rh-positive or Rh-negative status. Antibody screen ("type and screen") is performed with recipient serum to discover agglutinating or nonagglutinating antibodies. It includes ABO and Rh typing, and screens the donor blood for common antibodies (both direct and indirect) such as Kell, Kidd, and Duffy. This takes approximately 30 to 45 minutes. The antiglobulin (Coomb's) test detects antibody or complement on human RBC membranes, and is used to evaluate for hemolysis.

■ Full cross match ("type and cross") means that the recipient's plasma is mixed with donor cells to check for compatibility, and no hemolysis or agglutination. This process takes approximately 5 minutes. Thus all four steps of a full type and cross match require approximately 45 to 60 minutes. Cross-matched blood is dedicated to that patient for a specific time period (usually 48-72 hours). After this time, the blood is returned to the general pool available to all.

Table 84–2   Commonly Used Blood Products in the ED

	Indications	Components	Administration	Comment
Whole blood	Exchange or autologous transfusion	Plasma (with its proteins), red blood cells, white blood cells, and platelets.	450 ml/U May be given more quickly due to lower hematocrit.	Contains antibodies, proteins, possible infectious components; higher risk of infection than PRBCs and transfusion reactions. Platelets, granulocytes, and labile clotting factors decrease after refrigeration.
Packed red blood cells (PRBCs)	To provide additional oxygen carrying capacity; and expand volume.	Red blood cells. Washed RBCs depleted of plasma may ↓ allergic/anaphylactic reactions. Leukocyte-reduced RBCs may ↓ febrile reactions and reduce alloimmunization.	240–300 ml/U (hematocrit 70%–80%). Delivery rate is limited by the high hematocrit. Refrigerated shelf-life is 35 d.	Given with normal saline through micro- or macrofiltration pore. Large transfusions may cause a dilutional coagulopathy (PRBCs have ↓ factors or platelets). Each unit of packed RBCs raises the hematocrit by approximately 3%. In children, 5 ml/kg of PRBCs should raise the hematocrit by 5%.
Fresh frozen plasma (FFP)	Serious acute bleeding from coagulation-factor deficits.	Whole blood without cellular components; 90% water. Contains albumin, fibrinogen, globulins and clotting proteins. Freezing preserves coagulation factors including II, V, VII, VIII, IX, X, XI, XIII, fibrinogen.	200–250 ml/U Give immediately after thawing. Give 2 to 4 units; marked abnormalities (PTT above twice normal) may require up to 8 units.	Same complications as whole blood. Type AB plasma has no anti-A or anti-B antibodies so it is the universal FFP donor. One unit of FFP ↑ all coagulation factor levels by 2%–3%. FFP takes at least 40 min to thaw.

Continued

Table 84–2 Commonly Used Blood Products in the ED—*cont'd*

	Indications	Components	Administration	Comment
Platelets	Low platelet count (<10,000-50,000) with active bleeding.	Mainly platelets with a small amount of plasma and a few red blood cells (RBCs)	40-70 ml/U Platelet transfusions should be done after consultation with a hematologist or the blood bank. Usually given as a six pack. Females of childbearing age should get RhoGAM if Rh-negative and getting Rh-positive platelets due to the risk of Rh-alloimmunization.	Spontaneous bleeding is unlikely with platelets above 10,000-20,000, so "prophylactic" platelet transfusions are unnecessary. In processes with increased platelet destruction (ITP, TTP, DIC) platelet infusion can be harmful; only transfuse if life-threatening hemorrhage. ↑ infectious complications due to room temperature storage (↑ bacteria growth). ↓ transfusion reactions because ↓ RBCs, WBCs, or plasma. Shelf life is only up to 5 d. Six-pack of platelets (or one apheresis unit) adds ~30,000/μL to the platelet count. Patients who have received multiple platelet transfusions may develop alloimmunization, so will benefit from single-donor platelets.

Table 84–2   Commonly Used Blood Products in the ED—*cont'd*

	Indications	Components	Administration	Comment
Cryoprecipitate	May be used when specific clotting factor concentrates are not available.	Fibrinogen, von Willebrand's factor and factors VIII and XIII	Volume: 15-20 ml One unit contains at least 80 IU of factor VIII Dose is based on fibrinogen levels, antithrombin III levels, and coagulation parameters; 1 unit per 7-10 kg of body weight.	Is an alternative treatment for patients with hemophilia A or von Willebrand's when specific factor concentrates are unavailable. ABO typing is preferred (but not crucial as very little plasma is present). Rh typing is not needed as there are no RBCs present. Not commonly recommended except when fibrinogen is needed.
RhoGAM	Indicated for Rh-negative pregnant women who may be bearing Rh-positive children. Should be given to women at risk for fetomaternal transplacental hemorrhage: bleeding in early pregnancy, ectompic, trauma with potential antepartum hemorrhage.	Rho(D) immune globulin derived from human plasma.	Dose is 50 µg via intramuscular (IM) injection for first-trimester bleeding and 300 micrograms for all others.	It suppresses the immune response of Rh-negative women to Rh-positive RBCs. May also be given in pregnant Rh-negative women getting Rh-positive platelet transfusions

Continued

Table 84–2   Commonly Used Blood Products in the ED—*cont'd*

	Indications	Components	Administration	Comment
Factor VIII	Hemophilia A patients with bleeding.	Factor VIII concentrate, once made from extraction of pooled human plasma, is now prepared using recombinant-DNA derived factor VIII. Recombinant factor VIII has minimal risk of viral contamination. Some preparations use a human albumin base.	Volume: 1-2 ml IV 1 unit/kg of factor VIII concentrate increases activity by ~2%. Minor bleeding (small joints) requires 20%-40% of normal factor VIII levels. Moderate bleeding (large joint, neck, oral cavity) requires 40%-60% of normal levels. Life-threatening bleeding (intracranial, intra-abdominal, pharyngeal) requires 60%-100% of normal levels.	HIV and hepatitis viral transmission are now negligible. Antibodies to factor VIII develop in up to 15% of recipients. Massive doses of factor VIII may overwhelm the antibody response; give immunosuppressives and plasmapheresis. Major hemophiliacs may have <1% intrinsic factor VIII activity while those with minor disease may have 40%-50%, and may only need factor VIII concentrate for life-threatening bleeding.

Complications of Transfusion Therapy

■ One of the biggest concerns patients have regarding transfusion therapy is the infection risk from serious diseases such as human immuno-deficiency virus and hepatitis. The risk of contracting such diseases is summarized in Table 84–3.

■ Massive transfusion is defined as transfusion of at least one blood volume within 24 hours (~12 units of packed RBCs in a 70-kg adult). Adverse consequences of massive blood transfusions include hemolysis, coagulopathy, hypothermia, electrolyte disorders ($\downarrow$ or $\uparrow$ K^+, $\downarrow$ Ca^{++}), and volume overload.

Table 84–3   Infection Risk from Transfusion Therapy

	Risk	Comment
Bacterial	Sepsis occurs 1 in ~300,000 – 2.5 million transfusions.	Platelets are the most likely component to have bacterial infections (minor infections occur 1 in 2500 transfusions). Platelet contamination most commonly with *Staphylococcus aureus*. Red blood cell contamination most commonly with *Yersinia enterocolitica*. The patient presents with sepsis, bacteremia, or other manifestation of transmitted bacterial infection.
HIV	1:200,000 to 1:2 million	Both antigen and antibody tested in blood.
Hepatitis	Hepatitis A: 1 in 1,000,000 Hepatitis B: 1 in 30,000 to 250,000 Hepatitis C: 1 in 30,000 to 150,000	Tests for HepBsAg and HepB Core Ab. Tests for Hep C antigen itself (nucleic amplification technique) have decreased transmission rates to 1 in 900,000.
HTLV types I and II	1:250,000 to 1:2 million	Can cause leukemia
CMV	70% of adults are CMV-positive	CMV-negative blood is reserved for immunocompromised patients and neonates. CMV is stored in leukocytes. Can be prevented using leukocyte-reduced blood components.

CMV, cytomegalovirus.

Teaching Points

Patients who are hemodynamically stable should have two large-bore intravenous catheters. Large-volume transfusion through a large-bore peripheral catheter is preferred to standard central venous catheters unless a large-bore (8 French) introducer catheter is used.

Type O blood is considered the "universal donor", and is used when blood is required immediately such as the unstable patient who has ongoing blood loss. Because of the relative scarcity of group O-negative blood, its use is restricted to women of childbearing age who are at risk for Rh immunization against subsequent pregnancies. Universal donor group O-positive blood is recommended in all other patients.

The five laboratory tests that reflect basic parameters essential for blood volume and hemostasis are: hemoglobin and hematocrit, platelet count, prothrombin time, activated partial thromboplastin time, and fibrinogen level.

Transfusion therapy has many complications. Current methods have significantly reduced the associated risk of infection. Any patient receiving a transfusion should be closely monitored for a transfusion reaction. Patients receiving massive red blood cell transfusions are at risk for hemolysis, coagulopathies, hypothermia, volume overload, and electrolyte abnormalities.

Suggested Readings

DeLoughery TG. Critical care clotting catastrophies. Crit Care Clin 2005;21:531–562.
Drews RE. Critical issues in hematology: anemia, thrombocytopenia, coagulopathy, and blood product transfusions in critically ill patients. Clin Chest Med 2003;24:607–622.

CHAPTER **85**

Body Fluid Exposure

GREG MILLER ■ DIANE M. BIRNBAUMER

Overview

The three most important agents to consider when health care workers (HCWs) are exposed to body fluids are the human immunodeficiency virus (HIV), the hepatitis B virus (HBV), and the hepatitis C virus (HCV) (Table 85–1).

Approximately 600,000 to 800,000 percutaneous injuries (needle sticks) occur per year in the United States, with 27 sticks/100 beds in teaching hospitals, and 18 sticks/100 beds in nonteaching hospitals. The needlestick rate is approximately 1/10,000 venipunctures.

Risk Factors and Prevention

■ Focused training in universal precautions reduces body fluid exposures. Needles should never be recapped. Safety equipment is proven to decrease the rates of needle sticks. Resheathable needles reduce percutaneous injury by 23%, hinged needle shields reduce percutaneous injury by 66%, and self-blunting needles with rounded tips that protrude through the used needle reduce percutaneous injuries by 76%.

■ The successful immune response rate to the three-shot hepatitis B vaccine series is 88%; this rate is lower in the elderly, obese, and smokers. Doses should be given with at least 2-month intervals between the doses, and the HCW should be tested for anti-HBs 1 to 2 months after the last dose. Initial nonresponders should repeat the series because they have a 30% to 50% chance of responding to the second series. A titer of greater than or equal to 10 mIU/ml indicates immunity. Routine booster doses are not currently recommended because studies show an effective long-term immune response for up to 10 years.

Initial Diagnostic Approach

■ See Figure 85–1.

■ The history should focus on the HCW, the exposure, and the source.

■ Regarding the HCW, ascertain serologic status with respect to HIV, HCV, and HBV; HBV vaccine status; response to HBV vaccine (if vaccinated); and, if the exposure was a splash, the quality of overlying skin (healthy vs. chapped or lacerated). These levels should be recorded for the worker prior to any incident, but blood can be drawn for current levels during care of the incident in the ED (at hours when employees' health clinics are closed). See Table 85–2.

■ Regarding the exposure, first determine whether it was a percutaneous exposure or a mucosal or splash exposure. Four factors make a needlestick high risk: the depth of the stick, whether there was visible blood, whether the needle had been in the source's vein or artery, and whether the source has advanced HIV. Hollow-bore needles filled with blood are higher risk than blunt needles. For mucosal exposures, determine the amount and type of fluid; if the fluid is other than blood, it should be ascertained whether blood might have contaminated the fluid (e.g., bloody vomitus, traumatic lumbar puncture).

■ Regarding the source, ascertain the serologic status for HIV, HBV, and HCV after obtaining informed consent. Ask if the source had any risk behaviors (IV drug use, sexual contact with a known positive partner) in

Table 85–1 Risk of transmission of different viral agents depending on method of exposure

	Exposure route based on type of virus	Risk of seroconversion
HIV	Percutaneous injury	0.3% per average-risk needlestick; no number available for high-risk needlestick
	Mucous membrane splash	0.09% per splash
	Through broken skin (chapped hands, dermatitis)	Case reports, thought to be less dangerous than mucous membrane exposure
	Intact skin splash	No cases known
	Human bite	Case reports
	Receptive anal intercourse	0.5 to 3% per encounter
	Penile-vaginal intercourse Male to female Female to male	 0.1% per encounter Less than 0.1% per encounter
	Receptive oral sex	0.01% per encounter
	Insertive oral sex	0.005% per encounter
	Sharing needles with injection drug use	0.67% per use
HBV	HBsAg positive, HBeAg negative	Clinical hepatitis: 1-6% Seroconversion: 23-37%
	HBsAg positive, HBeAg positive	Clinical hepatitis: 22-31% Seroconversion: 37-62%
	Intact skin splash	No cases known
HCV	Percutaneous injury	Seroconversion 1.8-10%
	Mucus membrane splash	Case reports
	Intact skin splash	No cases known
	Human bite	Case report
	Sexual contact	0.1% per year of sexual contact
	Exposure fluid	**Risk of seroconversion**
	CSF, peritoneal fluid, synovial fluid, pleural fluid, pericardial fluid, amniotic fluid, human bite	Risk unknown, but considered infectious
	Feces, nasal secretions, saliva, sputum, sweat, tears, urine, vomitus	Considered non-infectious unless contaminated by blood

Percutaneous injury in unimmunized health care workers.

Table 85–2   Serologic tests for HIV, HBV, and HCV

	Test	Time to become positive	Notes
HIV	Rapid HIV	Up to 6 months after exposure	Results in 10-30 minutes 99.9% sensitive 98.9% specific
	ELISA	Up to 6 months after exposure	99.3% sensitive, 99.7% specific
	Western blot	Up to 6 months after exposure	Confirms positive ELISA
HBV	HBsAg	1-10 weeks after exposure	Presence implies infection; disappearance implies clearance of virus
	Anti-HBs	Months after exposure	If no HBsAg detected, then anti-HBs presence implies immunity; vaccine response is adequate if anti-HBs titer >10 mIU/mL
HCV	Anti-HCV HCV RNA	10 weeks after exposure	Initial screening test Only used to verify a positive anti-HCV, to exclude false-positives; not an initial screening test

the past 3 months; these sources may be infected but may not have seroconverted, which might result in falsely negative test results. Individual states have different laws about drawing HIV levels on unconscious patients, or what to do if the patient refuses to have a level drawn. There are great institutional variations as well. Some EDs will not perform levels because of the difficulties in providing counsel and other appropriate follow-up. Decisions about postexposure prophylaxis (PEP) can then be based on this information instead of waiting for confirmatory Western blot tests. If the source is HIV-positive, it is important to know the medication history, the viral load, how advanced the HIV is (terminal HIV infection is higher risk), and any history of drug-resistance.

■ Wounds should be cleansed thoroughly with soap and water. There is no evidence to support or refute the use of disinfectants. Mucus membranes should be thoroughly flushed with water.

■ Initially, the HCW should have the following studies drawn: HBV, HCV, HIV serologies, liver function tests, and, if not already done, anti-HBs antibody to assess response to HBV vaccine series. Women should be tested for pregnancy. If HIV PEP is to be started, a complete blood count, renal function, and hepatic function tests should be assessed before initiating therapy.

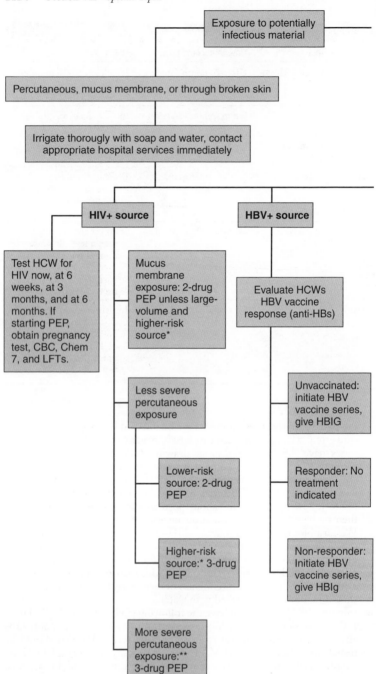

Figure 85–1. Algorithm for an approach to health care worker with occupational exposure. *Higher-risk source: symptomatic HIV, AIDS, acute seroconversion, viral load >1500.

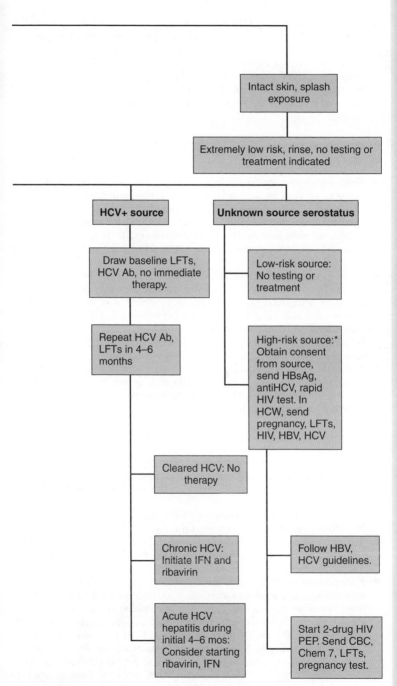

Figure 85–1. *cont'd* **More severe: hollow needle, deep puncture, visible blood on device, or needle previously in source's artery/vein.

- Follow-up testing for HIV should be performed at 6 weeks, 12 weeks, and 6 months. HIV testing should be done sooner if there are any symptoms consistent with acute retroviral syndrome, such as low-grade fevers, pharyngitis, lymphadenopathy, or maculopapular rash. Follow-up testing for HCV should consist of HCV antibody testing and alanine transaminase (ALT) activity drawn 4 to 6 months after the exposure. Any positive HCV antibody test result should be confirmed with supplemental testing.

Emergency Department Management Overview
General

- Several resources exist to help guide treatment. An interactive Web site (www.needlestick.mednet.ucla.edu) gives recommendations based on case-specific information. The National Clinicians' PEP Hotline (telephone no. 888-448-4911) can be consulted for complicated cases, online at www.ucsf.edu/hivcntr. Resources for hepatitis include a recorded message at the hotline (888) 443-7232, and a website at www.cdc.gov/hepatitis.
- HCWs exposed to HBV or HCV do not need to take special precautions to prevent transmission to sex partners, and they may get pregnant or continue breastfeeding. However, they should not donate blood or organs until it is clear they have not been infected. HCWs exposed to HIV should use condoms with their sexual partners, avoid pregnancy and breastfeeding, and not donate blood or organs. No special restrictions should be placed on exposed HCWs' work routine.
- Remember the psychosocial aspects of treatment. Post-traumatic stress disorder has been reported after needlestick. In one study, most HCWs who experience needlesticks report acute severe distress, and some quit their jobs as a result of the exposure.

Human Immunodeficiency Virus

- PEP decreases the risk of seroconversion by 81% when started within hours after the exposure. Double or even triple therapy is recommended, depending on the risk associated with the exposure (Tables 85–3 and 85–4).
- There are 21 reported instances of PEP failure, possibly relating to large inoculums, viral resistance, or short duration of PEP.
- Treatment should be individualized with the help of an infectious disease specialist; however, starting a basic regimen should not be delayed while waiting for expert consultation.
- Fifty percent of HCWs experience adverse symptoms on PEP, and 33% stop taking it due to those symptoms. Side effects of nausea and diarrhea from the drug regimen of ZDV and lamivudine (LTC) are common. Pancytopenia, hepatitis, pancreatitis, and nephrolithiasis have been reported with the use of protease inhibitors (PIs). Severe drug rashes can occur, evolving to Stevens Johnson's syndrome or Toxic epidermal necrolysis. PIs can cause hyperglycemia, and inhibit clearance of drugs metabolized in the liver while increasing clearance of oral contraceptives.

Table 85–3 Postexposure Prophylaxis for HIV

Exposure Type	Source of Exposure		
	HIV+, Class 1	HIV+, Class 2	Unknown HIV Status
Less severe percutaneous	Basic two-drug PEP	Expanded three-drug PEP	Generally no PEP warranted; if risk factors for HIV, two-drug PEP
More severe percutaneous	Expanded three-drug PEP	Expanded three-drug PEP	Generally no PEP warranted; if risk factors for HIV, two-drug PEP
Small-volume mucosal	Consider basic two-drug PEP	Basic two-drug PEP	Generally no PEP warranted; if risk factors for HIV, two-drug PEP
Large-volume mucosal	Basic two-drug PEP	Expanded three-drug PEP	Generally no PEP warranted; if risk factors for HIV, two-drug PEP

HIV, human immunodeficiency virus; PEP, postexposure protection.
Class 1: asymptomatic HIV or viral load < 1500.
Class 2: symptomatic HIV, AIDS, acute seroconversion, or viral load >1500.
More severe: hollow needle, deep puncture, visible blood on device, or needle previously in source's artery/vein.
Small-volume: a few drops.
Adapted from US Centers for Disease Control and Prevention. Updated U.S. Public Health Service guidelines for the management of occupational exposures to HBV, HCV, and HIV and recommendations for postexposure prophylaxis. MMWR Recomm Rep 2001;50:1–67.

When indinavir, a PI, is used, the HCW must be cautioned to drink six 8-oz glasses of water per day to avoid nephrolithiasis.

Hepatitis B Virus

- PEP is a combination of hepatitis B immune globulin (HBIG) and hepatitis B vaccine series depending on the patient's HBV vaccine status. PEP decreases risk by at least 75% when given within 1 week. Ideally it should be given within hours.
- The vaccine and the HBIG should be administered at two different sites.

Hepatitis C Virus

- Unlike HBIG, postexposure HCV IG is not effective.
- In cases of HCV exposure or infection, the recommendations regarding IFN and ribavirin are: (a) for patients with exposure, PEP is not recommended because there is no evidence that it prevents seroconversion;

Table 85–4   **Example Regimens for HIV Postexposure Prophylaxis**

	Recommended	Alternative
Basic two drug: two NRTIs	Zidovudine 600 mg PO BID plus lamivudine 150 mg PO BID	Lamivudine 150mg PO BID plus stavudine 40 mg PO BID Or Didanosine 400 mg daily, stavudine 50 mg PO BID
Expanded three drug	Basic regimen plus one of the following: Indinavir 800 mg PO TID Or Nelfinavir 750 mg PO TID Or Efavirenz 600 mg PO QHS Or Abacavir 300 mg PO BID	Ritonavir, saquinavir, amprenavir, delavirdine, lopinavir should only be used in consultation with experts

BID, *twice daily; HIV, human immunodeficiency virus; NRTI, nucleoside reverse transcriptase inhibitor; PEP, postexposure prophylaxis.*
Adapted from US Centers for Disease Control and Prevention. Updated U.S. Public Health Service guidelines for the management of occupational exposures to HBV, HCV, and HIV and recommendations for postexposure prophylaxis. MMWR Recomm Rep 2001;50:1–67.

(b) in patients with acute hepatitis C, data indicate interferon helps clear more patients at this stage than if started in chronic patients; nonetheless (c) patients with chronic hepatitis C are the only patients for whom interferon and ribavirin are currently approved.

Special Situations
Pediatrics

- Children may require PEP after sexual assault or accidental percutaneous exposure. The same criteria apply to children as to adults for initiating PEP; however, this should be done in consultation with a pediatric infectious disease specialist to recommend the best PEP regimen.
- Infants have the unique vector of HIV transmission through breast milk. The overall risk of HIV transmission is approximately 10-20%, with individual exposures estimated at 0.001%, and there are no reports of conversion after a single exposure to infected breast milk.

Nonoccupational Postexposure Prophylaxis

- Prophylaxis may be offered in nonoccupational situations such as sexual exposures or sharing needles for recreational drug use.
- The U.S. Centers for Disease Control and Prevention (CDC) recommends using two- or three-drug HIV PEP for people who have infrequent exposures, and present within 72 hours of a potential HIV exposure (for example, a sexual assault victim or an injection drug user who does

not usually share needles). PEP should not be given for people who present after 72 hours, or for people with recurrent risk for transmission, such as serodiscordant couples who have regular unprotected sex, or injection drug users who regularly share needles.

Community-Acquired Needlestick

■ PEP is not routinely recommended, though exceptions might be made if the needle were visibly contaminated with blood or found in an area with a high HIV seroprevalence.

Teaching Points

Exposure to body fluids is an occupational hazard of all health care workers.

It cannot be stressed enough that the usual cause is lack of compulsive wearing of protective gear; lack of compulsive handling of sharps, and lack of compulsive disposal of used intravenous equipment.

When suturing lacerations, it is the responsibility of the physician to dispose of all needles, scalpels, and suture materials; these must not be left for someone else to dispose on the laceration tray, or at the patient's bedside. When drawing blood, or starting intravenous access, it is the operator's responsibility to handle the needles with care. When undertaking a procedure that is likely to produce contamination such as thoracostomy or reduction and fixation of open fractures, it is prudent to double glove, and to be persistent in reducing the risk of puncture.

It has been shown that when the patient is a known HIV patient, medical personnel are more careful in their handling of sharps. It is only prudent to treat all unknown patients as if they were HIV positive.

Suggested Readings

Gerberding JL. Occupational exposure to HIV in health care settings. N Engl J Med 2003;348:826–833.

Update on emerging infections: news from the Centers for Disease Control and Prevention. Ann Emerg Med March 2002;39:319–328.

US Centers for Disease Control and Prevention. Updated U.S. Public Health Service guidelines for the management of occupational exposures to HBV, HCV, and HIV and recommendations for postexposure prophylaxis. MMWR Recomm Rep 2001;50:1–67.

US Centers for Disease Control and Prevention. Antiretroviral postexposure prophylaxis after sexual, injection-drug use, or other non-occupational exposure to HIV in the United States. MMWR 2005;54:1–20.

CHAPTER 86

Disaster

KELLY R. KLEIN ■ BRUNO PETINAUX

Overview

A disaster represents an untoward event, natural or human made, which overwhelms existing resources. Due to the unpredictable nature of disasters, hospitals, and communities must be ready for all hazards. Hospital responsibilities are not limited to the treatment of the immediately injured, but expand out to the community in general (Box 86–1).

Four Components of Disaster Response
Mitigation Phase

■ This represents steps to avoid or lessen the impact any given disaster may have on the facility and community using a risk and vulnerability assessment.

> **BOX 86–1   Overview of Hospital Responsibilities During a Disaster**
>
> - Staff: Timely and appropriate information, disease prophylaxis, family safety
> - Patients: Timely and appropriate information, personal safety, overall patient care
> - Visitors: Timely and appropriate information, personal safety
> - Community: Timely and appropriate information, education
> - State: Mutual aid agreements with other hospitals and regions for patient transfer, care, volunteers, credentialing
> - National: Members of the National Disaster Medical System (NDMS)*

*A section within the U.S. Department of Homeland Security, Federal Emergency Management Agency, Response Division, Operations Branch, and is responsible for supporting federal agencies in the management and coordination of the federal medical response to major emergencies and federally declared disasters. Support includes medical response to a disaster area in the form of teams, supplies, and equipment; patient movement from a disaster site to unaffected areas of the nation; definitive medical care at participating hospitals in unaffected areas.

Preparation Phase

■ This phase of a disaster response moves the mitigation phase from a prophylactic phase to a planning phase (i.e., operational and organizational preparation).

Response Phase

■ This phase represents the actual operation of a disaster plan to meet the needs of staff, patients, visitors, and the community at large during a disaster. The Hospital Emergency. Incident Command System (HEICS) is an emergency management system designed for hospitals. The HEICS uses a logical management structure, defined responsibilities, clear reporting channels, and a common nomenclature to help unify hospitals with other emergency responders.

Recovery Phase

■ This phase is probably the lengthiest process (days to years for full recovery).
  ■ Information needed to determine the hospital's response to a disaster is listed in Table 86–1.
  ■ The response phase considerations for the emergency department (ED) for a nonhospital evacuation situation are summarized in Table 86–2.

Table 86–1 Information Needed to Determine a Hospital's Response to Disaster	
Type of incident	**Natural or man made**
Number and type of victims expected to receive	Age group, specialty diseases (burns, blast injuries, infectious diseases, etc.)
Presence of contaminants	Decontamination procedures at the scene, need for antidotes
Modes of arrival	Privately owed vehicle, buses, emergency medical services
Timing of transport	All at once, stages
Complexity of care needed	Ventilators, critical care, special populations (burn), minor problems (that will occur in much greater numbers than major problems, and can rapidly overwhelm a facility so that it can no longer respond to a major problem).
Current utilization of existing hospital resources	Number of personnel available; number of beds; radiology/laboratory/pharmacy capacity, security staff available, supplies on hand
Potential impact of disaster on hospital directly	Building security and safety, utility supply, staff supply, communications

Table 86–2 ED Considerations for Disaster Response Phase	
Disaster event	The type of event and magnitude of injuries. The need for decontamination, isolation, prophylaxis, and evacuation.
Disaster patients	Probably most disaster patients will arrive on foot, and not be seriously injured. The more serious victims will probably be trapped at the site of the disaster scene, require extrication and transport, and may be the last to arrive at any facility. In an industrial chemical or radiation event, most patients will not have been decontaminated prior to coming to the hospital.
ED patients	Admitted ED patients seen before the disaster event should be sent immediately to another part of the hospital without further workup. Other ED patients without a disposition decision should either be discharged from the ED to complete workup after the disaster has been controlled, or admitted to another part of the hospital without further workup if it is deemed that they are too ill for safe discharge. Although often not deemed minor by the patient who has sustained the problem, patients with minor problems will always outnumber major ones. In most disaster situations, people are more willing to wait for care when they realize there are more complicated patients requiring care. Nevertheless, without planning, it will still be easy to overwhelm any facility with minor problems. Preparations should be made to care for these patients outside of the immediate ED area.
ED administration and staff	An administrative person in the ED with no direct patient care responsibilities is assigned to be in charge of the ED disaster response, and is in direct communication with the incident commander for the disaster management of the hospital. This person cannot and should not attempt to control everything; responsibilities must be delegated. An established call back system with complete and up-to-date contact information of all staff members makes it much easier to contact individuals in an emergency. Alternative methods of communicating with staff should be considered. In the case of mega emergencies, such as a hurricane or earthquake, it may not be possible to obtain any outside assistance for hours to days. ED facilities may even need to be relocated to another area of the hospital due to facility damage. There is a lag after a disaster before an effective response can be mounted, but victims often arrive before even the best plan can be implemented, and in fact, may be the means by which the ED and hospital discover the disaster. It is useful to keep a log during any event to help improve the disaster team future responses.

Table 86–2   ED Considerations for Disaster Response Phase—*cont'd*

> Any disaster situation has the potential to cause significant psychological impact on employees and patients.
>
> There may be a delay before additional food becomes available, so plan for feeding your staff in addition to your patients for several days.
>
> A public relations office separate from disaster care areas should be established to communicate and control the media.

An external disaster is a situation that occurs outside the hospital, somewhere in the community, when there is a disproportionate amount of staff and resources to care for incoming ED patients or victims. In an internal disaster, there is a potential need to evacuate existing patients to another facility or other area of the hospital due to problems incurred to the structure of the facility such as from fire, tornado, flood, or explosion. A natural disaster or man-made disaster can be both internal and external. An example is a massive hurricane with flooding such as what happened with Hurricane Katrina in 2005. Hospitals were faced with victims from the flood as well as needing to evacuate their facility due to flood damage, and the lack of basic resources of food, electricity, and water.

Triage for Mass Casualty Events

■ Triage is derived from the French meaning "to sort." It is used as a way to quickly assess and prioritize patients for treatment.

■ MASS triage is a simple technique for rapidly sorting a large number of patients at the scene into their initial triage category before an individual assessment is performed: Move, Assess, Sort and Send. In the MOVE stage, victims who are able are asked to move to a designated area, those unable to ambulate are asked to move an arm or a leg. Those who do neither are "ASSESSED" first. The START triage is applied at the "Assess" stage of MASS Triage. Patients are then "SORTED" into their respective triage categories, and "SENT" to the appropriate designated area for medical care.

■ The START triage system allows the triage officer to make treatment priority determinations without taking vital signs (Figure 86–1). To keep track of patients and their severity categories, utilize a tagging system that is color coded to assign priority.

■ In nondisaster situations, the most critical patients are cared for first, and with the greatest intensity of effort. In disaster situations, it is often necessary to delay care to some critical patients who are likely to die despite all care, so as to avoid the loss of otherwise more salvageable patients who are initially deemed less serious. Triage designation is not static, and can change based upon reassessment by the Triage Officer.

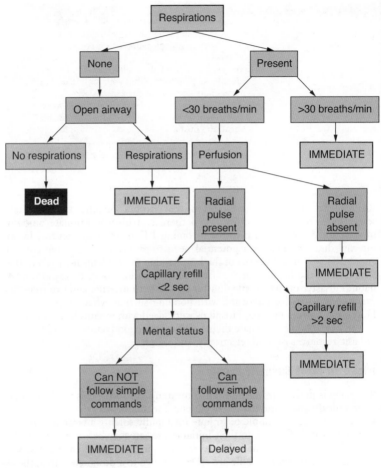

Figure 86–1. Start TRIAGE.

Decontamination

The decision on whether to initiate decontamination may be based on the following information:

- What was the contaminant?
- How was the exposure sustained?
- How long was the exposure?
- What signs and symptoms are now present? Will rescue personnel be contaminated by patients (e.g., patients with chemical contamination from insecticide will often contaminate the rescue workers who touch them without having personal protective gear)?

- Has the patient been decontaminated before transport?
- Is there an antidote available for this exposure?
- What kind of decontamination might be necessary?
- What do content experts advise? Experts include the local hazardous material team, Chemtrec (1-800-424-9300), Poison Control Centers (1-800-222-1222), Material safety data sheet (MSDS), labels, and experts.

There are two goals when dealing with decontamination: removal of the material to prevent further harm to the patient, and protection of hospital workers and treatment areas from secondary contamination. The location for a large decontamination area should be flexible, and can change during the event. Decontamination should be performed using appropriate personal protective equipment (PPE) to minimize the chance of worker exposure. There are four levels of PPE:

- Level A: Self-contained breathing apparatus (SCBA) enclosed in a vapor- and liquid-impervious suit. This is used when the concentrations of oxygen and the chemical are unknown.
- Level B: SCBA not fully enclosed in an impervious suit.
- Level C: Filtered air with a vapor- and liquid-resistant suit. There must be normal oxygen levels in the area. Level C is recommended for hospital decontamination personnel.
- Level D: Normal work uniform. Universal precautions with or without a N-95 mask.
- Refer to Figure 86–2 for an example decontamination scheme.

Chemical, Biologic, Radiologic, Nuclear, Explosive Events
Chemical Events

These will affect a fixed group of people quickly. Issues for the first responder and the first receivers are decontamination to prevent secondary contamination, treatment, and the control of patients who probably have had no exposure, but are frightened. Nonevent acute medical emergencies also occur, so it requires good planning to identify and separate these patients from the event medical problem (e.g., a bystander who is having a heart attack). Initially, neither the victims, nor the rescue personnel, nor the ED personnel will know what substance is involved, and it may take special information gathering from the industrial site of the disaster. Assessment of the patient with an unknown chemical exposure is summarized in Figure 86–3. Treatment options are discussed in the Table 86–3. PPE for Staff should be Level C or higher until patient is decontaminated.

Biologic Events

People who have been exposed to a biologic event will present hours to days to weeks after the exposure. Most of the diseases will present with rash, cough, or flulike symptoms (Figure 86–4). Epidemiology is very important, and should be assessed early to predict an area of spread. Unless announced by a terrorist, or in the case of disease weapons as obvious as hemorrhagic

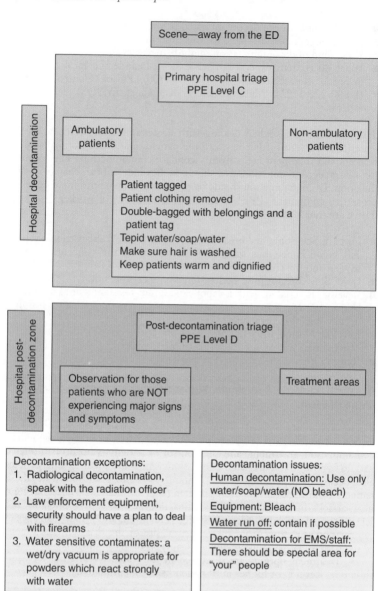

Figure 86–2. ED decontamination schema.

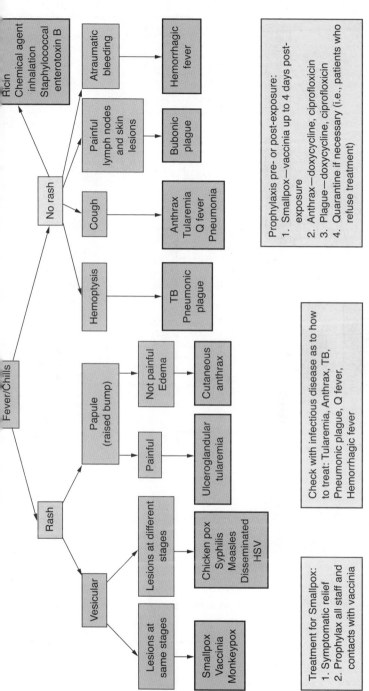

Figure 86–3. Algorithm for an unknown chemical exposure.

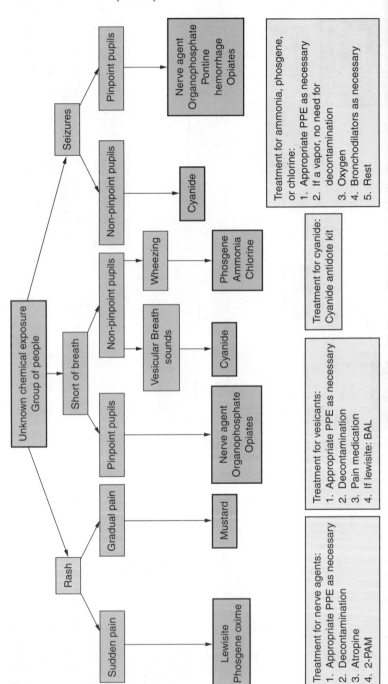

Table 86–3	Chemical Exposure Treatment	
Chemical Agent	**Decontamination**	**Treatment**
Nerve Agent/ organophosphate	PPE level C	Atropine 2 mg IV q5min until secretions dry up 2-PAM 600 mg IV over 30 min Diazapam 5-10 mg IV for seizures
Cyanide	N/A	Lilly kit Amyl nitrate crush one to two ampules Sodium nitrite 300 mg IV (10 ml of 3% solution) Sodium thiosulfate 12.5 g IV (50 ml of 25% solution)
Vesicants	PPE level C	Pain control British antilewisite (lewisite only)
Choking agents	N/A	Oxygen Bronchodilators as necessary Watch for pulmonary edema
Riot control agents	PPE level C	Bronchodilators as necessary

IV, intravenous; N/A, not applicable; PPE, personal protective equipment.

fever or smallpox, a biologic event will not be obvious. However, there a few clues that should tip you off to a biologic event:

- Severe disease in a previously healthy population
- Multiple people with the same complaint who have been at the same event or in the same area
- An endemic of a disease at the wrong time of the year
- Disease linked to a vector not endemic to the area
- An unusual number of severe or rapidly fatal diseases in a population
- An increased number of ill or dead animals
- An increased number of patients with severe pneumonia, sepsis syndrome, sepsis with coagulopathy, fever with rash, or cranial nerve palsies

There are very few of these diseases that are contagious, but in the initial stages, you will not know. PPE should be level D with universal precautions and N-95 mask. Treatment options are included in Table 86–4.

Radiologic Events

Radiologic events are relatively easy and quickly detected through the use of a Geiger counter. Nausea, vomiting, diarrhea, headache, weakness, and lymphocytopenia are all symptoms that may be attributed to a wide range of causes. Given the potential for radiation exposure, however, these symptoms may be important indications of acute radiation syndrome (ARS, see Table 86–5). The initial radiation injury happens to the patient at exposure.

Table 86–4   Biologic Exposure Treatment

Agent	Treatment	Prophylaxis	Contagion
Smallpox	AIRBORNE ISOLATION	Universal precaution with N-95 mask or higher	Yes, HIGH
Severe acute respiratory syndrome (SARS)	AIRBORNE ISOLATION Symptomatic treatment	Universal precaution with N-95 mask or higher Quarantine	Yes, HIGH
Anthrax	Doxycyline 100 mg IV q12h or ciprofloxacin 400 mg IV q12h	Universal precaution Doxycycline Ciprofloxicin	NO
Pneumonic Plague	Streptomycin 1 g IV or Gentamicin 5 mg/kg IV or Doxycycline 100 mg IV or Ciprofloxacin 400 mg IV	Universal precaution with N-95 mask or higher Doxycycline or ciprofloxacin	Yes, HIGH
Tularemia	Streptomycin 1 g IV or Gentamicin 5 mg/kg IV or Docycycline 100 mg IV or Ciprofloxacin 400 mg IV	Universal precaution Doxycycline or ciprofloxacin	NO
Q fever	Tetracycline 500 mg PO or Doxycycline 100 mg PO	Universal precaution Wait 8-12 d after exposure to start antibiotics Tetracycline or doxycycline	NO
Hemorrhagic Fevers	AIRBORNE ISOLATION Symptomatic treatment Consider ribavirin after consulting infectious disease	Universal precaution with N-95 or higher	Yes, HIGH
Botulism	RESPIRATORY SUPPORT Antitoxin available from CDC and some state health departments	Universal precaution NONE	NO

CDC, U.S. Centers for Disease Control and Prevention; IV, intravenous

Table 86–5 Acute Radiation Syndrome

Syndrome	Dose*	Prodromal Stage	Latent Stage	Manifest Illness Stage	Recovery
Hematopoietic (bone marrow)	>0.7 Gy (>70 rad) mild symptoms may occur as low as 0.3 Gy (30 rad)	• Symptoms are anorexia, nausea, and vomiting. • Onset occurs 1 h to 2 d after exposure. • Stage lasts for minutes to days.	• Stem cells in bone marrow are dying, although patient may appear and feel well. • Stage lasts 1 to 6 weeks.	• Symptoms are anorexia, fever, and malaise. • Drop in all blood cell counts occurs for several weeks. • Primary cause of death is infection and hemorrhage. • Survival decreases with increasing dose. • Most deaths occur within a few months after exposure.	• In most cases, bone marrow cells will begin to repopulate the marrow. • There should be full recovery for a large percentage of individuals from a few weeks up to two years after exposure. • Death may occur in some individuals at 1.2 Gy (120 rad). • The LD50/60‡ is about 2.5-5 Gy (250-500 rad)
Gastrointestinal (GI)	>10 Gy (>1000 rad) some symptoms may occur as low as 6 Gy (600 rad)	• Symptoms are anorexia, severe nausea, vomiting, cramps, and diarrhea. • Onset occurs within a few hours after exposure. • Stage lasts about 2 days.	• Stem cells in bone marrow and cells lining GI tract are dying, although patient may appear and feel well. • Stage lasts less than 1 week.	• Symptoms are malaise, anorexia, severe diarrhea, fever, dehydration, and electrolyte imbalance. • Death is due to infection, dehydration, and electrolyte imbalance. • Death occurs within 2 weeks of exposure.	• The LD100‡ is about 10 Gy (1000 rad)

Continued

Table 86–5 Acute Radiation Syndrome—*cont'd*

Syndrome	Dose*	Prodromal Stage	Latent Stage	Manifest Illness Stage	Recovery
Cardiovascular (CV)/central nervous system (CNS)	>50 Gy (5000 rad) some symptoms may occur as low as 20 Gy (2000 rad)	• Symptoms are extreme nervousness and confusion; severe nausea, vomiting, and watery diarrhea; loss of consciousness; and burning sensations of the skin. • Onset occurs within minutes of exposure. • Stage lasts for minutes to hours.	• Patient may return to partial functionality. • Stage may last for hours but often is less.	• Symptoms are return of watery diarrhea, convulsions, and coma. • Onset occurs 5-6 hours after exposure. • Death occurs within 3 days of exposure.	• No recovery is expected.

LD50/60, the dose necessary to kill 50% of the exposed population in 60 days; LD100, the dose necessary to kill 100% of the exposed population.
*The absorbed doses quoted here are "gamma equivalent" values. Neutrons or protons generally produce the same effects as gamma, beta, or X-rays but at lower doses. If the patient has been exposed to neutrons or protons, consult radiation experts on how to interpret the dose.
From Centers for Disease Control and Prevention. Available at http://www.bt.cdc.gov/radiation/arsphysicianfactsheet.asp. Last accessed April 21, 2006.

Irradiated patients are exposed to radioactive substances that travel through the patient's body, and do not deposit or leave behind any contamination, much like receiving an x-ray study. Such patients do not represent a contamination risk. Contaminated patients are those who have radiological particles on their person, such as contaminated dust after a radiological device explosion. Such patients will need to be decontaminated. These patients can be recognized using a Geiger counter at the initial triage point. Removal of clothing can easily eliminate up to 90% of contamination. Removal of clothing and showering with soap and water generally constitute the essence of decontamination. Should contaminated patients have wounds; these will also have to be decontaminated. The adage of time, distance, and shielding remains true for externally contaminated patients. Internally contaminated patients are those who may have inhaled or eaten contaminated material. They may or may not be externally contaminated as well. Initially, patients should be triaged on the basis of their traumatic injuries, and not because of their radiation injuries.

Radiological Decontamination Considerations

- PPD level D with N-95 mask to prevent particles from being inhaled
- Provide all staff members with radiation dosimeters
- Ensure frequent rotation of staff to minimize exposure time
- No eating or drinking in the decontamination area
- Radiologic officer with Geiger counter
- Protect patient's airway from inhalation of particles
- Catch water run off
- Decontamination order: wounds, orifices, highly contaminated areas, low level of contaminated skin areas
- After decontamination, resurvey the patient with a Geiger counter
- After decontamination level D, PPE is appropriate
- Discuss treatment options with appropriate resources. such as local radiation resources, Radiation Emergency Assistance Center/Training Site (REAC/TS), or Poison Control Centers

Medical and Sampling Considerations for Radiologic Events

- Nausea and vomiting is an indicator of radiation dose
- Emergency surgery needs to be performed within 12 to 24 hours, or must be delayed for 2 to 3 months
- Radioactive shrapnel should be removed with a long forceps, and placed in a lead container. It should be double bagged, and removed from the area.
- Determine the possibility of internal contamination: nasal swabs (label bags for each nare, swab should be DRY), oropharyngeal swabs, complete blood count with differential count every 2 hours for the first 24 hours, then every 24 hours, 24-hour urine/fecal collection.

Radiation Risk Exposure

- Risk to the responder/receiver is limited by *time*, *distance* and *shielding*. There has NEVER been a case of responder radiation injury during the treatment of a radiation contaminated patient.

Table 86–6 Radiologic Treatment

Radioactive Material	Treatment for Exposure only	Treatment for Contamination Inhalation/Wound/Ingestion
Radioactive iodine	None	Potassium iodine
Uranium	None	Bicarbonate
Plutonium	None	DTPA
Americium	None	DTPA
Cobalt-60	None	DTPA
Cesium	None	Prussian blue
Tritium	None	Water

DTPA, diethylenetriaminepentaacetate.

Radiologic Exposure Treatment

- Treatment options are briefly summarized in Table 86–6.
- Patients with ARS should be treated as follows: (1) Patients with nausea and vomiting should be given a centrally acting anti-emetic; (2) If there has been gastrointestinal ingestion, whole bowel irrigation is appropriate; (3) If there has been inhalation, then pulmonary lavage in the operating room has been used with success.
- In any hospital there should be people comfortable with radiation issues, such as a radiation-oncology physician, radiologists, or a designated radiation officer, who are resources for decontamination and treatment. Psychological support for employees and their families is very important. All treatment and decontamination staff should be wearing personal dosimeters INSIDE there outer clothing layers.

Teaching Points

Due to the unpredictable nature of disasters, emergency physicians must be ready for all hazards, and be familiar with the hospital disaster plan at their facility, including evacuation strategies and contingency plans in the event the hospital becomes unsafe or inoperable.

Treatment priorities in a disaster situation differ significantly from day-to-day operations. The goal is to do the greatest good for the greatest number of people instead of exhausting resources to save one critically ill patient. Triage is a dynamic process requiring constant reassessment.

The presentation of victims depends greatly on the type of disaster event. Victims of a biologic event may present to different facilities with a wide variety of symptoms hours to days to weeks after the exposure. Victims of chemical events typically present quickly, each with a similar constellation of symptoms. Safety of health care workers is critical in the care of any disaster victim, and patients must be decontaminated prior to entering the facility. Symptoms from radiation illness may not be apparent on initial presentation; however, if present, may be an indication of a potentially fatal dose of radiation.

Every disaster has a tremendous psychological impact on victims, families, and health care workers.

Suggested Readings

Arnold, JL, Halpern P, Tsai MC, Smithline H. Mass casualty terrorist bombings: a comparison of outcomes by bombing type. Ann Emerg Med 2004;43:263–273.

Burgess JL, Kirk M, Borron SW, Cisek J. Emergency department hazardous materials protocol for contaminated patients. Ann Emerg Med 1999;34;205–212.

Burgess JL. Hospital evacuations due to hazardous materials incidents. Am J Emerg Med 1999;17:50–52

Hick JL, Hanfling D, Burstein JL, Markham J, Macintyre AG, Barbera JA. Protective equipment for health care facility decontamination personnel: regulations, risks, and recommendations. Ann of Emerg Med 2003;42:370–380.

Hick JL, Penn P, Hanfling D, Lappe M, O'Laughlin D, et al. Establishing and training health care facility decontamination teams. Ann Emerg Med 2003;42:381–390.

Hick, JL, Hanfling D, Burstein JL, DeAtley C, Barbisch D, et al. Health care facility and community strategies for patient care surge capacity. Ann Emerg Med 2004;44:253–261.

Hogan DE, Waeckerle JF, Dire DJ, Lillibridge SR. Emergency department impact of the Oklahoma City terrorist bombing. Ann Emerg Med 1999;34:160–167.

Schultz CH, Mothershead JL, Field M. Bioterrorism preparedness, I: the emergency department and hospital. Emerg Med Clin North Am

CHAPTER **87**

EKG Interpretation and Pacemakers

Brian Alan Krakover ■ Purvi Shah

Overview

The electrocardiogram (EKG) is a graphic recording of the electrical activity of the heart. Normally the cardiac stimulus is generated in the sinoatrial (SA) node in the right atrium (RA), and spreads through the RA and left atrium (LA). It continues through the atrioventricular (AV) node and the bundle of His, which comprise the AV junction. It then passes into the left ventricle (LV) and right ventricle (RV) by way of the left and right bundle branches (continuations of the bundle of His), and finally to the ventricular muscle cells through the Purkinje fibers.

The EKG can give clues to coronary perfusion, pulmonary disease states, electrolyte disturbances, and drug toxicity. Any patient with an abnormally low or fast heart rate should have an EKG ordered to evaluate for the presence of conduction abnormalities and dysrhythmias.

The EKG should be interpreted systematically to avoid missing subtle but critical findings. In this chapter we will review the systematic approach to EKG interpretation.

Standard 12-Lead Electrocardiogram

- The four limb electrodes of the standard 12-lead EKG make up six leads (I, II, III, aVR, aVL, and aVF), which are oriented in the frontal (coronal) plane. Leads I, II, and III are termed *limb leads*. The fourth electrode located on the right extremity serves as an electrical ground. The augmented leads, aVR, aVL, and aVF are unipolar leads whereas lead I, II, and III are bipolar leads. Lead aVR stands alone, and has an orientation opposite the other limb and augmented leads. The six precordial leads (V_1, V_2, V_3, V_4, V_5, and V_6) are oriented in the horizontal (transverse) plane. Each precordial lead represents the cardiac electrical activity from that perspective.
- ***Lead placement for adult patients.*** Placement is summarized in Table 87–1.
- ***For pediatric patients.*** Leads V_4R and V_3R should also be recorded. These are mirror images of their left-sided counterparts. The chest of the tiny infant may not accommodate all the precordial leads; in such cases, the following array is recommended: V_3R or V_4R, V_1, V_3, and V_6. Limb lead placement is as in adults.
- Calibration refers to the amplitude of the waveforms on the tracing, and is usually set at of 10 mm/mV. The standardization mark at the extreme left side of the tracing is 10 mm tall (1 mV = 10 mm). Paper speed usually is usually set at 25 mm/s.
- Each small box on the EKG paper is 1 mm². Because the paper speed is usually 25 mm/s, each unit (horizontally) represents 0.04 second (25 mm/s × 0.04 s = 1 mm). Every five boxes correspond to 0.2 seconds

---

Table 87–1   Lead Placement for Standard 12-Lead EKG

	Electrode	Electrode Placement
Limb electrodes	RA	Right arm
	LA	Left arm
	RL	Right leg
	LL	Left leg
Precordial leads	V_1	Right sternal border, fourth ICS
	V_2	Left sternal border, fourth ICS
	V_3	Midway between V_2 and V_4
	V_4	Left midclavicular line, fifth ICS
	V_5	Left anterior axillary line, same horizontal level as V_4
	V_6	Left midaxillary line, same horizontal level as V_4 and V_5

EKG, electrocardiogram; ICS, intercostal space; LA, left atrium, RA, right atrium.

(5 × 0.04 = 0.2). A 1-mV signal produces a deflection of 10-mm amplitude (1 mV = 10 mm). The height of a wave is usually recorded in millimeters, not millivolts.

■ A positive (upward) deflection appears in any lead if the wave of depolarization spreads toward the positive pole of that lead. For example, if the ventricular stimulation is directed to the left, a positive deflection (R wave) is seen in lead I. A negative (downward) deflection appears in any lead if the wave of depolarization spreads toward the negative pole of that lead (or away from the positive pole). For example, if the ventricular stimulation is directed entirely away from the positive pole of any lead, a negative QRS complex (QS deflection) is seen. If the mean depolarization path is directed at right angles (perpendicular) to any lead, a small biphasic deflection (consisting of positive and negative deflections of equal size) is usually seen.

Basic Electrocardiogram Interpretation

■ *General.* When the sinus node is pacing the heart (sinus rhythm), the P wave (atrial stimulation or depolarization) always precedes the QRS complex (ventricular stimulation or depolarization) because the atria are electrically stimulated first. The ST segment and T wave represent the return of stimulated ventricular muscle to the resting state (ventricular repolarization). The normal P (sinus) wave rate is 60 to 100 beats per minute (bpm) with less than 10% variation. The maximum rate for a sinus tachycardia is 220 – age. A variation in rate of more than 10% may be due to a sinus arrhythmia. Essential components for EKG interpretation are discussed in the following sections. Measurements of these basic components are summarized in Table 87–2 and illustrated in Figure 87–1.

■ *P wave.* This represents an atrial depolarization, which is initiated by the sinus node in the right atrium. The atrial depolarization path therefore spreads from right to left and downward toward the AV junction. The positive pole of lead II points downward in the direction of the left leg whereas the positive pole of lead aVr points upward in the direction

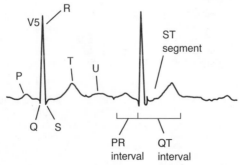

Figure 87–1. Components of the electrocardiogram waveform.

Table 87–2 Basic EKG Interpretation

	Evaluation	Examples of Abnormalities
Heart rate (HR)	Regular HR: 300 divided by number of large (0.2 s) boxes between two successive R waves; 1500 divided by number of small (0.04 s) boxes between successive R waves Irregular HR: Count number of cardiac cycles every 6 s and multiplying this number by 10. The top of the EKG paper is scored with vertical marks every 3 s.	>100 bpm is a tachycardia <60 bpm is a bradycardia. Look for hidden p waves. If the ventricular rate is ≅150 bpm, consider atrial flutter
Rhythm	Normal sinus rhythm: p wave at regular intervals before each QRS	Sinus rhythm with extra beats: PAC or PVC Ectopic (nonsinus) rhythm: atrial fibrillation, flutter, ventricular tachycardia, AV junctional escape rhythm
P wave and PR interval	P waves: height <2.5 mm and width <0.11 sec (<3 mm wide in all leads). PR interval is the beginning of P wave to the beginning of QRS complex. Normal 0.12–0.2 s.	Tall, peaked P waves may be a sign of right atrial overload (P pulmonale). Wide P waves are seen with left atrial abnormality. Small P waves (hyperkalemia). Uniformly prolonged: first degree AV block. Short PR, sinus rhythm, wide QRS and delta wave: Wolff-Parkinson-White syndrome. Short PR, retrode p waves (negative in lead II): ectopic atrial or AV junctional pacemaker) PR depression and ST elevation: pericarditis
QRS width (interval), QT interval (QT$_c$), QRS voltage and axis	Normally the QRS width is 0.1 s (100 ms) or less in all leads. The rate-corrected QT (QT$_c$) is obtained by dividing the actual QT by the square root of the RR interval (both measured in seconds). Normally the QT$_c$ is less than or equal to 0.44 s. Normally the left ventricle is electrically predominant over the right ventricle. As a result, prominent negative (S) waves are produced in the right chest leads, and tall positive (R) waves are seen in the left chest leads.	Prolonged with bundle branch blocks (Table 87–3), toxic conduction delays (hyperkalemia and drugs), beats of ventricular origin (PVC, ventricular escape beats, pacemaker), WPW. Drugs: quinidine, procainamide, disopyramide, sotalol, amiodarone, propafenone, flecainide, phenothiazine, tricyclic antidepressants. ↑ QT interval: see Table 87–4. ↓ QT interval: hypercalcemia and

Table 87-2 Basic EKG Interpretation—cont'd

	This is an estimation of the mean QRS axis in the frontal plan. The normal QRS axis lies between −30 degrees and +100 degrees. Lead I and II: if QRS complex in both leads is positive, the axis must be normal.	Look for signs of LVH or RVH (Table 87-5). Thin-chested people and young adults may show tall voltage without LVH. Causes for low voltage of the QRS complex. See Table 87-6 for axis calculation. Extreme axis deviation is abnormal and indicates a bundle branch block, ventricular hypertrophy, or pulmonary embolism.
R wave progression	Should see normal increase in the R/S ratio occurs as you move across the chest (V_1 to V_6).	Poor R wave progression (small or absent R waves in leads V_1 to V_3) may be seen in myocardial infarction (MI), altered lead placement, LVH, chronic lung disease, left bundle branch block.
q waves, ST segments, T and U waves	Q waves are normally seen in lead aV_R. Small "septal" q waves (<0.04 s) are normal in V_4 to V_6 and in one or more of leads I, aV_L, II, III, and aV_F. ST segment is normally isoelectric. T waves are positive in leads with a positive QRS complex; T waves may be normally negative in lead III even in the presence of a vertical QRS axis; negative in lead aV_R. U wave is a small deflection sometimes seen just after the T wave; usually in the same direction as the T wave.	Septal infarction may produce q waves of 0.02 s. The criteria for depth of abnormal q waves depends on the lead: lead I, >10% of QRS amplitude; leads II and aVF, >25%; aVL = 50% of R wave amplitude; V_2 through V_6 > 25% of R wave amplitude. The most concerning cause for ST segment abnormalities is myocardial ischemia. However, multiple other causes exist. See Table 87-7 and 87-8. See Table 87-9 for localization of the site of ischemia or infarction. See Table 87-7 for causes of T wave abnormalities. Prominent U waves may be a sign of hypokalemia, drug effect (quinidine, phenothiazine), after cerebral vascular accidental. A negative U wave and positive T wave may be seen with LVH with myocardial ischemia.

bpm, beats per minute; EKG, electrocardiogram; LVH, left ventricular hypertrophy; PAC, premature atrial contraction; PVC, premature ventricular contraction; RVH, right ventricular hypertrophy.

of the right shoulder. In normal sinus rhythm, atrial depolarization is directed toward lead II (upward P wave), and away from lead aVr (downward P wave).

- **PR interval.** Represents the time it takes for the stimulus to spread through the atria, and pass through the AV junction.
- **QRS width.** The QRS width, or interval, represents the time required for a stimulus to spread through the ventricles (ventricular depolarization). When the initial deflection of the QRS complex is negative (below the baseline), it is called a Q wave. The first positive deflection in the QRS complex is called an *R wave*. A negative deflection following the R wave is called an *S wave*. Occasionally the QRS complex contains more than two or three deflections. In such cases the extra waves are called R′ (R prime) waves if they are positive, and S′ (S prime) waves if they are negative. Initial depolarization of the ventricular septum is from left to right. This produces a small (septal) r wave in the right chest leads, and a small (septal) q wave in the left chest leads. The ventricular conduction system is trifascicular, consisting of the right bundle branch and the left bundle branch. The left bundle branch is further divided into anterior and posterior fascicles. Blockage of just the left anterior fascicle produces left anterior fascicular block (hemiblock) with left axis deviation (LAD). Blockage of just the left posterior fascicle produces left posterior fascicular block (hemiblock) with right axis deviation (RAD). Bifascicular block indicates blockage of any two of the three fascicles. A left bundle branch block signifies blockage of both the anterior and posterior fascicles of the left bundle. Complete heart block occurs when all three fascicles are blocked (trifascicular block). Bundle branch block criteria are summarized in Table 87–3.
- **The QT interval.** Measured from the beginning of the QRS complex to the end of the T wave. The QT interval depends on the heart rate. As the heart rate increases (RR interval shortens), the QT normally shortens; as the heart rate decreases (RR interval lengthens), the QT interval lengthens. The QTc is a more accurate measurement. Causes for QT prolongation are summarized in Table 87–4.
- **U waves.** This represents the last phase of ventricular repolarization. Normally the direction of the U wave is the same as that of the T wave.
- **Chamber hypertrophy.** There are multiple causes for the atria or ventricles to become enlarged. Common causes and determination of chamber hypertrophy are summarized in Table 87–5.
- **Axis determination.** The axis is the general direction of the electrical impulse (QRS complex) through the heart. It is usually directed to the bottom left. LAD is an abnormal extension of the mean QRS axis found in persons with an electrically horizontal heart, and RAD is an abnormal extension of the mean QRS axis in persons with an electrically vertical heart. The three methods used to calculate axis determination is summarized in Table 87–6.
- **ST segment.** The ST segment is that portion of the EKG cycle from the end of the QRS complex to the beginning of the T wave. The very beginning of the ST segment (actually the junction between the end of the QRS complex and the beginning of the ST segment) is sometimes called the J point.

Table 87–3 Bundle Branch Block Criteria

Right bundle branch block (RBBB)	"Complete" RBBB has a QRS duration >0.12 s. The second half of the QRS is oriented rightward and anteriorly because the right ventricle is depolarized after the left ventricle. Terminal R' wave in lead V_1 (usually see rSR' complex) indicating late anterior forces. Terminal S waves in leads I, aVL, V_6 indicating late rightward forces. Terminal R wave in lead aVR indicating late rightward forces.
Left bundle branch block (LBBB)	"Complete" LBBB has a QRS duration >0.12 s The second half of QRS is oriented leftward and posteriorly because the left ventricle is depolarized after the right ventricle. Terminal S waves in lead V_1 indicating late posterior forces Terminal R waves in lead I, aVL, V_6 indicating late leftward forces; usually broad, monophasic R waves are seen in these leads. Poor R progression from V_1 to V_3 is common.
Left anterior fascicular block	Left axis deviation in frontal plane, usually –45 to –90 degrees. rS complexes in leads II, III, aVF. Small q-wave in leads I or aVL. R-peak time in lead aVL >0.04s , often with slurred R wave downstroke. QRS duration usually <0.12 s unless coexisting RBBB. Usually see poor R progression in leads V_1-V_3, and deeper S waves in leads V_5 and V_6. May mimic LVH voltage in lead aVL, and mask LVH voltage in leads V_5 and V_6.
Left posterior fascicular block	Right axis deviation in the frontal plane (usually > +100 degrees) rS complex in lead I qR complexes in leads II, III, aVF, with R in lead III > R in lead II QRS duration usually <0.12 s unless coexisting RBBB Must first exclude other causes of right axis deviation such as cor pulmonale, pulmonary heart disease, pulmonary hypertension, etc.

LVH, left ventricular hypertrophy.

■ *T wave.* A normal T wave has an asymmetric shape; its peak is closer to the end of the wave than to the beginning. When it is negative, it descends slowly, and abruptly rises to the baseline. The asymmetry of the normal T wave contrasts with the symmetry of T waves in certain abnormal conditions such as myocardial infarction (MI) and hyperkalemia.

Table 87–4	Causes for QT Prolongation
Cardiac	Myocardial ischemia or infarction (occurs with deep T wave inversions) Myocarditis Bradyarrhythmias (especially high-grade atrioventricular block)
Neurologic	Cerebrovascular injury
Electrolyte abnormalities	Hypocalcemia Hypokalemia Hypomagnesemia
Drugs	Class I or III antidysrhythmic agents (e.g., quinidine, procainamide, disopyramide, sotalol, and amiodarone) Psychotropic agents (e.g., phenothiazines, tricyclic antidepressants, tetracyclic agents, and haloperidol) Others: terfenadine, bepridil, certain antibiotics (e.g., erythromycin and pentamidine), and cisapride (in high doses)
Environmental	Hypothermia
Congenital	Romano-Ward's syndrome (autosomal dominant) Jervell and Lange-Nielsen's syndrome (autosomal recessive with congenital deafness)
Other	Liquid-protein diets Starvation Arsenic poisoning

- *Assessing for signs of ischemia or infarction.* The classic changes of myocardial necrosis (Q waves), injury (ST elevation), and ischemia (T wave inversion) may all be seen during acute infarction. In recovery, the ST segment is the earliest change that normalizes, then the T wave; the Q wave usually persists. Therefore, the age of the infarction can be roughly estimated from the appearance of the ST segment and T wave. The ST segment elevations (and reciprocal ST depressions) are the earliest EKG signs of infarction, and are generally seen within minutes of the infarct. Tall, positive (hyperacute) T waves may also be seen at this time. The presence of pathologic Q waves in the absence of ST and T wave abnormality generally indicates prior or healed infarction. The variable shapes of ST segment elevations seen with acute MI are illustrated in Figure 87–2. Transient elevations are also seen with Prinzmetal's angina. ST segment elevations persisting for several weeks after an acute MI may be a sign of a ventricular aneurysm. Acute transmural ischemia can cause reciprocal ST segment depression. For example, anterior wall ischemia may be associated with reciprocal ST depression in the inferior leads and visa versa. There are several other significant conditions that also manifest on an EKG with ST segment abnormalities, such as pericarditis, and early repolarization (Tables 87–8). Localization of ischemic or infarction on an EKG is summarized in Table 87–9. Acute coronary syndrome is discussed in Chapter 22.

Table 87–5 Ventricular Hypertrophy

	EKG Findings	Other Findings	Example Pathology
Right atrium	Tall P wave (>2.5 mm). Width of the P wave is normal (<0.12 s)	May be seen with RVH	Pulmonary disease Congenital heart disease
Left atrium	Wide P wave with duration of 0.12 s or more (may not actually represent chamber enlargement but conduction delay). Amplitude may be normal or increased.	May be seen with LVH	Valvular heart disease Hypertensive heart disease Cardiomyopathy Coronary artery disease
Right ventricle	Tall R waves in the right chest leads, and the R wave may be taller than the S wave in lead V_1	Right axis deviation. Right ventricular strain: T wave inversions in leads V_1 to V_3	Congenital heart disease Pulmonary hypertension Mitral stenosis Pulmonary embolism (strain pattern)
Left ventricle	Sum of the depth of the S wave in lead V_1 (S_{V1}) and the height of the R wave in either lead V_5 or V_6 (R_{V5} or R_{V6}) exceeds 35 mm (3.5 mV). An R wave of 11-13 mm (1.1-1.3 mV) or more in lead aV_L	ST-T changes (strain): asymmetric appearance, with a slight ST segment depression, broadly inverted T wave; tall R waves. Axis deviation: usually horizontal; left axis deviation (i.e., an axis 30 degrees or more negative) may be present. QRS complex: may become wider and eventually develop bundle branch block pattern.	Systemic hypertension Aortic stenosis Aortic regurgitation Mitral regurgitation Dilated cardiomyopathy

EKG, electrocardiogram; LVH, left ventricular hypertrophy; RVH, right ventricular hypertrophy.

Table 87–6   Example of Axis Calculation

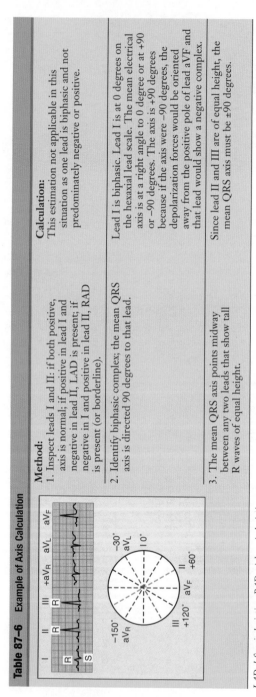

Method:	Calculation:
1. Inspect leads I and II: if both positive, axis is normal; if positive in lead I and negative in lead II, LAD is present; if negative in I and positive in lead II, RAD is present (or borderline).	This estimation not applicable in this situation as one lead is biphasic and not predominately negative or positive.
2. Identify biphasic complex; the mean QRS axis is directed 90 degrees to that lead.	Lead I is biphasic. Lead I is at 0 degrees on the hexaxial lead scale. The mean electrical axis is at a right angle to 0 degree or at +90 or –90 degrees. The axis is +90 degrees because if the axis were –90 degrees, the depolarization forces would be oriented away from the positive pole of lead aVF and that lead would show a negative complex.
3. The mean QRS axis points midway between any two leads that show tall R waves of equal height.	Since lead II and III are of equal height, the mean QRS axis must be ±90 degrees.

LAD, left axis deviation; RAD, right axis deviation.
(From Goldberger AL. *Clinical Electrocardiography: A Simplified Approach* (6th ed). St. Louis, MO: Mosby, 1999, p 46.)

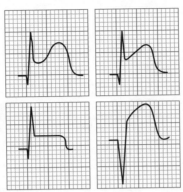

Figure 87–2. Variable shapes of ST segment elevations seen with acute myocardial infarctions. *(From Goldberger A. Clinical Electrocardiography: A Simplified Approach (6th ed). St. Louis, MO: Mosby, 1999, p 84.)*

Systematic Approach to the 12-Lead Electrocardiogram Rhythm Analysis

The four steps to EKG rhythm interpretation are listed follow (Table 87–2 shows normal values). Always compare the current EKG to any previous EKGs if available.

1. Determine the atrial and ventricular rhythm and rate. A normal rate is between 60 and 100 bpm. A bradycardia is a rate slower than 60 bpm, and tachycardia is a rate above 100 bpm. Determine the atrial and ventricular rates separately if they are different from each other. Determine the regularity or irregularity of the rhythm. Irregular rhythms should be described as totally irregular (*irregularly* irregular, as in atrial fibrillation) or regular with periods of irregularity (*regularly* irregular, as in atrial bigeminy).

2. Determine the P wave axis, duration, and morphology to provide information about the focus of origin of the atrial rhythm and whether the atria are being depolarized in an antegrade or retrograde manner. When sinus rhythm is present, the normal P wave is always negative in lead aVR and positive in lead II. However, if the pacing stimulus is coming from the AV junction (and not the sinus node), the atria are stimulated in a retrograde fashion and atrial depolarization spreads upward, toward lead aVR and away from lead II. In this situation, lead aVR may show a positive P wave and lead II a negative P wave. If the atrial rhythm is sinus, the P wave morphology and duration can suggest the presence of atrial enlargement or hypertrophy or interatrial conduction delay.

3. Identify the relationship of the P wave to the QRS complex. Is there one P wave for each QRS complex? Do the P waves precede or follow the QRS complexes? If the P wave follows the QRS complex, is it inverted in the inferior leads (II, III, and aVF) and positive in aVR, signifying retrograde atrial depolarization? What is the PR interval? Is it constant, or does it change?

Table 87–7	Differential for T Wave, Q wave, and ST Segment Abnormalities	
	Causes	**Normal Variants or Artifacts**
Q wave	Myocardial injury or infiltration Ventricular hypertrophy or enlargement Conduction abnormalities	Normal-variant septal Q waves in leads V_1, V_2, aV_L, III, and aV_F
T wave inversion	Myocardial ischemia or infarction (symmetric) Subacute or old pericarditis Myocarditis Myocardial contusion (from trauma) Subarachnoid hemorrhage (deep T waves) Mitral valve prolapse Digitalis effect (scooped or downsloping) Ventricle hypertrophy or BBB Wolff-Parkinson-White preexcitation pattern Ventricular pacing	T wave inversions may be seen normally in leads with a *negative QRS complex* (e.g., in lead aV_R). In adults, the T wave may be normally inverted in lead V_1 and sometimes inverted in lead V_2.
Peaked T waves	Myocardial ischemia Hyperkalemia Cerebrovascular hemorrhage LVH or LBBB Acute pericarditis	Early repolarization
ST depression	Myocardial ischemia or infarction (reciprocal changes) Ventricular hypertrophy Mitral valve prolapse (some cases) CNS disease Intraventricular conduction abnormalities Drugs (e.g., digoxin) Metabolic condition (e.g., hypokalemia)	Pseudo-ST-depression (wandering baseline due to poor skin-electrode contact) Physiologic J-junctional depression with sinus tachycardia (most likely due to atrial repolarization) Hyperventilation-induced ST segment depression
ST elevation	Myocardial ischemia Acute pericarditis (PR depression common) LVH or LBBB (lead V_1-V_2 or V_3 only) Left ventricular aneurysm (persistent STE after MI) Ventricular paced rhythm (resembles LBBB pattern) Myocardial injury Hyperkalemia (leads V_1 and V_2 only) Hypothermia (J wave or Osborne wave)	Slight deviations (generally less than 1 mm) may be normal. "Early repolarization": usually concave upwards of initial ST segment (begins J point), notching or slurring of terminal QRS complex, symmetric and concordant T waves of large amplitude, widespread distribution of STE. J point elevation is usually less than 3.5 mm. STE is greatest in mid- to left precordial leads. No q waves, reciprocal changes.

LBBB, left bundle branch block; LVH, left ventricular hypertrophy; RVH, right ventricular hypertrophy; RBBB, right bundle branch block.

Table 87–8   Comparison of Common Causes of ST Elevation

Electrocardiogram Finding	Acute Pericarditis	Myocardial Infarction	Early Repolarization
ST segment shape	Concave upward	Convex upward	Concave upward
Q waves	Absent	Present	Absent
Reciprocal ST segment changes	Absent	Present	Absent
Location of ST segment elevation	Limb and precordial leads	Area of involved artery	Precordial leads
ST/T ratio in lead V_6	>0.25	N/A	<0.25
Loss of R wave voltage	Absent	Present	Absent
PR segment depression	Present	Absent	Absent

N/A, not applicable.

Table 87–9   Localizing the Site of Ischemia or Infarction

Location	Leads	ST Segment
Anterior	V_3, V_4, and sometimes V_2	Elevation
Anteroseptal	V_1 through V_3, and sometimes V_4	Elevation
Septal	V_1 and V_2	Elevation
*Lateral	I, aV_L, V_5, and V_6	Elevation
Inferior	II, III, and aV_F	Elevation
Right ventricular	V_{4R}	Elevation
*Posterior	V_8 and V_9 V_1 through V_3	Depression

Posterior or lateral myocardial infarction may cause a tall R wave in V_1.

4. Determine the QRS axis, duration, amplitude, and morphology. Rhythms originating above the ventricles have a narrow complex and normal morphology unless bundle-branch block is present (wide QRS complex). QRS complexes originating from ventricular tissue are broad and bizarre.

Common Dysrhythmias
Isolated Ectopic Beats

- *Premature atrial contractions (PACs).* Although definitive causes are unknown, precipitating factors appear to include stress, fatigue, drugs/alcohol, tobacco, and caffeine. They may occur more in patients with chronic lung disease and ischemic heart disease. They occur in all age groups. Ectopic atrial pacemakers fire before the sinus node fires. On EKG, ectopic P waves occur prior to the next sinus beat, and have a different shape as compared with the P wave of the sinus wave. The ectopic P waves may or may not show conduction delays with respect to the QRS complex. There is no compensatory pause before the next beat since this represents a normal cycle. PACs need no treatment; treat the underlying disease if there is one. Avoidance of the precipitating factor such as caffeine is effective.

■ *Premature ventricular contractions (PVCs).* PVCs are among the most common dysrhythmias. They may occur in normal hearts, as well as those with serious organic heart disease. They may be due to an easily reversible cause such as hypokalemia, hypomagnesemia, and certain drugs. Beta-blocker therapy is sometimes used in patients with frequent PVCs and bothersome symptoms, or when they represent an underlying coronary artery disease. Individuals with PVCs may be asymptomatic, or they may complain of palpitations. PVCs occur before the next normal beat is expected. They usually precede the sinus P wave. They are aberrant in appearance. The QRS complex is abnormally wide (usually 0.12 seconds or more), and the T wave and QRS complex usually point in opposite directions. There is usually a compensatory pause before the next normal beat. Uniform PVCs have the same appearance in any lead, and arise from the same anatomic site (focus). By contrast, multiform PVCs have different morphologies in the same lead. The R on T refers to PVCs that are timed so that they fall near the peak of the T wave of the preceding normal beat. Those falling on the T wave are noteworthy in that they may precipitate ventricular tachycardia (VT) or ventricular fibrillation (VF). Two PVCs in a row are referred to as a *pair* or *couplet*. Three or more PVCs in a row are, by definition, VT. Ventricular bigeminy is a repetitive grouping of one normal beat and one PVC. The sequence of two normal beats with a PVC is ventricular trigeminy.

Tachycardias

■ *General.* Narrow QRS complex tachycardias are supraventricular in origin, and wide QRS complex tachycardias may be either supra-ventricular (with aberrant conduction), or ventricular, although in the absence of data to suggest otherwise, it is best to assume that the dysrhythmia is VT. The four major classes of a supraventricular tachydysrhythmia include sinus tachycardia, paroxysmal supraventricular tachycardia (PSVT), atrial flutter, and atrial fibrillation. Causes of wide QRS complex tachycardias include VT (three or more consecutive pre-mature ventricular complexes at a rate of 100 bpm) or a supraventricular tachycardia, atrial fibrillation or flutter, with aberrant ventricular conduction usually caused by a bundle branch block or atrioventricular bypass tract (Wolff-Parkinson-White [WPW] preexcitation pattern). Factors used to differentiate between VT and a supraventricular tachycardia with aberrancy are listed in Table 87–10. If the patient is unstable, (falling blood pressure, ischemic chest pain, altered mentation) cardiovert if the patient has a pulse, and defibrillate if there is no pulse. The advanced cardiac life support (ACLS) algorithm for tachycardic rhythms is reviewed in Chapter 6.

Table 87–10   Ventricular Tachycardia vs. Supraventricular Tachycardia with Aberrant Conduction

	Ventricular Tachycardia	Supraventricular Tachycardia with Aberrancy
Clinical features	Age 50 y or older	Age 35 y or less
History of coronary artery disease	Yes	No
Valvular heart disease	Mitral valve prolapse	Mitral valve prolapse
History	Ventricular tachycardia	Supraventricular tachycardia
Physical examination	Cannon A waves Variation in arterial pulse Variable first heart sound	
Electrocardiogram	Fusion beats Atrioventricular dissociation QRS >0.14 s Extreme left atrial deviation	None P waves followed by QRS QRS <0.14 s Normal axis
Response to vagal maneuvers	None	Slow response, or terminates
QRS Patterns	V_1: R, qR, RS V_6:S, rS, qR	rsR' qRs

- *Sinus tachycardia.* This rhythm is characterized by gradual increases and decreases in rate, with typical sinus P waves preceding each QRS complex. In an adult, the rate rarely exceeds 200 bpm. There are gradual increases and decreases in rate. There are many common benign causes for a sinus tachycardia such as pain, anxiety, exertion, drugs that increase sympathetic tone (e.g., cocaine) or block vagal tone (e.g., atropine and other anticholinergic agents). More serious causes must be considered such as dehydration, hypoxia (pulmonary embolism), myocardial ischemia, or anemia.
- *Paroxysmal supraventricular tachycardia (PSVT).* The major types of PSVT are described in Figure 87–3. There is no age or disease predisposition for most cases of AV nodal reentry tachycardias although it is seen more often in women, and can be associated with rheumatic heart disease, acute pericarditis, acute MI (AMI), mitral valve prolapse, or with one of the preexcitation syndromes such as WPW. PSVT also occurs in infants. Nonre-entrant supraventricular tachycardia (SVT) may be associated severe cardiac or pulmonary disease including AMI, chronic lung disease, alcoholic intoxication, or administration of certain medications. In SVT, there is a sudden onset of a rapid, narrow complex regular rhythm. The p waves may not be visible or may be inverted. The patient

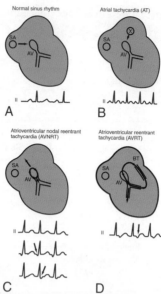

Figure 87-3. Major types of paroxysmal supraventricular tachycardia. *A,* The reference is normal sinus rhythm. *B,* With atrial tachycardia (*AT*), a focus (*X*) outside the sinoatrial (*SA*) node fires off automatically at a rapid rate. *C,* With atrioventricular (*AV*) nodal reentrant tachycardia (*AVNRT*) the cardiac stimulus originates as a wave of excitation that spins around the AV nodal (junctional) area. As a result, retrograde P waves may be buried in the QRS, or appear immediately before or just after the QRS complex (arrows) because of nearly simultaneous activation of the atria and ventricles. *D,* A similar type of reentrant (circus-movement) mechanism may occur with a bypass tract (*BT*) of the type found in Wolff-Parkinson-White syndrome. This mechanism is referred to as atrioventricular reentrant tachycardia. Note the negative P wave (*arrow*) in lead II, somewhat after the QRS complex. (With AVRT the P wave in lead II may be negative, flat, or positive.) *(From Goldberger A. Clinical Electrocardiography: A Simplified Approach (6th ed). St. Louis, MO: Mosby, 1999, p 148.)*

is aware of sudden onset of rapid palpitations with or without symptoms of chest discomfort, dizziness, or syncope. PSVT is commonly treated with vagal maneuvers, adenosine, beta–blockers, or calcium channel blockers. WPW is the most common accessory pathway syndrome, and causes preexcitation of the ventricles. These patients are prone to dysrhythmias, especially PSVT. The hallmark of this syndrome is paroxysmal tachycardia at a very rapid rate (150-300 bpm) due to loss of the normal conduction delay at the AV node. Characteristic features of WPW on an EKG include a short PR interval (<0.12 second), QRS duration greater than 0.10 second, and a slurred upstroke to the QRS complex, referred to as a *delta wave.* The short PR interval is the result of the absent AV node conduction delay, and the delta wave occurs because of early activation of the ventricular myocardium. Although the QRS complex is typically prolonged, it can vary and be near normal. Patients with the WPW syndrome often have one or more of the classic features missing on EKG especially if a sinus rhythm is present at the time of evaluation. Any tachycardia in an adult at a rate greater than 200 bpm suggests an accessory pathway syndrome. All AV nodal blocking drugs (especially calcium channel and β-adrenergic blockers, but also digoxin and adenosine) are contraindicated in patients with WPW who have a wide-complex QRS or irregular tachycardia (regardless of QRS duration). These agents may create a faster ventricular response pathway and potentially enhanced conduction through the accessory path. Procainamide or amiodarone are the drugs of choice for these patients. The Lown-Ganong-Levine syndrome is a rare accessory pathway syndrome associated with paroxysmal tachycardia, a short PR interval, and a normal QRS complex. The treatment parallels that for the WPW syndrome.

- *Atrial fibrillation (AF).* This dysrhythmia is a major cause of thromboembolism, and may cause impaired LV function primarily due to uncontrolled ventricular rates. Most patients complain of shortness of breath and fatigue; complaints of palpitations are surprisingly uncommon. AF is the result of chaotic depolarization of atrial tissues, and may be paroxysmal or chronic. Fibrillatory waves are seen on the EKG accompanied by an irregularly irregular QRS pattern. The QRS complexes are usually narrow, unless an underlying bundle branch block is present. The goals of treatment in atrial fibrillation are to control ventricular rate, to prevent thromboembolism, and to both convert to and maintain sinus rhythm. Beta-blockers, calcium-antagonists (verapamil and diltiazem), and digitalis (digoxin) are the usual drug choices for rate control in AF. Options for rhythm control include cardioversion or pharmacotherapy with class I and class III anti-dysrhythmic agents (see Chapter 90.3). Any precipitant for AF should be treated (Box 87–1).
- *Atrial flutter.* Atrial flutter characterized by rapid atrial rates of approximately 280 to 340 bpm. The ventricular response may be rapid with a fixed ratio of the atrial rate. The EKG typically shows prominent atrial activity with a *saw-tooth* pattern. The most common clinical presentation is with a regular tachycardia of 150 bpm, and any tachycardia that is fixed at this rate should be considered atrial flutter. Acute management of atrial flutter does not differ significantly from that of atrial fibrillation.
- *Ventricular tachycardia (VT).* VT is a run of three or more consecutive premature ventricular contractions. Sustained VT is potentially life-threatening because most patients are not able to maintain an adequate blood pressure at rapid ventricular rates, and the condition may degenerate into ventricular fibrillation, causing immediate cardiac arrest. A wide-complex tachycardia of unknown etiology should be treated as VT. The ventricular complexes have the same appearance in a single lead whereas in polymorphic VT, they are variable. The heart rate is faster than 100 bpm. The ACLS algorithm for the management of VT is outlined in detail in Chapter 6. VT should not be confused with an

---

BOX 87–1   Causes of Atrial Fibrillation

- Ischemic heart disease
- Valvular heart disease (most commonly mitral valve)
- Pericarditis
- Hyperthyroidism
- Sick sinus syndrome
- Myocardial contusion
- Acute ethanol intoxication (holiday heart syndrome)
- Hypertensive heart disease
- Cardiomyopathy
- Cardiac surgery
- Catecholamine excess
- Pulmonary embolism
- Congestive heart failure (also a result of atrial fibrillation)
- Re-entry phenomena (Wolff-Parkinson-White syndrome)
- Idiopathic

---

accelerated idioventricular rhythm (AIVR). In AIVR, the heart rate is usually between 50 and 100 bpm. AIVR is commonly associated with AMI, and may be a seen with reperfusion after thrombolytic therapy. It is short lived and does not require any specific therapy.

Bradycardias

- **General.** Bradycardia is usually defined as a heart rate of less than 60 bpm. This may be normal in healthy well-conditioned individuals. The two primary causes of pathologic bradycardia include depression of the dominant pacemaker (i.e., the sinus node) or a conduction system block. The rhythms seen with subsidiary pacemakers during SA and AV nodal block are called *escape* rhythms, as they provide a physiologic escape from no impulse generation (asystole). Emergent treatment is required only when the rate is less than 50 bpm with evidence of hypoperfusion or if the rhythm carries a high risk of progression to complete block.

- **Sinus bradycardia.** This is a regular rhythm at a rate of fewer than 60 bpm with a normal consistent P wave morphology and PR interval duration. This pattern may be found in healthy adults or during sleep. Other causes include hypothermia, excessive parasympathetic or diminished sympathetic stimulation (often from drug therapy), and carotid sinus hypersensitivity. Sinus bradycardia may be seen in the early stages of an acute inferior wall MI, due to parasympathetic stimulation. A sinus dysrhythmia is similar to sinus bradycardia except for the varying but normal ventricular rate. These are often due to respiratory variation and no treatment is required. Sinus bradycardia usually requires no treatment unless the patient is symptomatic, or it is the result of an underlying condition such as hypothermia or acute myocardial ischemia.

- **Sinoatrial (SA) block and escape rhythms.** Absent atrial depolarization (missing p waves) due to failure of the sinus node to generate an impulse, failure of impulse conduction out of the SA node, or failure of the impulse to activate the atria. SA block can be the result of ischemia, hyperkalemia, increased vagal tone, or drug therapy (including beta-blockers, calcium channel blockers, and digitalis). Incomplete SA block is diagnosed when an occasional P wave is dropped from the normal P-QRS-T sequence on the EKG. Complete SA block (or sinus arrest) manifests as no P waves on the surface EKG. Usually, a lower pacemaker will assume control in complete SA block. If this pacemaker is within the AV node, the QRS complex will be narrow, and an *idiojunctional* escape rhythm at a rate of 45 to 60 bpm is seen. Pacemakers within the His-Purkinje system usually result in a wide-complex *idioventricular* escape rhythm at a rate of 30 to 45 bpm. Treatment of SA block is based on symptoms, with atropine (aside from the setting of digitalis toxicity) and temporary pacing used if needed.

- *Atrioventricular (AV) block or dissociation.* AV block is the result of impaired conduction through the atria, AV node, or proximal His-Purkinje system. First-and second-degree AV block represent an incomplete conduction disturbance, whereas third-degree block indicates complete AV conduction interruption. Atropine and isoproterenol may improve conduction for type I second-degree AV block. Pharmacologic treatment for type II second-degree and third degree AV block is not indicated. Transcutaneous or transvenous pacing is often required, and emergent consultation with cardiology should be sought. Isorhythmic AV dissociation and complete heart block can be confused. Isorhythmic AV dissociation is usually a benign dysrhythmia but may reflect conduction disease or drug toxicity (e.g., digitalis, diltiazem, verapamil, and beta-blockers). Complete heart block is a critical dysrhythmia requires pacemaker therapy. In both, the atria and ventricles beat independently, but with complete heart block the ventricular rate is much slower than the atrial (sinus) rate. AV conduction blocks are summarized in Table 87–11.

- *Sick-sinus syndrome.* This is a group of cardiac rhythm disturbances characterized by abnormalities of the sinus node that can have alternating bradycardia and tachycardia. Causes include ischemia, systemic inflammatory disease, connective tissue diseases, nodal blocking medications, digoxin, or quinidine toxicity.

Table 87–11   Conduction Blocks: First Degree, Second Degree (Mobitz Type 1 or 2), Third Degree

Heart Block	PR Interval
First degree	>0.20 ms
Second degree: Mobitz type 1	Increasing until QRS dropped (Wenckebach)
Second degree: Mobitz type 2	PR interval constant, intermittent loss of QRS
Third degree	Dissociation of P-wave from QRS complex

Table 87–12 Five-Letter Pacemaker Code

Letter 1	Letter 2	Letter 3	Letter 4	Letter 5
Chamber paced	Chamber sensed	Sensing response	Programmability	Antitachycardia functions
A = atrium	A = atrium	T = triggered	P = simple	P = pacing
V = ventricle	V = ventricle	I = inhibited	M = multiprogrammable	S = shock
D = dual	D = dual	D = dual (A and V inhibited)	R = rate adaptive	D = dual (shock + pace)
O = none	O = none	O = none	C = communicating	O = none

Electronic Pacemakers

■ When a patient's conduction system fails and medications fail, implantable pacemakers help maintain functional cardiac rhythms. Leads are usually placed in either the atria or ventricles or both depending on the location of the dysfunction. On the EKG, pacer function is noted as small upward spikes, indicating depolarization. The five-letter pacemaker codes are summarized in Table 87–12.

Causes of Pacemaker Malfunction
Failure to Capture

■ Lead disconnection, break, or displacement
■ Exit block
■ Battery depletion

Undersensing

■ Lead displacement
■ Inadequate endocardial lead contact
■ Low-voltage intracardiac p waves and QRS complexes
■ Lead fracture

Oversensing

■ Sensing extracardiac signals: myopotentials
■ T wave sensing

Inappropriate Rate

■ Battery depletion
■ Ventriculoatrial (VA) conduction with pacemaker-mediated tachycardia
■ 1:1 response to atrial dysrhythmias

Teaching Points

The EKG tracing can give clues to coronary perfusion, pulmonary disease states, electrolyte disturbances, and drug toxicity. Any patient with a significantly low or fast heart rate should have an EKG ordered to evaluate for the presence of conduction abnormalities and dysrhythmias.

Any EKG should be interpreted systematically to avoid missing subtle but critical findings. Rhythm interpretation involves a careful evaluation of the p wave and QRS complex, and the relationship of both to each other.

Clues for the presence of ischemic changes include a careful evaluation for the presence of q waves, and the presence of ST segment or T wave changes. Efforts should be made to obtain a prior EKG for comparison. There are multiple other causes for ST segment and T wave changes.

Suggested Readings

Goldberger AL. Clinical Electrocardiography: A Simplified Approach (6th ed). St. Louis, MO: Mosby, 1999.

Josephson ME, Zimetbaum P et al. The bradyarrhythmias: disorders of sinus node function and AV conduction disturbances. In Fauci A, Braunwald E, Kasper, D et al. (editors). Harrison's Principles of Internal Medicine (4th ed). 1998, pp 1253–1261.

Niemann JT. Implantable cardiac devices. In: Marx JA, Hockberger RS, Walls RM (editors) Rosen's Emergency Medicine: Concepts and Clinical Practice (6th ed). Philadelphia: Mosby, 2006.

Wang K, Asinger RW, Marriott HJL. Current concepts: ST-segment elevation in conditions other than acute myocardial infarction. N Engl J Med 2003;349:2128–2135.

Yealy DM, Delbridge TR. The dysrhythmias. In: Marx JA, Hockberger RS, Walls RM (editors) Rosen's Emergency Medicine: Concepts and Clinical Practice (5th ed). St. Louis, MO: Mosby, 2002, pp 1053–1098.

Zimetbaum PJ, Josephson ME. Current concepts: use of the electrocardiogram in acute myocardial infarction. N Engl J Med 2003;348:933–940.

CHAPTER **88**

Electrolyte Abnormalities

COREY M. SLOVIS ■ PATRICK MEEHAN

Overview

Electrolyte abnormalities are very common in clinical practice. Some require immediate correction to avoid potential disaster, whereas others can be more slowly corrected. The presentation of electrolyte emergencies ranges from asymptomatic to profound mental status changes to life-threatening dysrhythmias.

Evaluation and management is directed at rapid intervention for life-threatening abnormalities while concomitantly identifying and treating the underlying cause of the problem. Dehydration is discussed in Chapter 26. Most asymptomatic patients can be discharged home safely with good outpatient follow-up. Any patient who presents with an altered mental status, concerning EKG changes, significant electrolyte abnormalities or underlying disease processes requires admission for further treatment and evaluation.

Specific Problems
Hypercalcemia

- *Background.* The causes of hypercalcemia are listed in Table 88–1. Primary hyperparathyroidism is the most common cause of hypercalcemia in outpatients, while malignancy is the most common cause of hypercalcemia in hospitalized patients. Hypercalcemia is the most common paraneoplastic complication of cancer. A common cause is metastatic cancer, and a common error is to assume that the patient is an end stage cancer patient, with no search for a treatable cause of hypercalcemia.
- *Clinical presentation.* Symptoms of hypercalcemia are often vague and nonspecific such as nonfocal abdominal pain, constipation, fatigue, diffuse aches and pains, or nausea and vomiting. The patient may have polyuria, or polydipsia. More severe elevations may result in profound dehydration, ileus, fecal impaction, hypotonia, ataxia, lethargy, confusion and coma. The patient may be hypertensive (increased vascular tone) or hypotensive (volume depletion). In addition, concomitant electrolyte abnormalities will frequently be present.
- *Diagnostic testing.* Standard electrolytes and renal function tests should be obtained. One can also order specific laboratory tests based on the possible underlying etiology like a phosphate level or other specific endocrine laboratories. Hypercalcemia is usually mild (<12 mg/dl) and

Table 88–1	Causes of Hypercalcemia
Malignant disease	Ectopic secretion of parathyroid hormone (carcinomas of the lung, breast, head and neck, T-cell lymphomas, and others), multiple myeloma, cancers metastatic to bone, 1,25-dihydroxyvitamin D excess (rare; lymphomas). This is the most common cause in hospitalized patients.
Endocrine/Metabolic	Hyperparathyroidism (most common in ambulatory patients), hyperthyroidism (by stimulation of osteoclastic bone resorption), adrenal insufficiency, milk-alkali syndrome, hypophosphatemia.
Infection and systemic disease	Granulomatous disease: sarcoidosis, tuberculosis, fungal disease.
Drug-induced	Vitamin A and D, thiazides, estrogens, lithium, aluminum intoxication; milk-alkali syndrome (excessive ingestion of calcium and absorbable antacids in conjunction with some degree of renal failure).
Immobilization	High bone turnover; Paget's disease.
Other	Acidosis can cause a mild hypercalcemia; alkalosis can cause a mild hypocalcemia.

asymptomatic, and rarely requires emergency treatment. Hypercalcemic crisis occurs in patients who have severe hypercalcemia (usually >14 mg/dl), is generally associated with prominent signs and symptoms, and requires immediate measures to lower the serum calcium. Prerenal azotemia may be noted. Characteristic EKG changes include shortening of the QT interval, and, to a lesser degree, prolongation of the PR interval and QRS widening. Rarely, severe hypercalcemia causes sinus bradycardia, bundle branch block, high-degree atrioventricular block, and even cardiac arrest.

■ *ED management.* Hypercalcemic patients should first have their "ABCs" secured. Any hypotension should be corrected with volume resuscitation. Once these basic steps have been performed, normal saline infusion at approximately 150-200 cc/hr (based on age, infirmity and renal function) should be initiated. Saline will block proximal reabsorption of calcium, and also cause significant caluresis. Once the patient is relatively euvolemic, the saline infusion should be supplemented by a titrated dose of a loop diuretic such as furosemide. Dosing should be adjusted to balance input and output. It has the additional benefit of blocking distal renal reabsorption of calcium, and is synergistic with saline's effects. Thiazide diuretics should not be used because they enhance distal absorption of calcium, and may worsen hypercalcemia. While this calcium excretion phase is occurring, electrolyte values, especially potassium and sodium, must be carefully monitored. Therapy for severe hypercalcemia should also include agents that reduce the mobilization of calcium from bone. Drugs that inhibit osteoclast-mediated bone resorption include the bisphosphonates, plicamycin, calcitonin, glucocorticoids, and gallium nitrate. The use of these adjunctive medicine therapies is tailored based on the underlying disease process. Dialysis can be used for patients with renal failure. The final step is to discover the underlying cause of the hypercalcemia. This is often done in conjunction with the patient's primary care physician, or an endocrinologist or other appropriate specialist. Patients with severe hypercalcemia, or who are symptomatic, should be admitted. Treatment is summarized in Table 88–2.

■ *Helpful hints and pitfalls.* These patients are at risk for nephrolithiasis and nephrocalcinosis. Hypercalcemia enhances the release of hydrochloric acid, gastrin, and pancreatic enzymes. Chronic hypercalcemia increases the risk of peptic ulcer disease and pancreatitis.

Hypocalcemia

■ *Background.* There are multiple causes of hypocalcemia (see Table 88–3). Only 1% of total body calcium is found in extracellular fluid (99% is found in the bones). Approximately half of the extracellular calcium is in the active ionized form, 40% is bound to albumin, and 10% is bound to anions like citrate. Extracellular calcium levels are normally maintained at 8.5-10.4 mg/dL. Total body calcium is controlled by a feedback system, in which parathyroid hormone (PTH) induces the bone and the kidneys to increase serum calcium levels, and vitamin D facilitates intestinal calcium absorption. Calcitonin lowers calcium by

Table 88–2   Treatment for Hypercalcemia

Goal in therapy	Intervention	Comment
Restore intravascular volume and correct electrolyte abnormalities	Normal saline for dehydration	May require up to 5 L per of normal saline. Hypokalemia and hypomagnesemia occur commonly, and these must be corrected.
Enhance calcium elimination	Saline diuresis Furosemide 10–40 mg IV every 6–8 h	Use diuretics after intravascular volume restored. Avoid thiazide diuretics.
Reduce osteoclastic activity	Biphosphonates: Etidronate 7.5 mg/kg over 4 h daily for 3–7 d Pamidronate 60 mg IV over 4 h (moderate) to 90-mg single 24-h IV infusion (severe cases) Zoledronate 4 mg IV over 15 minutes	Side effects: Increased creatinine and phosphate (etidronate), hypophosphotemia, leucopenia (pamidronate)
	Mithramycin 25 μg/kg IV over 4 h	Serum calcium levels decrease within 12 h Side effects: Neurotoxic, hepatotoxic, thrombocytopenia
	Calcitonin 4 IU/kg SQ or IM every 12 hours	Most rapid onset of action but only a modest reduction in calcium. Side effects: Nausea, abdominal cramping, flushing, allergy (rare)
	Gallium nitrate 100 mg/m²/d IV for 5 d in 1 L of NS or D5W	Associated with renal toxicity
	Glucocorticoids (hydrocortisone 200–300 mg/d)	Effective in patients with hypercalcemia due to hematologic malignancy, granulomatous disorders, or vitamin D intoxication.

D5W, 5% dextrose in water; IM, intramuscular; IV, intravenous; NS, normal saline; SQ, subcutaneous.

Table 88–3 Causes of Hypocalcemia	
Cause	**Example**
Parathyroid hormone deficiency	Hereditary (idiopathic), postsurgical, hypomagnesemia, neonatal hypocalcemia, DiGeorge's syndrome (abscence of the parathyroids)
Vitamin D deficiency	Malabsorption syndromes, liver disease, poor diet, lack of exposure to sunlight, antiseizure medications.
Parathyroid hormone resistance	Hypomagnesemia
$1,25(OH)_2$ D insufficiency or resistance	Chronic renal failure, hyperphosphatemia, vitamin D—dependent rickets, oncogenic osteomalacia
Other	Acute pancreatitis, citrated blood transfusion, osteoblastic metastases, acute rhabdomyolysis, acute renal failure, Foscarnet, radioactive dyes containing ethylenediaminetetraacetic acid (EDTA)

inducing renal, bone, and gastrointestinal losses. Hypocalcemia can be caused by any medication, surgery, trauma, infection, or inflammatory process that adversely affects GI absorption of calcium, PTH production or sensitivity, renal sparing of calcium, or liver production of albumin. Hypocalcemia can also be caused by alcohol abuse, pancreatitis, and associated electrolyte abnormalities such as hypomagnesemia. States of increased bone or cell breakdown (such as rhabdomyolysis, tumor lysis, or metastatic bone disease), or inadequate calcium replacement (such as rapid blood transfusion or hemodialysis) can also cause hypocalcemia.

- **Clinical presentation.** The patient may present with peri-oral or finger paresthesias, muscle cramps, tetanic contractions, generalized weakness, fatigue, altered mental status, irritability, confusion, hallucinations, seizures, shortness of breath, bronchospasm, laryngospasm, angina, hypotension, congestive heart failure, QT prolongation, or ventricular dysrhythmias. Chronic hypocalcemia can also cause cataracts, dry skin, and pruritus. Patients may have Chvostek's sign (the examiner taps the facial nerve and elicits facial or eye muscle twitching) or Trousseau's sign (the examiner inflates the blood pressure cuff to 20 mmHg above the systolic blood pressure for three minutes, and induces carpal spasms).

- **Diagnostic testing.** Calcium levels should be checked immediately in any patient with suspected hypocalcemia. A serum calcium level less than 8.5 mg/dL or an ionized calcium level less than 2.0 mmol/L is considered hypocalcemia. A whole blood ionized calcium level should be drawn in an unheparinized syringe, and rapidly analyzed to avoid changes in pH and anion chelation. Magnesium, potassium, and phosphate levels should also be obtained, as concurrent electrolyte abnormalities occur frequently. The PTH should also be checked if the underlying etiology is uncertain,

Table 88–4   Calcium Repletion

Drug	Dose	Elemental Calcium
Calcium chloride	5-10 ml IV over 5-10 min (faster in a "code")	272 mg (13.6 mEq)
Calcium gluconate	10-30 ml IV over 5-30 min	92 mg (4.5 mEq)
Calcium carbonate	1 g (up to 2 g) by mouth per day divided two to four times daily	1 g = 400 mg

IV, intravenous.

but results are unlikely to be available to the emergency physician. Total plasma calcium is affected by the patient's albumin level. The clinician can calculate the corrected calcium level according to the following formula: Corrected Ca (mg/dL) = measured total Ca (mg/dL) + 0.8 (serum albumin [g/dL]). However, this formula may be inaccurate in the elderly patient. The free (ionized) calcium level is not affected by the albumin level, so an ionized calcium level is always more accurate and better to obtain. An EKG should also be obtained to evaluate for a prolonged QT interval, and the patient should be placed on a monitor to evaluate for any dysrhythmias.

- *ED management.* Treatment is based on the patient's clinical status. An asymptomatic patient can often be treated with oral calcium supplementation such as calcium carbonate. A symptomatic patient should be given intravenous calcium replacement (at least 100-300 mg of elemental calcium over 5-30 minutes). This dosage raises the ionized level to 0.5-1.5 mmol and lasts 1-2 hours. In a code situation, or if a central line is in place, 5-10 ml of calcium chloride can be given IV. Otherwise, calcium gluconate 10-30 cc can be given IV over 5-10 minutes. This medication is less caustic to the veins, and can be given peripherally. Calcium repletion is summarized in Table 88–4. Adverse effects of IV calcium include nausea, vomiting, flushing, hypertension, and bradycardia. Calcium should be given cautiously in patients with respiratory failure, acidosis, severe hyperphosphatemia, or those on digitalis.
- *Helpful hints and pitfalls.* Any patient with concern for hypocalcemia should have an ionized calcium level.

Hyperkalemia

- *Background.* The most common causes are spurious, renal failure, acidosis, cell death (e.g., rhabdomyolysis, crush injury, tumor, lysis), and medication related. The most common cause of hyperkalemia is spurious: hemolysis occurring during or after the blood draw resulting in a false elevation in serum potassium. The intracellular concentration of potassium is 140 to 155 mEq/L, and the extracellular concentration is 3.5 to 5 mEq/L in the steady state. This gradient between inside and outside the cell is the key determinant of the resting membrane potential. Transcellular pumps, most importantly the Na-K ATPase pump, contribute to potassium's steady state.

- **Clinical presentation.** Based on the serum potassium, the etiology of the hyperkalemia, and the underlying co-morbid conditions, the patient may be completely asymptomatic, complaining of fatigue, malaise, or nausea; or have fluid overload, difficulty breathing, or cardiac arrest.

- **Diagnostic testing.** Standard laboratory evaluation should include electrolytes and renal function studies. Many hospital laboratories can report a serum potassium level more quickly from a blood gas analysis than from a chemical laboratory electrolyte analysis. Hyperkalemia is defined as potassium level greater than 5.0 mEq/L. Three classic EKG changes are seen as potassium levels rise. Tall, often peaked, T-waves are usually seen as potassium rises to 5.5 to 6 mEq/L. As the potassium level rises above 6.5 mEq/L, the PR interval prolongs and the P wave disappears. Once the potassium level approaches 8 mEq/L, the QRS begins to widen. The result of this progression is cardiac arrest with a sine wave or asystole as the underlying rhythm (Figure 88–1).

- **ED management.** Treatment of hyperkalemia can be divided into phases: 1) stabilizing the membrane potential, 2) driving potassium into the cell, and 3) removing potassium from the body (Table 88–5). Patients should be placed on a cardiac monitor, especially if they are ill-appearing, or have EKG changes. The underlying cause should be treated.

Hypokalemia

- **Background.** The five most common causes of hypokalemia are listed in Table 88–6. Significant hypokalemia may cause cardiac dysrhythmias due to potassium's effect on the action potential, and is almost always associated with hypomagnesemia.

- **Clinical presentation.** Hypokalemia is usually asymptomatic; however, it can be associated with nonspecific complaints including weakness, fatigue, constipation, muscle pain (manifest as excruciating cramps), and its most severe non-cardiac complication, rhabdomyolysis. It can also cause depression. Signs and symptoms of neuromuscular dysfunction usually occur when the serum potassium level is less than 2.5 mEq/L. This includes paresthesias, depressed deep tendon reflexes, fasciculations, muscle weakness, irritability and confusion. Muscular paralysis may occur with serum levels below 2.0 mEq/L.

- **Diagnostic testing.** Similar to hyperkalemia. Hypokalemia is defined as a potassium level less than 3.5 mEq/L. A magnesium level should be checked, as it is difficult to correct low potassium levels in the presence of hypomagnesemia. The EKG changes associated with hypokalemia include decreased T-wave amplitude, U-waves, prolongation of the Q-T interval, dysrhythmias (premature ventricular contractions, ventricular tachycardia, and torsades de points), and non-specific T wave and S-T interval changes.

- **ED management.** One way to estimate potassium needs is via the relationship that every 0.3 mmol decrease in the serum potassium level reflects up to 100 mmol reduction in total body stores. Hypokalemic patients may appear to rapidly normalize their serum potassium levels,

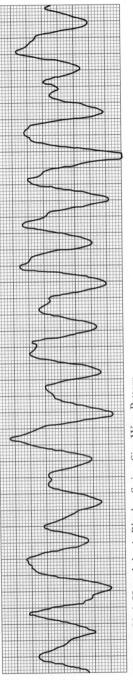

Figure 88–1. Hyperkalemia Rhythm Strip - Sine Wave Pattern.

Table 88–5 Treatment for Hyperkalemia

Phase	Intervention	Comment
Stabilizing the membrane	Calcium chloride: 13.6 mEq per 10-ml ampule IV. More potent and sclerosing to the veins because of its higher calcium concentration. Calcium gluconate: 4.6 mEq per 10-ml ampule IV. Can be given peripherally without likelihood of sclerosis.	Calcium infusion does not change the serum potassium level. Instead, it recreates the electrical gradient across the cell membrane. Short duration of action in the range of 5-20 min, and is used to stabilize patients as other therapies are begun. Calcium chloride needs to be given through central line, but can be given via peripheral vein in life-threatening emergencies ignoring the risk of vein damage if this is the only IV access site.
Driving potassium into the cell	Glucose and insulin: two ampules of 50% dextrose followed immediately by 10 units of regular insulin IV.	Insulin drives glucose into the cell, and also indirectly drives potassium intracellularly; sodium is pushed out. This is the fastest and most effective way to drive potassium into the cell, but it is only transient. Can lower serum potassium in minutes, and will lower serum potassium levels by 0.5 to 1.0 mEq in 1 h. May also induce subsequent hypoglycemia.
	Bicarbonate: 50-150 mEq IV over 30 to 60 min.	Bicarbonate does not work in nonacidotic patients, and should be reserved for acidotic hyperkalemic patients such as those with uremic acidosis. Bicarbonate's mechanism of action makes use of electrolyte shifts due to the change in serum pH. As a patient becomes less acidotic from the alkaline bicarbonate, hydrogen ions move out of the cell, and potassium ions are subsequently driven into the cell by a hydrogen/potassium exchange pump.

Table 88–5 Treatment for Hyperkalemia—*cont'd*

Phase	Intervention	Comment
	Beta-agonists: nebulization via mask with nebulized albuterol (10-20 mg).	Beta agonists stimulate the sodium-potassium ATPase pump. By stimulating this pump, sodium is moved out of the cell, and potassium is pumped inward. This will drop the serum potassium by 0.5 mEq/L.
Removing potassium from the body	Normal saline infusion coupled with furosemide	The patient must be able to produce urine.
	Kayexalate 30-60 g	This is an ion exchange resin, which binds to potassium. It must be combined with sorbital when given orally to be effective. Each gram binds 0.5-1 mEq of potassium.
	Dialysis	The most effective way to remove potassium from the body. Hemodialysis can remove up to 50 mEq/L of potassium per hour. Severely hyperkalemic patients with marginal or no renal function should be emergently dialyzed as soon as possible.

IV, intravenous.

Table 88–6	Five Major Causes of Hypokalemia
Renal losses	Diuretic use, steroid excess, metabolic alkalosis, antibiotics, diabetic ketoacidosis, renal tubular acidosis, alcohol abuse
Increased nonrenal losses	Sweating, diarrhea, vomiting, fistula
Decreased intake	Alcoholism, malnutrition
Intracellular shifts	Hyperventilation, drugs (insulin, beta-agonist, theophylline)
Endocrine	Cushing's disease,* diabetic ketoacidosis, Bartter's syndrome**

*Mineralocorticoid excess accelerates distal tubular potassium secretion.
**Defect causing an incomplete reabsorption of sodium chloride by the thick ascending limb of Henle resulting in increased delivery of sodium to the collecting duct and net salt wastage.

only to lose the vast majority of this administered potassium in their urine over the next 12-24 hours if magnesium is not combined with potassium therapy. There are several types of potassium salts: potassium chloride, phosphate, and bicarbonate. Potassium chloride is the most commonly used. PO replacement is always safer and easier than IV. If IV infusion is necessary, a rate of 10 meq/hr is considered very safe, while 20 meq/hr is usually safe. Doses greater than 20 mEq/hr should be given in a monitored setting through a central venous access site. Also, the more rapid the IV potassium infusion, the more likely that the solution will burn as it is infused. This can be alleviated to by adding 10 cc of 1% lidocaine to the IV solution.

- *Helpful hints and pitfalls.* Because potassium is an intracellular cation, a low serum potassium level reflects a much greater total potassium deficit. Because up to 50% of administered potassium is excreted in the urine, correction of large deficits may require several days.

Hypermagnesemia

- *Background.* The two main causes of clinically significant hypermagnesemia are iatrogenic magnesium overload and renal failure. Modest elevations may be seen in familial hypocalciuric hypercalcemia, with lithium ingestion, and during volume depletion.
- *Clinical presentation.* Initially, patients may present with nausea, flushing, headache, and diminished deep tendon reflexes (DTR's). More severe hypermagnesemia can lead to lethargy, hypotension, bradycardia, nonspecific EKG changes, muscle paralysis, loss of DTR's, respiratory failure (depressed respirations and apnea due to muscle paralysis), complete heart block, and cardiac arrest. As noted above, some patients with hypermagnesemia may present with renal failure as well, and may have corresponding signs and symptoms.
- *Diagnostic testing.* A serum magnesium should be checked immediately in symptomatic patients. Usually, patients begin to manifest symptoms

of hypermagnesemia at serum levels above 4 mEq/L. Magnesium concentration greater than 5 mEq/L causes a prolonged PR interval as well as increased QRS duration and QT interval. Complete heart block and cardiac arrest may occur at concentrations greater than 15 mEq/L. Hypermagnesemia causes a suppression of PTH secretion, and therefore can be associated with hypocalcemia.

■ *ED management.* Most stable or asymptomatic patients with hypermagnesemia can be treated with cessation of magnesium therapy only. However, any unstable patients or those in renal failure may require hemodialysis (or peritoneal dialysis). As a temporizing measure in sick patients while dialysis is being arranged, intravenous calcium (100-300 mg of elemental calcium) can be given as a magnesium antagonist (see Table 88–4).

■ *Helpful hints and pitfalls.* Magnesium is the ingredient in many over the counter laxatives and antacids.

Hypomagnesemia

■ *Background.* There are many causes of hypomagnesemia. Most causes are related to or dietary, gastroenterologic, renal, drugs, or endocrine-metabolic etiologies. See Table 88–7.

■ *Clinical presentation.* Patients may present with muscle cramping, diffuse weakness, palpitations, vertigo, ataxia, depression, seizures, or rarely, altered mental status. Patients with hypomagnesemia also commonly have hypokalemia and hypocalcemia.

■ *Diagnostic testing.* Patients begin to manifest symptoms of hypomagnesemia at serum levels below 1.8 mEq/L. Most of the total body magnesium is intracellular, and therefore a low serum magnesium level

Table 88–7 Causes of Hypomagnesemia	
Dietary	Alcoholism, malnourishment, and chronic diseases
Gastrointestinal	Malabsorption syndromes such as celiac sprue, bowel resection, radiation changes, chronic diarrhea, laxative abuse, inflammatory bowel disease, or gastrointestinal tumors
Renal	Acute tubular necrosis, postobstructive diuresis, renal tubular acidosis, or glomerulonephritis
Drug induced	Diuretics such as thiazides or loop diuretics, cisplatin, pentamidine, digitalis, aminoglycosides, or amphotericin B
Endocrine/metabolic	Diabetic ketoacidosis, alcoholic ketoacidosis, syndrome of inappropriate antidiuretic hormone, hypoparathyroidism
Other	Cirrhosis, rapid intravenous fluid resuscitation, hungry bone syndrome, primary aldosteronism, pregnancy or lactation

may not reflect the degree of total body hypomagnesemia. An ionized magnesium level is a more accurate measure of hypomagnesemia if available. Patients may have non-specific EKG changes, including ST and T wave abnormalities and widened QRS intervals.

■ *ED management.* A stable patient with hypomagnesemia can be treated with a loading dose of magnesium sulfate 2 grams IV over 10-60 minutes, and then 1-2 grams per hour until serum levels have normalized. An unstable patient can be given the 2 grams loading dose within one minute, and then 1-2 grams every minute for 5 minutes up to a total of 4-6 grams, until symptoms have resolved or a therapeutic effect is obtained, or levels have normalized. Adverse effects include diarrhea, respiratory depression, decreased deep tendon reflexes, renal insufficiency, heart block in digitalized patients, hypertension or asystole. Most asymptomatic patients with hypomagnesemia can be discharged home safely with good outpatient follow-up. Magnesium gluconate oral supplementation can be given at 500-1000 mg per day PO divided TID (or Magnesium oxide 400-800 mg PO Q day) if the patient is only mildly hypomagnesemic and asymptomatic.

Hypernatremia

■ *Background.* Adults with hypernatremia almost always have a total body water deficit. Hypernatremia is predominantly a disease of the elderly, and is most often seen in those who require others to provide them with water such as infants, intubated patients, those with severe cerebral palsy, and mental retardation.

■ *Clinical presentation.* Patients are usually older or debilitated, and often have significant comorbidities. Their presentation varies based on the degree of hypernatremia and dehydration, as well as their underlying comorbidities. This condition can also be seen in children with congenital renal diabetes insipidus who are prevented from drinking water freely (e.g., in school, where a teacher doesn't understand the child needs water at all times).

■ *Diagnostic testing.* Hypernatremia is defined as serum sodium concentration above 145 mEq/L.

■ *ED management.* Correction of hypernatremia follows similar guidelines as that of hyponatremia. The goal rate of change should be about 0.5 meq/hr with a daily goal of 10-12 meq/L. However, if a patient is hypotensive, blood pressure normalization takes priority over slow sodium correction. Normal saline should be used to restore hemodynamic stability, and then the next focus is the slow correction of the electrolyte disturbance. The final management goal is to treat the underlying cause.

■ *Helpful hints and pitfalls.* The central nervous system initially adapts to hypernatremia with brain shrinkage, and then subsequently the brain begins to make solutes. This intracellular solute gain helps increase the brain's osmolarity, and helps to restore the lost brain cell volume. Due to this relative hyperosmolarity, however, too rapid correction of the hypernatremia with hypotonic fluids can cause cerebral edema resulting in worsening mental status, coma, and death.

Hyponatremia

- *Background.* Sodium is the predominant extracellular cation that governs the movement of water among three major compartments: intracellular, interstitial, and intravascular. In order to determine the cause of hyponatremia, it is helpful to clinically assess the extracellular volume of the patient (see Table 88–8). Pseudohyponatremia is a falsely low serum sodium reading caused by the presence of other osmolar particles in the serum.
- *Clinical presentation.* The vast majority of patients with hyponatremia are only relatively symptomatic, and do not require emergent therapy. Some patients with more pronounced or chronic hyponatremia develop headache, nausea or confusion. Patients with severe hyponatremia can present with seizures, altered mental status, or coma. Presenting symptoms are largely based on the degree of hyponatremia, as well as how acutely the hyponatremia developed.
- *Diagnostic testing.* Serum electrolytes and osmolarity can be helpful in differentiating the various etiologies. Hyponatremia is defined as a serum sodium concentration of less than 135 mEq/L. The measured sodium value should be corrected in the presence of significant hyperglycemia. To calculate the corrected sodium level, add 1.6 mEq/L to the measured sodium for every 100 mg/dl of glucose above 100.
- *ED management.* Treatment can be complicated and dangerous if not done correctly. The means of correcting the hyponatremia is dependent on the reason for the hyponatremia in the first place (see Table 88–8). Patients with hyponatremia and dehydration readily respond to normal saline infusion. Hypotensive, dehydrated patients should be aggressively volume resuscitated with normal saline, but once hemodynamically stable, the infusion rate should be slowed down, and the serum sodium levels frequently checked to allow for a sodium rise of only 0.5 meq/hr or 10 meq/day (see Chapter 26). It is essential to determine the underlying cause for the patient's electrolyte imbalance. In general patients with hyponatremia with increased total body water, including the syndrome of inappropriate antidiuretic hormone production (SIADH), psychogenic polydipsia, and beer potomania respond to free water restriction. Hyponatremic patients with excess total body water and sodium respond to lasix, water restriction, and management of the underlying disease process. For documented hyponatremic patients with significant neurological symptoms, such as seizures, severe altered mental status, or coma, aggressive therapy is necessary to avoid permanent neurological deficits and even death from cerebral edema. In these patients, the target rate of correction is 1.5 to 2 mEq/L per hour with 3% hypertonic saline for the first 3 to 4 hours, or more briefly, if symptoms improve. The maximum rise of serum sodium concentration should still not exceed 10 mEq/L in the first 24 hours. An initial infusion rate can be estimated by multiplying the patient's body weight in kilograms by the desired rate of increase in serum [Na+] in milliequivalents per liter per hour. For example, in a 70-kg patient, an infusion of 3% NaCl at 70 mL/hour increases serum [Na+] by approximately 1 mEq/L per hour and an infusion of 35 mL/hour increases serum [Na+] by about 0.5 mEq/L per

Table 88-8 Classification of Hyponatremia Based on Extracellular Volume

	Causes	Diagnostics	Treatment
Pseudo-hyponatremia	High protein, hyperlipidemia, hyperglycemia, or laboratory error	Measurement of the serum sodium by direct potentiometry prevents this problem. Correction of serum sodium in the setting of hyperglycemia: add 1.6 mEq/L for every 100-mg/dl rise in the serum glucose over 100 mg/dl.	None
Hyponatremia with decreased extracellular volume	Patients with dehydration (decreased extracellular volume). Must differentiate whether the sodium loss is due to renal losses (diuretic use, mineralocorticoid deficiency, renal tubular acidosis, and salt-wasting nephropathy), or whether the patient has become dehydrated due to increased sweating, vomiting, diarrhea, third spacing, or other fluid losses.	A low urine sodium suggests that the body is trying to hold onto sodium (<20 mEq/L) as is the case with dehydration, whereas a high urine sodium (>20 mEq/L) suggests that the kidneys are wasting sodium.	Correct volume deficit with isotonic normal saline (0.9%), which is hypertonic compared to the patient's serum.
Hyponatremia with normal extracellular volume	Patients have elevated total body water (but a normal extracellular volume and no edema). SIADH: Results from excess anti-diuretic hormone production; usually caused by lung masses or infections, CNS disorders (including head trauma,) and drugs (including thiazides, oral hypoglycemics, narcotics).	Other potential causes of euvolemic hyponatremia (e.g., hypoadrenalism, hypothyroidism, renal failure) should be ruled out before the diagnosis of SIADH can be made. Patients with euvolemic hyponatremia have a urinary sodium concentration greater than 20 mEq/L.	Fluid restriction, and treat underlying cause. Lithium and demeclocycline, which inhibits the action of ADH, can also be used.

Table 88-8   Classification of Hyponatremia Based on Extracellular Volume—*cont'd*

	Causes	Diagnostics	Treatment
	ADH works in the kidneys to conserve water (and block diuresis). Psychogenic polydipsia: Results from patients drinking excessive quantities of fluid with relatively low sodium contents. Patients who drink excessive amounts of beer (beer potomania) have a similar presentation.	The capacity of the kidneys to excrete free water in the urine is overwhelmed. The urine in patients with psychogenic polydipsia is maximally dilute.	Fluid restriction and treat underlying cause.
Hyponatremia with increased extracellular volume	Sodium is retained but water retention exceeds that of sodium. These are the edematous patients with CHF, liver failure, and renal failure.	There is decreased effective renal perfusion resulting in secretion of ADH and aldosterone. Patients with CHF or liver failure typically have a urine sodium below 10 mEq/L, and those with renal failure have a concentration above 20 mEq/L.	ADH and aldosterone are effective for most patients. Diuretics may increase water excretion, however sodium excretion is also increased. Dialysis may be required for renal failure.

ADH, antidiuretic hormone; CHF, congestive heart failure; CNS, central nervous system; SIADH, syndrome of inappropriate antidiuretic hormone.

hour. Another method is described in Chapter 26 under "Hyponatremic Volume Depletion". The patient's serum sodium values should be followed closely with levels drawn approximately every 2-3 hours.

■ *Helpful hints and pitfalls.* Care must be taken to avoid too rapid correction that can result in Central Pontine Myelinolysis (also called the Osmotic Demyelinating Syndrome). This syndrome has been seen in patients whose sodium levels have risen by more than 10 meq/day. Patients can develop severe neurologic impairments including deep coma, flaccid paralysis, cranial nerve palsies, and a "locked-in" syndrome. This essentially irreversible syndrome usually progresses to death.

Hyperphosphatemia

■ *Background.* The most common cause of hyperphosphatemia is renal failure. Phosphate is normally excreted in the urine. The phosphate remains normal until the creatinine clearance falls below 30 ml/min. Other causes are acute phosphate overload or increased phosphate reabsorption. Acute phosphate overload is usually due to tissue breakdown such as tumor lysis syndrome, rhabdomyolysis, lactic acidosis, diabetic ketoacidosis, marked hemolysis, or iatrogenic overdose. Increased tubular reabsorption of phosphate by the kidneys occurs in patients due to hypoparathyroidism, tumor calcinosis, or bisphosphonate treatment. Pseudohyperphospatemia is due to interference with analytical methods, and is seen in patients with multiple myeloma, hyperlipidemia, hemolysis, and hyperbilirubinemia.

■ *Clinical presentation.* Patients may present with multiple different complaints, some of which may be related to associated electrolyte abnormalities, particularly hypocalcemia. In most cases, the symptoms of hyperphosphatemia are overshadowed by the signs and symptoms of the underlying disorder, such as rhabdomyolysis or hemolysis. Chronic hyperphosphatemia in renal failure can lead to a high calcium phosphate product, and result in metastatic calcifications in joints, tissues, and arteries.

■ *Diagnostic testing.* Hyperphosphatemia (>5.0 mg/dl) is rare in patients with normal renal function. Due to the frequency of associated electrolyte abnormalities, a serum calcium, potassium, and magnesium level should also be checked.

■ *ED management.* Acute severe hyperphosphatemia can cause symptomatic hypocalcemia, and should be treated as discussed in the section on hypocalcemia. Hyperphosphatemia usually resolves within 6 to 12 hours on its own in a patient with intact renal function. Phosphate excretion can be increased by IV normal saline infusion, although this can further exacerbate associated hypocalcemia. Acetazolamide, a carbonic anhydrase inhibitor, can also be given at a dose of 15 mg/kg IV. Hemodialysis may be indicated in patients with hyperphosphatemia and symptomatic hypocalcemia, particularly if renal failure is present. Patients who are asymptomatic with chronic hyperphosphatemia and renal failure may be managed on low phosphate diet and phosphate binders (e.g., calcium carbonate or Tums), but these medications are usually initiated by the internist or nephrologists.

Hypophosphatemia

- *Background.* The most common causes of hypophosphatemia are due to intracellular shifts, gastroenterological losses, or renal losses (see Table 88–9).
- *Clinical presentation.* Patients may present with multiple different complaints, some of which are often related to associated electrolyte abnormalities. Also, symptoms may be precipitated by glucose infusion, which drives phosphate into cells. Signs and symptoms of severe hypophosphatemia include weakness, confusion, respiratory muscle weakness, hypercarbia, congestive heart failure, hypotension, myalgias and rhabdomyolysis.
- *Diagnostic testing.* Hypophosphatemia has traditionally been classified as mild (2.5 to 2.8 md/dl), moderate (1.0 to 2.5 mg/dl), or severe (<1.0 mg/dl). Usually, patients begin to manifest symptoms of hypophosphatemia at serum levels below 1.0 mg/dL. Due to the frequency of associated electrolyte abnormalities, a serum calcium, potassium, and magnesium level should also be checked.
- *ED management.* Since hypophosphatemia often presents concurrently with hypokalemia, phosphate repletion is often given with potassium repletion. Phosphorous (K-Phos or Neutra-Phos) can be given 250-500 mg PO BID for stable or asymptomatic patients. Symptomatic, unstable, or severely hypophosphatemic patients (<1.5 mg/dL) should be given 0.08-0.16 mmol/kg IV (0.6-0.9 mg/kg/hr) over 6 hours.

Special Considerations
Pediatrics

- Pediatric patients deserve special mention. Infant seizures may be due to sodium abnormalities or hypocalcemia. Hyponatremia is second only to febrile seizures as a cause for first-time seizures in an infant. Water intoxication and gastrointestinal losses are the most common causes. Hyponatremia may also cause lethargy, decreased deep tendon reflexes (DTR), vomiting, or acute respiratory failure. Hypernatremia may also cause seizures and altered mental status in the young infant. Free water loss (e.g., diarrhea with high sodium replacement fluid) results in hypovolemic hypernatremia, and accounts for most cases seen in the

Table 88–9 Causes of Hypophosphatemia	
Intracellular shifts	Respiratory alkalosis, hyperglycemia
Gastrointestinal losses	Malabsorption or malnutrition (especially with alcohol abuse), vitamin D deficiency, protracted vomiting or diarrhea, nasogastric suctioning, phosphate binding antacids.
Renal losses	Diuresis, renal tubular acidosis, hyperosmolar states (e.g., diabetic ketoacidosis), hyperparathyroidism, aldosteronism, or glucocorticoid administration.

ED. Poor oral intake can also cause hypernatremia. These infants have increased DTRs, tetany, tonic spasm, tremulousness, rigidity, and a high pitched cry.

- Hypocalcemia is one of the common abnormalities in the newborn period. It is defined as a level <6 mg/dL in preterm newborns, <7 mg/dl in term newborns, and <8 mg/dl in a term infant older than 1 week. These infants also present with jitteriness and seizures. The majority have concomitant hypomagnesemia that must be corrected in order to correct the hypocalcemia. Causes include dietary intake and Vitamin D deficiency or resistance. It is more common in infants of diabetic mothers and preterm infants.

- In infants, phosphorus levels as high as 7.4 mg/dl are considered normal.

Teaching Points

Fluid and electrolyte disturbances are common problems. As with all metabolic diseases, the signs and symptoms are difficult to recognize, by both patient and physician, and the patient often appears more ill than the presenting complaints would suggest. It is rare for these disturbances to develop suddenly, and they are therefore difficult to repair quickly. Most of these patients will therefore require hospital admission.

The extreme ranges of imbalance are seen in very critically ill patients, and while total correction must be slow, immediate interventions may prevent death from dysrhythmia or shock.

Electrolyte imbalances rarely occur in isolation, so it is useful to always check levels of all of the electrolytes. Renal function should be assessed, and disturbances aggressively sought in any patient with chronic renal disease.

Suggested Readings

Adrogué HJ, Madias NE. Hyponatremia. New Engl J Med 2000;342:1581–9.
Adrogué HJ, Madias NE. Hypernatremia. New Engl J Med 2000;342:1493–9.
Bushinsky DA, Monk RD. Calcium. Lancet 1998;352:306-11.
Claudius I, Fluharty C, Boles R. The emergency department approach to newborn and childhood metabolic crisis. Emerg Med Clin North Am 2005;23:843–83.
Gennari FJ. Hypokalemia. N Engl J Med 1998;339;451–57.
Halperin ML, Kamel KS. Potassium. Lancet 1998;352:135–40.
Kumar S, Berl T. Sodium. Lancet 1998;352:220–28.

CHAPTER 89

Emergency Medical Services

JOHN PETTINI

Importance of Prehospital Care

- The importance of prehospital care in the chain of survival cannot be overstated. The key to insuring a quality emergency medical system (EMS) system is physician involvement with prehospital colleagues. Emergency physicians should be advocates for their local prehospital system, and be actively involved in its ongoing development.

Governance of Prehospital Care

- EMS systems are governed locally by regional medical directors. Medical directors usually are emergency medicine physicians who have experience in prehospital care, or are fellowship trained in EMS. In large systems, there may be multiple associate medical directors. Regional systems implement prehospital treatment protocols in accordance with the scope of practice allowed by the state level regulations.
- The medical director has a contractual agreement with an administrative authority to implement patient care protocols, ensure continuing education, provide system oversight through quality assurance and improvement, and handle system complaints and remediation of providers. Protocols serve as pre-established practice guidelines that define the standard of care for most illnesses or injuries encountered in the prehospital setting. Protocols may include standing orders for particular clinical situations and operational issues, such as hospital destination policies, termination of resuscitation, and patient transport refusal.
- In the United States, EMS is delivered by a multitude of different interests such as the fire service, area hospitals, private for-profit contractors, and volunteer agencies.

Types of Medical Direction

- Protocol-driven medical direction consists of standing orders covering most common medical and trauma encounters is the norm. These standing orders are considered *off-line medical direction*.
- Protocols usually have decision points where it may be necessary to confer with a physician directly such as in the case of field termination of resuscitation. Direct communication by telephone or radio with a base station physician is termed *online medical direction*. Most systems operate with this combination of offline and online medical direction.
- Field supervision of EMS was pioneered in the early development of advanced life support systems. The role of the physician in the field is still

being defined; most EMS systems operate without field physicians in the United States.

Training Levels of Emergency Medical Services Providers

EMS providers generally fall into two tiers of ability: basic and advanced life support.

- *Emergency medical technician (EMT) basic.* The scope of practice of an EMT includes basic physical examination skills, nondefinitive airway control, emergency childbirth, splinting, spinal immobilization, cardio-pulmonary resuscitation, and defibrillation with an automated defibrillator. In some systems Epi pens and intramuscular glucagon can be used. Training is usually completed in 200 hours with annual continuing education and recertification.
- *EMT paramedic.* The scope of practice of an EMT paramedic includes basic and intermediate skills, plus extensive training in advanced cardiac life support (ACLS) and trauma life support. Skills include advanced airway techniques including endotracheal intubation and surgical airway IV fluids, medication administration, and 12-lead electrocardiograms (EKGs). Training is usually between 1000 and 1500 hours.

Some systems, particularly in rural areas, may use providers whose training is between the EMT basic and paramedic levels. These intermediate providers may be allowed to start IVs, administer fluids, and perform endotracheal intubation.

Air Transport

- Most areas of the country are covered by emergency helicopter response services. The role of helicopters is to transport the sickest patients quickly from the scene to definitive care. Their benefit is felt the most in remote rural areas where ground transport takes many hours, and the helicopter provides a quick means of providing advanced life support to a system that only has basic life support.
- Emergency physicians should consider air transport in urban and suburban areas with critical patients when traffic may prolong ground transportation.
- Additionally, many helicopters are staffed with critical care registered nurses capable of caring for patients on balloon pumps and multiple infusion medications, which may not be within the scope of paramedic training.

Regional Communications and Coordination

- Centralized, regional communication centers are common in populated areas. An effective communication system is critical for ensuring the delivery of quality and expeditious care in the prehospital environment. Essential components include public information, and education programs regarding general access to emergency medical services (e.g., dialing 911); technology to ensure rapid access and communications;

trained emergency medical dispatchers capable of call prioritization, allocation of available resources, and providing emergency patient care instructions before EMS arrival; and communication between pre-hospital care providers and hospital personnel. In disasters, these same centers function to appropriately distribute patients on the basis of available resources.

Prehospital Medical Care

Prehospital care providers respond to a variety of medical situations, and often function in an austere environment with limited resources compared with the capabilities of a functioning ED. Scene safety and personal protective equipment are critical to any prehospital response. Patient care priorities for common EMS responses are discussed in the following sections.

■ *Respiratory emergencies.* Basic measures to secure a patient's airway, including manual maneuvers (e.g., chin lift, jaw thrust), oral and naso-pharyngeal devices, and the use of a bag-valve-mask (BVM), are used by EMT basic providers. Advanced interventions used by paramedic providers may include endotracheal intubation, the use of alternative adjuncts (e.g., blind-insertion airway device, laryngeal mask airway), or very rarely, even surgical cricothyrotomy. Rapid-sequence intubation (RSI) regimens are commonly used by air medical services but are only used by a small number of ground prehospital providers. It is not possible to make every prehospital care system the equivalent of an ED, thus RSI in the field appears to be too dangerous to utilize, and pediatric intubation is such a rare event, that in most systems it is preferable to avoid it, and instead use BVM for these patients. Many advanced programs have protocols for the initial medical management of common respiratory diseases such as bronchospasm from asthma, chronic obstructive pulmonary disease (albuterol, terbutaline), or anaphylaxis (diphenhydramine, epinephrine, steroids).
■ *Cardiac emergencies.* All prehospital providers are trained in basic cardiac life support. Defibrillators are traditionally used by paramedics who are capable of rhythm interpretation. Automatic external defibrillators (AEDs) are now in widespread use by emergency responders and laypersons with little or no knowledge of cardiac arrest. Twelve-lead EKGs are becoming more common in the prehospital environment. Some systems are capable of transmitting a copy of the EKG to the receiving hospital prior to arrive resulting in shorter times to intervention (thrombolytic administration or catheterization laboratory admission). Medications used for ACLS are available for use by paramedic providers. Thrombolytic therapy is not currently being used in the prehospital environment, but may have a role in rural areas with long transport times.
■ *Trauma.* The primary goal for prehospital care for major trauma is rapid transport to the nearest hospital capable of managing such injuries. Most interventions for traumatic injuries should be performed while en route to the hospital in an effort to reduce on-scene time. The priorities of prehospital care include airway management (including intubation

if needed), control of external bleeding, immobilization of the spine, needle decompression of suspected tension pneumothorax, and splinting of major extremity fractures. Prehospital IV crystalloid resuscitation of bluntly injured patients is recommended, but aggressive IV fluid administration is discouraged in patients with penetrating injury unless the patient manifests severe shock or prolonged transport (more than 30 minutes) is expected.

Patient Transfers

■ Prehospital care providers are often involved in the transfer of a patient from one hospital facility to another. The Emergency Medical Treatment and Active Labor Act mandates that unstable patients should not be transferred to another facility at the request of a managed care organization unless the transferring hospital is incapable of providing standard care, and the receiving hospital does have the capability to manage the condition and foreseeable complications. If the patient is transferred, the risk and benefits of the transfer must be clearly documented, informed consent should be obtained from the patient or family, appropriate equipment and personnel for transportation should be arranged, treatment and stabilization should be initiated, the receiving facility should accept the patient, and the appropriate patient records should be sent to the receiving facility.

Teaching Points

Emergency physicians should be familiar with the capabilities and written protocols of local EMS providers. Although functioning in a much more austere environment, prehospital care can make a vital difference in the outcome of critically ill patients. ED personnel should take the time to obtain as much historical information from EMS providers on arrival to the ED as this is often the only information available.

Suggested Readings

Bailey ED, Wydro GC, Cone DC. Termination of resuscitation in the prehospital setting for adult patients suffering nontraumatic cardiac arrest. National Association of EMS Physicians Standards and Clinical Practice Committee. Prehospital Emergency Care 2000;4:190–195.

Blackwell TH. Principles of emergency medical systems. In: Marx JA, Hockberger RS, Walls RM (editors). Rosen's Emergency Medicine: Concepts and Clinical Practice (6th ed). Philadelphia: Mosby, 2006, pp 2984–2993.

Fowler R, Pepe PE. Prehospital care of the patient with major trauma. Emerg Med Clin North Am 2002;20:953–974.

Hopson LR. Guidelines for withholding or termination of resuscitation in prehospital traumatic cardiopulmonary arrest: joint position statement of the National Association of EMS Physicians and the American College of Surgeons Committee on Trauma. J Am Coll Surg 2003;196:106–112.

McCabe CJ, Warren RL Trauma: an annotated bibliography of the recent literature—2003. Am J Emerg Med 2004;22:405–424.

CHAPTER 90

Pharmacology

90.1 Analgesia and Sedation

Adam Wos ■ Paul Ishimine ■ Tom Catron

Procedural Sedation and Analgesia (PSA)

- PSA refers to the use of analgesic, dissociative, and sedative agents to relieve pain and anxiety associated with diagnostic and therapeutic procedures.
- A directed history and physical examination should precede every PSA to assess for underlying medical problems, specifically addressing airway and cardiovascular function. The need for preprocedural fasting, and the duration of this fasting state, remains controversial.
- PSA should generally involve two experienced individuals, one to monitor sedation, and the other to actually perform the procedure. PSA should be done in a dedicated area with adequate monitoring equipment (pulse oximetry, blood pressure and cardiac monitoring), and resuscitative equipment (oxygen, bag valve mask, suction, drug reversal agents). Capnometry may be helpful if available. Agents for PSA often have a narrow therapeutic index, and should be given in small doses and titrated to a desired effect. After completion of the procedure, the patient should be alert and oriented or at baseline mental status with stable vital signs prior to discharge. The patient should leave with a reliable adult who can observe the patient for post-procedural complications. The patient should not drive.
- The key to procedural safety is the ability to watch the patient while the procedure is being performed. Thus, if there are no personnel available to monitor the patient, the procedure is best deferred, or performed somewhere else, such as an operating theatre where effective monitoring can be achieved.
- See Table 90.1–1 for commonly used analgesia and sedative agents.
- Reversal agents for benzodiazepines (flumazenil) and narcotics (nalaxone) are discussed in Chapter 72.

Table 90.1–1 Analgesic and Sedative Agents

Drug name	Adult dose (A), Pediatric (P) dose	Side effects	Comments
		Narcotics	
Codeine	A: 15-60 mg PO/SC/IM P: 0.5-1 mg/kg PO/SC/IM	Euphoria, sedation, constipation, GI upset	Commonly used in combination with acetaminophen or aspirin. Antitussive effects
Fentanyl (Duragesic, Sublimaze)	A: 2 mcg/kg IM or slow IV, or intranasal, 25–100 mcg/hr transdermally P (>1y): 1-2 mcg/kg IM/IV	Respiratory depression, facial pruritis, chest wall rigidity (rare, with rapid administration)	Peak within minutes, duration 20–40 minutes, no histamine release. Few hemodynamic effects. Chest wall rigidity reversed with naloxone.
Hydromorphone (Dilaudid)	A: 2-4 mg PO, 0.5-2 mg IM/IV/SC, 3 mg PR P: 0.03–0.08 mg/kg PO or 0.015 mg/kg IV	Respiratory depression, histamine release can lead to pruritis and hypotension, nausea, vomiting	More potent than morphine with less histamine release Duration of action 3-4 hrs Antitussive effect
Hydrocodone (Lortab, Lorcet, Norco, Vicoden, Vicoprofen)	A: 5-10 mg PO P: 0.2 mg/kg PO (of hydrocodone)	Causes more drowsiness and dizziness than codeine, but fewer GI side effects.	Prodrug of hydromorphone. Commonly used in combination with acetaminophen or ibuprofen. Antitussive effect.
Meperidine (Demerol)	A: 50-150mg IM/IV/SC/PO P: 1-1.5 mg/kg IM/IV/SC/PO	Hypotension, histamine release, respiratory depression, tremors, seizures, nausea, vomiting, euphoria, neuroleptic malignant syndrome with MAOI	Duration up to 2 hrs Abuse potential Rarely used for PSA IM preferred over IV and SC Normeperidine (meperidine metabolite) is associated with seizures
Morphine (Avinza, Roxinal, MS Contin, others)	A: 2.5-10 mg IV/IV/SC, 10-30mg PO P: 0.05-0.2 mg/kg slow IV/SC/IM, 0.2-0.5 mg/kg PO	Respiratory depression, histamine release with pruritis and hypotension, nausea, vomiting	IV dose peak in 10-30 minutes, duration up to 4 hours Erratic oral absorption

Drug Name	Adult dose (A), Pediatric (P) / dose	Side Effects	Comments
Oxycodone (Percocet, Percodan, Roxicet)	A: 10 mg PO P: 0.05-0.15 mg/kg PO (of oxycodone)	Hypotension Respiratory depression	Commonly used in combination with acetaminophen or aspirin. Less nauseating than codeine.
Other Analgesic Agents			
Ibuprofen (Motrin, Advil, others)	A: 200-800 mg PO q 8 hours P: 5-10mg/kg PO q 8 hours	GI irritation and bleeding, platelet inhibition, renal failure	Commonly prescribed anti-inflammatory
Indomethacin (Indocin)	A: 25-50 mg PO/PR tid	Gastrointestinal irritation Platelet inhibition Renal failure	Highly effective anti-inflammatory Not recommended in the elderly due to increased adverse reactions Used in neonates to close a patent ductus arteriosus
Ketorolac (Toradol)	A: 15-60 mg IV/IM q 6 hours or 30 mg IV; 10 mg PO q 4-6 hours P: 0.5 mg/kg IM to max 30 mg	GI irritation and bleeding, platelet inhibition, renal failure	Often effective in renal colic Duration of treatment not to exceed 5 days due to GI side effects Renal dosing required
Naproxen (Aleve, others)	A: 250-500 mg PO bid P: 5-7 mg/kg PO bid	Gastrointestinal irritation Platelet inhibition Renal failure	Increased dosing interval compared to others.
Acetylsalicylic acid (Ecotrin, others)	A: 325-650 mg PO q 4-6 hours	GI irritation/bleeding Irreversible platelet inhibition Hypersensitivity	Anti-inflammatory properties seen at higher doses. Avoid in pediatric fever due to association with Reye's syndrome.
Acetaminophen (Tylenol, others)	A: 325-1000mg PO/PR P:10-15mg/kg PO/PR	Hepatic necrosis in severe overdose	Analgesic of choice in children with viral infections or varicella Lacks anti-inflammatory action

Continued

Table 90.1–1 Analgesic and Sedative Agents—*cont'd*

Drug name	Adult dose (A), Pediatric (P) dose	Side effects	Comments
		Sedative Agents	
Methohexital (Brevital)	A: 1-1.5 mg/kg IV P: Not commonly used for PSA	Oversedation, respiratory depression, apnea, hypotension, myoclonus, thrombophlebitis	Onset in 1 min when given IV Clinical recovery rapid Proconvulsant unlike other barbiturates No analgesic properties
Pentobarbital (Nembutal)	A: 100 mg IV, up to 500 mg P: 2-6 mg/kg IM/PO (max 100 mg); 1-3 mg/kg IV	Respiratory depression and apnea, hypotension	Rarely used for adult PSA Sedative of choice in many centers for pediatric sedation
Thiopental (Pentothal)	A: 50-100 mg IV; up to 5mg/kg for induction P: 0.5-2 mg/kg IV	Respiratory depression and apnea, hypotension	Rapid onset and recovery similar to methohexital. No analgesic properties. Anticonvulsant activity.
Midazolam (Versed)	A: 1-2 mg IV (up to 5 mg), 2 mg IM P: 0.25-1 mg/kg PO (max 20 mg), 0.2-0.5 mg/kg intranasal, 0.5 mg/kg PR, 0.1-0.2 mg/kg IM 6 mos to 5 yrs: 0.05-0.1 mg/kg IV, titrate up to max 6 mg 6-12 yrs: 0.025-0.05 mg/kg IV, to max 10 mg	Respiratory depression, minimal cardiovascular, depression, paradoxical excitability occasionally seen especially in children	Most common benzodiazepine for PSA Peak effect 2-3 min when given IV No analgesic properties, needs to be given with an analgesic for painful procedures

Drug name	Adult dose (A), Pediatric (P) dose	Side effects	Comments
Etomidate (Amidate)	A: 0.1-0.3 mg/kg IV P: 0.1-0.3 mg/kg IV (but not well studied in children for PSA)	Pain on injection Respiratory depression Myoclonus Nausea and vomiting Transient adrenal suppression	Rapid onset and recovery. No analgesic effects. Minimal effects on cardiovascular system and intracranial pressure. Myoclonic jerks fairly common that can be mistaken for seizures.
Ketamine (Ketalar)	A: 1-2 mg/kg slowly, then 0.25 to 0.5 mg/kg IV q 5-10 min. P: 10 mg/kg PO 30 min. prior; IV: 1-2 mg/kg @ 0.5 mg/kg/min, IM: 3 – 4 mg/kg; 0.5 mg/kg incremental doses if initial dose is inadequate	Salivation and bronchorrhea Elevation in HR, BP, and myocardial O2 consumption ↑ICP or IOP Transient laryngospasm, apnea or respiratory depression Hallucinatory "emergence reactions"	Dissociative sedation, with preservation of cardiopulmonary function and airway protective reflexes Potent bronchodilator Occasionally given with atropine or glycopyrrolate to avoid hypersalivation Midazolam frequently used in older children and adults to blunt emergence reactions
Nitrous oxide	20-50% concentration administered with oxygen	Nausea, dizziness, euphoria, Laughter	Given by self-administered demand valve mask; requires cooperative patient Rapidly absorbed, peak effect in 5 min, wears off shortly after discontinuation Airway reflexes, hemodynamic status, and respirations remain intact .
Propofol (Diprivan)	Adults < 50y: 0.5-1 mg/kg IV bolus over 30 sec, q 10 seconds then 0.1 to 0.2 mg/kg prn. Elderly: half of the above dose P: 1 mg/kg IV bolus with a 0.5 mg/kg titration dose	Potent respiratory depression and sudden apnea Hypotension by negative inotropy and venodilatation Antiemetic properties Pain at injection site	Lipid soluble, given IV only. Onset of action in 1 minute. Clinical recovery 5-15 minutes after bolus or drip. Inconsistent amnestic effects.

ICP: intracramial pressure; IOP: intraocular pressure

90.2 Antimicrobial Therapy

Amy Kahn

- The decision to use a particular antibiotic ideally is determined by culture isolation of the offending organism, and the sensitivity of this organism to a particular antibiotic. However, this information is usually not available in the ED.
- Empiric antibiotic therapy can be life-saving, and should be started as soon as possible in the ED.
- The choice of which agent to use should always be based on the most likely involved organism and local resistance patterns.
- See Table 90.2–1 for a description of commonly used antibiotics.
- See Table 90.2–2 and 90.2–3 for common problems requiring antibiotics therapy in the ED.

90.3 Cardiovascular Pharmacology

Brenna M. Farmer ■ Chuck Seamens

- This section will summarize the most common cardiovascular drugs used in the ED.
- See Table 90.3–1 for drugs used in acute coronary syndrome. Thrombolytic therapy is reviewed in Chapter 90.5.
- See Table 90.3–2 for inotropic and vasopressor agents.
- See Table 90.3–3 for antidysrhythmic agents.
- See Chapter 39 for medications used to treat hypertension.

90.4 Gastrointestinal Pharmacology

- Gastrointestinal complaints such as nausea, vomiting, diarrhea, and constipation are common in the ED.
- See Tables 90.4–1 through 90.4–3 for agents used to treat these symptoms.
- Refer to Chapter 23 for agents used to treat constipation.

Table 90.2–1 Common Antimicrobial Therapy

	Mechanism of Action	Specific Drugs	Comment
Penicillin (PCN)	Binds to penicillin binding proteins and blocks cross linking of cell wall.	**1st generation** benzathine penicillin (Bicillin L-A): 1.2 million units IM; peds < 27 kg 0.3–0.6 MU, > 27kg 0.9 MU. penicillin G: 250,000-400,-000 units/kg/day IV divided q4-6 hours. penicillin V (Pen-Vee K): 200-500 mg PO quid; peds 25-50 mg/kg/day divided bid or qid.	Covers most streptococci and oral anaerobic coverage
		2nd generation Dicloxacillin: 250-500 mg PO qid; peds 12.5-25 mg/kg/day divided qid. nafcillin: 1-2 g IM/IV q4 hours; peds 150-200 mg/kg/day divided q4-6 hours. oxacillin: 1-2 g IM/IV q4-6 hours; peds 150-200 mg/kg/day divided q4-6 hours.	Covers most streptococci and *Staph aureus*; penicillinase resistant
		3rd generation amoxicillin: 250-500 mg PO tid; peds 40 mg/kg/day PO divided tid or 45 mg/kg/day PO divided bid. amoxicillin-clavulanate (Augmentin) : 500-875 mg PO bid or 250-500 mg PO tid; peds dose similar to amoxicillin. ampicillin: 1-2 g IV q4-6 hours; peds 50-400 mg/kg/day IM/IV divided q 4-6 hours. ampicillin-sulbactam (Unasyn): 1.5-3 g IM/IV q 6 hours; peds 100-400 mg/kg/day of ampicillin divided q6 hours.	Aminopenicillins; covers most streptococci and gram negatives. β-lactamase inhibitors (clavulanate, sulbactam) added to increase antibacterial spectrum. Higher dose of 80 mg/kg/day divided bid or tid for otitis media.

Continued

Table 90.2–1   Common Antimicrobial Therapy—*cont'd*

	Mechanism of Action	Specific Drugs	Comment
		4th generation piperacillin-tazobactam (Zosyn): 3.375-4.5 g IV q6 hours; peds 240 mg/kg/day of piperacillin IV divided q 8 hours. ticarcillin-clavulanate (Timentin): 3.1 g IV q 4-6 hours; peds 50 mg/kg (up to 3.1 g) IV q4-6 hours.	Covers *Pseudomonas*.
Cephalosporins	Binds to PCN binding proteins and blocks cross linking of cell wall (less susceptible to β-lactamase than penicillins)	**1st generation** cefazolin (Ancef): 1 g IM/IV q 6-8 hours; peds 25-50 mg/kg/day divided q 6-8 hours. cephalexin (Keflex): 250-500 mg PO qid; peds 25-50 mg/kg/day divided q 6-8 hours.	Covers gram positive, including *Staph aureus* and basic gram negative.
		2nd generation cefaclor (Ceclor): 250-500 mg PO tid, peds 20-40 mg/kg/day PO divided tid. cefotetan (Cefotan): 1-2 g IM/IV q 12 hours; peds 20-40 mg/kg IV q 12 hours. cefoxitin (Mefoxin): 1-2 g IM/IV q 6-8 hours; peds 80-160 mg/kg/day IV divided q 4-8 hours. cefuroxime (Zinacef): 750-1500 mg IM/IV q8 hours; peds 50-100 mg/kg/day IV divided q6-8 hours. (Ceftin): 250-500 mg PO bid; peds 20-30 mg/kg/day divided bid.	Improved gram negative coverage with some anaerobes. Less *Staph aureus* coverage.

Mechanism of Action	Specific Drugs	Comment
	3rd generation cefdinir (Omnicef): 14 mg/kg/day up to 600 mg/day PO divided qd or bid. cefixime (Suprax): 400 mg PO qd or 200 mg PO bid; single dose of 400 mg PO for gonorrhea; peds 8 mg/kg/day divided qd-bid. cefotaxime (Claforan): 1-2 g IM/IV q6-8 hours; peds 50-180 mg/kg/day IM/IV divided q4-6 hours. ceftazidime (Fortaz): 1 g IM/IV or 2 g IV q8-12 hours; peds 30-50 mg/kg IV q 8 hours. ceftriaxone (Rocephin): 1-2 g IM/IV q 24 hours, single dose 125 mg IM (250 mg for PID) for gonorrhea; peds 50-75 mg/kg/day up to 2 g q 12-24 hours IV (up to 1 g IM), 100 mg/kg/day IV for meningitis.	Improved gram negative and some pseudomonal coverage. Less *Staph aureus* coverage.
	4th generation cefepime (Maxpime): 0.5-2 g IM/IV q 12 hours; peds 50 mg/kg IV q 8-12 hours.	Similar to 3rd generation with better pseudomonal coverage. Has anti-staphylococcal activity of 1st generation.
Carbapenums Binds to PCN binding proteins, and blocks cross linking of cell wall.	imipenem-cilastin (Primaxin): 250-1000 mg IV q 6-8 hours; peds > 3 month 15-25 mg/kg IV q 6 hours. meropenem (Merrem IV): 1 g IV q 8 hours; peds 20-40 mg/kg up to 2 g IV q 8 hours.	Headache, fever, diarrhea, nausea, hepatic enzyme elevations
Fluoro-quinolones Inhibits DNA gyrase (topoisomerase II) thus inhibiting DNA replication	**2nd generation** ciprofloxacin (Cipro): 250-750 mg PO bid; 200-400 mg IV q 8-12 hours; 100 mg PO bid for simple UTI or Cipro XR 500 mg PO qd. norfloxacin (Noroxin): 400 mg PO bid x 3 days for simple UTI. ofloxacin (Floxin): 200-400 mg IV/PO q 12 hours.	Covers gram negative including *Pseudomonas*; *Staph aureus*, but not good coverage of pneumococcus; some atypicals

Continued

Table 90.2–1 Common Antimicrobial Therapy—cont'd

	Mechanism of Action	Specific Drugs	Comment
		3rd generation levofloxacin (Levaquin): 250-750 mg PO/IV qd.	Covers gram negative including *Pseudomonas*; covers *Staph aureus* and pneumococcus; extended spectrum for atypical pneumonias.
		4th generation gatifloxacin (Tequin): 400 mg IV/PO; 400 mg PO single dose for simple UTI. gemifloxacin (Factive): 320 mg PO qd x 5-7 days. moxifloxacin (Avelox): 400 mg PO/IV qd x 5-14 days.	Similar to 3rd generation; better pneumococcus coverage
Macrolides	Inhibits protein synthesis by binding to the 50S ribosomal subunit	erythromycin ethyl succinate (EES, Eryped): 400 mg PO qid; peds 30-50 mg/kd/day divided qid. erythromycin ethyl succinate + sulfisoxazole (Pediazole): 50 mg/kg/day based on EES dose PO divided tid or qid. erythromycin lactobionate (Erythrocin IV): 15-20 mg/kg/day (max 4 g) divided q 6 hours; peds 15-50 mg/kg/day divided q 6 hours.	Drug of choice for *Mycoplasma pneumoniae*, *Legionella pneumophila*, diphtheria, pertussis, *Chlamydia trachomatis* pneumonia or conjunctivitis, and bacillary angiomatosis. Increased incidence of hepatotoxicity with the estolate salt. GI symptoms common with oral dose. IV administration is associated with phlebitis.
		azithromycin (Zithromax): 500 mg IV qd; 500 mg PO day 1 and 250 mg PO qd to total 5 days; peds 10 mg/kg up to 500 mg qd for 5 days.	Better GI tolerance and activity against gram negative aerobes and *Neisseria spp.* Commonly used for a wide variety of acute upper and lower respiratory tract infections

Table 90.2–1 Common Antimicrobial Therapy—*cont'd*

	Mechanism of Action	Specific Drugs	Comment
		clarithromycin, (Biaxin): 250–500 mg PO bid; Biaxin XL 1000 mg PO qd with food; a single 1 g PO dose for *Chlamydia trachomatis*. peds 7.5 mg/kg PO bid;	Better GI tolerance. Commonly used for a wide variety of acute upper and lower respiratory tract infections. Same coverage as erythromycin but better activity than erythromycin against most staphylococci and streptococci.
Tetracyclines	Inhibits protein synthesis by binding to the 30S ribosomal subunit	doxycycline: 100 mg PO bid on day 1, then 50 mg PO bid. minocycline: 200 mg IV/PO initially, then 100 mg q 12 hours. tetracycline: 250–500 mg PO qid.	Broad gram-positive and gram-negative coverage; also *Mycoplasma, Rickettsia, Chlamydia, Plasmodium falciparum,* and syphilis. First choice for rare disease: plague, brucellosis, cholera Photosensitivity, GI distress Contraindications: children (discolors teeth and inhibits bone growth).
Aminoglycoside	Inhibits protein synthesis by binding to initiation complex.	amikacin: 15 mg/kg up to 1500 mg/day IM/IV divided q 8-12 hours or 15 mg/kg q 24 hours. gentamicin: 3-5 mg/kg/day IM/IV divided q 8 hours or 5-7 mg/kg IV q 24 hours; peds 2-2.5 mg/kg q 8 hours.	Wider-spectrum againts gram-negatives such as *Acinctobacter, E. coli, Klebsiella, Enterobacter, Pseudomonas, Shigella,* and *Serratia.*

Continued

Table 90.2–1 Common Antimicrobial Therapy—*cont'd*

	Mechanism of Action	Specific Drugs	Comment
		tobramycin: 3-5 mg/kg/day IM/IV divided q 8 hours or 5-7 mg/kg IV q 24 hours; peds 2-2.5 mg/kg q 8 hours.	May cause nephrotoxicity, ototoxicity, vertigo, ataxia. amikacin: peak 20-35 mcg/ml, trough < 5 mcg/mL. gentamicin and tobramycin: peak 5-10 mcg/ml, trough <2 mcg/ml
Clindamycin	Inhibits protein synthesis by binding to the 50S ribosomal subunit	600-900 mg IV q 8 hours, IM if < 600 mg or 150-450 mg PO qid; peds 20-40 mg/kg/day IV divided q 6-8 hours or 8-25 mg/kg/day PO divided tid.	Active against most gram-positive aerobic cocci and anaerobes. Adverse effects include pseudomembranous colitis, fever, diarrhea
Vancomycin	Inhibits cell wall synthesis by blocking polymerization of glycoprotein	1 g IV q12, each dose over 1 hour; peds 10-15 mg/kg IV q 6 hours. For clostridium difficile diarrhea: 40-50 mg/kg/day (max 500 mg/day) PO divided qid for 7-10 days.	Highly active against most gram-positives including MRSA. Adverse effects include flushing, nephrotoxicity, ototoxicity
Trimethoprim-Sulfmethoxazole (TMP-SMX)	Inhibits two steps in the bacterial folic acid synthesis pathway	1 tab PO bid double strength (160 mg/800 mg) or single strength (80 mg/400 mg); peds 5 ml suspension/10 kg (up to 10 ml)/dose PO bid.	Active against *S. aureus*, group A streptococcus, *E. coli*, *Klebsiella*, *Pneumocystic carinii*. May cause hypersensitivity, hemolysis in G6PD deficiency Contraindicated: infants, pregnancy, severe renal disease or hepatic dysfunction

Table 90.2-1 Common Antimicrobial Therapy—*cont'd*

	Mechanism of Action	Specific Drugs	Comment
Metronidazole	Interferes with helical structure of DNA	1 g or 15 mg/kg IV load then 500 mg or 7.5 mg/kg IV/PO q 6 hours (max 4 g/day); peds 7.5 mg/kg IV q 6 hours. For C. difficile: 500 mg PO tid; peds 10-15 mg/kg/dose PO.	Active against most obligate anaerobic bacteria and many protozoa. May cause headache, disulfiram-like reaction with alcohol
Aztreonam	Binds to penicillin binding proteins; blocks cross linking of cell wall	0.5-2 g IM/IV q 6-12 hours; peds 30 mg/kg q 6-8 hours.	Primarily active against gram-negatives including *Pseudomonas*. May cause rash, nausea, diarrhea
Rifampin	Inhibition of DNA polymerase	10 to 20 mg/kg (600 mg maximum) in a single daily administration. Prophylaxis for Neisseria meningitides: 600 mg PO bid × 2 days; peds (> 1 month) 10 mg/kg (up to 600 mg) PO bid; peds (< 1 month) 5 mg/kg PO bid × 2 days.	Active against *M. tuberculosis*, some gram negative and gram-positive. Used for community required MRSA.
Linezolid	Protein synthesis inhibitors	400-600 mg IV/PO q 12 hours; peds 10 mg/kg IV/PO q 8 hours.	Used for MRSA Slow IV infusion > 30 minutes.

Table 90.2–2 Common ED Problems Requiring Outpatient Antibiotics

Indication	Antibiotic (see dosing above)	Duration	Comments
Bite wound	amoxicillin/clavulanate	5 days (dog) 10 days (cat) 10 days(human)	Non-infected bites.
Bronchitis	amoxicillin/clavulanate, azithromycin, clarithromycin, fluoroquinolone	3–10 days	Antibiotics are given only for patients with underlying lung disease such as a COPD exacerbation. Use fluoroquinolone with enhanced activity against *S. pneumo*.
Cellulitis	cephalexin, amoxicillin/clavulanate, azithromycin/clarithromycin, clindamycin	5–10 days	Uncomplicated cases. Consider treating for community acquired MRSA (CA MRSA) if it is prevalent in the area or patient population you are treating. A typical case is a rapid onset of a skin infection that the patient often attributes to a "spider bite" without actually visualising an insect bite. Treatment options for CA MRSA include TMP/SMX + rifampin, clindamycin, high dose levofloxacin; IV vancomycin or linezolid for severe cases.
Cystitis	trimethoprim/sulfmethoxazole DS, ciprofloxacin, levofloxacin	3 days	Treatment of uncomplicated cystitis.
	cephalexin	7 days	
Influenza	amantidine	5 days	Treats influenza A only
	oseltamivir	5 days	Treats influenza A and B

MRSA, methicillin-resistant Staph aureus

Table 90.2–2   Common ED Problems Requiring Outpatient Antibiotics—*cont'd*

Indication	Antibiotic (see dosing above)	Duration	Comments
Otitis media	amoxicillin, amoxicillin/clavulanate, cefdinir	7–10 days	If no recent antibiotics, treat with amoxicillin high dose.
Pharyngitis	penicillin VK, benzathine penicillin, clindamycin, erythromycin, clarithromycin	10 days	2nd generation cephalosporins can also be used.
	azithromycin	5 days	
Pneumonia (outpatient)	azithromycin	5 days	Many patients with pneumonia will require admission.
	clarithromycin, levofloxacin	7–14days	
Pelvic Inflammatory Disease	levofloxacin plus metronidazole	14 days	Consider hospitalization for peritonitis, pregnancy, non-compliance or ill-appearing patient.
	ceftriaxone	X 1 and	
	doxycycline	14 days	
Syphilis	benzathine penicillin G 2.4 mU IM	X1	Primary or secondary syphilis only; if PCN allergic, use doxycycline 100 mg PO bid for 14 days. Neurosyphilis is treated with pen G 3-4 mU q 4 hour for 10-14 days. These patients require admission.

Refer to: HIV related infections: Chapter 37, "HIV"
Sexually transmitted disease: Chapter 67, "Infectious Disease"
Pelvic inflammatory disease and vaginitis: Chapter 68, "Obstetrics and Gynecology"

Table 90.2–3 Initial Antibiotics for ED Problems Requiring Hospital Admission

Indication	Empiric Antibiotic	Comments
Cellulitis (severe, diabetic, or failure of outpatient treatment)	cefazolin, cefotaxime, clindamycin, piperacillin-tazobactam	Vancomycin for MRSA. Meropenem or imepenum for severe limb threatening infection.
Cholecystitis	piperacillin/tazobactam, ticarcillin-clavulanate, 3rd generation cephalosporin + metronidazole	Ceftriaxone is associated with biliary sludge. One third of patients will require decompression.
Endocarditis	vancomycin, gentamcin	Add rifampin for prosthetic valve
Meningitis	ceftriaxone or cefotaxime plus vancomycin	Add ampicillin to cover listeria if < 3 months or >50 or alcoholic. Use ampicillin and cefotaxime in a neonate
Necrotizing Fasciitis	penicillin G plus clindamycin; ceftriaxone; imepenum	All require emergent surgical debridement
Neutropenic Fever	a carbapenum or extended-spectrum antipseudomonal cephalosporin (e.g., cefepime), or piperacillin/tazobactam as monotherapy. vancomycin	Should be bactericidal for gram-negative pathogens, particularly *P. aeruginosa* Vancomycin should be considered as initial therapy only in patients at high risk of serious gram-positive pathogen infection.
Open Fracture	cefazolin	Add gentamicin for contaminated wound
Osteomyelitis	nafcillin or cefazolin (hematogenous) cefepime (contiguous)	Add vancomycin for possible MRSA.
Peritonitis	cefotaxime, piperacillin/tazobactam, levoquin + metronidazole, imepenum, or ampicillin + metronidazole + gentamycin (severe)	Must cover both gram negative aerobic and anaerobic bacteria.

Table 90.2–3 Initial Antibiotics for ED Problems Requiring Hospital Admission—*cont'd*

Indication	Empiric Antibiotic	Comments
Pneumonia	cefotaxime plus azithromycin, levofloxacin, cefepime	All patients with community acquired pneumonia should have coverage with a macrolide or fluoroquinolone for atypical organisms. Use cefepime or meropenem for ICU patients
Pyelonephritis	ciprofloxacin levofloxacin, or ceftriaxone cefotaxime, ampicillin + gentamycin	Rule out obstructive uropathy if hypotensive.
Sepsis	imipenem-cilastin + vancomycin piperacillin/tazobactam	Depends on suspected cause: intra-abdominal (see peritonitis), pyelonephritis. Vancomycin is used to cover MRSA. Use ceftriaxone if concerned for meningococcaemia. Consider activated protein C for patients in shock (ICU only)
Sepsis (pediatric)	See Chapter 79	
Septic arthritis	nafcillin, cefotaxime	For empiric therapy of septic joint
	ceftriaxone	For gonococcal arthritis

MRSA, methicillin-resistant Staphylococcus aureus.
Refer to: HIV related infections: Chapter 37, "HIV"
    Sexually transmitted disease: Chapter 67, "Infectious Disease"
    Pelvic inflammatory disease and vaginitis: Chapter 84, "Obstetrics and Gynecology"

Table 90.3–1 Drugs for Acute Coronary Syndrome

	Dose	Comments
ASA	162–325 mg PO (crushed or chewed)	Has been proven to decrease mortality.
Clopidogrel (Plavix)	300–600 mg PO initially, then 75 mg PO qd	Give to all patients who have ACS that are ASA allergic.
Unfractionated heparin (UFH)	60–70 U/kg IV bolus (max 5000 U) and 12–15 U/kg/h infusion (max 1000 U/h)	Maintain partial thromboplastin time (PTT) 60–80 seconds. Added to antiplatelet therapy with ASA or clopidogrel.
Low molecular weight heparin (LMWH)	Enoxaparin 30 mg IV x 1 then 1 mg/kg SC bid	An alternative to UFH in ACS. Reserved for those patients with either non–ST-segment elevation myocardial infarction or high-risk unstable angina. Enoxaparin is preferable to UFH as an anticoagulant in patients who develop unstable angina or ST elevated MI (UA/STEMI) in the absence of renal failure and unless CABG is planned within 24 hours. Added to antiplatelet therapy with ASA or clopidogrel.
IIB/IIIA inhibitors	Abciximab (Reopro): 0.25 mg/kg bolus, then 0.125 µg/kg/min infusion (max–10 µg/min) eptifibatide (Integrilin): 180 µg/kg bolus then 2.0 µg/kg/min tirofiban (Agrastat): 0.4 µg/kg/min for 30 minutes (equals 0.2 µg/kg bolus), then 0.1 µg/kg/min	Eptifibatide or tirofiban should be administered to patients who experience continuing ischemia, an elevated troponin, or high-risk features when percutaneous coronary intervention (PCI) is not planned. Administer a platelet GP IIB/IIA antagonist to patients in whom catheterization and PCI are planned.
Nitroglycerin	0.4 mg SL q 5 min x 3 doses 10–20 mcg/min IV, titrate up by 10–20 mcg/min IV prn	Avoid in patients with a right ventricular infarction, severe aortic stenosis, or on oral phosphodiesterase 5 (PDE5) inhibitors such as Viagra as this drug can cause severe hypotension in these patients.

Table 90.3–1 Drugs for Acute Coronary Syndrome—*cont'd*

	Dose	Comments
Morphine	1-5 mg IV	Relief of pain and anxiety is believed to decrease adrenergic outflow thereby decreasing myocardial oxygen demand. Major side effects include hypotension, respiratory depression, and nausea, sometimes requiring the use of antiemetics.
Beta blocker	Metoprolol 5 mg IV q 5 min × 3 doses	Can decrease mortality by reducing myocardial oxygen demand by reducing heart rate, systemic arterial pressure, and myocardial contractility. Contraindications include cardiogenic shock, active airway compromise caused by reactive airway disease—asthma or COPD—acute congestive heart failure (CHF), and atrioventricular block. Patients with cocaine-induced chest pain should not receive pure beta-blockers due to the potential for unopposed alpha receptor stimulation.
Calcium channel blockers	Diltiazem: 180 mg PO qd (max 360mg); 20 mg IV for rapid afib. Verapamil: 40-80 mg PO tid or qid (max 480 mg/day) or 2.5-5 mg IV for rapid afib.	For unstable angina or NSTEMI with continuing ischemia when beta-blockers are contraindicated. The nondihydropyridines, such as verapamil and diltiazem, have more effect on slowing atrioventricular and sinus node conduction, thereby decreasing oxygen demand by decreasing contractility, heart rate, and afterload, which may impart benefit.
ACE inhibitor	Captopril (short acting) 25 mg PO q 6 hours	Should be initiated after the patient has demonstrated hemodynamic stability, usually within the first 36 hours. Highly recommended in patients who experience left ventricular systolic dysfunction, CHF, or diabetes when hypertension persists despite treatment with nitroglycerin and a beta-blocker.

ACS, acute coronary syndrome; BID, twice daily; CHF, congestive heart failure; COPD, chronic obstructive pulmonary disease; max, maximum; NSTEMI, non ST elevated MI; QD, daily; QID, four times daily; SC, subcutaneous; TID, three times daily.

Table 90.3–2 Inotropic and Vasopressor Agents

Drug	Mechanism of Action	Indications	Dose
Dopamine Intropin	Low dose: dopaminergic receptors, dilates mesenteric and renal vessels. Intermediate dose: beta 1 effects. High dose: adds alpha effects.	Shock – usually first line.	Low: 2-5 mcg/kg/min Interm.: 5-10 mcg/kg/min High: 10-50 mcg/kg/min All doses are I.V. and should be titrated for effect
Dobutamine Dobutrex	Beta-1 selective synthetic catecholamine.	Cardiogenic shock, pulmonary edema, chronic CHF with refractory symptoms.	Start 2-20 mcg/kg/min IV and titrate for effect
Norepinephrine Levophed	Sympathomimetic with alpha-1 > beta-1 effects to increase blood pressure.	Shock (especially in cases of refractory shock – added to dopamine or dobutamine).	Start at 8-12 mcg/min IV and titrate for effect
Epinephrine Adrenalin	Nonselective sympathomimetic.	Cardiac Arrest (See ACLS Protocols). Anaphylaxis. Asthma.	Cardiac arrest: 1 mg IV Bolus Anaphylaxis or asthma: 0.1-0.5 mg SC/IM q 10 min x 2 doses for moderate cases or 1-4 mcg/min IV for severe cases
Phenylephrine Neo-Synephrine	Alpha agonist.	Shock.	50 mcg boluses for severe hypotension, then 100-180 mcg/min. The usual dose once BP is stabilized is 40-60 mcg/min.

Table 90.3–2 Inotropic and Vasopressor Agents—*cont'd*

Drug	Mechanism of Action	Indications	Dose
Vasopressin	Acts like endogenous ADH on the V1 receptor to cause vasoconstriction.	Cardiac Arrest. Shock.	Cardiac arrest: 40 units IV x 2 doses Q 3 min. Shock: 0.01–0.1 units/min IV infusion
Digitalis Digoxin Lanoxin Digitek Lanoxicaps	Acts as a Na-K ATPase inhibitor, leading to positive inotropy. It also enhances vagal activity in the AV node and decreases the ventricular rate.	Atrial fibrillation. CHF. Cardiogenic shock. Valvular heart disease.	Digoxin maintenance: 0.125–0.25mg PO QD Rapid atrial fibrillation : load 0.5mg IV then 0.25 mg × 2 doses
Phophodiesterase (PDE) Inhibitors Inamrinone (Amrinone) Milrinone (Primacor)	Inhibits PDE isoenzyme III (found in cardiac and vascular smooth muscle) which causes calcium influx during the action potential; increases cardiac output; reduces pulmonary capillary wedge pressure; and reduces peripheral vascular resistance.	Cardiogenic shock. Pulmonary edema with hypotension. Acute exacerbation of congestive heart failure.	Inamrinone 0.75mg mg/kg bolus over 2 min then 5–10 mcg/kg/min IV infusion Milrinone Load 50mcg/kg IV over 10 min, then 0.375–0.75mcg/kg/min IV infusion

Table 90.3–3 Antiarrhythmic Agents

Class Drug	Mechanism of Action	Indications	Dose	Comments
Class 1A Procainamide	Sodium channel blocker which prolongs the QT interval and prolongs repolarization.	Ventricular tachycardia, Supraventricular tachycardias	Load 17 mg/kg at a maximum rate of 20 mg/min (or 20-50mg/min in life-threatening ventricular tachycardias); stop when the dysrhythmia is suppressed, hypotension develops, or the QRS widens more than 50%. Daily dose is usually 500-1250 mg PO Q6H.	Usually used after amiodarone or lidocaine in refractory ventricular tachycardias. Prodysrhythmic. Can cause a lupus-like syndrome, should be avoided in patients with prolonged QT syndrome or hypotension
Class 1B Lidocaine	Sodium channel blocker. Shortens repolarization.	Ventricular Dysrhythmias	Ventricular Fibrillation 1-1.5 mg/kg IV Bolus Ventricular Tachycardia 1 mg/kg IV, then 0.5 mg IV Q 8-10 min PRN until maximum of 3 mg/kg.	Has become second line for ventricular dysrhythmias (amiodarone is first line in ACLS). Prodysrhythmic. Can cause paresthesias, tremors, nausea, hearing changes, slurred speech, seizures, coma, and death
Class 1C Flecainide	Sodium channel blocker. Little effect on repolarization.	Ventricular dysrhythmias Supraventricular dysrhythmias.	Load 50 mg PO Q12H; may increase by 50 mg Q12H every 4 days to a maximum dose of 300mg total per day.	Used in patients with no structural heart disease. Can cause hypotension and bradycardia; oral paresthesias, nausea, vomiting, or blurry vision.
Propafenone	See above.	See above.	Start 150 mg PO Q8H; may increase to 225 mg PO Q8H in 3-4 days.	

Class Drug	Mechanism of Action	Indications	Dose	Comments
Class 2 Metoprolol	Beta Blockers -Beta 1 selective	Tachydysrhythmias that originate above the AV node Hypertension ACS	5 mg IV Q5-15 min × 3 doses; 50 mg PO BID or 100 mg PO QD and increase as needed for effect to a maximum of 450 mg per day	Used for rate control of atrial fibrillation in pts with a history of coronary artery disease. Can cause bradycardia, hypotension, myocardial depression, reduced exercise tolerance, sedation, sleep disturbances, depression, hypoglycemia, or bronchospasm in patients with asthma or emphysema.
Propanolol (non-selective)	-Non-selective gents with Beta 2 blocker properties can cause bronchospasm	See above.	1 mg IV Q 2 min to maximum of 2 doses in 4 hours; 20-40 mg PO BID or 60-80 mg PO QD	
Class 3 Amiodarone	Potassium channel blocker which prolongs the action potential and refractory period, and depresses SA and AV node	-Ventricular tachydysrhythmias -Atrial tachydysrhythmias	-Ventricular Fibrillation dose: 300 mg I.V. bolus -Dose for other life-threatening tachydysrhythmias: 150 mg I.V over 10 minutes, then 1 mg/min × 6 hours, then 0.5 mg/min × 18 hours. -Oral loading dose: 800-1600 mg PO QD × 3 weeks, then 400-800 mg PO QD × 3 weeks then 200-400 mg PO QD	First line drug for ventricular fibrillation or tachycardia. Potentiates the effects of digoxin and warfarin. Contraindicated in patients with a marked bradycardia or second or third degree heart block without a pacemaker. It is prodysrhythmic, and can cause hypotension, pulmonary fibrosis, paresthesias.
Class 4 Diltiazem	Calcium channel blocker which increases the refractory period and slows conduction through the AV node	Rate control for tachycardias originating above the AV node Hypertension Angina	20 mg IV Bolus Q 15 min × 2 doses PRN, then start 5-15 mg/hr IV infusion; many oral preparations available, including 120-240mg QD extended release.	First line for atrial fibrillation and atrial flutter with rapid ventricular response unless the patient has coronary artery disease with a poor ejection fraction, hypotension, bradycardia, or AV block. May cause lower extremity edema.

Continued

Table 90.3-3 Antiarrhythmic Agents—*cont'd*

Class Drug	Mechanism of Action	Indications	Dose	Comments
Miscellaneous				
Adenosine	Enhanced K+ conductance and inhibition of Ca++ influx increases the AV nodal refractory period	Paroxysmal supraventricular tachycardia	6 mg IV bolus followed by rapid fluid bolus in large bore peripheral IV or central IV, due to short half-life (<10 seconds); 12 mg IV bolus dose may be given in 1-2 minutes and repeated another time if necessary.	First line for paroxysmal supraventricular tachycardia. Causes a transient asystole and AV block, hypotension, flushing, shortness of breath, chest burning, feeling of impending doom, headache, and paresthesias (the patient should be warned of this prior to administration).
Atropine	Antimuscarinic which inhibits acetylcholine to block vagal activity	Bradycardias: sinus, AV block	0.5-1 mg IV bolus Q 3-5 min to a maximum of 0.04 mg/kg (see ACLS protocols); peds 0.02 mg/kg/dose	Not for third degree AV block. Can cause tachycardias.
Magnesium	Calcium antagonist	Torsades de Pointes	2-4 grams IV. May repeat as needed for effect while monitoring for signs of toxicity.	First line therapy for Torsades de pointes; also used for prolonged QT syndromes, pre-eclampsia, eclampsia, tocolysis, and asthma. Can cause hypotension, loss of reflexes, and pulmonary edema in high doses.

ACLS, advanced cardiac life support; ACS, acute coronary syndrome; AV, atrioventricular; IV< intravenous; max., maximum; P, pediatric; PO, by mouth; QD, daily.

Table 90.4–1   Acid Blocking Medications

	Dose	Comment
Histamine Receptor Antagonists		
Nizatidine	150 mg bid	Competitive inhibitors of histamine for the H_2 receptor on parietal cells, and reduce, both the volume of gastric juice and its hydrogen ion concentration. Dosages of all these agents should be reduced in patients with renal failure. Side effects are rare and include somnolence, dizziness, confusion, cardiac conduction abnormalities, gynecomastia (cimetidine)
Famotidine	20 or 40 mg bid	
Cimetidine	800 mg bid or 400 mg qid	
Ranitidine	150 mg bid	
Proton Pump Inhibitors		
Omeprazole	20–40 mg qd	Irreversibly binds to stimulated proton pumps to block secretion of hydrogen ions. Hepatically metabolized. Side effects are minimal. Significantly higher doses required in Zollinger-Ellison syndrome.
Rabeprazole	20 mg qd	
Lansoprazole	15 mg qd; 30 mg po for erosive esophagitis	
Pantoprazole	40 mg qd	
Other		
Misoprostol (Cytotec)	200 μg 4 times a day with food	Causes inhibition of gastric acid secretion, increased secretion of mucus and bicarbonate, and stimulation of mucosal blood flow. Only used for prevention of NSAID-induced gastric ulcers in high-risk patients. Should not be used in any female patient of childbearing age who is not using contraception (abortifacient).
Sucralfate	1 g 4 times a day given 30 to 60 minutes before meals.	Binds to epithelial cells; especially to ulcerated surfaces; provides a protective layer that inhibits further acid damage.

Table 90.4–2 Common Antiemetics

Drug	Example	Dose	Route of Administration	Adverse Effects	Frequently prescribed for
Antihistamines Anticholinergics	Meclizine (Antivert) Scopolamine	25 mg QD–TID 1.5 mg	PO Transdermal	Sedation Blurred vision, dry mouth, sedation, confusion, constipation, urinary retention	Vertigo, motion sickness Motion sickness
Neuroleptics dopamine antagonists	Promethazine (Phenergan) Prochlorperazine (Compazine) Droperidol (Inapsine)	12.5–25 mg q 4–6 h 5–10 mg q 6–8 h 0.625–1.25 mg q 4–6 h	PO/IM/IV PO/PR IM/IV	Sedation, restlessness, dystonia, extrapyramidal effects, anticholinergic effects, and QT prolongation	Many causes of nausea/vomiting
Prokinetics	Metoclopramide (Reglan)	5–10 mg q 6–8 h	PO/IM/IV	Sedation and extrapyramidal effects	Gastroparesis
Serotonin antagonists	Ondansetron (Zofran)	4–8 mg q 6–8 h	IM/IV	Headache	Head injury, pediatric patients

IM, intramuscular; IV, intravenous; PO, by mouth; PR, per rectum; TID, three times daily; QD, daily.

Table 90.4–3 Common Antidiarrheal Agents*

Drug	Adult Dose	Pediatric dose	Comments
Bismuth subsalicylate (Pepto-Bismol, Kaopectate)	2 tabs or 30 ml PO q30min to 1 hour up to 8 doses per day	3-6 years: 5 ml 6-9 years: 10 ml	Has antidiarrheal effects through an antisecretory salicylate moiety, and its antibacterial properties make it useful as prophylaxis in travelers' diarrhea. Risk of Reye's syndrome in children. May cause blackened stools.
Diphenoxylate + atropine (Lomotil)	2 tabs or 10 ml PO qid.	For children > 2 years: 0.3-0.4 mg/kg/day PO div qid	Works by slowing intraluminal flow of liquid, facilitating intestinal absorption. Cheaper than loperamide but has central opiate effects and may have cholinergic side effects. May facilitate the development of HUS in patients infected with enterohemorrhagic
Loperamide (Immodium)	4 mg PO initially, then 2 mg PO after each unformed stool; maximum of 16 mg/day.	13-20 kg: 1 mg tid 20-30 kg: 2 mg PO bid > 30 kg: 2 mg PO tid	Same mechanism as diphenoxylate. May facilitate the development of HUS in patients infected with enterohemorrhagic *E coli*.

HUS, hemolytic uremic syndrome.

For use in afebrile patients with nonbloody stools. Patients should increase their fluid intake while taking antimotility agents because these agents may cause fluid pooling in the intestine, and mask fluid losses.

90.5   Thrombolytic Therapy

Shamai A. Grossman   ■   Sam Shen

General Principles of Thrombolytic Therapy

■ Thrombolytics are a class of drugs used to break down clots found in acute myocardial infarction, acute ischemic strokes, and thromboembolic disease such as pulmonary embolism (PE) and deep venous thrombo- embolism (DVT). The clinical benefit of dissolving clots must be weighed with the complication of bleeding. Several of the thrombolytic agents approved by the Food and Drug Administration in the United States for clinical use include the following: Streptokinase (Streptase, Kabikinase), Alteplase (t-PA, Activase), Reteplase (Retavase), Tenecteplase (TNKase).

■ Blood clots are formed when fibrinogen is converted to fibrin, which cross-links to form a clot. Plasmin is an enzyme that breaks down the clot by disrupting fibrin. Thrombolytics work by coverting plasminogen to plasmin, which then takes apart fibrin in the blood clot. As the clot breaks apart, blood flow is restored.

■ Although there are many thrombolytic agents in use and under devel- opment, the more commonly used ones are listed in Table 90.5–1. The drugs differ in their indications, half-life, and administration. The most important complication is hemorrhage. The incidence of anaphylaxis is one per thousand.

■ The specific indications for acute myocardial infarction include patients with chest pain suggestive of an acute myocardial infarction up to 12 hours after symptom onset and either: ST elevation (>1 mm in two contiguous leads) or a new left bundle branch block. See Table 90.5–2. Acute coronary syndrome is discussed in Chapter 22. Cardiovascular pharmacology is reviewed in Chapter 90.3.

■ The specific indications for reperfusion of stroke include clinical diag- nosis of ischemic stroke, onset of symptoms or signs within three hours prior to the administration of the agents, and the absence of hemorrhage as the cause of the ischemic stroke. See Box 90.5–1. A detailed discussion of stroke is located in Chapter 56.

■ The specific indications for thromboembolic disease (e.g., pulmonary embolism) are hypotension with pulmonary embolism, severe hypoxemia, right ventricular dysfunction, or extensive deep venous thromboembolism.

■ Approximately 20-30 percent of patients are ineligible for thrombolytic therapy. Age greater than 75 is no longer a major contraindication for therapy. Menstruation is not a contraindication to thrombolytic therapy.

Generic Name	Trade Name	Use	Dose	Comments
Streptokinase	Streptase, Kabikinase	Acute myocardial infarction (AMI), PE, DVT	AMI: 1.5 million units over 60 minutes PE: 3 million units over 24 hours DVT: 250,000 unit bolus, then 100,000 units/hour for 24-72 hours depending on location	Onset of action: immediate Half-life: 83 minutes
Alteplase	t-PA, Activase	AMI, Ischemic stroke, PE	AMI: >67kg; 100mg total dose over 1.5 hours; infuse 15 mg over 1-2 minutes, 50 mg over 30minutes, then remaining over 60 minutes. If <67kg, 1.25 mg/kg; infuse 15 mg over 1-2 minutes, then 0.75 mg/kg (not to exceed 50 mg) over next 30 minutes, followed by 0.5 mg/kg (not to exceed 35 mg) over next 60 minutes. Load 0.09 mg/kg bolus over 1 minute, followed by 0.81 mg/kg as continuous infusion over 60 minutes PE: I.V.: 100mg over 2 hours	Stroke: Maximum dose 90 mg Half-life: 5 minutes
Reteplase	Retavase	AMI	10 units over 2 minutes followed by a second dose 30 minutes later of 10 units	Onset of action: 30-90 minutes Half-life 13-16 minutes
Tenecteplase	TNKase	AMI	Weight-based dosing. Administer over 5 seconds. <60kg: 30 mg dose 60 to <70kg: 35 mg 70 to <80kg: 40 mg 80 to <90kg: 45 mg > = 90kg: 50 mg	Half-life: 90-130 minutes

AMI, acute myocardial infarction.
All agents are given intravenously.

Table 90.5–2	Thrombolytic Therapy in Acute Myocardial Infarction
Indications	Patients with ST-segment elevation myocardial infarction (STEMI) with symptom onset of less than 12 hours previously
	ST-segment elevation in at least two contiguous leads or new/presumably new left bundle branch block
	Primary PCI is not immediately available
Absolute Contraindications	Active internal bleeding
	Previous hemorrhagic stroke
	Other cerebrovascular events within one year
	Suspected aortic dissection
Relative Contraindications	Known bleeding diathesis (liver dysfunction or current use of anticoagulants
	Nonhemorrhagic stroke more than one year previously
	Chronic hypertension (systolic blood pressure >170 mmHg)
	Prior central venous or noncompressible puncture, pregnancy, aortic dissection, or neoplasm
	Prolonged cardiopulmonary resuscitation (>10 minutes)
	Head injury or trauma within two weeks
	Recent surgery (less than two weeks)
Complications	The predominant complication is bleeding, and hemorrhagic stroke is the most concerning morbidity. The most common site of spontaneous bleeding is the gastrointestinal tract. The rate of intracerebral bleeding is 1-2%, while the rate of non-intracerbral bleeding is up to 30%. Approximately 5% of patients require transfusions. Allergic reaction is also the cause of considerable morbidity with thrombolytic therapy.

BOX 90.5–1   Criteria for Intravenous Thrombolytic Therapy for Acute Stroke

Inclusion

Ischemic stroke within 3 hours of symptom onset

Age >17 years old

Exclusion

Symptom onset >3 hours

Rapidly improving neurologic deficits

A head CT scan shows hemorrhage

Suspicion of subarachnoid hemorrhage

Stroke, intracranial or intraspinal surgery, or serious head trauma in past 3 months

Major surgery or serious trauma in past 14 days

GI or GU hemorrhage in past 21 days

Arterial puncture at noncompressible site, or lumbar puncture in past 7 days

History of intracranial hemorrhage

Known intracranial neoplasm, arteriovenous malformation, or aneurysm

Uncontrolled hypertension at time of treatment

Seizure at stroke onset

Platelets < 100,000/mm

Current use of anticoagulants with PT > 15 sec

Use of heparin within 48 hours

Glucose < 50 or > 400 mg/dl

90.6 Respiratory Pharmacology

- Refer to Chapter 24 and Chapter 52 for a discussion of common problems causing respiratory complaints.
- Table 90.6–1 summarized medications commonly used in the treatment of asthma and chronic obstructive pulmonary disease. Table 90.6–2 reviews medications often used for the symptomatic treatment of cough and congestion.

Table 90.6–1 Medications for Obstructive Airway Disease Exacerbations

	Mechanism of Action	Specific Drug	Dose	Comments
Anti-cholinergic	Antagonize acetylcholine at the postganglionic parasympathetic receptor. This causes a decrease in vagally mediated bronchoconstriction occurring primarily in the central airways.	Ipratropium bromide	Add 0.5 mg of ipratropium nebulized or MDI	Onset is 20 minutes Maximal effect in 1 to 2 hours. Minimal side effects and include tremors and dry mouth. More commonly used for COPD exacerbations; used in asthma patients with poor initial response to β-agonists.
β-agonist	Increase in cyclic AMP. Causes rapid relaxation of bronchial smooth muscles, inhibition of the release of inflammatory mediators, and improvement in mucociliary clearance	Albuterol	2.5 to 5.0 mg of nebulized albuterol q 20 minutes for 3 doses or as a continuous nebulization treatment	For acute exacerbation. Can cause tremors, palpitations, tachycardia, headache, mild hypokalemia, and nausea and vomiting.
		Salmeterol	For patients 12 years of age and older: 2 inhalations (42 mcg) twice daily (morning and evening, approximately 12 hours apart).	Long acting, for maintenance. Used to prevent asthma attacks. They are not used to relieve an attack that has already started.
		Terbutaline	A: 0.25 mg in adults SC given every 20 minutes × 3 P: 0.01 mg/kg to a maximum of 0.3 mg	Used for severe asthmatics. Has no added benefit over aerosolized treatment. Use for severe exacerbations or if unable to use either a nebulizer or MDI. Primarily cardiovascular side effects (increased heart rate and blood pressure). Use with caution in patients with a history of cardiovascular disease.
		Epinephrine	A: 0.3–0.5 cc SC in adults	Similar to terbutaline

	Mechanism of Action	Specific Drug	Dose	Comments
Steroids	Causes inhibition of recruitment of inflammatory cells and inhibition of release of proinflammatory mediators and cytokines from activated inflammatory and epithelial cells.	Prednisone	A: 40 to 60 mg/day PO for 5-10 days P: 1-2 mg/kg PO for 5 days, max dose of 60 mg/day	Should be given within 1 hour of ED presentation if not relieved by β-agonist treatment Most routes of administration of systemic steroids seem to be equivalent. Inhaled steroids for the long-term control. Minimal side effects with short term use.
		Methyl-prednisolone	A: 80-125 mg IV P: 1 mg/kg for	Can be reserved for the severe asthmatic in extremis. May also use dexamethasone, 1.7 mg/kg IM.
Other Agents	Mechanism unknown but may cause decreased uptake of calcium by bronchial smooth muscle cells, which may lead to bronchodilatation	Magnesium	1.2 to 2 g IV over 20 min	Used in severe asthmatics. Onset in 2 to 5 minutes. Side effects include hypotension, malaise, warm sensation, and flushing. Monitor for cardiac arrhythmias, neurologic abnormalities, and renal failure.
	Stimulates the release of catecholamines causing bronchodilatation	Ketamine	1 to 2 mg/kg IV at a rate of 0.5 mg/kg/min initially prior to intubation, then 3 µg/kg/min IV	Used mostly in pediatric patients with acute asthma exacerbations. Good choice for induction agent for intubation. Side effects include hypersecretion and postemergence hallucinations. It is contraindicated in patients with ischemic heart disease, hypertension, preeclampsia, and increased intracranial pressure

Table 90.6–2 Common Medications for Cough and Cold Symptoms

		Dose	Comment
Antitussives and expectorants	Benzonatate (Tessalon Pearls)	100-200 mg PO tid	Swallow whole; numbs mouth.
	Dextramethorphan	10-20 mg PO q 4 hours or 30 mg PO q 6-8 hours.	Side effects may include nausea, vomiting, and constipation. Serious toxicity may arise if dextrometorphan is taken with some monoamine oxidase inhibitors (MAOIs) such as serotonin syndrome. Avoid alcohol, antihistaminic drugs, and antidepressants.
	Guaifenesin	100-400 mg PO q4 hours; 100-200 mg/dose if 6-12 y/o; 50-100 mg/dose if 2-5 y/o.	May cause nausea and vomiting, and rarely, dizziness, headaches, or a rash
Decongestant	Pseudoephedrine	60 mg PO q 4-6 hours; peds 30 mg/dose if 6-12 y/o, 15 mg/dose if 2-5 y/o.	Avoid if severe heart disease or markedly elevated blood pressure. Taking MAIOs inhibitors may increase the blood pressure.
Antihistamine	Chlorpheniramine (Chlor-Trimeton)	4 mg PO q 4-6 hours (max 24 mg/day)	May cause significant drowsiness, especially in patients taking MAIO drugs, alcohol, or anti-depressants. They should be used with caution in patients with bronchial asthma or glaucoma. Urinary retention is a common anticholinergic adverse effect.
	Clemastine (Tavist)	1.34 mg PO bid; max 8 mg/day.	
	Fexofenadine (Allegra)	60 mg PO bid or 180 mg PO qd; peds 30 mg PO bid if 6-12 y/o.	
	Loratadine (Claritin)	If > 6 y/o 10 mg PO qd; 2-5 y/o give 5 mg PO qd.	

BID, twice daily; PO, by mouth; TID, three times daily; QD, daily.

CHAPTER 91

Emergency Procedures

Eugene W. Hu ▪ Benjamin K. Wakamatsu ▪ Dustin D. Smith

Overview

This chapter will review common procedures performed in the emergency department (ED).

There are two general types of consent: implied and informed. Implied consent covers necessary lifesaving procedures that it is presumed any reasonable person would wish to have. In a patient who maintains decision-making capacity, implied consent is presumed in low-risk situations such as the patient who requires suturing of a hand laceration, and holds an arm steady to facilitate the procedure. An example of a patient who does not have this capacity would be an unconscious individual with a life-threatening problem who requires emergent interventions.

Informed consent involves patients with decision-making capacity, and requires that they are given all the pertinent facts regarding the risks and benefits of a particular procedure, understands them, and voluntarily agrees to undergo the procedure. This is documented with a consent form, and is part of the medical record. Procedures requiring this type of consent include procedural sedation, lumbar puncture, and sometimes (may be institutionally dependent) central venous access.

Personal protective equipment should be worn for all procedures, and may include a gown, glove, and masks depending on exposure risk.

Several procedures will be covered elsewhere in this book: airway (see Chapter 5); joint reductions and splinting (see Chapter 17); local anesthesia and nerve blocks, suturing (see Chapter 94); nasal packing (see Chapter 64); dorsal slit for phimosis and paraphimosis reduction (see Chapter 47); excision of thrombosed hemorrhoid (see Chapter 48); and ophthalmology (see Chapter 69).

Conscious sedation is discussed in Chapter 90.1.

The following procedures will be reviewed in this chapter:
91.1   Central Venous Access
91.2   Umbilical Vein Catheterization
91.3   Intraosseous Infusion
91.4   Saphenous Vein Cutdown
91.5   Pericardiocentesis

91.1 Central Venous Access

Central Venous Access

Indications	Contraindications: (Relative)
Rapid fluid resuscitation in the absence of large peripheral IV	Bleeding diatheses
	Distorted Anatomy
Venous access in patients with poor peripheral access	Suspected injury to the vascular structure
Administration of parenteral nutrition	Skin lesions and infections
Administration of solutions irritating to peripheral lines (e.g., $CaCl$, KCl)	Factors predisposing to sclerosis at the site (i.e., vasculitides, history of radiation therapy, long term venous access at the site)
Advanced monitoring techniques (e.g., central venous pressure)	
Access for hemodialysis	
Access for transvenous pacemakers	

Complications of Central Venous Access

General	Subclavian and Internal Jugular Cannulation	Femoral Vein Cannulation
Arterial puncture	Air embolization	Bladder perforation
Catheter embolization	Delayed myocardial	Bowel perforation
Cellulitis	perforation	Peritonitis
Guidewire embolization	Hemothorax	
Formation of an	Hemomediastinum	
arteriovenous fistula	Hematoma	
Misplaced catheter	Hydrothorax	
Nerve palsy (e.g.,	Hydromediastinum	
brachial plexus)	Pneumothorax	
Osteomyelitis (e.g.,		
clavicle)		
Sepsis		
Thrombophlebitis		
Thrombosis		

Procedure
Subclavian Vein Cannulation, Infraclavicular Approach (Figure 91–1)

1. Place the patient in the supine position in 15 to 30 degrees of Trendelenburg, with the head in neutral position, and the ipsilateral arm abducted.
2. Sterilely prepare, and drape the infraclavicular area.
3. The most common entry site is inferior to the junction between the middle and medial thirds of the clavicle.
4. Anesthetize the skin and the subcutaneous structures including the periosteum of the clavicle near the sternoclavicular junction.
5. Direct the bevel of the needle inferomedially.
6. Advance the needle into the skin, passing just deep to the clavicle, aiming just superior to the sternoclavicular junction. Aspirate the syringe at all times.
7. Vessel entry usually occurs at 3 to 4 cm of needle length.
8. Proceed as per the Seldinger technique described later in this section.
9. After both successful and unsuccessful cannulation attempts, auscultate lung sounds bilaterally. Obtain a chest radiograph to confirm proper line placement, and to ensure there is no evidence of a pneumothorax prior to using the line.

Subclavian Vein Cannulation, Supraclavicular Approach (Figure 91–2)

1. Place the patient in the supine position in 15 to 30 degrees of Trendelenburg, with the head turned slightly to the contralateral side.
2. Sterilely prepare and drape the supraclavicular area.

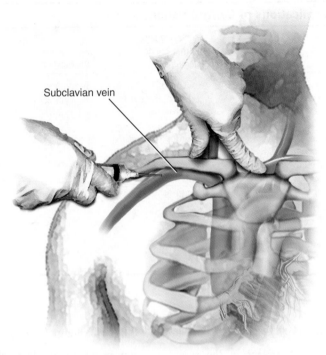

Subclavian vein

Figure 91–1. Subclavian vein cannulation: infraclavicular approach. Hand position during subclavian venipuncture. *(Reproduced from Linos D, Mucha P, von Heerden J: Subclavian vein: a golden route. Mayo Clin Proc 1980;5:318.)*

3. The entry site is 1 cm lateral to the clavicular head of the sterno-cleidomastoid muscle and 1 cm superior to the clavicle.
4. Anesthetize the skin at this area.
5. Direct the bevel of the needle medially.
6. Advance the needle into the skin, aiming at the angle formed between the lateral aspect of the clavicular head of the sternocleidomastoid muscle and the clavicle. The needle should also be angled superficially, 10 degrees to the coronal plane. Aspirate the syringe at all times.
7. Vessel entry usually occurs at 2 to 3 cm of needle length.
8. Proceed as per the Seldinger technique described later in this section.
9. After both successful and unsuccessful cannulation attempts, auscultate lung sounds bilaterally. Perform a chest radiograph to confirm proper line placement, and to ensure there is no evidence of a pneumothorax prior to using the line.

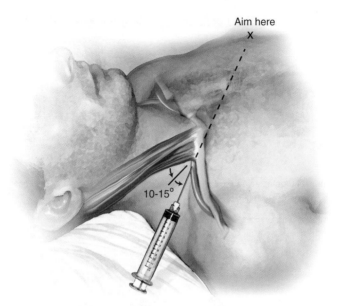

Figure 91–2. Subclavian vein cannulation: supraclavicular approach. For the supraclavicular approach, the needle is inserted above and behind the clavicle, bisecting the angle made by the clavicle and the lateral border of the sternocleidomastoid muscle (clavisternomastoid angle). The point of entry is 1 cm lateral to the clavicular head of the muscle and 1 cm posterior to the clavicle. The needle traverses an avascular plane, puncturing the junction of the subclavian and internal jugular vein behind the sternoclavicular joint. The right side is preferred because of a direct route to the superior vena cava and the absence of the thoracic duct. The needle is directed 45 degrees from the sagittal plane and 10 to 15 degrees upward from the horizontal plane, aiming toward the contralateral nipple. Note that the vein is just posterior to the clavicle at this juncture. *(Reproduced from Roberts JR, Hedges JR [editors]. Clinical Procedures in Emergency Medicine [4th ed]. Philadelphia: Elsevier, 2005, p 429.)*

Internal Jugular Vein Cannulation, Central Approach (Figure 91–3)

1. Place the patient in the supine position in 15 to 30 degrees of Trendelenburg, with the head turned slightly to the contralateral side to expose the landmarks.
2. Sterilely prepare and drape the neck.
3. The entry site is the apex of the triangle formed by the two heads of the sternocleidomastoid muscle and the clavicle.
4. Palpate the carotid artery pulsations.
5. Anesthetize the skin lateral to the carotid pulse.
6. Direct the bevel of the needle superficially.

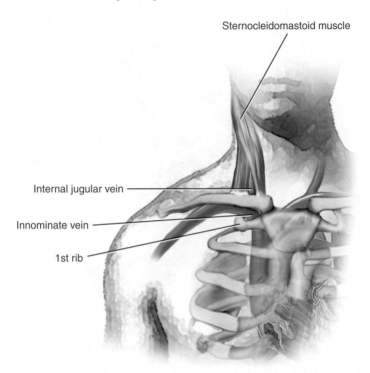

Sternocleidomastoid muscle

Internal jugular vein

Innominate vein

1st rib

Figure 91–3. Internal jugular vein cannulation: central approach. The internal jugular vein is located between the sternal and clavicular heads of the sternocleidomastoid. The needle is introduced at the apex of the triangle formed by the clavicle and the sternal and clavicular heads of the sternocleidomastoid, and is directed caudally at a 30- to 40-angle to the skin. *(Reproduced from Roberts JR, Hedges JR [editors]. Clinical Procedures in Emergency Medicine [4th ed]. Philadelphia: Elsevier, 2005, p 430.)*

7. Advance the needle into the skin, lateral to the carotid pulse, entering at an angle of 30 to 40 degrees to the skin, aiming for the ipsilateral nipple. Aspirate the syringe at all times.
8. Vessel entry usually occurs at 1 to 1.5 cm of needle length. Do not advance more than 5 cm.
9. Proceed as per the Seldinger technique described later in this section.
10. After both successful and unsuccessful cannulation attempts, auscultate lung sounds bilaterally. Perform a chest radiograph to confirm proper line placement, and to ensure there is no evidence of a pneumothorax prior to using the line.

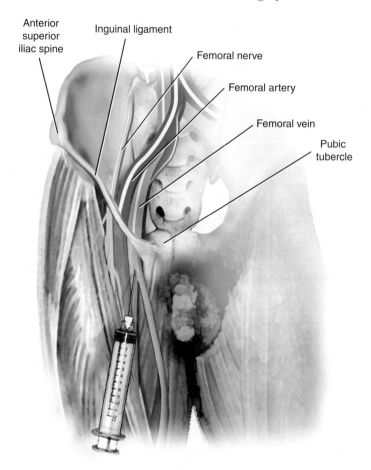

Figure 91–4. Femoral vein anatomy. The needle should be introduced caudal to the inguinal ligament. The femoral vein is *medial* to the femoral artery. *(Reproduced from Rosen P, Chan TC, Vilke GM, Stembach G. Atlas of Emergency Procedures. St. Louis, MO: Mosby, 2001, p 86.)*

Femoral Vein Cannulation (Figure 91–4)

1. Place the patient in the supine position.
2. Sterilely prepare and drape the femoral area.
3. Palpate the femoral pulse, usually located between the middle and medial thirds of an imaginary line between the anterior superior iliac spine and the pubic tubercle.
4. Anesthetize the skin.

5. The entry site is just medial to the femoral pulse, approximately 1.5 cm inferior to the inguinal ligament.
6. Direct the bevel of the needle superficially.
7. Advance the needle into the skin at a 45-degree angle to the skin, aiming towards the umbilicus. Aspirate the syringe at all times.
8. Proceed as per the Seldinger technique described later in this section.

Seldinger Technique

1. Once a flash of nonpulsatile, dark blood is obtained, and is easily aspirated, the needle is presumably in the venous lumen. Remove the syringe, and occlude the hub of the needle with a gloved finger. This is to prevent an air embolus.
2. Pass the guide wire into the needle, advancing until at least a quarter of the total length has passed.
3. Remove the needle, maintaining a hold on the guide wire at all times.
4. Incise the skin next to the guide wire using the scalpel. Direct the sharp edge of the scalpel away from the guide wire to avoid cutting the wire. The incision should be roughly equal to the width of the catheter, and extend just past the dermis.
5. Feed the guide wire into the tapered end of the dilator.
   While maintaining a hold on the guide wire, advance the dilator into the skin using a gentle twisting motion. The dilator should be advanced until it is within the vessel lumen.
6. Remove the dilator, maintaining a hold on the guide wire at all times.
7. Feed the guide wire into the distal aspect of the catheter.
   While maintaining a hold on the guide wire advance the catheter into the skin until the desired depth is achieved.
   For a femoral line, it may be advanced fully.
   Proper position of the subclavian and internal jugular catheters leaves the catheter tip approximately 2 cm below the manubriosternal junction, in the superior vena cava.
8. If using a multiple-lumen catheter, the guide wire should be fed into the distal port and the hub of the distal lumen should be uncapped. Most central line kits are marked "distal" or have a brown colored cap on the distal lumen port. The hubs of the other lumens should remain capped.
9. Remove the guide wire and occlude the hub of the catheter with a gloved finger.
10. Attach a syringe to the hub and aspirate, ensuring easy flow of venous blood.
11. Flush the lumen with saline and cap the catheter.
12. Suture the catheter in place, affixing it to the skin.
13. Cleanse the skin and place a sterile dressing.
14. Sterilely dress the site.

Pearls and Pitfalls for Central Venous Access

Ultrasound guided central venous line placement minimizes complications.

Hold onto the guide wire at all times! An entire guide wire may be lost into the vessel lumen, and may embolize.

Always aspirate with the syringe when advancing and retracting the needle.

The right side approach for subclavian and internal jugular lines is preferred over the left. It is a more direct route, the apex of the lung is lower, and it avoids the left-sided thoracic duct.

If subclavian cannulation is to be attempted in the setting of a penetrating chest wound, the vein on the ipsilateral side of the wound should be cannulated to avoid the possibility of bilateral pneumothoraces.

In the setting of a bleeding diathesis, the preferred order of approach is femoral, internal jugular, and lastly subclavian due to complications or difficulties in compressing the vessels for hemostasis.

Never force a guide wire into position. It should pass easily if the needle is correctly placed.

Never forcefully remove a guide wire. This may shear the wire and cause a guide wire embolus. If encountering difficulty removing the wire, remove both the wire and needle together.

91.2 Umbilical Vein Catheterization

Umbilical Vein Catheterization

Indications	Contraindications: Relative	Complications
Emergency vascular access of a neonate without other vascular access	Necrotizing enterocolitis Omphalitis Omphalocele Peritonitis Vascular compromise of the lower extremities	Air embolism Bleeding Catheter embolization Hepatic necrosis Infection Malpositioned catheter Vascular insufficiency Vessel perforation

Procedure

1. Flush the catheter with the heparinized saline.
2. Attach the three-way stopcock to the catheter.

3. Place the neonate under the radiant warmer.
4. Cleanse the umbilical stump.
5. Drape the umbilical area.
6. Place a purse-string suture or umbilical tape 1 cm distal to the junction between the skin of the abdominal wall and the umbilical cord.
7. Cut the cord with the scalpel distal to the suture.
8. Identify the umbilical vessels. The single large, thin-walled vein is usually at the 12 o'clock position. The two smaller, thick-walled arteries are usually at the 4 and 8 o'clock positions.
9. Insert the catheter into the lumen of the umbilical vein. Catheter: 3.5-French for neonates <1500 g, 5-French for neonates >1500 g
10. Advance the catheter 1 cm past the point where there is good blood return, approximately 4 to 5 cm into the vein. This includes the length of the umbilical stump.
11. Tighten the purse-string suture or umbilical tape to secure the catheter.
12. Dress the catheter site.
13. Obtain a radiograph of the site prior to using the catheter.

Pearls and Pitfalls for Umbilical Vein Catheterization

After cutting the umbilical cord, the vein may keep bleeding, but the arteries will usually constrict, reducing or eliminating arterial bleeding.

In the emergent setting, placement into the inferior vena cava is not recommended as placement into the portal vein may not be avoided.

91.3 Intraosseous Infusion

Intraosseous infusion

Indications	Contraindications	Complications
Emergent vascular access in the absence of intravenous access	**Absolute**: fracture through the bone of choice; cellulitis, infection, or burn over insertion site **Relative**: recent intraosseous puncture through the same bone; osteogenesis imperfecta; osteoporosis	Cellulitis Compartment syndrome Epiphyseal injury Fat embolus Fluid or medication extravasation Fracture Incomplete penetration of the bone Needle blockage Osteomyelitis Through-and-through penetration of the bone

Procedure

1. Select the entry site (Figure 91–5). The most common site in pediatric patients up to 5 years of age is the proximal tibia, 1 to 3 cm distal to the tibial tuberosity on the flat medial aspect of the bone. The most common site in adults is the medial aspect of the distal tibia, just proximal to the medial malleolus and posterior to the greater saphenous vein.
2. Prep the skin overlying the entry site with the cleansing solution.
3. Anesthetize the skin and periosteum.
4. Hold the intraosseous needle firmly in the palm of the dominant hand with the index finger along the needle approximately 1 cm from the bevel to serve as a stop. The interosseus needle has a stylet, and the size is 13 to 20 gauge.
5. At the entry site, angle the needle away from the nearest joint space.
6. Advance the needle with a twisting motion, applying steady pressure on the bone.
7. Penetration of the cortex results in a sudden decrease in resistance as the needle moves into the marrow space.
8. Remove the stylet.
9. Connect the syringe, and aspirate blood and marrow to confirm positioning.
10. Infuse several milliliters of saline, and observe for any signs of extravasation. If there is resistance to the infusion, withdraw the needle several millimeters, and reattempt. If there is continued resistance, remove the needle and use another location.
11. Disconnect the syringe, and connect infusion tubing.
12. Tape the needle and tubing in place.
13. Apply the protective shield over the needle and secure it in place.
14. Obtain a radiograph of the site to ensure no evidence of fracture or of radiographically evident malposition.

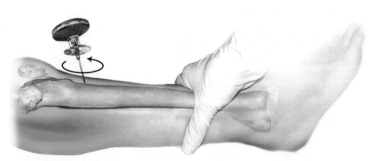

Figure 91–5. Intraosseous needle insertion. (*Reproduced from Rosen P, Chan TC, Vilke GM, Stembach G. Atlas of Emergency Procedures. St. Louis, MO: Mosby, 2001, p 99.*)

Pearls and Pitfalls for Intraosseous Infusion

Aspiration of blood may be unsuccessful in cardiac arrest and other shock states.

Aspirated blood may be used for blood type and cross matching, blood urea nitrogen, creatinine, glucose, and calcium levels. A complete blood count will not be reliable.

The clinical response to medication or fluid administration through an intraosseous site should be equivalent to infusion through an intravenous site.

Administration of high-dose epinephrine through an intraosseous line may decrease bone marrow blood flow, obligating the need for pressurized infusion afterwards.

91.4 Saphenous Vein Cutdown

Saphenous Vein Cutdown

Indications	Contraindications (Relative)	Complications
Venous access in the absence of other alternative means of vascular access	Existence of a less invasive alternative means of vascular access Coagulopathy Infection over the site Injury proximal to the site	Arterial laceration Catheter embolization Catheter misplacement Hematoma Infection Nerve laceration Phlebitis

Procedures (Figure 91–6)

1. Identify the landmarks. The saphenous vein cutdown is usually performed at the distal aspect of the leg, 1 cm anterior to the medial malleolus. Alternative sites are: 1-4 cm distal to the knee just posterior to the tibia on the medial aspect of the leg or 4 cm distal to the inguinal ligament, just distal to the femoral triangle.
2. Place a venous tourniquet if possible.
3. Prepare and drape the skin area.
4. Administer the local anesthetic.
5. Using a No. 11 blade scalpel make a transverse skin incision through all skin layers until subcutaneous fat is viewed.
6. Bluntly dissect through the subcutaneous tissue using the curved hemostat. The spreading motion of the hemostat should be parallel to the course of the vein (i.e., longitudinal) perpendicular to the transverse incision.

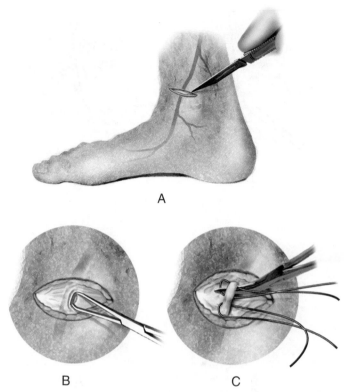

Figure 91–6. *A,* Make a transverse incision at the level of the medial malleolus between the apex of the malleolus and the anterior tibialis tendon. Dissect through the subcutaneous tissue and insert the hemostat on the medial side of the incision with the tip pointing downward until there is contact with the periosteum. *B,* Turn the tip upward and exit at the lateral aspect of the incision. The vein will lie on within the tissue overlying the hemostat. *C,* Clear the vein of the adjacent tissue by blunt dissection. Grasp a 3-0 absorbable suture with the hemostat and pass it under the vein.

7. Expose and isolate the vein, freeing it from surrounding tissue. Use the tissue spreader to help maintain exposure.
8. Pass proximal and distal suture ties under the vein, approximately 1 to 3 cm apart.
9. Tie the distal ligature to occlude the vein. Leave the ends of the ligature long.
10. Gently elevate and stretch the vein until it is flat.
11. Make a flap incision over the superior surface of the vessel between the two ties using a No. 11 scalpel, cutting approximately one-third to one-half of its diameter. The incision should not be through and through.

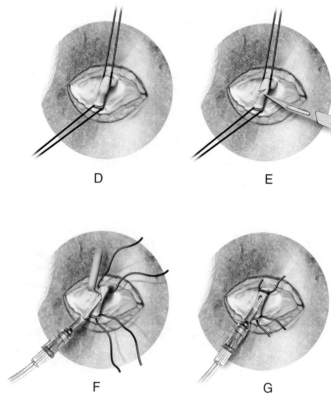

Figure 91–6. *cont'd D,* Cut the suture as shown and tie the distal suture to ligate the vessel distally. *E,* Raise the vein by lifting the sutures and make a flap incision on the anterior wall of the vessel with a no. 11 scalpel. *F,* Pull the vein taught by gentle traction on the distal and proximal suture Advance a catheter into the vessel using the vein pick. *G,* Tie the proximal suture around the portion of the vein containing the catheter. *(Reproduced from Rosen P, Chan TC, Vilke GM, Stembach G. Atlas of Emergency Procedures. St. Louis, MO: Mosby, 2001, p 90–93.)*

12. Place the intravenous catheter (8 French or 10 gauge) through the venous incision directed cephalad. An alternative is to first thread the catheter through a separate stab incision just distal to the skin incision, and then through the incision in the vein.
13. Tie the proximal suture to secure the catheter.
14. Allow the catheter to back-bleed to remove any air within it.
15. Connect the intravenous tubing to the catheter.
16. Remove the tourniquet.
17. Close the skin using the nylon sutures.
18. Dress the skin and secure the intravenous tubing with gauze and tape.

Pearls and Pitfalls for Saphenous Venous Cutdown

In the ankle area, the saphenous vein runs alongside the saphenous nerve. Transection at this area produces a sensory deficit to a small area along the medial aspect of the foot.

A traditional cutdown with ligatures sacrifices the saphenous vein. A minicutdown or modified cutdown may preserve the vein.

91.5 Pericardiocentesis

Pericardiocentesis

Indications	Contraindications (Relative)	Complications
Relief of cardiac tamponade	Alternative treatment modalities available.	Air embolism
Diagnosis of the etiology of a pericardial effusion	Coagulopathy	Coronary vessel laceration
		Development of tamponade
		Dysrhythmia
		Hemopericardium
		Myocardial laceration
		Pneumothorax

Procedure

1. Consider premedicating the patient with atropine to help prevent vasovagal reactions.
2. Attach the syringe to the needle.
3. If possible, elevate the head of the bed so that the patient's chest is at a 45-degree angle.
4. Prepare and drape the desired entry site.
5. Administer local anesthetic.
6. Use one of the approaches described below for needle insertion. The needle should be 18 gauge, and 7.5 to 12.5 cm in length. Using an ultrasound probe increases the safety of the procedure, and improves the success in aspirating the pericardial fluid.
7. If the pericardiocentesis is positive and a catheter must be left in place: pass a guide wire through the needle; remove the needle while maintaining a constant hold on the guide wire; pass the dilator over the guide wire to create a tract and then remove the dilator; pass the catheter over the guide wire, and remove the guide wire; place the stopcock on the catheter, and secure the catheter in place.
8. Obtain a chest radiograph to evaluate for any evidence of pneumothorax.

Subxiphoid (Paraxiphoid) Approach

1. The entry site is between the xiphoid process and the left costal margin.
2. The needle is directed at a 30- to 45-degree angle to the skin, aimed at either the left shoulder (most common), left scapula tip, sternal notch, right shoulder, or right scapular tip. The subxiphoid approach is likely to injure the thin-walled right atrium when one aims for the left shoulder. Aiming for the left shoulder directs the needle toward either the left ventricle or the anterior wall of the right ventricle.
3. Advance the needle, aspirating every 1 to 2 mm, until blood or fluid is obtained, or cardiac pulsations are felt.

Parasternal Approach

1. The entry site is in the fifth intercostal space immediately lateral to the sternum.
2. The needle is inserted perpendicular to the skin over the superior border of the rib.
3. Advance as described in step 3 of the subxiphoid approach listed above.

Apical Approach

1. Palpate the point of maximal impulse (PMI).
2. The entry site is 1 cm lateral to one intercostal space below the PMI.
3. Advance as described in step 3 of the subxiphoid approach.

Pearls and Pitfalls for Pericardiocentesis

In the emergency department, pericardiocentesis should only be performed under emergent circumstances, i.e., pericardial tamponade. Otherwise, echocardiography or CT scanning should be used to confirm the presence of the effusion, and the procedure is performed under fluoroscopic or ultrasound guidance.

Multiple studies have demonstrated that the traditional subxiphoid approach has a higher rate of myocardial injury. The parasternal and apical approaches are associated with higher rates of pneumothorax.

There is no agreed-upon best approach for aiming the needle in the subxiphoid approach. When aiming for the right shoulder, the right atrium may be injured. When aiming for the right scapular tip, the needle is expected to travel parallel to the right side of the heart with less of a chance to injure a coronary vessel or the myocardium.

Blood in the pericardial cavity is usually predominantly clotted. If 20 ml of blood is easily aspirated, usually the needle is in the right ventricle.

91.6 Emergency Pacing

Emergency Pacing

Indications	Contraindications
*Symptomatic bradycardia or atrioventricular block Asystole (immediately after onset) Overdrive pacing of ventricular tachycardia or paroxysmal supraventricular tachycardia (PSVT) Sinus arrest Sick sinus syndrome	Severe hypothermia: pacing may result in ventricular fibrillation

*Symptomatic refers to syncope, presyncope, hypotension, angina, pulmonary edema, or evidence of decreased cerebral perfusion

Complications of Cardiac Pacing

General	Transcutaneous	Transvenous
Dysrhythmias Failure to capture	Discomfort or pain Failure to capture due to pacer pad placement, patient girth, or pericardial effusion Failure to diagnose underlying ventricular fibrillation Interference with cardiac monitoring Interference with monitoring pulses	Catheter displacement Catheter misplacement Catheter fracture Changes to pacing threshold from drug effects, fibrosis, inflammation, metabolic changes, physiologic changes Complications associated with central venous line placement Loose lead Postpacer syndrome due to decreased ventricular filling from atrial contraction Ventricular perforation with hemopericardium or cardiac tamponade

Procedure
Transcutaneous Pacing

1. Place the anterior pacer pad over the left anterior chest wall at the point of maximal impulse.
2. Place the posterior pacer pad on the patient's back, directly opposite the anterior pad.
3. If using a separate EKG monitor with output adapter, place the leads.
4. Administer intravenous analgesics or benzodiazepines as needed for patient comfort.
5. For bradyasystolic dysrhythmias, synchronous pacing is preferred, usually at a rate of 60 to 70 beats per minute. Activate the transcutaneous pacer, and slowly increase the output from the minimal setting until capture is achieved. Pacing should be continued at approximately 1.25 times the threshold for capture. In bradyasystolic arrest, the output may be initially set to the maximum, and decreased when capture is achieved.
6. Adjust the heart rate as necessary to maintain the desired blood pressure or mental status.
7. Reposition the pacer pads if necessary for capture (deactivate the device first).
8. Consider placing a transvenous pacer if still unable to capture.
9. For overdrive pacing of ventricular tachycardia or PSVT: Asynchronous pacing consisting of short bursts of 6 to 10 beats at a time is applied at a rate 20 to 60 beats per minute higher than the intrinsic heart rate. For VT, the usual rate applied will be 200 beats per minute. For PSVT, the usual rate applied will be 240 to 280 beats per minute.

Transvenous Pacing with EKG Guidance

1. If using a catheter with a balloon, inflate the balloon to check for leaks, then deflate.
2. Attach EKG monitor leads to the patient.
3. Attach a chest lead (usually V_1 or V_5) to the distal (negative) terminal of the pacing catheter with an alligator clip if using EKG guidance (Figure 91–7).
4. Select the insertion site. The right internal jugular vein has the most direct route to the superior vena cava, and is the preferred site. The left subclavian vein is preferred over the right subclavian for similar reasons.
5. Place an introducer sheath using the Seldinger technique as described in 91.1. The introducer sheath should be 7.5 French in size to accommodate a 3 to 5 French pacing catheter. A 14 gauge angiocath may also be used. If the introducer is too large, blood will leak between the pacing catheter and the introducer.
6. Advance the pacing catheter 10 to 12 cm into the vein, past the distal end of the introducer sheath.
7. When the catheter is in the superior vena cava, the EKG chest lead monitor should demonstrate negative deflections for both P waves and QRS waves. Inflate the balloon.
8. Advance the catheter.

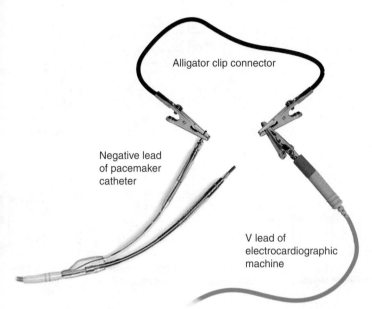

Figure 91–7. Using alligator clips to connect the *negative* lead of the pacemaker catheter to the V lead of an electrocardiographic machine. *(Reproduced from Roberts JR, Hedges JR [editors]. Clinical Procedures in Emergency Medicine [4th ed]. Philadelphia: Elsevier, 2005, p 289.)*

9. Monitor the chest lead tracing as the catheter advances. As it travels into the right atrium, the P wave deepens. As it traverses the atrium, the P wave gradually become upright. As it passes the tricuspid valve into the right ventricle, the P wave will become smaller, and the QRS complex will deepen. If it passes into the inferior vena cava, the P wave and QRS complex will both decrease in amplitude (Figure 91–8).
10. When the catheter is in the right ventricle, deflate the balloon.
11. Advance the catheter until it is in contact with the ventricular wall. The chest lead monitor will show ST segment elevation. If instead the P wave again inverts and the QRS segment becomes smaller, the tip may have drifted into the pulmonary artery. In this case, withdraw the catheter and then readvance.
12. When the catheter tip is in contact with the endocardium, disconnect the EKG lead from the pacing catheter, and connect it to the appropriate lead on the patient.
13. Connect the positive and negative leads to the proper terminals on the pacing generator.
14. Set the pacer to synchronous pacing mode.
15. Set the pacer rate to 80 beats per minute, or up to 10 beats per minute higher than the intrinsic ventricular rhythm, whichever is higher.
16. Set the pacer output initially to maximum (usually 20 mA), and decrease it when capture is achieved. Set the output to 1.5 to 2 times the

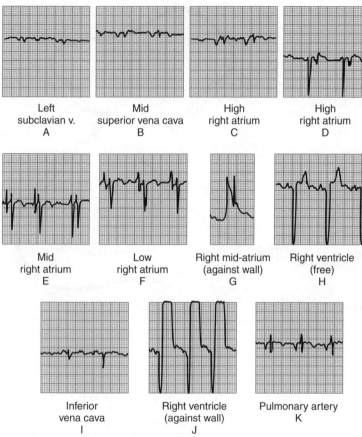

Figure 91–8. A–K. Intracardiac electrocardiography: Electrical signals of atrial and ventricular depolarization and repolarization from different vascular and intracardiac locations. *(A–F and H–K from Bing OH, McDowell JW, Hantman J, et al: Pacemaker placement by electrocardiographic monitoring. N Engl J Med 287:651, 1972. G from Goldberger E: Treatment of Cardiac Emergencies, 3rd ed. St. Louis, CV Mosby, 1982, p 252.)*

threshold output required for capture. The usual setting will be approximately 5 mA.
17. If capture is not achieved, the catheter may need to be repositioned.

Transvenous Pacing without EKG Guidance

1. Place the introducer sheath as described in Transvenous Pacing with EKG Guidance.

2. Advance the pacing catheter 10 to 12 cm into the introducer sheath.
3. Inflate the balloon.
4. Connect the catheter to the pacing generator.
5. Set the pacer to synchronous pacing mode.
6. Set the pacing rate to twice the intrinsic heart rate.
7. Set the pacer output to 0.2 mA.
8. Set the pacer to sense but not to pace.
9. Advance the catheter.
10. On entering the right ventricle, the pacer should sense the intrinsic heart beat.
11. Deflate the balloon.
12. Increase the pacer output to maximum.
13. Advance the pacer to capture the ventricle. If capture is not achieved after advancing another 10 cm, withdraw the catheter and readvance.
14. Decrease the pacer output to determine the threshold for capture. Set the output to 1.5 to 2 times the threshold output required for capture. The usual setting will be approximately 5 mA.

Transvenous Pacing in Patients with Decreased or No Forward Blood Flow

1. Transcutaneous pacing is preferred in emergent situations.
2. The right internal jugular vein should be selected as this offers the most direct route into the right ventricle.
3. The pacer should be placed as in transvenous pacing without EKG guidance explained above, but the balloon tip should not be inflated as blood flow will not adequately direct the catheter tip into the right ventricle.
4. The pacer should be set to asynchronous mode.

Pearls and Pitfalls for Cardiac Pacing

There is minimal risk of electrical injury to healthcare providers during transcutaneous pacing. Chest compressions may be continued.

Separate defibrillator pads or paddles, if used, should be placed at least 2 to 3 cm away from transcutaneous pacer pads.

If a transvenous pacemaker catheter causes ectopy, it should be withdrawn until the ectopy stops and then readvanced.

When withdrawing a pacing catheter with a balloon tip, always deflate the balloon first.

91.7 Tube Thoracostomy

Tube Thoracostomy		
Indications	**Contraindications**	**Complications**
Pneumothorax greater than 15- 20 %	Absolute: none	Persistent pneumothorax
Symptomatic pneumothorax of any size	Relative: bleeding or coagulation abnormalities; active skin infection at site of procedure	Lung parenchyma injury
Hemothorax		Cardiac injury
Persistent pleural effusion		Large-vessel injury with hemorrhage
Empyema		Cardiac dysrhythmias
Post needle thoracostomy		Infection

Procedure (Figure 91–9)

1. Position the patient in the supine position. Use a 12 to 28 French chest tube for air and a 34 to 40 French tube for fluid drainage.
2. Locate the fourth or fifth intercostal space between the anterior axillary and mid axillary line. The tube will be placed over the rib to avoid the neurovascular bundle (remember to stay lateral to the pectoral muscles).
3. Tape the patient's arm above the patient's head to assist in spreading the ribs.
4. Prepare the skin with gauze soaked in povidone iodine, and drape with sterile towels.
5. Prepare the chest tube by placing a Kelly clamp transversely at the tapered distal end of the tube (this prevents blood from dripping out when the tube is placed into the chest). Then place a second Kelly clamp at the proximal tip of the chest tube parallel to the long axis (to support the tube during placement into the chest.)
6. Anesthetize the skin one intercostal space below the chosen tube insertion site. Load a syringe with 10-ml of lidocaine. With the 25- or 27-gauge needle make a large skin wheel 2 to 3 cm in diameter. Advance the needle to the rib above while aspirating. Anesthetize the periosteum and tissue while withdrawing the needle.
7. Anesthetize the deep tissues next. Load the syringe again with 20-ml of lidocaine. Insert the needle at the skin wheel, and find the rib above again. Walk the needle up the rib drawing back as you advance. You will be able to withdraw air when the pleural space is encountered. Withdraw the needle slightly and inject all 20-ml of lidocaine to provide anesthesia to the parietal pleura.
8. Using the scalpel make a 2- to 3-cm horizontal skin incision over the chosen rib.

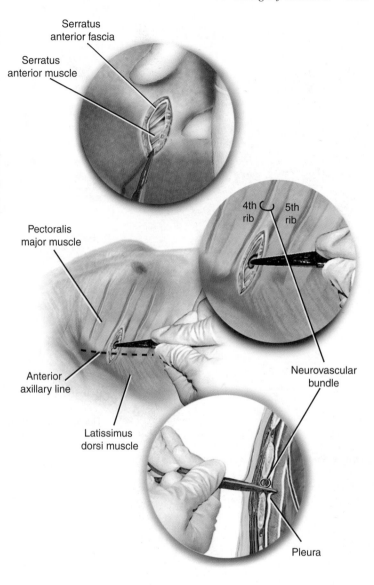

Serratus
anterior fascia

Serratus
anterior muscle

Pectoralis
major muscle

4th
rib

5th
rib

Anterior
axillary line

Neurovascular
bundle

Latissimus
dorsi muscle

Pleura

A.

Figure 91–9. Tube thoracostomy. *A,B.* Make a 2- to 3-cm incision over the fifth rib at the anterior axillary line. Dissection should be caudad, over the top of the fourth or fifth rib. Using a closed clamp or scissors, with index finger approximately 1- to 2 inches from sharp end, bluntly penetrate the parietal pleura with a steady firm pressure. Open the instrument wide after penetrating the pleura, and remove it with the instrument still open wide. Insert a gloved finger though the opening to verify position and absence of adhesions or abdominal organs.

Continued

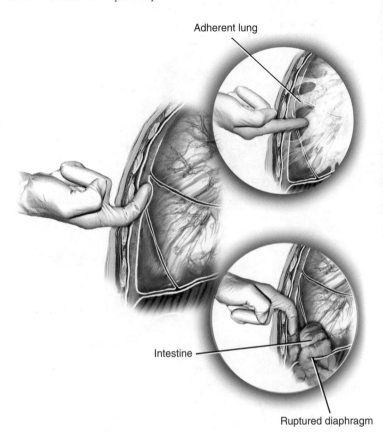

Adherent lung

Intestine

Ruptured diaphragm

B

Figure 91–9. Tube thoracostomy. *cont'd.*

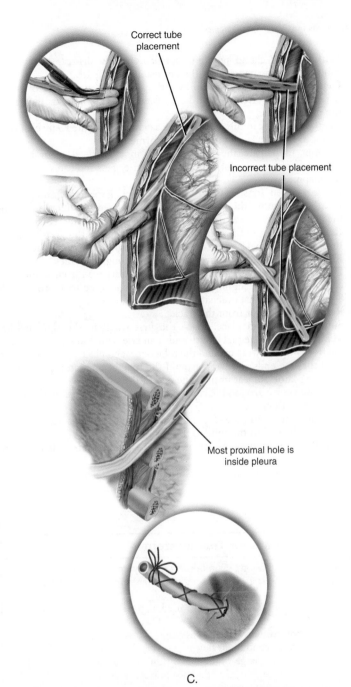

Correct tube placement

Incorrect tube placement

Most proximal hole is inside pleura

C.

Figure 91–9. *cont'd, C,* Guide the chest tube in place by sliding it over the inserted fingers. Direct the tube posteriorly and cephalad until all of the holes are within the thoracic cavity, then secure the tube. *(Reproduced from Rosen P, Chan TC, Vilke GM, Stembach G. Atlas of Emergency Procedures. St. Louis, MO: Mosby, 2001, p 41–43.)*

9. With a Kelly clamp pointed cephalad, bluntly dissect through the subcutaneous tissue to reach the periosteum of the rib.

10. Gently guide the Kelly clamp over the rib, and penetrate through the parietal pleura. There should be a *pop*, and escape of air or fluid from the pleural space.

11. Keep your finger in the pleural space as you remove the Kelly clamp (so as not to lose the track you have just formed).

12. Attempt to palpate the lung and the inner parietal pleural tissue. Palpation of intestine or other abdominal organs indicates rupture of the diaphragm.

13. Guide a closed Tonsil clamp though the track. Expand the entry site by forcefully opening the clamp (remember to keep the fulcrum outside the actual pleural space to maximize the spreading of the tissue).

14. Keep your finger in the pleural space as you remove the Tonsil clamp.

15. Insert the proximal end of the chest tube using the previously placed Kelly clamp to guide it above the rib and through the track.

16. Disengage the Kelly clamp, and continue to advance the chest tube in a cephalad direction angling posteriorly. Advance tube to approximately 8-cm beyond the last evacuation hole on the tube.

17. Remove your finger from the track.

18. Suture the tube in place. Place the first stitch in the skin incision (remember to have equal length ends), and tie with 4 square knots. Take the free ends and wrap around the tube once, and place a surgeon's knot. Take the free ends and wrap around the tube again, and place another surgeon's knot. Repeat until at the end of the suture.

19. Wrap Xeroform around the chest tube, and apply to the skin. Cover the xeroform with gauze.

20. Tape the gauze and tube to the skin using the benzoin as needed.

21. Connect the end of the tube to the Pleur-evac.

22. Tape the connection point between the chest tube and the Pleur-evac to ensure no air leaks.

23. Obtain a chest radiograph to ensure proper placement.

Pearls and Pitfalls for Thoracostomy

In the setting of a tension pneumothorax (i.e., hypotension due to pneumothorax), insert a 14-gauge angiocatheter perpendicular to the skin, in the fourth intercostal space laterally. A 20-gauge, 1-inch angiocatheter or over-the-needle catheter should be used on patients weighing less than 40 kg.

A needle thoracostomy necessitates a tube thoracostomy.

If a sudden large continuous flow of blood is seen coming out of the chest tube, consider a large vessel injury. If this occurs, do not remove the chest tube, clamp the tube, tape the tube in place, and call surgery for an emergent operative thoracotomy.

91.8   Thoracotomy

Thoracotomy		
Indications	**Contraindications**	**Complications**
Penetrating chest trauma with signs of life in the field or emergency department Blunt chest trauma with signs of life Cardiac tamponade (consider peri-cardiocentesis first) Hemothorax with greater than 800 ml initial output and 50 ml every 10 min after	Blunt trauma with no signs of life in the field	Phrenic nerve injury Coronary artery injury Infection Myocardial injury, especially the atria

Procedure
General

1. Locate the fifth rib and the fourth intercostal space. Perform a left anterolateral thoracotomy.
2. At the fourth intercostals space just above the fifth rib make a firm, definitive cut through the skin, pectoralis and serratus muscles using the scalpel. The cut should begin 2-cm lateral to the sternum and end just beyond the posterior axillary line (Figure 91–10A).
3. Briefly hold mechanical ventilation at expiration.
4. Using the Mayo or Metzenbaum scissors, push through the intercostal muscle just above the fifth rib, and cut along the rib to expose the pleural cavity (Figure 91–10B).
5. Insert the rib spreader. The handle of the spreader should be directed posteriorly, and the blades should be initially closed. Turn the handle of the rib spreader so that the two blades separate to expose the underlying structures (Figure 91–10C).

Intrathoracic Procedures

1. Pericardiotomy (Figure 91–10D): Locate the phrenic nerve running superior-inferior along the pericardium, and avoid damaging underlying structures. Grasp the anterior pericardium with forceps, and using the scissors, make a nick in the pericardium parallel to the phrenic nerve. Using the scissors in a very shallow angle, extend the incision from the

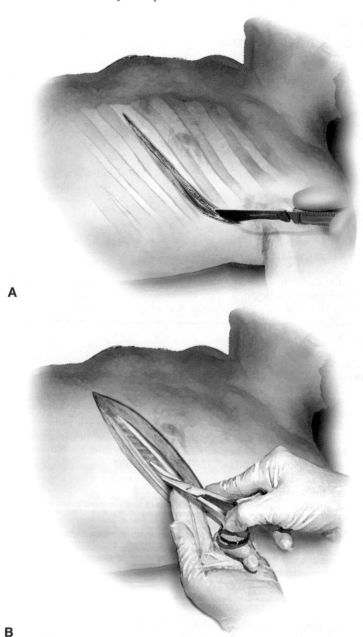

A

B

Figure 91–10. Thoracotomy. **A:** At the fourth intercostals space just above the fifth rib make a firm, definitive cut through the skin pectoralis and serratus muscles using the scalpel. The cut should begin 2-cm lateral to the sternum and end just beyond the posterior axillary line. **B:** Using the Mayo or Metzenbaum scissors, push through the intercostal muscle just above the fifth rib and cut along the rib to expose the pleural cavity.

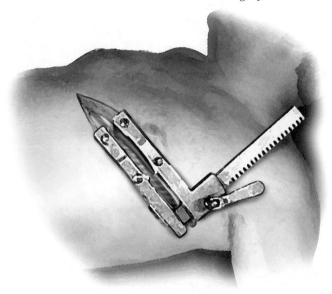

C

D

Figure 91–10. *cont'd,* **C:** Insertion of the rib spreader. The handle of the spreader should be directed posteriorly and the blades should be initially closed. Turn the handle of the rib spreader so that the two blades separate to expose the underlying structures. **D:** Incision of the pericardial sac. Locate the pericardium and identify the phrenic nerve running in a superior-inferior direction. Open the pericardium by grasping the tissue with a toothed forcep and make nick with a scalpel, being careful to avoid the phrenic nerve. Extend the incision in a cephalocaudad direction using blunt tipped scissors.

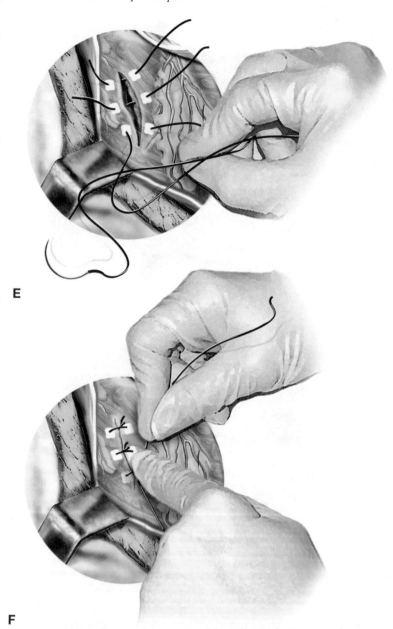

E

F

Figure 91–10. *cont'd,* **E:** Cardiorrhaphy for penetrating injury to the heart. A finger may be inserted into the wound as a temporizing measure. A cardiovascular suture can be used to close the wound temporarily. Teflon pledgets should be used to avoid causing further laceration to the friable myocardium. Be careful not to place sutures through coronary arteries. *(Reproduced from Rosen P, Chan TC, Vilke GM, Stembach G. Atlas of Emergency Procedures. St. Louis, MO: Mosby, 2001, p 55DE.)*

apex of the heart to the root. Clear any blood clots and the heart may be delivered from the pericardium.

2. Controlling cardiac hemorrhage (Figures 91–10E and F): If there is an obvious cardiac puncture or laceration, a finger can be placed to occlude the wound. Temporary repair of the wound may be attempted using suture with Teflon or Gore-Tex pledgets. If suturing is not feasible, a Foley catheter can be inserted into the wound, inflated, and pulled gently to occlude the wound.

3. Direct cardiac compression (Figure 91–10D): Can be done with or without a pericardiotomy. The left hand is cupped around the right ventricle, the right hand and fingers should be held firm to form a paddle. A gentle clapping motion is made with the hands remembering to compress from the apex towards the root.

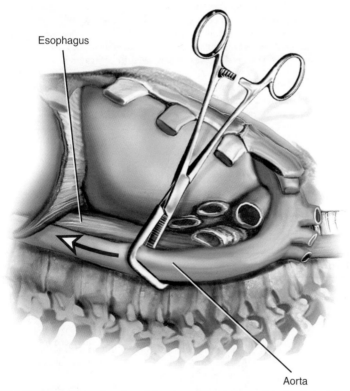

Esophagus

Aorta

Figure 91–11. Cross-clamping of the aorta. After the aorta is isolated, the left index finger can be flexed around the aorta and a DeBakey, curved Kelly, or a Satinsky aortic clamp can be guided to clamp the aorta. The aorta is a pulsatile (but pulsations may be absent in cardiac arrest), muscular structure directly anterior to the esophagus. *(Reproduced from Rosen P, Chan TC, Vilke GM, Stembach G. Atlas of Emergency Procedures. St. Louis, MO: Mosby, 2001, p 59D.)*

4. Aortic cross clamping (Figure 91–11): Locate the aorta by sliding your left hand along the posterior thoracic cage towards the midline. The aorta is anterior to the vertebral bodies. A nasogastric tube in the esophagus will help to differentiate the aorta and the esophagus. The aorta can be compressed against the vertebral bodies with the fingers or an aortic tamponade device. To formally clamp the aorta, the aorta must first be bluntly dissected free from the esophagus and the mediastinal pleura. Once free, the left index finger can be flexed around the aorta, and a DeBakey, curved Kelly or a Satinsky aortic clamp can be guided to clamp the aorta.

Pearls and Pitfalls for Thoracotomy

The patient should be intubated with the lungs deflated while the thorax is being opened to avoid injury to the lungs.

A nasogastric tube should be passed into the stomach to help differentiate the esophagus and the aorta.

Be aware that the internal mammary arteries may be cut by the primary incision or by the scissors. The vessel may need to be ligated if bleeding actively.

When trying to locate the aorta, it is imperative that care be taken while the hand is advanced along the posterior thorax to prevent injury to the operator due to rib fractures.

91.9 Thoracentesis

Thoracentesis

Indications	Contraindications	Complications
Pleural effusion: diagnostic or therapeutic	Absolute: none Relative: bleeding or coagulation abnormalities Active skin infection at site of procedure Mechanical ventilation Minimal fluid presence (<1cm of fluid on lateral decubitus radiograph)	Pneumothorax Bleeding Pain Infection Abdominal organ injury Cough Vasovagal event Tumor seeding

Procedure

1. Position the patient sitting upright with the back exposed.
2. Percuss the chest for dullness.
3. Mark a level one to two rib spaces below the superior point of the percussed dullness. This entry point for the needle should be half way between the midscapular line and the posterior axillary line. The entry point should never be below the eighth intercostal space (approximately 1 to 2 cm below the tip of the scapula) (Figure 91–12).
4. A large area should be sterilized with povidone iodine and then sterilely draped
5. Using the 20-ml syringe and a 25-gauge needle, infiltrate the skin, periosteum and the parietal pleura with 1% lidocaine. Pass the needle above the rib to avoid the intercostal neurovascular bundle, and aspirate as the needle is advanced.
6. Advance the anesthetic needle while aspirating until pleural fluid is obtained. The depth of the needle should be noted as the needle is removed.
7. Prepare for the thoracentesis: For diagnostic thoracentesis, assemble the 18- or 22-gauge needle and the 60-ml syringe. For therapeutic thoracentesis, assemble the over-the-needle catheter with a 20-ml syringe. Next connect the three way stop cock to the 60-ml syringe in

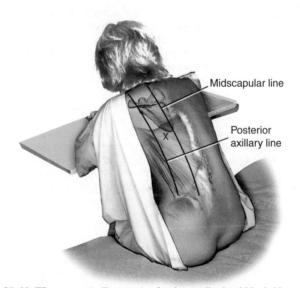

Figure 91–12. Thoracentesis. Entry point for the needle should be half way between the midaxillary line and the posterior axillary line. The entry point should never be below the eighth intercostal space (approximately 1-2 cm below the tip of the scapula). *(Reproduced from Rosen P, Chan TC, Vilke GM, Stembach G. Atlas of Emergency Procedures. St. Louis, MO: Mosby, 2001, p 37.)*

one port and the sterile tubing to another. Attach the other end of the tubing to the fluid collector, and place the fluid collector aside. The three-way stop cock lever should be set to allow flow to the syringe.

8. Advance the needle to the same depth as the anesthetic needle while aspirating. If using one of the over-the-needle catheters, use the scalpel to nick the skin to allow easier passage of the needle.

9. When the pleural fluid is obtained, stop advancing the needle. If using a hypodermic needle, grasp the needle at the skin to stabilize it. If using the over-the-needle catheter, point the needle caudally, and while holding the syringe and needle stable, advance the catheter. Remove the needle, and cover the hub of the catheter immediately with your finger to prevent air leaking into the pleural cavity. Connect the three-way stopcock to the catheter.

10. Withdraw the fluid into the syringe. If the stopcock method is being used, adjust the stopcock lever to close the tubing port, and withdraw fluid using the 60-ml syringe port. When the 60-ml syringe is full, adjust the stopcock to close the thoracentesis needle port, and expel the fluid into the specimen collector through the stopcock tubing connection.

11. Turn the stopcock lever to close the tubing side again, and repeat steps 9 and 10 as needed until the patient is symptomatically improved or 1 L is removed, whichever occurs first.

12. Once the procedure is done, remove the needle or catheter, and cover with sterile bandages.

13. Send the fluid for analysis of lactate dehydrogenase, glucose, protein, specific gravity, cell count, differential, crystals, Gram's stain, aerobic/anaerobic cultures, Acid-fast/fungal culture and stain. If an exudate is suspected, amylase, triglycerides, cholesterol, complement, rheumatoid factor, immunoelectrophoresis, carcinoembryonic antigen, cytology, lupus erythematosus cells, and pH should also be ordered. See Appendix 1 for pleura fluid analysis.

14. Routine postprocedure chest radiographs are not necessary if the patient is asymptomatic. A chest radiograph should be obtained in patients who require multiple needle passes, are at risk for adhesions, have aspiration of air, or develop any new symptoms during or after the procedure. Other indications include patients with severe underlying lung disease, and patients who are receiving mechanical ventilation as they are at risk for future decompensation from expansion of a small asymptomatic pneumothorax.

Pearls and Pitfalls for Thoracentesis

The height of the effusion is located clinically by dullness to percussion and a decrease in tactile fremitus. Never rely on the chest radiograph to determine the level of effusion as the radiographic level changes with patient positioning and respiration.

A lateral decubitus chest radiograph is used to identify free pleural fluid. If the distance between the inside of the thoracic cavity and the outside of the lung is less than 10 mm, the pleural effusion is not likely to be clinically significant, and, in any case, will be difficult to sample by thoracentesis.

A dry thoracentesis occurs if there is no pleural effusion, incorrect point of entry is chosen, or it the needle is too short for a large patient. If the patient has suffered no complications from the failed attempt, the thoracentesis can be attempted again after re-localization of the pleural effusion.

If air is obtained from the thoracentesis, this may represent entry into the lung parenchyma. Usually a pneumothorax caused by thoracentesis is small, and can be managed conservatively without a thoracostomy. If the patient has no new symptoms, the procedure can be reattempted.

Remove the necessary amount of pleural fluid (usually 100 ml for diagnostic studies), but do not remove more than 1500 ml of fluid at any one time because of increased risk of pulmonary edema or hypotension (pneumothorax from needle laceration of the visceral pleura is also much more likely to occur if an effusion is completely drained).

91.10 Lumbar Puncture

Lumbar Puncture (LP)

Indications	Contraindications	Complications
Diagnosis of central nervous system infection	Infection in the soft tissues at the puncture site	Bleeding
Altered level of consciousness	Increased intracranial pressure from space-occupying lesion	Introduction of infection
Diagnosis of subarachnoid hemorrhage	Lateralizing neurologic signs	Spinal headache
Therapeutic treatment of pseudotumor cerebri	Signs of uncal herniation	Implantation of epidermoid tumor
		Herniation
		Neurologic damage

Procedure (Figure 91–13)

1. Position the patient in either the lateral decubitus position or upright sitting position. Have the patient's knees drawn up towards the chest. The lateral decubitus position allows for more accurate measurement of opening pressure. While in the lateral decubitus position, use pillows to keep the head and spine aligned. The patient's shoulders and hips should be kept perpendicular to the table.
2. Identify the proper landmarks: palpate the posterior-superior iliac crests bilaterally, and draw an imaginary line between them. This line should

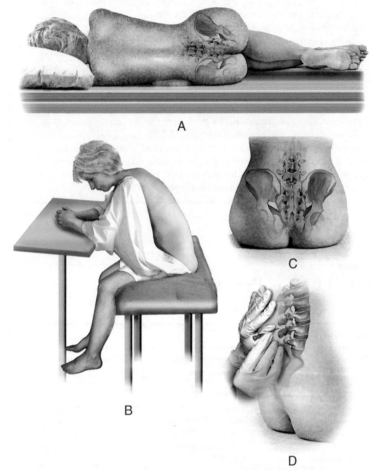

Figure 91–13. Lumbar puncture. *A,* Lateral decubitus position. *B,* Upright, with the patient leaning over, placing arms on a table, Mayo stand or chair. *C,* At the level of the iliac crests, palpate the spinous processes and locate the intervertebral space at this level (usually the L-3 to L-4 space). *D,* Puncture the skin with the spinal needle, aiming midline toward the umbilicus. *(Reproduced from Rosen P, Chan TC, Vilke GM, Stembach G. Atlas of Emergency Procedures. St. Louis, MO: Mosby, 2001, p 157.)*

approximately cross the L-4 spinous process. In adults, the lumbar puncture (LP) should be performed in the midline from the L-2/L-3 interspace to the L-5/S-1 interspace. In infants, the LP should be performed at the L-4/L-5 or L-5/ S-1 interspace. Note or mark the area of your planned entry.

3. Put on sterile gloves. All of the following steps should be performed in sterile fashion.
4. Cleanse the skin with the antiseptic solution in a circular motion starting at the desired point of entry and widening with each successive motion to cover the area of skin that will not be covered with a sterile drape during the procedure. Repeat twice.
5. Drape the patient. Leave approximately a 10×10-cm area surrounding the site of skin entry exposed.
6. Allow the antiseptic solution to dry.
7. Anesthetize the skin at your entry site with a skin wheal.
8. Anesthetize the deeper subcutaneous tissues.
9. Use a 20- or 22- gauge spinal needle (with stylet) for adults, and 25- or 27-gauge needle in infants. Hold the spinal needle with the thumbs and index fingers of both hands for stability. Direct the bevel of the needle laterally in relation to the patient.
10. Insert the spinal needle through the skin at the midline sagittal plane, and angle it towards the patient's umbilicus while staying in the longitudinal axis.
11. Pass the spinal needle deeper into the subcutaneous tissues, frequently removing the stylet to assess for cerebrospinal fluid (CSF) return, indicating entry into the subarachnoid space. Often a pop is felt when the ligamentum flavum is penetrated.
12. If bone is encountered, withdraw the needle to the skin, and ensure that the needle is in the midline. Re-angle the needle superiorly or inferiorly as necessary.
13. When CSF returns, connect the manometer and stopcock to the spinal needle to measure opening pressure. The zero marking on the manometer should be at the level of the spinal needle to ensure that the pressure reading is accurate.
14. Collect sufficient fluid, usually one milliliter in each of four tubes, labeled 1 through 4 in succession.
15. Remove the spinal needle, and place pressure at the entry site.
16. Cleanse the skin, and place a clean dressing over the entry site.

Pearls and Pitfalls for Lumbar Puncture

Correct coagulopathies prior to performing LP. Monitor afterwards for the possible development of a spinal epidural hematoma.

Use an adequate amount of anesthetic. For most LPs, you will use more than is provided in commercial LP trays.

A small change in the angle of entry of the spinal needle at the skin may result in a large variation of needle position by the time the tip reaches the depth of the subarachnoid space.

In the event of a traumatic tap in which the blood does not clear, repeat the LP with a fresh spinal needle in a more superior interspace if possible.

91.11 Paracentesis

Paracentesis		
Indications	**Contraindications: absolute**	**Complications**
New-onset ascites	Severe uncorrected coagulopathy	Abdominal wall hematoma
Tense ascites	Infection over the entry site	Bladder perforation
Diagnosis of infection	Hematoma over the entry site	Gastrointestinal perforation
	Dilated veins over the entry site	Infection
		Intraperitoneal hemorrhage
		Persistent fluid leak
		Vessel perforation

Procedure (Figure 91–14)

1. Ensure that the patient has ascites via physical examination or imaging confirmation.
2. To decrease the chance of bladder perforation, have the patient void. Catheterize the patient if necessary.
3. Place the patient either in the supine or the lateral decubitus position.
4. Select the appropriate site of entry. The preferred site is 2 cm inferior to the umbilicus in the midline through the linea alba. If the patient has scarring or infection in this area, the alternative is either lower quadrant of the abdomen, 4 to 5 cm superior and slightly medial to the anterior superior iliac spine, lateral to the rectus sheath. If using the lower quadrant with the patient in the lateral decubitus position, the dependent lower quadrant is used.
5. Prepare the skin overlying the entry site with the antiseptic cleansing solution.
6. Sterilely glove, and place the drapes around the entry site.
7. Anesthetize the entry site.
8. Retract the skin over the entry site approximately 1 to 2 cm caudally.
9. Use an 18 gauge needle for therapeutic paracentesis, and 20- or 22-gauge needles for diagnostic paracentesis. Holding the paracentesis needle perpendicular to the skin, insert it into the entry site while aspirating.
10. Advance the needle slowly until ascitic fluid is flowing. Release retraction on the skin.
11. Withdraw fluid using the 50-ml syringe, or connect the connecting tubing and vacuum bottles if withdrawing larger amounts of fluid.
12. Fill the specimen tube with ascitic fluid for laboratory analysis.
13. When the desired amount of fluid has been removed, withdraw the needle and place a bandage over the entry site. See Appendix 1 for peritoneal fluid analysis.

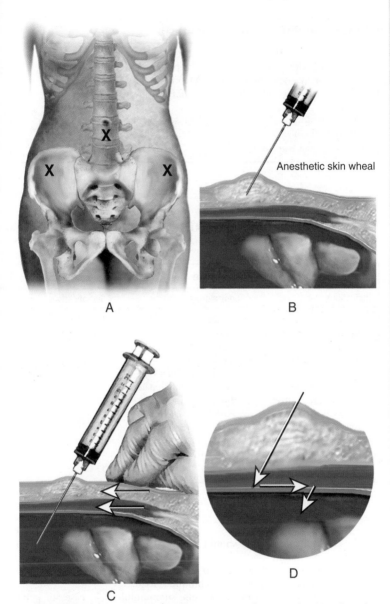

Anesthetic skin wheal

A

B

C

D

Figure 91–14. Paracentesis. *A,* Site for paracentesis: lower quadrant just lateral to the rectus muscle (avoiding epigastric vessels) or midline a few centimeters below the umbilicus where depended ascites is usually detected. *B,* Inject a small wheal at the site. *C,* Direct the angiocatheter into the site at a 70- to 90-degree angle to the skin. *D,* Z-track: Apply slight traction on the skin when first entering to form a z-track through the skin and subcutaneous tissue to help seal the needle tract and prevent leakage once the angiocatheter is removed. *(From Rosen P, Chan TC, Vilke GM, Sternbach G. Atlas of Emergency Procedures. St. Louis, MO: Mosby, 2001, p 113.)*

Pearls and Pitfalls for Paracentesis

If using an angiocatheter, the paracentesis needle may be removed, and fluid may be withdrawn through the angiocatheter.

Patients may be positioned in the lateral decubitus position with the paracentesis performed either in the midline or in the dependent lower quadrant.

Retraction of the skin during needle insertion allows for creation of a Z tract when the needle is removed and the skin slides back to its original position. This theoretically minimizes ascites leakage.

91.12 Diagnostic Peritoneal Lavage (DPL)

Diagnostic Peritoneal Lavage

Indications	Contraindications	Complications
In trauma, rapid determination of intraperitoneal hemorrhage or of solid and hollow organ injury or diaphragmatic injury. Treatment of hypothermia by lavage of peritoneum with warm fluids.	Absolute: clinical mandate for emergent laparotomy. Relative: midline abdominal surgery, obesity, coagulopathy, abdominal wall infection, pelvic fracture (lavage interpretation only), second or third trimester pregnancy	Bowel perforation Vascular injury Infection

Procedure

1. The stomach and bladder should preferably be decompressed to prevent inadvertent injury.
2. The patient is placed supine, and administered sedation and analgesia as appropriate especially if open technique is used.
3. Site: infraumbilical in most patients, supraumbilical in cases of pelvic fracture or pregnancy.
4. Local anesthesia (1% lidocaine *with* epinephrine) should be infiltrated liberally into the area for incision and dissection.
5. The semi-open and open techniques are described in Figure 91–15.
6. The closed technique is described in Figure 91–16.

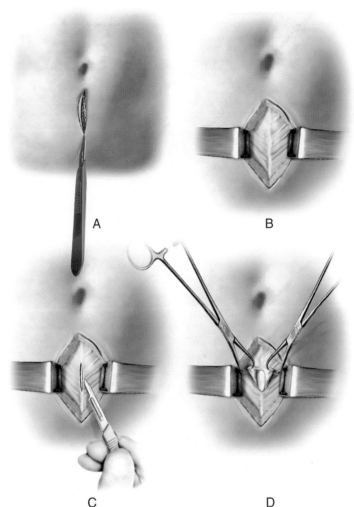

A

B

C

D

Figure 91-15. Diagnostic peritoneal lavage: open and semi-open technique.
A, After bladder decompression (generally by Foley catheter placement), a 4- to
6-cm-long vertical infraumbilical incision is made with a no. 11 scalpel. *B,* Blunt
dissection using Army-Navy retractors is carried down to the *rectus fascia*. Crossing
bands of crural fibers may be seen. *C,* A 2- to 3-mm incision is made through the
rectus fascia in the midline (*linea alba*) with a no. 15 scalpel. *D,* Towel clips grasp each
side of the *rectus fascia*, which is lifted prior to insertion of the trocar and diagnostic
peritoneal lavage (DPL) catheter.

Continued

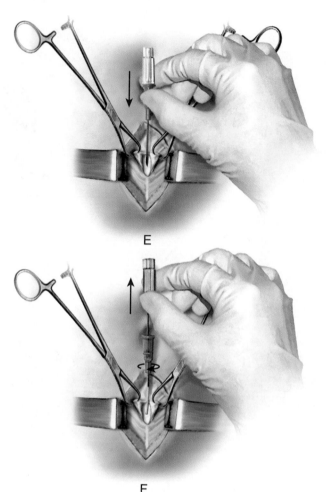

E

F

Figure 91–15. *cont'd,* Diagnostic peritoneal lavage: open and semi-open technique. *E,* The trocar (or stylet) with DPL catheter is passed at a 45-degree caudad angle into the fascial opening and through the peritoneum. Note that in the fully open method, the incision in the *rectus fascia* is extended, the peritoneum is directly visualized and incised, and the catheter alone is placed into the peritoneal cavity. *F,* As soon as the peritoneum has been entered, only the catheter is gently advanced into the peritoneal cavity while the trocar (or stylet) is withdrawn. It is often helpful to advance the catheter with a slight twisting motion, and to direct it toward either the right or left pelvic gutter. *(From Roberts JR, Hedges JR [editors]. Clinical Procedures in Emergency Medicine [4th ed]. Philadelphia: Elsevier, 2005, p 848.)*

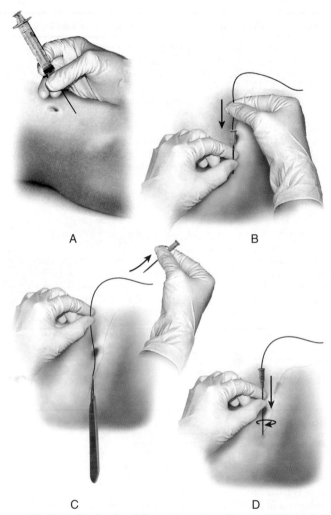

A

B

C

D

Figure 91–16. *A,* For the closed diagnostic peritoneal lavage (DPL) method using a guide wire (Seldinger technique), the needle is inserted into the peritoneal cavity in the midline just below the umbilicus, and aimed slightly caudad. After penetration through the skin the needle will pass through the anterior fascia, the posterior fascia, and then the peritoneum. *B,* The flexible guide wire is passed through the needle and into the peritoneal cavity. Ideally, the wire should be directed toward the right or left pelvic gutter. The needle is withdrawn while the wire is stabilized with the operator's free hand at all times. *C,* A stab incision is made with a No. 11 scalpel immediately below the wire to permit easier passage of the DPL catheter. *D,* The DPL catheter is directed over the wire and into the peritoneal cavity using a slight twisting motion. The wire is stabilized by the operator at all times, and removed after catheter placement. The catheter should be directed toward the right or left pelvic gutter when advanced. *(From Roberts JR, Hedges JR [editors]. Clinical Procedures in Emergency Medicine [4th ed]. Philadelphia: Elsevier, 2005, p 849.)*

Pearls and Pitfalls for Diagnostic Peritoneal Lavage

Diagnostic peritoneal lavage (DPL) is considered positive if you obtain: Gross blood or succus entericus on initial aspiration, more than 100,000/mm^3 of red blood cells on lavage fluid, more than 500/mm^3 white blood cells, lavage fluid vegetable fibers.

In pregnancy, the supraumbilical approach and open technique should be used.

Disadvantages of DPL include the invasiveness, risk of complications over noninvasive diagnostic measures (computed tomography [CT scan] or focused abdominal sonography in trauma [FAST] examination), inability to detect retroperitoneal injuries, high rate of nontherapeutic laparotomies, and low specificity.

For blunt trauma in the hemodynamically unstable patient, a positive DPL indicates the need for an immediate celiotomy. In the hemodynamically stable patient, however, the DPL criteria are too sensitive and nonspecific. A DPL is typically not required, and a CT scan of the abdomen is indicated in these situations.

In penetrating trauma, the RBC threshold indicating the need for celiotomy is lowered to 5000 RBC/mm^3. See Chapter 14 for further discussion of DPL results.

Prophylactic antibiotics are not indicated for routine DPL because local and systemic infections are rare.

91.13 Arthrocentesis

Arthocentesis

Indications	Contraindications	Complications
Joint infection is suspected or diagnosis is uncertain Pain relief and increase range of motion Removal of hemarthrosis	Absolute: skin infection over entry site. Relative: uncorrected coagulopathy, bleeding diatheses, joint prosthesis (consult orthopedics), bacteremia	Infection Bleeding

Procedure

1. The location and positioning for the most common joint aspirations is listed in Table 91–1.
2. Locally infiltrate the area selected using a 25-gauge needle with 2 to 10 ml of local anesthetic; do not hit the bone.
3. Prepare and drape the site in a sterile fashion.

Continued

Location	Positioning	Technique	Illustration
Knee	Supine position with the knee in extension or slight flexion with a towel roll behind the knee.	Identify an area at the intersection of the proximal pole of the patella and either the medial or lateral edge of the patella. Enter the joint with an 18-gauge needle. Be careful not to strike the underside of the patella	
Ankle	Supine position with the foot in a moderate amount of plantar flexion.	Dorsiflex the foot to locate the anterior tibialis tendon anteriorly. Also identify the joint line between the tibia and the talus. Enter the joint with a 20-gauge needle between the tibialis anterior tendon and the extensor hallicus longus tendon at the joint line. Avoid scraping the talus and do not direct the needle downward toward the heel.	
Metatarsal-phalangeal joint	Supine position with toe flexed 15 to 20 degrees to increase target area.	Locate the joint space between the distal portion of the metatarsal and proximal portion of the proximal phalynx. Enter the joint with a 22-gauge needle. Avoiding the extensor tendon (in midline and palpable by extending the toes).	

Table 91–1 Joint Aspiration Techniques—*cont'd*

Location	Positioning	Technique	Illustration
Shoulder	Sitting position with shoulder externally rotated.	Locate the humeral head anteriorly. Entry will be just medial to this, and just lateral and inferior to the coracoid process. Direct the 20- or 22-gauge needle from an anterior approach. It should be aimed in a posterior, lateral, and slightly superior direction until the joint space is entered.	
Elbow	Place the arm on a firm surface with the elbow flexed 90 degrees with the thumb up.	Make sure the effusion is in the joint and not an olecranon bursitis. Palpate the radial head by passively supinating and pronating the forearm. Palpate a small hollow area between the radial head and the lateral epicondyle of the humerus. Extending the elbow may help identify this small gap. Enter this site laterally with a 20- or 22-gauge needle.	
Wrist	Supine position.	Identify the entry site on the dorsal surface of the wrist by flexing and extending the wrist. Enter the joint space with a 22-gauge syringe at the radiocarpal junction, in the hollow space just distal and ulnar to Lister's tubercle (bump on the distal radius). Avoid the anatomic snuff box.	

*From Ro> D Ch TC Kb Cl> l 3 Tl> M

4. Enter the skin with an 18- or 20-gauge needle attached to a syringe. Aspirate gently while advancing the needle. Stop advancing when there is easy flow of joint fluid into the syringe. Avoid using excessive negative pressure on the syringe as this will pull the synovium over the needle bevel and prevent flow.
5. For traumatic hemarthroses, optionally inject 0.25% bupivicaine into the joint area before removing the needle for short term pain control. (Example: inject up to 15 ml into the knee joint for an acute tear of the anterior cruciate ligament).
6. Remove the needle. Send aspirate for Gram's stain, culture and sensitivity, cell count, crystals if infection or inflammation is suspected. Joint fluid interpretation is located in Appendix 1.

Pearls and Pitfalls for Arthrocentesis

The ankle is the joint that is most likely to become infected requiring meticulous attention to aseptic technique.

If infection is suspected, and only a few drops of joint fluid are available, the study of choice is a Gram's stain.

Steroids should not be injected into a joint that may be infected.

If corticosteroids (e.g., triamcinolone) are injected into a joint, warn the patient about a painful *steroid flare* 24 hours after the procedure. The patient can be treated with anti-inflammatory medications, splinting, and rest, and should be cautioned to avoid sports for 5 days.

After the arthrocentesis is complete, a long-acting anesthetic agent (bupivicaine 0.25%) may be injected to provide temporizing comfort. The needle is left in place, and the syringes are changed.

91.14 Nasogastric Tube Placement

Nasogastric Tube Placement

Indications	Contraindications	Complications
Gastric distention/ aspiration of gastric contents	Cribriform plate injury/other facial or basilar skull fractures	Bronchial placement Epistaxis Intracranial placement
Recurrent vomiting	Severe coagulopathy	Perforation of pharynx/Pneumonia/
Gastrointestinal bleeding	Esophageal strictures Alkali ingestion	bronchus/alveoli Pneumothorax Tube-induced hypersalivation

Procedure

1. Position the patient: The awake patient should be in the high Fowler position (sitting upright at 90 degrees). The comatose or sedated patient may be supine.
2. Estimate the insertion distance of the tube:

    (distance between the xiphoid process and the earlobe)
    + (distance between the earlobe and the tip of the nose) + 15 cm.

3. Assess the patient's nares for patency; use the larger naris.
4. Administer topical vasoconstrictor to the nares and anesthetic to the nasopharynx and oropharynx at least 5 minutes before insertion of tube.
5. Lubricate the tube.
6. Insert the tube into the naris directed posteriorly. Do not direct it superiorly along the bridge of the nose.
7. Advance the tube with gentle pressure posteriorly, reposition to the other naris if necessary.
8. After passage into the oropharynx, allow the patient to rest briefly if necessary.
9. Continue advancing the tube into the esophagus.
10. Helpful tips: Have the patient sip water through a straw during this portion. Flexion of the neck may facilitate passage into the esophagus. Withdraw into the oropharynx for excessive coughing, gagging, or condensation within the tube during exhalation (as this may be evidence the nasogastric tube has passed into the trachea). Advance the tube to the predetermined depth after entrance into the esophagus.
11. Confirm placement. Instill 20 ml of air while listening over the stomach. Aspirate gastric contents, or administer 15 ml of normal saline through the tube and then aspirate.
12. Secure the tube with tape or a butterfly bandage.

Pearls and Pitfalls for Nasogastric Tube Insertion

Nasogastric tube placement is safe in the presence of esophageal varices unless the patient has had recent variceal banding. Nasogastric lavage is more of a diagnostic test than a treatment for gastrointestinal bleeding (GIB). Applied alone, an NGT cannot be expected to alter outcomes in patients with confirmed GIB.

Obtain radiograph when in doubt of placement.

91.15 Urethral Catheterization

Urethral Catheterization		
Indications	**Contraindications**	**Complications**
Collect urine for urinalysis	Suspected urethral trauma	Urethral trauma
Monitor urine output	Perineal hematoma	Formation of false lumen
Evaluate post voiding urine volumes		Hematuria
Instill contrast media		Urethral stricture
Relieve obstruction		Infection

Procedure

1. Easiest to have the patient in the supine position.
2. Put on the sterile gloves.
3. Obtain a 14 or 16 French urethral catheter in adults. Sterilely prepare the catheter by testing the balloon by filling with 10-ml normal saline by syringe. Deflate and lubricate the catheter tip.
4. Drape around the groin.
5. In men, grasp the penis with your non dominant hand, and position it perpendicular to the body. The foreskin should be retracted in uncircumcised men. In women, retract the labia minor to expose the urethra. The non dominant hand will now be the non sterile hand.
6. Using your sterile hand, use the forceps to dip the cotton balls in the povidone-iodine, and clean the skin around the meatus, wiping away from the meatus.
7. Insert the catheter into the urethra. In men, advance the catheter to the hub of the Y connector. In women, advance until urine is encountered and seen in the tube, then advance the catheter 5 cm more.
8. Inflate the balloon with 10 ml of normal saline.
9. Secure the catheter to the inner thigh with tape.

Pearls and Pitfalls for Urinary Catheterization

There should be minimal resistance at the external sphincter, and placement should not require significant force.

Inflation of the balloon should not cause pain. If pain or hematuria is experienced, deflate the balloon, and remove the Foley.

In trauma patients, a rectal examination should be done before the Foley is placed. A high riding prostate, blood at the urethral meatus, or significant pelvic injury requires a retrograde urethrogram to rule out urethral disruption.

91.16 Vaginal Delivery

Vaginal Delivery		
Indications	**Contraindications**	**Complications**
Active labor with eminent delivery	Absolute: None for eminent delivery Relative: Placenta previa Previous cesarean delivery Prolapsed umbilical cord	Breech presentation Shoulder dystocia Birth trauma Vaginal and cervical laceration Postpartum hemorrhage

Procedure (Figure 91–17)

1. Position the patient in the dorsal lithotomy position.
2. Gown up and glove sterilely. Absolute sterility is not necessary.
3. Clean the vulva, perineum, and anus with povidone-iodine in the anterior to posterior direction.
4. With the right hand support the perineum by slightly elevating the baby's head anteriorly (pushing up rostrally and anteriorly with a towel at the perineum).
5. With the left hand, place the pad of the thumb and the first three fingers on the head of the baby to help control the rate of expulsion.
6. When the head is delivered ask the patient to stop pushing.
7. Use the bulb syringe to aspirate the nostrils and mouth.
8. Check for a nuchal cord. If the baby has a nuchal cord, attempt to reduce. If unable to reduce, clamp the umbilical cord at the neck with two Kelly clamps approximately 1 cm apart, and with the scissors, cut between the clamps. Reduce the cord from the baby's neck.
9. Grasp the head firmly between the palms of both hands. Firmly and gently pull the head down to deliver the anterior shoulder.
10. Now gently pull the head up to deliver the posterior shoulder.
11. Hold both sides of the baby with your arms parallel to the baby's body. Cup the baby's head in your hand to maintain a secure grip as the baby is being delivered.
12. Hold the baby slightly lower than the umbilical cord briefly before clamping the cord.
13. Clamp the cord several centimeters from the baby's abdomen. Place the second clamp 2 cm distal and cut between the clamps.
14. The baby should be dried and warmed in an incubator.
15. Deliver the placenta. Place the left hand just above the pubic symphysis, and apply gentle upward pressure. This allows palpation and support of the uterus.

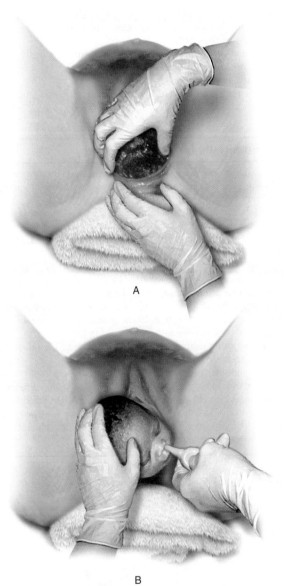

Figure 91–17. *A,B*. Vaginal delivery. With the right hand support the perineum by slightly elevating the baby's head anteriorly (pushing up rostrally and anteriorly with a towel at the perineum). With the left hand, place the pad of the thumb and the first three fingers on the head of the baby to help control the rate of expulsion. When the head is delivered ask the patient to stop pushing. Use the bulb syringe to aspirate the nostrils and mouth.

16. Gentle traction should be placed on the umbilical cord. The delivery of the placenta is eminent when there is a brief rush of blood and lengthening of the cord.
17. Deliver the placenta into the bowl, and examine to verify that it is intact to ensure nothing is retained in the uterus.
18. Massage the uterus vigorously.
19. Survey for tears and lacerations of the cervix, vagina, and perineum.
20. Repair any lacerations with 2-0 Vicryl.

Pearls and Pitfalls for Vaginal Delivery

Prophylactic antibiotics for group B streptococcus (GBS) are indicated for GBS bacteriuria during current pregnancy, positive GBS screening culture during current pregnancy (unless a planned cesarean delivery, in the absence of labor or amniotic membrane rupture, is performed), or unknown GBS status and any of the following: delivery at less than 37 weeks of gestation, amniotic membrane rupture 18 hours, intrapartum temperature 38.0° C).

Postpartum hemorrhage management: Oxytocin 20 to 40 units diluted in 1000 ml of normal saline to be infused at a titrated rate with goal of preventing uterine atony, or oxytocin 10 units IM.

Postpartum hemorrhage caused by uterine inversion may be controlled by gently placing a fist in the mother's vagina, and using the fingers to push laterally before directing the fist toward the fundus.

If heavy meconium is noted at delivery of the head, immediate suction is necessary to prevent aspiration.

In cases of shoulder dystocia, the posterior shoulder should be rotated anteriorly and upward, with application of suprapubic pressure to deliver the anterior shoulder. If this is unsuccessful, continue rotation anteriorly to deliver the posterior shoulder. A generous episiotomy may be required.

Vaginal delivery in the ED should be avoided for breech delivery if possible.

91.17 Incision and Drainage

Incision and Drainage		
Indications	**Contraindications**	**Complications**
Soft tissue abscess	No absolute contraindications. Relative contraindications in which incision and drainage in an operating room should be considered include very large abscesses, inability to achieve adequate local anesthesia or procedural sedation, abscesses of the hand (other than felons).	Injury to underlying structures during incision. Endocarditis if not given prophylaxis

Procedure

1. Position the patient for optimal exposure.
2. Locate the fluctuant area of the abscess.
3. Prep the skin with gauze soaked in povidone iodine (optional step as sterility cannot be maintained for the procedure).
4. Anesthetize beyond the entire length of the fluctuance.
5. Make an incision that extends the entire length of the fluctuance (sometimes an elliptical incision is helpful for complete drainage, and to promote healing).
6. Drain the cavity, and use the curved Kelly's or equivalent to gently sweep into the abscess cavity to break down loculations. If cultures are to be taken insert the culture swab at this step.
7. Irrigate the abscess cavity with normal saline.
8. Insert the packing gauze gently into the cavity so that packing adheres to the walls of the abscess cavity.
9. Dress the wound generously.

Pearls and Pitfalls for Abscess Drainage
Use caution with underlying structures when draining an abscess. Antibiotic prophylaxis is recommended for patients at risk of endocarditis. Antibiotics are not needed after a successful incision and drainage. Indications for antibiotics include immunocompromised states or extensive cellulitis.

CHAPTER 92

Radiology

J. SCOTT STEPHENS ■ DANIEL S. MOORE

Overview

This chapter will primarily review imaging modalities used in the ED to evaluate the head, face, chest, abdomen, and extremities. Normal examples of the most common imaging studies are provided.

Almost all computed tomography (CT scan) studies are done with helical acquisition. A few studies, such as some noncontrast head CT scans and high-resolution CT scan of the chest, are still acquired with nonhelical (sequential) technique. Contrast related issues that may influence the ability to perform a CT scan in the ED are summarized in Table 92–1.

Magnetic resonance imaging (MRI) is rarely ordered emergently from the ED. Common indications include evaluating patients for possible cerebral aneurysm, acute stroke, or spinal cord compression. Contraindications for MRI may include the presence of a cardiac pacemaker or implanted cardiac defibrillator (ICD), aneurysm clips, metal in the orbit, or an implanted medical device such as a nerve stimulator or medication pump. This list continues to change, and should not substitute for thorough individual screening of the patient by qualified MRI personnel.

Images can be acquired in one of three orientations: axial, coronal, and sagittal (Figure 92–1). CT scan imaging typically uses the axial orientation. Coronal CT scan imaging is most commonly used to better visualize the orbits. All three orientations are used in MRI, and are available with CT scans using sophisticated reconstruction techniques.

Radiation exposure is always a concern in pregnancy, and is summarized in Box 92–1.

Emergency ultrasound is an important imaging modality used by emergency physicians, and is discussed in Chapter 93.

Head
Head CT Scan

- A head CT scan is commonly ordered in the ED for patients with complaints of headache, alterations in mental status, head trauma, and neurologic complaints such as stroke.

Table 92–1	Common IV Contrast–Related Issues Used for CT Scan in the ED
Metformin	For those patients taking metformin, stop the medication at the time of contrast administration, and for 48 h thereafter.
Pregnancy	Contrast should be avoided in pregnant women particularly during the first trimester unless the benefit clearly outweighs the potential risk. If the patient is breastfeeding, the milk should be removed with a pump, and discarded prior to contrast administration and afterward for 12-24 h.
Allergic reactions	Minor reactions such as urticaria are fairly common. Serious anaphylactoid type reactions are rare, and the overall risk of death is less than 1/130,000. Although a prior reaction is the best indicator of a future reaction, the risk remains low (8%-25%). Recurrent life-threatening reactions are extremely rare. Pretreating patients at risk is safe, and has been proven to be effective in preventing minor reactions. It delays the study (at least 12 h), but has not been proven to reduce major reactions. Prednisone 40 mg orally 24, 12, and 2 h before contrast administration is one pretreatment regimen. Alternatively, give methylprednisolone 32 mg orally 12 and 2 h before contrast administration. Nonionic contrast (preferably isotonic) should be used. Allergy to shellfish is not a risk factor for reaction to iodinated contrast agents.
Nephropathy	A baseline creatinine greater than 1.5 mg/dl should raise concern for giving IV contrast. The prime risk for contrast induced nephropathy is pre-existing renal dysfunction. For patients at increased risk, if time allows and clinically appropriate, the patient should be hydrated with intravenous normal saline. The use of an iso-osmolar contrast agent (Visipaque) has also been shown to decrease the risk of nephropathy in small studies. *N*-acetylcysteine (NAC) 600 mg orally twice daily reduces nephropathy in people who have baseline renal impairment, and who are given radiocontrast.

CT scan, computed tomography; ED, emergency department; IV, intravenous. (From Bettmann, Michael A. Frequently Asked Questions: Iodinated Contrast Agents.RadioGraphics 2004;24:S3–S10.)

■ Brain anatomy in a noncontrast head CT scan is reviewed in Figures 92–2. See Chapters 9 (epidural hematoma, subdural hematoma), 35 (brain abscess, subarachnoid hemorrhage), and 56 (stroke) for examples of pathology seen on a CT scan. Calcifications and acute blood appear white, whereas cerebrospinal fluid appears black. Intra-axial lesions are within the brain or spinal cord. Extra-axial lesions are outside of the brain, and include the meninges, ventricles, and skull.

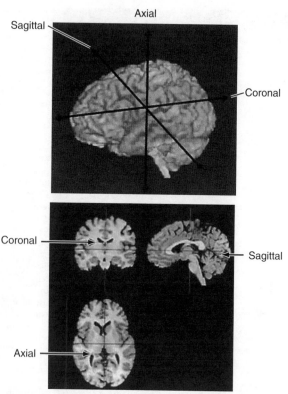

Figure 92–1. Image orientation. These figures were generated using the BioImage Suite software package. Images courtesy of Papademetris X, Jackowski M, Rajeevan N, Constable RT, and Staib LH. BioImage Suite: An integrated medical image analysis suite, Section of Bioimaging Sciences, Dept. of Diagnostic Radiology, Yale School of Medicine. http://www.bioimagesuite.org.

- A simplified approach to reviewing a head CT scan begins with the 4 Bs: grossly look **B**ilaterally (evaluating for symmetry), evaluate for **B**lood, abnormalities in the **B**rain itself, and the **B**one. Next evaluate the fluid-filled spaces (the cisterns and ventricles) and air-filled spaces (sinuses and mastoid air cells) (Table 92–2). Extracranial tissues should also be assessed (soft tissues, and orbits). Remember that cerebrospinal fluid (CSF) is secreted by the choroid plexus within each of the four ventricles. CSF flows from the two lateral ventricles into the third ventricle, through the aqueduct of Sylvius, into the midline fourth ventricle, and then enters the subarachnoid space. Expanded areas of the subarachnoid space are called cisterns.
- The role of contrast enhanced head CT scans in current practice is primarily limited to situations in which MRI is not readily available or is contraindicated. In general, contrast is used when there is a concern for an infectious or neoplastic process. Otherwise, if the noncontrast CT scan of the head shows no abnormalities, the likelihood of a significant finding on post–contrast-enhanced imaging is very low.

BOX 92–1 Radiation in Pregnancy

The golden rule: The mother's health is the primary concern. There is increased risk primarily of mental retardation, growth retardation, microcephaly, or intrauterine demise in a first-trimester fetus exposed to doses greater than 1 rad. A CT scan of the abdomen or pelvis, a CT scan of the lumbar spine, fluoroscopic studies, and studies involving multiple radiographs of the abdomen, pelvis, or lumbar spine can routinely exceed a fetal dose of 1 rad of ionizing radiation. When the radiation dose exceeds 1 rad, a radiation physicist should become involved to more accurately estimate fetal dose.

Rule number two: Always keep the radiation dose as low as reasonably achievable. The fetus should be shielded from the radiation to the greatest degree possible, and the study should be altered to reduce the exposure as much as possible, while still providing the necessary information. For studies other than single or two view radiograph examinations, obstetrics and radiology should be consulted if time and the clinical situation allow.

For renal colic, the preferred protocol is to begin with renal ultrasound to evaluate for obstruction with included images of the bladder using color Doppler to evaluate for the ureteral jets. If this is inconclusive, a *one-shot IVP (intravenous pyelogram)* is performed. This generally involves two to three radiographs. A CT scan is rarely of additional benefit.

Brain MRI

- An MRI of the brain may be ordered from the ED to rule out an acute stroke, cerebral aneurysm (when combined with MR angiography [MRA]), or other mass lesion. MRI has almost entirely supplanted contrasted CT scans of the head.
- For stroke, diffusion-weighted imaging can reveal most stokes within hours of onset. Generally noncontrast CT scans are performed initially to exclude hemorrhage or large infarcts with a high risk of hemorrhagic conversion. The patient is then treated according to the findings and an MRI is performed as soon as possible to confirm the diagnosis, evaluate the extent of infarction, and to help determine the cause.

Face
Maxillofacial CT Scan

- A maxillofacial CT scan is typically ordered for patients with trauma, soft-tissue infection (e.g., orbital cellulitis), or mass lesion involving the face. With the exception of the Panorex and mandible films, radiograph studies of the face are rarely ordered because a CT scan is far more accurate. The tradeoff is an increased radiation dose.
- Direct coronal images are acquired by placing the patient's neck in flexion, and tilting the gantry. When the patient's neck is immobilized (such as with trauma), or the patient cannot cooperate for proper

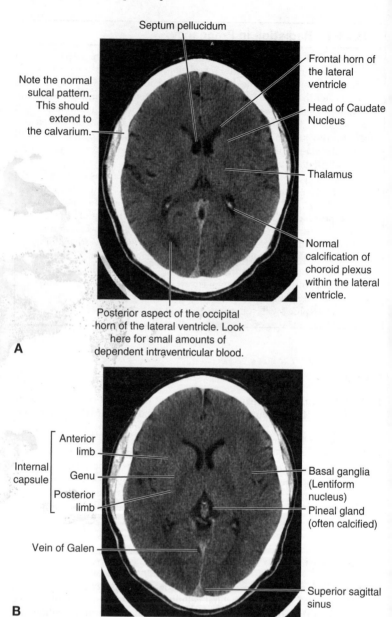

Septum pellucidum

Frontal horn of the lateral ventricle

Head of Caudate Nucleus

Thalamus

Normal calcification of choroid plexus within the lateral ventricle.

Note the normal sulcal pattern. This should extend to the calvarium.

Posterior aspect of the occipital horn of the lateral ventricle. Look here for small amounts of dependent intraventricular blood.

A

Internal capsule
Anterior limb
Genu
Posterior limb

Basal ganglia (Lentiform nucleus)

Pineal gland (often calcified)

Vein of Galen

Superior sagittal sinus

B

Figure 92–2. A–F: Noncontrast axial head computed tomography: normal anatomy.

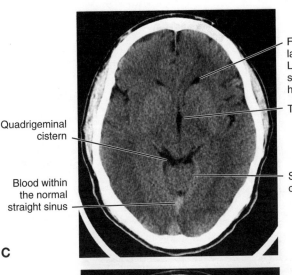

Frontal horn of lateral ventricle. Look here for signs of early hydrocephalus.

Third ventricle

Quadrigeminal cistern

Superior vermis of the cerebellum

Blood within the normal straight sinus

C

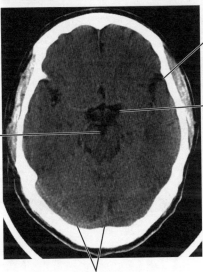

Interpeduncular cistern. This should always be visualized. If it is not it may be filled with subarachnoid blood.

Sylvian fissure. Search closely here for subarachnoid blood.

Suprasellar cistern. As the name implies, it sits just above the sella. It resembles a five point star in shape, and is a center point for the circle of willis. It is the most likely location for subarachnoid blood from a leaking anterior circulation aneurysm to collect.

Blood in the normal venous confluence and transverse sinus

D

Figure 92–2. *continued*

positioning, indirect reconstructions are often performed from the axial data. This is not as helpful as direct coronal imaging, but sometimes must suffice.

■ Facial anatomy on a noncontrast CT scan is reviewed in Figure 92–3. See Chapter 10 for a detailed discussion of facial fractures.

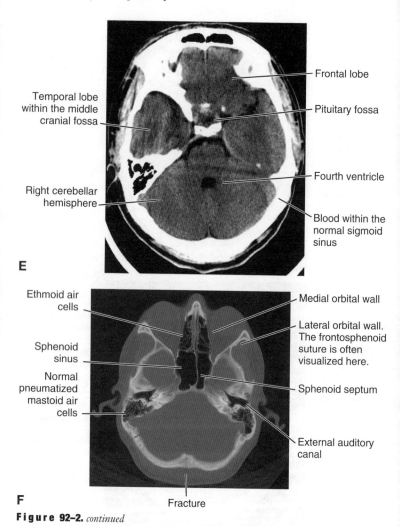

Frontal lobe

Temporal lobe within the middle cranial fossa

Pituitary fossa

Right cerebellar hemisphere

Fourth ventricle

Blood within the normal sigmoid sinus

E

Ethmoid air cells

Medial orbital wall

Lateral orbital wall. The frontosphenoid suture is often visualized here.

Sphenoid sinus

Normal pneumatized mastoid air cells

Sphenoid septum

External auditory canal

F

Fracture

Figure 92–2. *continued*

■ Evaluation of a CT scan of the face should include the soft tissues, paranasal sinuses, bones, and orbits. Use the soft-tissue window settings to evaluate the soft tissues and orbits. Use the bone window settings to evaluate the sinuses and bones. Search for fractures or blood layering within the sinuses. Blood within a sinus is a very strong indicator of fracture although some fractures may not be clearly visualized. Although air-fluid levels can be seen with nontraumatic sinus disease, on soft-tissue window settings, acute blood will typically have a higher density than simple fluid. Always evaluate the region of the cribriform plate as a disruption can lead to CSF leaks as well as intracranial spread of

Table 92–2	**Head CT Scan Evaluation**
	Abnormalities Found on Head CT Scan
Blood	Extra-axial blood may be due to subdural, epidural, subarachnoid, or intraventricular bleeding. An example of intra-axial bleed is an intracerebral hematoma. Acute blood is white. Blood is isodense within 1 week. Blood in the sphenoid sinus indicates a basilar skull fracture.
Brain	Any asymmetry such as the presence of a mass (tumor or abscess), contusion, mass effect, stroke, air, or abnormal gray-white matter differentiation. Loss of the differentiation occurs with cerebral edema. Effacement (compression of the sulci) is often the earliest evidence of increased intracranial pressure, edema, or hydrocephalus. Most cerebral infarcts are not detectable by noncontrast CT scans within the first 12-24 h. Focal areas of low density likely represent one of the following: air, fat, edema, encephalomalacia, or tumor. Encephalomalacia refers to a focal area of dead brain that has been resorbed leaving, for lack of a better description, a hole in the brain. A very common example are the small lacunar infarcts (lacunar means a small cavity). Air within the cranium is usually from fracture (either open fracture or fracture into an air filled sinus or cavity), or from a recent surgical procedure.
Bone	Any fracture, displacement, or lesion.
Cisterns	Any blood or decreased patency in any of the four cisterns: circummesencephalic, suprasellar, quadrigeminal, sylvian. This is the most likely location for subarachnoid blood from a leaking aneurysm to collect.
Ventricles	Any asymmetry or dilatation in one of the four interconnected ventricles in the brain. If the ventricles are enlarged, but the sulci are effaced (compressed), there is hydrocephalus. If all of the ventricles are enlarged, and the sulci are diffusely enlarged, the cause is likely atrophy with ex vacuo effect on the ventricles.
Air-filled spaces	Look for the presence of trauma, fluid, or inflammation. Fractures through the sinuses or mastoid air cells can result in intracranial pneumocephalus. Penetrating trauma can also cause this. An airfluid level in the sphenoid sinus or mastoid air cells are indirect evidence of a basilar skull fracture.

CT scan, computed tomography.

infections. Using the bone window settings, search for fractures or foreign bodies. Medial orbital wall fractures and fractures through the orbital floor are common injuries to the orbit. The coronal images (see Figure 92–4) are most helpful for evaluating the orbital floor and roof for herniation, and possible entrapment of orbital fat or muscles. Orbital roof fractures can cause intracranial injury as well. The orbital septum is

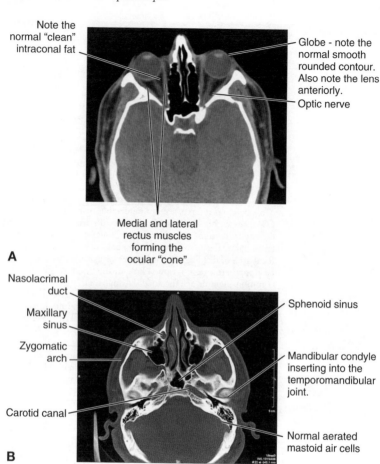

Note the normal "clean" intraconal fat

Globe - note the normal smooth rounded contour. Also note the lens anteriorly.

Optic nerve

Medial and lateral rectus muscles forming the ocular "cone"

A

Nasolacrimal duct

Maxillary sinus

Zygomatic arch

Carotid canal

Sphenoid sinus

Mandibular condyle inserting into the temporomandibular joint.

Normal aerated mastoid air cells

B

Figure 92–3 (A–B). Noncontrast axial facial computed tomography: normal anatomy.

a band of fibrous tissue that courses roughly between the anterior most aspect of the medial and lateral orbital walls. The septum separates the orbital contents from the eyelids and surrounding facial tissues that are prone to infection. The septum is sometimes visible on MRI; however, its location can be estimated on CT scan. Air posterior to the septum is referred to as intraorbital emphysema, and is abnormal.

■ For evaluation of maxillofacial trauma, contrast is only needed when there is concern for vascular injury in which case CT angiography (different contrast injection rate with thinner sections) should be performed. Contrast should be administered for the evaluation of infectious or neoplastic processes.

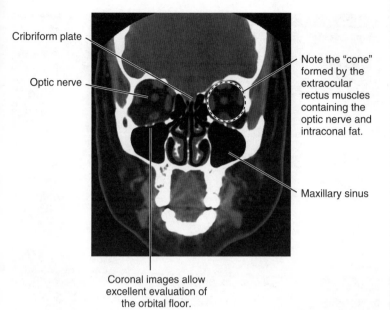

Cribriform plate

Optic nerve

Note the "cone" formed by the extraocular rectus muscles containing the optic nerve and intraconal fat.

Maxillary sinus

Coronal images allow excellent evaluation of the orbital floor.

Figure 92–4. Noncontrast facial CT: normal anatomy, coronal view.

Chest
Chest Radiographs

- Radiographs of the chest are typically ordered for patients with respiratory and cardiac complaints. A portable anteroposterior (AP) chest radiograph is needed for patients too sick to leave the ED, but the quality of such images is less optimal than the two-view PA and lateral study of the chest.
- Special views of the chest include lordotic views to better visualize the apex of the lungs, lateral decubitus (patient on one side) to determine the presence of free layering fluid, and oblique views (rib series) to detect rib fractures.
- Chest anatomy on a normal AP and lateral radiographs of the chest are summarized in Figure 92–5.
- A simplified approach to reviewing a chest radiograph is summarized in Table 92–3.

Chest CT Scans

- The caveat for CT angiography (CTA) is that the patient must be able to hold a breath for 30 seconds to 1 minute, there must be excellent intravenous access (at least 20 gauge not in the hand, foot, or wrist), and the patient's weight must not exceed the CT scan table limit (usually

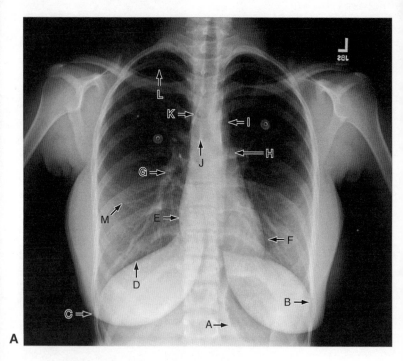

A

A - Air within the stomach.
B - Lateral costophrenic angle.
C - Soft tissue contour of the right breast. Note how the
    lower lungs appear whiter than the upper lungs.
    This is due to the overlying soft tissues attenuating
    the x-rays.
D - Right hemidiaphragm. Both hemidiaphragms should
    be well visualized. If they are not, suspect disease
    within the corresponding lower lobe.
E - Right heart border (right atrium). If the right heart
    border is not clearly visualized, there is likely
    disease within the right middle lobe.
F - Left heart border (left atrial appendage and left
    ventricle). If the left heart border is not clearly
    visualized, suspect disease within the lingula.
G - Right pulmonary artery.
H - Main pulmonary artery.
I - Aortic arch (knob). The space between H and I is the
    aortopulmonary window. It should always be seen,
    and if it is not, suspect a mass or lymphadenopathy.
J - Carina.
K - Right paratracheal stripe.
L - Posterior rib (3rd).
M - Anterior rib (4th).

Figure 92–5. Chest radiograph. *A,* Posteroanterior (PA) radiograph.

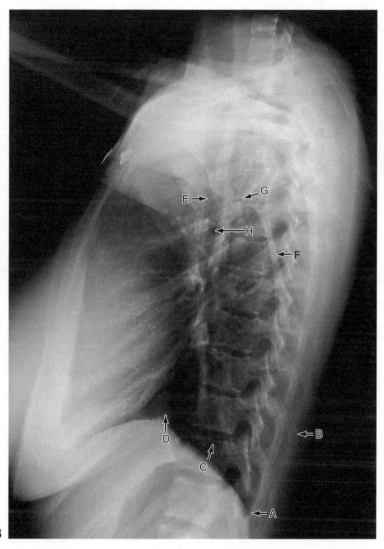

A - Posterior costophrenic angle.
B - Posterior right rib. The right ribs appear larger than the left due to magnification.
C - Spine. The spine should gradually become less dense towards the lung bases due to less structural overlap. If the lower spine is less dense than the upper spine, an infiltrate may be present in the lower lung or pleural space.
D - Inferior vena cava.
E - Trachea.
F - Scapula.
G - Aortic arch.
H - Left mainstem bronchus.

Figure 92–5. *B,* Lateral radiograph.

Table 92–3 Simple Approach to Evaluating a Chest Radiograph

*A*irway	Look for tracheal deviation consistent with a tension pneumothorax.
*B*reathing (lungs)	Consolidation may be due to edema, blood, pus, mucous, or neoplasm. A silhouette sign occurs if an area of lung becomes nonaerated (i.e., collapsed or consolidated), the densities of the structure and adjacent nonaerated lung become similar, and the structure becomes no longer visible (e.g., disease within the right middle lobe obscures the right heart border). Air bronchograms occur when portions of the lung become nonaerated, and these bronchi are no longer surrounded by air, but rather soft-tissue or water density. This causes them to become visible on the radiograph.
	Congestive heart failure: increased interstitial markings, increased vascularization, peribronchial cuffing, Kerley B lines, and alveolar edema.
	Atelectasis is volume loss. The only clear direct sign of a lobar atelectasis is displacement of the interlobar fissures toward the collapsed portions of lung. The atelectatic areas will usually appear more opaque than the surrounding aerated lung. A common cause of a moderate to large area of atelectasis (i.e., lobar collapse) is an obstructing neoplasm.
	Pneumothorax: end expiratory views are clearer. Look for an absence of lung markings or deep sulcus sign (see Diaphragms).
*B*ones	Evaluate for rib fractures or other bony pathology.
*C*ardiovascular	Assess the cardiac silhouette. A portable anteroposterior (AP) chest radiograph done on expiration makes the heart size appear bigger. Evaluate for aortic injury such as a widened mediastinum, inability to visualize the normal aortic knob, and descending thoracic aorta.
*D*iaphragms	Evaluate for free air underneath the diaphragm, flattening (e.g., chronic obstructive pulmonary disease), asymmetry, and loss of the costophrenic angle (e.g., effusion) or if the air collects in the costophrenic angle, the so-called "deep sulcus sign" may be visualized. This is when the costophrenic angle appears elongated extending along the lateral aspect of the abdomen.
*E*xtra tubes	Endotracheal tube: The end of the tube should be 2-4 cm above the carina.
	Tracheostomy: The tube should be located one half the distance from the stoma to the carina.
	Central line: A central venous catheter should be located above the right atrium; a pulmonary artery catheter should be located not more than 3-5 cm from the midline.
	Nasogastric tube: The nasogastric tube should be in the stomach (not the gastroesophageal junction), and should not be coiled up in the esophagus or trachea.
	Chest tube: For a pneumothorax, the tip should be directed posteriorly and superiorly, toward the apex. For an effusion, the tip of the tube should be directed inferiorly and posteriorly. The proximal side port in both situations should be within the chest cavity.

about 350 lb). Even technically poor studies can usually identify large emboli in the main or proximal segmental vessels.

■ Normal chest CT scan anatomy is illustrated in Figure 92–6. Pulmonary embolism and aortic dissection are two common diagnoses that are evaluated with an emergent CT scan of the chest (Figures 92–7a and 92–7b).

Abdomen
Abdominal Radiograph Films

■ The imaging evaluation of a patient with acute abdominal signs or symptoms may begin with radiograph examination to evaluate for bowel obstruction or free intraperitoneal air.

■ The *KUB* is a radiograph of the abdomen taken in a supine position centered on the region of the *K*idneys, *U*reter, and *B*ladder. It is not the ideal study in a patient with acute abdominal pain. The *acute abdominal series* is a series of three radiographs: an erect AP view of the chest, a supine AP view of the abdomen, and an erect AP view of the abdomen. A left-side–down lateral decubitus view can be substituted for the erect view in patients who cannot sit up. The upright (or decubitus) view is essential because large amounts of free intraperitoneal air can be impossible to recognize on a supine film. Also, air/fluid levels cannot be visualized on a supine film. The upright chest also allows for detection of intrathoracic processes that can mimic abdominal pathology clinically.

■ Bowel gas patterns seen on radiograph films of the abdomen are illustrated in Figure 92–8. See Chapter 18 for a small bowel obstruction as seen on plain film.

Abdominal CT Scan

■ A CT scan of the abdomen and pelvis is the study of choice for most acute abdominal conditions. Common exceptions include suspected cholelithiasis/cholecystitis and gynecologic processes that are better evaluated with ultrasound.

■ Oral contrast with dilute barium suspension or an iodinated water-soluble contrast agent should be used whenever feasible. The main exception is evaluation for traumatic injury in which delaying the examination for oral contrast is not appropriate. Oral contrast is particularly essential in thin patients and children because the lack of intra-peritoneal fat makes separation of bowel from pathology very difficult. It is important to allow appropriate time (about 3 hours) for the contrast to pass into the appendix and colon before scanning. An oral bolus should be given about 30 minutes before scanning to adequately opacify the stomach and duodenum. Rectal administration of contrast is occasionally needed as well.

■ Intravenous contrast is used for most studies. The main exception is renal colic studies in which intravenous contrast (particularly contrast excreted by the kidneys into the ureters) may cause obscuration of small calcifications. Significant pathology (particularly tumors of the liver, spleen, or pancreas) can easily go undetected on non–contrast-enhanced studies. Therefore, contrast should be utilized whenever possible.

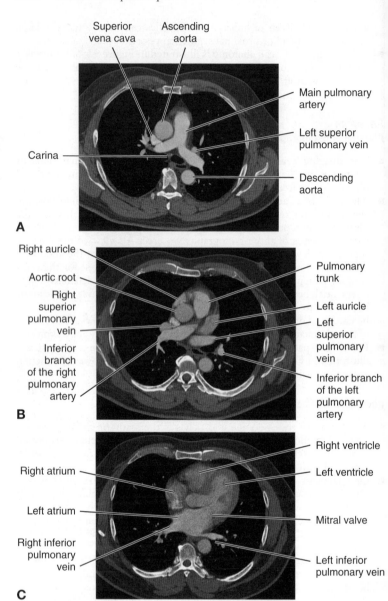

Figure 92–6. A–C Contrast-enhanced axial computed tomography of the chest: normal anatomy.

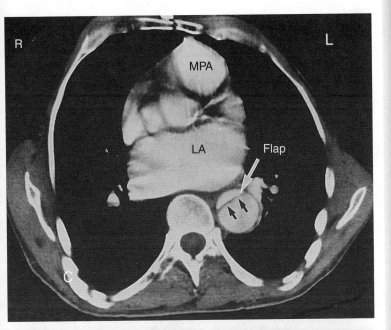

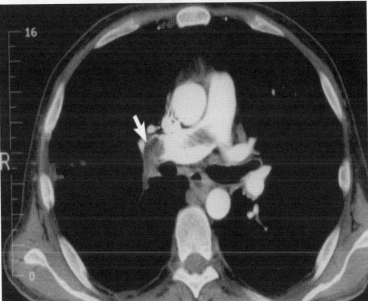

Figure 92–7. *A,* Chest CT in patient with an aortic dissection. The key imaging finding needed to diagnose aortic dissection is the intimal flap (arrow). This is a thin membrane separating the true and false lumens. It represents the aortic intima which is displaced and separated from the aortic media by the dissecting hematoma. *(From Mettler, FA. Essentials of Radiology, 2nd ed., 2005 Saunders, page 148, figure 5-33b.)* *B,* Chest CT revealing a pulmonary embolism. Large clot (arrow) obstructing the right main pulmonary artery. *(From Mettler, FA. Essentials of Radiology, 2nd ed., 2005 Saunders, page 137, figure 5-18c.)*

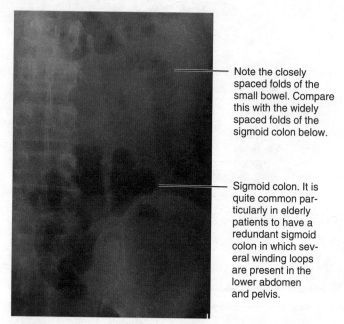

Note the closely spaced folds of the small bowel. Compare this with the widely spaced folds of the sigmoid colon below.

Sigmoid colon. It is quite common particularly in elderly patients to have a redundant sigmoid colon in which several winding loops are present in the lower abdomen and pelvis.

Figure 92–8. Abdominal plain film showing the colon and small bowel.

- Abdominal and pelvic anatomy of a contrast CT scan study is reviewed in Figure 92–9. See Chapter 18 for CT scan imaging examples of an abdominal aneurysm, appendicitis, and diverticulitis.

Extremities

- Plain films of the extremities are often obtained to rule out a fracture. A minimum of two perpendicular views must be ordered, usually in an AP and lateral projection, unless emergent intervention is required (e.g., immediate reduction of a dislocation in the presence of neuro-vascular compromise). Additional oblique views may be ordered.
- Most fractures in adults traverse the cortical surface. Plain films should be carefully evaluated for the presence of a cortical break. In contrast, impaction injuries may present with increased bone density representing compressed fractured bone. The fracture margins of an acute fracture are sharp or ill-defined and not well corticated.
- Refer to Chapter 17 (Extremity Trauma) for terminology used to describe fractures, special views of the extremities on plain film, and a brief discussion of common fracture types.
- Other concerning bone findings that may be visualized on plane films include bone tumors and osteomyelitis. Sclerotic or lytic bone lesions are concerning for a bone tumor. Metastatic bone lesions are more common in patients older than 40 years. A helpful mnemonic for remembering

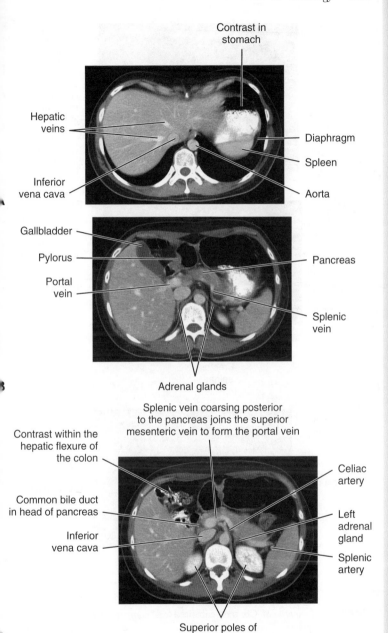

Figure 92–9. (A-J) Contrast-enhanced axial computed tomography of the abdomen and pelvis.

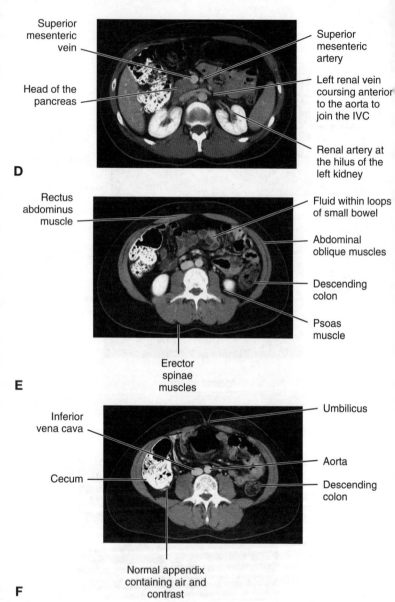

Superior mesenteric vein

Head of the pancreas

D

Superior mesenteric artery

Left renal vein coursing anterior to the aorta to join the IVC

Renal artery at the hilus of the left kidney

Rectus abdominus muscle

Fluid within loops of small bowel

Abdominal oblique muscles

Descending colon

Psoas muscle

Erector spinae muscles

E

Inferior vena cava

Cecum

Umbilicus

Aorta

Descending colon

Normal appendix containing air and contrast

F

Figure 92–9. *continued.* Contrast-enhanced axial computed tomography of the abdomen and pelvis.

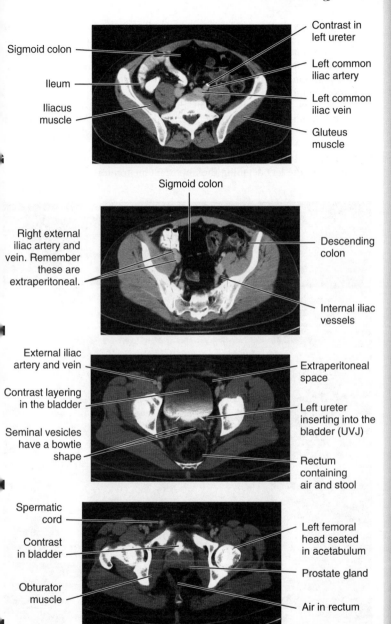

Figure 92–9. *continued.* Contrast-enhanced axial computed tomography of the abdomen and pelvis.

malignancies that metastasize to bone is *BLT and a kosher pickle*, which stands for the following: breast, lung, thyroid, kidney, and prostate. Plain films are not helpful early in the course of osteomyelitis, and will not show any abnormality for up to 2 weeks. Findings include soft-tissue swelling, bone destruction, and periosteal reaction. A bone scan or MRI is more helpful, especially early on.

■ A CT scan imaging is used in the evaluation of complicated joint fractures, but is seldom needed emergently in the ED. MRI is of limited use in the evaluation of acute extremity injury, but may be helpful in the evaluation of joint trauma or avascular necrosis.

■ Figures 92–10 through 92–15 show common normal plain film images ordered in the ED detailing the important anatomical findings.

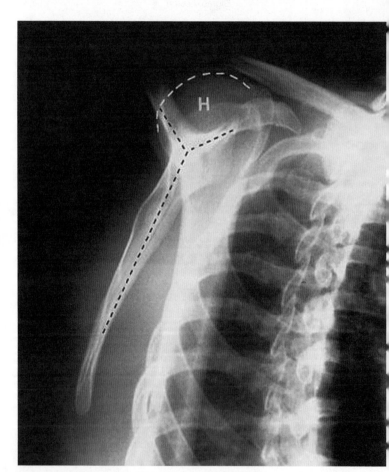

Figure 92–10. Normal oblique "Y" view of the shoulder. On this view, the elements of the scapula form a Y, and the humeral head should overlap the intersecting arms of the Y. *(From Mettler. Essentials of Radiology, 2nd ed. Philadelphia: Saunders, 2005.)*

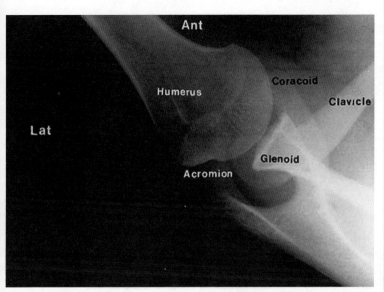

Figure 92–11. Normal axillary view of the shoulder. *(From Mettler. Essentials of Radiology (2nd ed). Philadelphia: Saunders, 2005.)*

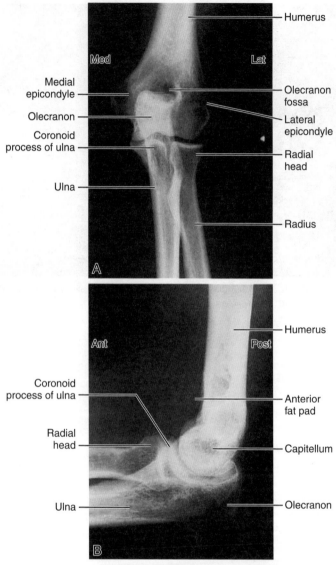

Figure 92–12. Normal anatomy of the elbow in the anteroposterior projection
(A) and in the lateral projection **(B)**. In the lateral projection, a normal elbow
should have an anterior humeral line, a radiocapitellar line, and absence of a large
anterior fat pad or any posterior fat pad. The anterior humeral line is an imaginary
line drawn on a lateral radiograph along the anterior surface of the humerus
through the elbow. Normally this line transects the middle third of the capitellum.
The radiocapitellar line is an imaginary line drawn through the midradial shaft and
should normally pass through the capitellum on any radiographic projection. *(From
Mettler. Essentials of Radiology, 2nd ed. Philadelphia: Saunders, 2005.)*

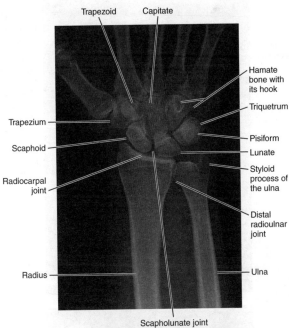

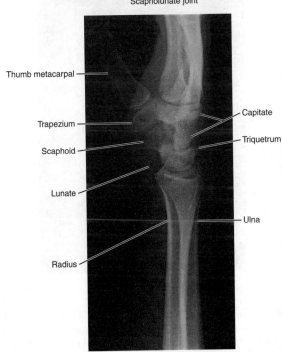

Figure 92–13. Normal anatomy of the wrist in anteroposterior (A) and lateral (B) projection.

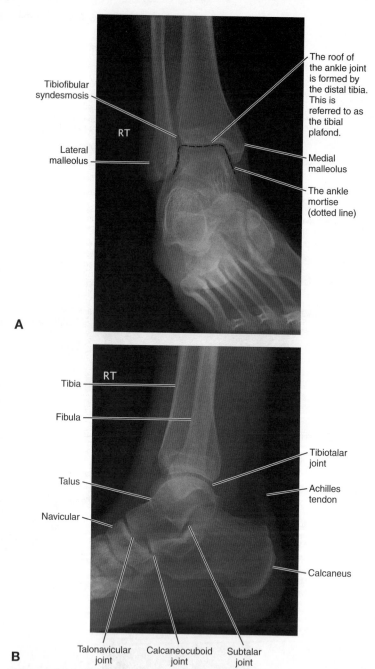

Figure 9-14. Normal anatomy of the ankle in anteroposterior (AP) **(A)** and lateral **(B)** projection. The AP view in this figure is a mortise view in which the ankle is positioned in approximately 10 to 15 of internal rotation. The purpose of this view is to evaluate articulations of the tibia and fibula with the talus. On a standard AP view, there is overlap of the lateral talus and distal fibula, limiting evaluation of this area.

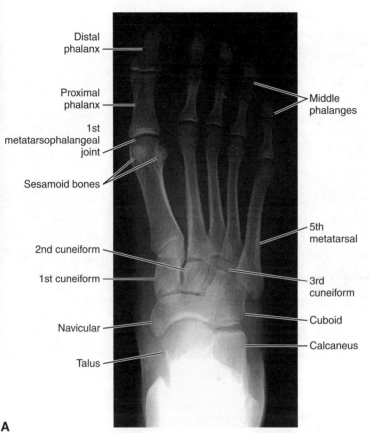

A

Figure 92–15. Normal anatomy of foot in the anteroposterior **(A)** and lateral **(B)** projection.

Continued

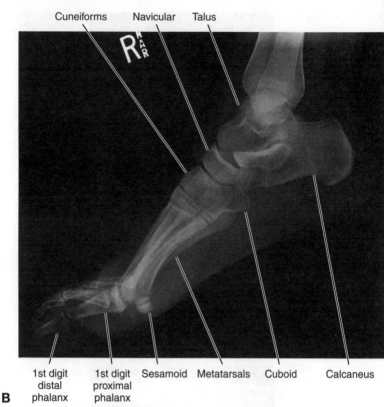

Cuneiforms   Navicular   Talus

R

1st digit distal phalanx   **1st digit proximal phalanx**   Sesamoid   Metatarsals   Cuboid   Calcaneus

B

Figure 92–15. *continued.* Normal anatomy of foot in the anteroposterior **(A)** and lateral **(B)** projection.

Suggested Readings

Bettmann MA. Frequently Asked Questions: Iodinated Contrast Agents. Radiographics 2004; 24:S3-S10.

Huda W, Slone RM. Review of Radiologic Physics, 2nd ed. Philadelphia: Lippincott Williams & Wilkins, 2003.

Mettler FA Jr. Essentials of Radiology, (2nd ed). Philadelphia: Saunders, 2005

Wiest PW, Roth CK. Fundamentals of Emergency Radiology. Philadelphia: Saunders, 2006.

CHAPTER 93

Emergency Ultrasound

CHALENE A. CORINALDI ■ ANDY KAHN ■ P. J. KONICKI

Overview

Bedside sonography is a rapid, noninvasive, portable, easily repeatable procedure that attempts to answer focused, clinical questions.

There are six primary indications for emergency ultrasound: detection of hemoperitoneum or hemopericardium, aortic aneurysm, pericardial effusion, intrauterine pregnancy, cholelithiasis, and hydronephrosis. Indications for emergency ultrasound use continue to change and rapidly expand.

Principles

- *Echogenicity.* Provides high-frequency sound waves (pulses) to obtain images of internal organs. These pulses can be absorbed, refracted, or reflected. The quantity and speed at which the pulses return determine what is displayed on the monitor. Describes how *bright* or *white* an image is relative to the surrounding tissue. Sound waves are conducted quickly through fluid producing a black (*anechoic*) image. In contrast, sound waves are conducted poorly through dense structures like bone, which produces a white (*hyperechoic*) image. The variable echoes produced depend on how fast sound is conducted through a particular tissue. Body habitus, bowel gas, subcutaneous emphysema, and air in tissue spaces all tend to obscure ultrasound images.
- *Transducer (probe).* The choice of probe depends on the type of study being performed. In general, lower frequency probes (2.5-5 MHz) are used to scan deeper structures (i.e., aorta, heart and kidney) and higher frequency probes (5-10+ MHz) are used for superficial structures (i.e., intercavitary, soft tissue, and vascular access). The indicator on each probe is directed by the sonographer to produce a particular scan plane. The basic scan planes are transverse, longitudinal (sagittal), coronal, and oblique (Table 93–1).
- The term *window* is used to describe the anatomic image produced, depending on where the ultrasound probe is placed on the patient's body. For example, common windows for imaging the heart in the ED include the subcostal (or subxiphoid) and the parasternal windows (Figures 93–1 through 93–3). The *axis* for a particular window can be changed by rotating the probe 90 degrees.

Table 93–1	Basic Scan Planes
Longitudinal	Indicator directed toward patient's head. A plane that runs from head to foot and would divide the patient into right and left halves.
Transverse	Indicator rotated 90 degrees from longitudinal. This plane divides the body into upper and lower portions and extends from side to side.
Oblique	Indicator between longitudinal and transverse.
Coronal	Indicator directed toward patient's head, but scanning from patient's sides (flank areas). This plane divides the patient into anterior and posterior halves.

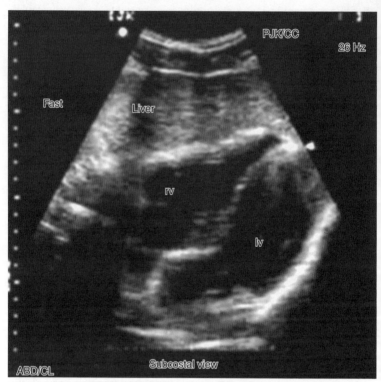

Figure 93–1. Subcostal view. Place probe in the subxyphoid area and angle upward under the costal margins toward the left shoulder.

Focused Assessment with Sonography for Trauma

- *Background.* Focused assessment with sonography for trauma (FAST) is the most common beside ultrasonographic application. A review of anatomy is helpful before scanning. The *pericardium* (subxyphoid) is a layer of tissue that surrounds and protects the heart. It consists of an outer fibrous

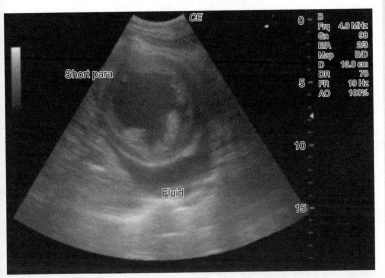

Figure 93–2. Short parasternal axis view revealing the left ventricle with surrounding effusion. The parasternal short view is obtained at the same parasternal window as the long view with the transducer now rotated 90 degrees so that the marker is toward the right hip. *(From Tang A, Euerle B. Emergency department ultrasound and echocardiography. Emergency Medicine Clinics of North America, 2005;23:1179–1194.)*

layer that attaches to the diaphragm, sternum, and ribs, and an inner, serous, layer that is adherent to the heart. The normal volume of pericardial fluid between these two layers is 20 ml (usually not visible). The *pleural space* is a potential space between the lung and pleura above the diaphragm. *Morrison's pouch* (right upper quadrant [RUQ]) is a potential space created by Glisson's capsule of the liver and Gerota's fascia of the kidney. Because it is the most dependent part of the upper peritoneal cavity, detection of free fluid is most sensitive in this area. *Paracolic gutters* are spaces between the kidneys and psoas muscles. The *splenorenal recess* (left upper quadrant [LUQ]) is the space between the spleen and the kidney. The bladder lies posterior to the symphysis pubis; the uterus and rectum are posterior to the bladder. The *cul de sac* (pelvis) refers to the rectovesical pouch in males and rectouterine pouch (pouch of Douglas). It is the most dependent part of the lower abdomen.

- **Indications.** Evaluation of patients with blunt or penetrating trauma of the torso for free intraperitoneal or pericardial fluid. Especially useful in unstable patients when computed tomography is not advisable and for trauma in pregnancy.
- **Technique.** There are four basic views used to identify free pericardial or intraperitoneal fluid. These include the subxyphoid (pericardial), RUQ (hepatorenal recess/Morrison's pouch), LUQ (splenorenal recess), and pelvis (cul de sac). Ultrasound is used to identify free fluid in these potential spaces (Table 93–2). A normal FAST scan on the initial evaluation

Table 93–2	Basic Views of the FAST Examination	
	Technique	**Abnormality**
Cardiac	The subxyphoid (also called subcostal, see Figure 93–1) is most commonly used. The pericardium is the thin white line surrounding the heart.	An abnormal scan demonstrates fluid (black) surrounding the heart.
RUQ view	Start with indicator toward patient's head. Place probe at the right mid to posterior-axillary line between the eleventh and twelfth ribs. Turn probe obliquely (indicator toward bed) to scan *between* the ribs. Sweep the area with the probe to visualize liver, kidney, paracolic gutter, and pleural space. Scan both in longitudinal and transverse. The white line above the liver is the diaphragm.	An abnormal scan demonstrates fluid (black) between liver and kidney (Morrison's pouch), in paracolic gutter, or pleural space (directly above diaphragm) (see Figure 93–4).
LUQ view	Start with indicator toward patient's head. Place probe at left posterior axillary line between the tenth and eleventh ribs. If the kidney is seen first, move probe cephalad to visualize the spleen. Turn probe obliquely (indicator toward the bed) to scan *between* ribs. Sweep the area with the probe to visualize spleen, kidney, paracolic gutter, and pleural space. Scan both in longitudinal and transverse.	An abnormal scan demonstrates fluid (black) between diaphragm and spleen, between the spleen and kidney, in paracolic gutter, or above diaphragm (pleural space) (see Figure 93–5).
Pelvis view	Start with indicator toward patient's head. Place probe midline on the lower abdomen just above symphysis pubis. If you do not see the bladder (well-circumscribed and fluid-filled) aim probe caudally toward patient's feet. Rotate probe 90 degrees counterclockwise to obtain transverse images. Use a sweeping motion with the probe while scanning to visualize the bladder, uterus, areas posterior to both. The bladder provides an acoustic window for better visualization. If a Foley catheter is placed prior to the exam, the Foley bag can be clamped or raised above the patient to re-introduce fluid into the bladder.	An abnormal scan demonstrates a hypo- or anechoic area (fluid) posterior to the bladder (see Figure 93–6).

FAST, focused abdominal sonography in trauma; LUQ, left upper quadrant; RUQ, right upper quadrant.

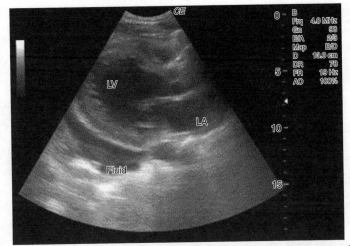

Figure 93–3. Long parasternal axis view of pericardial effusion. The parasternal window is located immediately to the left of the sternum in the second, third, or fourth intercostal space. The transducer is oriented along the long axis of the heart, from the right shoulder to the left hip, with the marker toward the left hip. The depth should be in the lower range because the heart is close to the anterior chest wall. LA, left atrium; LV, left ventricle. *(From Tang A, Euerle B. Emergency department ultrasound and echocardiography. Emergency Medicine Clinics of North America, 2005;23:1179–1194.)*

does *not* mean there is no free fluid. Blood can take time to accumulate so *repeat* the examination when there is the clinical probability of intraperitoneal injury, or if the patient condition worsens. Use the 2.5- to 3.5-MHz curvilinear probe (see Figures 93–1 through 93–6).

- *Limitations.* Unable to visualize less than 200 ml of fluid. Poor identification of solid organ, bowel, diaphragm, and retroperitoneal injury. Cannot distinguish ascites from blood. Limited examination with obesity and subcutaneous emphysema.

Vascular Applications: Aortic Aneurysm

- *Background.* The abdominal aorta is a retroperitoneal structure that lies anterior to the lumbar spine. It enters the abdominal cavity at T-12 (subxyphoid), and bifurcates at the level of the umbilicus. It is shorter than 3 cm and tapers distally. The main branches are the celiac trunk, superior mesenteric artery, renal arteries, inferior mesenteric artery, and common iliac arteries. The inferior vena cava lies to the right of the aorta and spine. The presence of an abdominal aortic aneurysm (AAA) is acurately determined with an ultrasound study.
- *Indication.* Suspected ruptured AAA. Rupture usually occurs in patients with diameters over 5 cm. Risk of rupture is directly related to the size of the aneurysm. With rupture the operative mortality is 50%.
- *Technique.* Use 2.5- to 3.5-MHz curvilinear probe. Landmarks: The *spine* (white with posterior shadow) is posterior and the *inferior vena*

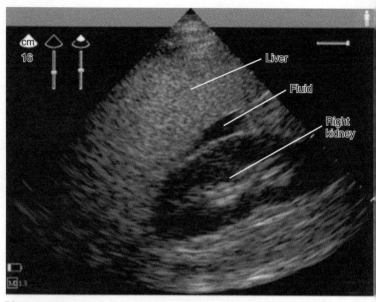

Figure 93–4. Free fluid in the hepatorenal interface (Morrison's pouch). (*From: Rose JS. Ultrasound in abdominal trauma. Emerg Med Clin North Am, 2004;22:581–599.*)

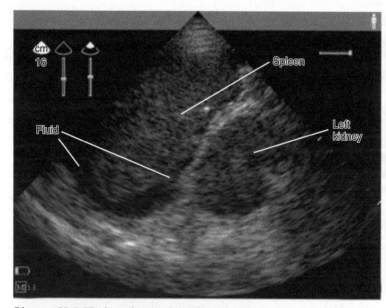

Figure 93–5. Fluid in splenorenal interface. Note that fluid in the subphrenic space is larger than in the splenorenal space due to the phrenicolic ligament. (*From: Rose JS. Ultrasound in abdominal trauma. Emerg Med Clin North Am, 2004;22:581–599.*)

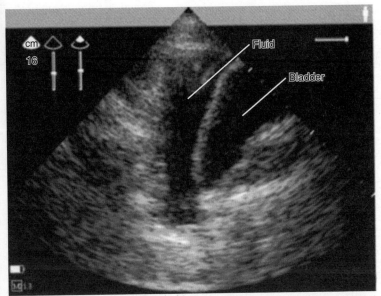

Figure 93–6. Longitudinal pelvic view with intraperitoneal fluid seen outside of the bladder. (*From: Rose JS. Ultrasound in abdominal trauma. Emerg Med Clin North Am, 2004;22:581–599.*)

cava (IVC) is adjacent to the aorta. A common error is to mistake the IVC for the aorta. You can distinguish the IVC (thinner wall) from the aorta (thicker wall) by compression (IVC collapses), having the patient "sniff" (IVC collapses), or using color-flow Doppler. To scan longitudinally place the probe in the subxyphoid area slightly to the left of midline (indicator to patient's head). Slowly move the probe inferiorly to scan the entire abdominal aorta from the diaphragm (subxyphoid area) to the bifurcation of the iliac arteries (near umbilicus). To scan transversely rotate indicator 90 degrees counterclockwise and repeat above. Scan and measure the aorta in both *longitudinal and transverse* planes. The normal abdominal aorta is less than 3 cm (outer-to–outer wall) and tapers distally. An aortic diameter over 3 cm *or* 1.5 times that of the proximal segment is considered to be an aneurysm (Figure 93–7).

- *Findings.* Aneurysm, mural thrombus, linear flap (dissection), true and false lumens, hemoperitoneum (suggests rupture), hydronephrosis (from compression of ureters).
- *Limitations. Unable to confirm rupture of aneurysm* due to poor visualization of retroperitoneal space, unable to evaluate proximal and distal extension of aneurysm. Views are obscured by bowel gas, body habitus, and free air.

Cardiac Applications

- *Indications.* Cardiac arrest, hypotension, acute chest pain, and trauma (refer to FAST section). Echocardiography is reliable in evaluating pericardial effusions. Lack of cardiac motion in asystole and pulseless

Thrombus

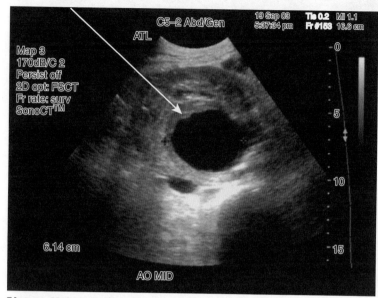

Figure 93–7. Transverse image of abdominal aortic aneurysm measuring 6.14 cm with thrombus. (*From: Barkin AZ, Rosen CL. Ultrasound detection of abdominal aortic aneurysm. Emerg Med Clin North Am 2004;22:675-82.*)

electrical activity (PEA) can be confirmed visually. Ejection fraction can also be estimated by bedside sonography, and can help distinguish between cardiogenic and septic shock in a hypotensive patient.

- ■ **Technique.** Use 2.5-MHz curvilinear or flat, phased array probe. If feasible, place patient in left lateral decubitus position with left hand under head for optimal images. Basic views used in the ED are listed in Table 93–3 (Figures 93–1, 93–2, 93–3, and 93–8).
- ■ **Findings.** Pericardial effusion (anechoic stripe around heart), pericardial tamponade (effusion, collapse of right ventricle in diastole, swinging heart), no cardiac motion (asystole, PEA), abnormal ventricular wall motion (myocardial ischemia, infarction, etc.), dilated or thickened cardiac chambers, ascending aortic aneurysm/dissection (aortic root >5 cm; possible linear flap; difficult to assess without transesophageal echocardiography), thrombus, vegetations, valvular abnormalities, pacemaker capture (visualizing contraction of ventricles with pacemaker spike) and location of trravenous pacer (should be in the right ventricle).
- ■ **Limitations.** Subcutaneous emphysema, pneumopericardium, large anteroposterior diameter (chronic obstructive pulmonary disease; COPD), chest wall deformities. Pitfalls: mistaking pericardial fat for pericardial fluid, and not recognizing, pericardial hematoma. Fat lies *anterior* to the heart, can look hypoechoic; fluid pools in *posterior* pericardial space; blood clot may be initially echogenic.

Table 93–3	**Basic Views of the Cardiac Examination**
Subxyphoid (subcostal)	Place probe in subxyphoid space with indicator to patient's left. Angle probe so that it is almost parallel to abdominal wall. Aim toward left shoulder. Best view to evaluate pericardial space, can see four chambers (see Figure 93–1).
Parasternal short	Rotate probe indicator 90 degrees clockwise to the patient's left shoulder (2 o'clock) from the PSL view. Visualize the left ventricle, mitral valve, left atrium, right ventricle, and aortic valve (see Figure 93–2).
Parasternal long (PSL)	Place probe on third to fourth intercostal space directly to the left of the sternum. Rotate probe indicator to right shoulder (10 o'clock). Visualize the left atrium, mitral valve, left ventricle, aortic valve, and aortic root (see Figure 93–3).
Apical four-chamber	Place probe on the fifth intercostal space (nipple line) with indicator toward patient's left. Angle probe toward patient's right shoulder. Visualize a coronal view of all four chambers of the heart (see Figure 93–8).

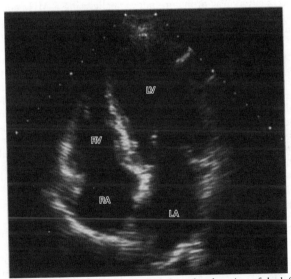

Figure 93–8. Normal, transthoracic, apical, four-chamber view of the left ventricle (LV) and right ventricle (RV) in a normal heart depicting the relationship between the LV and RV, with the LV being normally larger than the RV, and the IVS bulging slightly toward the RV. *(From Beaulieu Y, Marik PE. Bedside ultrasonography in the ICU (Part 1). Chest 2005;128:881–895.)*

Obstetric and Gynecologic Applications

- **Background.** The uterus lies posterior to the bladder. The fundus either rests superiorly on the bladder (anteverted) or points posteriorly (retroverted). The nonpregnant uterus is usually shorter than 7 cm in length and the ovaries are smaller than 3 cm. Fallopian tubes are usually not visualized by ultrasound. The cul de sacs lie anterior and posterior (pouch of Douglas) to the uterus. The adnexa contain ovaries and iliac vessels. Ovaries are oval-shaped structures in the adnexa with peripheral hypoechoic follicles. For optimal views, the full bladder is used as a window in the transabdominal examination and the bladder is emptied for the endovaginal examination.

- **Indications.** Establish location of pregnancy and fetal heart rate in the symptomatic first trimester pregnant patient or asymptomatic pregnant patient with risk factors for ectopic pregnancy, detection of fetal cardiac movement in patients in their second or third trimester, and evaluation of pregnant trauma patients. Early intrauterine pregnancy (IUP) is demonstrated by a gestational sac surrounded by a double decidual (DD) layer in the endometrial cavity, a yolk sac, or a fetal pole. Transabdominally, a gestational sac can be seen as early as 5.5 to 6 weeks. Endovaginally at 4.5 to 5 weeks. An IUP should be visualized at a beta-human chorionic gonadotropin (β-hCG) level of 1000 IU/L. Cardiac motion may be seen at 6 weeks.

- **Technique.** Pelvic ultrasound can be performed transabdominally using 3.5-MHz curvilinear probe or endovaginally using 5-MHz endovaginal probe. Transabdominal scanning should be performed on pregnant trauma patients with vaginal bleeding due to possible placenta abruption. For endovaginal scanning, place cover on endovaginal probe (gel in condom or glove covering probe and on outside of cover). Gently insert probe into the vagina or ask patient to insert probe (Table 93–4).

- **Findings.** Gestational sac, double decidual sign, yolk sac, fetal pole (Figure 93–9), cardiac activity, free fluid in cul de sacs, adnexal masses, or fluid. Other findings may include ovarian cysts, uterine hypo or hyper-echoic masses (fibroids), fluid in fallopian tubes (hydro or pyosalpinx), or tubo-ovarian abscess.

- **Limitations.** Early gestations (unable to see gestational sac), inability to visualize all ectopic pregnancies, fibroids, or intrauterine devices (IUDs) that obscure views.

Hepatobiliary Applications

- **Background.** The gallbladder (GB) has a fundus, body, and neck. It connects directly to the cystic duct, which joins the common hepatic duct to form the common bile duct (CBD). The CBD runs anterior to the portal vein and to the right of the hepatic artery. The CBD empties into the duodenum. Main portal triad consists of the portal vein, CBD, and hepatic artery.

- **Indications.** Suspected biliary etiology for abdominal pain (cholelithiasis, cholecystitis).

- **Technique.** Longitudinal, transverse with 3.5-MHz probe. Place probe longitudinally in subxyphoid area and slowly move it laterally along the

Table 93–4 Technique for Gynecology Ultrasound

	Plane	Technique
Transabdominal (uses bladder as a window)	Longitudinal	Place probe in midline just superior to symphysis pubis; indicator to patient's head. Visualize bladder (triangular) and uterus directly posterior to bladder. A hyperechoic endometrial stripe is oriented longitudinally in the nonpregnant patient. In the pregnant patient an intrauterine pregnancy is represented by a gestational sac in the endometrial cavity, double decidual sign, yolk sac, or fetal pole. Use sweeping motions from right to left to evaluate entire uterus and adnexa. Look for fluid between uterus and bladder (anterior cul de sac), posterior to uterus (pouch of Douglas), and adnexal masses/fluid.
	Transverse	Rotate probe 90 degrees counterclockwise. Should see bladder, then ureters posterior to bladder, and adnexa laterally. Sweep caudal and cephalad from fundus of uterus to cervix. Endometrial stripe is oriented horizontally. Measure fetal heart rate (B/M mode).
Endovaginal (empty bladder)	Longitudinal	Obtained when the indicator is facing the ceiling. Visualize uterus by sweeping probe anteriorly/posteriorly and adnexa by sweeping probe laterally.
	Transverse	Obtained by rotation of indicator 90 degrees counterclockwise. Visualize uterus from fundus to cervix. Sweep probe laterally, anteriorly and posteriorly to visualize adnexa. Look for endometrial gestational sac, fluid in cul de sacs, adnexal masses/fluid. Measure fetal heart rate (B/M mode).

inferior costal margin until GB is seen. Keep probe angled up towards the shoulder. If having difficulty visualizing the GB, ask the patient to inhale and hold a deep breath to bring the GB down from under the costal margins. Positioning the patient on the left side may also facilitate visualization of the gall bladder (GB and bowel gas descends). Once the GB is found, rotate the probe, keeping the GB visualized to obtain *longitudinal* and *transverse* views. *The classic view* is that of the main lobar

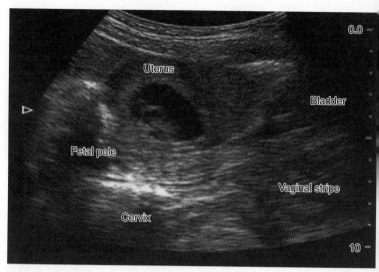

Figure 93–9. Intrauterine pregnancy. Transabdominal sagittal view shows bladder anteriorly, vaginal stripe posteriorly, and fetal pole within a gestation sac located in the anteverted uterus. *(From Tang A, Euerle B. Emergency department ultrasound and echocardiography. Emergency Medicine Clinics of North America, 2005;23:1179–1194.)*

fissure (hyperechoic line) connecting the neck of GB to the right portal vein. *Short of gallstones, this is the only confirmation that the gallbladder is the object being scanned.* Scan in both planes. Gallstones usually appear echogenic with posterior acoustic shadowing (dark area beneath stones). If the gallstones are very small, there may be no shadowing. A gallstone-filled bladder commonly reveals a WES (wall echo shadow) sign, which appears as an anechoic stripe of bile between an echogenic anterior wall and a posterior echogenic line of stones with significant posterior shadowing. Look for signs of *cholelithiasis*: gallstones, sludge (dependent gray material within GB), and *cholecystitis*: stone plus dilated transverse GB (>5 cm), thickened anterior GB wall (>4 mm), pericholecystic fluid, a positive sonographic Murphy's sign (probe compression at fundus of the GB elicits pain and blocks inhalation). Cholecystitis is still primarily a *clinical* diagnosis. To view the *portal triad*, place the probe in the right epigastric area aimed toward the right shoulder. This will give you a *longitudinal view* of the portal vein with the hepatic artery and the CBD directly above. Rotate the probe 90 degrees counterclockwise to get a *transverse* image of the portal vein, CBD (anterolateral), and hepatic artery (anteromedial). This is the classic "Mickey Mouse" sign where the left "ear" is the CBD, right "ear" is the hepatic artery, and the "face" is the portal vein. The normal CBD usually measures (inner to inner wall) less than one tenth of the patient's age, and up to 1 cm for those with a history of cholecystectomy.

- *Findings.* Gallstones, sludge, impacted stone, a dilated GB, a thickened anterior GB wall, pericholecystic fluid, a dilated common bile duct (suggests stone in duct), a positive sonographic Murphy's sign. Other findings include folds and polyps (do not move with repositioning).

■ *Limitations.* Mistaking the bowel or a vessel for the GB, wall thickening can be caused by a contracted GB (recent, <4 hours since last oral intake or other disease states [i.e., ascites, liver disease]), air in biliary tree or bowel gas obscuring views, ascites mimicking cholecystitis, and difficulty visualizing CBD stones.

Renal Applications

■ *Background.* The kidneys are retroperitoneal. The normal renal cortex is hypoechoic when compared to surrounding tissue (liver, spleen), and the renal sinus is hyperechoic. When the urinary tract is obstructed, hydronephrosis is observed as a dilated renal pelvis and separation of calyces. Hydronephrosis is graded from minimal (I) to severe (III). Renal stones are highly echogenic with posterior acoustic enhancement.

■ *Indications.* Renal colic; detection of hydronephrosis

■ *Technique.* Using 3.5-MHz probe, scan both kidneys coronally from the upper to the lower poles in longitudinal and transverse planes. Also scan the bladder. Place a probe longitudinally in the midaxillary line. To obtain a transverse view, rotate the probe 90 degrees away from the midline. The normal kidney is 9 to 12 cm in length.

■ *Limitations.* Inability to detect the cause of obstruction and ureteral stones; false positives with full bladder, masses, cysts, blood vessels.

Other Applications

■ Other common emergency ultrasound procedures are briefly discussed below. Other advanced applications are listed in Table 93–5.

■ *Intravenous line placement.* Ultrasound gel is first placed into a sterile cover or glove, then a linear probe (7.5 MHz) is inserted. Sterile lubricant

Table 93–5   Other Applications of Ultrasound Used by Emergency Medicine Physicians

Vascular (Doppler)	Deep venous thrombosis
Cardiac	Left ventricular function in hypotensive states or cardiac arrest
Testicular	Hydrocele, epididymitis, torsion, trauma
Intra-abdominal	Appendicitis
Orbital	Retinal detachment, hematoma, optic nerve measurements correlating with intracranial pressure
Musculoskeletal	Fractures, fracture reduction, arthrocentesis
Airway	Endotracheal tube placement
Obstetric	Second- and third-trimester bleeding to detect placenta previa

(i.e., Surgilube) is placed between the glove and patient. Veins usually are larger and more compressible compared to adjacent arteries. Color-flow Doppler can be used to confirm vascular structures by detection of blood flow, and to distinguish the pulsatile flow of arteries from that of veins. The needle appears as a hyperechoic (white) structure appearing in the field of view during the dynamic technique. The remaining techniques for insertion of peripheral, internal jugular, and femoral lines are the same. The exception to this is subclavian vein catheterization. This is done via a supraclavicular approach. The skin puncture site for subclavian vein access is approached at 1 cm lateral to the sternal notch and 1 cm superior to the clavicle. The probe is inferior to the needle and angled caudally. The number of attempts and time to central venous access is improved with ultrasound guidance.

■ *Abscess detection and incision.* The linear probe can detect abscesses as hypoechoic or anechoic collections with possible posterior acoustic enhancement. Color-flow Doppler may also show increased blood flow to the surrounding area due to hyperemia and inflammation. Abscesses can be measured, and extent of drainage assessed.

■ *Foreign body detection and removal.* Wooden foreign bodies are usually radiolucent on plain films. They can appear hyperechoic with shadowing in an ultrasound study, and may be removed using ultrasound assistance by a static or dynamic technique.

■ *Thoracentesis.* Anechoic pleural fluid can be distinguished from the echogenicity of the diaphragm (white) and lung tissue (gray, mobile). Pleural fluid appears anechoic and a needle can be visualized during the procedure.

■ *Paracentesis.* Abdominal organs, floating bowel, and area of maximal anechoic fluid are visualized to safely place a needle for drainage of ascitic fluid.

■ *Pericardiocentesis.* Pericardial fluid appears anechoic. Ultrasound is used to detect the area with maximal fluid, and the needle entry can be visualized during the procedure. Saline can be injected to localize a needle in the pericardial space.

Teaching Points

Ultrasound technology has become a useful tool in the practice of emergency medicine. It was initially introduced for some very focused clinical assessments such as the presence of hemoperitoneum, an abdominal aortic aneurysm, a pericardial effusion, or an ectopic pregnancy. There are many other useful clinical questions to answer with ultrasound studies, such as its utility for diagnosis of cholecystitis, abscesses, foreign bodies, appendicitis, venous extremity thrombosis, as well as to assist in the performance of many EM procedures, such as central line placement. As ultrasonography becomes a familiar tool for the emergency physician to use, more and more usage will be defined for its role in emergency medicine.

Suggested Readings

Beaulieu Y, Marik PE. Bedside ultrasonography in the ICU (Part 1). Chest 2005;128:881–895.

Ma OJ, Mateer JR. Emergency Ultrasound. New York: McGraw-Hill, 2003.

Tang A, Euerle B. Emergency department ultrasound and echocardiography. Emergency Medicine Clinics of North America, 2005;23:1179–1194.

CHAPTER **94**

Wound Care

Suneet Singh ■ Nikolas Mendrygal ■ Lynn P. Roppolo

Overview

The vast majority of traumatic lacerations present to the emergency department (ED), and are managed by emergency physicians. The primary goals of intervention are to maintain function, minimize scarring, and prevent infection.

There are three types of closure performed in the ED. Closure by *primary intention* is closure of a wound in the ED at the time of presentation (i.e., suturing). *Delayed primary closure* (also known as tertiary intention) is closure of the wound 3 to 5 days after initial presentation (before the formation of granulation tissue), to decrease the risk of infection. *Secondary intention* is healing of an open wound that has loss of tissue or infection such that tissue surfaces cannot be approximated. The wound is usually not sutured closed. Granulation tissue is allowed to form, followed by a large scar formation. Epithelium ultimately grows over the scar tissue.

There are four tissue layers in most traumatic lacerations: epidermis, dermis, subcutaneous, and fascia. The epidermis and dermis are treated as one layer in regard to wound care. Closure of this layer provides the wound with most of its strength. The subcutaneous layer consists primarily of adipose tissue and adds little to wound strength. The fascial layer involves deeper structures. The fascia is a specialized connective tissue layer that surrounds muscles, bones, and joints. Wounds involving the fascial layer are complex wounds that often require a multi-layered closure.

Wound healing is a gradual but complex process that begins with epithelization that occurs within 48 hours. This creates a barrier over the wound that prevents outside contamination. It is estimated that only 60% of the wound's optimal tensile strength is achieved by 4 months.

This chapter will focus on common lacerations presenting to the ED. Other types of wound care are discussed in other chapters. Abscess drainage is described in Chapter 91. High-pressure injection injuries and hand infections requiring surgical drainage are discussed in Chapter 17.

Initial Diagnostic Approach

- ***General.*** Assess the ABCs (*a*irway, *b*reathing, and *c*irculation) using advanced cardiac life support (ACLS; see Chapter 6) and advanced trauma life support (ATLS; see Chapter 8) guidelines described previously. In regards to the wound, initially perform a rapid assessment of the injury, and manage emergent conditions expeditiously (i.e., hemorrhage control, fracture reduction for vascular compromise, etc.)

- ***History.*** Evaluate for the presence of any host factors that may have an adverse effect on wound healing such as old age, diabetes, immuno-compromised state, malnutrition, or coagulopathy. Determine the exact time that the injury occurred. To minimize the risk of infection, wounds on the extremity should be closed within 6 to 10 hours. Wounds in highly vascular areas such as the face and scalp can be closed without increased infection risk as long as 24 hours after injury. Each patient should be considered individually as the number of hours that has elapsed before a wound can be closed is not clearly defined. The mechanism of injury is essential to identify the potential for other injuries (e.g., fractures, tendon laceration), wound contamination, or foreign bodies (e.g., glass, teeth). Crush injuries result in more devitalized tissue, and are more prone to infection. Inquire about tetanus immunization and allergies (i.e., anesthetic agents, antibiotics, latex). If the injury involves an upper extremity, the dominant hand should be noted. Determine if any prehospital care was provided (cleansing, irrigation, hemostasis control). Early wound cleaning may prevent proliferation of bacteria contaminating the wound, and should be taken into consideration in patients with a delayed presentation to the ED. If the injury involves a bite wound, obtain a detailed history of the source of the bite and the potential need for rabies prophylaxis.

- ***Physical examination.*** Perform a more thorough wound evaluation complete with a detailed motor and neurovascular examination. Most wounds require local anesthesia in order to thoroughly examine and clean the area. Note the presence of wound contamination, devitalized tissue, foreign bodies, and involvement of deeper structures. For extremity injuries, active and passive range of motion should be performed of the injured area while the wound is being explored to completely identify injury to underlying structures (e.g., tendons). Elements that should be included in the physical examination of any wound are summarized in Table 94–1. The hand examination is summarized in Table 94–2.

- ***Plain films.*** Obtain when radio-opaque foreign bodies (Chapter 33) are suspected to be within the wound. Order radiographs even if foreign bodies are removed on initial examination to ensure smaller or hidden objects are not still present. Also assesses for underlying fractures, which, if present, are considered open fractures requiring emergent intervention. Last, evaluate for gas in the soft tissues, which may be

Table 94–1	**Physical Examination of Wounds**
Length	In centimeters or inches; measure it.
Location	Anatomical location; be as precise as possible. Diagrams may help.
Wound edges	Clean or untidy.
Depth	Superficial, partial thickness, full thickness, muscle, or bone.
Contamination and foreign bodies	A full evaluation may not be possible until the wound is fully prepared. See Chapter 33 for Foreign Bodies.
Tendon injury	A full evaluation may not be possible until the wound is fully prepared. Perform full range of motion of the injured part, and note the integrity of any visible tendons.
Fractures or dislocation	May be obvious on physical examination or on radiograph. The presence of this in association with an open wound is an orthopedic emergency (see Chapter 17).
Sensory	Should be done before the administration of anesthesia. Checking sensation to light and soft touch is all that is needed. Check two-point discrimination in hand injuries (normal 1-6 mm).
Motor	Full range of motion of the affected area should be evaluated. If pain is a limiting factor, local and systemic analgesia should be administered first.
Vascular	Check capillary refill, palpate pulses, or use the Doppler to assess blood flow (including digital pulsations for hand injuries). Apart from the absence of any signal, arterial injury may be suggested by a change in the usual triphasic quality of the Doppler pulse to a biphasic or monophasic wave form as the pulse is "damped" by partial occlusion. Perform the Allen's test on the hand (see Appendix 2).

secondary to an infection caused by a gas-forming organism (i.e., *Clostridia* species).

- *Ultrasound.* An ultrasound study is a useful adjunctive tool for quick bedside assessment for foreign bodies. This modality can also assess for radiolucent objects such as wood.
- *Computed tomography (CT scan).* A CT scan is not commonly required, but can be used if foreign bodies are suspected, especially if small and of similar density to soft tissues.

Emergency Department Management Overview
General

- The ABCs always take precedence to managing any wound.

Table 94–2 **Examination of the Hand**

Nerve	Motor	Sensory*
Radial nerve	Extend the wrist	Dorsal first web space
Median nerve	Oppose the tips of the thumb with index finger or little finger as if holding a teacup.	Volar tip of the index finger
Ulnar nerve	Abduct and adduct the fingers	Volar tip of the little finger

Evaluation of Intrinsic Muscles	Muscle Function
Touch the tip of the thumb to the tip of the little finger	Thenar muscles
Abduction and adduction of fingers	Interossei muscles
Flex the MCP and extend the PIP and DIP	Lumbricals
Oppose the thumb and radial side of the index finger to form a circle while the examiner uses one finger to pull the disrupt the circle.	Abductor pollicis muscle

Evaluation of Extrinsic Muscles	Tendon Function
Bend the tip of the thumb	Flexor pollicis longus
Bend the DIP of each finger while the examiner holds the PIP of that finger in extension	FDP
Bend the PIP of each finger while the examiner hold the other fingers in extension (to block function of FDP)	FDS
Flex the wrist	Flexor carpi ulnaris, flexor carpi radialis, and palmaris longis
Abduct the thumb	Abductor pollicis longus and brevis
Extend the wrist against resistance	Extensor carpi radialis longus and brevis
Extend and adduct (ulnar deviate) the wrist	Extensor carpi ulnaris
Place hand palm down and elevate the thumb	Extensor pollicis longus

DIP, distal interphalangeal; FDP, flexor digitorum profundus; FDS, flexor digitorum superficialis; MCP, metacarpophalangeal; PIP, proximal interphalangeal.
*Because some overlap occurs between various sensory nerves, it is preferable to test sensation in those areas least likely to have dual innervation.

Medications

- *Analgesia and sedation.* Systemic pain relief with oral or intravenous (IV) opioids for severe pain. Avoid nonsteroidal anti-inflammatory drugs (NSAIDs) if ongoing hemorrhage is an issue. Local anesthesia is discussed in subsequent sections. For larger wounds, multiple wounds necessitating wound management, or patients experiencing a significant amount of preprocedural anxiety, procedural sedation with an anxiolytic, analgesic, and amnestic agents may help provide a better environment to manage the wounds, and thus enhance better patient care and satisfaction (see Chapter 90.1). For more extensive or complicated wounds (e.g., arterial, tendon injuries), repair should be performed in the operating room under general anesthesia by a qualified consultant. For pediatric patients, restraints may be required to supplement other techniques used to facilitate patient cooperation (i.e., analgesia, conscious sedation, anesthesia, distraction, parental involvement). A papoose board or similar restraint is often needed. The need for restraint should be explained to both the parents and child.

- *Local anesthesia.* The extent of the injury will determine the particular agent and method utilized. True allergy to local anesthetics is rare, and usually involves the anesthetic's preservative. If a true allergy does exist, a local anesthetic from a different class or 1% diphenhydramine should be used. The common amide anesthetics include lidocaine, mepivicaine, and bupivacaine. The two common esters include procaine and tetracaine. An easy way to remember this is that the generic name of all amides contain the letter "I" twice. Topical anesthetic agents are used mostly with children. TAC (tetracaine 0.25%-0.5%, adrenaline 0.025%-0.05%, cocaine 4%-11.8%) is the original topical anesthetic used. Due to the cocaine component, it has occasionally been associated with dysrhythmias, seizures, and cardiac arrest. LET (lidocaine 4%, epinephrine 0.1%, tetracaine 0.5%) has a better safety profile. Avoid using it on large wounds and mucous membranes to minimize toxicity from the anesthetic agents. Apply 1 to 3 ml onto the wound and wound edges with a cotton-tipped applicator. The gel formulation does not need to be covered but the solution formulation does. It is usually effective within 20 minutes, at which time the skin around the wound appears blanched due to the effect of epinephrine. Most wounds can be managed with infiltration of lidocaine 1% locally into the noncontaminated wound margins. Depending upon the site of injury, lidocaine with premixed epinephrine may be used for better hemostasis in highly vascular areas such as the scalp and oral cavity. Epinephrine should not be used on the eyes, ears, nose, fingers, toes, nipples, or genitalia. See Tables 94–3 and 94–4 for dosing of local anesthetics commonly used in the ED. To minimize the pain associated with local infiltration, use the smallest needle and inject slowly. A 25 or 27 gauge should be used. Buffered lidocaine has been shown to be less painful, and is prepared by using a 10:1 ratio of 1% lidocaine to 0.9 mEq/L sodium bicarbonate. Infiltrating through the wound margins (and not through the overlying skin) is recommended, and may also be less painful. If the wound is contaminated or infected, a field block or infiltration through healthy intact skin is preferable. Wipe intact skin with isopropyl alcohol or povidone-iodine

Table 94–3 Comparison of Common Local Anesthetic Agents

| Drug | Plain Solution | | | With Epinephrine |
	Concentration, %	Maximum Dose,* mg/kg	Duration	Maximum Dose,* mg/kg
Short duration Procaine	0.5, 1, 2	7	20-30 min	10
Moderate duration Lidocaine	0.5, 1, 2	5	1.5 h	7
Mepivacaine	0.5, 1, 2	5-7	3 h	10
Long duration Bupivacaine	0.25, 0.5	2.5†	3 to 6 h	3-5

*Maximum doses are controversial and irrelevant because toxicity is caused by the free, unbound form and not the total dose given or the plasma peak concentration. Epinephrine prolongs the duration of action and decreases systemic absorption.

†The dose of bupivacaine should not exceed 400 mg in a 24-h period. Systemic toxicity is much higher than other topical agents due to high potency and protein binding.

Table 94–4 Calculation of Anesthetic Doses

Anesthetic Dose,%	Strength, mg/ml
0.25	2.5
0.5	5
1	10
2	20

solution prior to infiltration. Always aspirate the needle just prior to injecting to avoid intravascular injection. Subsequent injections of anesthetic should overlap a region that was just anesthetized to minimize pain associated with puncturing the skin or subcutaneous tissue. Regional nerve blocks provide the added benefit of not further distorting the wound architecture, providing a broader area of anesthesia, and causing less discomfort in areas in which local infiltration would be very painful (Table 94–5).

- *Antibiotics.* May be administered to reduce wound infections, though no evidence exists of its efficacy. Prophylactic antibiotics should be given for heavily contaminated wounds, bite or puncture wounds, prevention of endocarditis, any association with an open joint or fracture, or an immunocompromised state. First-generation cephalosporins, such as cefazolin 1-2 g IV every 6 to 8 hours, will cover for staphylococcal and streptococcal organisms. For contaminated open fractures, gentamycin can be added for gram-negative coverage. For nonbite wounds, the duration of antibiotic prophylaxis is generally 3 to 7 days with an oral agent such as cephalexin 500 mg four times per day. Penetrating wounds generally require a broad-spectrum antibiotic to select for organisms particular to the individual injury (e.g., amoxicillin-clavulanate for animal

Nerve	Area Affected	Technique	Image
Digital	Isolated finger. For the thumb and fifth, all four digital nerves (two volar, two palmar) must be blocked. The second through fourth digits are supplied by only the palmar branch except for the skin of the proximal dorsal digit.	The digital nerves are located at the 2, 4, 8, and 10 o'clock in relationship to the bone. Inject on the dorsal (preferred due to thinner skin and less pain) or volar surface. Inject 0.5-1.0 ml on each side of digit in the web space.	 Needle redirected without withdrawal from the skin Second puncture site anesthetized
Radial	Dorsum of lateral hand and first through third and lateral half of fourth digits proximal to DIP	Inject lateral to the palpable artery at the level of the palmar crease. Inject 2 to 5 ml at the depth of the artery. Inject 5 ml in a SQ field block from the initial point of injection to the dorsal midline.	 Superficial radial nerve
Median	Volar surface of radial distribution plus distal to DIP	Insert the needle perpendicularly on the radial border of the palmars logis tendon just proximal to the proximal wrist crease. Advance slowly until a pop is felt as the needle penetrates the retinaculum. Inject 3 to 5 ml of anesthetic.	 Flexor carpi radialis, Median nerve, Flexor digitorum superficialis, Palmaris longus tendon

Continued

Table 94–5 Regional Blocks—*cont'd*

Nerve	Area Affected	Technique	Image
Ulnar	Medial half of fourth and all of fifth digit volar and dorsal plus medial aspect of hand	Lateral approach (preferred): insert needle on the ulnar aspect of the wrist at the proximal palmar crease, and direct horitontally under the flexor carpi ulnaris (FCU) toward the ulnar bone. Inject 3 to 5 ml of anesthetic as the needle is slowly withdrawn. Inject an additional 5 ml of anesthetic from the lateral border of the FCU tendon to the dorsal midline.	
Supraorbital/ Supratrochlear	Forehead superficial to the eyebrow and lateral to the lambdoid suture.	Inject 3-6 ml of anesthetic deep and parallel to the eyebrow to reach both medial (supratrochlear) and lateral (supraorbital) branches.	

Table 94-5 Regional Blocks—*cont'd*

Nerve	Area Affected	Technique	Image
Infraorbital	Cheek from lower eyelid to upper lip and lateral aspect of nose, lateral side of the face	Inject 2-3 ml at anesthetic either directly percutaneous or intraoral (more prolonged) at the upper premolar tooth. Use topical anesthetic for intraoral route.	Infraorbital nerve
Mental	Lower lip and chin	Inject 1-2 ml of anesthetic either directly percutaneous or intra-oral (less painful) at the lower second premolar. Use topical anesthetic for intra-oral route.	Mental nerve

Digital block: (From Roberts: *Clinical Procedures in Emergency Medicine* [4th ed]. Philadelphia: WB Saunders, 2004, p 581.)
Radial nerve block: (From Roberts: *Clinical Procedures in Emergency Medicine* [4th ed]. Philadelphia: WB Saunders, 2004, p 577.)
Ulnar/Median nerve block: (From Roberts: *Clinical Procedures in Emergency Medicine* [4th ed]. Philadelphia: WB Saunders, 2004, p 575.)
Color face block picture: (From Miller: *Miller's Anesthesia* [6th ed]. New York: Churchill Livingstone, 2005; Wedel OJ, Horlocker TT: *Nerve Blocks, Appendix Color Atals. In: Miller RM. Miller's anesthesia* (6th ed). Philadelphia: Elsevier, 2005, plate 1.)
Lammers RL, Trolt TT: *Methods of wound closure. In: Roberts JR, Hedges JR. Clinical Procedures in Emergency Medicine* (4th ed). Philadelphia: Saunders, 2004, pp 575-581.

Table 94–6 Recommendations Tetanus Prophylaxis in Wound Management

History of tetanus toxoid administration	Clean, minor wounds		All other wounds**	
	Tetanus toxoid*	Immuno-globulin	Tetanus toxoid*	Immunoglobulin
Unknown or < 3 doses	Yes	No	Yes	Yes (250IU HTIG*** or 3000 IU equine tetanus antitoxin)
> 3 doses	No, unless >10 years since last dose	No	No, unless >5 years since last dose	No

Tetanus and diphtheria toxoids, adsorbed (for adult use). For children <7 years old, DTP (DT, if pertussis vaccine is contraindicated) is preferred to tetanus toxoid alone. For persons >=7 years old, Td is preferred to tetanus toxoid alone.
**All other wounds contaminated with dirt, feces, and saliva; puncture wounds; avulsions; and wounds resulting from missiles, crushing, burns, and frostbite.*
***HTIG: Human tetanus immunoglobulin*

bites and fluoroquinolone for penetrating injury through athletic shoes, etc.). Topical antibiotics should be applied for the first 3 days (until epithelization occurs) on all wounds closed with sutures or staples to minimize infection. These agents also prevent adherence of the dressing to the wound, and reduce the formation of the crust that develops which separates the wound edges.

- **Tetanus.** Current recommendations are listed in Table 94–6. Be sure that the booster and immunoglobulin are not administered into the same anatomic site.

- **Rabies.** Immunoprophylaxis requires both passive immunization with antibody (immune globulin) and active immunization with vaccine (Table 94–7). Both parts of this treatment must be given, even when treatment is delayed. Human rabies immune globulin (HRIG) 20 IU/kg should be administered as soon after the bite as possible. If possible, the entire dose of HRIG should be infiltrated into and around the wound(s). Any remaining volume should be injected intramuscularly at a site distant from the vaccine. Local or state agencies should be contacted first to determine the need for postexposure prophylaxis (PEP). If immediate consultation is required and local agencies are unavailable, emergency physicians can call the Division of Viral and Rickettsial Diseases at the Centers for Disease Control and Prevention (CDC) at 404-639-1050 during business hours, and at 404-639-2888 on nights, weekends, and holidays.

Wound Preparation

- **Sterile vs. clean technique.** Wound care in the emergency department is handled under sterile conditions utilizing sterile gloves, needles, laceration repair kits, sutures, and so forth.

Table 94–7   Determining the Need for Rabies Prophylaxis

Animal Type	Evaluation and Disposition of Animal	Postexposure Prophylaxis Recommendations
Dogs, cats, and ferrets	Healthy and available for 10-d observation	Persons should not begin prophylaxis unless animal develops clinical signs of rabies
	Rabid or suspected rabid	Immediately vaccinate
	Unknown (e.g., escaped)	Consult public health officials
Skunks, raccoons, foxes, and most other carnivores; bats	Regarded as rabid unless animal proven negative by laboratory tests[‡]	Consider immediate vaccination
Livestock, small rodents, lagomorphs (rabbits and hares), large rodents (woodchucks and beavers), and other mammals	Consider individually	Consult public health officials Bites of squirrels, hamsters, guinea pigs, gerbils, chipmunks, rats, mice, other small rodents, rabbits, and hares almost never require antirabies postexposure prophylaxis

(From CDC. Human rabies prevention—United States, 1999: recommendations of the Advisory Committee on Immunization Practices [ACIP], MMWR 1999;48:1.)

- *Hemostasis.* Direct pressure is the best method to control bleeding. If the bleeding is arterial, only attempt ligation if it is a minor peripheral vessel on an extremity. Never attempt blind clamping with hemostats as this can create tissue ischemia and damage vital structures such as a tendon, nerve, or artery. If the bleeding vessel can be visualized, establish proximal control with a 5-0 absorbable suture. If the vessel is not seen, sutures placed using the figure-of-eight suture technique can be attempted to obtain hemostasis. Only in extreme circumstances can a blood pressure cuff be applied proximal to the wound and inflated approximately 30 mmHg higher than the systolic pressure for 30 minutes to tourniquet the bleed. Ensure that the tourniquet is not on longer than 1 hour because longer ischemia times are associated with tissue necrosis. If bleeding cannot be controlled, surgery should be consulted.
- *Irrigation.* Good evidence exists that the key to prevention of wound infections is copious high pressure irrigation. Normal saline is generally considered the irrigant of choice. Tap water can also be used as an irrigant. Do not use hydrogen peroxide or iodine because these can actually impair local host resistance to microbes as well as damage tissue directly. Dilute povidone-iodine solution (1%) does not have any advantage over tap water or normal saline. In general, irrigate with at

least 50 to 100 ml per centimeter of laceration into the wound through a 19- to 20-gauge needle or angiocatheter attached to a 50-ml syringe to generate a pressure of 15 to 25 pounds per square inch (psi). Commercial devices that use high-pressure pulsatile flow should be used cautiously as they can paradoxically create tissue ischemia if administered too closely to the wound. Significantly contaminated wounds may require more irrigation fluid and higher pressures.

- *Hair.* Hair should only be removed by clipping as shaving may increase risk for infection. Hair should not be removed from the eyebrows as there is a chance that it may not grow back.
- *Foreign body removal.* All foreign bodies must be removed, especially if they are easy to remove with little risk for complication. Other foreign bodies that should be removed include reactive materials such as wood; any contaminated object such as dirt, rock, and clothing; foreign bodies in the foot; any impingement upon neurovascular structures or joints; or impairment of function. The risk of removing a foreign body must be balanced against the benefit of removing it. A deep, inert foreign body may not be worth the risk associated with removing it (see Chapter 33).
- *Debridement.* This involves removing all obvious debris and necrotic tissue from the wound that can increase the risk for infection. Devitalized tissue should be removed to establish clean wound edges prior to closure. Tissue loss should be minimized if possible especially on the face. Use a 15-blade scalpel or a pair of iris scissors for debridement. Gentle scrubbing may be effective in older wounds.

Wound Closure

- Depending upon the mechanism and time elapsed before the patient's arrival at the ED, the initial decision is to determine if the wound should heal via primary intention (immediate reapproximation), delayed primary closure (reapproximation after waiting 3-5 days), or secondary intention (no reapproximation).
- In delayed primary closure, the wound is prepared, debrided, and irrigated in the same manner as for immediate closure. The wound should then be packed to prevent it from closing on its own (i.e., wet-to-dry dressing). If on an extremity, the injury should be splinted and dressed, and appropriate wound care instructions should be given. The patient should return for a wound check and packing change in 24 hours, and instructed to follow up in another 72 hours for definitive repair. In 4 to 6 days after the initial injury, the dressing is removed, which debrides the wound. If there is good granulation tissue and no signs of infection, a no. 15 blade scalpel is used to remove the granulation tissue before suturing. If granulation tissue has not formed, the closure is considered a delayed primary closure. If granulation tissue has formed, this is considered a secondary closure. It is safe, and probably easier to do a delayed primary closure. The wound can then be irrigated and sutured. Follow-up and suture removal are the same as for primary closure.
- Types of sutures are listed in Table 94–8. General suturing principles are listed in Table 94–9. Common suture techniques used in the ED are summarized in Table 94–10. In general, skin and tendons are repaired with nonabsorbable sutures, and deeper tissues are repaired with

Table 94–8   Common Suture Material in the Emergency Department

	Suture Material	Indications
Absorbable sutures	Chromic gut	Intraoral lacerations Vascular ligation Muscle repair
	Polydioxanone (PDS)	Muscle repair and dermal approximation. Can be used for intraoral mucosa.
	Vicryl	For subcutaneous and mucosal closures.
Nonabsorbable sutures	Silk	Easy to handle and comfortable for the patient. Good for the lips, nose, or nipples.
	Nylon	Commonly used for skin closure.
	Polypropylene (Prolene)	Commonly used for skin closure especially in hair covered areas due to the blue color contrast.

Table 94–9   General Suturing Principles

Repair all layers	This will help minimize scarring, eliminate dead space, decrease tension on the wound, and promote healing. Once fascial layers are reapproximated, the subcutaneous (SC) is sutured. This is the fatty and fibrous SC tissue (hypodermis).
Evert wound edges	For better cosmetic results. The needle should be perpendicular to the skin with each bite and follow the arc of the needle. Go deeper than wide. Enter the opposite wound margin at the same level. Horizontal or vertical mattress sutures can improve inversion. Never place mattress sutures on the face.
Suture placement	For lengthy wounds, start in the middle to avoid a dog ear. Make sure all sutures are equidistant from the wound edge and each adjacent suture. The distance between each suture varies on the location and the patient (e.g., 5-10 mm on the scalp, 2-4 mm on the face). Make sure the knot lies flat. Pull knots off to the side of the wound margin. Avoid suturing too tightly. Subcutaneous sutures should not have long suture tails left in the wound.
Other	Be gentle in handling tissue with forceps to avoid causing further injury.

Table 94-10 Common Suture Techniques

	Technique	Use	Image
Simple interrupted	Sutures are placed equidistant from one another until the wound is completely approximated.	Most common technique. If one stitch in the closure fails, the remaining stitches continue to hold the wound together	
Simple continuous	The first suture is placed similar to the simple interrupted fashion. The difference lies in that the needle is not cut off, but instead is continually re-introduced across the entire length of the wound until ultimately being tied off at the end. Each bite is made at a 45-degree angle to the wound margin, but the complete suture is perpendicular to it. The last loop is placed just beyond the end of the wound, and the suture is tied, with the last loop used as a "tail" in the process of tying the knot.	Used for clean wounds that are under little or no tension and are on flat, immobile skin surfaces in patients who have no medical conditions that would impair healing.	
Horizontal mattress	After the initial needle throw across the two sides of the wound, the suture is not tied off. The needle is re-inserted just adjacent to the location at which it has just exited, and then comes back across the wound to come out adjacent to the initial throw. The two ends of the suture are now adjacent and can be tied off.	Ideal for areas that have redundant tissue (web space of the hand, elbow) or are under tension. Mattress sutures are typically not placed on the face.	

Table 94–10 Common Suture Techniques—*cont'd*

Technique	Use	Image
Vertical mattress	Best technique for wound edge eversion. Ideal for areas that have redundant tissue (web space of the hand, elbow) or are under tension. Mattress sutures are typically not placed on the face.	
	The first needle throw is large and deep as it crosses the two sides of the wound. After this throw, the needle is then reversed, re-enters the side it has just exited, but is now more proximal while remaining in-line with the initial throw. This subsequent throw is both smaller and more superficial as it comes back across the wound to exit adjacent yet within the area of the initial larger bite. The suture is then tied off.	
Subcutaneous (buried knot)	For deeper lacerations to approximate the SC layer	
	The initial needle throw is deep within the dermal layer and exits more superficially at the epidermal-dermal junction on the same side of the wound. The next needle throw is directly across at the same depth on the opposite side of the wound and is placed at the epidermal-dermal junction. The needle exits deeper within the dermis such that the ensuing knot is now buried within the deeper layers of the dermis. The suture may be placed obliquely rather than vertically to facilitate knot tying. Avoid long tails but should be long enough to prevent unraveling.	

Continued

Table 94–10 Common Suture Techniques—*cont'd*

	Technique	Use	Image
Figure-of-eight	The most common approach is illustrated to the right. The area to be sutured is divided into four quadrants (a–d). Enter in at "a" through the skin through the SC tissue to the other side at point "b." Cross over the wound diagonally to point "c" and go through the SC tissue to cross to the other side at point "d." Tie this end of the suture with the original end at point "a."	For wounds with friable tissue, or to tamponade bleeding	

(Reproduced from Roberts: *Clinical Procedures in Emergency Medicine* (4th ed). Philadelphia: WB Saunders, 2004, pp 670, 674, 678.)

absorbable sutures. All sutures are sized by diameter with smaller ones being designated by more "O's" (i.e., 5-O suture is smaller than 4-O). Keep in mind that the longer the sutures stay in, the more scarring from the suture itself. Depending upon the material, the suture can be monofilament or braided. Monofilament sutures (e.g., nylon, polypropylene, polydioxanone [PDS], plain gut and chromic gut) have less tissue reactivity (i.e., lower inflammatory reaction rates and less associated infections), but are weaker. Braided sutures are stronger, but are more prone to bacterial overgrowth. Differing means of suture placement exist, and which to use is determined by considering wound location, wound edge characteristics, and tissue tension. Recommended sizes of sutures and removal guidelines are listed in Table 94–11. Special techniques for suturing are described in Table 94–12.

- The management of bite wounds is summarized in Table 94–13. Evaluate all bite wounds for injuries to deep structures, such as tendons, joint capsules, blood vessels, nerves, and bone. Meticulous cleansing, irrigation, and debridement are necessary. Tetanus and rabies prophylaxis are discussed in Table 94–6 and 94–7.
- Alternatives to suturing include tissue adhesives, staples, and tape (steri-strips) and are summarized Table 94–14. The wound should be cleaned and irrigated in the same manner as for sutures.
- Skin avulsions can be treated with gelfoam or a nonadhering gauze pressure dressing such as adaptic or xeroform. Larger avulsions can be repaired by excision of the wound margins with extension and undermining. Plastic surgery may need to be consulted for more extensive wounds.
- Closing a wound loosely is occasionally discussed as an option in the treatment of contaminated wounds. This choice is rarely, if ever, utilized. The loosely closed wound approximates the tissue margins enough to allow the wound to seal itself completely within 48 hours. The infection

Table 94–11   Suture Size and Removal Guidelines

Location	Suture Size	Removal (days)
Scalp	4-0, 5-0	5-8
Face	5-0, 6-0	3-5
Chest/abdomen	3-0, 4-0	7-10
Back	3-0, 4-0	10-12
Upper extremity: joint surface	3-0, 4-0	10-12
Upper extremity: nonjoint surface	4-0, 5-0	7-10
Lower extremity: joint surface	3-0, 4-0	12-14
Lower extremity: nonjoint surface	3-0, 4-0	7-10

*Steri-strips should be applied to nonhairy areas after removal

Table 94–12 Special Suturing Techniques

	Suture	Anesthesia	Recommendations for Closure
Face	6-0 nonabsorbable for the skin (Prolene preferred in hairy areas due to blue color). 5-0 or 6-0 absorbable for deeper structures.	Depending on the area: local infiltration; superior orbital, supratrochlear, or inferior orbital block.	Debridement should be conservative to preserve normal facial structures. Palpate for any fractures. Do not shave the eyebrows. Lacerations that follow natural skin lines and creases will have a less noticeable scar (Figure 94–1). Approximation of the dermis with a SC stitch or a combination of SC and subcuticular stitches should bring the edges together or within 1-2 mm of apposition.
Nose	6-0 nonabsorbable for the skin; 5-0 or 6-0 absorbable for deeper structures.	An infraorbital block on the affected side, combined with a supratrochlear block and local wound infiltration.	Conservative debridement due to minimal redundant tissue present. Avoid directly suturing the cartilage as this may predispose to infection and necrosis. Most nasal fractures do not need reduction before soft tissue repair. The margins of the perichondrium should be apposed to bring the edges of the cartilage together. Through-and-through lacerations require a layered closure; the mucosa should be closed with fine absorbable suture, followed by approximation of any fractured cartilage with similar suture; irrigate after closure of each layer. Intranasal lacerations should be repaired by ENT. Drain septal hematomas with a vertical incision, nasal packing, prophylactic antibiotics, and refer to ENT.

	Suture	Anesthesia	Recommendations for Closure
Ear	Fine absorbable suture for perichondrial layer.	Form a wheal with lidocaine (no epinephrine) about the entire base of the ear; anesthetizes all but the external canal and concha (direct infiltration required).	Conservative debridement should be performed. The cartilage should be apposed by placing a suture in the perichondrium and dermis. Skin coverage is important to prevent drying, necrosis, and infection of the cartilage. If there is skin tissue loss, a small amount of cartilage may be removed for better skin coverage. A pressure dressing should be applied to prevent bleeding (wet cotton balls to support the ear followed by a circumferential dressing around the head). Any auricular hematoma requires drainage with an 18-gauge needle to prevent cartilage necrosis and deformation known as a "cauliflower ear". Use prophylactic antibiotics for any possible contamination due to the avascularity of the cartilage.
Buccal mucosa (cheek)	6-0 nonabsorbable for the skin; 5-0 or 6-0 absorbable for deeper structures.	Infraorbital nerve block and local infiltration.	Larger wounds (>2 cm) tend to trap food or may interfere with chewing surfaces of the teeth. Through and through lacerations should have a layered closure from the inside out. Irrigation may be repeated after the inner mucosal layer is closed. The integrity of Stensen's duct from the parotid gland must be determined: dry the inner mucosa, press on the parotid gland, and look for the appearance of saliva at the duct opening. A lacerated duct should be referred to ENT for repair. Evaluate for the integrity of the facial nerve lateral to a imaginary line dropped vertically from the lateral canthus of the eye; these injuries should be repaired by an ENT.

Continued

Table 94–12 Special Suturing Technique—*cont'd*

	Suture	Anesthesia	Recommendations for Closure
Lip	Absorbable 4.0 or 5.0 suture for mucosal surfaces. Nonabsorbable 5.0 or 6.0 suture for dermal surface.	Regional anesthesia if the vermillion border is involved with an infraorbital block for the upper lip or a mental block for the lower lip. Local injection may distort anatomy.	Misalignment of 1 mm in the vermillion border can have adverse cosmetic consequences. Minimal debridement is needed as the lip is highly vascular and heals well. If over 25% of the lip is missing, consult ENT for repair. The first stitch should approximate the vermillion border. For through-and-through lacerations: close the muscular/fibrous layer and inner mucosa first and the dermal surface last.
Tongue	Absorbable 4.0 or 5.0 suture.	Local infiltration, inferior alveolar nerve block (see Chapter 61) or a lingual nerve block (inject 0.5–1.0 ml of anesthetic into the base of the tongue posterior and medial to the most distant molar) can be performed.	Wounds larger than 2 cm or bisect the tongue should be repaired. After irrigation, grasp the tongue with gauze, towel clamp, or ring forceps. Tie the sutures loosely as the tongue tends to swell, which can be minimized with a single dose of decadron (0.6 mg/kg) or cold application (i.e., ice).
Scalp	Nonabsorbable 3-0 nylon or polypropylene suture on a large needle. Separate closure of the galea can be done with an absorbable 3-0 or 4-0 suture.	Local infiltration. Combine with epinephrine for bleeding.	Galeal lacerations need to be closed to ensure control of bleeding and protect against the spread of infection. The galea is firmly attached to the underside of the SC fascia, and is rarely identified as a distinct layer in a wound. Rule out underlying fracture by digital or instrument palpation (if concerned for glass). The scalp can be closed with a single layer of sutures that incorporates the skin, SC fascia, and the galea. Blood clots and foreign bodies should be removed. Scalp hair does not need

Table 94–12 Special Suturing Technique—*cont'd*

	Suture	Anesthesia	Recommendations for Closure
			to be shaved but can be clipped. For bleeding: add epinephrine to local anesthetic, direct pressure, ligate small vessels with a 5-0 Vicryl suture, place a figure-of-eight suture, and expedite closure. A scalp tourniquet may also be used temporarily.
Subungal hematoma	None, unless associated with a nail bed laceration	A nerve block is not necessary for trephination.	Subungal hematomas: trephinate if <50% of the nail plate surface; remove nail plate if >50%. Obtain radiographs to rule out a fracture; trephination will convert a closed fracture to an open one. For trephination, use a heated large bore needle or battery powered, fine-tipped cautery device, and only insert through the nail plate until blood appears.
Nail bed laceration	6-0 absorbable suture such as vicryl for nail	A digital block is useful for most nail bed injuries.	Proximal or longitudinal lacerations require removal of entire nail plate. A digital tourniquet may be briefly applied. The nail plate does not need to be placed under the eponychium for the new nail plate to grow, which happens in 60–90 d. Remove the nail plate with closed iris scissors, and advance under the distal nail plate, gently opening to dissect the nail plate from the nail bed. After the nail plate is dissected away from the nail folds, remove it. The points of the scissors should be kept pointing toward the nail plate.

ENT, ear, nose, and throat; SC, subcutaneous.

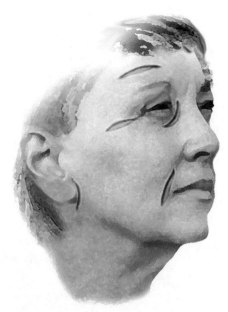

Figure 94–1. Lacerations following natural skin lines (shown here) heal with a less noticeable scar than those that are oblique or perpendicular to natural lines (or wrinkles). *(From Roberts JR, Hedges J. Clinical Procedures in Emergency Medicine (4th ed). Philadelphia: Elsevier, 2004, p 680.)*

risk when using this method is the same as when closing the wound traditionally.

■ Wounds involving deeper structures such as tendons, joints, and nerves require consultation. The one exception is extensor tendon injuries that can be closed primarily in the ED. Repair of lacerated extensor tendons can be delayed for up to 72 hours to still be considered for primary closure. If repair is delayed, care in the ED should still include copious wound irrigation, skin closure, splint application, and referral to a hand specialist. A 4-0 nonabsorbable suture should be used to repair a lacerated extensor tendon. The suture techniques for repair are demonstrated in Figure 94–2.

■ If the wound cannot be closed without excessive skin tension, consider surgical consultation for more advanced wound closure techniques (i.e., rotational skin flaps, skin grafts).

Postprocedure Care

■ Apply topical antibiotic ointment and oral antibiotics as described in the preceding sections. Facial and scalp wounds only require topical antibacterial ointment unless there is potential for hematoma formation that will require a pressure dressing for 1 to 3 days.

■ The dressing over a wound consists of a nonadherent layer adjacent to the wound (or just topical antibiotic ointment), gauze sponges to absorb

	Infection Risk	Wound Closure Indications	Infection Prophylaxis
Cat	Up to 50% infection rate due to deep penetrating of teeth; most common organism is *Pasteurella multicida* which causes a rapidly progressive cellulitis within 24 h.	On the face only.	Antibiotics effective against *P. multicida* include amoxicillin/clavulanate, penicillin, tetracycline, quinolones, second- and third-generation cephalosporins, and trimethoprim-sulfamethoxazole. Oral first-generation cephalosporins, dicloxacillin, vancomycin, erythromycin, and clindamycin may not be effective.
Dog	10% infection rate but is worse on the hands; most are polymicrobial; *P. multicida* is less common.	Most can be closed primarily if <8 h old, are not deep puncture wounds, and not infected. Copious irrigation and debridement is required. Smaller bites or puncture wounds should be left open.	Antibiotics are recommended for high risk injuries such as hand wounds, heavy contamination, significant tissue destruction, >8 h old, tendon or joint involvement, or patients with an immunocompromised state. Include coverage for *P. multicida* and anaerobes.
Human	50% incidence of infection after hand bites. Usually polymicrobial with *S aureus*, *Streptococcus* species, and anaerobes (*Eikenella corrodens*) being the most common	All closed fist injuries should undergo local meticulous exploration to rule out involvement of deeper structures. Bites on the hand should be left open. Bites to the face can be closed primarily. Through-and-through lacerations of the lip from a tooth puncture may require a layered closure, but are at high risk of infection. Bites to other areas may need to be left open, or closed with delayed primary closure.	Indicated for all but the most superficial wounds. Choices include second-generation cephalosporin, amoxicillin-clavulanate, erythromycin, azithromycin, clarithromycin, fluoroquinolones, or clindamycin. Infected human bites, especially to the hand, require admission for IV antibiotics. Human bites are not a risk for HIV unless a there is exposure to a significant amount of blood.

CDC, US Centers for Disease Control and Prevention; HIV, human immunodeficiency virus; IV, intravenous;

Table 94–14 Alternatives to Suturing

	Advantages and Uses	Disadvantages	Application
Tissue adhesives Examples: Octylcyanoacrylate (Dermabond, Ethicon) and n-butyl-2-cyanoacrylate (Indermil)	Ease of use, decrease pain, less time to apply, no follow-up needed for suture removal, possesses some antimicrobial properties against gram-positive organisms. Used for short clean wounds that are not under tension.	Less tensile strength, adhesive may seep into the wound causing a foreign body reaction, irrigation and debridement may be less aggressive since local anesthesia is often not needed.	Should never be applied within wounds. Approximate wound edges with the fingers or forceps. Three to four layers of adhesive should be painted over opposed wound edges, extending at least 5 mm beyond edges of the wound (long axis). Hold wound edges together for at least 30 s. Aftercare: avoid application of ointments; do not soak in water or scrub; wash gently after 24 h, no dressing required.
Staples	Faster repair, lower cost, decreased tissue reactivity. Used for linear lacerations with sharp, straight edges on the scalp, extremities, or trunk.	Should not be used on the face, neck, hands or feet. Deep sutures may be required to decrease tension. May not be used in deep scalp lacerations with active bleeding.	Approximate the wound edges prior to application. Aftercare: similar to sutures.
Tape	Faster repair, lower cost, decreased tissue reactivity. Can be used to close a wound primarily or for additional support of a wound after suture or staple removal.	Cannot be used in areas under tension.	Used for superficial straight lacerations under little tension. May be used for friable skin tears in the elderly. The skin must be clean and dry. Apply benzoin on the skin (but not in the wound) prior to application to improve adherence. The tape will fall off after a few days.

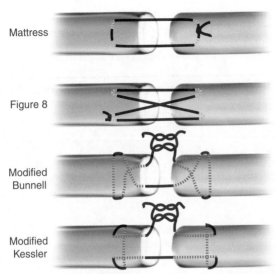

Mattress

Figure 8

Modified Bunnell

Modified Kessler

Figure 94–2. Suture techniques used in extensor tendon repair. *(From Newport ML, Williams CD. Biomechanical characteristics of extensor tendon suture techniques. J Hand Surg 1992;17:1117.)*

any drainage, and an outer wrapping such as Kerlix gauze. Epithelization occurs faster if the wound is kept moist for 48 hours.
- Compression dressings should also be placed over areas with dead space that may accumulate blood such as the ear and web space of the hand.
- The initial dressing should be kept in place for at least 24 hours. The wound should not be allowed to get wet for the first 48 hours, and should not be immersed in water (i.e., dish washing, baths, or water sports), until the wound is healed (i.e., sutures are removed). The wound should be kept clean and dry. Transparent adhesive dressings such as Opsite can also be used.

Disposition

- *Consultation.* Consultation with the appropriate surgical subspecialty is indicated for extensive or high risk injuries. As mentioned previously, wounds involving deeper structures such as tendons, joints, vessels, and nerves require consultation. Consultation should also be done for foreign bodies that are difficult to remove, complex lacerations requiring extensive time for repair, and high pressure injection injuries. The particular consultant will be dependent upon the anatomic location of the injury. Early consultation is mandatory for open fractures, suspicion of clostridial gangrene, or suspicion of necrotizing fasciitis.
- *Admission.* Admission is seldom needed but may be warranted for high-risk injuries in which the patient may be susceptible to systemic illness or other complication stemming from the injury.
- *Discharge.* Most patients seen in the ED for wound care will be discharged. Ensure the patient has close follow-up with a physician within

24 to 48 hours for a wound evaluation. The patient should be instructed to return to the ED for signs of infection such as redness, warmth, purulent drainage, or severe pain. A summary of discharge instructions including the time for suture removal are listed in Box 94–1.

BOX 94–1 Discharge Instructions for Laceration Repair

Elevating the injured extremity and use of cold compresses for at least 48 h to decrease swelling.

Nonfacial wounds should be dressed in a bulky dressing: Do not remove for 24-48 h.

After 48 h, keep the wound clean and dry. Wash the area with several times a day with soap and water.

Avoid prolonged immersion in water (e.g., swimming or dishwashing).

Antibacterial ointment should be applied to all facial wounds after each cleansing.

Avoid strong sun exposure especially to facial wounds.

Return to the emergency department for signs of infection: purulent drainage, increased redness or red streaking, swelling, worsening pain, fever, chills.

Suture removal is as follows: face (3-5 d), scalp (5-8 d), torso (7-10 d), upper extremity (10-12 d*), lower extremity (10-14 d*). Steri-strips will then be applied to nonhairy areas.

Sutures in areas involving a joint surface such as the knee or elbow should be left in longer.

Teaching Points

One of the most common reasons for going to an ED is to have an acute wound repaired. The techniques for doing this require time and patience, and if done properly will leave optimal scars that will not require subsequent plastic surgical repair.

While both the patient and the physician would prefer to utilize a primary closure, this should not be carried out in the contaminated wound, or if there is an unknown degree of contamination.

Wound repair should be accompanied by sufficient analgesia, and for extensive wounds, especially in children or adults who cannot cooperate, conscious sedation will lead to a more humane experience and an improved cosmesis.

Prophylactic antibiotics are reserved for special circumstances, and all wounds should have the tetanus status updated. Prophylactic rabies treatment can be ascertained with the help of the local Public Health Department.

The patient need not know the degree of training and expertise required to obtain a good wound repair, but is entitled to having the best cosmetic outcome possible.

Suggested Readings

Crystal CS, Blankenship RB. Local anesthetics and peripheral nerve blocks in the emergency department. Emerg Med Clin N Am 2005;23:477-502.

Lammers RL, Trott AT Methods of wound closure. In: Roberts JR, Hedges JR (editors). Clinical Procedures in Emergency Medicine (4th ed.). Philadelphia: Saunders, 2004, pp. 655-693.

Appendix 1 Quick Reference

Amy Kahn

A. Metric Conversions
   Temperature (Celsius to Fahrenheit):
   $T_C = (5/9) * (T_F - 32)$
   $T_F = (9/5) * (T_C + 32)$

Table 1A	Temperature Conversions		
°C	°F	°C	°F
35.0	95.0	38	100.4
36.0	96.8	38.5	101.3
36.5	97.7	39	102.2
37.0	98.6	39.5	103.1
37.5	99.5	40.0	104.0

Weight:	1 kilogram (kg) = 2.2 pound (lb)
	1 lb = 0.454 kg
	1 ounce = 28.4 gram
Volume:	1 teaspoon = 5 ml
	1 tablespoon = 15 ml
	1 fluid ounce = 30 ml
	1 cup = 240 ml
	1 pint = 473 ml
	1 quart = 946 ml
Length:	1 cm = 0.394 inch
	1 inch = 2.54 cm

B. Common Laboratory Studies

Table 1B Common Laboratory Studies

Category	Laboratory	Reference Range	Comments
Hematology	WBC	$4.5-11 \times 10^3$ per uL	Increase may indicate infection, tissue necrosis, inflammation, malignancy, stress, medications (e.g., steroids, epinephrine). Decrease may indicate immunosuppresion, overwhelming infection, viral infection.
	Hemoglobin	M: 13.5-17.5 g/dL F: 12-16 g/dL	If decreased: use MCV to differentiate between microcytic, normocytic, and macrocytic anemia. Macrocytic → folate or B12 deficiency, malabsorption, hypothyroidism, liver disease. Normocytic → blood loss, anemia of chronic disease. Microcytic → iron deficiency, thalassemia, lead, chronic disease.
	Hematocrit	M; 39-49% F: 35-45%	If increased: polycythemia, hemoconcentration, CHF, COPD, congenital heart disease.
	Platelets	$150-450 \times 10^3$ per uL	Increased risk of spontaneous bleeding at <20,000. Increased (thrombocytosis): in acute infection, splenectomy, malignancy, chronic inflammation, acute hemorrhage, polycythemia vera, myeloproliferative disorders. Decreased: sepsis, DIC, high volume blood transfusion, immunologic, hypersplenism, malignancy, medications, liver disease, artificial heart valve. In thrombotic thrombocytopenic purpura (TTP), platelet counts are often < 20,000 with hemolytic anemia but normal coagulation studies.
	Neutrophil	57-67%	Also known as segs, polys, or PMNs- primary defense against bacterial infection and stress. Most commonly elevated with bacterial infection; multiple other causes such as tissue necrosis (e.g., cancer, burns, trauma, myocardial infarction), metabolic disorders, hemorrhage, hemolysis, and myeloproliferative disorders. Leukopenia may be due to sepsis, defect in bone marrow production, drug effects, or cytotoxic agents. Neutropenia is defined as a neutrophilic granulocyte count of less than 1500/mm³ and is calculated as follows: absolute neutrophil count: WBC × (% bands + % mature neutrophile) × 01

Table 1B Common Laboratory Studies—*cont'd*

Category	Laboratory	Reference Range	Comments
	-mature -bands	54-62% 3-5%	A "left shift" refers to an increase in the percentage of mature neutrophils and in the number of immature, newly released neutrophils, known as bands. The normal band to PMN ratio is 0.1 : 0.3. Infection and steroid administration can increase the number of bands.
	Lymphocytes	22-33%	Increased in viral infections, bacterial infection (TB), leukemia, Hodgkin's lymphoma, multiple myeloma, inflammatory disorders.
	Monocytes	3-7%	May be elevated with infections (TB, viruses, infectious mononucleosis, parasites, rickettsial), inflammation, malignancy.
	Eosinophils	1-3%	May be elevated in allergy, parasitic infections, fungal infection, collagen vascular disease, dermatological disease, inflammatory bowel disease, hypereosinophilic syndromes.
	Basophils	0-1%	Elevation associated with leukemia, myeloproliferative disorders, infection and inflammation, chronic allergy.
Sed Rate (ESR)		M: <15 mm/hour F: <20 mm/hour	Elevated in infection, inflammation, autoimmune disorders – important in diagnosis of temporal arteritis. Nonspecific finding. If elevated but no evidence of disease on clinical presentation, can be evaluated as an outpatient. Significant elevations (> 100 mm/h) requires a thorough ED evaluation.
C-reactive protein		< 8 mg/L	Increased in infection (bacterial > viral), tissue injury or necrosis, and inflammatory disorders.
Reticulocyte		0.5 – 2.8%	Increased: hemolytic anemia, post hemorrhage, treatment for anemia. Decreased: bone marrow failure, renal failure, chronic disease, hypothyroid.

Continued

Table 1B Common Laboratory Studies—*cont'd*

Category	Laboratory	Reference Range	Comments
Coagulation	PT	11-15 seconds	Elevated in disorders of the extrinsic & common coagulation pathway and in warfarin use
	aPTT	20-35 seconds	Elevated in disorders of the intrinsic & common coagulation pathway and in heparin use
	Bleeding Time	2-7 minutes	Used to assess platelet function
	Thrombin Time	6.3-11.1 seconds	Used in evaluation of hypercoagulability or bleeding
	Fibrinogen	200-400 mg/dL	Used in evaluation of DIC: fibrinogen is decreased and fibrin degradation products (FDP) are increased.
	FDP	<10 ug/mL	Used to evaluate DIC and in the evaluation of suspected DVT or PE.
	D-Dimer	<0.5 ug/mL	May be helpful if PE probability is low.
Chemistry	Sodium	135-145 mEq/L	Correction for glucose: measured Na + [$1.5 \times$ (glucose − 150)/100]
	Potassium	3.5-5.1 mEq/L	Hemolysis is a common cause for elevation.
	Chloride	98-106 mEq/L	Elevations occur with hypernatremia, low anion gap state, or normal anion gap metabolic acidosis. Decreased in metabolic alkalosis (increased bicarbonate)
	Bicarbonate	22-29 mEq/L	Decreases in metabolic acidosis, gastrointestinal loss, or from renal failure or renal tubular acidosis (retention of acid or impaired production of HCO_3). Increased with loss of gastric acid, volume contraction, exogenous HCO_3, hypokalemia, hypercapnea, hyperaldosteronism, hypoparathyroidism.
	BUN	7-18 mg/dL	Elevated from increased protein or decreased renal clearance.
	Creatinine	0.6-1.2 mg/dL	Elevated from decreased renal clearance or increased creatinine load (e.g., massive trauma, rhabdomyolysis, large protein intake).
	Glucose	70-115 mg/dL	Values detected by reagent strips may be higher than plasma levels in anemic patients.

Category	Laboratory	Reference Range	Comments
	Ionized Calcium	4.65-5.28 mg/dL	This is the more physiologically active component.
	Magnesium	1.3-2.1 mEq/L	Important to correct magnesium when trying to correct a low K+.
	Phosphorus	2.7-4.5 mg/dL	Low levels may occur with prolonged hyperventilation, but do not cause true phosphate depletion.
Abdominal labs	Albumin	3.5-5.5 g/dL	Decreased due to impaired synthesis (e.g., malnutrition, malabsorption, hepatic dysfunction), or to losses (e.g., ascites or protein-losing nephropathy or enteropathy). Prealbumin is considered to be a better early indicator of change in nutritional status.
	Protein, total	6-8 g/dL	Elevated in dehydration, sarcoidosis, collagen-vascular diseases, multiple myeloma, Waldenström's macroglobulinemia. Decreased in malnutrition, cirrhosis, nephrosis, low-protein diet, overhydration, malabsorption, pregnancy, severe burns, neoplasms, chronic diseases.
	Aspartate aminotransferase (AST)	15-40 U/L	ALT is more specific for liver disease. Aminotransferase levels are seldom greater than 500 units in obstructive jaundice, cirrhosis, and alcoholic liver disease; levels may be in the thousands in disorders causing
	Alanine aminotransferase (ALT)	8-40 U/L	extensive hepatic necrosis such as acute hepatitis and hepatic ischemia from shock. If the ALT is less than 300, an AST/ALT ratio of greater than 2 is suggestive of alcoholic liver disease. Other causes for elevation: myocardial infarction, pericarditis, CHF, infectious mononucleosis, renal infarction, and acute pancreatitis.
	Alkaline phosphatase	50-120 U/L	Mostly derived from the liver, bone, and small intestine; also in WBCs and placenta. Isoenzyme determination can identify the source. Elevations of hepatic origin are due to biliary obstruction, cholestatic hepatitis, infiltrative liver disease, drug reactions, and canalicular obstruction in hepatitis.
	γ-Glutamyl transferase (GGT)	8-50 U/L	Dramatic increases in GGT typically indicate liver disease. More likely to be elevated in maintenance drinkers of alcohol than in binge drinkers. Medications may cause an increase.

Continued

Table 1B Common Laboratory Studies—*cont'd*

Category	Laboratory	Reference Range	Comments
	Lactate dehydrogenase (LDH)	120-240 U/L	Highly nonspecific test of hepatocellular damage. Moderately elevated in *Pneumocystis carinii* pneumonia. LD isoenzymes may be useful in determining the source of injury. Isoenzyme LDH-1 is found in RBCs and is elevated in hemolysis.
	Bilirubin, total Bili, conjugated (direct)	0.2-1 mg/dL 0-0.2 mg/dL	Indirect bilirubinemia (unconjugated) is usually due to hemolysis or defect in hepatic conjugation (enzyme defect or hepatocyte damage) and occurs when the unconjugated fraction is > 1.2 mg/dl and the conjugated component is < 20% of the total. Direct hyperbilirubinemia (conjugated) is due to bile obstruction or hepatocellular damage that allows conjugation but not secretion (cholestasis). It occurs when the indirect portion is < 20% of the total. Renal excretion of bilirubin occurs in the presence of biliary tree obstruction or hepatic disease.
	Amylase	25-125 U/L	Poor specificity for pancreatitis
	Lipase	10-140 U/L	Better test for the diagnosis of pancreatitis
Cardiac Enzymes	CPK	Male: 29-90 U/L Female: 10-70 U/L	The majority is found in skeletal muscle.
	CPK-MB fraction percent of total CPK	0-4%	CK-MB comprises up to 5% of skeletal muscle, and can be elevated in noncardiac disease states. CPK-MB isoenzymes can also be released with cardiac trauma, defibrillation, and myocarditis. It peaks slightly earlier than does total CPK, and normalizes within 72 hours of elevation.
	Troponin I	<0.1 mg/L	This is more specific for myocardial injury than troponin T2.

Category	Laboratory	Reference Range	Comments
Urinalysis	Color	Clear yellow	Red or red-brown urine may be due to hematuria, myoglobinuria, rifampin, urobilinogen, bilirubin, porphyria, pigment in beets and blackberries, or medications (e.g., phenytoin, phenothiazine, metronidazole).
	Specific gravity	1.001-1.035	Elevated in volume depleted states. Significant elevations after administration on iodinated contrast media or mannitol.
	pH	4.5-8.0	Usually more acidic. Highly alkaline urine suggests urinary tract infection with a urea-splitting organism such as *Proteus* or *E. coli*. Alkaline urine also present with renal tubular acidosis, sodium bicarbonate or acetazolamide, vomiting, metabolic alkalosis, and chronic renal failure, but also seen with hypokalemia. Acidic urine present with acidosis, high protein diet, diarrhea, and dehydration.
	Protein	Negative	Increased in glomerular diseases, infections, tubular disorders and exercise. Albumin is more readily detected than globulins. The presence of Bence-Jones proteins may be missed.
	Blood	Negative	Menstruating females should have a catheterized specimen. Bleeding anywhere in the urinary tract will produce hematuria. Myoglobinuria presents with positive blood but negative RBCs on microscopy.
	Glucose	Negative	Elevations in urine suggests a serum glucose > 170 mg/dL. May be elevated in normal individuals after a high glucose beverage.
	Ketones	Negative	Increased in ketoacidosis. Dipstick urinalysis measures acetoacetic acid or acetone but not beta-hydroxybutyrate.
	Leukocyte esterase	Negative	Positive in most urinary infections.
	Nitrite	Negative	Positive in most gram-negative urinary infections. A negative test does not rule out infection.
	Bilirubin	Negative	Mostly seen with liver and biliary disease. Complete biliary obstruction is suggested when the bilirubin is positive but the urobilinogen is negative.

Continued

Table 1B Common Laboratory Studies—*cont'd*

Category	Laboratory	Reference Range	Comments
	Urobilinogen	Negative	Seen in hemolysis and cirrhosis. May also be due to suppression of gut flora from antibiotics.
	Crystals	Negative	Uric acid and calcium oxalate may be present in an normal urinalysis. Calcium oxalate may be seen with nephrolithiasis.
	Casts	RBC cast: none WBC cast: none Epithelial: occasional Hyaline: occasional	Hyaline casts are seen in causes of proteinuria, dehydration, or exercise. RBC casts are seen in glomerulonephritis. WBC casts are present in pyelonephritis.
	Microbiology	RBCs: 0-3/hpf WBCs: 0-4/hpf Epithelial: occasional	RBCs are concerning for glomerular injury, stones, inflammation or neoplasm. WBC > 5/hpf are concerning for infection. An adequate specimen should have < 5/hpf.
	Spot urine for electrolytes	Chloride Potassium Sodium	< 10 mmol/L: chloride-sensitive metabolic alkalosis. > 20 mmol/L: chloride-resistant metabolic alkalosis. < 10 mmol/L: hypokalemia from extrarenal causes. > 10 mmol/L: renal wasting of potassium. < 20 mmol/L: volume depletion, prerenal azotemia. 20-40 mmol/L: indeterminate > 40 mmol/L: acute tubular necrosis, adrenal insufficiency, renal salt wasting, SIADH.
Arterial blood gas	pH $PaCO_2$ PaO_2 HCO_3 Base excess	7.35-7.45 35-45 mmHg 80-100 mmHg 21-27 mEq/L ±2 mEq/L	Measured value. Measured value. Measured value. Calculated value. Quantity of acid/alkali needed to return to normal pH in vitro. Calculated value.

Table 1B Common Laboratory Studies—*cont'd*

Category	Laboratory	Reference Range	Comments
Miscellaneous	Cortisol (random)	> 18 µg/dl	In a stressful clinical situation, levels < 18 µg/dl implies decreased cortisol production.
	Lactate	< 2 mmol/L	The blood specimen should be immediately transported on ice. Level of more than 5 mmol/L and a pH of less than 7.35 are seen in critically ill patients and have a very poor prognosis.
	TSH	0.3-3.5 mU/L	Used in routine screening for thyroid dysfunction.
	Free T4	0.8-2.0 ng/dl	Serum free T4 levels, inconjunction with serum thyroid-stimulating hormone (TSH) levels, are routinely used for the diagnosis of suspected hypothyroidism or hyperthyroidism. This has largely replaced the FTI assay.
	Free T3	2.5-6.0 pg/ml	Not as helpful as free T4 levels in diagnostic evaluation.

Table 1C Analysis of Cerebrospinal Fluid

Test	Normal value	Significance of abnormality
Cell count	<5 WBC/mm³ <1 PMN/mm³ <1 eosinophil/mm³	Increased WBC counts are seen in all types of meningitis and encephalitis; increased PMN count suggests bacterial pathogens.
Gram's stain	No organism	Offending organism identified 80% of time in bacterial meningitis, 60% if patient pretreated with antibiotics.
Turbidity	Clear	Increased turbidity with leukocytosis, blood, or high concentration of microorganisms.
Xanthochromia	None	Presence of RBCs in spinal fluid for 4 hr before lumbar puncture; occasionally caused by traumatic tap.
CSF-to-serum glucose ratio	0.6:1	Depressed in pyogenic meningitis or hyperglycemia.
Protein	15–45 mg/dl	Elevated with acute bacterial or fungal meningitis; also elevated with vasculitis, syphilis, encephalitis, neoplasms, and demyelination syndromes.
India ink stain	Negative	Positive in one third of cases of cryptococcal meningitis.
Cryptococcal antigen	Negative	90% accuracy for cryptococcal disease.
Lactic acid	<35 mg/dl	Elevated in bacterial and tubercular meningitis.
Bacterial antigen tests	Negative	>95% specific for organism tested; up to 50% false-negative rate.
Acid-fast stain	Negative	Positive in 80% of cases of tuberculous meningitis if >10 ml of fluid.

CSF, Cerebrospinal fluid; PMN, polymorphonuclear; WBC, white blood cell.

From: Lavoie FW, Saucier JR. Central nervous system infections. In: Marx JA, Hockberger RS, Walls RM (editors), Rosen's Emergency Medicine: Concepts and Clinical Practice (6th ed). Philadelphia: Mosby. 2006, p 1711.

Table 1D	Common Tests for Pleural Fluid Analysis*
Test	**Analysis of result**
Albumin	Serum albumin minus the pleural fluid albumin. If >1.2 g/dL, the patient likely has a transudative effusion.
Protein and lactate dehydrogenase (LDH)	Calculate pleural fluid to serum ratio for protein and for LDH.** If protein ratio is >0.5 or LDH ratio is > 0.6, most consistent with an exudate. Also considered to be an exudate if > 2/3 x (upper limit of normal for serum LDH level).
Glucose	A low glucose concentration (<60 mg/dL) may be due to an empyema, ruptured esophagus, complicated parapneumonic infection, malignancy, rheumatoid arthritis, or tuberculosis. These diagnoses are not excluded by a high or normal pleural fluid glucose.
White blood count (WBC)	If >1000 cells/mm^3, may be from infection or inflammatory process. Counts may reach levels >10,000 cells/mm^3, most commonly with parapneumonic effusions. A predominance of PMNs indicates an acute process affecting the pleural surface, such as infection or pulmonary infarct. A predominance of mononuclear cells is consistent with a more chronic pleural process.
Red blood cells (RBC)	A grossly bloody pleural effusion or RBC count of >100,000 cells/mm^3 is suggestive of trauma, malignancy, or pulmonary infarction.

*Once a fluid is classified as transudative, it typically requires no further fluid analysis, and therapy is directed at the underlying cause of the effusion (CHF, nephrosis, etc.). Undiagnosed exudates, at a minimum, should have pleural fluid sent for cell count with differential, Gram's stain, culture, cytology, and glucose.

**$\dfrac{\text{pleural fluid level (of protein or LDH)}}{\text{serum level (of protein or LDH)}}$

Table 1E	Peritoneal Fluid Analysis
Test	**Analysis of result**
WBC PMN	Greater than 250 WBC cells/mm^3 with greater than 50% PMNs is strongly suggestive of spontaneous bacterial peritonitis. The most valuable method for detecting infection is a culture, and one should be sent in blood culture bottles.
RBC	Increased RBC usually from traumatic tap. Blood-to-ascites albumin difference of < 1.1 g/dL is useful for the detection of malignant ascites.
albumin	Calculate the serum-ascites albumin concentration gradient (difference of albumin level between serum and ascites fluid). If >1.1 g/dL suggests portal HTN (e.g., cirrhosis, alcoholic hepatitis, portal vein thrombosis, cardiac ascites) and <1.1 g/dL suggests non-portal HTN causes of ascites (e.g., peritoneal carcinomatosis, tuberculous peritonitis, nephrotic syndrome, or pancreatic ascites).
Miscellaneous:	Other tests include total protein, glucose, LDH, amylase Low glucose suggests infection. A protein level > 2.5g suggests non-portal HTN. Evaluate for opportunistic infections such as tuberculosis in immunosuppressed patients. Cytology should be sent to evaluate for malignancy. Triglyceride and bilirubin levels may be sent if the gross appearance of ascites fluid suggests increased levels.

Table 1F Synovial Fluid Analysis

Condition	Gross Appearance	WBC/mm³	PMN's	Glucose	Crystals	Culture
Normal Joint Fluid	Clear	<200	<25	90-100	None	neg
Degenerative Joint Disease	Clear	<4000	<25	90-100	None	neg
Traumatic	Bloody, Straw Colored	<4000	<25	90-100	None	neg
Pseudogout	Turbid	2000-50000	>75	80-100	Positively birefringent rhomboid shaped	neg
Gout	Turbid	20000-100,000	>75	80-100	Negatively birefringent needle shaped	neg
Septic Arthritis	Purulent/turbid	>50000	>75	<50	None	Organism specific
Rheumatoid Arthritis/ Seronegative Arthropathies	Turbid/clear	2000-50000	50-75	~75	None	neg

Table 1G Drug Levels

Antibiotics	P (Peak) and T (Trough)
Amikacin	P: 25.0-35.0 µg/ml T: 5.0-7.5 µg/ml
Gentamicin/tobramycin	P: 5.0-8.0 µg/ml T: 1.0-2.0 µg/ml
Gentamicin/tobramycin (24-h dosing and normal renal function) Vancomycin	P: > 10 µg/ml T: 1.0-2.0 µg/ml P: 20.0-40.0 1.0-2.0 µg/ml T: 5.0-10.0 1.0-2.0 µg/ml

Other Drugs	Therapeutic Level
Acetaminophen	10-20 µg/ml
Carbamazepine	8-12 µg/ml
Digoxin	0.8-2.0 ng/ml
Lidocaine	1.5-6.5 µg/ml
Lithium	0.6-1.2 mmol/L
Phenobarbital	15.0-40.0 µg/ml
Phenytoin (total)	10.0-20.0 µg/ml
Procainamide	4.0-10.0 µg/ml
N-acetylprocainamide (NAPA-active metabolite of procainamide)	5.0-30.0 µg/ml
Quinidine	3.0-5.0 µg/ml
Salicylate	20-30 µg/ml
Tacrolimus	5.0-15.0 ng/ml
Theophylline	5.0-15.0 µg/ml
Valproic acid	50.0-100.0 µg/ml

Table 1H   Common Equations and Calculations

Aa gradient (in mmHg)	• $(FiO_2 \times 713) - (PaCO_2/0.8) - PaO_2$ • $150 - (PaCO_2/0.8) - PaO_2$ (On room air)
ABG	• General Rule: Δ 10mmHg $PaCO_2 = \Delta$ 0.08 pH
Acute Lung Injury (ALI) Ratio	• PaO2/FiO2 (ALI present if <300, ARDS present if <200)
Anion Gap	• $Na - (Cl + HCO_3)$ Normal range is 8-16
Anion Gap Delta	• Delta gap = normal gap − anion gap
Body Water Deficit	• Deficit (in liters) = $0.6 \times$ weight (in kg) $\times$ [(Na/140) − 1]
Body Surface Area	• BSA = [(height in cm $\times$ weight in kg)/3600]^2
Creatinine Clearance (24 hour urine) (in mg/mL)	• = [urine Cr (mg/dL) $\times$ urine volume (mL)]/ [plasma Cr (mg/dL) $\times$ time (min)] • renal impairment: normal >100, mild 40-60, moderate 10-40, severe <10
Glomerular Filtration Rate (Cockcroft–Gault Method)	• GFR (male) = [(140-age) $\times$ weight(kg)]/ [72 $\times$ serum creatinine] • GFR (female) = GFR (male) $\times$ 0.85 • Use same values as above for renal impairment
Fractional Excretion of Sodium	• FENa (%) = [urine Na $\times$ serum Cr]/ [urine Cr $\times$ serum Na] $\times$ 100 • FENa < 1 $\rightarrow$ pre-renal, FENa > 1 $\rightarrow$ renal
Ideal Body Weight	• Males: IBW (in kg) = (height in meters)^2 $\times$ 23 • Females: IBW (in kg) = (height in meters)^2 $\times$ 21.5
Maintenance Fluid Rate (pediatrics)	• 0-10 kg = 4 cc/kg/hr • 10-20 kg = 40 cc/hr + 2cc/kg/hr (for each kg over 10 kg) • Above 20 kg = 60 cc/hr + 1 cc/kg/hr (for each kg over 20 kg)
Mean arterial pressure (MAP)	• MAP = DBP + (SBP − DBP)/3 • Normal value N70-110
Osmolality (serum)	• Calculated osmolality (mOsm/kg) = (2 $\times$ Na) + (BUN/2.8) + (Glucose/18) • Normal is 285-295 mosm/kg H_2O
Osmolar Gap	• Gap = measured osmolality (serum) − calculated osmolality
Parkland Burn Equation	• Fluid required in first 24 hr = (% BSA burned) $\times$ (weight in kg) $\times$ (4 mL) • $^1/_2$ over first 8 hours, other $^1/_2$ over subsequent 16 hours
Urine Anion Gap (use when serum anion gap is normal in patient with acidosis)	• UAG = urine sodium + urine potassium − urine chloride • Normal range is -10 to 10 • < - 10 suggests non-renal cause for acidosis • >10 suggest renal cause for acidosis

Appendix 2 Physical Examination Findings

Scott B. Murray ■ Heather S. Hammerstedt ■ Sean P. Kelly

Table 2A	Glasgow Coma Scale	
Response	**Score**	***Significance* and Further Details**
Eye Opening	4	*Intact reticular activating system*
Spontaneous	3	Only opens eyes when instructed
To verbal command	2	Only opens eyes to painful stimuli
To pain	1	Does not open eyes
None		
Verbal Ability		
Oriented, conversant	5	*Intact cerebral cortex*
Disoriented, conversant	4	Normal, well-articulated speech but disoriented.
Inappropriate words	3	Random, but comprehensible words
Incomprehensible sounds	2	Groaning, no comprehensible words
No verbalization	1	No sound generated
Motor Response		
Obeys verbal commands	6	*Intact cerebral cortex and corticospinal tract*
Localizes painful stimuli	5	Attempts to remove painful stimuli
Withdraws to painful stimuli	4	Purposely moves away from painful stimuli
Decorticate response to pain	3	Abnormal flexion response to painful stimuli
Decerebrate response to pain	2	Abnormal extension response to painful stimuli
No response	1	*Loss of medullary function or cervical cord injury*

Table 2B	Cranial Nerves
Cranial Nerve	**Function**
I: Olfactory nerve	Sense of smell
II: Optic nerve	Vision
III: Oculomotor nerve	Oculomotor function via motor fibers to levator palpebrae, superior rectus, medial rectus, inferior rectus, and inferior oblique muscles. Pupillary constriction via parasympathetic fibers to constrictor pupillae and ciliary muscles
IV: Trochlear nerve	Motor supply to the superior oblique muscle
V: Trigeminal nerve	Motor supply to muscles of mastication and to tensor tympani Sensory to face, scalp, oral cavity (including tongue and teeth)
VI: Abducens nerve	Motor supply to the lateral rectus muscle
VII: Facial nerve	Motor supply to muscles of facial expression. Parasympathetic stimulation of the lacrimal, submandibular, and sublingual glands. Sensation to the ear canal and tympanic membrane
VIII: Vestibulocochlear nerve	Hearing and balance
IX: Glossopharyngeal nerve	General sensation to posterior third of tongue. Taste for posterior third of tongue. Motor supply to the stylopharyngeus
X: Vagus nerve	Motor to striated and muscles of the pharynx, larynx and tensor (veli) palatine. Motor to smooth muscles and glands of the pharynx, larynx, thoracic and abdominal viscera. Sensory from larynx, trachea, esophagus, thoracic and abdominal viscera
XI: Spinal accessory nerve	Motor supply to the sternocleidomastoid and trapezius muscles
XII: Hypoglossal nerve	Motor supply to the intrinsic and extrinsic muscles of the tongue

Physical Examination	Technique	Indicates
Finger-to-nose	The patient touches his nose, then extends the arm and touches the examiner's finger. This is repeated several times with the eyes open, then with the eyes closed. Both sides are tested for comparison.	Dysmetria (past-pointing with the finger) indicates an ipsilateral cerebellar lesion.
Heel-to-shin	While lying supine on the bed, the patient places his or her heel just below the knee on the opposite side, and slides it down the shin to the top of the foot. This process is repeated as rapidly as possible for 10 s on each side.	Abnormal results in the heel-to-shin test indicate an ipsilateral cerebellar lesion.
Rapid alternating movements	The patient places his or her hand in the opposite hand or on his or her knee and turns it over repeatedly as fast as he or she can for 10 s. The process is repeated on the other side.	Asymmetric dysdiadochokinesia (the inability to perform rapid alternating movements) indicates an ipsilateral cerebellar lesion. Note that patients with other movement disorders such as Parkinson's disease may have symmetric dysdiadochokinesia
Romberg test	The patient stands still with eyes open and heels together. The examiner should stand in close proximity in case the patient starts to fall. The patient then closes his or her eyes and the examiner notes if the ataxia worsens.	A true positive Romberg occurs when ataxia is present at baseline (even while the patient's eyes are open). When the eyes are closed, the ataxia worsens. The Romberg test is negative if the ataxia does not worsen. Patients need two out of three working inputs to the cortex to achieve balance (visual confirmation of position, non-visual confirmation of position from proprioception and vestibular input, and a normal cerebellum). A positive Romberg implies that the patient has a cerebellar abnormality and is depending on proper visual input to maintain balance. Closing the eyes brings out the deficit more severely. Technically, if no gait or truncal ataxia is present at baseline, the Romberg test does not really apply.

Table 2D   Minimental Status Examination

Question	Points
"What is the year? Season? Date? Day of the week? Month?"	0-5
"Where are we? State? Country? Town? Hospital floor?"	0-5
"I'd like to test your memory; say these words: boat, cucumber, wire"	0-3
"Begin with 100 and count backwards by 7." (Answers = 93, 86, 79, 72, 65)	0-5
"Can you name the three objects I named before?"	0-3
"Name these items" and point to a pencil and a watch	0-2
"Repeat the following: 'No ifs, ands, or buts.'"	0-1
"Take a paper in your right hand, fold it in half, and put it on the floor."	0-3
Tell the patient to "Read and obey the following" and write "CLOSE YOUR EYES."	0-1
"Write a sentence."	0-1
Draw interlocking pentagons and have patient copy it.	0-1

Patient score <22 points = organic disorder likely; patient score >22 points = organic disorder unlikely.

Table 2E   Strength Testing Scale

Score	Strength
0	No strength
1	Slight contraction, but no movement
2	Able to move without gravity
3	Able to resist gravity
4	Able to resist examiner, but not full strength
5	Full strength

Table 2F   Deep Tendon Reflexes Grading Scale

Score	Reflexes
0	Absent
1	Decreased, but present
2	Normal
3	Brisk (excessive)
4	Clonus

Table 2G   Reflex Nerve Roots

Score	Nerve Roots (Afferent, Efferent)
Achilles	S1, S2 "Buckle my shoe"
Patellar	L3, L4 "Kick the door"
Biceps	C5, C6 "Pick up sticks"
Triceps	C7, C8 "Lay 'em straight"
Pupils	CN 2, CN 3
Corneal	CN 5, CN 7
Gag	CN 9, CN 10

Table 2H Abnormal Lung Sounds and Pulmonary Physical Examination Findings

Finding	Description	Pathology
Crackles	Fine or coarse, sound like hair rubbing against the stethoscope	Pulmonary edema, pneumonia, pulmonary fibrosis
Rales	Coarse crackles	Pulmonary edema, pneumonia, pulmonary fibrosis
Wheezes	Usually expiratory, prolonged, and high pitched	Asthma, COPD
Rhonchi	Low-pitched wheezes	Asthma, COPD
Pleural Friction Rub	Inspiratory and expiratory, coarse, grating, rubbing sound	Pleural inflammation, effusion, or infarction
Mediastinal Crunch (Hamman's sign)	Crackles heard over the mediastinum, which correspond to heartbeats instead of respirations	Pneumomediastinum
Stridor	A predominately inspiratory wheeze, loudest over the trachea	Airway obstruction, croup, foreign body, tracheal stenosis
Broncophony	The spoken words "ninety nine" sound abnormally loud and clear	Pneumonia
Egophony	"Eee" to "ay" changes	Pneumonia
Whispered Pectoriloquy	The whispered words "ninety nine" or "1-2-3" sound abnormally loud and clear	Pneumonia
Tactile fremitus	Spoken words more easily felt (by the examiner's hand on the chest wall) than normal	Pneumonia
Hyper-resonance to percussion	Percussion of the chest is more tympanitic than normal	Pneumothorax
Dullness to percussion	Percussion of the chest is much more dull than normal	Hemothorax, pleural effusion

COPD, *chronic obstructive pulmonary disease.*

Table 2I Cardiac Murmur Intensity

Grade	Description of Murmur
I	Faint
II	Quiet, but identifiable with the stethoscope on the chest
III	Moderately loud
IV	Loud
V	Very loud, can be heard with the stethoscope partly off the chest
VI	Very loud, can be heard with the stethoscope entirely off the chest

Table 2J   Other Cardiovascular Examination Measurements

Exam	Description
Measuring jugular venous pressure (JVP)	The patient should have the head of the bed elevated approximately 30-45 degrees. The examiner should adjust the bed until the distension of the jugular vein is visible. Note that if the patient is too horizontal, the JVP may not be visible because the jugular vein is distended all the way past the mandible. If the patient is too vertical, the JVP may not be visible because the distension is below the sternal notch. The examiner should measure the vertical distance from the sternal notch (which is always approximately 5 cm above the heart, regardless of the angle of the head of the bed). A visible JVP at greater than 4 cm above the sternal notch is considered pathologic.
Measuring a pulsus paradoxus	Under normal conditions, a patient's blood pressure and pulse may decrease with respiratory inspiration by as much as 10 mm Hg due to increased intrathoracic pressure and venous return. A pulsus paradoxus is present if the blood pressure decrease is over 10 mm Hg during inspiration. The examiner should inflate the blood pressure cuff above the systolic blood pressure and slowly deflate it until the first Korotkoff sounds are heard during expiration (signifying the peak systolic pressure). The examiner should note this blood pressure reading. The cuff is then deflated slowly again until Korotkoff sounds are heard throughout the respiratory cycle, during inspiration and expiration. This is the lowest systolic blood pressure. Normally, this difference is 3-4 mm Hg. A difference of greater than 10 mm Hg is pathologic. If the pulsus paradoxus is severe enough, it may also be possible to palpate a reduced peripheral pulse during inspiration.
Measuring ankle brachial index (ABI)	The examiner should measure the highest systolic blood first pressure reading in each arm by recording the Doppler sound heard at the radial artery as the cuff is deflated. The greatest of the two arm pressures should be used for calculating the ABI. The examiner should measure the highest systolic blood pressure reading in each leg by placing the cuff on the calf and recording the first Doppler sound heard at the dorsalis pedis (DP) and the posterior tibial (PT) artery as the cuff is deflated. The highest arm pressure divided by the highest left ankle pressure (either DP or PT) gives the ABI for the left leg. And the highest arm pressure divided by the highest right ankle pressure (either DP or PT) gives the ABI for the right leg.
Allen's test	Exsanguinate the hand by elevation while the patient's hand is held in a clenched fist. The health care provider places his or her thumbs over the radial and ulnar arteries, at the wrist. The patient is then asked to extend the fingers. The palm should appear blanched or pale. The provider then releases the thumb over one of the arteries and the palm should become pink within 2-5 s if the artery is patent. This is then repeated for the other artery.

Table 2K	Ankle Brachial Index (ABI) Measurement Interpretation	
ABI	**Medical Interpretation in Evaluating Peripheral Vascular Disease and Arterial Occlusion**	**Surgical Interpretation in Evaluating Penetrating Trauma to the Extremity**
>0.9	Normal	Normal; significant vascular injury unlikely; may be observed
<0.9	Peripheral vascular disease is present	Abnormal; consider angiography, duplex, or operative exploration by trauma or vascular surgeon
<0.8	Claudication may occur with exercise	Same as 0.9
<0.4	Claudication may be present at rest	Need urgent surgical repair
<0.25	Severe peripheral artery disease is present and gangrene could result	Revascularization probably not possible, patient may need an amputation

Table 2L	Physical Examination Signs in the Patient with Abdominal Pain	
Sign	**Technique**	**Indicates**
Murphy's sign	Palpation of the RUQ causes the patient to halt deep inspiration due to pain	Acute cholecystitis
Obturator's sign	Internal rotation of the flexed right hip causes RLQ pain	Acute appendicitis
Ileopsoas's sign	Thigh flexion against resistance causes RLQ pain	Acute appendicitis
Rovsing's sign	Palpation of the LLQ causes RLQ pain	Acute appendicitis
Fluid wave	An assistant places his or her hands along the midline of a supine patient (to stop wave transmission through fat). The examiner taps one flank and feels for transmission of the wave to the opposite flank.	Ascites
Shifting dullness	The examiner percusses and finds the border of tympany (air) and dullness (fluid) to percussion. The patient lays on a side, and the process is repeated. Shifting dullness is present if the border between tympany and dullness moves significantly	Ascites

LLQ, left lower quadrant; RLQ, right lower quadrant; RUQ, right upper quadrant.

Appendix 3   Documentation

Craig Reece Brockman II

The medical record is a legal document used to communicate patient care information. Documentation is important to any medical practice. Charts don't have to be encyclopedic, but should be focussed with most attention to revealing thought processes, patient course through the ED, procedures, and disposition. It is also used to bill for the services provided by the treating physician. It is this last purpose that will be discussed here from the perspective of the emergency physician. The three elements of the medical record are history, physical examination, and medical decision making.

Medical decision making (MDM) is the most nebulous of the three elements. Document all of your interpretations of tests, procedures, consultations, repeated examinations, and the emergency department (ED) course the MDM section takes care of itself. Essential components of medical decision making are summarized in the Box 3A. Components of the history and physical examination are listed in Table 3A.

Critical Care Documentation

- Medicare's clinical criteria for critical care is as follows:
  High probability of sudden clinically significant or life-threatening deterioration in a patient's condition that requires the highest level of physician preparedness to intervene urgently.
- Critical care billing is related to time spent: the physician must document the amount of time spent as reimbursement is "per minute." Activities that count for critical care include: time spent at the bed side, time spent reviewing test results, time spent discussing care with nursing or medical staff (consultants, etc.), time spent documenting on the patient (writing the chart), time spent gathering history from someone other than the patient, and time spent discussing care/prognosis with the family. Activities that do not count in adding up critical care time include

---

BOX 3A   Medical Decision Making

- Record all tests ordered
- Record, at a minimum, all abnormal test results
- Record interpretations for those studies on which you based your course of treatment
- List treatment options and more importantly, the patient's response to that treatment (deteriorate, stabilize, improve)
- Record consultations and relevant information discussed
- Record the disposition and condition of the patient on discharge/transfer
- Document all procedures

anything not related to treatment of the patient, and time spent performing separately billable procedures (e.g., cardiac pulmonary resuscitation, intubation, chest tube, monitor interpretation, pulse oximetry interpretation, and any other procedures).

Teaching institutions

■ Teaching attending physicians must document that they saw and examined the patient, that they agree with the resident's history, physical, diagnosis, and plan (or document any differences). Critical care can only be billed for critical care time spent by the teaching physician (i.e., time the teaching physician was present).
■ The teaching physician must be present for the procedure, and must document their presence during the proceduce.
■ In the academic setting, the teaching physician is the only person who may bill for critical care time.

Other Documentation

■ *Procedures.* Document each procedure as these are billed separately.
■ *Pulse oximetry interpretation.* A few private insurance companies will pay for pulse oximetry readings. Recording an interpretation (normal, hypoxic, borderline) of the result as the percent number is not enough. If hypoxic, the plan to correct the hypoxia must be apparent in the chart (supplemental oxygen, nebulizer treatments, etc.).
■ *Electrocardiogram (EKG) interpretation.* This is often billed for by cardiology, but a few private insurance companies will pay the ED physician as well. The physician must document three different aspects of the reading or interpretation and document "interpreted by me."
■ *Cardiac monitor and rhythm strip interpretation.* This is a separate charge from EKG interpretation. The cardiac monitor must be ordered to charge for the interpretation.
■ *Radiograph interpretations.* Like EKG interpretations, radiograph interpretation is usually billed by the radiologist, but a few private insurance companies will pay the ED physician for an interpretation. Again, the ED physician must document "interpreted by me."

Levels of Service

■ The levels of service used in the ED for billing and coding purposes are summarized in Table 3C. Most patients seen in the ED will be in the last two categories ("detailed" and "comprehensive").
■ Tips for documenting a *comprehensive* history and physical examination (Level 5 chart) are listed in Table 3B. Accurately document to this level when in doubt.

Table 3A	**Components of the History and Physical Examination**
History of present illness (HPI)	Location, quality, severity, associated signs and symptoms, timing, context (at rest, with exertion, after lifting a weight), duration, modifying factors. If the patient is unable to give a history, document this, and the reason why (altered mental status, critical nature of patient, patient intubated, etc)
Past history, family, social history (PFSH)	Past history (medical and surgical history, medications, allergies), family history (diseases related to current complaint), social history (drugs/alcohol/tobacco, marital status, living arrangement, occupation, sexual history)
Review of Systems (ROS)	Constitutional (fever, chills, weight loss); eyes (vision changes, photophobia, eye pain, diplopia); ear, nose and throat (sore throat, earache, rhinorrea, congestion); cardiovascular (chest pain, palpitations, edema); respiratory (cough, shortness of breath); gastrointestinal (abdominal pain, nausea, vomiting, diarrhea, constipation); genitourinary (dysuria, discharge or lesions); musculoskeletal (joint pain, back pain, neck pain); integumentary (rash, ulcers, wounds); neurological (headache, seizure, dizziness, weakness, numbness); psychiatric (depression, anxiety, suicidal ideation, hallucinations); endocrine (polyuria, polydipsia); hematologic/lymphatic (swollen glands, bleeding, bruising); immunologic (allergies, immunosupression)
Physical Examination	Body area: head, face, neck, chest, abdomen, back, genitals, extremities. Organ system: constitutional (fevers, chills); eyes/ears/nose/throat, respiratory, cardiovascular, gastrointestinal, genitourinary, musculoskeletal, skin, neurologic, psychiatric, hematologic/lymphatic immunologic

Table 3B	**Summary of Documentation for "Comprehensive" or Level 5 Chart***
HPI	Chief complaint, four or more descriptors (e.g., location, quality, severity, associated signs and symptoms, timing, context, duration, modifying factors)
PFSH	Past history, plus a family or social history (2 of 3)
ROS	10 systems (use of "all other systems reviewed are negative" is acceptable as long as a 10 system review was actually done)
Physical examination	Eight systems: General (WD, WN in NAD), cardiac, pulmonary, abdominal, skin (color, temperature, hydration), psychiatric (orientation, memory, affect), and two more based on complaint

HPI, *history of present illness; NAD, no apparent distress; PFSH, past history, family and social history; ROS, review of systems; WD, well developed; WN, well nourished.*
*See Table 3C

Table 3C   Documentation Requirements Based on Level of Service

Levels of Service	HPI	ROS	PFSH	Physical Examination	Example
1. Problem focused	Brief (one to three descriptors)	Not required	Not required	One body area/organ system	Medication refill
2. Expanded problem focused	Brief (one to three descriptors)	Problem Pertinent (one system)	Not required	Two to four body areas/ organ systems	Upper respiratory infection, otitis media
3. Expanded problem focused	Brief (one to three descriptors)	Problem pertinent (one system)	Not required	Two to four body areas/ organ systems	Pharyngitis, corneal abrasion
4. Detailed	Extended (four or more descriptors)	Extended (two to nine systems)	Pertinent (one of the three)	Five to seven body areas/ organ systems	Laceration fracture pneumonia
5. Comprehensive	Extended (four or more descriptors)	10 systems	Two of the three	Eight or more body areas/ organ systems	Congestive heart failure, appendicitis

HPI, history of present illness; PFSH, past history, family and social history; ROS, review of systems.

Appendix 4 Evidence-Based Medicine

Richard Ismach ■ Samuel Luber

In practice, Evidence-Based Medicine [EBM] comprises the tools to find and apply up-to-date evidence to the care of your patients. Skills you will need include efficient literature searching, critical appraisal of the articles you find, and the application of Bayesian probability revision to clinical medicine. Box 4A shows the classic approach to practicing EBM.

Critical Appraisal

While all evidence is imperfect, even the best evidence must be interpreted in light of the individual patient, the physician's experience, and the recognition that study populations may differ from the patient for whom you are caring. Even when a study is of good quality, it may not apply to other patient populations or in other situations. Before you apply the results of biomedical research to a patient, you should assess the validity of the study and the applicability of the results to your patient. Although critical appraisal can be very involved and sophisticated, some common-sense rules adapted from the Centre for Evidence-Based Medicine will help you quickly evaluate studies of diagnostic tests (Box 4B) or treatments (Box 4C).

Diagnostic Questions

Differential diagnosis in emergency medicine emphasizes potential threats to life and limb. The same principles of diagnosis apply in all fields of medicine. Starting with a pretest probability, we use a test result to yield a post-test probability. If the post-test probability is high enough, we say that we have ruled in a diagnosis. If it is low enough, we say that we have ruled out a diagnosis. You can remember the meaning of various test characteristics using a 2×2 table, as in Figure 4A. The following are definitions of common statistical terms used in EBM in studies involving diagnostic tests:

BOX 4A   The Five Steps of Evidence-Based Medicine

- Convert a clinical problem into an answerable question
- Search the literature for answers to the question
- Evaluate the quality of the evidence you find
- Apply the evidence, along with your patient's values and your own judgment, to patient care
- Evaluate your own effectiveness and efficiency at practicing evidence-based medicine

BOX 4B Critical Appraisal of Studies of Diagnostic Tests

- Was there an independent, blind comparison with a "gold" standard of diagnosis?
- Was the diagnostic test evaluated in an appropriate spectrum of patients (like those in whom it would be used in practice)?
- Was the gold standard applied regardless of the diagnostic test result?
- For a clinical decision rule, was it validated in a second, independent group of patients?
- Is the diagnostic test available, affordable, accurate, and precise in your setting?
- Can you generate a sensible estimate of your patient's pre-test probability?
- Will the resulting post-test probabilities affect your management and help your patient?

BOX 4C Critical Appraisal of Studies of Treatments

- Was the assignment of patients to treatments randomized?
- Was the randomization list concealed?
- Was follow-up sufficiently long and complete?
- Were all patients analyzed in the groups to which they were randomized (intention to treat)?
- Were patients and clinicians kept "blind" to treatment?
- Were the groups treated equally, apart from the experimental treatment?
- Were the groups similar at the start of the trial?
- Is your patient so different from those in the study that its results cannot apply?
- Is the treatment feasible in your setting?
- Does this treatment suit your patient's values, preferences, and circumstances?

Sensitivity
- The probability that a test result is positive when given to a group of patients with the target disorder. A sensitive test will have few false negatives. A phrase to help remember this is *SnNOut:* If a sensitive test is negative, the disease is ruled out. Sensitivity is calculated as follows:
  - Sensitivity = True positives/(true positives + false negatives)

Specificity
- The probability that a test result is negative when given to a group of patients without target disorder. A specific test has few false positives. A phrase to help remember this is *SpPIn:* If a specific test is positive, the disease is ruled in. × Specificity is calculated as follows:
  - Specificity = True negatives/(true negatives + false positives)

Figure 4A. 2×2 table.

Likelihood Ratios

■ These more current test characteristics reflect both sensitivity and specificity, and are most often given separately as the likelihood for a positive test (LR+) and that for a negative test (LR-). The positive likelihood ratio (LR+) is the likelihood that a given test result would be expected in a patient with the target disorder compared with the likelihood that that same result would be expected in a patient without the target disorder. A good LR- is less than or equal to 0.1, and a good LR+ is 10 or higher.

Predictive Value

■ Predictive value is a test characteristic that is less commonly used.

■ The positive predictive value (PPV) is the probability that an individual has the target disorder given a positive test result. It is calculated by: True positives/(true positives + false positives)

■ The negative predictive value (NPV) is the probability that an individual has the target disorder given a negative test result. It is calculated by: True negatives/(true negatives + false negatives)

■ Since these probabilities depend heavily on the prevalence of the target disorder being tested for, most experts believe their application is limited.

Pretest Probability

■ Pretest probability is the same as prevalence within a study of a diagnostic test. Other sources of pretest probability include epidemiologic studies, Department of Health Data, or clinical experience. The pretest probability influences the ability of a test to predict the probability of disease. Even if a test has excellent sensitivity and specificity, which is very rare since they vary inversely for virtually all biologic tests, a test used in a patient with a low pretest probability will have poor predictive value.

Post-Test Probability

■ Post-test probability is the proportion of patients with that particular test result who have the target disorder. One can use the LR to calculate post-test probability by use of a nomogram developed by Fagan (Figure 4B). A straight line joining the patient's pretest probability of a particular disease and the LR for the test result points to the post-test probability of that disease.

Bayesian Probability Revision

■ The Bayesian probability revision is what underlies our use of diagnostic information. Conceptually, we multiply our pretest probability by our test result to get a post-test probability. In fact, to do this numerically requires converting the pretest probability into the pretest odds, then multiplying by the likelihood ratio to get the post-test odds, and then finally converting back into a post-test probability. This can be done quickly and easily using nomograms or special calculators (both on-line and on personal digital assistant applications). Usually, the only reason to actually calculate a post-test probability is as a teaching example. In real life, the inputs rest on too many hard-to-measure assumptions, and a numeric result gives an unrealistic illusion of precision. The idea, however, is crucial.

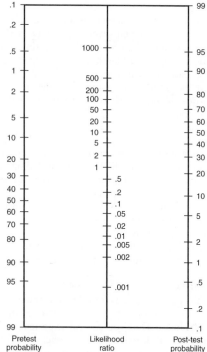

Figure 4B. Fagan nomogram. (From Fagan TJ. Nomogram for Bayes' theorem. N Engl J Med 1975;293:257.)

Treatment Questions

Treatment can also be thought of as a stochastic process—one where our reasoning should take account of probability. For any given treatment—say a drug for the treatment of glaucoma—there is a certain probability that it will be beneficial. That is, only some patients will respond as desired. There is also a certain probability that the treatment will harm the patient. Definitions of common statistical terms used in EBM in studies involving treatment.

   Number needed to treat (NNT) is the number of patients that must be treated for one patient to have the desired outcome. It is easily calculated: NNT = 1/ARR, where ARR is the absolute risk reduction. If 25% of control patients die and 10% of treated patients die, ARR = 15% and NNT = 7. A low NNT means the treatment is very effective; a large NNT means it is rarely effective.

   Number needed to harm (NNH) is completely analogous—down to the calculations—with NNT. The difference is in the nature of the outcome: desirable or undesirable.

Decision analysis allows a more formal approach to balancing the pros and cons of different treatment strategies. Best approached with special software, it involves using a decision tree with estimated probabilities for branches and relative utilities for each outcome. *Utility* is a number ranging from 0 (worst outcome) to 1.0 (best outcome). A variation is cost-benefit analysis, where economic costs are emphasized. These are often reported in terms of the cost per *quality-adjusted life-year* (QALY), and costs much over $100,000/QALY appear exorbitant.

Appendix 5 Emergency Medicine Web Resources

James Killeen ■ Jeremy Peay

General Emergency Medicine Sites	
ERSTAT	EMERGENCY DEPARTMENT. Favorite sites from the home page of Emergency Medicine at the Rehoboth McKinley Christian Hospital. http://www.erstat.com
National Center for Emergency Medicine Informatics	Emergency medicine (EM) resources at the National Center for Emergency Medicine Informatics (NCEMI), which is a multicenter not-for-profit institute, include more than 100 different tools to help with clinical emergency medicine, medical education, medical research, and EM management. Clinical calculators, reference materials, medical search engines, online books, electrocardiogram archives, radiographs, links to other emergency medicine sites, and much more. http://www.ncemi.org/
Emergency Medicine Learning and Resource Center	Site dedicated to promoting and advancing emergency medicine, disaster management, prehospital emergency care, and public health by providing education and research activities. www.emlrc.org
MD Choice	A privately held company founded by academic physicians and backed by private venture capital. MDchoice.com is the result of new technology combined with the content of several medical Web sites including NetMedicine.com, Physician's Choice, and EMBBS.com (The Emergency Medicine and Primary Care Home Page). http://www.mdchoice.com
McGill Faculty of Medicine: Emergency Medicine Links	http://www.mcgill.ca/emergency/links/

Evidence-Based Medicine	
BestBETS	Provides rapid evidence-based answers to real-life clinical questions. http://www.bestbets.org/
UpToDate	A comprehensive, evidence-based clinical information site that requires a subscription, but is an excellent resource of current knowledge in internal medicine. http://www.uptodate.com/
Evidence-Based Emergency Medicine at the New York Academy of Medicine	An excellent resource for emergency-based medicine topics related topics with links to several other sites including the User's Guides to the Medicine Literature. http://www.ebem.org
Textbooks and Reference Materials	
EMedicine	An online emergency medicine textbook. http://www.emedicine.com/emerg
MD Consult	An excellent resource for medical reference book, journals, clinics, guidelines, and drug information. www.mdconsult.com
Merck Medicus	Huge compendium of free medical resources; registration is required, but free. http://www.merckmedicus.com
Practice Guidelines	
American College of Emergency Physicians (ACEP)	These ACEP board-approved documents describe the College's policies on the clinical management of presenting symptoms, specific illnesses or injuries. http://www.acep.org/webportal/PracticeResources/ClinicalPolicies/
Agency for Health Care Policy and Research (AHCPR)	The AHCPR offers clinical care guidelines. http://www.ahcpr.org
National Guideline Clearinghouse	A public resource for evidence-based clinical practice guidelines. www.guideline.gov
Picture Archives	
EDPicture	Rapidly search all the sites below and more with a single tool! http://www.ncemi.org/edpicture/index.htm
Dermatology Atlas	http://dermatlas.med.jhmi.edu/derm/
Dermatology Images	A large set of dermatologic photos from the University of Iowa. http://tray.dermatology.uiowa.edu/DermImag.htm
Radiology Image Links	http://www.radiologyeducation.com/

Radiology Images	Medical cases with associated radiographs or computed tomography images. http://www.mdchoice.com/xray/xrx.asp
Medical Images	Medical cases with associated photographs. Cases include subject reviews and questions. http://www.mdchoice.com/photo/photos.asp

Emergency Medicine Cases

EKG Cases	Interesting electrocardiogram case of the month. http://www.mdchoice.com/ekg/ekg.asp
Emergency Medicine CyberSchool from Mount Sinai Medical Center	http://www.mssm.edu/emergmed/cschool.htm
Trauma.ORG	Moulage scenarios from the United Kingdom. http://www.trauma.org/resus/moulage/moulage.html
Trauma Surgery Site LA-USC	Good Slide show for visual clues. http://www.surgery.usc.edu/clerkship/educationalslides.html
Trauma X-Ray Collection Liverpool Hospital	Great collection of trauma films. http://www.swsahs.nsw.gov.au/livtrauma/education/xray.asp

Organizations

American Academy of Emergency Physicians	Home page of the American Academy of Emergency Physicians, whose membership is limited to board-certified emergency physicians. http://www.aaem.org
American College of Emergency Physicians	Home page of the American College of Emergency Physicians. http://www.acep.org/
Society of Academic Emergency Medicine	Home page of the Society for Academic Emergency Medicine (SAEM). The mission of the SAEM is to foster emergency medicine's academic environment in research, education, and health policy through forums, publications, interorganizational collaboration, policy development, and consultation services for teachers, researchers, and students. http://www.saem.org
American Board of Emergency Medicine	The American Board of Emergency Medicine (ABEM) site has information regarding upcoming examinations and information about ABEM. http://www.abem.org
Emergency Medicine Residents' Association	The Emergency Medicine Residents' Association Web site provides information for medical students interested in emergency medicine and current emergency medicine residents. http://www.emra.org

Index